T0213357

Register Now for Online Access to Your Book!

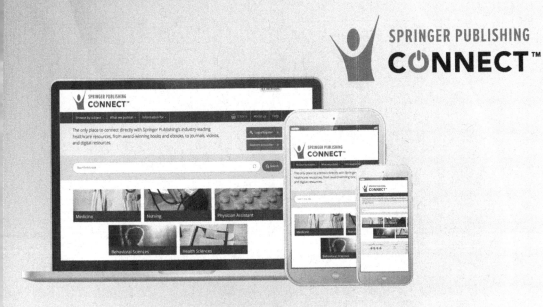

SPRINGER PUBLISHING
CONNECT™

Your print purchase of *Essentials of Clinical Radiation Oncology, Second Edition,* **includes online access to the contents of your book**—increasing accessibility, portability, and searchability!

Access today at:
http://connect.springerpub.com/content/book/978-0-8261-6909-9
or scan the QR code at the right with your smartphone. Log in or register, then click "Redeem a voucher" and use the code below.

> GYJP4AN9

Scan here for quick access.

Having trouble redeeming a voucher code?
Go to https://connect.springerpub.com/redeeming-voucher-code

If you are experiencing problems accessing the digital component of this product, please contact our customer service department at cs@springerpub.com

The online access with your print purchase is available at the publisher's discretion and may be removed at any time without notice.

Publisher's Note: New and used products purchased from third-party sellers are not guaranteed for quality, authenticity, or access to any included digital components.

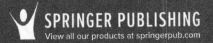

SPRINGER PUBLISHING
View all our products at springerpub.com

ESSENTIALS OF CLINICAL RADIATION ONCOLOGY

ESSENTIALS OF CLINICAL RADIATION ONCOLOGY

Second Edition

Editors

Sarah M. C. Sittenfeld, MD
Assistant Professor
Department of Radiation Oncology
University of Cincinnati
Cincinnati, Ohio

Matthew C. Ward, MD
Adjunct Assistant Professor
Department of Radiation Oncology
Levine Cancer Institute
Atrium Health
Charlotte, North Carolina

Rahul D. Tendulkar, MD
Associate Professor
Cleveland Clinic Lerner College of Medicine
Staff Physician
Cleveland Clinic Foundation
Cleveland, Ohio

Gregory M. M. Videtic, MD, CM, FRCPC
Professor of Medicine
Cleveland Clinic Lerner College of Medicine
Staff Physician
Department of Radiation Oncology
Cleveland Clinic Foundation
Cleveland, Ohio

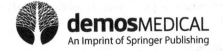
demosMEDICAL
An Imprint of Springer Publishing

Springer Publishing Company, LLC
11 West 42nd Street, New York, NY 10036
www.springerpub.com
connect.springerpub.com/

Acquisitions Editor: David D'Addona
Compositor: Exeter Premedia Services Private Ltd.

ISBN: 978-0-8261-6908-2
ebook ISBN: 978-0-8261-6909-9
DOI: 10.1891/9780826169099

21 22 23 24 25 / 5 4 3 2 1

Medicine is an ever-changing science. Research and clinical experience are continually expanding our knowledge, in particular our understanding of proper treatment and drug therapy. The authors, editors, and publisher have made every effort to ensure that all information in this book is in accordance with the state of knowledge at the time of production of the book. Nevertheless, the authors, editors, and publisher are not responsible for any errors or omissions or for any consequence from application of the information in this book and make no warranty, expressed or implied, with respect to the content of this publication. Every reader should examine carefully the package inserts accompanying each drug and should carefully check whether the dosage schedules therein or the contraindications stated by the manufacturer differ from the statements made in this book. Such examination is particularly important with drugs that are either rarely used or have been newly released on the market.

Library of Congress Cataloging-in-Publication Data

Names: Sittenfeld, Sarah M. C., editor. | Ward, Matthew C., 1986- editor. |
 Tendulkar, Rahul D., editor. | Videtic, Gregory M. M., editor.
Title: Essentials of clinical radiation oncology / editors, Sarah M.C.
 Sittenfeld, Matthew C. Ward, Rahul D. Tendulkar, Gregory M.M. Videtic.
Description: Second edition. | New York : Demos Medical Publishing, [2022]
 | Includes bibliographical references and index.
Identifiers: LCCN 2021017425 (print) | LCCN 2021017426 (ebook) | ISBN
 9780826169082 (paperback) | ISBN 9780826169099 (ebook)
Subjects: MESH: Neoplasms--radiotherapy | Handbook
Classification: LCC RC271.R3 (print) | LCC RC271.R3 (ebook) | NLM QZ 39
 | DDC 616.99/40642--dc23
LC record available at https://lccn.loc.gov/2021017425
LC ebook record available at https://lccn.loc.gov/2021017426

Sarah M. C. Sittenfeld: 0000-0002-2771-4914
Matthew C. Ward: 0000-0002-8423-890X

Contact sales@springerpub.com to receive discount rates on bulk purchases.

Publisher's Note: **New and used products purchased from third-party sellers are not guaranteed for quality, authenticity, or access to any included digital components.**

Printed in the United States of America.

To the enduring commitment of past, present, and future residents in the pursuit of knowledge, without whom this work would not have been possible.

CONTENTS

Contributors   *xiii*
Preface   *xvii*
About the Format of This Book   *xix*

I. CENTRAL NERVOUS SYSTEM

1. Glioblastoma   **3**
   Aditya Juloori, Jennifer S. Yu, and Samuel T. Chao

2. Anaplastic Gliomas   **11**
   Shireen Parsai, Martin C. Tom, and Samuel T. Chao

3. Low-Grade Gliomas   **17**
   Martin C. Tom and Erin S. Murphy

4. Meningioma   **25**
   Martin C. Tom, David J. Schwartz, and Abigail L. Stockham

5. Primary Central Nervous System Lymphoma   **33**
   Ian W. Winter, Samuel T. Chao, and Erin S. Murphy

6. Pituitary Adenoma   **39**
   Zachary Mayo and John H. Suh

7. Trigeminal Neuralgia   **47**
   Bindu V. Manyam, Vamsi Varra, and Samuel T. Chao

8. Vestibular Schwannoma   **53**
   Winston Vuong, Jeffrey A. Kittel, and John H. Suh

9. Uveal Melanoma   **61**
   Martin C. Tom, Gaurav Marwaha, John H. Suh, and Arun D. Singh

10. Spine Tumors   **69**
    Sarah S. Kilic, Ehsan H. Balagamwala, and Samuel T. Chao

II. HEAD AND NECK

11. Oropharynx Cancer   **79**
    Shireen Parsai, Aditya Juloori, Nikhil P. Joshi, and Shlomo A. Koyfman

12. Oral Cavity Cancer   **91**
    Kailin Yang, Bindu V. Manyam, and Neil M. Woody

13. Nasopharyngeal Cancer   **99**
    Christopher W. Fleming, Shireen Parsai, and Nikhil P. Joshi

14. Laryngeal Cancer   **107**
    Aditya Juloori, Shauna R. Campbell, and Shlomo A. Koyfman

15. Salivary Gland Tumors   **115**
    Sarah S. Kilic, Martin C. Tom, Shlomo A. Koyfman, and Nikhil P. Joshi

16. Carcinoma of Unknown Primary of the Head and Neck   123
    Monica E. Shukla and Jeffrey A. Kittel

17. Postoperative Radiation for Head and Neck Cancer   131
    Timothy D. Smile and Carryn M. Anderson

18. Thyroid Cancer   139
    James R. Broughman and Nikhil P. Joshi

19. Sinonasal Tumors   145
    Timothy D. Smile and Neil M. Woody

III. SKIN

20. Nonmelanoma Skin Cancer   155
    Ian W. Winter, Neil M. Woody, and Shlomo A. Koyfman

21. Malignant Cutaneous Melanoma   167
    Sarah S. Kilic, Aditya Juloori, and Nikhil P. Joshi

22. Mycosis Fungoides   175
    Vamsi Varra, Matthew C. Ward, and Gregory M. M. Videtic

IV. BREAST

23. Early-Stage Breast Cancer   183
    Kailin Yang, Rahul D. Tendulkar, and Chirag Shah

24. Locally Advanced Breast Cancer   207
    Christopher W. Fleming, Yvonne D. Pham, and Rahul D. Tendulkar

25. Ductal Carcinoma In Situ   219
    Timothy D. Smile, Rahul D. Tendulkar, and Chirag Shah

26. Recurrent Breast Cancer   229
    Ian W. Winter, Camille A. Berriochoa, and Chirag Shah

V. THORACIC

27. Early-Stage Non–Small-Cell Lung Cancer   239
    Sarah S. Kilic, Gaurav Marwaha, Kevin L. Stephans, and Gregory M. M. Videtic

28. Stage III Non–Small-Cell Lung Cancer   249
    Aditya Juloori, Matthew C. Ward, and Gregory M. M. Videtic

29. Small-Cell Lung Cancer   257
    Camille A. Berriochoa and Gregory M. M. Videtic

30. Mesothelioma   269
    Sarah M. C. Sittenfeld, Bindu V. Manyam, and Gregory M. M. Videtic

31. Thymoma   275
    Christopher W. Fleming, Jonathan M. Sharrett, and Gregory M. M. Videtic

VI. GASTROINTENTINAL

32. Esophageal Cancer   283
    Camille A. Berriochoa and Gregory M. M. Videtic

33. Gastric Cancer   293
    Bindu V. Manyam, Kevin L. Stephans, and Gregory M. M. Videtic

34. Hepatocellular Carcinoma   303
    Shauna R. Campbell, Neil M. Woody, and Kevin L. Stephans

35. Pancreatic Adenocarcinoma   311
    James R. Broughman and Ehsan H. Balagamwala

36. Rectal Cancer   325
    Ian W. Winter, Ehsan H. Balagamwala, and Sudha R. Amarnath

37. Anal Cancer   339
    Kristine Bauer-Nilsen, Aditya Juloori, and Sudha R. Amarnath

38. Cholangiocarcinoma   347
    Christopher W. Fleming, Shauna R. Campbell, and Kevin L. Stephans

VII. GENITOURINARY

39. Low-Risk Prostate Cancer   355
    Timothy D. Smile and Rahul D. Tendulkar

40. Intermediate- and High-Risk Prostate Cancer   373
    Rahul D. Tendulkar, Bindu V. Manyam, and Omar Y. Mian

41. Post-Prostatectomy Radiation Therapy   387
    James R. Broughman, Camille A. Berriochoa, and Rahul D. Tendulkar

42. Bladder Cancer   395
    Winston Vuong, Omar Y. Mian, and Rahul D. Tendulkar

43. Testicular Cancer   403
    Zachary Mayo, Ehsan H. Balagamwala, and Rahul D. Tendulkar

44. Penile Cancer   411
    Rahul D. Tendulkar, Rupesh Kotecha, and Omar Y. Mian

45. Urethral Cancer   419
    Rahul D. Tendulkar, Rupesh Kotecha, and Omar Y. Mian

46. Renal Cell Carcinoma   423
    Sarah M. C. Sittenfeld and Rahul D. Tendulkar

VIII. GYNECOLOGIC

47. Cervical Cancer   429
    Sudha R. Amarnath, Monica E. Shukla, and Sheen Cherian

48. Uterine Cancer: Endometrial Cancer and Uterine Sarcoma   439
    Shireen Parsai, Sarah M. C. Sittenfeld, Michael Weller, and Sudha R. Amarnath

49. Vulvar Cancer   455
    Ahmed Halima and Sudha R. Amarnath

50. Vaginal Cancer   463
    Camille A. Berriochoa and Sudha R. Amarnath

IX. HEMATOLOGIC

51. Adult Hodgkin's Lymphoma   471
    Matthew C. Ward and Sheen Cherian

52. Aggressive Non-Hodgkin's Lymphoma   481
    James R. Broughman, Matthew C. Ward, and Chirag Shah

53. Indolent Non-Hodgkin's Lymphoma   493
    Christopher W. Fleming, Aryavarta M. S. Kumar, and Matthew C. Ward

54. Multiple Myeloma and Plasmacytoma   499
    Kailin Yang and Sheen Cherian

X. SARCOMAS

55. Soft Tissue Sarcoma   505
    Shauna R. Campbell, Jonathan M. Sharrett, Jacob G. Scott, and Chirag Shah

XI. PEDIATRIC

56. Medulloblastoma   519
    Timothy D. Smile, Camille A. Berriochoa, and Erin S. Murphy

57. Ependymoma   531
    Matthew C. Ward, John H. Suh, and Erin S. Murphy

58. Brainstem Glioma   537
    Sarah M. C. Sittenfeld, Jason W. D. Hearn, and John H. Suh

59. Craniopharyngioma   545
    Martin C. Tom, Timothy D. Smile, and Erin S. Murphy

60. Rhabdomyosarcoma   549
    Shauna R. Campbell, Samuel T. Chao, and Erin S. Murphy

61. Neuroblastoma   557
    Charles Marc Leyrer and Erin S. Murphy

62. Wilms Tumor   569
    James R. Broughman and Erin S. Murphy

63. Ewing's Sarcoma   575
    Kailin Yang, Ehsan H. Balagamwala, and Erin S. Murphy

64. Pediatric Hodgkin's Lymphoma   581
    Sarah M. C. Sittenfeld and Erin S. Murphy

65. Miscellaneous CNS Pediatric Tumors   589
    Shauna R. Campbell and Erin S. Murphy

XII. METASTASES AND PALLIATIVE RADIOTHERAPY

66. Brain Metastases   595
    Shauna R. Campbell, Martin C. Tom, and John H. Suh

67. Bone and Spine Metastasis   607
    Ehsan H. Balagamwala, Samuel T. Chao, and Andrew D. Vassil

68. Malignant Spinal Cord Compression   *615*
     Camille A. Berriochoa and Bindu V. Manyam

69. Superior Vena Cava Syndrome   *621*
     Kailin Yang and Gregory M. M. Videtic

70. Palliative Radiotherapy   *625*
     Matthew C. Ward and Justin J. Juliano

71. Oligometastatic Disease   *631*
     Ian W. Winter, Ehsan H. Balagamwala, and Martin C. Tom

XIII. BENIGN DISEASES

72. Radiation Therapy for Benign Diseases   *639*
     Ahmed Halima and Chirag Shah

Abbreviations   *645*
Index   *667*

CONTRIBUTORS

Sudha R. Amarnath, MD, Assistant Professor of Medicine, Department of Radiation Oncology, Taussig Cancer Center, Cleveland Clinic Foundation, Cleveland, Ohio

Carryn M. Anderson, MD, Clinical Associate Professor, Department of Radiation Oncology, University of Iowa Hospitals & Clinics, Iowa City, Iowa

Ehsan H. Balagamwala, MD, Assistant Professor, Department of Radiation Oncology, Taussig Cancer Center, Cleveland Clinic Foundation, Cleveland, Ohio

Kristine Bauer-Nilsen, MD, Resident Physician, Department of Radiation Oncology, Taussig Cancer Center, Cleveland Clinic Foundation, Cleveland, Ohio

Camille A. Berriochoa, MD, Radiation Oncologist, Department of Radiation Oncology, Saint Alphonsus Regional Medical Center, Boise, Idaho

James R. Broughman, MD, Resident Physician, Department of Radiation Oncology, Taussig Cancer Center, Cleveland Clinic Foundation, Cleveland, Ohio

Shauna R. Campbell, DO, Staff Physician, Department of Radiation Oncology, Taussig Cancer Center, Cleveland Clinic Foundation, Cleveland, Ohio

Samuel T. Chao, MD, Professor, Department of Radiation Oncology, Rose Ella Burkhardt Brain Tumor and Neuro-oncology Center, Cleveland Clinic Foundation, Cleveland, Ohio

Sheen Cherian, MD, MSc, MRCP, FRCR, DABR, Assistant Professor, Cleveland Clinic Lerner College of Medicine, Staff Physician, Department of Radiation Oncology, Taussig Cancer Center, Cleveland Clinic Foundation, Cleveland, Ohio

Christopher W. Fleming, MD, Associate Staff, Department of Radiation Oncology, Maroone Cancer Center, Cleveland Clinic Florida, Weston, Florida

Ahmed Halima, MD, Resident Physician, Department of Radiation Oncology, Taussig Cancer Center, Cleveland Clinic Foundation, Cleveland, Ohio

Jason W. D. Hearn, MD, Assistant Professor, Department of Radiation Oncology, University of Michigan, Ann Arbor, Michigan

Nikhil P. Joshi, MD, Assistant Professor, Department of Radiation Oncology, Rush University Medical Center, Chicago, Illinois

Justin J. Juliano, MD, Radiation Oncologist, Department of Radiation Oncology, New York Oncology Hematology, Clifton Park, New York

Aditya Juloori, MD, Assistant Professor, Department of Cellular and Radiation Oncology, University of Chicago, Chicago, Illinois

Sarah S. Kilic, MD, Resident Physician, Department of Radiation Oncology, Taussig Cancer Center, Cleveland Clinic Foundation, Cleveland, Ohio

Jeffrey A. Kittel, MD, Radiation Oncologist, Radiation Oncology Associates, Ltd.; Department of Radiation Oncology, Aurora St. Luke's Medical Center, Milwaukee, Wisconsin

Rupesh Kotecha, MD, Chief of Radiosurgery, Director of CNS Metastasis, Department of Radiation Oncology, Miami Cancer Institute, Baptist Health South Florida; Associate Professor, Department of Radiation Oncology, FIU Herbert Wertheim College of Medicine, Miami, Florida

Shlomo A. Koyfman, MD, Assistant Professor, Department of Medicine, School of Medicine, Case Comprehensive Cancer Center, Case Western Reserve University, Cleveland, Ohio

Aryavarta M. S. Kumar, MD, PhD, Assistant Professor, Department of Radiation Oncology, Louis Stokes Cleveland VA Medical Center, Cleveland, Ohio

Charles Marc Leyrer, MD, Assistant Professor, Department of Radiation Oncology, Wake Forest Baptist Health, Winston-Salem, North Carolina

Bindu V. Manyam, MD, Radiation Oncologist, Department of Radiation Oncology, Allegheny Health Network Cancer Institute, Pittsburgh, Pennsylvania

Gaurav Marwaha, MD, Assistant Professor and Residency Program Director, Department of Radiation Oncology, Rush University Medical Center, Chicago, Illinois

Zachary Mayo, MD, Resident Physician, Department of Radiation Oncology, Taussig Cancer Center, Cleveland Clinic Foundation, Cleveland, Ohio

Omar Y. Mian, MD, PhD, Staff, Department of Radiation Oncology, Taussig Cancer Center, Cleveland Clinic Foundation, Cleveland, Ohio

Erin S. Murphy, MD, Associate Professor, Department of Radiation Oncology, Taussig Cancer Center, Cleveland Clinic Foundation, Cleveland, Ohio

Shireen Parsai, MD, Radiation Oncologist, Department of Radiation Oncology, OhioHealth Riverside Methodist Hospital, Columbus, Ohio

Yvonne D. Pham, MD, Radiation Oncologist, Therapeutic Radiologists, Inc. (TRI, P.A.), Kansas City, Missouri

David J. Schwartz, MD, Director, Staten Island Radiation Oncology, Staten Island, New York

Jacob G. Scott, MD, DPhil, Staff Physician-Scientist, Department of Radiation Oncology, Taussig Cancer Center, Cleveland Clinic Foundation, Cleveland, Ohio

Chirag Shah, MD, Director of Breast Radiation Oncology, Department of Radiation Oncology, Taussig Cancer Center, Cleveland Clinic Foundation, Cleveland, Ohio

Jonathan M. Sharrett, DO, Radiation Oncologist, Spokane Cyberknife and Summit Cancer Centers, Spokane, Washington

Monica E. Shukla, MD, Assistant Professor, Department of Radiation Oncology, Medical College of Wisconsin, Milwaukee, Wisconsin

Arun D. Singh, MD, Professor of Ophthalmology, Director of Department of Ophthalmic Oncology, Cole Eye Institute, Cleveland Clinic Foundation, Cleveland, Ohio

Sarah M. C. Sittenfeld, MD, Assistant Professor, Department of Radiation Oncology, University of Cincinnati, Cincinnati, Ohio

Timothy D. Smile, MD, Resident Physician, Department of Radiation Oncology, Taussig Cancer Center, Cleveland Clinic Foundation, Cleveland, Ohio

Kevin L. Stephans, MD, Associate Professor, Department of Radiation Oncology, Taussig Cancer Center, Cleveland Clinic Foundation, Cleveland, Ohio

Abigail L. Stockham, MD, Consultant and Assistant Professor, Department of Radiation Oncology, Mayo Clinic, Rochester, Minnesota

John H. Suh, MD, Chairman, Department of Radiation Oncology, Taussig Cancer Center, Cleveland Clinic Foundation, Cleveland, Ohio

Rahul D. Tendulkar, MD, Associate Professor, Department of Radiation Oncology, Taussig Cancer Center, Cleveland Clinic Foundation, Cleveland, Ohio

Martin C. Tom, MD, Assistant Professor, Department of Radiation Oncology, Miami Cancer Institute, Baptist Health South Florida; Herbert Wertheim College of Medicine, Florida International University, Miami, Florida

Vamsi Varra, MD, Intern, Department of Internal Medicine, University Hospitals Cleveland Medical Center, Cleveland, Ohio

Andrew D. Vassil, MD, Staff Physician, Department of Radiation Oncology, Taussig Cancer Center, Cleveland Clinic Foundation, Cleveland, Ohio

Gregory M. M. Videtic, MD, CM, FRCPC, Professor of Medicine, Cleveland Clinic Lerner College of Medicine; Staff Physician, Department of Radiation Oncology, Cleveland Clinic Foundation, Cleveland, Ohio

Winston Vuong, MD, Resident Physician, Department of Radiation Oncology, Taussig Cancer Center, Cleveland Clinic Foundation, Cleveland, Ohio

Matthew C. Ward, MD, Adjunct Assistant Professor, Department of Radiation Oncology, Levine Cancer Institute, Atrium Health, Charlotte, North Carolina

Michael Weller, MD, Staff Physician, Department of Radiation Oncology, Taussig Cancer Center, Cleveland Clinic Foundation, Cleveland, Ohio

Ian W. Winter, MD, Resident Physician, Department of Radiation Oncology, Taussig Cancer Center, Cleveland Clinic Foundation, Cleveland, Ohio

Neil M. Woody, MD, MS, Assistant Professor, Department of Radiation Oncology, Taussig Cancer Center, Cleveland Clinic Foundation, Cleveland, Ohio

Kailin Yang, MD, PhD, Resident Physician, Department of Radiation Oncology, Taussig Cancer Center, Cleveland Clinic Foundation, Cleveland, Ohio

Jennifer S. Yu, MD, PhD, Staff, Department of Radiation Oncology, Department of Cancer Biology, Burkhardt Brain Tumor and Neuro-oncology Center, Cleveland Clinic Foundation; Associate Professor, Program Leader, Developmental Therapeutics Program, Co-Leader, Cancer Stem Cell Working Group, Case Comprehensive Cancer Center, Cleveland, Ohio

PREFACE

Essentials of Clinical Radiation Oncology was born out of the long-standing tradition in the Cleveland Clinic Radiation Oncology Residency program of preparing yearly "handouts" summarizing the most recent and high-yield data to complement the formal teaching curriculum. As recent graduates of the Cleveland Clinic residency program, we attest to their value not only in learning the basics of radiation oncology but in our continued education as independent clinicians. It was with great pride that we shared the hard work of decades of residents with the broader radiation oncology community in the publication of our first edition, and we were pleased to receive validation of its worth from a diverse group of readers.

The field of radiation oncology is continually evolving, as developing data inform new treatment paradigms or updates established ones. With the second edition of *Essentials of Clinical Radiation Oncology,* we aim to keep pace with the changing clinical environment by providing readers with the most up-to-date studies and treatment approaches. In addition to incorporating new data throughout, we have included several new chapters to help comprehensively cover the broadest range of clinical topics.

While much has changed in the field over the past several years, the outstanding dedication of current Cleveland Clinic Radiation Oncology residents, recent graduates, and current faculty to education has remained strong. Without them, this update would not have been possible. It is with deep gratitude to these many coauthors and on their behalf that we now offer this present edition to the radiation oncology community. As with the first edition, we appreciate readers' suggestions and welcome any feedback via Twitter. We trust this resource will prove valuable to all practitioners in their continued efforts to provide excellent patient care.

Sarah M. C. Sittenfeld, MD (@SarahSittenfeld)
Matthew C. Ward, MD (@MCWardMD)
Rahul D. Tendulkar, MD (@RTendulkarMD)
Gregory M. M. Videtic, MD, CM, FRCPC, FACR, FASTRO

ABOUT THE FORMAT OF THIS BOOK

The intention of this book is to serve as a resource for all levels of practitioners, from medical students to practicing physicians. Therefore, the reader will find clinically pertinent details starting from basic epidemiology and culminating in an evidence-based approach to important and up-to-date clinical questions. The front matter of each chapter contains information about the disease and its natural history. This includes a summary of the American Joint Committee on Cancer 8th edition staging system (or other relevant risk-stratification systems), printed in an abbreviated format intended for physician understanding. Next, general Treatment Paradigms are included in the midpart of each chapter to give the reader an overview of the role of each anticancer modality in the multidisciplinary care of the patient. Finally, the highlight of this resource is the Evidence-Based Q&A format of clinical studies presented to guide the reader through the most pertinent literature. Each study is block-quoted from the source with a quick-access citation to the original reference in combination with a condensed summary intended to highlight the pertinent findings. It should be noted that our intention with this book is to provide a manual of information useful to the clinician, rather than to be "prescriptive" in terms of staging, radiation delivery, or chemotherapy dosing. Our hope is that this format provides an efficient yet thorough method for practitioners to develop a deeper understanding of a disease and the current state of its treatment.

I ■ CENTRAL NERVOUS SYSTEM

1 ■ GLIOBLASTOMA

Aditya Juloori, Jennifer S. Yu, and Samuel T. Chao

QUICK HIT ■ GBM is the most common primary brain tumor in adults. GBM has a poor prognosis with a median survival of ~14 months. Treatment is maximal safe resection with neurologic preservation followed by adjuvant chemoRT. The standard RT dose is 60 Gy with TMZ given 75 mg/m² daily concurrently and 150 to 200 mg/m² adjuvantly for days 1 to 5 of a 28-day cycle for 6 to 12 months as tolerated. RT field is typically 46 Gy to T2/FLAIR edema and then additional 14 Gy boost to resection cavity and T1 contrast enhancement, generally with a 2-cm CTV expansion. The most common site of treatment failure is local progression. For older or frail patients, options include palliative care, short-course RT ± TMZ, or TMZ alone (particularly for MGMT methylated patients).

EPIDEMIOLOGY: Most common (80%) primary malignant brain tumor in adults.[1] Incidence: Three to four cases per 100,000 or about 10,000 cases/year in the United States. Median age at diagnosis is 64 and the male-to-female ratio is approximately 1.5:1.[2]

ANATOMY: Diffusely infiltrative tumor that grows along white matter tracts. Location is dependent on amount of white matter: 75% are supratentorial (31% temporal, 24% parietal, 23% frontal, 16% occipital), <20% multifocal, 2% to 7% multicentric, 10% present with positive CSF cytology.[3]

PATHOLOGY: Cell of origin is the supporting glial cells of CNS. WHO 2016 update[4] now defines three distinct types: glioblastoma, IDH-wild-type; glioblastoma, IDH-mutant; and glioblastoma, NOS (see the Genetics section for details on IDH1). Other rare variants include giant cell glioblastoma, gliosarcoma, or epithelioid glioblastoma. Diagnosis of a WHO grade IV glioma requires the pathognomonic finding of "pseudopalisading" necrosis OR at least three MEAN criteria: high mitotic index, endothelial proliferation, nuclear atypia, or necrosis.

GENETICS

MGMT Gene Methylation: O^6-methylguanine-DNA methyltransferase is located on chromosome 10q26. Its purpose is to repair alkylation of guanine at the O^6 position. When the promoter undergoes epigenetic silencing by methylation, the gene is downregulated. The Hegi study (see Evidence-Based Q&A) defined its prognostic and predictive value.

IDH1 Mutation: Present in ~10% of GBM and associated with increased age and secondary tumors that developed from previous low-grade gliomas.[4] IDH1 mutation is an independent positive prognostic factor (MS 27.4 months for IDH1-mutant vs. 14 months for IDH1-wild-type).[5]

EGFRv3 Variant: In-frame deletion of exons 2 to 7 of the *EGFR* gene affecting 801 base pairs and is an independent predictor of a poor prognosis with standard chemoRT.[6]

BRAF V600E Mutation: Same variant as in melanoma, but seen commonly in giant cell and epithelioid glioblastomas and lower grade gliomas.[7]

ATRX: Alpha-thalassemia/mental retardation syndrome x-linked gene (*ATRX*) is a gene that is involved in chromatin regulation. A mutation in ATRX is frequently seen in patients with grade II/III astrocytomas as well as patients with secondary GBM.[8–10]

See Chapter 3 for a discussion of 1p19q codeletion.

CLINICAL PRESENTATION: Headache, cognitive changes, seizure, motor weakness, nausea/vomiting, visual loss, sensory loss, language disturbance, dysphagia, papilledema, gait disturbance, intracranial bleed.

WORKUP: H&P with neurologic exam. Fundoscopic exam (if suspicious of increased intracranial pressure).

Labs: CBC to establish baseline for CHT.

Imaging: MRI brain with and without gadolinium (heterogeneous enhancement, central necrosis, surrounding edema; T1 hypointense and T2 edema hyperintense).

Biopsy: Stereotactic or open biopsy with genetic assessment as earlier.

PROGNOSTIC FACTORS: Clinical factors as established by Li et al.[11]: KPS, age, extent of resection. MGMT status, IDH1 status. See Table 1.1 [12] for RTOG RPA.

Table 1.1: RPA Classification for Glioblastoma Multiforme			
RPA Class	Defining Variables	MS (mos)	OS at 1, 3, and 5 Yrs
III	<50 y/o and KPS ≥90	17.1	70%, 20%, 14%
IV	<50 y/o and KPS <90 ≥50 y/o, KPS ≥70, resection, and working	11.2	46%, 7%, 4%
V + VI	≥50 y/o, KPS ≥70, resection, and not working ≥50 y/o, KPS ≥70, biopsy only ≥50 y/o, KPS <70	7.5	28%, 1%, 0%

Source: From Li J, Wang M, Won M, et al. Validation and simplification of the Radiation Therapy Oncology Group recursive partitioning analysis classification for glioblastoma. *Int J Radiat Oncol Biol Phys.* 2011;81(3):623–630. doi:10.1016/j.ijrobp.2010.06.012; Walker MD, Alexander E, Jr., Hunt WE, et al. Evaluation of BCNU and/or radiotherapy in the treatment of anaplastic gliomas: a cooperative clinical trial. *J Neurosurg.* 1978;49(3):333–343. doi:10.3171/jns.1978.49.3.0333

TREATMENT PARADIGM

Surgery: Primary treatment is maximal safe surgical resection with neurologic preservation. For technically unresectable tumors, a biopsy is warranted to obtain tissue. Various tools may be applied to improve safety of resection such as intraoperative ultrasound/MRI, functional mapping (phase reversal, direct brain stimulation, awake anesthesia). To evaluate the extent of resection, obtain a contrast-enhanced MRI within 72 hours of surgery (ideally 24–48 hours) to avoid confounding with subacute blood products.

Chemotherapy: As established in the Stupp trial, daily use of TMZ 75 mg/m^2 concurrently during RT course, including weekends. This is followed by adjuvant TMZ for d1–5 of 28-day cycle for 6 to 12 months, starting at 150 mg/m^2 and escalated as tolerated to 200 mg/m^2. Major side effects of TMZ are constipation, thrombocytopenia, and neutropenia. Patients treated with TMZ require prophylaxis against pneumocystis pneumonia and can be given daily DS trimethoprim/sulfamethoxazole or alternatively, two pentamidine inhalation treatments during the RT course. TMZ is a prodrug converted to MTIC, which alkylates DNA. Only 5% to 10% of methylation events yield the O^6-methylguanine, but if the methyl group is not removed prior to cell division, the adducts are highly cytotoxic (see MGMT earlier).

Radiation

Indications: Adjuvant RT improves OS vs. observation or CHT alone after surgery (see the following studies) and is indicated in all patients of sufficient functional status to tolerate treatment.

Dose: 60 Gy/30 fx is standard. For older or frail individuals, various hypofractionated schemes have been investigated (see the following studies). In the palliative setting, RT is superior to best supportive care in terms of OS.

Toxicity: Acute: Fatigue, headache, exacerbation of presenting neurologic deficits, alopecia, nausea, cerebral edema. Late: Cognitive changes, radiation necrosis, hypopituitarism, cataracts, vision loss (rare and location-dependent).

Procedure: See *Handbook of Treatment Planning in Radiation Oncology*, Chapter 3.[13]

■ **EVIDENCE-BASED Q&A**

■ **What is considered optimal surgery for glioblastoma?**

Lacroix, MDACC (*J Neurosurg 2001*, **PMID 11780887**): RR showing improved OS with ≥98% resection in better prognostic patients (young, good KPS, no MRI evidence of necrosis). GTR also limits chance of cerebral edema during RT. **Conclusion: GTR improved OS in select patients compared with no clear benefit to STR.**

■ **What are the contraindications to GTR?**

Eloquent/inaccessible areas involved (brainstem, motor cortex, language centers, etc.), significant infiltration past midline, periventricular or diffuse lesions, medical comorbidities.

■ **How did we arrive at the current standard RT dose?**

The BTCG 69-01[12] and 1981 SGSG[14] studies demonstrated a doubling of survival with adjuvant RT over best supportive care. Dose escalation was beneficial to 60 Gy/30 fx, but there was no benefit to escalating to 70 Gy. A subsequent University of Michigan experience[15] showed that escalating to 90 Gy still resulted in 90% in-field failures and increase in toxicity. Thus 60 Gy/30 fx is considered the standard dose for GBM. A recent single-arm phase I study from the University of Michigan has shown promising median OS of 20.1 months with safe dose escalation to 75 Gy/30 fx along with concurrent and adjuvant TMZ.[16] This has raised the question again about the potential benefit of dose escalation in the TMZ era and has in part led to the ongoing NRG BN001 trial.

■ **What chemotherapies have been used after surgery?**

Historically, nitrosoureas were utilized, until a meta-analysis of PRTs of RT vs. RT + nitrosoureas showed only modest 1-year OS benefit.[17] BCNU was the RTOG standard of care for many years. BCNU wafers (Gliadel) were investigated in a phase III trial of RT ± BCNU wafers: MS improved to 13.9 months vs. 11.8 months.[18] However, the survival advantage was possibly driven by grade III patients, and a subsequent 2007 meta-analysis suggested BCNU wafers are not effective or cost-effective for glioblastoma.[19]

■ **What trial defines the current standard of care in GBM management?**

RT + concurrent and adjuvant TMZ is the standard of care based on the Stupp trial.

Stupp, EORTC 26899/NCIC (*NEJM* **2005, PMID 15758009**; *Lancet Oncol* **2009, PMID 19269895**): PRT of 573 patients with GBM, ages 18 to 70 with ECOG PS 0 to 2. All patients received EBRT 60 Gy/30 fx, and were randomized to RT alone or chemoRT with concurrent TMZ 75 mg/m² d1–7 q1week and then adjuvant TMZ 150 to 200 mg/m² d1–5 q4weeks × 6C. 80% received full course; 40% received full 6 cycles of adjuvant TMZ. OS and PFS were significantly improved (see Table 1.2) with the benefit holding across all subgroups and MGMT status as the strongest prognostic and predictive factor. **Conclusion: Concurrent chemoRT and adjuvant TMZ established as standard of care for GBM.**

Table 1.2 : Stupp Trial Results, Including 2009 Update (All Differences Are Statistically Significant)				
	MS	2-Yr PFS	2-Yr OS	5-Yr OS
RT	12.1 mos	1.8%	10.9%	1.9%
RT + TMZ	14.6 mos	11.2%	27.2%	9.8%

■ **What is the impact of MGMT status on the prognosis for GBM and their response to TMZ?**

MGMT silencing is both prognostic (better outcome regardless of treatment) and predictive (better response to a specific treatment—TMZ in this case) for GBM.

Hegi (*NEJM* **2005, PMID 15758010**): Subset analysis of 206 GBM patients in the Stupp trial, 45% of whom had epigenetic silencing of MGMT by methylation. Regardless of TMZ use, MGMT methylation was associated with improved OS (MS 15.3 vs. 11.8 months). Survival in methylated patients treated with RT + TMZ vs. RT alone was 21.7 months vs. 15.3 months ($p = .007$) and 2-year OS was 46% vs. 23% ($p = .007$). In nonmethylated patients, MS difference between the groups was NS (12.7 vs. 11.8 months); however, 2-year OS was significant (13% vs. 2%). **Conclusion: MGMT methylation is both prognostic and predictive for response to TMZ.** *Comment: The use of TMZ in unmethylated patients is controversial; some feel the subset was underpowered and patients may still benefit.*

■ **Is there any benefit to increasing the dose density of TMZ?**

Gilbert, RTOG 0525 (*JCO* 2013, PMID 24101040): PRT of 833 patients treated 60 Gy/30 fx with daily TMZ (75 mg/m²) randomized to adjuvant Stupp regimen (150–200 mg/m² × 5 days) vs. adjuvant TMZ 75 to 100 mg/m² × 21 days q4w × 6 to 12 cycles. Increasing the number of days that patients received TMZ did not improve OS or PFS, regardless of methylation status. However, the study did confirm the prognostic significance of MGMT methylation, with improved OS (21.2 vs. 14 months, $p < .0001$). **Conclusion: MGMT methylation is prognostic, but dose-dense TMZ was not beneficial.**

■ **Is there any role of hyperfractionation in GBM?**

RTOG 8302[20] and RTOG 9006[21] examined this question and showed no benefit to hyperfractionated RT compared to standard fractionation in patients with malignant glioma.

■ **Does a radiosurgery boost improve disease control for GBM patients?**

Souhami, RTOG 9305 (*IJROP* 2004, PMID 15465203): PRT of GBM patients with KPS ≥70 and unifocal, enhancing, well-demarcated, ≤4 cm lesion randomized to RT + BCNU ± upfront SRS (15–24 Gy, depending on size). MS was 13.5 months in SRS arm vs. 13.6 months in standard arm. **Conclusion: There is no role for an upfront SRS boost in GBM.**

■ **Is there a role for a brachytherapy boost in malignant gliomas?**

Two PRTs showed no improvement in overall survival with brachytherapy boost including using I-125 implant prior to EBRT or after EBRT in malignant gliomas.[22,23]

■ **What is the role of WBRT in GBM?**

WBRT can be considered for multifocal disease/subependymal spread, or poor performance patients (KPS <60), with comparable outcomes (MS ~7 months) to limited volume RT.[24,25]

■ **What is the basis for the treatment volumes used during standard chemoRT?**

After standard treatment, over 80% of recurrences occur within a 2-cm margin of the contrast-enhancing lesion seen on CT or MRI at original diagnosis.[26] Thus high-dose treatment volume typically includes a 2-cm CTV expansion of the resection cavity and any residual enhancing tumor, as used in RTOG protocols. Though peritumoral edema seen on T2 and FLAIR MRI sequences is typically targeted in the low-dose PTV, retrospective single-institution reviews have suggested that there are no increased rates of local recurrence when peritumoral edema is not specifically targeted during radiation treatment.[27] In fact, EORTC protocols for GBM do not include targeting of edema volumes.[26]

■ **Is there a benefit to the addition of bevacizumab to TMZ?**

Gilbert, RTOG 0825 (*NEJM* 2014, PMID 24552317): PRT in 637 GBM patients treated with the Stupp regimen with or without bevacizumab 10 mg/kg q2 weeks × 12 cycles after RT. Patients stratified by MGMT methylation status. Prespecified coprimary end points were OS and PFS. Use of bevacizumab did not improve MS (15.7 vs. 16.1 months). Although PFS was increased with use of bevacizumab (10.7 vs. 7.3 months, $p = .007$), this did not meet the prespecified end point of $p < .004$. Bevacizumab group was also associated with increased hypertension, VTE events, intestinal perforation, and neutropenia. **Conclusion: No improvement in OS with addition of bevacizumab to standard RT + TMZ; there was a modest PFS benefit, but this did not reach predefined target for statistical significance.**

Chinot, AVAGLIO Study (*NEJM* 2014, PMID 24552318): PRT of 921 patients with GBM treated with Stupp regimen with or without biweekly bevacizumab 10 mg/kg q2 weeks. OS was not statistically improved 16.8 vs. 16.7 months. PFS was statistically improved to 10.6 from 6.2 months with addition of bevacizumab. However, higher grade III toxicity was observed in the bevacizumab arm 66.8% vs. 51.3%.

■ What are TTF and is there a benefit in GBM?

Polarization occurs in cells during the spindle formation process in mitosis. Alternating electric fields can be used to disrupt this normal polarization, thus inhibiting cell division. The FDA-approved NovoTTF-100A (Optune) is a device a patient wears on their head along with an attached portable battery pack that emits alternating electric fields.

Stupp (*JAMA* 2017, PMID 29260225): PRT of 695 patients with GBM treated with chemoRT (Stupp regimen) and then randomized to either conventional adjuvant TMZ or TTF + TMZ. MFU 40 months, minimum follow-up 24 months. TTF significantly improved OS (20.9 months vs. 16.0 months, *p* < .001) and PFS (6.7 m vs. 4.0 m, *p* < .001) with use of TTF + TMZ. Mild to moderate skin toxicity underneath the transducer arrays occurred in 52% of patients who received TTF vs. no patients who received TMZ alone. **Conclusion: NovoTTF + adjuvant TMZ as part of Stupp protocol is associated with a 5-month OS benefit.**

MANAGEMENT OF OLDER/FRAIL PATIENTS WITH GBM

■ What is the role of RT over best supportive care?

Radiation therapy improves OS over best supportive care in older patients with good KPS.

Keime-Guibert, France (*NEJM* 2007, PMID 17429084): PRT of 81 patients ≥age 70 (all KPS ≥70) with newly diagnosed AA or GBM randomized to RT 50.4 Gy/28 fx vs. best supportive care after biopsy/resection. MS improved with RT (29.1 vs. 16.9 weeks, *p* = .002). No difference between the arms in terms of QOL or cognition. Trial closed early after interim analysis demonstrated improved OS with use of RT. **Conclusion: RT plays an important role in improving OS in GBM patients even in the older population, without decline in QOL or measured cognitive function.**

■ Is hypofractionation comparable to standard fractionation for older-adult/poor performance status GBM patients?

Multiple trials have demonstrated the efficacy of hypofractionated, shortened regimens for select patients who are not receiving systemic therapy. An important caveat is that these trials generally have not taken into account genetic markers and thus it is unknown what the durability of control is compared to standard therapy for those with favorable genetic profiles. Prospectively validated regimens include 40 Gy/15 fx, 34 Gy/10 fx, and 25 Gy/5 fx.

Roa, Canadian (*JCO* 2004, PMID 15051755): PRT of 100 patients ≥60 y/o randomized to 60 Gy/30 fx vs. 40 Gy/15 fx (no CHT), MS was 5.1 months for standard vs. 5.6 for shorter course RT (NS); shorter course arm required less steroid use at end of treatment (49% vs. 23%); 26% patients stopped long-course RT vs. 10% in short-course arm. **Conclusion: In patients older than 60 who are not receiving systemic therapy, there is no difference in OS between 40 Gy/15 fx and standard fractionation.**

Roa, IAEA (*JCO* 2015, PMID 26392096): PRT of 98 older/frail patients (age ≥50 and KPS 50–70 or age ≥65 with KPS ≥50) with GBM randomized to 25 Gy/5 fx vs. 40 Gy/15 fx. No CHT given. Patients receiving 25 Gy/5 fx had noninferior OS compared to those receiving 40 Gy/15 fx, and no difference in PFS or QOL. **Conclusion: Short-course RT delivered in 1 week (25 Gy/5 fx) is a treatment option for older and/or frail patients with newly diagnosed GBM.**

■ Can TMZ be substituted for RT in elderly patients?

TMZ alone is a noninferior option compared to standard RT in older patients and may be preferred over RT alone in patients with MGMT promoter methylation.

Wick, NOA-08 (*Lancet Oncol* 2012, PMID 22578793): PRT of 373 patients with AA (11%) or GBM (89%), age >65 and KPS ≥60 randomized to (a) TMZ alone (100 mg/m² for 7 days, alternating with 7 days off, for as long as tolerated) vs. (b) standard RT alone (60 Gy/30 fx). OS for patients receiving TMZ alone was noninferior to those receiving standard RT (8.6 months vs. 9.6 months). Patients with MGMT promoter methylation had improved OS compared to unmethylated patients. Patients with MGMT methylation had significantly improved EFS with receipt of TMZ compared to RT. Patients without methylation had significantly improved EFS when receiving RT compared to TMZ. **Conclusion: TMZ alone is noninferior to standard RT alone in this older patient population. MGMT promoter methylation is an important prognostic factor and may be predictive for appropriate treatment regimen.**

Malmström, Nordic Trial (*Lancet* 2012, PMID 22877848): PRT of 342 patients with GBM and age >60 randomized to CHT alone (TMZ 200 mg/m² d1–5 of 28-day cycle for up to 6 cycles) vs. 60 Gy/30 fx vs. 34 Gy/10 fx. MS significantly improved for patients receiving TMZ alone (8 months) vs. standard RT (6 months) but not vs. hypofractionated RT (7.5 months). For patients >70, survival was improved in both the TMZ and hypofractionated arms compared to standard fractionation. **Conclusion: Older patients had a detriment in OS when receiving standard RT compared to TMZ alone. Use of TMZ alone or hypofractionated RT should be considered standard in the elderly population, especially if over age 70.**

■ **Should TMZ be added to short-course RT?**

Perry, EORTC 26062 (*NEJM* 2017, PMID 28296618): PRT of patients with age ≥60 with newly diagnosed GBM were treated with 40 Gy/15 fx and randomized to no systemic therapy vs. 3 weeks concurrent TMZ and monthly adjuvant TMZ up to 12 cycles. RT + TMZ significantly improved OS compared to RT alone (9.3 vs. 7.6 months, $p = .0001$). PFS was improved as well (5.3 vs. 3.9 months, $p < .0001$). OS improved in MGMT methylated (13.5 vs. 7.7 months, $p = .0001$) but not statistically significant in unmethylated patients (10 vs. 7.9 months, $p = .055$). **Conclusion: There is an OS benefit to the addition of TMZ to RT even for those receiving a hypofractionated regimen. Patients with MGMT methylation benefit most from RT + TMZ with a ~6-month improvement in OS.**

RECURRENT/PROGRESSIVE GBM

■ **What are the options when there is disease recurrence?**

Recurrence is common with 80% of recurrences within 2-cm of primary.[26] Options include re-resection, ± carmustine wafer placement, bevacizumab, and TTF.

■ **Is re-irradiation an option for progression?**

Fokas (*Strahlenther Onkol* 2009, PMID 19370426): RR of 53 patients with recurrent GBM. Demonstrated MS of 9 months after re-RT with median dose of 30 Gy in median dose/fx of 3 Gy; only KPS <70 predicted for poor survival. Well tolerated with no acute or late toxicity >2. **Conclusion: Hypofractionated RT is safe and feasible for re-irradiation of GBM.**

■ **What is the role of pulsed-reduced dose-rate re-irradiation to minimize toxicity?**

The inverse dose-rate effect may allow for reassortment of tumor cells while the treatment is delivered, perhaps leading to increased tumor kill with decreased toxicity due to normal tissue repair.

Adkison, Wisconsin (*IJROBP* 2011, PMID 20472350): RR of 103 patients (86 with GBM) with pulsed reduced dose-rate re-RT. RT was delivered slowly at 0.0667 Gy/min to a median dose of 50 Gy. Four of 15 patients had significant RT necrosis on autopsy. MS for GBM patients after pulsed reduced dose-rate RT was 5.1 months. **Conclusion: Pulsed-reduced dose-rate RT appears safe in the re-irradiation setting in order to treat larger volumes to a higher dose.**

■ **Is bevacizumab effective for recurrent GBM?**

Bevacizumab is beneficial in improving PFS as a second-line therapy with or without re-irradiation; however, it is associated with a higher rate of toxicity.

Wong (*JNCCN* 2011, PMID 21464145): Meta-analysis of 15 trials (mainly phase II data) with a total of 548 patients treated with bevacizumab at recurrence. MS was 9.3 months 6% complete response, 49% partial response, and 29% stable disease.

Friedman, BRAIN Trial (*JCO* 2009, PMID 19720927): A total of 167 patients with recurrent GBM were randomized to bevacizumab or bevacizumab + irinotecan. MS 9 months in each arm; however, significantly worse grade III toxicities with use of combination therapy.

REFERENCES

1. Ostrom QT, Gittleman H, Fulop J, et al. CBTRUS statistical report: primary brain and central nervous system tumors diagnosed in the United States in 2008–2012. *Neuro Oncol.* 2015;17(Suppl 4):iv1–iv62. doi:10.1093/neuonc/nov189
2. Thakkar JP, Dolecek TA, Horbinski C, et al. Epidemiologic and molecular prognostic review of glioblastoma. *Cancer Epidemiol Biomarkers Prev.* 2014;23(10):1985–1996. doi:10.1158/1055-9965.EPI-14-0275
3. Smith MA, Freidlin B, Ries LA, Simon R. Trends in reported incidence of primary malignant brain tumors in children in the United States. *J Natl Cancer Inst.* 1998;90(17):1269–1277. doi:10.1093/jnci/90.17.1269
4. Louis DN, Perry A, Reifenberger G, et al. The 2016 World Health Organization classification of tumors of the central nervous system: a summary. *Acta Neuropathologica.* 2016;131(6):803–820. doi:10.1007/s00401-016-1545-1
5. Sanson M, Marie Y, Paris S, et al. Isocitrate dehydrogenase 1 codon 132 mutation is an important prognostic biomarker in gliomas. *J Clin Oncol.* 2009;27(25):4150–4154. doi:10.1200/JCO.2009.21.9832
6. Pelloski CE, Ballman KV, Furth AF, et al. Epidermal growth factor receptor variant III status defines clinically distinct subtypes of glioblastoma. *J Clin Oncol.* 2007;25(16):2288–2294. doi:10.1200/JCO.2006.08.0705
7. Kleinschmidt-DeMasters BK, Aisner DL, Birks DK, Foreman NK. Epithelioid GBMs show a high percentage of BRAF V600E mutation. *Am J Surg Pathol.* 2013;37(5):685–698. doi:10.1097/PAS.0b013e31827f9c5e
8. Jiao Y, Killela PJ, Reitman ZJ, et al. Frequent ATRX, CIC, FUBP1 and IDH1 mutations refine the classification of malignant gliomas. *Oncotarget.* 2012;3(7):709–722. doi:10.18632/oncotarget.588
9. Kannan K, Inagaki A, Silber J, et al. Whole-exome sequencing identifies ATRX mutation as a key molecular determinant in lower-grade glioma. *Oncotarget.* 2012;3(10):1194–1203. doi:10.18632/oncotarget.689
10. Liu XY, Gerges N, Korshunov A, et al. Frequent ATRX mutations and loss of expression in adult diffuse astrocytic tumors carrying IDH1/IDH2 and TP53 mutations. *Acta Neuropathol.* 2012;124(5):615–625. doi:10.1007/s00401-012-1031-3
11. Li J, Wang M, Won M, et al. Validation and simplification of the Radiation Therapy Oncology Group recursive partitioning analysis classification for glioblastoma. *Int J Radiat Oncol Biol Phys.* 2011;81(3):623–630. doi:10.1016/j.ijrobp.2010.06.012
12. Walker MD, Alexander E, Jr., Hunt WE, et al. Evaluation of BCNU and/or radiotherapy in the treatment of anaplastic gliomas: a cooperative clinical trial. *J Neurosurg.* 1978;49(3):333–343. doi:10.3171/jns.1978.49.3.0333
13. Videtic GMM, Woody N, Vassil AD, eds. *Handbook of Treatment Planning in Radiation Oncology,* 3rd ed. Demos Medical; 2020. doi:10.1891/9780826168429
14. Kristiansen K, Hagen S, Kollevold T, et al. Combined modality therapy of operated astrocytomas grade III and IV: confirmation of the value of postoperative irradiation and lack of potentiation of bleomycin on survival time: a prospective multicenter trial of the Scandinavian Glioblastoma Study Group. *Cancer.* 1981;47(4):649–652. doi:10.1002/1097-0142(19810215)47:4<649::AID-CNCR2820470405>3.0.CO;2-W
15. Chan JL, Lee SW, Fraass BA, et al. Survival and failure patterns of high-grade gliomas after three-dimensional conformal radiotherapy. *J Clin Oncol.* 2002;20(6):1635–1642. doi:10.1200/JCO.2002.20.6.1635
16. Tsien CI, Brown D, Normolle D, et al. Concurrent temozolomide and dose-escalated intensity-modulated radiation therapy in newly diagnosed glioblastoma. *Clin Cancer Res.* 2012;18(1):273–279. doi:10.1158/1078-0432.CCR-11-2073
17. Fine HA, Dear KB, Loeffler JS, et al. Meta-analysis of radiation therapy with and without adjuvant chemotherapy for malignant gliomas in adults. *Cancer.* 1993;71(8):2585–2597. doi:10.1002/1097-0142(19930415)71:8<2585::AID-CNCR2820710825>3.0.CO;2-S
18. Westphal M, Hilt DC, Bortey E, et al. A phase 3 trial of local chemotherapy with biodegradable carmustine (BCNU) wafers (Gliadel wafers) in patients with primary malignant glioma. *Neuro Oncol.* 2003;5(2):79–88. doi:10.1093/neuonc/5.2.79
19. Garside R, Pitt M, Anderson R, et al. The effectiveness and cost-effectiveness of carmustine implants and temozolomide for the treatment of newly diagnosed high-grade glioma: a systematic review and economic evaluation. *Health Technol Assess.* 2007;11(45):iii–iv, ix–221. doi:10.3310/hta11450
20. Werner-Wasik M, Scott CB, Nelson DF, et al. Final report of a phase I/II trial of hyperfractionated and accelerated hyperfractionated radiation therapy with carmustine for adults with supratentorial malignant gliomas. Radiation Therapy Oncology Group Study 83-02. *Cancer.* 1996;77(8):1535–1543. doi:10.1002/(SICI)1097-0142(19960415)77:8<1535::AID-CNCR17>3.0.CO;2-0
21. Scott CB, Curran WJ, Yung WKA, et al. Long term results of RTOG 90-06: a randomized trial of hyperfractionated radiotherapy to 72.0 Gy and carmustine vs standard RT and carmustine for malignant glioma patients with emphasis on anaplastic astrocytoma (AA) patients. *Proc Am Soc Clin Oncol.* 1998;17(Abstract 1546):401a.
22. Laperriere NJ, Leung PM, McKenzie S, et al. Randomized study of brachytherapy in the initial management of patients with malignant astrocytoma. *Int J Radiat Oncol Biol Phys.* 1998;41(5):1005–1011. doi:10.1016/S0360-3016(98)00159-X

23. Selker RG, Shapiro WR, Burger P, et al. The Brain Tumor Cooperative Group NIH Trial 87-01: a randomized comparison of surgery, external radiotherapy, and carmustine versus surgery, interstitial radiotherapy boost, external radiation therapy, and carmustine. *Neurosurgery.* 2002;51(2):343–355; discussion 355–347. doi:10.1227/00006123-200208000-00009

24. Kita M, Okawa T, Tanaka M, Ikeda M. Radiotherapy of malignant glioma: prospective randomized clinical study of whole brain vs local irradiation. *Gan No Rinsho Japan J Cancer Clin.* 1989;35(11):1289–1294.

25. Shapiro WR, Green SB, Burger PC, et al. Randomized trial of three chemotherapy regimens and two radiotherapy regimens and two radiotherapy regimens in postoperative treatment of malignant glioma. Brain Tumor Cooperative Group Trial 8001. *J Neurosurg.* 1989;71(1):1–9. doi:10.3171/jns.1989.71.1.0001

26. Niyazi M, Brada M, Chalmers AJ, et al. ESTRO-ACROP guideline "target delineation of glioblastomas". *Radiother Onco.* 2016;118(1):35–42. doi:10.1016/j.radonc.2015.12.003

27. Chang EL, Akyurek S, Avalos T, et al. Evaluation of peritumoral edema in the delineation of radiotherapy clinical target volumes for glioblastoma. *Int J Radiat Oncol Biol Phys.* 2007;68(1):144–150. doi:10.1016/j.ijrobp.2006.12.009

2 ■ ANAPLASTIC GLIOMAS

Shireen Parsai, Martin C. Tom, and Samuel T. Chao

QUICK HIT ■ WHO grade III gliomas are referred to as anaplastic gliomas. While historically considered more aggressive than grade II gliomas, molecular classification has allowed for more granular prognostication among subgroups. Anaplastic gliomas include anaplastic oligodendroglioma (AO) IDH-mutant and 1p19q codeleted, anaplastic astrocytoma (AA) IDH-mutant, and AA IDH-wild-type. The general treatment paradigm includes maximal safe surgical resection followed by adjuvant RT and CHT. The randomized trials that established a survival benefit from CHT used PCV. However, concurrent and adjuvant TMZ is given more often and is still subject to ongoing study. An improved understanding of genomics is rapidly informing the clinical behavior and treatment.

EPIDEMIOLOGY: Grade III gliomas account for 25% of high-grade gliomas; the majority are AAs.[1] AOs account for 0.4% and AAs 1.7% of newly diagnosed gliomas.[2] Oligodendrogliomas are more common in younger patients.[3]

RISK FACTORS: Previous ionizing radiation.[4] Genetic syndromes (<5% of gliomas) associated with gliomas include NF1 (17q, café au lait spots, Lisch nodules, neurofibroma, optic glioma, astrocytoma), NF2 (22q, bilateral acoustic neuroma, glioma, meningioma, ependymoma), tuberous sclerosis (ash-leaf macules, subependymal giant cell astrocytoma, gliomas), Li–Fraumeni syndrome, and von Hippel–Lindau (hemangioblastoma).[1]

ANATOMY: Most arise in the cerebral hemispheres. The frontal lobe is more common than parietal/temporal, which is more common than occipital. Cerebellar tumors are uncommon.[1,2]

PATHOLOGY: Histologic subtypes include AA and AO. WHO grading is classically based on the presence of two of the following criteria (MEAN): high **m**itotic index, **e**ndothelial proliferation, nuclear **a**typia, or **n**ecrosis.[5] WHO grade I: benign, none. Grade II: low grade, one feature. Grade III: anaplastic, two features. Grade IV: malignant, three to four features or necrosis.[1] Currently, WHO classification is now performed by integrating the phenotypic and genetic/mutational signatures. See Chapter 3 for an expanded discussion of the 2016 WHO CNS classification update and the cIMPACT updates, which will inform the next WHO update.

GENETICS: Oligodendrogliomas are molecularly defined per the 2016 WHO CNS classification by allelic loss of the 1p and 19q chromosome arms ("1p19q codeletion") as well as IDH mutation. AOs carry a relatively favorable prognosis of ~14 years.[6] *ATRX* loss and *TP53* mutation is characteristic of astrocytoma (but not required for diagnosis) and is mutually exclusive with 1p19q codeletion. AAs with an IDH mutation have an intermediate prognosis of 5.5 years.[6] AAs without an IDH mutation have a prognosis similar to that of glioblastoma of ~1.5 years.[6] See Chapter 3 for an expanded discussion on genetic mutations and how they are used for integrated glioma classification.

CLINICAL PRESENTATION: Headache and seizures are the most common symptoms. Other symptoms may include memory loss, motor weakness, visual symptoms, language deficit, and cognitive and personality changes. In general, size and location dictate presenting symptoms.[1]

WORKUP: H&P with neurologic exam.

Labs: CBC, pregnancy test in young females, other basic labs prior to CHT.

Imaging: MRI with gadolinium contrast. Anaplastic gliomas are typically hypointense on T1 with heterogeneous enhancement with gadolinium (up to one third may not enhance). Following surgical resection, obtain a postoperative MRI within 72 hours (ideally 24–48 hours) to determine the extent of resection and residual disease.[1]

Pathology: Must obtain tissue diagnosis by biopsy or surgical resection.

PROGNOSTIC FACTORS

Patient-Related: Historically, an RPA by the RTOG classified patients based on factors such as age (<50 vs. ≥50), KPS (<90 vs. 90–100), mental status changes, and duration of symptoms (>3 months better than >3 months).[7–9] The most favorable RPA class (<50 y/o with AA and normal mental status) demonstrated an MS of 58.6 months.

Tumor-Related: AO has a better prognosis compared to AA. The following molecular genetic alterations are positive prognostic factors: IDH mutations, 1p19q codeletion, and MGMT promoter methylation.[1,6,10,11]

Treatment-Related: Extent of surgical resection.[9]

NATURAL HISTORY: Anaplastic gliomas, like other gliomas, are locally aggressive and frequently cause symptoms related to local progression and edema of surrounding tissue by alterations in permeability of blood–brain barrier.[1,12]

TREATMENT PARADIGM

Surgery: Maximal safe resection with neurologic preservation is standard. See Chapter 1 for further details.

Chemotherapy: Randomized trials including RTOG 9402 and EORTC 26951 have established a survival benefit with the addition of PCV CHT to RT for IDH-mutant anaplastic gliomas (PCV: lomustine, procarbazine, and vincristine). The addition of adjuvant TMZ to RT improves OS for IDH-mutant AAs. TMZ vs. PCV is currently being compared on the CODEL trial for AOs. Some institutions favor TMZ over PCV given that it is better tolerated. TMZ is given 75 mg/m^2 daily with RT including weekends, followed by 150 to 200 mg/m^2 daily on days 1 through 5 of 28-day cycles, with the first cycle beginning 28 days after the completion of RT. Up to 12 cycles of adjuvant TMZ are administered. Subgroup analyses have demonstrated no benefit with the addition of CHT for IDH-wild-type AAs.

Radiation

Indications: Adjuvant RT improves overall survival after surgery compared to observation or CHT alone and is indicated for all high-grade gliomas.

Dose: The most common dose is 59.4 Gy/33 fx per trials discussed in the following.

Toxicity: Common acute side effects may include fatigue, headache, alopecia, skin erythema, nausea, memory changes, or cerebral edema. Late effects are dependent on tumor location but may include radiation necrosis, memory/cognitive changes, hearing loss, optic neuritis, cataracts, hypopituitarism.

Procedure: See *Handbook of Treatment Planning in Radiation Oncology,* Chapter 3.[13]

■ EVIDENCE-BASED Q&A

■ What is the role of RT in the management of anaplastic gliomas?

The role of RT was initially established in the 1970s and 1980s due to a survival benefit.

Walker (*J Neurosurg* 1978, PMID 355604): 303 patients with anaplastic gliomas randomized to one of four arms: (a) best supportive care, (b) BCNU alone, (c) RT alone, (d) RT + BCNU. RT was delivered as 50 to 60 Gy to the whole brain. MS was 14 weeks, 18.5 weeks, 35 weeks, and 34.5 weeks, respectively.

■ What is the role of CHT in addition to RT?

Two landmark studies from RTOG and EORTC established the utility of adding CHT (PCV) to RT in anaplastic gliomas. Subsequent subset analyses have shed light on the importance of molecular markers.

Cairncross, RTOG 9402 (*JCO* **2006, PMID 16782910; Update** *JCO* **2013, PMID 23071247; Subset** *JCO* **2014, PMID 24516018)**: PRT of 291 patients newly diagnosed with AO/AOA randomized after surgery to four cycles PCV *prior* to RT vs. RT alone. PCV was administered every 6 weeks. RT started within 6 weeks of completion of CHT. A dose of 59.4 Gy/33 fx was given: 50.4 Gy/28 fx to the resection cavity and any T2 abnormality + 2 cm and then a 9 Gy/5 fx boost to the resection cavity and any T1 postcontrast enhancement plus 1 cm; 79% of "RT alone" patients eventually received CHT (PCV or TMZ); only 46% of PCV + RT patients received all four cycles of CHT. Original analyses in 2006 did not demonstrate a survival benefit with chemoRT as compared to RT alone for the entire cohort (4.7 years vs. 4.6 years, respectively). However, on subset analysis in 2014, patients with IDH-mutated tumors lived longer after chemoRT as compared to those with RT alone. Within the IDH-mutated subgroup, patients with 1p19q codeletion lived the longest. For patients with IDH-wild-type, chemoRT did not increase survival compared to RT alone.

Table 2.1: Results of Cairncross RTOG 9402, 2014 Subset Analysis

	RT + PCV (MS, yrs)	RT alone (MS, yrs)	*p* value
All patients	4.6	4.7	NS
IDH-mutated, 1p19q codeleted	14.7	6.8	.01
IDH-mutated, 1p19q intact	5.5	3.3	.045
IDH-wild-type	1.8	· 1.3	NS

van den Bent, EORTC 26951 (*JCO* **2006, PMID 16782911; update** *JCO* **2013, PMID 23071237)**: PRT of 368 patients newly diagnosed with AO/AOA randomized after surgery to RT followed by PCV x 6C vs. RT alone. Patients received RT within 6 weeks of surgery. A dose of 59.4 Gy/33 fx was given: 45 Gy followed by 14.4 Gy boost. Six cycles of PCV were started within 1 month of completing RT and administered every 6 weeks. Thirty-eight percent of PCV patients discontinued CHT prematurely; 82% of RT alone patients received CHT (PCV > TMZ + others) at recurrence; 55% of RT + PCV patients received salvage CHT (TMZ > PCV + others). On post hoc path review, one third of patients were found to have GBM; MFU 140 months. OS significantly improved among the entire group with PCV: 42.3 vs. 30.6 months. Significant improvements in PFS noted in both 1p19q codeleted (157 vs. 50 months) and 1p19q intact (15 vs. 9 months). No long-term difference in QOL reported after PCV. IDH mutation and 1p19q codeletion were independently significant on multivariate prognostic model. MGMT methylation status was not an independent prognostic factor of survival.

Table 2.2: 2013 Results of EORTC 26951 for Anaplastic Gliomas

	RT + PCV (MS, yrs)	RT Alone (MS, yrs)	*p* value
All patients	3.5	2.6	.018
1p19q codeleted	Not reached	9.3	.059
1p19q intact	2.1	1.8	.185

■ **What is the management of AAs?**

Though often categorized with AOs and AOAs, it is important to note that histologic AAs were not enrolled on either RTOG 9402 or EORTC 26951. Instead, the standard of care of chemoRT is derived from historical malignant glioma trials, of which AAs constituted a minority of patients. They also made up a small minority of the patients on the Stupp trial (see Chapter 1), from which the modern treatment paradigm is generally extrapolated. The only modern prospective randomized evidence in AAs comes from RTOG 9813. However, the contemporary definition of AA uses molecular markers, and subset analyses of RTOG 9402 or EORTC 26951 showed benefit to PCV for AA with IDH mutation.

Chang, RTOG 9813 (*Neuro Oncol* **2017, PMID 27994066)**: PRT of 196 patients with AA or AOA (<25% oligo component) and KPS ≥60 was randomized to RT with concurrent and adjuvant TMZ vs. RT and nitrosourea (either BCNU or CCNU); RT was 59.4 cGy/ 33 fx. No difference in survival between arms (3.9 vs. 3.8 years, *p* = .36). The RT + NU arm had a significantly higher rate of worse overall grade ≥3 toxicity (75.8% vs. 47.9%, *p* < .001). **Conclusion: RT + TMZ was not beneficial compared to RT + nitrosourea but was better tolerated.**

■ **What is the role of TMZ for anaplastic gliomas?**

Despite the survival advantage demonstrated with PCV in patients with AOs and AOAs, many substitute TMZ as it is easier to administer and generally better tolerated. RTOG 0131, NOA-04, and the early results of CATNON all suggest this is a reasonable substitution.

Vogelbaum, RTOG 0131 (*J Neuroncol* 2015, PMID 26088460): Phase II, single-arm trial including 48 patients undergoing TMZ x 6C followed by concurrent RT + TMZ (if disease progression seen on CT/MRI scans every 8 weeks while on pre-RT TMZ). RT 59.4 Gy/33 fx. MFU 8.7 years, median PFS 5.8 years, MS not reached. 1p19q status available in 37 cases. OS and PFS not reached for codeleted patients. Four patients (10%) achieved complete response. **Conclusion: Pre-RT TMZ followed by concurrent RT and TMZ is indirectly comparable to PCV followed by RT.**

Wick, NOA-04 (*JCO* 2009, PMID 19901110; Update *Neuro Oncol* 2016, PMID 27370396): PRT of 318 patients with anaplastic glioma randomly assigned 2:1:1 (A:B1:B2) to receive (A) RT 54 to 60 Gy, (B1) PCV, or (B2) TMZ. In arm A, patients received CHT after progression, and in arm B1 or B2, patients received RT after progression. The primary end point was TTF defined as progression after RT and one CHT in either sequence. The initial results reported in 2009 did not identify any difference in TTF, PFS, or OS between primary CHT compared to RT. This was confirmed with report of long-term results in 2016. The study also identified IDH1 mutation as a positive prognostic factor with a stronger impact as compared to 1p19q codeletion or MGMT methylation. Subset analysis demonstrated that AOs (IDH-mutant, 1p19q codeleted) had improved PFS with PCV vs. TMZ, suggesting PCV may be more effective in this subset.

van den Bent, EORTC CATNON (*Lancet* 2017, PMID 28801186; Update *Lancet* 2021, PMID 34000245): Phase III PRT of 748 patients with newly diagnosed anaplastic glioma with *1p19q intact* randomized to 1 of 4 arms: (a) RT (59.4 Gy/33 fx) alone, (b) RT + concurrent TMZ, (c) RT alone + adjuvant TMZ, or (d) RT + concurrent and adjuvant TMZ. Stratified based on MGMT methylation, age, 1p loss of heterozygosity, presence of oligodendroglial elements, and performance status. Interim analysis with MFU 27 months and 99% enrollment at the time of analysis. HR for OS with *adjuvant* TMZ 0.65 (SS). 5-year OS 55.9% with adjuvant TMZ, 44.1% without adjuvant TMZ. Adjuvant TMZ improved PFS 42.8 vs. 19.0 months (*p* < .05). MGMT methylation was prognostic for OS but not predictive of improved outcome to adjuvant TMZ at this stage. At second interim analysis with MFU 55.7 months, futility of concurrent TMZ was declared (MS 66.9 months with concurrent TMZ vs. 60.4 months without). Adjuvant TMZ improved OS vs. not adjuvant TMZ (MS 82.3 months vs. 46.9 months). **Conclusion: Adjuvant TMZ, but not concurrent TMZ, improved PFS and OS for 1p19q intact anaplastic gliomas.**

Jaeckle, CODEL (*Neuro Oncol* 2020, PMID 32678879): PRT of 36 patients with 1p19q codeleted WHO grade III oligodendrogliomas randomized to RT (59.4 Gy) alone, RT with concurrent and adjuvant TMZ, or TMZ alone in the initial CODEL design. With 7.5-year follow-up, PFS was shorter with TMZ alone compared to the RT arms (HR 3.12, 95% CI: 1.26–7.69, p = .014). The comparison was underpowered to determine OS differences. No differences were observed in neurocognitive decline. **Conclusion: Patients with 1p19q codeleted AOs had significantly shorter PFS when treated with TMZ alone compared to RT arms. The CODEL trial is now redesigned to compare RT + PCV vs. RT + TMZ, and is ongoing.**

REFERENCES

1. Halperin EC, Wazer DE, Perez CA, Brady LW. *Perez and Brady's Principles and Practice of Radiation Oncology*, 6th ed. Lippincott Williams; 2013.
2. Ostrom QT, Cioffi G, Gittleman H, et al. CBTRUS Statistical report: primary brain and other central nervous system tumors diagnosed in the United States in 2012–2016. *Neuro Oncol.* 2019;21(Suppl 5):v1–v100. doi:10.1093/neuonc/noz150
3. Morgan LL. The epidemiology of glioma in adults: a "state of the science" review. *Neuro-oncol.* 2015;17(4):623–624. doi:10.1093/neuonc/nou358
4. Braganza MZ, Kitahara CM, Berrington de Gonzalez A, et al. Ionizing radiation and the risk of brain and central nervous system tumors: a systematic review. *Neuro Oncol.* 2012;14(11):1316–1324. doi:10.1093/neuonc/nos208
5. Marquet G, Dameron O, Saikali S, et al. Grading glioma tumors using OWL-DL and NCI Thesaurus. *AMIA Annu Symp Proc.* 2007;508–512.

6.   Cairncross JG, Wang M, Jenkins RB, et al. Benefit from procarbazine, lomustine, and vincristine in oligodendroglial tumors is associated with mutation of IDH. *J Clin Oncol.* 2014;32(8):783–790. doi:10.1200/JCO.2013.49.3726

7.   Lamborn KR, Chang SM, Prados MD. Prognostic factors for survival of patients with glioblastoma: recursive partitioning analysis. *Neuro Oncol.* 2004;6(3):227–235. doi:10.1215/S1152851703000620

8.   Curran WJ Jr, Scott CB, Horton J, et al. Recursive partitioning analysis of prognostic factors in three Radiation Therapy Oncology Group malignant glioma trials. *J Natl Cancer Inst.* 1993;85(9):704–710. doi:10.1093/jnci/85.9.704

9.   Gorlia T, Delattre JY, Brandes AA, et al. New clinical, pathological and molecular prognostic models and calculators in patients with locally diagnosed anaplastic oligodendroglioma or oligoastrocytoma: a prognostic factor analysis of European Organisation for Research and Treatment of Cancer Brain Tumour Group Study 26951. *Europ J Cancer.* 2013;49(16):3477–3485. doi:10.1016/j.ejca.2013.06.039

10. Wick W, Hartmann C, Engel C, et al. NOA-04 randomized phase III trial of sequential radiochemotherapy of anaplastic glioma with procarbazine, lomustine, and vincristine or temozolomide. *J Clin Oncol.* 2009;27(35):5874–5880. doi:10.1200/JCO.2009.23.6497

11. van den Bent MJ, Carpentier AF, Brandes AA, et al. Adjuvant procarbazine, lomustine, and vincristine improves progression-free survival but not overall survival in newly diagnosed anaplastic oligodendrogliomas and oligoastrocytomas: a randomized European Organisation for Research and Treatment of Cancer phase III trial. *J Clin Oncol.* 2006;24(18):2715–2722. doi:10.1200/JCO.2005.04.6078

12. Gramatzki D, Dehler S, Rushing EJ, et al. Glioblastoma in the Canton of Zurich, Switzerland revisited: 2005 to 2009. *Cancer.* 2016;122(14):2206–2215. doi:10.1002/cncr.30023

13. Videtic G, Woody, N. *Handbook of Treatment Planning in Radiation Oncology*, 3rd ed. Demos Medical Publishing, LLC; 2020.

3 ■ LOW-GRADE GLIOMAS

Martin C. Tom and Erin S. Murphy

QUICK HIT ■ WHO grade I to II gliomas are commonly referred to as LGGs, which are an uncommon and heterogeneous group of primary brain tumors presenting primarily in younger adults or children. Molecular and genomic factors have improved prognostic and predictive stratification. Mutation in the enzyme IDH has emerged as the most informative genomic change and confers a favorable prognosis. Ongoing studies seek to define management based on molecular classification, but established treatment paradigms remain largely based on clinical factors and require patient-specific decision-making. Following maximal safe surgical resection, options include observation, RT, CHT, or combined chemoRT. RT dose is typically 45 to 54 Gy. CHT consists of either TMZ or PCV.

Table 3.1: General Postoperative Treatment Paradigm for LGGs

Classification	Risk Factors	Postoperative Management
Grade I gliomas	GTR	• Observation
	STR	• Observation • RT
Grade II; oligodendroglioma, IDH-mutant and 1p19q codeleted or Grade II; diffuse astrocytoma, IDH-mutant	Low risk*	• Observation
	High risk†	• RT → PCV • RT → TMZ • RT + TMZ → TMZ • Observation in select patients
Grade II; diffuse astrocytic glioma, IDH-wild-type, with molecular features of glioblastoma, WHO grade IV	NA	• RT → PCV • RT + TMZ → TMZ • RT alone

RT dose is 45–54 Gy at 1.8 Gy/fx; treatment paradigms defined based on clinical and molecular characteristics. Consider 60 Gy/30 fx for diffuse astrocytic glioma, IDH-wild-type, with molecular features of glioblastoma, WHO grade IV.
*Low risk per RTOG 9802 defined as age <40 and GTR.
†High risk per RTOG 9802 defined as age ≥40 or STR; per RTOG 0424, defined as ≥3 risk factors (age ≥40, tumor ≥6 cm, tumor crossing midline, preoperative NFS >1, astrocytoma histology).

EPIDEMIOLOGY: Approximately 22,456 cases of primary neuroepithelial tumors occur in the United States annually, of which approximately 11% are grade I and 14% are grade II.[1]

RISK FACTORS: Ionizing radiation and genetic syndromes including NF-1 (17q, café au lait spots, Lisch nodules, neurofibromas, optic gliomas, and astrocytomas), NF-2 (22q, bilateral acoustic neuromas, meningiomas, ependymomas, gliomas), tuberous sclerosis (ash-leaf macules, hamartomas, angiofibromas, periungual fibromas, subependymal giant cell astrocytoma, gliomas), or Li–Fraumeni syndrome (TP53 mutation, gliomas, sarcomas, breast cancer, leukemia, adrenocortical carcinomas).

ANATOMY: Typically, LGGs arise from the supratentorial cortex. Brainstem gliomas and optic pathway gliomas, when biopsied, are often classified as low grade and are discussed elsewhere.

PATHOLOGY: Gliomas represent a group of tumors with characteristics of neuroglial cells (astrocytes or oligodendrocytes). LGGs represent a heterogeneous group of WHO grade I (noninfiltrative) and grade II (infiltrative/diffuse) glial neoplasms.

WHO Grading: Grading is based on the presence of the following histologic features: high mitotic index, endothelial proliferation, nuclear atypia, or necrosis ("MEAN" mnemonic).

2016 WHO CNS Classification Update[2]: In addition to histology, the 2016 classification uses molecular markers to better define CNS tumors, which supersedes traditional histopathologic classification for diffuse gliomas (see Figure 3.1). Although WHO grade is still used, molecular classification has made the distinction between grades II and III (anaplastic) gliomas less apparent. Thus, some now categorize grade II and III gliomas as "lower grade gliomas."

Oligodendroglioma, IDH-Mutant and 1p19q Codeleted: Median OS >10 years.[3] Favorable prognosis and response to CHT. Characterized by IDH mutation and 1p19q codeletion.

Diffuse Astrocytoma, IDH-Mutant: Median OS typically >10 years,[4] characterized by IDH mutation with ATRX loss, TP53 mutation, 1p19q intact.[3] Prognosis is less favorable than oligodendroglioma, IDH-mutant and 1p19q codeleted.

Diffuse Astrocytoma, IDH-Wild-Type: Median OS ~2 years, less common, characterized by lack of an IDH 1 or 2 mutation.[3] To better define this subset of histologic WHO grade II and III tumors, which behave akin to grade IV tumors, additional criteria have been added—lack of an IDH 1 or 2 mutation AND one of the following: EGFR amplification, combined whole chromosome 7 gain and whole chromosome 10 loss, or TERT promoter mutation.[5] In the upcoming WHO classification, it is expected that tumors that meet this criteria will be classified as glioblastoma, IDH-wild-type.[6]

Gemistocytic Astrocytoma, IDH-Mutant: Median OS typically <4 years,[7] high risk for malignant transformation and treated as WHO grade III glioma. Histology shows large, densely packed gemistocytes.

Grade I Tumors

Pilocytic Astrocytoma: Slow growing, often cystic tumor in children and young adults demonstrating Rosenthal fibers. Enhances on MRI due to degenerative hyalinization of blood vessels. BRAF is a driver mutation. Malignant transformation rare. Commonly located in the posterior fossa.

Pleomorphic Xanthoastrocytoma: Large, peripheral tumor frequently with leptomeningeal involvement. Often benign despite aggressive histologic appearance.

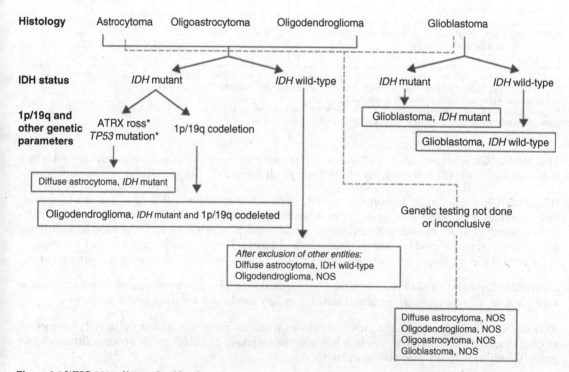

Figure 3.1 WHO 2016 glioma classification.
*Characteristic but not required for diagnosis.
Source: From Louis DN, Perry A, Reifenberger G, et al. The 2016 World Health Organization classification of tumors of the central nervous system: a summary. *Acta Neuropathol.* 2020;131(6):803–820. doi:10.1007/s00401-016-1545-1

Subependymal Giant Cell Astrocytoma: Well-defined tumor typically along lateral ventricles.

Ganglioglioma: Composed of both neoplastic neurons and astrocytes, commonly in temporal lobe, indolent course.

Genetics

IDH1 and IDH2 Mutations: Present in majority of WHO grade II gliomas, favorable prognosis compared to IDH-wild-type.[8] IDH mutations are uncommon in pediatric gliomas and grade I tumors.

1p19q Codeletion: Defining feature of oligodendroglioma, favorable prognosis.[8]

TP53 Mutation and/or ATRX Mutation: Characteristic of IDH-mutated astrocytomas, ATRX mutation is mutually exclusive from 1p19q codeletion;[9] less favorable prognosis than 1p19q codeletion.

TERT Promoter Mutation: Among IDH-wild-type LGG, it confers a poor prognosis, whereas among IDH-mutant LGG, it confers a favorable prognosis.[10]

MGMT Methylation: Associated with improved OS among high-risk LGG treated with RT + TMZ.[11–13]

BRAF: BRAF V600E mutation is present in ganglioglioma, pilocytic astrocytoma, and pleomorphic xanthoastrocytoma.[14] KIAA1549-BRAF fusion is observed in the majority of pilocytic astrocytomas.[15]

CDKN2A/B Homozygous Deletion: Associated with poor prognosis. It is expected that in the updated WHO classification, presence of CDKN2A/B homozygous deletion in an IDH-mutant astrocytoma will be classified as astrocytoma, IDH-mutant, WHO grade IV.[6]

H3 K27M Mutation: Associated with poor prognosis. Present in the majority of pediatric midline gliomas.[16]

H3 G34 Mutation: Associated with poor prognosis akin to WHO grade IV. Present in diffuse gliomas of the cerebral hemispheres, IDH-wild-type, in children and young adults.[6]

CLINICAL PRESENTATION: Depends on location, but most commonly presents as a transient neurologic disturbance or seizure (seizure in >80% of LGG compared to 70% and 50% in anaplastic and GBM, respectively[17]). Most commonly nonenhancing hemispheric lesion (~20% do enhance[18]), rarely mass effect. Best seen on T2 MRI (hypointense on T1, nonenhancing with gadolinium). Calcifications may be present, most commonly in oligodendrogliomas, and may be more common with 1p19q codeletion.[19] Of note, pilocytic astrocytomas enhance via a different mechanism than anaplastic astrocytomas and GBM (degenerative hyalinization of blood vessels).

WORKUP: H&P, neurologic exam, neurocognitive testing, EEG if seizures. MRI with and without contrast. Functional MRI if in critical region. Establish preoperative neurocognitive baseline through testing if possible. Obtain tissue via a maximal safe resection, with biopsy only if a resection is not possible. In general, obtain a postoperative MRI within 72 hours of surgery (ideally 24–48 hours) to determine the extent of surgical resection/residual disease and avoid confounding by blood products.

PROGNOSTIC FACTORS: There is no consensus definition of low-risk and high-risk patients. Prior to the advent of molecularly defined subgroups, various cooperative groups have defined risk factors differently based on clinical factors. Pignatti combined EORTC trials and established five poor prognostic factors: age ≥40, astrocytoma histology, tumor ≥6 cm, tumor crossing midline, and preoperative neurologic deficits.[16] RTOG 9802 stratified patients based on age and resection status, with those <40 achieving a GTR composing the low-risk group. Seizure at presentation is a positive prognostic factor as it is associated with the presence of an IDH mutation.[20] Another combined EORTC/RTOG/NCCTG analysis by Gorlia identified four externally validated factors: neurologic deficit at presentation, <30 weeks since first symptoms, astrocyte histology, and tumor >5 cm.[21] Note that age was not prognostic in this analysis. Molecular markers have since been found to be more important predictors of outcome, but it is likely that both molecular and clinical characteristics contribute to outcomes[22] (see Genetics).

NATURAL HISTORY: Varies widely depending on histology, prognostic factors, and molecular markers. However, most patients with grade II gliomas eventually deteriorate from tumor recurrence (typically occurring at the original site). At recurrence, up to 70% of tumors have undergone malignant transformation (i.e., WHO grade III/IV).[19] Grade I gliomas can be cured with complete resection.

TREATMENT PARADIGM: Most patients are recommended maximal safe resection followed by post-operative MRI to evaluate extent of resection. Low-risk patients may be observed, whereas high-risk patients are typically recommended adjuvant chemoRT. While there is no consensus definition for low or high risk, generally low-risk patients are <40 years old and achieve GTR (per RTOG 9802) or have fewer Pignatti risk factors (see Prognostic Factors). Current trials are designed using molecular classification as distinct entities.

Surgery: Generally required to establish a diagnosis and debulk the tumor for those with extensive neurologic symptoms. There are no trials directly assessing extent of resection in LGG; however, degree of resection is a strong prognostic factor.[23] The low-risk arm from RTOG 9802 showed significant correlation between amount of residual tumor on imaging and recurrence.[24] IDH-mutant astrocytomas appear to benefit from greater extent of resection, whereas the impact for IDH-mutant oligodendrogliomas is less clear.[25-27]

Observation: Following surgery, observation is an option for low-risk patients. This was supported by the "Non-Believers Trial" (as discussed in the following) and the phase II portion of RTOG 9802, which defined low-risk patients as those <40 years old achieving a GTR. However, close follow-up is crucial as RTOG 9802 showed a greater-than-50% risk of progression at 5 years in low-risk patients undergoing observation. RTOG 0925 may provide more insight on the role of observation for low-risk patients.

Chemotherapy: The use of adjuvant CHT (and chemoRT) in LGG continues to evolve. Patients with high-risk features may be chosen for immediate post-op therapy. RTOG 9802 (phase III) investigated adjuvant RT followed by 6 cycles of PCV, whereas RTOG 0424 (phase II) evaluated RT with concurrent and adjuvant TMZ for 12 months. Both regimens have activity in LGG, but level I evidence (RTOG 9802) exists only for PCV. However, many institutions favor TMZ over PCV given better tolerance and ease of administration. EORTC 22033-26033 showed that dose-dense TMZ alone did not result in superior PFS compared to RT alone. However most favor combined modality therapy at the time of postoperative treatment.

Radiation

Indications: High-risk patients should undergo adjuvant chemoRT as established by RTOG 9802 (high-risk patients defined as age ≥40 or <40 years old following STR).

Dose: Doses of 45 to 54 Gy are acceptable.[22] No benefit to escalating dose from 45–50.4 Gy to 59.4–64.8 Gy, as discussed in the following. RTOG 9802 and RTOG 0424 used 54 Gy/30 fx.

Toxicity: Acute: Fatigue, headache, exacerbation of presenting neurologic deficits, alopecia, nausea, cerebral edema, side effects related to chemotherapy. Late: Cognitive changes, radiation necrosis, hypopituitarism, cataracts, vision loss (rare and location dependent).

■ **EVIDENCE-BASED Q&A**

▪ **Does early surgical resection improve outcomes compared to watchful waiting?**

Retrospective studies favor up-front maximal safe resection. However, no prospective trials are available to answer this question.

Jakola, Norwegian University Hospitals (*JAMA* 2012, PMID 23099483): Population-based study of surgical resection (and extent) compared to observation, chosen by patient's residential address. In hospital A, patients were biopsied and observed (50% ultimately underwent resection), but in hospital B an early resection was performed. OS significantly better with early surgical resection (5-yr OS 60% vs. 74%, *p* = .01), favoring early resection. Fewer patients achieved resection if delayed (89% vs. 59%). **Conclusion: Early resection is warranted if safe and feasible.**

▪ **Is it safe to observe patients after surgery and save RT for progression?**

Yes, but the ideal population to observe is unclear in the genomic era, and routine observation is associated with reduced PFS and increased seizure rates.

van den Bent, EORTC 22845 "Non-Believers Trial" (*Lancet* 2005, PMID 16168780): PRT of 311 patients (WHO PS 0–2) with LGG after surgery randomized to immediate RT (54 Gy/30 fx) vs. observation with RT at progression. Included astrocytoma (50%), oligodendroglioma (13%), mixed (13%), and incompletely resected pilocytic astrocytomas (1%). Greater than 90% resection in 42%, 50% to 89% resection in 20%, and <50% resection or biopsy in 38%. Sixty-five percent of patients in observation arm eventually received RT. Survival after first recurrence was better in patients who were observed up front (3.4 vs. 1 yr), likely due to RT salvage. Malignant transformation 70%, equal between arms. **Conclusion: Immediate (vs. delayed) RT improved PFS and decreased seizure rate, but did not improve OS.**

Table 3.2: Results of EORTC "Non-Believers Trial"					
	MS	5-Yr OS (%)	Median PFS	5-Yr PFS (%)	Seizures at 1 Yr (%)
Observation	7.4 yrs	65.7%	3.4 yrs	34.6%	41%
Post-op 54 Gy/30 fx	7.2 yrs	68.7%	5.3 yrs	55.0%	25%
p value	.872		<.0001		.0329

Shaw, RTOG 9802 Phase II (*J Neurosurg* 2008, PMID 18976072): Phase II portion, postsurgery, observed 111 patients <40 y/o who achieved GTR and reported 5-year OS of 93% and 5-year PFS of 48%. GTR was determined by neurosurgeon at time of surgery. Review of post-op MRI revealed that 59% of patients had <1 cm residual disease (26% recurrence), 32% had 1- to 2-cm residual disease (68% recurrence), 9% had >2 cm residual disease (89% recurrence). Poor prognostic factors included large tumor size (≥4 cm), astrocytoma or mixed oligoastrocytoma histology, and residual disease ≥1 cm by MRI. **Conclusion: LGG in patients <40 y/o following GTR have >50% risk of progression at 5 years and should be closely followed with consideration of adjuvant treatment.**

■ **Does RT dose escalation improve outcomes?**

Despite early retrospective data supporting a benefit, two trials have failed to confirm a role for dose escalation.[28]

Karim, EORTC 22844 "Believers Trial" (*IJROBP* 1996, PMID 8948338): PRT of 379 patients with supratentorial low-grade astrocytomas, oligodendrogliomas, and mixed oligoastrocytoma, ages 16 to 65, KPS ≥60, randomized to 45 Gy/25 fx vs. 59.4 Gy/33 fx after any degree of resection. Radiation necrosis risk 2.5% vs. 4% at 2 years. **Conclusion: No difference in 5-year OS (59% vs. 58%) or PFS (50% vs. 47%) with dose escalation.**

Shaw, RTOG 9110 (*JCO* 2002, PMID 11980997; update Breen *Neuro Oncol* 2020, PMID 32002556): PRT of 203 patients with supratentorial grade 1 to 2 astrocytoma, oligodendroglioma, or mixed oligoastrocytoma randomized to 50.4 Gy/28 fx vs. 64.8 Gy/36 fx, following any degree of resection. No improvement with high-dose RT in 15-year OS (22.4%) vs. low-dose RT (24.9%, *p* = .98) or 15-year PFS (high dose, 15.2% vs. low dose, 9.5%; *p* = .71). **Conclusion: No difference in 5-year OS (64% vs. 72%) with higher rate of severe radiation necrosis seen with high-dose arm (5% vs. 2%). Ninety-two percent of failures were in field.**

■ **How do tumor progression and RT affect cognition?**

One reason to delay RT is to avoid the initial neurocognitive effects of treatment, but this is associated with reduced PFS (see "Non-Believers Trial"), which may also affect cognition. Analysis of RTOG 9110 showed stable MMSE scores for most patients and improvement in MMSE for those with lower baseline scores.[29] *Analysis of RTOG 9802 showed improved MMSE scores with the addition of CHT.*[30] *However, MMSE may not be as reliable in evaluating neurocognitive function as more formal testing. A more extensive analysis of 20 patients in RTOG 9110 used formal cognitive testing and showed stable neurocognitive function up to 5 years after RT.*[26] *RT dose escalation may worsen QOL as analysis of the "Believers Trial" showed that patients who received dose escalation reported worse QOL than conventional RT doses.*[30]

■ **Does adjuvant chemoRT improve outcomes compared to adjuvant RT alone?**

The addition of PCV to RT nearly doubles survival in high-risk patients.

Shaw, RTOG 9802 Phase III (*JCO* 2012, PMID 22851558; Update Buckner *NEJM* 2016, PMID 27050206): Phase III component of the phase II/III trial, which randomized 251 unfavorable risk patients (age >40 or <40 y/o achieving only STR) with LGG (WHO grade II astrocytoma, oligodendroglioma, and mixed oligoastrocytoma in 26%, 42%, and 32%) to RT alone vs. RT followed by 6 cycles of PCV. RT dose was 54 Gy/30 fx to the T2 MRI signal + 2 cm block margin. The addition of PCV improved OS vs. RT alone (13.3 vs. 7.8 years, HR: 0.59, $p = .003$). Favorable prognostic variables for both OS and PFS included receipt of PCV and oligodendroglioma histology. Exploratory analysis of patients with IDH1 mutation demonstrated significantly longer OS (13.1 vs. 5.1 years). Power insufficient to investigate IDH1-wild-type. PCV grade 3 to 4 toxicity 67%. **Conclusion: The addition of PCV to RT almost doubles OS in high-risk patients.**

Table 3.3: Final Results of RTOG 9802 Phase III Component				
	MS	10-Yr OS (%)	Median PFS	10-Yr PFS (%)
RT alone	7.8 yrs	41	4 yrs	21
RT followed by PCV	13.3 yrs	62	10.4 yrs	51
p value	.003		<.001	

Bell, RTOG 9802 Genomic Analysis (*JCO* 2020, PMID 32706640): This post hoc genomic analysis of RTOG 9802 grouped patients by the WHO 2016 molecular classification and found the addition of PCV was associated with improved PFS and OS among both IDH-mutant subgroups, but not the IDH-wild-type group.

Table 3.4: Genomic Analysis of RTOG 9802 Phase III Component					
	IDH-Mutant, 1p19q codel		IDH-Mutant, 1p19q noncodel		IDH-Wild-Type	
	mOS	mPFS	mOS	mPFS	mOS	mPFS
RT alone	13.9 yrs	5.8 yrs	4.3 yrs	3.3 yrs	~1.9 yrs	~0.7 yrs
RT followed by PCV	NR	NR	11.4 yrs	10.4 yrs	~1.9 yrs	~0.7 yrs
p value	0.029	<0.001	0.013	0.003	0.94	0.41

■ **Is treatment with TMZ similar to PCV?**

Level I data support the addition of PCV to RT, which improves OS compared to adjuvant RT alone. However, PCV is toxic and more difficult to administer than TMZ. Many therefore give TMZ, extrapolating from high-grade glioma data. This question is being addressed in the ongoing CODEL study, a phase III trial randomizing patients with 1p19q codeletion (either LGG or AG) to adjuvant RT followed by PCV vs. RT + TMZ followed by TMZ.

Fisher, RTOG 0424 (*IJROBP* 2015, PMID 25680596; Update *IJROBP* 2020, PMID 32251755): Single-arm phase II trial of high-risk LGG (WHO grade II astrocytomas, oligodendrogliomas, and mixed oligoastrocytoma) treated with RT (54 Gy/30 fx) with concurrent daily TMZ followed by 12 cycles of monthly TMZ. Patients must have had ≥3 risk factors of the following: age ≥40, tumor ≥6 cm, tumor crossing midline, preoperative NFS >1, astrocytoma histology; 129 patients eligible with MFU 9 years; 3-year OS 73.5% comparing favorably to historical rate of 54% ($p < .001$) and higher than hypothesized rate of 65%; 3-year PFS 59% and grade 3/4 toxicity in 44%/10%. Median OS 8.2 years and median PFS 4.5 years. **Conclusion: Long-term results with TMZ are favorable, but equivalency of TMZ and PCV remains unknown.**

■ **Are there subsets of patients who can be treated initially with CHT alone?**

Given the long and variable natural history of LGG and relatively younger patient population, studies have evaluated whether RT can be deferred to avoid toxicity. EORTC 22033-26033 found that TMZ alone was not superior in terms of PFS compared to RT alone in high-risk LGG, and also found no difference in HRQOL or impaired cognitive dysfunction. Although not directly comparable, it should be noted that the median PFS of 39 months (TMZ alone) and 46 months (RT alone) in the EORTC study was far less than the median PFS of 10.4 years (RT + PCV) in RTOG 9802. Longer follow-up and OS outcomes from EORTC 22033-26033 are awaited.

Baumert, EORTC 22033-26033 (*Lancet Oncol* 2016, PMID 27686946): PRT of 477 patients with LGG, age ≥18, ≥1 high-risk feature (age >40, size >5 cm, progressive disease, tumor crossing midline, neurologic symptoms) randomized to RT alone (50.4 Gy/28 fx) vs. dose-dense TMZ alone (75 mg/m^2 days 1–21 of a 28-day cycle, maximum 12 cycles). Stratified by 1p deletion, contrast enhancement, age ≥40, ECOG ≥1. Primary end point PFS. Median PFS 46 months for RT alone vs. 39 months for TMZ alone (p = .22). OS not reached. Exploratory analysis showed IDH mutation/1p19q non-codeleted had longer PFS if treated with RT alone vs. TMZ alone (p = .0043), but no difference for IDH-mutated/1p19q codeleted or IDH-wild-type. Grade 3 to 4 hematologic toxicity <1% RT vs. 14% TMZ, moderate/severe fatigue 3% RT vs. 7% TMZ, grade 3 to 4 infections 1% RT vs. 3% TMZ. **Conclusion: TMZ alone does not result in superior PFS compared to RT alone in high-risk LGG. OS end point and further data maturation for molecular subtypes awaited.**

Reijneveld, EORTC 22033-26033 HRQOL (*Lancet Oncol* 2016, PMID 27686943): HRQOL and global cognitive functioning evaluated in the preceding study (LGG treated with RT alone vs. TMZ alone) using EORTC questionnaire and MMSE. No difference in HRQOL at 36 months between RT alone vs. TMZ alone (p = .98). No difference in impaired cognitive function at baseline (13% in RT vs. 14% TMZ) or at 36 months after treatment (8% in RT vs. 6% TMZ). **Conclusion: HRQOL and global cognitive function (by MMSE) did not differ in LGG patients treated with RT alone vs. TMZ alone.**

REFERENCES

1. Ostrom QT, Cioffi G, Gittleman H, et al. CBTRUS statistical report: primary brain and other central nervous system tumors diagnosed in the United States in 2012–2016. *Neuro Oncol.* 2019;21(Suppl 5):v1–v100. doi:10.1093/neuonc/noz150

2. Louis DN, Perry A, Reifenberger G, et al. The 2016 World Health Organization classification of tumors of the central nervous system: a summary. *Acta Neuropathol.* 2016;131(6):803–820. doi:10.1007/s00401-016-1545-1

3. Bell EH, Zhang P, Shaw EG, et al. Comprehensive genomic analysis in NRG oncology/RTOG 9802: a phase III trial of radiation versus radiation plus procarbazine, lomustine (CCNU), and vincristine in high-Risk low-Grade glioma. *J Clin Oncol.* 2020;38(29):3407–3417. doi:10.1200/JCO.19.02983

4. Reuss DE, Mamatjan Y, Schrimpf D, et al. IDH mutant diffuse and anaplastic astrocytomas have similar age at presentation and little difference in survival: a grading problem for WHO. *Acta Neuropathol.* 2015;129(6):867–873. doi:10.1007/s00401-015-1438-8

5. Brat DJ, Aldape K, Colman H, et al. cIMPACT-NOW update 3: recommended diagnostic criteria for diffuse astrocytic glioma, IDH-wildtype, with molecular features of glioblastoma, WHO grade IV. *Acta Neuropathol.* 2018;136(5):805–810. doi:10.1007/s00401-018-1913-0

6. Louis DN, Wesseling P, Aldape K, et al. cIMPACT-NOW update 6: new entity and diagnostic principle recommendations of the cIMPACT-Utrecht meeting on future CNS tumor classification and grading. *Brain Pathol.* 2020;30(4):844–856. doi:10.1111/bpa.12832

7. Okamoto Y, Di Patre PL, Burkhard C, et al. Population-based study on incidence, survival rates, and genetic alterations of low-grade diffuse astrocytomas and oligodendrogliomas. *Acta Neuropathol.* 2004;108(1):49–56. doi:10.1007/s00401-004-0861-z

8. Cancer Genome Atlas Research Network, Brat DJ, Verhaak RG, et al. Comprehensive, integrative genomic analysis of diffuse lower-grade gliomas. *N Engl J Med.* 2015;372(26):2481–2498. doi:10.1056/NEJMoa1402121

9. Reuss DE, Sahm F, Schrimpf D, et al. ATRX and IDH1-R132H immunohistochemistry with subsequent copy number analysis and IDH sequencing as a basis for an "integrated" diagnostic approach for adult astrocytoma, oligodendroglioma and glioblastoma. *Acta Neuropathol.* 2015;129(1):133–146. doi:10.1007/s00401-014-1370-3

10. Eckel-Passow JE, Lachance DH, Molinaro AM, et al. Glioma groups based on 1p/19q, IDH, and TERT promoter mutations in tumors. *N Engl J Med.* 2015;372(26):2499–2508. doi:10.1056/NEJMoa1407279

11. Bell EH, Zhang P, Fisher BJ, et al. Association of MGMT Promoter Methylation status with survival outcomes in patients with high-risk glioma treated with radiotherapy and temozolomide: an analysis from the NRG oncology/RTOG 0424 trial. *JAMA Oncol.* 2018;4(10):1405–1409. doi:10.1001/jamaoncol.2018.1977

12. Thon N, Eigenbrod S, Kreth S, et al. IDH1 mutations in grade II astrocytomas are associated with unfavorable progression-free survival and prolonged postrecurrence survival. *Cancer.* 2012;118(2):452–460. doi:10.1002/cncr.26298

13. Watanabe T, Katayama Y, Yoshino A, et al. Aberrant hypermethylation of p14ARF and O6-methylguanine-DNA methyltransferase genes in astrocytoma progression. *Brain Pathol.* 2007;17(1):5–10. doi:10.1111/j.1750-3639.2006.00030.x

14. Olar A, Sulman EP. Molecular markers in low-grade glioma-toward tumor reclassification. *Semin Radiat Oncol.* 2015;25(3):155–163. doi:10.1016/j.semradonc.2015.02.006

15. Jones DT, Kocialkowski S, Liu L, et al. Tandem duplication producing a novel oncogenic BRAF fusion gene defines the majority of pilocytic astrocytomas. *Cancer Res.* 2008;68(21):8673–8677. doi:10.1158/0008-5472.CAN-08-2097

16. Mosaab A, El-Ayadi M, Khorshed EN, et al. Histone H3K27M mutation overrides histological grading in pediatric gliomas. *Sci Rep.* 2020;10(1):8368. doi:10.1038/s41598-020-65272-x

17. Gunderson LL, Tepper JE, Bogart JA. *Clinical Radiation Oncology,* 4th ed. Elsevier; 2016.

18. Lote K, Egeland T, Hager B, et al. Prognostic significance of CT contrast enhancement within histological subgroups of intracranial glioma. *J Neurooncol.* 1998;40(2):161–170. doi:10.1023/a:1006106708606

19. Jenkinson MD, du Plessis DG, Smith TS, et al. Histological growth patterns and genotype in oligodendroglial tumours: correlation with MRI features. *Brain.* 2006;129(7):1884–1891. doi:10.1093/brain/awl108

20. Reichenthal E, Feldman Z, Cohen ML, et al. Hemispheric supratentorial low-grade astrocytoma. *Neurochirurgia (Stuttg).* 1992;35(1):18–22. doi:10.1055/s-2008-1052239

21. Gorlia T, Wu W, Wang M, et al. New validated prognostic models and prognostic calculators in patients with low-grade gliomas diagnosed by central pathology review: a pooled analysis of EORTC/RTOG/NCCTG phase III clinical trials. *Neuro Oncol.* 2013;15(11):1568–1579. doi:10.1093/neuonc/not117

22. Etxaniz O, Carrato C, de Aguirre I, et al. IDH mutation status trumps the Pignatti risk score as a prognostic marker in low-grade gliomas. *J Neurooncol.* 2007;135(2):273–284. doi:10.1007/s11060-017-2570-1

23. Aghi MK, Nahed BV, Sloan AE, et al. The role of surgery in the management of patients with diffuse low grade glioma: a systematic review and evidence-based clinical practice guideline. *J Neurooncol.* 2015;125(3):503–530. doi:10.1007/s11060-015-1867-1

24. Shaw EG, Berkey B, Coons SW, et al. Recurrence following neurosurgeon-determined gross-total resection of adult supratentorial low-grade glioma: results of a prospective clinical trial. *J Neurosurg.* 2008;109(5):835–841. doi:10.3171/JNS/2008/109/11/0835

25. Wijnenga MMJ, French PJ, Dubbink HJ. et al. The impact of surgery in molecularly defined low-grade glioma: an integrated clinical, radiological, and molecular analysis. *Neuro Oncol.* 2018;20(1):103–112. doi:10.1093/neuonc/nox176

26. Patel SH, Bansal AG, Young EB, et al. Extent of surgical resection in lower-grade gliomas: differential impact based on molecular subtype. *AJNR Am J Neuroradiol.* 2019;40(7):1149–1155. doi:10.3174/ajnr.A6102

27. Kavouridis VK, Boaro A, Dorr J, et al. Contemporary assessment of extent of resection in molecularly defined categories of diffuse low-grade glioma: a volumetric analysis. *J Neurosurg.* 2019;1–11. doi:10.3171/2019.6.JNS19972

28. Shaw EG, Daumas-Duport C, Scheithauer BW, et al. Radiation therapy in the management of low-grade supratentorial astrocytomas. *J Neurosurg.* 1989;70(6):853–861. doi:10.3171/jns.1989.70.6.0853

29. Brown PD, Buckner JC, O'Fallon JR, et al. Effects of radiotherapy on cognitive function in patients with low-grade glioma measured by the folstein mini-mental state examination. *J Clin Oncol.* 2003;21(13):2519–2524. doi:10.1200/JCO.2003.04.172

30. Prabhu RS, Won M, Shaw EG, et al. Effect of the addition of chemotherapy to radiotherapy on cognitive function in patients with low-grade glioma: secondary analysis of RTOG 98-02. *J Clin Oncol.* 2014;32(6):535–541. doi:10.1200/JCO.2013.53.1830

4 ■ MENINGIOMA

Martin C. Tom, David J. Schwartz, and Abigail L. Stockham

QUICK HIT ■ Meningiomas are the most common primary brain tumors in adults, representing approximately 40% of all primary brain tumors with ~30,500 cases per year in the United States, 80% of which are WHO grade I.[1-3] Asymptomatic grade I meningiomas can be observed, whereas maximal safe surgical resection is otherwise the standard of care for lesions that are surgically accessible. The extent of surgical resection and grade of meningioma determine initial postsurgical approach (see Table 4.1). Recurrent meningiomas are generally managed with re-resection followed by RT when no previous RT has been administered. Unresectable meningiomas are managed with fractionated RT or SRS, depending on grade, size, and location. Similar strategies are employed in the setting of spinal meningiomas (approximately 10% of cases). While the vast majority of meningiomas are benign, they may ultimately cause significant morbidity and mortality. Particularly in young patients, the likelihood and morbidity of recurrence must be weighed against the potential long-term sequelae of RT to the brain. Grade II meningiomas have an intermediate prognosis, while grade III meningiomas are aggressive with high recurrence and mortality rates. Recurrent meningiomas have higher subsequent recurrence rates than newly diagnosed meningiomas, adding further complexity to management decisions.

TABLE 4.1: RT Dose Guidelines for Meningioma

Extent of Resection	WHO Grade I	WHO Grade II	WHO Grade III
GTR	Observe	EBRT 54–59.4 Gy/30–33 fx	60–66 Gy/30–33 fx
STR	Observe OR EBRT 54 Gy/30 fx OR SRS 12–14 Gy	59.4–60 Gy/30–33 fx	60–66 Gy/30–33 fx
Recurrent disease	Consider further resection + EBRT 54 Gy/30 fx OR SRS 12–14 Gy	Consider further resection + 59.4–60 Gy/30–33 fx OR SRS 16 Gy	Consider further resection 60–66 Gy/30–33 fx OR SRS 18–24 Gy (based on size)
Unresectable disease	EBRT 54 Gy/30 fx OR SRS 12–14 Gy	59.4–60 Gy/30–33 fx OR SRS 16 Gy	60–66 Gy/30–33 fx OR SRS 18–24 Gy (based on size)

EPIDEMIOLOGY: 30,551 cases per year in the United States; approximate 1-, 5-, and 10-year survival rates are 80%, 65%, and 58%, respectively (decreased survival rate with increasing age). Incidence increases with age (especially >65).[1] There is approximately a 2:1 female predominance though males are slightly more likely to have atypical or malignant meningiomas.[1,2]

RISK FACTORS: Older age, ionizing radiation, NF2, MEN1, exogenous/endogenous hormones, elevated BMI, decreased physical activity, increased height (women), uterine fibroids, and breast cancer.[2,4-10] The degree to which estrogen exposure is an independent risk factor from BMI, decreased physical activity, increased height, uterine fibroids, and breast cancer is unclear.

ANATOMY: Arises from the arachnoid layer of the meninges between the dura mater and pia mater, commonly at sites of high density of arachnoid villi and associated arachnoid cap cells. Most frequently noted at supratentorial sites of dural reflection, such as at the cerebral convexity (~20%) and parafalcine/parasagittal (~25%), along the sphenoid wing (~20%) and skull base (resulting in decreased surgical accessibility), intraventricular and suprasellar region, and olfactory groove (~10%) and in the posterior fossa most commonly along the petrous bone (~10%).

PATHOLOGY: Classified by the WHO into three grades: WHO grade I (benign), WHO grade II (atypical, yet still benign), and WHO grade III (malignant).

TABLE 4.2: Summary of WHO Grading for Meningiomas				
WHO Grade	**Frequency**	**Subtypes**	**Characteristics**	**Recurrence After GTR**
Grade I	80%	Meningothelial Fibroblastic Transitional Psammomatous Angiomatous Microcystic Secretory Metaplastic Lymphoplasmacyte-rich	Psammoma bodies Cellular whorls Calcifications	7%–25%
Grade II	18%	Chordoid Clear cell Atypical	≥4 mitoses/10 HPF, brain invasion OR ≥3 features below: • Hypercellularity • Small cells w/ high nuclear:cytoplasm ratio • Prominent nucleoli • Patternless/sheet-like growth • Foci of spontaneous necrosis	29%–52%
Grade III	2%	Anaplastic Papillary Rhabdoid	≥20 mitoses/10 HPF and/or • Carcinomatous features • Sarcomatous features • Melanomatous features • Loss of usual growth pattern • Brain invasion • Abundant mitoses with atypia • Multifocal necrotic foci	50%–94%

GENETICS: Genetic mutations are common, but the clinical impact of mutations is evolving. DNA methylation profiling and other molecular signatures are promising to better risk-stratify meningiomas.[11] Relevant molecular alterations include TERT, PIK3CA, POLR2A, SMO, KLF4, AKT1, TRAF7, NF2, and SUFU.[12]

CLINICAL PRESENTATION: May be asymptomatic. If symptomatic: headaches, seizure, altered cognition, focal neurologic deficit—these are further detailed in Table 4.3 (data modified from Raizer).[13]

TABLE 4.3: Common Presenting Symptoms of Meningioma Based on Location
Parasagittal: motor and/or sensory changes
Frontal: personality change, avolition, executive dysfunction, disinhibition, urinary incontinence, Broca's aphasia
Temporal: memory changes, Wernicke aphasia (left), aprosody (right), olfactory symptoms including seizures
Cavernous sinus: CN symptoms (nerves III, IV, V1–V2, VI pass through the cavernous sinus), decreased visual acuity, impaired extraocular motion with resultant diplopia, numbness
Occipital lobe: visual field deficit
Cerebellopontine angle: unilateral deafness/decreased hearing, facial numbness, facial weakness
Optic nerve sheath: ipsilateral decreased visual acuity/blindness, exophthalmos, ipsilateral pupillary dilation nonreactive to direct light but with retained consensual contraction
Sphenoid wing: cranial neuropathy, seizures
Tentorium: extra-axial compression with associated occipital/parietal/cerebellar symptoms
Foramen magnum: paraparesis, urinary/anal sphincter dysfunction, tongue atrophy ± fasciculation
Spinal canal: back pain, Brown-Séquard (hemispinal cord) syndrome

WORKUP: H&P with attention to the neurologic exam, head CT, MRI brain to evaluate for a well-circumscribed, classically homogeneously enhancing extra-axial mass with a dural tail (present in more than half of meningiomas—may also be present in patients with chloroma, lymphoma, and sarcoidosis). Meningiomas are T1 isointense and CT isodense with normal brain parenchyma unless contrast is administered, underscoring the importance of IV contrast when possible. Evaluate for bone invasion and/or reactive hyperostosis. Modest perilesional edema may be present; this is more frequently encountered with rapidly enlarging atypical and/or malignant meningiomas as well as convexity or parasagittal meningiomas. Extensive perilesional edema is a relative contraindication to SRS as patients may have considerable posttreatment edema following treatment of convexity meningiomas.

PROGNOSTIC FACTORS: Poorer prognosis with increasing grade, decreasing extent of resection, proliferative index (Ki-67) >1%, brain invasion, age <45, chromosomal abnormalities involving 14 and 22, aggressive clinical behavior, p53 overexpression.[14-20]

NATURAL HISTORY: Approximately 1 to 2 mm of growth annually for grade I meningiomas. Most failures occur locally, and local progression can further aggravate associated neurologic symptoms. Marginal failure around the meninges is possible, particularly with high-grade meningioma.

TREATMENT PARADIGM

Observation: Observation may be appropriate for incidentally discovered small, asymptomatic meningiomas. Observation is also appropriate for WHO grade I tumors following GTR and may be considered following STR as well. Surveillance with MRI is recommended annually for patients with WHO grade I meningiomas undergoing observation to assess need for treatment.

Surgery: Standard is maximal safe surgical resection. Often requires craniotomy, but for sphenoid wing/skull base lesions, endoscopic surgery may be indicated. Simpson grade correlates with local failure (Table 4.4). Postoperative brain MRI should be obtained within 48 hours of surgery.

TABLE 4.4: Simpson Grading System for Meningioma Resection		
Grade	Extent of Resection	Recurrence Rate at 5 Years (%)
0	GTR, including dural attachment and bone plus stripping of 2–4-cm dura	0
1	GTR, including dural attachment and any abnormal bone	9
2	GTR, with coagulation instead of resection of dural attachment	19
3	GTR of meningioma without resection or coagulation of dural attachment	29
4	Subtotal resection	44
5	Tumor debulking or decompression only	N/A

Chemotherapy: No primary role for CHT. Although medical therapy is nonstandard, 2020 NCCN guidelines suggest patients with radiographic progression may benefit from bevacizumab to prevent rapid neurologic deterioration.[21]

Radiation

Dose: WHO grade I meningiomas generally are treated to 50.4 Gy/28 fx or 54 Gy/30 fx. WHO grade II meningiomas are treated to 59.4 Gy/33 fx or 60 Gy/30 fx. WHO grade III meningiomas are treated to 60–66 Gy/30–33 fx. See RTOG 0539 for common dosing strategy. SRS dose, when feasible, is 12 to 14 Gy for grade I tumors. When surrounding tissues allow, 16 Gy for grade II tumors may be considered as well as RTOG 9005 dosing for grade III tumors (18–24 Gy). Brachytherapy is utilized at select institutions for multiply recurrent meningiomas.

Procedure: See *Handbook of Treatment Planning in Radiation Oncology*, Chapter 3.[22]

■ EVIDENCE-BASED Q&A

■ Do incidentally discovered meningiomas require aggressive intervention?

Incidentally appreciated meningiomas may not require additional intervention. In at least one study, more than half of patients' meningiomas demonstrated no growth at 5 years. These patients may be followed with imaging at 3 to 6 months and then annually thereafter if no growth is appreciated.[23]

■ What is the optimal first-line management in the treatment of meningiomas?

Maximal safe surgical resection provides the greatest opportunity for minimizing recurrence rates. The extent of resection is graded according to the Simpson grading system, which was the foundational study in meningioma.[24]

Mayo Clinic (*Mayo Clin Proc* 1998, PMID 9787740): RR of 581 patients treated with initial resection. GTR in 80%. The 5- and 10-year PFS was 88% and 75% for GTR but only 61% and 39% for less than GTR. Perioperative mortality was 1.6%. A matched cohort analysis suggested nontrivial increase in morbidity and mortality from meningioma and/or treatment. Many of the risk factors for recurrence we use today were noted in this study. *Comment: Used an older data set. Surgical techniques, radiographic evaluation, and perioperative care may have improved since that time.[16]*

■ What is the role of RT in the management of WHO grade I meningiomas?

GTR (Simpson 1–3) is generally considered definitive, and patients may be followed with surveillance imaging. However, with longer follow-up, recurrence rates as high as 20%, 40%, and 60% have been reported at 5, 10, and 15 years, likely reflecting modern imaging capabilities.[16,25–27] RT is typically reserved for salvage for these patients. For those with STR (Simpson 4–5), recurrence rates of 40% at 5 years and 60% at 10 years can be reduced to those of GTR (approximately halved) with adjuvant RT doses >50.4 Gy.[28,29]

■ What is the role of RT in the management of WHO grade II meningiomas?

Adjuvant RT is generally recommended after GTR and strongly recommended after STR. Adjuvant RT after GTR of a WHO grade II meningioma is 54 Gy per RTOG 0539. After STR of a WHO grade II, adjuvant RT to 59.4 Gy/33 fx or 60 Gy/30 fx is recommended to minimize risk of LR based on multiple retrospective series.[30–34] Without RT, LR rates of up to 60% at 5 years and CSS of only 70% at 10 years have been observed.[25,35] Following GTR (Simpson 1–2), 5-year PFS is roughly doubled, from approximately 40% to 80% with adjuvant RT.[31,36] Following STR, adjuvant RT is strongly recommended due to high recurrence rates.

■ Can RT margins be reduced in patients with WHO grade II meningioma treated with IMRT?

Although RTOG 0539 used at least a 1-cm CTV expansion for WHO grade II meningiomas, retrospective data suggest a 5-mm CTV and a 3-mm PTV may be used without undue risk of LR.[26]

■ What is the role of RT in the management of WHO grade III meningiomas?

Adjuvant RT is necessary regardless of resection extent. WHO grade III meningiomas are relatively rare, with less than 300 cases per year in the United States.[1] As such, decisive data are lacking, although it is clear that OS is relatively poor with a generally accepted mean of >3 years.[27] A minimum dose of 60 Gy is recommended.[30–32,37,38]

■ Are there prospective data to guide the treatment of meningiomas in the modern era?

Rogers, RTOG 0539 (Low Risk, *ASTRO* 2016, LBA 7; Intermediate Risk, *J Neurosurg* 2018, PMID 28984517; High Risk, *IJROBP* 2020, PMID 31786276): RTOG 0539 was the first prospective trial guiding the use of RT for meningiomas. Three risk groups were defined: low, intermediate, and high (see **Table 4.5**). **Conclusion: This trial supports observation for low-risk patients and 54 Gy for intermediate-risk patients. WHO grade I patients s/p STR may warrant adjuvant RT (crude failure rate 40%).**

TABLE 4.5: RTOG 0539 Summary

Risk Group	Definition	EBRT Dose	Target Volume	Outcomes
Low (n = 63)	WHO grade I meningioma s/p GTR or STR	Observation	N/A	5-yr PFS: 86.1% 5-yr LF: 12.5% (preliminary)
Intermediate (n = 48)	WHO grade II meningioma s/p GTR Recurrent WHO grade I meningioma	54 Gy/30 fx	Tumor bed + 1 cm CTV, reduced to 5 mm around barriers	3-yr PFS: 93.8% 3-yr LF: 4.1%
High (n = 51)	WHO grade III meningioma (any resection) WHO grade II meningioma s/p STR Recurrent WHO grade II meningioma	60 Gy/30 fx (HD PTV) with simultaneous low-dose PTV 54 Gy	HD PTV: gross tumor + resection bed + 1 cm LD PTV: gross tumor + resection bed + 2 cm	3-yr PFS: 59.2% 3-yr LF: 31.1% 3-yr OS: 78.6%

Weber, EORTC 22042-26042 (*Radiother Oncol* 2018, PMID 29960684): Single-arm phase II study of 56 patients with grade II meningioma s/p GTR and RT 60 Gy/30 fx designed to show 3-year PFS >70%. With MFU 5.1 years, 3-year PFS was 88.7% and OS was 98.2%. Late grade ≥3 toxicity was 14.3%. **Conclusion: Grade II meningioma s/p GTR and 60 Gy/30 fx results in PFS of 88.7%.** *Note: Observational cohorts of grade II meningiomas s/p STR and grade III meningiomas s/p any extent of resection have not yet been reported.*

▪ How frequently should patients be surveyed following treatment for meningioma?

For WHO grades I and II or unresected meningiomas, the 2020 NCCN guidelines recommend surveillance imaging with contrast-enhanced MRI at 3, 6, and 12 months, then every 6 to 12 months for 5 years, then every 1 to 3 years thereafter as clinically indicated. More frequent imaging may be required for WHO grade III and for any grade treated for recurrence or with CHT.

▪ Should patients previously treated with RT be screened for meningioma?

No. The incidence of clinically relevant meningioma in patients with a history of cranial RT is approximately 3% at 30 years from the time of RT.[33] The incidence of any meningioma in patients with no history of cranial RT may be as high as approximately 13% at 10 years.[34] The incidence may reach 20% in patients with previous cranial RT who undergo screening with MRI at 20 years following RT.[36] The estimated risk of neoplastic transformation from modern, highly conformal or SRS techniques is low at approximately 1 in 1,000.[39] Therefore, a multidisciplinary working group in the United Kingdom has advised against screening as the risks of anxiety from serial MRI examinations and potential knowledge of an asymptomatic (and sometimes unresectable) tumors outweigh the benefits.[40]

▪ What dose of SRS should be used to treat meningioma and what are the outcomes?

Similar to brain metastases, SRS dose depends on the volume being treated and the dose to adjacent critical structures. Mean doses generally have ranged from 16 to 24 Gy, depending on location, with >20 Gy associated with higher rates of LC.[16,41,42] Maximal dose for cavernous sinus meningiomas is 12 to 14 Gy, with doses >18 Gy associated with unacceptable CN toxicity.[43–45] Fractionated SRT with BED >50 Gy may decrease toxicity rates for patients in whom critical structures limit SRS dose.[46] Most SRS series report excellent LC, with 10-year rates ranging from >90% for WHO grade I to >60% for WHO grades II and III.[41,47–49]

▪ What is meningiomatosis and how should it be managed?

Meningiomatosis is commonly associated with NF or MEN syndromes. Treatment should be coordinated in a multidisciplinary fashion, with surgery given primary consideration due to concerns of secondary malignancy induction. RT is indicated for surgically unresectable or recurrent lesions.[50]

REFERENCES

1. Ostrom QT, Gittleman H, Fulop J, et al. CBTRUS Statistical Report: primary brain and central nervous system tumors diagnosed in the united states in 2008–2012. *Neuro Oncol.* 2015;17 Suppl 4:iv1–iv62. doi:10.1093/neuonc/nov189
2. Wiemels J, Wrensch M, Claus EB. Epidemiology and etiology of meningioma. *J Neurooncol.* 2010;99(3):307–314. doi:10.1007/s11060-010-0386-3
3. Marosi C, Hassler M, Roessler K, et al. Meningioma. *Crit Rev Oncol Hematol.* 2008;67(2):153–171. doi:10.1016/j.critrevonc.2008.01.010
4. Asgharian B, Chen YJ, Patronas NJ, et al. Meningiomas may be a component tumor of multiple endocrine neoplasia type 1. *Clin Cancer Res.* 2004;10(3):869–880. doi:10.1158/1078-0432.CCR-0938-3
5. Jhawar BS, Fuchs CS, Colditz GA, Stampfer MJ. Sex steroid hormone exposures and risk for meningioma. *J Neurosurg.* 2003;99(5):848–853. doi:10.3171/jns.2003.99.5.0848
6. Benson VS, Pirie K, Green J, et al. Lifestyle factors and primary glioma and meningioma tumours in the Million Women Study cohort. *Br J Cancer.* 2008;99(1):185–190. doi:10.1038/sj.bjc.6604445
7. Johnson DR, Olson JE, Vierkant RA, et al. Risk factors for meningioma in postmenopausal women: results from the Iowa Women's Health Study. *Neuro Oncol.* 2011;13(9):1011–1019. doi:10.1093/neuonc/nor081
8. Wiedmann M, Brunborg C, Lindemann K, et al. Body mass index and the risk of meningioma, glioma and schwannoma in a large prospective cohort study (The HUNT Study). *Br J Cancer.* 2013;109(1):289–294. doi:10.1038/bjc.2013.304
9. Niedermaier T, Behrens G, Schmid D, et al. Body mass index, physical activity, and risk of adult meningioma and glioma: A meta-analysis. *Neurology.* 2015;85(15):1342–1350. doi:10.1212/WNL.0000000000002020
10. Custer BS, Koepsell TD, Mueller BA. The association between breast carcinoma and meningioma in women. *Cancer.* 2002;94(6):1626–1635. doi:10.1002/cncr.10410
11. Sahm F, Schrimpf D, Stichel D, et al. DNA methylation-based classification and grading system for meningioma: a multicentre, retrospective analysis. *Lancet Oncol.* 2017;18(5):682–694. doi:10.1016/S1470-2045(17)30155-9
12. Suppiah S, Nassiri F, Bi WL, et al. Molecular and translational advances in meningiomas. *Neuro Oncol.* 2019;21 (Suppl 1):i4–i17.
13. Raizer J. Meningiomas. *Curr Treat Options Neurol.* 2010;12(4):360–368. doi:10.1007/s11940-010-0081-x
14. Anvari K, Hosseini S, Rahighi S, et al. Intracranial meningiomas: prognostic factors and treatment outcome in patients undergoing postoperative radiation therapy. *Adv Biomed Res.* 2016;5:83. doi:10.4103/2277-9175.182214
15. Durand A, Labrousse F, Jouvet A, et al. WHO grade II and III meningiomas: a study of prognostic factors. *J Neurooncol.* 2009;95(3):367–375. doi:10.1007/s11060-009-9934-0
16. Stafford SL, Perry A, Suman VJ, et al. Primarily resected meningiomas: outcome and prognostic factors in 581 Mayo Clinic patients, 1978 through 1988. *Mayo Clin Proc.* 1998;73(10):936–942. doi:10.4065/73.10.936
17. Pasquier D, Bijmolt S, Veninga T, et al. Atypical and malignant meningioma: outcome and prognostic factors in 119 irradiated patients. A multicenter, retrospective study of the Rare Cancer Network. *Int J Radiat Oncol Biol Phys.* 2008;71(5):1388–1393. doi:10.1016/j.ijrobp.2007.12.020
18. Yang SY, Park CK, Park SH, et al. Atypical and anaplastic meningiomas: prognostic implications of clinicopathological features. *J Neurol Neurosurg Psychiatry.* 2008;79(5):574–580. doi:10.1136/jnnp.2007.121582
19. Cai DX, Banerjee R, Scheithauer BW, et al. Chromosome 1p and 14q FISH analysis in clinicopathologic subsets of meningioma: diagnostic and prognostic implications. *J Neuropathol Exp Neurol.* 2001;60(6):628–636. doi:10.1093/jnen/60.6.628
20. Vranic A, Popovic M, Cor A, et al. Mitotic count, brain invasion, and location are independent predictors of recurrence-free survival in primary atypical and malignant meningiomas: a study of 86 patients. *Neurosurgery.* 2010;67(4):1124–1132. doi:10.1227/NEU.0b013e3181eb95b7
21. NCCN Clinical Practice Guidelines in Oncology: Central Nervous System Cancers 3.2020. National Comprehensive Cancer Network; 2020. https://www.nccn.org/professionals/physician_gls/pdf/cns.pdf. Accessed September 24.
22. Videtic GMM. *Handbook of Treatment Planning in Radiation Oncology,* 3rd ed. Demos Medical; 2020. doi:10.1891/9780826168429
23. Yano S, Kuratsu J, Kumamoto Brain Tumor Research G. Indications for surgery in patients with asymptomatic meningiomas based on an extensive experience. *J Neurosurg.* 2006;105(4):538–543. doi:10.3171/jns.2006.105.4.538
24. Simpson D. The recurrence of intracranial meningiomas after surgical treatment. *J Neurol Neurosurg Psychiatry.* 1957;20(1):22–39. doi:10.1136/jnnp.20.1.22
25. Komotar RJ, Iorgulescu JB, Raper DM, et al. The role of radiotherapy following gross-total resection of atypical meningiomas. *J Neurosurg.* 2012;117(4):679–686. doi:10.3171/2012.7.JNS112113
26. Press RH, Prabhu RS, Appin CL, et al. Outcomes and patterns of failure for grade 2 meningioma treated with reduced-margin intensity modulated radiation therapy. *Int J Radiat Oncol Biol Phys.* 2014;88(5):1004–1010. doi:10.1016/j.ijrobp.2013.12.037
27. Perry A, Scheithauer BW, Stafford SL, Lohse CM, Wollan PC. "Malignancy" in meningiomas: a clinicopathologic study of 116 patients, with grading implications. *Cancer.* 1999;85(9):2046-2056. doi:10.1002/(SICI)1097-0142(19990501)85:9%3C2046::AID-CNCR23%3E3.0.CO;2-M
28. Miralbell R, Linggood RM, de la Monte S, et al. The role of radiotherapy in the treatment of subtotally resected benign meningiomas. *J Neurooncol.* 1992;13(2):157–164. doi:10.1007/BF00172765

29. Rogers L, Barani I, Chamberlain M, et al. Meningiomas: knowledge base, treatment outcomes, and uncertainties. A RANO review. *J Neurosurg.* 2015;122(1):4–23. doi:10.3171/2014.7.JNS131644

30. Sughrue ME, Sanai N, Shangari G, et al. Outcome and survival following primary and repeat surgery for World Health Organization Grade III meningiomas. *J Neurosurg.* 2010;113(2):202–209. doi:10.3171/2010.1.JNS091114

31. Boskos C, Feuvret L, Noel G, et al. Combined proton and photon conformal radiotherapy for intracranial atypical and malignant meningioma. *Int J Radiat Oncol Biol Phys.* 2009;75(2):399–406. doi:10.1016/j.ijrobp.2008.10.053

32. Hug EB, Devries A, Thornton AF, et al. Management of atypical and malignant meningiomas: role of high-dose, 3D-conformal radiation therapy. *J Neurooncol.* 2000;48(2):151–160. doi:10.1023/A:1006434124794

33. Friedman DL, Whitton J, Leisenring W, et al. Subsequent neoplasms in 5-year survivors of childhood cancer: the Childhood Cancer Survivor Study. *J Natl Cancer Inst.* 2010;102(14):1083–1095. doi:10.1093/jnci/djq238

34. Muller HL, Gebhardt U, Warmuth-Metz M, et al. Meningioma as second malignant neoplasm after oncological treatment during childhood. *Strahlenther Onkol.* 2012;188(5):438–441. doi:10.1007/s00066-012-0082-7

35. Aghi MK, Carter BS, Cosgrove GR, et al. Long-term recurrence rates of atypical meningiomas after gross total resection with or without postoperative adjuvant radiation. *Neurosurgery.* 2009;64(1):56–60; discussion 60. doi:10.1227/01.NEU.0000330399.55586.63

36. Banerjee J, Paakko E, Harila M, et al. Radiation-induced meningiomas: a shadow in the success story of childhood leukemia. *Neuro Oncol.* 2009;11(5):543–549. doi:10.1215/15228517-2008-122

37. Dziuk TW, Woo S, Butler EB, et al. Malignant meningioma: an indication for initial aggressive surgery and adjuvant radiotherapy. *J Neurooncol.* 1998;37(2):177–188. doi:10.1023/A:1005853720926

38. Kaur G, Sayegh ET, Larson A, et al. Adjuvant radiotherapy for atypical and malignant meningiomas: a systematic review. *Neuro Oncol.* 2014;16(5):628–636. doi:10.1093/neuonc/nou025

39. Niranjan A, Kondziolka D, Lunsford LD. Neoplastic transformation after radiosurgery or radiotherapy: risk and realities. *Otolaryngol Clin North Am.* 2009;42(4):717–729. doi:10.1016/j.otc.2009.04.005

40. Sugden E, Taylor A, Pretorius P, et al. Meningiomas occurring during long-term survival after treatment for child-hood cancer. *JRSM open.* 2014;5(4):2054270414524567. doi:10.1177/2054270414524567

41. Kano H, Takahashi JA, Katsuki T, et al. Stereotactic radiosurgery for atypical and anaplastic meningiomas. *J Neurooncol.* 2007;84(1):41–47. doi:10.1007/s11060-007-9338-y

42. Choi CY, Soltys SG, Gibbs IC, et al. Cyberknife stereotactic radiosurgery for treatment of atypical (WHO grade II) cranial meningiomas. *Neurosurgery.* 2010;67(5):1180–1188. doi:10.1227/NEU.0b013e3181f2f427

43. Lee JY, Niranjan A, McInerney J, et al. Stereotactic radiosurgery providing long-term tumor control of cavernous sinus meningiomas. *J Neurosurg.* 2002;97(1):65–72.

44. Spiegelmann R, Cohen ZR, Nissim O, et al. Cavernous sinus meningiomas: a large LINAC radiosurgery series. *J Neurooncol.* 2010;98(2):195–202.

45. Skeie BS, Enger PO, Skeie GO, et al. Gamma knife surgery of meningiomas involving the cavernous sinus: long-term follow-up of 100 patients. *Neurosurgery.* 2010;66(4):661–668; discussion 668–669.

46. Arvold ND, Lessell S, Bussiere M, et al. Visual outcome and tumor control after conformal radiotherapy for patients with optic nerve sheath meningioma. *Int J Radiat Oncol Biol Phys.* 2009;75(4):1166–1172. doi:10.1016/j.ijrobp.2008.12.056

47. Lee JY, Niranjan A, McInerney J, et al. Stereotactic radiosurgery providing long-term tumor control of cavernous sinus meningiomas. *J Neurosurg.* 2002;97(1):65–72. doi:10.3171/jns.2002.97.1.0065

48. Spiegelmann R, Cohen ZR, Nissim O, et al. Cavernous sinus meningiomas: a large LINAC radiosurgery series. *J Neurooncol.* 2010;98(2):195–202. doi:10.1007/s11060-010-0173-1

49. Skeie BS, Enger PO, Skeie GO, et al. Gamma knife surgery of meningiomas involving the cavernous sinus: long-term follow-up of 100 patients. *Neurosurgery.* 2010;66(4):661–668; discussion 668-669. doi:10.1227/01.NEU.0000366112.04015.E2

50. Wentworth S, Pinn M, Bourland JD, et al. Clinical experience with radiation therapy in the management of neurofi-bromatosis-associated central nervous system tumors. *Int J Radiat Oncol Biol Phys.* 2009;73(1):208–213. doi:10.1016/j.ijrobp.2008.03.073

5 ■ PRIMARY CENTRAL NERVOUS SYSTEM LYMPHOMA

Ian W. Winter, Samuel T. Chao, and Erin S. Murphy

QUICK HIT ■ PCNSL accounts for about 4% of primary brain tumors with common occurrence in the immunosuppressed population. Treatment options include MTX-based CHT ± consolidation with WBRT, Ara-C ± etoposide, or high-dose CHT followed by autologous SCT. Careful patient selection and clinical trial availability often determine therapy (Table 5.1).

Table 5.1: General Treatment Paradigm for Primary CNS Lymphoma	
Induction Phase	**Consolidation Phase After Complete Response**
MTX-based CHT	Observation
	WBRT to 23.4 Gy/13 fx (higher dose or boost if <CR)
	Ara-C ± etoposide
	High-dose CHT + ASCT

EPIDEMIOLOGY: PCNSL accounts for about 4% of primary brain tumors, with a yearly age-adjusted incidence of 4 per million.[1] In the mid-1990s, the incidence rose significantly but since then has declined due to improvements in the management and incidence of HIV/AIDS. However, the incidence rate within immunocompetent older adults has risen in the past decade.[2] The median age of diagnosis is in the 60s.[3] It is considered an AIDS-defining illness, and those with an HIV infection have a 3,600-fold increased risk of developing PCNSL.[2] In this population, EBV infection is associated with PCNSL development.

RISK FACTORS: Congenital or acquired immunodeficiency: HIV infection, iatrogenic immunosuppression, severe combined immunodeficiency, Wiskott–Aldrich syndrome, ataxia–telangiectasia, or common variable immunodeficiency. In immunocompetent patients, the risk factors are less established. It is unclear if autoimmune disease is considered a true risk factor.[4]

ANATOMY: Presentations include intracranial, leptomeningeal, periventricular, vitreous, and/or spinal lesions. Location in order of decreasing frequency: frontal lobe, parietal lobe, temporal lobe, basal ganglia, corpus callosum, cerebellum, brainstem, insula, occipital lobe, and fornix.[3] Twenty percent of cases involve the eyes (commonly bilateral) and about 1% have isolated spinal cord involvement, typically involving the lower cervical or upper thoracic regions.[5]

PATHOLOGY: The large majority (90%–95%) of PCNSL are diffuse large B-cell lymphomas, with the other 5% to 10% composed of Burkitt, lymphoblastic, marginal zone, or T-cell lymphoma. Neoplastic B lymphocytes are classically described by "perivascular cuffing" with expression of CD20, CD19, CD22, BCL-6, and IRF4/MUM1; markers of B-cells, germinal center B-cells, and late germinal center B-cells, respectively.[5]

CLINICAL PRESENTATION: The clinical presentation is highly variable depending on location of disease (see Table 5.2). The majority of patients present with a single lesion (66%). Nonspecific symptoms include confusion, lethargy, headaches, focal neurologic deficits, neuropsychiatric symptoms, increased intracranial pressure, or seizures.[5] In a small percentage of patients (10%–15%), gastrointestinal symptoms or respiratory illness may be seen before manifestation of neurological symptoms.[3]

Table 5.2: Presentation of Primary CNS Lymphoma by Location	
Primary cerebral lymphoma	Focal deficits (70%), neuropsychiatric symptoms (43%), increased intracranial pressure (33%), seizures (14%)[3]
Primary leptomeningeal lymphoma	Cranial neuropathies (58%), spinal symptoms (48%), headache (44%), leg weakness (35%), ataxia (25%), encephalopathy (25%), bowel and bladder dysfunction (21%)[6]
Primary intraocular lymphoma	Ocular complaints (62%), behavioral/cognitive changes (27%), hemiparesis (14%), headache (14%), seizures (5%), ataxia (4%), visual field deficit (2%)[7]
Primary spinal lymphoma	Myelopathies[8]
Neurolymphomatosis	Painful neuropathies including sensorimotor or pure sensory neuropathy, and pure motor neuropathy[9]

WORKUP: The International PCNSL Collaborative Group[10] recommends the following: H&P with complete neurologic and lymphatic exam including peripheral lymph nodes and testicular exam. Mini-Mental State Exam. Document performance status. Ophthalmologic and slit-lamp exam.

Labs: LDH, liver function tests, renal function tests, HIV status. Lumbar puncture (at least 1 week after surgery) with assessment of CSF cytology, total protein, cell count, glucose, beta-2 microglobulin, immunoglobulin heavy gene rearrangement, and flow cytometry.[6]

Imaging: Contrast-enhanced MRI brain; if spinal symptoms are present, MRI spine. CT chest, abdomen, pelvis with IV contrast or whole body PET/CT scan. Consider testicular ultrasound in men over age 60 or patients who have positive findings on physical exam.

Biopsy: Stereotactic needle biopsy is standard. Needle biopsy is preferred to surgical resection due to less risk and no clinical benefit with surgical resection. An ocular biopsy or CSF cytology can also be used for diagnosis.[7] Bone marrow biopsy is also indicated. If biopsy is nondiagnostic in the context of steroids, discontinue steroids and rebiopsy or repeat CSF evaluation at progression.[11]

PROGNOSTIC FACTORS: No formal staging system exists for PCNSL, but multiple prognostic systems have been described, as in the following tables (Tables 5.3 & 5.4).

Table 5.3: IELSG Score for Primary CNS Lymphoma[12]			
Number of Risk Factors	2-Yr OS: All Patients	2-Yr OS (With High-Dose MTX)	Risk factors: age >60, ECOG PS >1, elevated LDH, elevated CSF protein concentration (45 mg/dL in patients ≤60 years old; 60 mg/dL if >60 years old), and involvement of deep structures of the brain (e.g., periventricular regions, basal ganglia, corpus callosum, brainstem, cerebellum)
0–1	80% ± 8%	85% ± 8%	
2–3	48% ± 7%	57% ± 8%	
4–5	15% ± 7%	24% ± 11%	

Table 5.4: MSKCC Prognostic Classification[13]		
Class 1: ≤50 yrs	MS 8.5 yrs	FFS 2 yrs
Class 2: >50 yrs, KPS ≥70	MS 3.2 yrs	FFS 1.8 yrs
Class 3: patients ≥50 yrs, KPS <70	MS 1.1 yrs	FFS 0.6 yrs

TREATMENT PARADIGM

Surgery: Biopsy alone is sufficient for diagnosis. Surgical resection is not indicated. PCNSL involvement is classically widespread and involves deep brain structures. Therefore, surgical resection is potentially risky and has not been shown to increase OS.[5]

Chemotherapy: CHT is considered the mainstay of treatment. High-dose MTX (3.5–8 g/m^2) is standard and can be administered as monotherapy (older adults) or more commonly as multidrug therapy. The ideal combination regimen has yet to be defined but may include MTX, rituximab, and various combinations of temozolomide, cytarabine, ifosfamide, procarbazine, and vincristine. After a complete response, consolidation therapy with Ara-C ± etoposide and ASCT are options.

Radiation

Indications: WBRT is used for consolidation after MTX-based CHT or for palliation. Historically, high-dose WBRT alone was the mainstay of treatment but is no longer considered the best long-term option for disease control. The utility of low-dose WBRT to 23.4 Gy/13 fx as consolidation approximately 3 to 5 weeks after CR remains controversial.[14] In patients >60 years old, WBRT in combination with MTX is concerning for neurotoxicity. It has yet to be determined if RT should be withheld in this patient population. Ocular RT can be considered for ocular involvement not responding to CHT. Consider WBRT for palliation in patients ineligible for CHT.

Dose: If WBRT is delivered after CR to CHT, standard is 23.4 Gy/13 fx. If PR, consider WBRT 30 to 36 Gy with boost to 45 Gy/25 fx.[11]

Toxicity: Acute: fatigue, headache, nausea, alopecia, skin erythema, high-frequency hearing loss, changes to hearing and taste, dry mouth. For ocular irradiation: dry eyes, less commonly retinal injury and cataracts. Late: Neurotoxicity changes such as short-term memory loss, verbal fluency/recall, gait changes, ataxia, Parkinson-like features, behavioral changes, and leukoencephalopathy.

Procedure: See *Handbook of Treatment Planning in Radiation Oncology,* Chapter 3.[15]

Medical: Traditionally, corticosteroids are held prior to biopsy unless medically necessary.[16] After biopsy, steroids can be used for quick alleviation of neurologic symptoms. Radiologic regression can be transiently seen with steroids in about 40%, which is suggestive but not diagnostic of PCNSL.

■ **EVIDENCE-BASED Q&A**

▓ **What is the role for radiation therapy alone for PCNSL?**

Historically, RT alone was the initial treatment for PCNSL. However, WBRT alone has shown little success in long-term disease control with high rates of local recurrence.

Nelson, RTOG 8315 (*IJROBP* 1992, PMID 1572835): Single-arm phase II of 41 patients treated with 40 Gy WBRT plus 20 Gy boost to tumor bed plus 2 cm margin. MS 12.2 months. 62% CR. The main location of relapse was at the local site of disease. High KPS and CR were associated with increased OS. **Conclusion: PCNSL shows a good response to WBRT alone, but local recurrence is common.**

▓ **Can combination CHT with WBRT improve outcomes when compared to WBRT alone?**

DeAngelis, RTOG 9310 (*JCO* 2002, PMID 12488408): Multicenter, single-arm phase II prospective study evaluating upfront MPV (methotrexate, procarbazine, vincristine) CHT combination with RT; 102 immunocompetent patients were enrolled; 5 cycles of MTX 2.5 g/m², vincristine, intra-Ommaya MTX, procarbazine, and consolidation WBRT followed by Ara-C. WBRT was 45 Gy (1.8 Gy/fx) in 63 patients, but due to late neurotoxicity seen with this dose, 16 patients who achieved CR after induction received 36 Gy (1.2 Gy/fx BID) for 15 days instead; 34% relapsed during follow-up period. Median PFS 24 months, MS 36.9 months. Between 45 Gy WBRT and 36 Gy hyperfractionated RT (1.2 Gy BID); there was no difference noted in PFS (24.5 months vs. 23.3 months; $p = .81$) and OS (37 months vs. 47.9 months; $p = .65$). Side effects of RT included the following: myelosuppression (63%) and delayed neurologic toxicities classified mostly as leukoencephalopathy (15%); 8 cases of the neurologic toxicities progressed to fatalities. **Conclusion: HD-MTX in combination with other agents improved survival compared to historical rates of RT alone. This CHT combination provides a high response rate, but in conjunction with WBRT there is a significant late risk of neurotoxicity.**

▓ **Is consolidation WBRT superior to CHT alone?**

Thiel (*Lancet Oncol* 2010, PMID 20970380): Phase III PRT to compare HD-MTX vs. HD-MTX plus WBRT; 551 patients received 6 cycles of HD-MTX and HD-MTX plus ifosfamide and were randomly assigned to immediate WBRT (45 Gy/30 fx of 1.5 Gy) or delayed WBRT. For patients with PR after

CHT, they received high-dose Ara-C or WBRT; 13% died during initial CHT. In addition, there was a high dropout rate, leaving 318 patients to be analyzed. In HD-MTX + WBRT patients, MS was 32.4 months and median PFS was 18.3 months. In patients who received CHT alone, the MS was 37.1 months and median PFS was 11.9 months. Neurotoxicity was higher in the WBRT group vs. the non-WBRT group in both clinical (49% vs. 26%) and neuroradiology (71% vs. 46%) assessment. **Conclusion: No statistically significant difference was found in OS or PFS between the WBRT + CHT and CHT alone, but the noninferiority end point of 0.9 was not met. Therefore, the study was unable to conclude if WBRT has an impact on OS when added to CHT. In addition, the neurotoxicity rates were greater in the WBRT cohort.** *Comment: A small percentage of patients were treated per protocol.*

■ **Can the dose of WBRT be reduced to avoid neurotoxicity but still maintain benefit?**

Morris, MSKCC Multi-Center Trial (*JCO* 2013, PMID 24101038): Single-arm phase II trial assessing consolidation with rd-WBRT 23.4 Gy and addition of rituximab to MPV; 45 Gy was delivered for those with PR. Of 52 patients, 31 achieved CR postinduction. Both CR and PR received Ara-C as consolidation after RT. In the rd-WBRT group, median PFS was 7.7 years, 5-year OS was 80%, and MS was not reached with an MFU of 5.9 years. For the entire cohort, median PFS was 3.3 years and MS was 6.6 years. No evidence of cognitive decline was observed, with the exception of motor speed. **Conclusion: rd-WBRT and Ara-C following R-MPV demonstrated good control with minimal neurotoxicity.**

■ **What is the role of temozolomide?**

Glass, RTOG 0227 (*JCO* 2016, PMID 27022122): Single-arm phase I/II trial of induction CHT (rituximab, TMZ, and MTX) followed by WBRT (36 Gy/30 fx at 1.2 Gy BID), followed by adjuvant TMZ. 53 patients treated in phase II portion. Primary end point 2-year OS. 2-year OS was 80.8% and PFS was 63.6%, significantly improved from historical controls; 66% of patients experienced grade 3 to 4 toxicities prior to WBRT, and 45% experienced grade 3 to 4 toxicities attributable to post-WBRT CHT. **Conclusion: Induction with rituximab, TMZ, and MTX followed by hyperfractionated WBRT is safe, with 2-year OS superior to that of historical controls.**

■ **Does low-dose WBRT improve PFS as compared to CHT alone?**

This is a question on the completed but not yet reported trial RTOG 1114. This trial delivers rituximab, methotrexate, procarbazine, vincristine, and cytarabine; randomizes to low-dose WBRT (23.4 Gy/13 fx) or no RT; and then delivers two additional cycles of cytarabine. The addition of WBRT is hypothesized to improve PFS, but this remains an open question.

■ **Is there a role for stem cell transplant with high-dose CHT?**

High-dose CHT plus autologous SCT has a role in both initial and salvage therapy for patients with PCNSL.[17,18] *However, more trials are needed to fully evaluate its potential. Two randomized trials have been designed to further test HCT + ASCT, CALGB 51101, and IELSG 32. CALGB 51101 examined consolidation HCT + ASCT vs. nonmyeloablative CHT; results are not yet reported.*

Ferreri, IELSG-32 (*Lancet Haematol* 2016, PMID 27132696 and *Lancet Haematol* 2017, PMID 29054815): International phase II study with double randomization investigating both MTX-based initial CHT and WBRT vs. HDT + ASCT as consolidation. For the first randomization, 227 HIV-negative patients with newly diagnosed PCNSL were randomized to MTX + cytarabine, MTX + cytarabine + rituximab, or MTX + cytarabine + rituximab + thiotepa; 219 patients were assessable with an MFU 30 months. CR rates for the 3 arms were 23%, 30%, and 49%, respectively, with arms 2 and 3 statistically significantly improved vs. arm 1, at the cost of greater hematologic toxicity in arm 3. For the second randomization, 118 patients with responsive or stable disease were randomized to WBRT 36 Gy (with a 9-Gy boost in patients with PR) or carmustine–thiotepa followed by ASCT. The primary end point was 2-year PFS. There were no significant differences in PFS between WBRT and ASCT (80% vs. 69%, $p = .17$). Hematologic toxicity was more common in the ASCT arm, and two patients died of infection. **Conclusion: WBRT and ASCT are both feasible and effective consolidation therapies following high-dose MTX-based induction therapy.**

■ How is response assessed in PCNSL?

According to the International PCNSL Collaborative group guidelines,[10] in order to assess response, MRI must be completed within 2 months of finishing treatment. LP and/or ophthalmologic exam must be completed if initially positive (Table 5.5).

Table 5.5: Response Criteria in PCNSL per International PCNSL Collaborative Guidelines[10]				
Response	**Steroid Use**	**Eye Exam**	**CSF**	**MRI**
CR	None	Normal	Negative	No enhancement
Unconfirmed CR	Any	Normal or minor abnormality	Negative	No enhancement or minor abnormality
PR	N/A	Decrease in vitreous cells/retinal infiltrate	Persistent or suspicious	≥50% decrease in enhancement
PD	N/A	New ocular disease	Recurrent or positive	≥25% increase or new lesion/site

■ What is the role of WBRT as salvage therapy?

WBRT provides an adequate option as salvage therapy for recurrent or refractory PCNSL. Other options include additional CHT or HDT + ASCT.

Nguyen (*JCO* 2005, PMID 15735126): Evaluation of 27 patients with tumor relapse or progression of a refractory tumor after primary CHT with HD-MTX. Salvage WBRT ± boost was delivered, with the majority (67%) of patients remaining on steroids. Median WBRT dose was 36 Gy (1.5 Gy/fx was most prevalent); 5 patients received a boost to a median dose of 10 Gy and 2 patients received an SRS boost of 12 or 16 Gy; 74% had either a CR ($n = 10$) or a PR ($n = 10$) to WBRT; 8 patients later progressed or recurred at a median 18.8 months post-WBRT. Delayed neurotoxicity was diagnosed in 3 patients, at a median of 25 months, with none resulting in death. **Conclusion: WBRT is an effective option in the salvage setting. For older patients, withholding WBRT until the time of progression may decrease neurotoxicity rates.**

REFERENCES

1. Hoffman S, Propp JM, McCarthy BJ. Temporal trends in incidence of primary brain tumors in the United States, 1985–1999. *Neuro Oncol.* 2006;8(1):27–37. doi:10.1215/S1522851705000323
2. Villano JL, Koshy M, Shaikh H, et al. Age, gender, and racial differences in incidence and survival in primary CNS lymphoma. *Br J Cancer.* 2011;105(9):1414–1418. doi:10.1038/bjc.2011.357
3. Bataille B, Delwail V, Menet E, et al. Primary intracerebral malignant lymphoma: report of 248 cases. *J Neurosurg.* 2000;92(2):261–266. doi:10.3171/jns.2000.92.2.0261
4. Schiff D, Suman VJ, Yang P, et al. Risk factors for primary central nervous system lymphoma: a case-control study. *Cancer.* 1998;82(5):975–982. doi:10.1002/(SICI)1097-0142(19980301)82:5<975::AID-CNCR25>3.0.CO;2-X
5. Ferreri AJ, Marturano E. Primary CNS lymphoma. *Best Pract Res Clin Haematol.* 2012;25(1):119–130. doi:10.1016/j.beha.2011.12.001
6. Taylor JW, Flanagan EP, O'Neill BP, et al. Primary leptomeningeal lymphoma: International Primary CNS Lymphoma Collaborative Group report. *Neurology.* 2013;81(19):1690–1696. doi:10.1212/01.wnl.0000435302.02895.f3
7. Grimm SA, McCannel CA, Omuro AM, et al. Primary CNS lymphoma with intraocular involvement: International PCNSL Collaborative Group Report. *Neurology.* 2008;71(17):1355–1360. doi:10.1212/01.wnl.0000327672.04729.8c
8. Flanagan EP, O'Neill BP, Porter AB, et al. Primary intramedullary spinal cord lymphoma. *Neurology.* 2011;77(8):784–791. doi:10.1212/WNL.0b013e31822b00b9
9. Grisariu S, Avni B, Batchelor TT, et al. Neurolymphomatosis: an International Primary CNS Lymphoma Collaborative Group report. *Blood.* 2010;115(24):5005–5011. doi:10.1182/blood-2009-12-258210
10. Abrey LE, Batchelor TT, Ferreri AJ, et al. Report of an international workshop to standardize baseline evaluation and response criteria for primary CNS lymphoma. *J Clin Oncol.* 2005;23(22):5034–5043. doi:10.1200/JCO.2005.13.524
11. NCCN. Clinical practice guidelines in oncology: central nervous system cancers. 2020;3.2020.
12. Ferreri AJ, Blay JY, Reni M, et al. Prognostic scoring system for primary CNS lymphomas: the International Extranodal Lymphoma Study Group experience. *J Clin Oncol.* 2003;21(2):266–272. doi:10.1200/JCO.2003.09.139

13. Abrey LE, Ben-Porat L, Panageas KS, et al. Primary central nervous system lymphoma: the Memorial Sloan-Kettering Cancer Center prognostic model. *J Clin Oncol*. 2006;24(36):5711–5715. doi:10.1200/JCO.2006.08.2941

14. Shah GD, Yahalom J, Correa DD, et al. Combined immunochemotherapy with reduced whole-brain radiotherapy for newly diagnosed primary CNS lymphoma. *J Clin Oncol*. 2007;25(30):4730–4735. doi:10.1200/JCO.2007.12.5062

15. Videtic GMM WN, Vassil AD. *Handbook of Treatment Planning in Radiation Oncology*, 3rd ed. Demos Medical; 2020. doi:10.1891/9780826168429

16. Ferreri AJ. How I treat primary CNS lymphoma. *Blood*. 2011;118(3):510–522. doi:10.1182/blood-2011-03-321349

17. Soussain C, Hoang-Xuan K, Taillandier L, et al. Intensive chemotherapy followed by hematopoietic stem-cell rescue for refractory and recurrent primary CNS and intraocular lymphoma: Societe Francaise de Greffe de Moelle Osseuse-Therapie Cellulaire. *J Clin Oncol*. 2008;26(15):2512–2518. doi:10.1200/JCO.2007.13.5533

18. Illerhaus G, Marks R, Ihorst G, et al. High-dose chemotherapy with autologous stem-cell transplantation and hyperfractionated radiotherapy as first-line treatment of primary CNS lymphoma. *J Clin Oncol*. 2006;24(24):3865–3870. doi:10.1200/JCO.2006.06.2117

6 ■ PITUITARY ADENOMA

Zachary Mayo and John H. Suh

> **QUICK HIT** ■ Pituitary adenoma can be observed in up to 17% of the population but is often asymptomatic and found incidentally by MRI or autopsy.[1,2] Symptoms may include visual impairment, headache, or hormonal aberrations. Treatment options include surgery, medication, or SRS/fractionated RT to relieve pressure on chiasm and correct hormonal abnormalities (Figure 6.1). When defining response to treatment in the literature, LC refers to radiographic response (size criteria), whereas remission/response refers to normalization of hormone secretion (complete or partial).

EPIDEMIOLOGY: Accounts for 10% to 15% of CNS neoplasms, and approximately 14,000 cases are diagnosed in the United States each year.[3] Typically diagnosed between 30 and 50 years of age. Male-to-female ratio 1:1, but females are more frequently symptomatic and have higher incidence rates until age 30, when pattern reverses; 70% are secretory.

RISK FACTORS: Personal or family history of colorectal cancer, surgically induced menopause.[4,5] Associated syndromes: MEN1 (mnemonic: 3 Ps; pituitary [25%], parathyroid, and pancreatic islet cell tumors), isolated familial somatotropinoma, Carney complex (spotty skin pigmentation, myxomas, endocrine overactivity, schwannomas).

ANATOMY: The pituitary gland lies within the concave sella turcica of the sphenoid bone. The anterior–posterior clinoid processes make up the anterior–posterior sella borders, respectively. The diaphragma sellae is a dural fold comprising the superior border and the cavernous sinus (contains internal carotid arteries and CN III, IV, V1, V2, VI) lies laterally. Embryologically, the anterior lobe (adenohypophysis) develops from Rathke's pouch and the posterior lobe (neurohypophysis) from the third ventricle. Pituitary adenomas arise in the anterior lobe, which secretes FSH, LH, ACTH, TSH, PRL, and GH (mnemonic: FLAT PiG). The posterior lobe secretes oxytocin and ADH.

PATHOLOGY: Mallory's trichrome staining can be used to identify functional adenomas. GH secreting adenomas are typically eosinophilic, ACTH secreting adenomas are basophilic, and nonfunctioning adenomas are chromophobic.[6,7]

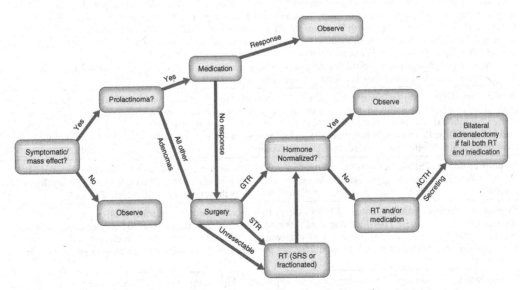

Figure 6.1 General treatment paradigm for pituitary adenoma.

CLINICAL PRESENTATION: Often an asymptomatic, incidental finding. Symptoms can manifest as endocrinopathies (see Table 6.1 for specific tumors) due to hormonal deficiency/hypersecretion, visual field deficits due to optic chiasm compression/involvement (bitemporal hemianopsia, homonymous hemianopsia, temporal quadrantanopia), or apoplexy (acute hemorrhage/infarction). Cavernous sinus invasion can cause CN palsies.

WORKUP: H&P with focus on CN exam and visual field testing.

Labs: CBC, CMP, baseline endocrine function. Examine respective secretory status with TSH, T3/T4, ACTH, 24-hour urinary free cortisol, PRL, IGF-1.

Imaging: T1-weighted MRI with gadolinium; best seen on coronal views. Adenomas are less vascular than normal pituitary (take up gadolinium to a lesser degree than normal pituitary gland), so they appear hypointense in early phase of DCE MRI.[1] Picoadenoma <0.3 cm, microadenoma <1 cm diameter, macroadenoma ≥1 cm, giant adenoma >4 cm. Skeletal survey if acromegaly is present.

Differential for Pituitary Mass

Neoplasms: Pituitary tumor, craniopharyngioma, meningioma, germ cell tumor, metastatic tumor, glioma, lymphoma, chordoma.

Benign: Pituitary hyperplasia (pregnancy, long-standing hypothyroidism/hypogonadism), Rathke's cleft cyst, arachnoid cyst, aneurysm, empty sella syndrome, inflammatory lesions (granuloma), abscess.

PROGNOSTIC FACTORS: Better prognosis with GTR. Worse prognosis with cavernous sinus invasion.[8] *Hardy grading:* 0: intrapituitary microadenoma with normal sella appearance; I: normal sella size with asymmetric floor; II: enlarged sella with intact floor; III: localized erosion of sella floor; IV: diffusely eroded sella floor.[9,10]

Table 6.1: Overview of Pituitary Adenoma Subtypes
Prolactinoma: Most common pituitary adenoma. First-line treatment is medical management with dopamine agonists (e.g., bromocriptine, cabergoline). Most patients have >50% reduction in PRL level with medication. Prolactin levels fall within first 2 to 3 weeks; 80% show >25% reduction in volume, with decrease in size beginning within 6 weeks. Surgery should be considered if dopamine agonist unsuccessful, in women wishing to become pregnant, or with pituitary apoplexy. Lower RT remission rate when RT given alone without medical management compared to other adenoma subtypes. SRS CR rate is 15% to 50% alone, but with medical management increases to 40% to 80% at 2 to 8 years. Fractionated RT alone CR rate is 25% to 50% and with addition of medical therapy increases to 80% to 100% at 1 to 10 years.[9]
Cushing's disease (ACTH): First-line treatment is surgery. Remission rate after surgery: 89% for microadenomas, 63% for macroadenomas, and 81% for macroadenomas where GTR anticipated.[11] Tumor extension beyond sella is predictive of nonremission and late recurrence. RT is the preferred second-line treatment over medical management. Fractionated RT remission rate is 50% to 80% with median time to remission 18 to 42 months. SRS with medical therapy leads to local control rates of 85% to 100% with median time of 7.5 to 33 months for ACTH normalization.[9] Bilateral adrenalectomy, which can lead to Nelson's syndrome (rapid enlargement of pituitary adenoma, muscle weakness, and skin hyperpigmentation due to melanocyte stimulating hormone), is a final salvage approach.
Acromegaly (GH): First-line treatment is surgery. For patients failing surgery, 50% to 60% show reduced GH/IGF-1 levels with somatostatin analogues (side effects: malabsorptive diarrhea, nausea/vomiting, gallbladder sludge, abdominal cramping). Remission rate of fractionated RT and SRS similar: 50% to 60% at 5 to 10 years, and 65% to 87% at 15 years.[9] GH receptor antagonist (pegvisomant) reduces IGF-1 levels (not GH) if other treatments fail. Side effects of pegvisomant: nausea/vomiting, flu syndrome, diarrhea, abnormal LFTs.
Hyperthyroidism (TSHoma): First-line treatment is surgery. Consider postoperative RT to higher dose of 54 Gy as TSHomas are locally aggressive and less responsive to RT. Medical therapy with somatostatin analogues, thyroid ablation, methimazole/propylthiouracil, which inhibits thyroperoxidase (converts T3 to T4).
Pituitary carcinoma: Extremely rare (0.2% of pituitary tumors). Frequently metastatic (CSF or systemic) with mean survival of 1.9 years.[1] First-line treatment is temozolomide, which is also used to treat *aggressive pituitary tumors*—not defined by histology but rather as locally aggressive and not controlled by surgery, RT, and medication. Low MGMT (immunohistochemistry, not promoter methylation) may be a predictive marker for treatment response.[12,13]
Nonsecretory/functioning: First-line treatment is surgery to relieve compression. RT recommended for STR or recurrence.[14] At least partial reduction in size expected in two thirds of cases. LC >90% at 10 yrs with RT.

TREATMENT PARADIGM

Observation: Most asymptomatic pituitary adenomas without lab abnormalities can be safely observed.

Surgery: Surgery is first-line treatment for all except prolactinoma and pituitary carcinoma.

Surgical Technique: (a) **TSS** performed in >95% cases. TSS has two approaches: sublabial (older technique) and transnasal (microscopic or endoscopic endonasal). Endoscopic is minimally invasive and improves surgical visualization, which may allow for more complete resection and reduced complications.[15] Complications include death (1%), meningitis, CSF leak, diabetes insipidus (6%), hemorrhage, stroke, visual deficit. (b) **Transcranial approach** for large tumors. LC approximately 95%, hormone normalization 70% to 80% short term, 40% long term. Evolution of surgical technique over time from transcranial to microscopic TSS to endoscopic TSS has improved outcomes (lower incidence of revision surgery, postoperative hemorrhage, diabetes insipidus, and panhypopituitarism).[16] Intraoperative MRI can improve extent of surgical resection for both microscopic and endoscopic TSS.[17]

Medical Management

Table 6.2: Medical Management of Secretory Pituitary Adenomas			
Hormone (Frequency)	Hormone Levels	Signs and Symptoms	Medical Therapy
Prolactin (30%)	High	Female: amenorrhea, oligomenorrhea, or infertility. Male: low libido or erectile dysfunction, galactorrhea, osteoporosis	Cabergoline, bromocriptine, quinagolide (not available in the United States)
	Low	Inability to lactate after delivery	No treatment currently available
Growth hormone (25%)	High	Gigantism (before puberty) Acromegaly (after puberty): thickening of bones in jaw, fingers, and toes; frontal bossing; macroglossia, hyperhidrosis, muscle weakness, glucose intolerance (50%), hypogonadism, cardiomegaly, fatigue, paresthesias, arthralgias, hypothyroidism	Octreotide, lanreotide, pegvisomant injection (expensive but more effective)
	Low	Infancy and childhood: growth failure Adults: loss of strength, stamina, bone density, and musculature, poor memory, depression	Recombinant human GH preparations (i.e., somatropin)
ACTH (15%)	High	Cushing's disease (not syndrome): central obesity, hypertension, glucose intolerance, hirsutism, easy bruising, striae, osteoporosis, psychologic changes, hypogonadism	Ketoconazole, mitotane, metyrapone
	Low	Hypoglycemia, dehydration, weight loss, weakness, tiredness, dizziness, low blood pressure, nausea/vomiting, diarrhea	Hydrocortisone
TSH (1%)	High	Hyperthyroidism, weight loss, anxiety, heat intolerance, palpitations, diaphoresis, irritability, muscle weakness. Graves' ophthalmopathy	Somatostatin analogue (octreotide, lanreotide), methimazole, propylthiouracil
	Low	Cold intolerance, constipation, weight gain, fatigue, anhidrosis, dry skin, brittle hair/fingernails, infertility, hyperprolactinemia, goiter	Levothyroxine

Radiation

Indications: Second-line therapy if STR s/p surgery, unresectable/inoperable, recurrence after surgery, and/or refractory to medical management. Discontinue medical management 1 month prior to RT and resume after RT completed. Improved response when RT delivered off medical therapy (may alter cell cycle and radiosensitivity)[18–21] as well as reduced hypopituitarism. Goal is to stabilize or reduce mass effect and normalize hormone levels (takes many years). Excellent LC of 90% to 100% in most studies regardless of RT technique and adenoma subtype. Smaller tumors have improved response and lower risk of hypopituitarism. *SRS vs. fractionated RT:* SRS preferred due to faster time to hormone normalization and patient convenience. Fractionated RT if tumor >3 cm or <3 to 5 mm from chiasm due to risk of visual deficits.[9] Risk for hypopituitarism high for both modalities (20% at 5 years; 80% at 10–15 years).[22] Panhypopituitarism occurs in 5% to 10% patients at 5 years.[9]

Dose: SRS: 14 to 20 Gy for nonsecretory tumors; 20 Gy or higher for secretory tumors.

Fractionated RT: 45 to 50.4 Gy/25 to 28 fx for nonsecretory; 50.4 to 54 Gy/28 to 30 fx for secretory.

Fractionated SRS: 17 to 21 Gy/3 fx, 22 to 25 Gy/5 fx for nonsecretory; 17.4 to 26.8 Gy/3 fx, 20 to 32 Gy/5 fx for secretory tumors.[23,24]

Re-irradiation: 35 to 49.6 Gy, median dose 42 Gy at 1.8 to 2 Gy/fx.[25,26]

(Note: Fractionated SRS and re-irradiation doses require further validation.)

Constraints: Optic pathway, maximum: 8 to 10 Gy (1 fx), 17.4 Gy (3 fx), 25 Gy (5 fx), 54 Gy (conventional fractionation).

Toxicity: Acute: Fatigue, headache, infection, alopecia, otitis. Late: hypopituitarism, radionecrosis, vision impairment, hearing loss, stroke (relative risk 2–4),[27–29] second malignancy (2% at 10–20 years).[30]

■ EVIDENCE-BASED Q&A

▪ What are the expected outcomes with SRS?

Kotecha, ISRS Guidelines (*Neuro Oncol* 2020, PMID 31790121): Meta-analysis of 35 retrospective studies of nonfunctioning pituitary adenomas treated with SRS (median 15 Gy, range: 5–35 Gy) or hypofractionated RT (median 21 Gy, range: 12–25 Gy in 3–5 fx). After SRS, 5- and 10-year LC was 94% and 83%, respectively. After hypofractionated RT, 5-year LC was 97%. Most common toxicity was hypopituitarism, estimated at 21%. **Conclusion: Both SRS and hypofractionated RT provide excellent LC for nonfunctioning pituitary adenomas.**

Sheehan, University of Virginia (*J Neurosurg* 2013, PMID 23621595): RR of 512 patients from 9 centers treated with GKRS for nonfunctioning pituitary adenomas to median dose of 16 Gy and treatment volume 3.3 cm.[31] Prior surgery in 70% of patients with cavernous sinus involvement and 33% with suprasellar extension; 3-year LC 98%, 5-year LC 95%, 10-year LC 85%. Smaller target size and absence of suprasellar extension associated with improved PFS. Post-SRS complications included the following: CN dysfunction in 9.3% (CN II: 6.6%; CN III: 1.36%; CN IV: 0.23%; CN V: 0.90%; CN VI: 0.45%; CN VII: 0.23%); hypopituitarism in 21.1% (cortisol: 9.9%; thyroid: 16.3%; gonadotropin: 8.3%; GH: 8.4%); 1.4% with diabetes insipidus; 6.6% with further tumor growth; 7.7% patients required further surgery or RT.

Minniti (*Radiat Oncol* 2016, PMID 27729088): Review of 92 SRS publications. Biochemical remission: GH (1,802 patients) 44% at MFU 59 months; ACTH (706 patients) 48% at 56 months; PRL (610 patients) 44% at 49 months. LC 95% regardless of adenoma subtype. Hypopituitarism in 24% at 5 years. Optic neuropathy 0% to 3% for Dmax <8 to 10 Gy to optic nerves/chiasm. CN dysfunction and brain necrosis <2%.

Hung (*J Neurosurg* 2019, PMID 31374549): RR of 289 patients with prolactinomas treated with SRS. Endocrine remission (off of dopamine agonist) rates were 28%, 41%, and 54% at 3, 5, and 8 years after SRS, respectively. Endocrine control (with dopamine agonist) in 63%. Tumor progression in 5%. Toxicity included 25% hormone deficiency and 3% visual complication.

Ding, (*Neurosurgery* 2019, PMID 29757421): RR of 371 patients with acromegaly treated with SRS. Rates of initial and durable endocrine remission at 10 years were 69% and 59%, respectively. The mean time to durable remission after SRS was 38 months. Biochemical relapse in 9% at a mean time of 17 months. Cessation of IGF-1 lowering medication prior to SRS was the only independent predictor of durable remission ($p = .01$).

■ **Is there a difference between time to endocrine response when comparing fractionated RT VS. SRS?**

Hormone normalization appears to occur faster after SRS in some series. Important to note that SRS cases usually have smaller volume tumors compared to fractionated RT cases, which may influence outcomes.

Kong, Korea (*Cancer* 2007, PMID 17599761): Compared outcomes of fractionated RT vs. SRS in 125 patients. Median time to CR was 63 months for fractionated RT vs. 26 months for SRS ($p = .007$). Overall CR rate was 26.2% at 2 years and 76.3% at 4 years. Similar LC in both arms.

■ **What are the expected outcomes with proton therapy for pituitary adenoma?**

Petit, Harvard (*Endocr Pract* 2007, PMID 18194929): RR of 22 patients treated for GH secreting adenoma with proton SRS. All had prior TSS. Median dose to tumor margin was 20 CGE. At MFU of 6.3 years, PR 95%, CR 59% with median time to CR of 42 months. New pituitary deficits requiring replacement hormones in 38% and 10% developed panhypopituitarism. No visual complications or cerebral necrosis.

Petit, Harvard (*J Clin Endocrinol Metab* 2008, PMID 18029460): RR of 38 patients (33 Cushing's, 5 Nelson's). All had prior TSS without biochemical cure, 4 patients with prior photon RT. All Nelson's syndrome patients had prior bilateral adrenalectomy. Median dose to tumor margin: 20 CGE. At MFU of 62 months, CR 52% for Cushing's, 100% for Nelson's. Median time to CR was 18 months; 52% developed new pituitary deficits requiring replacement hormones at a median time of 27 months with 6% experiencing panhypopituitarism. No visual complications, CVA, or secondary tumors.

Wattson, Harvard (*IJROBP* 2014, PMID 25194666): RR of 144 patients treated with 3D-conformal passive scattered proton therapy using 2 to 5 beams. Median dose to tumor margin: 20 CGE. LC 98% at MFU of 43 months. New hypopituitarism developed at a median time of 40 months with larger target volume predictive of hypopituitarism (HR: 1.3, $p = .004$); 3-year hypopituitarism rate 45%, 5-year rate 62%; 4 patients developed temporal lobe seizures. No CVA or secondary malignancies at MFU 4.3 years. See Table 6.3 for biochemical CR results.

Table 6.3: Biochemical Outcomes After Proton Therapy for Secretory Pituitary Adenoma				
Syndrome	N	3-Yr CR (%)	5-Yr CR (%)	Median Time to CR (mos)
Cushing's	74	54	67	32
Nelson's	8	63	75	27
Acromegaly	50	26	49	62
Prolactinoma	9	22	38	60
TSHoma	3	0	33	51

■ **What is the risk of secondary malignancy with RT for pituitary adenoma?**

Pollock, Mayo Clinic (*IJROBP* 2017, PMID 28333013): RR of 188 patients treated with GKRS. Median dose was 18 Gy to tumor margin. No secondary malignancy or malignant transformation reported at MFU of 8.5 years (5–22.3).

Minniti, Royal Marsden (*J Clin Endocrinol Metab* 2005, PMID 15562021): RR of 462 patients who received fractionated RT; 76% received conventional three-field RT to 45 Gy/25 fx. At MFU of 12 years, 11 patients developed secondary brain tumors (5 meningiomas, 4 high-grade astrocytomas,

1 meningeal sarcoma, 1 PNET). Cumulative risk 2% at 10 years, 2.4% at 20 years. Relative risk 10.5 compared to normal population.

REFERENCES

1. Suh JH, Chao ST, Murphy ES, Weil RJ. Pituitary tumors and craniopharyngiomas. In: Gunderson LL, Tepper JE, eds. *Clinical Radiation Oncology.* 4th ed. Elsevier; 2015:502–520. doi:10.1016/B978-0-323-24098-7.00029-0
2. Ezzat S, Asa SL, Couldwell WT, et al. The prevalence of pituitary adenomas: a systematic review. *Cancer.* 2004;101(3):613–619. doi:10.1002/cncr.20412
3. Ostrom QT, Cioffi G, Gittleman H, et al. CBTRUS statistical report: primary brain and other central nervous system tumors diagnosed in the United States in 2012–2016. *Neuro Oncol.* 2019;21(Suppl 5):v1–v100. doi:10.1093/neuonc/noz150
4. Hemminki K, Försti A, Ji J. Incidence and familial risks in pituitary adenoma and associated tumors. *Endocr Relat Cancer.* 2007;14(1):103–109. doi:10.1677/ERC-06-0008
5. Schoemaker MJ, Swerdlow AJ. Risk factors for pituitary tumors: a case-control study. *Cancer Epidemiol Biomarkers Prev.* 2009;18(5):1492–1500. doi:10.1158/1055-9965.EPI-08-0657
6. Kovacs K, Horvath E. Tumors of the pituitary gland. In: Hartmann WH, Sobin LH, eds. *Atlas of Tumor Pathology.* Armed Forces Institute of Pathology; 1986.
7. Asa SL. Tumors of the pituitary gland. In: *Atlas of Tumor Pathology.* American Registry of Pathology Press; 2011.
8. Diri H, Ozaslan E, Kurtsoy A, et al. Prognostic factors obtained from long-term follow-up of pituitary adenomas and other sellar tumors. *Turk Neurosurg.* 2014;24(5):679–687. doi:10.5137/1019-5149.JTN.9140-13.1
9. Loeffler JS, Shih HA. Radiation therapy in the management of pituitary adenomas. *J Clin Endocrinol Metab.* 2011;96(7):1992–2003. doi:10.1210/jc.2011-0251
10. Di Ieva A, Rotondo F, Syro LV, et al. Aggressive pituitary adenomas--diagnosis and emerging treatments. *Nat Rev Endocrinol.* 2014;10(7):423–435. doi:10.1038/nrendo.2014.64
11. Johnston PC, Kennedy L, Hamrahian AH, et al. Surgical outcomes in patients with Cushing's disease: the Cleveland clinic experience. *Pituitary.* 2017. doi:10.1007/s11102-017-0802-1
12. Bengtsson D, Schröder HD, Andersen M, et al. Long-term outcome and MGMT as a predictive marker in 24 patients with atypical pituitary adenomas and pituitary carcinomas given treatment with temozolomide. *J Clin Endocrinol Metab.* 2015;100(4):1689–1698. doi:10.1210/jc.2014-4350
13. McCormack AI, Wass JA, Grossman AB. Aggressive pituitary tumours: the role of temozolomide and the assessment of MGMT status. *Eur J Clin Invest.* 2011;41(10):1133–1148. doi:10.1111/j.1365-2362.2011.02520.x
14. Sheehan J, Lee CC, Bodach ME, et al. Congress of neurological surgeons systematic review and evidence-based guideline for the management of patients with residual or recurrent nonfunctioning pituitary adenomas. *Neurosurgery.* 2016;79(4):E539–E540. doi:10.1227/NEU.0000000000001385
15. Kabil MS, Eby JB, Shahinian HK. Fully endoscopic endonasal vs. transseptal transsphenoidal pituitary surgery. *Minim Invasive Neurosurg.* 2005;48(6):348–354. doi:10.1055/s-2005-915635
16. Linsler S, Quack F, Schwerdtfeger K, Oertel J. Prognosis of pituitary adenomas in the early 1970s and today-Is there a benefit of modern surgical techniques and treatment modalities? *Clin Neurol Neurosurg.* 2017;156:4–10. doi:10.1016/j.clineuro.2017.03.002
17. Pala A, Brand C, Kapapa T, et al. The Value of Intraoperative and Early Postoperative Magnetic Resonance Imaging in Low-Grade Glioma Surgery: A Retrospective Study. *World Neurosurg.* 2016;93:191–197. doi:10.1016/j.wneu.2016.04.120
18. Sheehan JP, Pouratian N, Steiner L, et al. Gamma Knife surgery for pituitary adenomas: factors related to radiological and endocrine outcomes. *J Neurosurg.* 2011;114(2):303–309. doi:10.3171/2010.5.JNS091635
19. Castinetti F, Nagai M, Dufour H, et al. Gamma knife radiosurgery is a successful adjunctive treatment in Cushing's disease. *Eur J Endocrinol.* 2007;156(1):91–98. doi:10.1530/EJE-07-0514
20. Pollock BE, Jacob JT, Brown PD, Nippoldt TB. Radiosurgery of growth hormone-producing pituitary adenomas: factors associated with biochemical remission. *J Neurosurg.* 2007;106(5):833–838. doi:10.3171/jns.2007.106.5.833
21. Pouratian N, Sheehan J, Jagannathan J, et al. Gamma knife radiosurgery for medically and surgically refractory prolactinomas. *Neurosurgery.* 2006;59(2):255–266; discussion 255–266. doi:10.1227/01.NEU.0000223445.22938.BD
22. Molitch ME. Diagnosis and treatment of pituitary adenomas: a review. *JAMA.* 2017;317(5):516–524. doi:10.1001/jama.2016.19699
23. Iwata H, Sato K, Nomura R, et al. Long-term results of hypofractionated stereotactic radiotherapy with CyberKnife for growth hormone-secreting pituitary adenoma: evaluation by the Cortina consensus. *J Neurooncol.* 2016;128(2):267–275. doi:10.1007/s11060-016-2105-1
24. Iwata H, Sato K, Tatewaki K, et al. Hypofractionated stereotactic radiotherapy with CyberKnife for nonfunctioning pituitary adenoma: high local control with low toxicity. *Neuro Oncol.* 2011;13(8):916–922. doi:10.1093/neuonc/nor055
25. Schoenthaler R, Albright NW, Wara WM, et al. Re-irradiation of pituitary adenoma. *Int J Radiat Oncol Biol Phys.* 1992;24(2):307–314. doi:10.1016/0360-3016(92)90686-C

26. Flickinger JC, Deutsch M, Lunsford LD. Repeat megavoltage irradiation of pituitary and suprasellar tumors. *Int J Radiat Oncol Biol Phys*. 1989;17(1):171–175. doi:10.1016/0360-3016(89)90385-4

27. Brada M, Burchell L, Ashley S, Traish D. The incidence of cerebrovascular accidents in patients with pituitary adenoma. *Int J Radiat Oncol Biol Phys*. 1999;45(3):693–698. doi:10.1016/S0360-3016(99)00159-5

28. Erridge SC, Conkey DS, Stockton D, et al. Radiotherapy for pituitary adenomas: long-term efficacy and toxicity. *Radiother Oncol*. 2009;93(3):597–601. doi:10.1016/j.radonc.2009.09.011

29. Sattler MG, Vroomen PC, Sluiter WJ, et al. Incidence, causative mechanisms, and anatomic localization of stroke in pituitary adenoma patients treated with postoperative radiation therapy versus surgery alone. *Int J Radiat Oncol Biol Phys*. 2013;87(1):53–59. doi:10.1016/j.ijrobp.2013.05.006

30. Minniti G, Traish D, Ashley S, et al. Risk of second brain tumor after conservative surgery and radiotherapy for pituitary adenoma: update after an additional 10 years. *J Clin Endocrinol Metab*. 2005;90(2):800–804. doi:10.1210/jc.2004-1152

31. McDowell BD, Wallace RB, Carnahan RM, et al. Demographic differences in incidence for pituitary adenoma. *Pituitary*. 2011;14(1):23–30. doi:10.1007/s11102-010-0253-4

7 ■ TRIGEMINAL NEURALGIA

Bindu V. Manyam, Vamsi Varra, and Samuel T. Chao

QUICK HIT ■ Trigeminal neuralgia, also referred to as "tic douloureux," is a rare condition characterized by episodic, debilitating pain of the face. It is typically unilateral and described as an electric or shock-like sensation.[1] First-line therapy is antiepileptic medication, such as carbamazepine or oxcarbazepine.[2] Second-line therapy for patients who are refractory to medical therapy include surgical procedures such as microvascular decompression, percutaneous balloon microcompression, radiofrequency rhizotomy, and radiation therapy using SRS.[3] Long-term follow-up demonstrates good outcomes of pain relief with SRS.[2]

EPIDEMIOLOGY: Trigeminal neuralgia is the most common facial pain syndrome, with an annual incidence of 15,000 cases in the United States.[4] Male-to-female ratio is 1:1.5.[5] It usually presents in the fifth through the seventh decades of life.[6]

RISK FACTORS: Trigeminal neuralgia is more common in women. Patients with multiple sclerosis are at higher risk for trigeminal neuralgia. Hypertension is a suggested risk factor due to the precipitation of tortuous vasculature, though this association is uncertain.[7]

ANATOMY: The trigeminal nerve (CN V) emerges from the midlateral surface of the pons, providing the sensory supply to the face and the motor supply to the muscles of mastication. The semilunar or Gasserian ganglion of the trigeminal nerve is located in Meckel's cave near the apex of the petrous part of the temporal bone. The three branches of the trigeminal nerve are as follows: **ophthalmic nerve (V1)**, which exits the superior orbital fissure and supplies the cornea, ciliary body, iris, lacrimal glands, conjunctiva, and skin of the upper face; **maxillary nerve (V2)**, which exits through foramen rotundum and supplies the pterygopalatine fossa, infraorbital canal, and the skin of the external nasal/superior labial face; and **mandibular nerve (V3)**, which exits through foramen ovale and supplies the teeth and gums of the mandible, skin of the temporal region, lower lip, muscles of mastication, and sensation of the anterior two thirds of the tongue.

ETIOLOGY: Etiologies include vascular compression of the trigeminal root (most common), benign tumors, malignancy, and multiple sclerosis.[1] Compression due to an ectatic loop of artery or vein is the etiology in 80% to 90% of cases. The compression usually occurs within a few millimeters of entry into the pons (also called the "root entry zone").[8]

CLINICAL PRESENTATION: The ICHD-3 defines the diagnostic criteria of classic trigeminal neuralgia as at least three attacks of unilateral facial pain occurring in one or more divisions of the trigeminal nerve without radiation beyond the trigeminal distribution and at least three of the following characteristics: (a) recurring paroxysmal attacks lasting from a fraction of a second to 2 minutes; (b) severe intensity; (c) electric-shock-like shooting, stabbing, or sharp in quality; and (d) at least three attacks precipitated by innocuous stimuli to the affected side of the face (some attacks may be, or may appear to be, spontaneous). There must not be clinical evidence of neurologic deficit and the condition should not be accounted for by another ICHD-3 diagnosis.[1] Of note, pain is typically within the V2 and/or V3 distribution, with V1 the least common distribution. Unlike other facial pain syndromes, trigeminal neuralgia does not usually wake patients from sleep. Involvement of the V1 distribution can also be associated with autonomic symptoms of lacrimation, conjunctival injection, and rhinorrhea.

WORKUP: Trigeminal neuralgia can be diagnosed based on the classic clinical features described. A careful dental exam should be performed. An MRI is indicated to identify etiologies, such as demyelinating lesions, a mass in the cerebellopontine angle, or an ectatic blood vessel. The CISS sequence is especially helpful in identifying aberrant vessels. If the patient is unable to get an MRI, a CT cisternogram can be obtained.

TREATMENT PARADIGM

Observation: Observation is appropriate for patients whose symptoms are tolerable and infrequent.

Medical: Antiepileptic drugs are first-line therapy.[9] More than 25% do not respond to medical therapy or have poor tolerance secondary to the associated toxicities of dose escalation necessary for adequate pain control. Carbamazepine (600–800 mg daily) is the first-line agent and has been shown to be effective in four randomized controlled trials.[10–13] Most common side effects include drowsiness, dizziness, nausea, and vomiting.[9] Leukopenia and aplastic anemia are rare but more serious complications. Second-line agents include clonazepam, gabapentin, lamotrigine, oxcarbazepine, and topiramate.[9]

Surgery: Typically used if patients have symptoms refractory to medical therapy.[3]

- Microvascular decompression (gold standard): Removal or separation of various vascular structures, usually an ectatic superior cerebellar artery, away from the trigeminal nerve.[14] About 70% of patients are pain free at 10 years.[15] Risk of complications include 0.2% perioperative mortality, 0.1% brainstem infarction, and 1% ipsilateral hearing loss.[2]
- Radiofrequency rhizotomy: Application of heat to the Gasserian ganglion, thought to selectively destroy pain impulses carried by unmyelinated or thinly myelinated fibers.[16] A heat probe is inserted through foramen ovale in cycles of 45 to 90 seconds at 60 to 90 °C.[17] About 75% are pain free at 14 years.[18]
- Glycerol rhizolysis: Injection of 0.1 to 0.4 mL of glycerol into the trigeminal cistern.[19] Provides instant pain relief; however, up to 92% have recurrence of symptoms at 6 years.[20]
- Balloon compression: Use of a Fogarty catheter to compress the Gasserian ganglion by inflating with 0.5 to 1.0 mL of contrast dye for 1 to 6 minutes.[21]

Radiation

Indications: SRS is a minimally invasive option that is preferred for patients with medically refractory disease who are not good candidates for surgery. Target is the proximal trigeminal root.

Dose: Typical SRS dose is 70 to 90 Gy in a single fraction prescribed to the 100% isodose line via a 4-mm shot directed at the root entry zone of the trigeminal nerve into the pons. Radiation causes axonal degeneration and necrosis.

Toxicity: Risks of complications include <10% facial numbness/paresthesia and <1% anesthesia dolorosa.[22] A nomogram developed by Lucas et al. quantifies the durability of pain relief and demonstrated that Burchiel pain type prior to treatment (defined as type 1, in which >50% of symptoms are episodic, or type 2, in which >50% of symptoms are constant), the BNI pain score after SRS, and post-SRS facial numbness were predictive of outcomes. Patients with type 1 Burchiel pain type, low BNI pain score after SRS, and absence of post-SRS facial numbness tend to have more durable pain relief.[23]

- **EVIDENCE-BASED Q&A**

MEDICAL THERAPY

- **What are the outcomes with carbamazepine?**

Wiffen (*Cochrane Database Syst Rev* **2011, PMID 21249671**): Meta-analysis of 15 PRTs and 629 patients with chronic neuropathic pain of different etiologies (trigeminal neuralgia, postherpetic neuralgia, etc.); 70% of patients reported some degree of improvement in pain, with an NNT of 1.7 (1.5–2.0); 66% of patients who received carbamazepine experienced at least one adverse event compared to 27% with placebo, though serious adverse events were not reported. **Conclusion: Carbamazepine is effective in the treatment of chronic neuropathic pain but is associated with higher rate of adverse events.**

SURGERY

- **How do microvascular decompression and partial sensory rhizotomy differ in outcomes?**

Zakrzewska (*Neurosurgery* **2005, PMID 5918947**): Survey of 245 patients who underwent microvascular decompression and 60 patients who underwent partial sensory rhizotomy (procedure in which the trigeminal nerve is severed). Overall satisfaction was 89% with microvascular decompression and 72% with partial sensory rhizotomy ($p < .01$). The final outcome was reported to be better than expected in 80% with microvascular decompression and in 54% with partial sensory rhizotomy ($p < .01$); 22% of these felt they were worse off after partial sensory rhizotomy. **Conclusion: Patient satisfaction is higher with microvascular decompression than partial sensory rhizotomy.**

STEREOTACTIC RADIOSURGERY

■ **What is the appropriate target volume for SRS, and does increasing the treatment volume improve outcomes?**

Flickinger, Pittsburgh/Mayo Clinic (*IJROBP* 2001, PMID 11567820): PRT of 87 patients treated with SRS randomized to a one-isocenter (n = 44) or two-isocenter (n = 43) technique; 75 Gy was prescribed to the maximum point. At an MFU of 26 months, complete pain relief (with or without medication) was 68%. Pain relief was identical between one- and two-isocenter SRS treatments. Improved pain relief was associated with younger age ($p = .025$) and fewer prior procedures ($p = .039$). Complications (numbness or paresthesias) correlated with the nerve length irradiated ($p = .018$). **Conclusion: Increasing the treatment volume to include longer nerve length does not significantly improve pain relief but may increase complications.**

■ **Does SRS dose escalation improve outcomes?**

Kotecha, Cleveland Clinic/Mid-Michigan (*IJROBP* 2016, PMID 27325473): RR of 870 patients from two institutions, divided into three groups based on treatment dose using GKRS and prescribed to the 100% isodose line: ≤82 Gy (352 patients), 83 to 86 Gy (85 patients), and ≥90 Gy (433 patients). The 4-year rates of pain response were 79%, 82%, and 92% in patients treated to ≤82 Gy, 83 to 86 Gy, and ≥90 Gy, respectively. Patients who received ≤82 Gy had an increased risk of treatment failure, compared to those who received ≥90 Gy (HR: 2.0, $p = .0007$). Treatment-related facial numbness was similar among those receiving ≥83 Gy. The rate of anesthesia dolorosa was 1%. **Conclusion: Dose escalation >82 Gy to the 100% isodose line may be associated with increased pain relief and duration of pain relief but at the expense of increased treatment-related facial numbness.**

■ **What are the outcomes with linear-accelerator-based radiosurgery for trigeminal neuralgia, and does increasing dose in linear-accelerator-based radiosurgery improve outcomes?**

Smith, UCLA (*IJROBP* 2011, PMID 21236592): RR of 179 patients treated with linear-accelerator-based radiosurgery for trigeminal neuralgia. Significant pain relief was noted at a mean of 28.8 months in 79% of the patients, with average time to pain relief of 1.92 months; 19% had recurrent pain at 13.5 months. Of the 28 patients treated with 70 Gy and 30% IDL touching brainstem, 64% had significant relief and 36% had numbness. Of the 82 patients treated with 90 Gy and 30% IDL touching brainstem, 79% had significant relief and 49% had numbness. Of the 59 patients treated with 90 Gy and 50% IDL touching brainstem, 88% had significant relief. **Conclusion: Increased radiation dose and greater volume of brainstem irradiation may improve patient-reported outcomes but may increase numbness and trigeminal dysfunction.**

■ **Can SRS be repeated for recurrent trigeminal neuralgia?**

Herman, University of Maryland (*IJROBP* 2004, PMID 15093906): RR of 18 patients who underwent repeat SRS for recurrent trigeminal neuralgia at a median time of 8 months after initial procedure. Median prescription dose was 75 Gy for first treatment and 70 Gy for second treatment. After initial SRS, pain responses reported were 50% excellent, 28% good, 6% fair, and 16% poor. After repeat SRS, 45% excellent, 33% good, 0% fair, and 22% poor pain responses were reported. New or increased facial numbness was reported in 11%. Repeat SRS resulted in a median 60% improvement in quality of life, and 56% of patients reported that the procedure was successful. **Conclusion: Repeat SRS provided similar rates of complete pain control as the first treatment and improvement in quality of life. However, repeat SRS was not effective for patients who had no response to the initial treatment.**

■ **What is the most cost-effective procedure for trigeminal neuralgia?**

Pollack, Mayo Clinic (*IJROBP* 2005, PMID 15951649): Prospective, cost-effectiveness study comparing microvascular decompression, glycerol rhizotomy, and SRS. The cost and outcomes of 153 procedures at a tertiary referral center were studied. Patients who underwent microvascular decompression had significantly better pain outcomes (85% and 78% at 6 and 24 months) compared with those who underwent glycerol rhizotomy (61% and 55% at 6 and 24 months, $p = .01$) and SRS (60% and 52% at 6 and 24 months, $p < .01$). There was no difference in outcome between glycerol rhizotomy and SRS ($p = .61$). The costs per quality-adjusted pain-free year were $6,342, $8,174, and $8,269 for glycerol rhizotomy, microvascular decompression, and SRS, respectively. The cost of glycerol rhizotomy was more than that of SRS due to the need for repeat procedures. **Conclusion: In patients who are medically operable, microvascular decompression may be the most efficacious and cost-effective procedure compared to glycerol rhizotomy and SRS.**

REFERENCES

1.   Headache Classification Committee of the International Headache Society. The international classification of headache disorders, 3rd edition (beta version). *Cephalalgia*. 2013:33(9):629–808. doi:10.1177/0333102413485658

2.   Gronseth G, Cruccu G, Alksne J, et al. Practice parameter: the diagnostic evaluation and treatment of trigeminal neuralgia (an evidence-based review): report of the quality standards subcommittee of the American academy of neurology and the European federation of neurological societies. *Neurology*. 2008;71(15):1183–1190. doi:10.1212/01.wnl.0000326598.83183.04

3.   Bennetto L, Patel NK, Fuller G. Trigeminal neuralgia and its management. *BMJ*. 2007;334(7586):201–205. doi:10.1136/bmj.39085.614792.BE

4.   Pope JE, Narouze S. Orofacial pain. In: *Essentials of Pain Medicine*, 3rd ed. W.B. Saunders; 2011:283–293. doi:10.1016/B978-1-4377-2242-0.00051-1

5.   Maarbjerg S, Gozalov A, Olesen J, Bendtsen L. Trigeminal neuralgia: a prospective systematic study of clinical characteristics in 158 patients. *Headache*. 2014;54(10):1574–1582. doi:10.1111/head.12441

6.   Ritter PM, Friedman WA, Bhasin RR. The surgical treatment of trigeminal neuralgia: overview and experience at the University of Florida. *J Neurosci Nurs*. 2009;41(4):211–214; quiz 215–216. doi:10.1097/JNN.0b013e3181aaaa9d

7.   Lin KH, Chen YT, Fuh JL, Wang SJ. Increased risk of trigeminal neuralgia in patients with migraine: a nationwide population-based study. *Cephalalgia*. 2015. doi:10.1177/0333102415623069

8.   Love S, Coakham HB. Trigeminal neuralgia: pathology and pathogenesis. *Brain*. 2001;124(Pt 12):2347–2360. doi:10.1093/brain/124.12.2347

9.   Attal N, Cruccu G, Haanpaa M, et al. EFNS guidelines on pharmacological treatment of neuropathic pain. *Eur J Neurol*. 2006;13(11):1153–1169. doi:10.1111/j.1468-1331.2006.01511.x

10. Campbell FG, Graham JG, Zilkha KJ. Clinical trial of carbazepine (tegretol) in trigeminal neuralgia. *J Neurol Neurosurg Psychiatry*. 1966;29(3):265–267. doi:10.1136/jnnp.29.3.265

11. Killian JM, Fromm GH. Carbamazepine in the treatment of neuralgia: use of side effects. *Arch Neurol*. 1968;19(2):129–136. doi:10.1001/archneur.1968.00480020015001

12. Nicol CF. A four year double-blind study of tegretol in facial pain. *Headache*. 1969;9(1):54–57. doi:10.1111/j.1526-4610.1969.hed0901054.x

13. Rockliff BW, Davis EH. Controlled sequential trials of carbamazepine in trigeminal neuralgia. *Arch Neurol*. 1966;15(2):129–136. doi:10.1001/archneur.1966.00470140019003

14. Jannetta PJ. Microsurgical management of trigeminal neuralgia. *Arch Neurol*. 1985;42(8):800. doi:10.1001/archneur.1985.04210090068018

15. Barker FG, Jannetta PJ, Bissonette DJ, et al. The long-term outcome of microvascular decompression for trigeminal neuralgia. *N Engl J Med*. 1996;334(17):1077–1084. doi:10.1056/NEJM199604253341701

16. Seegenschmiedt H. *Radiotherapy for Non-Malignant Disorders: Contemporary Concepts and Clinical Results*. Springer Publishing Company; 2008.

17. Tang Y-Z, Yang L-Q, Yue J-N, et al. The optimal radiofrequency temperature in radiofrequency thermocoagulation for idiopathic trigeminal neuralgia: a cohort study. *Medicine*. 2016;95(28):e4103–e4106. doi:10.1097/MD.0000000000004103

18. Taha JM, Tew JM Jr, Buncher CR. A prospective 15-year follow up of 154 consecutive patients with trigeminal neuralgia treated by percutaneous stereotactic radiofrequency thermal rhizotomy. *J Neurosurg*. 1995;83(6):989–993. doi:10.3171/jns.1995.83.6.0989

19. Lopez BC, Hamlyn PJ, Zakrzewska JM. Systematic review of ablative neurosurgical techniques for the treatment of trigeminal neuralgia. *Neurosurgery*. 2004;54(4):973–982: discussion 973–982. doi:10.1227/01.NEU.0000114867.98896.F0

20. Deer TR, Leong MS, Buvanendran A. American Academy of Pain Medicine. *Comprehensive Treatment of Chronic Pain by Medical, Interventional, and Integrative Approaches: The American Academy of Pain Medicine Textbook on Patient Management.* Springer Publishing Company; 2013.

21. de Siqueira SR, da Nobrega JC, de Siqueira JT, Teixeira MJ. Frequency of postoperative complications after balloon compression for idiopathic trigeminal neuralgia: prospective study. *Oral Surg Oral Med Oral Pathol Oral Radiol Endod.* 2006;102(5):e39–e45. doi:10.1016/j.tripleo.2006.03.028

22. Nurmikko TJ, Eldridge PR. Trigeminal neuralgia: pathophysiology, diagnosis and current treatment. *Br J Anaesth.* 2001;87(1):117–132. doi:10.1093/bja/87.1.117

23. Lucas JT, Jr., Nida AM, Isom S, et al. Predictive nomogram for the durability of pain relief from gamma knife radiation surgery in the treatment of trigeminal neuralgia. *Int J Radiat Oncol Biol Phys.* 2014;89(1):120–126. doi:10.1016/j.ijrobp.2014.01.023

8 ■ VESTIBULAR SCHWANNOMA

Winston Vuong, Jeffrey A. Kittel, and John H. Suh

QUICK HIT ■ Vestibular schwannoma, previously called "acoustic neuroma," is a slow-growing, benign tumor of the cerebellopontine angle that typically presents with unilateral hearing loss. Treatment options include observation, microsurgical resection, and RT (SRS or fractionated). SRS is generally prescribed up to 13 Gy and conventional fractionation to 45 to 54 Gy. Tumor control outcomes appear equivalent between those of surgery and RT, but RT may minimize impact on QOL.

EPIDEMIOLOGY: Incidence is approximately 0.6 to 1.9/100,000, making up 8% of intracranial tumors. Incidence is increasing with increased utilization of diagnostic imaging.[1,2] Median age at diagnosis is 50 to 55, and incidence increases with age.[1,3]

RISK FACTORS: Increasing age, NF2 (96% of patients with NF2, often bilateral), NF1 (5% of patients with NF1, unilateral), childhood exposure to RT (RR 1.14/Gy).[4]

ANATOMY: VS typically arises from the vestibular portion of CN VIII and is unilateral in 90% of cases. CN VIII arises from the junction of the pons and medulla, enters the internal auditory foramen along with the facial nerve (CN VII), and then divides into the vestibular and cochlear nerves. The cochlear nerve runs to the spiral ganglion and innervates the spiral organ of Corti and the cochlea. The vestibular nerve runs to the vestibular ganglion and splits into three branches. The superior branch innervates the utricle and the superior and lateral semicircular ducts. The inferior branch innervates the saccule and the posterior branch innervates the posterior semicircular duct. VS arises with equal frequency in the superior and inferior branches and rarely in the cochlear nerve. It tends to occur in the vestibular region of the foramen, where the nerve acquires a Schwann cell sheath, although it can sometimes arise from or grow into the CPA.

PATHOLOGY: VS is composed of atypical proliferations of Schwann cells, which are found lining peripheral nerves. Histopathologically, they are similar to other peripheral schwannomas and are composed of alternating zones of dense and sparse cellularity, termed "Antoni A" and "Antoni B," respectively. IHC demonstrates S100 positivity.[5] Malignant degeneration is extremely rare.

GENETICS: Biallelic inactivation of NF2 on chromosome 22, which produces the tumor suppressor merlin, is common in sporadic VS and is the cause of bilateral VS in NF2.[6]

CLINICAL PRESENTATION: Hearing loss (95%; only two thirds are aware of it; average duration ~4 years although 16% develop sudden hearing loss), tinnitus (63%; average duration ~3 years), vestibular symptoms (61%; often mild to moderate, nonspecific, and fluctuating; average duration ~2 years), headache (12%; most often occipital), trigeminal symptoms (9%; typically facial numbness/hyperesthesia/pain; average duration ~1 year), facial nerve symptoms (6%; typically facial weakness, less commonly taste disturbance; average duration ~2 years), and other symptoms from brainstem compression (ataxia, hydrocephalus, dysarthria, dysphagia, hoarseness) are uncommon.[7] The House–Brackmann and Gardner–Robertson scales are common metrics of facial paralysis and hearing loss, respectively (Tables 8.1 and 8.2).

WORKUP: H&P including Weber and Rinne tests to evoke asymmetric sensorineural hearing loss and CN exam, audiometry; consider BAER testing (BAER/ABR; 60% to 90% sensitive with lower sensitivity for small tumors; 60%–90% specific).[8] Vestibular testing is uncommon.

Imaging: MRI of the brain with contrast is the gold standard for diagnosis. High-resolution CT with IV contrast if unable to obtain MRI. MRI shows isointense or slightly hypointense signal to brain on T1, typically with homogeneous contrast enhancement although occasional cystic degeneration can be seen.[9] Classic finding is "ice-cream cone" shape with widening of the porus acusticus.[10] Differential includes VS, meningioma, glomus tumor, ependymoma, facial or trigeminal schwannoma, epidermoid cyst, metastasis.

Table 8.1: House–Brackmann Facial Paralysis Scale[11]	
Grade I	Normal
Grade II	Mild dysfunction (slight weakness, normal symmetry at rest)
Grade III	Moderate dysfunction (obvious but not disfiguring weakness, synkinesis) with normal symmetry at rest Complete eye closure with maximal effort Good forehead movement
Grade IV	Moderately severe dysfunction (obvious and disfiguring asymmetry, significant synkinesis) Incomplete eye closure Moderate forehead movement
Grade V	Severe dysfunction (barely perceptive motion)
Grade VI	Total paralysis

Table 8.2: Gardner–Robertson Hearing Loss Scale[12]	
Grade I	Good–excellent (70%–100% speech discrimination)
Grade II	Serviceable (50%–69%)
Grade III	Nonserviceable (5%–49%)
Grade IV	Poor (1%–4%)
Grade V	None

PROGNOSTIC FACTORS: Baseline level of hearing loss, growth rate >2.5 mm/yr, and delay in diagnosis.[13–16] Initial tumor size is not prognostic.[15] Patients with growth rate >2.5 mm/yr have decreased rates of hearing preservation (32% vs. 75%, $p < .0001$) and decreased median time to total hearing loss (7.0 vs. 14.8 years, $p < .0001$).[15,16]

STAGING: VSs are not staged but can be graded on the Koos grading scale (Table 8.3).[17]

Table 8.3: Koos Grading Scale for VS[17]	
Grade I	Intracanalicular
Grade II	Tumor extending into the posterior fossa, with or without an intracanalicular component, without touching the brainstem
Grade III	Tumor extending into the posterior fossa, compressing the brainstem, but not shifting it from the midline
Grade IV	Tumor extending into the posterior fossa, compressing the brainstem, and shifting it from the midline

TREATMENT PARADIGM

Table 8.4: General Probability of Hearing Preservation in Favorably Selected Patients[18]			
	2 Yrs	5 Yrs	10 Yrs
Observation	>75% to 100%	>50% to 75%	Insufficient data
SRS	>75% to 100%	>50% to 75%	>25% to 50%
Surgery	>25% to 50%	>25% to 50%	>25% to 50%

Favorably selected patients include small- to medium-sized sporadic VS, good–excellent speech discrimination (Gardner–Robinson Grade I).

Observation: Consider observation with MRI every 6 to 12 months in patients without baseline hearing loss and stability or slow rate of growth. Observation is especially favored in older patients with significant comorbidities. Indications for treatment vary but can include >2.5 mm growth/year and new onset or worsening of symptoms. Patients undergoing observation should be counseled that they have a risk of hearing loss without treatment (see Table 8.4). Current consensus guidelines suggest annual imaging at least up to 5 years with possible longer duration of follow-up up to 10 years.[18,19]

Surgery: In general, surgery has excellent results for resection of the entire tumor but can have poor outcomes with hearing preservation. Hearing preservation is most likely when the tumor is <1.5 to 2 cm in size.[20] Other major morbidities include CSF leaks, tinnitus, headaches, and facial paralysis.[21] Surgery is still the most common treatment for VS and is especially considered for younger patients, larger tumors, tumors causing mass effect or dizziness, cystic tumors, and small anatomically favorable tumors with good hearing.[22] There are three main surgical approaches for resection (see Table 8.5).[21-23] The goal of resection is to maximize tumor removal while minimizing morbidity.

Table 8.5 Surgical Techniques for VS

Approach	Pros	Cons
Retrosigmoid/suboccipital	Possible hearing conservation and facial nerve sparing	Associated with increased risk of CSF leaks and HA
Translabyrinthine	Possible preservation of facial function	No hearing preservation, a fat graft is required, and the sigmoid sinus is more prone to injury
Middle fossa	Possible hearing conservation for small tumors (≤1.5 cm)	Facial nerve more vulnerable to injury, dural lacerations likely in older patients, may cause trismus from temporalis muscle injury

Chemotherapy: There is generally no role for systemic therapy, although bevacizumab has shown response in rare progressive situations associated with NF2.[24]

Radiation: Several options for treatment with RT exist. SRS (with GKRS or LINAC-based radiosurgery), FSRT, and proton beam RT have been used. RT is appropriate when the tumor is <3 to 4 cm in size or when surgery is not an option or refused.[25]

SRS: Doses above 12.5 to 13 Gy are associated with increased morbidity with regard to facial paralysis, trigeminal neuralgia, and hearing loss.[26,27] Long-term results show >95% control with minimal morbidity or impact on QOL. Impact on hearing preservation and relative differences between treatment modalities appears to vary with time.[28,29] In a series of 440 patients with long-term follow-up, one patient (0.3%) developed malignant transformation.[30]

FSRT: Treatments can range from 20 Gy/4 fx to 57.6 Gy/32 fx. Typical hypofractionated dose is 25 Gy/5 fx and 45 to 54 Gy/25 to 30 fx for conventional fractionation. Controversy exists whether FSRT is superior to SRS, but it is recommended with larger tumors (>3–4 cm) in an effort to spare adjacent normal structures such as the brainstem and cochlea.

Procedure: See *Handbook of Treatment Planning in Radiation Oncology*, Chapter 3.[31]

■ **EVIDENCE-BASED Q&A**

▪ **What are the outcomes of treatment with surgical resection for patients with VS?**

Surgical resection is generally technically achievable with high rates of control.[20] The risk of significant complications is low. There may be a lower rate of complications with maximal safe resection, allowing for residual tumor rather than attempted GTR in all patients.[21] However, patients who undergo STR are at a higher risk of recurrence than patients who undergo GTR or NTR.[32]

Samii, Germany (*Neurosurgery* 1997, PMID 8971819): RR of 1,000 consecutive patients with VS resected by suboccipital approach between 1978 and 1993; 98% of tumors were completely removed.

Anatomic preservation of the facial nerve and the cochlear nerve was achieved in 93% and 68%, respectively. Major neurologic complications included tetraparesis in one patient, hemiparesis in 1%, lower cranial nerve palsies in 5.5%, and cerebrospinal fluid fistulas in 9.2%. There were 11 deaths (1.1%) occurring at 2 to 69 days postoperatively.

Carlson, Mayo Clinic (*Laryngoscope* 2012, PMID 22252688): RR of 203 patients treated at a single institution. Patients were classified by GTR, NTR, or STR; 144 patients underwent GTR, 32 NTR, and 27 STR; 12 patients (6%) had a recurrence at a mean of 3.0 years after surgery; 5-year RFS was estimated at 91%. Patients who received STR were 9 times more likely to fail than patients undergoing NTR or GTR. No significant difference between patients with NTR and GTR was noted. Patients with nodular enhancement on initial post-op MRI had a 16-times higher risk of recurrence compared to patients with linear patterns.

■ **How does SRS compare with observation?**

SRS appears to have limited impact on QOL compared to observation.[33]

Breivik, Norway (*Neurosurgery* 2013, PMID 23615094): Prospective cohort study of patients who underwent GKRS (113) or observation (124). Patients underwent GKRS with small tumors (<20 mm) after growth was observed by referring physician (*n* = 31), by patient choice (*n* = 26), or with tumors >20 mm who refused surgery. GKRS dose was 12 Gy to the tumor periphery. Serviceable hearing was lost in 76% of patients on observation and 64% with GKRS (NS). Patients treated with GKRS had significantly less need for future treatment. Symptoms and QOL did not differ between groups. **Conclusion: GKRS appears to prevent the need for further treatment and appears not to significantly impact rates of hearing loss, symptoms, or QOL compared to observation.**

■ **How does RT compare with microsurgical resection?**

Generally, studies have shown equivalent tumor control with SRS compared to microsurgical resection with generally better functional outcomes and less impact on QOL with SRS.[28,34–36] *However, there is no consensus on the optimal management. The ideal population of patients for each modality overlaps (small tumors with preserved hearing) but surgery may be preferred in larger tumors, especially in patients with mass effect.*

Pollock, Mayo Clinic (*Neurosurgery* 2006, PMID 16823303): Prospective cohort study of 82 patients with unilateral <3 cm VS undergoing surgical resection (*n* = 36) or GKRS (*n* = 46). GKRS mean dose was 12.2 Gy to tumor margin; mean maximum dose, 26.4 Gy. No difference in tumor control (100% vs. 96%, *p* = .50). GKRS patients had better facial nerve preservation at 3 months (100% vs. 69%, *p* < .001), 1 year (100% vs. 69%, *p* < .001), and last f/u (100% vs. 75%, *p* < .01). GKRS patients had better hearing preservation at 3 months (77% vs. 5%, *p* < .001), 1 year (63% vs. 5%, *p* < .001), and last f/u (63% vs. 5%, *p* < .001). GKRS patients had better physical functioning, energy, and pain at 3 months, 1 year, and last f/u. **Conclusion: Similar tumor control with GKRS or surgery but less morbidity with GKRS.**

Maniakas, Montreal (*Otol Neurotol* 2012, PMID 22996165): Meta-analysis of 16 studies comparing microsurgical resection and SRS. Overall, SRS showed significantly better long-term hearing preservation rates than microsurgery (70% vs. 50%, respectively, *p* < .001). Crude rates of long-term tumor progression were not significantly different between SRS and microsurgery (3.8% and 1.3%, respectively).

■ **What are the long-term results of SRS?**

Long-term results for SRS show excellent LC. However, with longer term follow-up, it appears that rates of hearing preservation may continue to decline.[29,30,37]

Hasegawa, Japan (*J Neurosurg* 2013, PMID 23140152): RR of 440 patients treated with GKRS between 1991 and 2000. MFU 12.5 years. Actuarial 5- and 10-year PFS was 93% and 92%, respectively. No patient failed >10 years after treatment. On MVA, significant brainstem compression, marginal dose ≤13 Gy, prior treatment, and female sex correlated with decreased PFS. Patients treated with ≤13 Gy had an increased rate of facial nerve preservation (100% vs. 97%); 10 patients (2.3%) developed delayed cyst formation. One patient (0.03%) developed malignant transformation.

Carlson, Mayo Clinic (*J Neurosurg* 2013, PMID 23101446): RR of 44 patients with long-term audiometric follow-up after SRS. SRS was given with 12 to 13 Gy to the periphery of the tumor. MFU 9.3

years; 36 patients developed nonserviceable hearing at mean of 4.2 years after SRS. Kaplan–Meier estimated rates of serviceable hearing at 1, 3, 5, 7, and 10 years following SRS were 80%, 55%, 48%, 38%, and 23%, respectively. MVA revealed that pretreatment ipsilateral pure tone average ($p < .001$) and tumor size ($p = .009$) were statistically significantly associated with time to nonserviceable hearing.

■ Can SRS be used for larger tumors (>3 cm)?

Yang, Pittsburgh (*J Neurosurg* 2011, PMID 20799863): RR of 65 patients with VS between 3 and 4 cm in one extracanalicular maximum diameter (median tumor volume 9 mL) who underwent GKRS; 17 patients (26%) had previously undergone resection; 2 years later, 7 tumors (11%) had grown; 18 (82%) of 22 patients with serviceable hearing before SRS still had serviceable hearing after SRS more than 2 years later; 3 patients (5%) developed symptomatic hydrocephalus and underwent placement of a VP shunt. In 4 patients (6%), trigeminal sensory dysfunction developed, and in 1 patient (2%) mild facial weakness (House–Brackmann Grade II) developed after SRS. In univariate analyses, patients who had a previous resection ($p = .010$), those with tumor volume >10 mL ($p = .05$), and those with Koos grade 4 tumors ($p = .02$) had less likelihood of tumor control after SRS.

■ How does fractionated RT compare WITH SRS?

Fractionation offers a theoretical radiobiologic advantage compared to single-fraction treatment, which should allow for improved sparing of normal structures. However, evidence for differences in outcome between SRS and five-fraction or longer treatment courses is limited to retrospective data and may only improve hearing preservation.[27,38,39]

Coombs, Heidelberg (*IJROBP* 2010, PMID 19604653): Prospective cohort study of 200 patients with 202 VS treated with either LINAC-based SRS ($n = 30$) or FSRT ($n = 172$). SRS dose was 13 Gy to 80% isodose line, and FSRT median dose was 57.6 Gy/32 fx. MFU 75 months. No difference in 5-year LC (96% overall). FSRT and SRS showed equivalent hearing preservation (76% at 5 years) for SRS dose ≤13 Gy. For SRS dose >13 Gy ($n = 11$), hearing preservation was significantly worse than FSRT. Both patients who developed trigeminal neuralgia in the SRS group were treated with >13 Gy. Rate of facial nerve weakness was 17% in the SRS group and 2% in the FSRT group. Only 1 patient treated with SRS to ≤13 Gy developed facial weakness. **Conclusion: SRS with doses ≤13 Gy is a safe and effective alternative to FSRT. FSRT should be reserved for larger lesions.**

Meijer, Netherlands (*IJROBP* 2003, PMID 12873685): RR of 129 consecutive patients treated with either single-fraction or five-fraction RT using LINAC-based SRS techniques. Patients were prospectively selected for single fraction if edentate and five fractions if dentate due to the immobilization device used. Single-fraction arm treated with 10 to 12.5 Gy and five-fraction arm treated with 20 to 25 Gy. Patients in the single-fraction arm were older (mean age 63 years vs. 49 years), but there were no other significant differences between groups. No significant differences in 5-year LC (100% vs. 94%), facial nerve preservation (93% vs. 97%), and hearing preservation (75% vs. 61%); 5-year trigeminal nerve preservation was significantly different (92% vs. 98%, $p = .048$) favoring the fractionated group.

REFERENCES

1. Babu R, Sharma R, Bagley JH, et al. Vestibular schwannomas in the modern era: epidemiology, treatment trends, and disparities in management. *J Neurosurg.* 2013;119(1):121–130. doi:10.3171/2013.1.JNS121370
2. Cioffi G, Yeboa DN, Kelly M, et al. Epidemiology of vestibular schwannoma in the United States, 2004–2016. *Neurooncol Adv.* 2020;2(1):vdaa135. doi:10.1093/noajnl/vdaa135
3. Propp JM, McCarthy BJ, Davis FG, Preston-Martin S. Descriptive epidemiology of vestibular schwannomas. *Neuro Oncol.* 2006;8(1):1–11. doi:10.1215/S1522851704001097
4. Shore-Freedman E, Abrahams C, Recant W, Schneider AB. Neurilemomas and salivary gland tumors of the head and neck following childhood irradiation. *Cancer.* 1983;51(12):2159–2163. doi:10.1002/1097-0142 (19830615)51:12<2159::AID-CNCR2820511202>3.0.CO;2-L
5. Sobel RA. Vestibular (acoustic) schwannomas: histologic features in neurofibromatosis 2 and in unilateral cases. *J Neuropathol Exp Neurol.* 1993;52(2):106–113. doi:10.1097/00005072-199303000-00002
6. Sughrue ME, Yeung AH, Rutkowski MJ, et al. Molecular biology of familial and sporadic vestibular schwannomas: implications for novel therapeutics. *J Neurosurg.* 2011;114(2):359–366. doi:10.3171/2009.10.JNS091135
7. Matthies C, Samii M. Management of 1000 vestibular schwannomas (acoustic neuromas): clinical presentation. *Neurosurgery.* 1997;40(1):1–9: discussion 9–10. doi:10.1227/00006123-199701000-00001

8. Doyle KJ. Is there still a role for auditory brainstem response audiometry in the diagnosis of acoustic neuroma? *Arch Otolaryngol Head Neck Surg.* 1999;125(2):232–234. doi:10.1001/archotol.125.2.232

9. Schmalbrock P, Chakeres DW, Monroe JW, et al. Assessment of internal auditory canal tumors: a comparison of contrast-enhanced T1-weighted and steady-state T2-weighted gradient-echo MR imaging. *AJNR Am J Neuroradiol.* 1999;20(7):1207–1213.

10. Vestibular Schwannomas: lessons for the neurosurgeonpart idiagnosis, neuroimaging, and audiology. *Contemp. Neurosurg.* 2011;33(20):6. doi:10.1097/01.CNE.0000408561.95604.01

11. House JW, Brackmann DE. Facial nerve grading system. *Otolaryngol Head Neck Surg.* 1985;93(2):146–147. doi:10.1177/019459988509300202

12. Gardner G, Robertson JH. Hearing preservation in unilateral acoustic neuroma surgery. *Ann Otol Rhinol Laryngol.* 1988;97(1):55–66. doi:10.1177/000348948809700110

13. Bakkouri WE, Kania RE, Guichard JP, et al. Conservative management of 386 cases of unilateral vestibular schwannoma: tumor growth and consequences for treatment. *J Neurosurg.* 2009;110(4):662–669. doi:10.3171/2007.5.16836

14. Stangerup SE, Tos M, Thomsen J, Caye-Thomasen P. Hearing outcomes of vestibular schwannoma patients managed with 'wait and scan': predictive value of hearing level at diagnosis. *J Laryngol Otol.* 2010;124(5):490–494. doi:10.1017/S0022215109992611

15. Sughrue ME, Kane AJ, Kaur R, et al. A prospective study of hearing preservation in untreated vestibular schwannomas. *J Neurosurg.* 2011;114(2):381–385. doi:10.3171/2010.4.JNS091962

16. Sughrue ME, Yang I, Aranda D, et al. The natural history of untreated sporadic vestibular schwannomas: a comprehensive review of hearing outcomes. *J Neurosurg.* 2010;112(1):163–167. doi:10.3171/2009.4.JNS08895

17. Koos WT, Day JD, Matula C, Levy DI. Neurotopographic considerations in the microsurgical treatment of small acoustic neurinomas. *J Neurosurg.* 1998;88(3):506–512. doi:10.3171/jns.1998.88.3.0506

18. Olson JJ, Kalkanis SN, Ryken TC. Congress of neurological surgeons systematic review and evidence-based guidelines on the treatment of adults with vestibular schwannomas: executive summary. *Neurosurgery.* 2017;82(2):129–134. doi:10.1093/neuros/nyx586

19. Goldbrunner R, Weller M, Regis J, et al. EANO guideline on the diagnosis and treatment of vestibular schwannoma. *Neuro Oncol.* 2020;22(1):31–45. doi:10.1093/neuonc/noz153

20. Gormley WB, Sekhar LN, Wright DC, et al. Acoustic neuromas: results of current surgical management. *Neurosurgery.* 1997;41(1):50–58: discussion 58–60. doi:10.1097/00006123-199707000-00012

21. Samii M, Matthies C. Management of 1000 vestibular schwannomas (acoustic neuromas): surgical management and results with an emphasis on complications and how to avoid them. *Neurosurgery.* 1997;40(1):11–21: discussion 21–13. doi:10.1097/00006123-199701000-00002

22. Carlson ML, Link MJ, Wanna GB, Driscoll CL. Management of sporadic vestibular schwannoma. *Otolaryngol Clin North Am.* 2015;48(3):407–422. doi:10.1016/j.otc.2015.02.003

23. Lanman TH, Brackmann DE, Hitselberger WE, Subin B. Report of 190 consecutive cases of large acoustic tumors (vestibular schwannoma) removed via the translabyrinthine approach. *J Neurosurg.* 1999;90(4):617–623. doi:10.3171/jns.1999.90.4.0617

24. Plotkin SR, Duda DG, Muzikansky A, et al. Multicenter, prospective, phase II and biomarker study of high-dose bevacizumab as induction therapy in patients with neurofibromatosis type 2 and progressive vestibular schwannoma. *J Clin Oncol.* 2019;37(35):3446–3454. doi:10.1200/JCO.19.01367

25. Yang H-C, Kano H, Awan NR, et al. Gamma Knife radiosurgery for larger-volume vestibular schwannomas. *J Neurosurg JNS.* 2011;114(3):801. doi:10.3171/2010.8.JNS10674

26. Mendenhall WM, Friedman WA, Buatti JM, Bova FJ. Preliminary results of linear accelerator radiosurgery for acoustic schwannomas. *J Neurosurg.* 1996;85(6):1013. doi:10.3171/jns.1996.85.6.1013

27. Combs SE, Welzel T, Schulz-Ertner D, et al. Differences in clinical results after LINAC-based single-dose radiosurgery versus fractionated stereotactic radiotherapy for patients with vestibular schwannomas. *Int J Radiat Oncol Biol Phys.* 2010;76(1):193–200. doi:10.1016/j.ijrobp.2009.01.064

28. Carlson ML, Tveiten OV, Driscoll CL, et al. Long-term quality of life in patients with vestibular schwannoma: an international multicenter cross-sectional study comparing microsurgery, stereotactic radiosurgery, observation, and nontumor controls. *J Neurosurg JNS.* 2015;122(4):833. doi:10.3171/2014.11.JNS14594

29. Carlson ML, Jacob JT, Pollock BE, et al. Long-term hearing outcomes following stereotactic radiosurgery for vestibular schwannoma: patterns of hearing loss and variables influencing audiometric decline. *J Neurosurg.* 2013;118(3):579–587. doi:10.3171/2012.9.JNS12919

30. Hasegawa T, Kida Y, Kato T, et al. Long-term safety and efficacy of stereotactic radiosurgery for vestibular schwannomas: evaluation of 440 patients more than 10 years after treatment with Gamma Knife surgery. *J Neurosurg.* 2013;118(3):557–565. doi:10.3171/2012.10.JNS12523

31. Videtic GMM, Woody NM. *Handbook of Treatment Planning in Radiation Oncology.* 3rd ed. Demos Medical; 2020.

32. Carlson ML, Van Abel KM, Driscoll CL, et al. Magnetic resonance imaging surveillance following vestibular schwannoma resection. *Laryngoscope.* 2012;122(2):378–388. doi:10.1002/lary.22411

33. Breivik CN, Nilsen RM, Myrseth E, et al. Conservative management or gamma knife radiosurgery for vestibular schwannoma: tumor growth, symptoms, and quality of life. *Neurosurgery.* 2013;73(1):48–56: discussion 56–47. doi:10.1227/01.neu.0000429862.50018.b9

34. Régis J, Pellet W, Delsanti C, et al. Functional outcome after gamma knife surgery or microsurgery for vestibular schwannomas. *J Neurosurg.* 2002;97(5):1091–1100. doi:10.3171/jns.2002.97.5.1091

35. Pollock BE, Driscoll CL, Foote RL, et al. Patient outcomes after vestibular schwannoma management: a prospective comparison of microsurgical resection and stereotactic radiosurgery. *Neurosurgery.* 2006;59(1):77–85: discussion 77–85. doi:10.1227/01.NEU.0000219217.14930.14

36. Maniakas A, Saliba I. Microsurgery versus stereotactic radiation for small vestibular schwannomas: a meta-analysis of patients with more than 5 years' follow-up. *Otol Neurotol.* 2012;33(9):1611–1620. doi:10.1097/MAO.0b013e31826dbd02

37. Lunsford LD, Niranjan A, Flickinger JC, et al. Radiosurgery of vestibular schwannomas: summary of experience in 829 cases. *J Neurosurg.* 2005;102 Suppl:195–199. doi:10.3171/sup.2005.102.s_supplement.0195

38. Andrews DW, Suarez O, Goldman HW, et al. Stereotactic radiosurgery and fractionated stereotactic radiotherapy for the treatment of acoustic schwannomas: comparative observations of 125 patients treated at one institution. *Int J Radiat Oncol Biol Phys.* 2001;50(5):1265–1278. doi:10.1016/S0360-3016(01)01559-0

39. Meijer OW, Vandertop WP, Baayen JC, Slotman BJ. Single-fraction vs. fractionated linac-based stereotactic radiosurgery for vestibular schwannoma: a single-institution study. *Int J Radiat Oncol Biol Phys.* 2003;56(5):1390–1396. doi:10.1016/S0360-3016(03)00444-9

9 ■ UVEAL MELANOMA

Martin C. Tom, Gaurav Marwaha, John H. Suh, and Arun D. Singh

QUICK HIT ■ Uveal melanoma (UM) is the most common form of ocular melanoma, with the uvea consisting of the iris, ciliary body, and choroid. It is unrelated to cutaneous melanoma and was historically managed with enucleation. Now, the standard of care for small- to medium-sized tumors is definitive RT with either episcleral plaque brachytherapy or charged particle RT, which offers >90% tumor control and useful vision-sparing. Larger tumors have less favorable tumor control and are managed with either charged particle RT or enucleation. Diagnosis is often made without biopsy by a well-trained ophthalmologist at an office exam with ultrasound assistance. It is imperative to rule out distant metastases on workup, particularly liver metastases, with dedicated CT/MRI.

Table 9.1: Treatment Paradigm of UM[1]	
Tumor Size	**Management**
Less than 3 risk factors*	Monitor
Diameter 5 to 18 mm and thickness <2.5 mm	Plaque brachytherapy[†] Particle beam RT[‡]
Diameter ≤18 mm and thickness 2.5 to 10 mm	Plaque brachytherapy[†] Particle beam RT[‡] Enucleation
Diameter >18 mm (any thickness) Or thickness >10 mm (any diameter) Or thickness >8 mm with optic nerve involvement (any diameter)	Particle beam RT[‡] Enucleation

*Risk factors: symptomatic, diameter >5 mm, thickness >2 mm, subretinal fluid or orange pigment, tumor within 3 mm of optic disc, US hollowness, absence of halo.
[†]Plaque brachytherapy: [106]Ru or ^{125}I to 85 Gy is commonly used.
[‡]Particle beam RT: 56 to 60 GyE in 4 daily fractions or up to 70 GyE in 5 fractions.
Source: From Uveal Melanoma. *NCCN Clinical Practice Guidelines in Oncology, 2.2020.* 2020.

EPIDEMIOLOGY: Uncommon, with 1,500 to 2,000 cases/year. Most common primary eye tumor in adults, often affects fair-skinned individuals (98%) with a median age of 62. Most common locations are choroid (85%–90%), ciliary body (5%–8%), and iris (3%–5%).[2]

RISK FACTORS: Vast majority are sporadic. However, the following factors may increase risk: fair iris/skin color, propensity to sunburn, UV exposure (questionable), oculodermal melanocytosis,[3–5] germline BAP1 mutation, dysplastic nevus syndrome, and NF-1.

ANATOMY: The posterior uvea is composed of the choroid (i.e., the retina's vascular support layer), which is where light-protective melanocytes reside. The anterior uvea is the iris of the eye and ciliary body (which controls accommodation and lens movement). The entire uveal tract lies beneath the sclera (the white fibrous protective layer of the eye).

PATHOLOGY: Uveal melanocytes arise from neural crest cells. The degree of pigmentation determines iris color. Pathologic types: spindle cell (best prognosis), mixed (majority of cases), and epithelioid (worst prognosis).

GENETICS: Unlike cutaneous melanoma, UM is not associated with BRAF gene mutations. GNAQ and GNA11 mutations are evident early in the tumorigenesis process; also increasing evidence of families with germline BAP1 mutations; and somatic mutations in EIF1AX and SF3B1.[6] Combination of monosomy 3 and 8q gain associated with metastasis. A 15-gene expression profile test is an accurate prognostic marker.[7]

CLINICAL PRESENTATION: Visual symptoms (distortion, visual field loss, scotomas, floaters), retinal detachment (larger tumors), and rarely pain/eye inflammation. One-third of patients are asymptomatic.

WORKUP: Ophthalmologists can make clinical diagnosis 95% of the time.[2] Diagnostic techniques should include the following: slit lamp, indirect ophthalmoscopy, fundus photography, transillumination, fluorescein angiography, and ocular ultrasound (for tumor height/diameter). Typical UMs are subretinal, brown, raised, and dome shaped. Internal extension of tumor results in a mushroom-shaped mass apparent on ultrasonography. Biopsy is indicated in clinically atypical tumors and is also helpful for prognostication.[4] Risk of seeding due to biopsy is rare.[8] Differential diagnosis includes metastases, benign nevus, hemangioma, retinal detachment. Metastatic evaluation: CT abdomen (MRI if highly concerned for liver metastases or if CT equivocal).

PROGNOSTIC FACTORS: Poor prognostic factors include epithelioid cell, large tumor, involvement of ciliary body, older age.

NATURAL HISTORY: The uvea lacks lymphatic channels; thus metastases from the uvea spread hematogenously to liver (90% of metastases), skin, and lungs. After RT, tumors tend to regress slowly over a few years. Useful vision (>20/200) is preserved in 50% of patients with tumor size and location being the main drivers for visual outcomes (i.e., >6 mm tumors and proximity to optic nerve/fovea predict for worse visual outcomes).

STAGING

Table 9.2: AJCC 8th Edition Staging (2017) for UM*				
	Iris Melanoma			
T1	**a** Limited to the iris, ≤3 clock hours in size	**N**	**a**	Metastasis in ≥1 regional LN
			b	No regional LNs, but discrete tumor deposits in orbit, not contiguous to the eye
	b Limited to the iris, >3 clock hours in size	**M1**	**a**	Distant metastasis, all ≤3.0 cm
	c Limited to the iris with secondary glaucoma	**M1**	**b**	Distant metastasis, largest 3.1 to 8 cm
T2	**a** Confluent with or extending into ciliary body without secondary glaucoma	**M1**	**c**	Distant metastasis, largest ≥8.0 cm
	b Confluent with or extending into ciliary body and choroid, without secondary glaucoma	**Group Staging**		
	c Confluent with or extending into the ciliary body, choroid, or both with secondary glaucoma	**I**	T1aN0M0	
		IIA	T1b-dN0M0, T2aN0M0	
			T2bN0M0, T3aN0M0	
			T2c-dN0M0, T3b-cN0M0, T4aN0M0 T3dN0M0, T4b-cN0	
			T4d-eN0M0	
			Any T, N1M0 or any T, any N, M1a-c	
T3	• Confluent with or extending into the ciliary body, choroid, or both with scleral extension	**IIB**		

(continued)

Table 9.2: AJCC 8th Edition Staging (2017) for UM* *(continued)*			
T4	a	Episcleral extension ≤5 mm in largest diameter	IIIA	
	b	Episcleral extension >5 mm in largest diameter	IIIB	
		Choroidal and ciliary body melanoma	IIIC	
T1	a	Size category 1 without ciliary body involvement and extracellular extension	IV	
	b	Size category 1 with ciliary body involvement		
	c	Size category 1 without ciliary body involvement but with extraocular extension ≤5 mm		
	d	Size category 1 with ciliary body involvement and extraocular extension ≤5 mm		
T2	a	Size category 2 without ciliary body involvement or extraocular extension		
	b	Size category 2 with ciliary body involvement		
	c	Size category 2 without ciliary body involvement, with extraocular extension ≤5 mm		
	d	Size category 2 with ciliary body involvement and extraocular extension ≤5 mm		
T3	a	Size category 3 without ciliary body involvement and extraocular extension		
	b	Size category 3 with ciliary body involvement		
	c	Size category 3 without ciliary body involvement, with extraocular extension ≤5 mm		
	d	Size category 3 with ciliary body involvement and extraocular extension ≤5 mm		
T4	a	Size category 4 without ciliary body involvement and extraocular extension		
	b	Size category 4 with ciliary body involvement		
	c	Size category 4 without ciliary body involvement but with extraocular extension ≤5 mm		
	d	Size category 4 with ciliary body involvement and extraocular extension ≤5 mm		
	e	Any size category with extraocular extension >5 mm		

*Because of the intricacy of the AJCC staging, in practice and in most studies, the COMS staging system is utilized. It is broken into three groups: small—1 to 3 mm in apical height and 5 to 16 mm across (>90% 5-yr OS); medium—3.1 to 8 mm in apical height and <16 mm across (80%–85% 5-yr OS); large—>8 mm in apical height or >16 mm across (60% 5-yr OS).

Table 9.3: Size Categories (Ciliary Body and Choroidal UM)

Thickness (mm)							
>15					4	4	4
12.1–15.0				3	3	4	4
9.1–12.0		3	3	3	3	3	4
6.1–9.0	2	2	2	2	3	3	4
3.1–6.0	1	1	1	2	2	3	4
≤3.0	1	1	1	1	2	2	4
	≤3.0	3.1 to 6.0	6.1 to 9.0	9.1 to 12.0	12.1 to 15.0	15.1 to 18.0	>18.0
	Largest Basal Diameter (mm)						

TREATMENT PARADIGM

Observation: Reasonable for asymptomatic T1a lesions, with close ophthalmic surveillance q3 to 6 months (treat for any growth or symptoms). NCCN guidelines recommend surveillance if fewer than 3 of the following risk factors are present: symptomatic, diameter >5 mm, thickness >2 mm, subretinal fluid or orange pigment, tumor within 3 mm of optic disc, US hollowness, absence of halo.[1]

Surgery: Enucleation was the historical standard of care, but in the 2000s, episcleral brachytherapy became the first-line treatment for small- to medium-sized (<10 mm in apical height) tumors and offered equivalent survival with vision-sparing capability. Particle beam RT or *enucleation* under general anesthesia with orbital implant continues to be used when brachytherapy is not feasible (i.e., for larger tumors, poor functional outcome predicted with brachytherapy). For select larger tumors, in an effort to avoid radiation side effects, fragmentation and vitreous cutter *endoresection* can be performed a few weeks postbrachytherapy.[4] Definitive, local resection (*exoresection*) may be feasible as well, in select anterior or large tumors. *Orbital exenteration* is utilized in the setting of massive orbital extension causing pain/blindness.

Chemotherapy: In stage IV disease, cytotoxic agents are of limited benefit, whereas dual checkpoint inhibition (nivolumab plus ipilimumab) provides modest benefit.[9] For isolated liver metastases, locally ablative therapies are employed (e.g., chemoembolization, metastatectomy, RFA, internal/external radiation).

Radiation

- *Episcleral brachytherapy* typically with ^{125}I or ^{106}Ru (more common in Europe and better for smaller tumors as it offers a more rapid dose falloff) radionuclides. The half-lives of ^{125}I and ^{106}Ru are 60 days and 374 days, respectively. Plaques are generally gold plated, with grooves in which radiation sources are glued or molded. The plaques come in a variety of shapes/sizes to accommodate critical vision structures. The plaques contain eyelets, which the ophthalmologist uses to suture the plaque onto the episcleral surface overlying the tumor with a 2 mm margin of safety, under general anesthesia. The ophthalmologist makes a conjunctival peritomy; then the globe is transilluminated and tumor outlined. Next, a dummy plaque is used to verify the proper position. Then, the radioactive plaque is placed. Dose is 85 Gy (at a dose rate of 0.6–1.05 Gy/h) prescribed to 5 mm from inner scleral surface unless the tumor is >5 mm, in which case prescription is to apex of tumor.[10] The plaque remains in place for 3 to 7 days, during which time the patient wears a lead eye shield. The plaque is removed by the ophthalmologist, and the patient returns home with bandages and pain medications.
- *Charged particle beam radiation* (56–60 GyE in 4 daily fractions or up to 70 GyE in 5 fractions). Most commonly with protons. Tantalum marker rings are surgically placed at the tumor borders for tumor delineation and to serve as fiducials, and multiple additional planning inputs are used for target delineation, including US, surgeon mapping, and CT/MRI. The optimal gaze direction to minimize dose to the cornea, lens, macula, and optic nerve is used.

Side effects: Acute: pain (brachy), rarely dry eye. Late: vasculopathy (driven by disc/fovea proximity), cataract formation (especially anterior tumors), maculopathy, retinopathy (most common side effect with brachy), optic neuropathy.

Other Modalities: Transpupillary thermotherapy is associated with high risk of local recurrence alone, but can easily be combined with brachytherapy as an adjunct. For radiation failures, transpupillary thermotherapy or repeat brachytherapy can be employed.[11]

■ EVIDENCE-BASED Q&A

SMALL TUMORS

■ Is it necessary to treat all small UMs?

No, risk of death is low provided patients are serially monitored with ophthalmologic exams. Significant growth on follow-up exams is an indication for treatment.

COMS Report No. 5, "Small" Choroidal Melanoma Series (*Arch Ophthalmol* 1997, PMID 9400787): Nonrandomized prospective study of 204 patients with small choroidal melanomas (i.e., 1–3 mm height and ≥5 mm in basal diameter). MFU was 92 months. Eight percent of patients were treated at study enrollment and 33% treated during follow-up. Tumor growth noted in 21% at 2 years and 31% at 5 years. Twenty-seven patients died; 6 from distant metastases. Five-year OS 94% and 8-year OS 85%. **Conclusion: Majority of patients with "small" choroidal melanomas (66%) may represent choroidal nevus and therefore can be closely monitored. Observation of small tumors may be appropriate until progression is noted.**

■ What factors determine the use of each isotope (^{125}I vs. ^{106}Ru)?

^{106}Ru offers a more rapid dose falloff than ^{125}I, which may aid in sparing critical vision structures in the management of smaller tumors (<5 mm) without compromising oncologic outcomes.

Takiar, MD Anderson (*PRO* 2015, PMID 25423888): RR of 107 patients treated with ^{125}I ($n = 67$) or ^{106}Ru ($n = 40$). ^{106}Ru: 5-year LC, PFS, and OS: 97%, 94%, and 92%, respectively. ^{125}I: 5-year LC, PFS, and OS: 83%, 65%, and 80%, respectively. In patients with apical tumor height ≤5 mm, PFS was slightly better for ^{106}Ru ($p = .02$). Enucleation-free survival was better in ^{106}Ru patients ($p = .02$) as were radiation retinopathy ($p = .03$) and cataracts ($p < .01$). **Conclusion: Both isotopes offer excellent local control for small UMs, though ^{106}Ru does so with reduced toxicity.**

MEDIUM TUMORS

■ How does the historical standard of enucleation compare with episcleral plaque brachytherapy?

No difference in overall survival. Eye- and vision-sparing with brachytherapy. In the rare event of radiation failure, patients can be salvaged effectively with enucleation.

COMS Report No. 28, "I-125 vs. Enucleation" (*Arch Ophthalmol* 2006, PMID 17159027): PRT of 1,317 patients with medium-sized choroidal melanomas (≥2.5–10 mm height and <16 mm in largest basal diameter)—enucleation vs. episcleral plaque brachytherapy with ^{125}I (85 Gy Rx dose). Exclusions: fovea/optic disc/ciliary body involvement; 13% of episcleral plaque patients were salvaged (due to tumor progression or RT complications) with enucleation by 5 years.

Table 9.4: Results of COMS 28 Trial of I-125 vs. Enucleation for Choroidal Melanoma						
	5- and 12-Yr OS	12-Yr DM	I-125 Arm	Median Visual Acuity	20/40 or Better	20/200 or Worse
Enucleation	81%/59%	17%	Baseline	20/32	70%	10%
I-125 plaque 85 Gy	82%/57%	21%	3 yrs after I-125	20/125	34%	45%
p value	NS	NS				

Conclusion: Episcleral plaque brachytherapy offers equivalent OS compared to enucleation. This PRT set the precedent for plaque brachytherapy as the standard of care in this patient population.

LARGE TUMORS

■ **What are the management options for large tumors that are not amenable to plaque brachytherapy?**

Plaque brachytherapy is limited by suboptimal dosimetry for large tumors, and by technical challenges for those in close proximity or surrounding the optic disc. Historically, enucleation was the standard. Neoadjuvant EBRT was assessed on COMS 15, but did not result in improved outcomes compared to enucleation alone. Charged particle RT does not suffer the limitations of plaque brachytherapy for large tumors, and is used as globe-sparing treatment with favorable outcomes.

COMS Report No. 15, "Large Tumors" (*Arch Ophthalmol* 2001, PMID 11346394): PRT of 1,003 patients with large choroidal melanomas (>16 mm in largest basal diameter regardless of height, or >10 mm in height regardless of diameter, or >8 mm in height if <2 mm from optic disc)—enucleation vs. preoperative 20 Gy/5 fx EBRT + enucleation. Preoperative EBRT did not increase complication rate, but did have fewer local recurrences (0 vs. 5). Distant metastases were most commonly seen in liver (93%), lung (24%), and bone (16%).

Table 9.5 Results of COMS 15 Trial of Neoadjuvant EBRT for Large UMs		
	5-Yr OS	**5-Yr DSS**
Enucleation alone	57%	72%
Pre-op EBRT 20 Gy + enucleation	62%	74%
p value	.32	.64

Papakostas, Proton RT Large Tumors (*JAMA Ophthalmol* 2017, PMID 29049518): RR of 336 patients with large tumors (as defined by COMS 15) treated with proton RT 70 CGE in 5 fx. Ten-year outcomes included tumor control, 87.5%; eye retention, 70.4%; melanoma-related morality, 48.5%; OS, 60.7%; visual acuity retention >20/200, 8.7%; ability to count fingers, 22.4%. A 1-mm increase in diameter was associated with 20% increased risk of melanoma-related mortality.

CHARGED PARTICLE RT

■ **How does plaque brachytherapy compare with charged particle irradiation?**

Charged particle RT, most commonly with protons, is the second most common treatment modality after plaque brachytherapy and has been used to treat UM for decades; 5-year estimates with proton RT treatment include LC, >90%; OS, 70% to 85%; DMFS, 75% to 90%; and DSS, 75% to 90%.[12] Advantages of using charged particle RT include the ability to treat larger tumors or those encircling the optic disc, where plaque brachytherapy is limited and enucleation is the alternative. Data from a meta-analysis and a single RCT using helium ions suggest charged particle RT is associated with improved local control rates compared to plaque brachytherapy, but at the expense of increased anterior eye complications.

Char, UCSF (*Ophthalmology* 1993, PMID 8414414): PRT of 184 patients randomized to helium ion 70 Gy/5 fx vs. episcleral plaque brachytherapy (^{125}I) for tumors <10 mm height and <15 mm diameter. Helium ion therapy had greater local control (100% vs. 83%), comparable survival, and fewer salvage enucleations (9% vs. 17%), however, with more anterior complications (dry eye, neovascular glaucoma, epiphora). **Conclusion: Compared to brachytherapy, helium ion therapy was associated with better local control and less salvage enucleation, but more anterior segment toxicity.**

Chang, Meta-analysis (*Br J Ophthalmol* 2013, PMID 23645818): Analysis of 49 studies reporting local failure after globe-conserving therapy. **Conclusion: Local failure rates vary by treatment modality.**

Table 9.6: Results of Meta-Analysis of Globe-Conserving Therapy for UM			
Modality	Weighted Mean Local Failure (%)	Weighted Mean Tumor Diameter (mm)	Weighted Mean Tumor Height (mm)
Brachytherapy (n = 3,868)	9.45	11.00	4.48
Charged particle RT (n = 7,043)	4.21	13.93	5.54
Photon RT (n = 542)	7.85	11.40	6.15
Surgery (n = 537)	18.60	12.96	7.98
Laser (n = 552)	20.80	7.00	2.50

▪ What is the optimal dose to treat UM with charged particle RT?

Only one RCT compared proton RT 50 CGE vs. 70 CGE both in 5 fx with similar outcomes. A recent survey demonstrated the most commonly used dose was 60 GyE in 4 fx.[13]

Gragoudas, Proton Dose (*Arch Ophthalmol* 2000, PMID 10865313): PRT of 188 patients with UM <15 mm diameter and <5 mm height randomized to proton RT 50 CGE vs. 70 CGE both in 5 fx generally over a 7-day period. At 5 years, LF and DM rates were similar at 2% to 3% and 7% to 8%, respectively. The proportion of patients with visual acuity of at least 20/200 were ~55% in both groups. Radiation maculopathy rates were also similar. Patients treated with 50 CGE had significantly less visual field loss. **Conclusion: Lower dose proton RT was not associated with improved visual acuity, but had less visual field loss. LF and DM rates were similar.**

OTHER OCULAR TUMORS

A number of other ocular tumors are treated with RT, though given the relative uncommonness, limited data are available. Conjunctival melanoma is distinct from UM and is primarily treated with wide local excision and adjuvant CHT, RT (brachytherapy or charged particle RT), and/or cryotherapy.[14] Other rare conjunctival tumors, such as squamous cell carcinoma, are managed similarly. Choroidal metastases are typically treated with palliative EBRT, but have been treated with brachytherapy and charged particle RT in select cases. Angiomas and retinal hemangiomas can be treated with surgery, laser therapy, cryotherapy, plaque brachytherapy, or charged particle RT.[15,16]

Retinoblastoma is the most common malignant primary intraocular tumor of childhood. EBRT was previously used as a globe-sparing treatment, but alternatives such as CHT (systemic and local) and other focal therapies (e.g., laser therapy, cryotherapy) with less secondary malignancy risk are now preferred. Plaque brachytherapy has been used for smaller tumors, but its use has similarly been replaced with other focal therapies with less side effects.[17] Currently, EBRT is typically reserved for progressive or persistent disease following CHT or focal treatment.

REFERENCES

1. Uveal Melanoma. *NCCN Clinical Practice Guidelines in Oncology*, 2.2020. 2020.
2. Aronow ME, Topham AK, Singh AD. Uveal Melanoma: 5-year update on incidence, treatment, and survival (SEER 1973-2013). *Ocul Oncol Pathol*. 2018;4(3):145–151. doi:10.1159/000480640
3. Weis E, Shah CP, Lajous M, et al. The association between host susceptibility factors and uveal melanoma: a meta-analysis. *Arch Ophthalmol*. 2006;124(1):54–60. doi:10.1001/archopht.124.1.54
4. Seregard S, Pelayes DE, Singh AD. Radiation therapy: uveal tumors. *Dev Ophthalmol*. 2013;52:36–57. doi:10.1159/000351055
5. Singh AD, Rennie IG, Seregard S, et al. Sunlight exposure and pathogenesis of uveal melanoma. *Surv Ophthalmol*. 2004;49(4):419–428. doi:10.1016/j.survophthal.2004.04.009
6. Field MG, Harbour JW. Recent developments in prognostic and predictive testing in uveal melanoma. *Curr Opin Ophthalmol*. 2014;25(3):234–239. doi:10.1097/ICU.0000000000000051
7. Onken MD, Worley LA, Char DH, et al. Collaborative Ocular Oncology Group report number 1: prospective validation of a multi-gene prognostic assay in uveal melanoma. *Ophthalmology*. 2012;119(8):1596–1603. doi:10.1016/j.ophtha.2012.02.017

8. Singh AD, Medina CA, Singh N, et al. Fine-needle aspiration biopsy of uveal melanoma: outcomes and complications. *Br J Ophthalmol.* 2016;100(4):456–462. doi:10.1136/bjophthalmol-2015-306921
9. Nathan P, Ascierto PA, Haanen J, et al. Safety and efficacy of nivolumab in patients with rare melanoma subtypes who progressed on or after ipilimumab treatment: a single-arm, open-label, phase II study (CheckMate 172). *Eur J Cancer.* 2019;119:168–178. doi:10.1016/j.ejca.2019.07.010
10. Marwaha G, Macklis RM, Singh AD, Wilkinson A. Brachytherapy. In: Singh AD, Pelayes DE, Seregard S, Macklis RM, eds. *Ophthalmic Radiation Therapy: Techniques and Applications.* Karger; 2013;29–35.
11. Bellerive C, Aziz HA, Bena J, et al. Local failure after episcleral brachytherapy for posterior uveal melanoma: patterns, risk factors, and management. *Am J Ophthalmol.* 2017;177:9–16. doi:10.1016/j.ajo.2017.01.024
12. Verma V, Mehta MP. Clinical outcomes of proton radiotherapy for uveal melanoma. *Clin Oncol (R Coll Radiol).* 2016;28(8):e17–e27. doi:10.1016/j.clon.2016.01.034
13. Hrbacek J, Mishra KK, Kacperek A, et al. Practice patterns analysis of ocular proton therapy centers: the international OPTIC survey. *Int J Radiat Oncol Biol Phys.* 2016;95(1):336–343. doi:10.1016/j.ijrobp.2016.01.040
14. Wong JR, Nanji AA, Galor A, Karp CL. Management of conjunctival malignant melanoma: a review and update. *Expert Rev Ophthalmol.* 2014;9(3):185–204. doi:10.1586/17469899.2014.921119
15. Singh AD, Nouri M, Shields CL, et al. Treatment of retinal capillary hemangioma. *Ophthalmology.* 2002;109(10):1799–1806. doi:10.1016/s0161-6420(02)01177-6
16. Mishra KK, Daftari IK. Proton therapy for the management of uveal melanoma and other ocular tumors. *Chin Clin Oncol.* 2016;5(4):50. doi:10.21037/cco.2016.07.06
17. Ortiz MV, Dunkel IJ. Retinoblastoma. *J Child Neurol.* 2016;31(2):227–236. doi:10.1177/0883073815587943

10 ■ SPINE TUMORS

Sarah S. Kilic, Ehsan H. Balagamwala, and Samuel T. Chao

> **QUICK HIT** ■ Chondrosarcomas and chordomas are rare spine and skull base tumors. Chondrosarcomas are usually low-grade, indolent cartilage-producing tumors that rarely metastasize, though high-grade or rare histologies can behave more aggressively. Surgery is the preferred management, and is usually curative. Most tumors are chemo- and radioresistant, with no major role for CHT, and RT is reserved for the incompletely resected or unresectable setting. Chordomas are locally destructive tumors that arise from remnants of the embryonic notochord. They most commonly occur in the skull base, spine, and sacrum. Optimal management of resectable lesions includes en bloc resection with adjuvant RT. Treatment of skull base chordomas is challenging due to delicate anatomic location, which mandates maximally safe resection followed by adjuvant RT, often using advanced techniques (protons, heavy ions) if available.

Table 10.1: General Treatment Paradigm for Chondrosarcomas and Chordomas

Chordoma, resectable	Complete surgical resection + adjuvant RT to ≥70 Gy if incomplete resection
Chondrosarcoma, low grade	Complete surgical resection; no role for CHT or RT
Chondrosarcoma, high grade or unconventional histology	Complete surgical resection; consider preoperative RT to 50.4 Gy if positive margins likely; consider post-op RT to 70 Gy for R1 resection, up to 78 Gy for R2 resection
Chordoma or chondrosarcoma, unresectable or incompletely resectable	Maximal safe resection + RT to >70 Gy; strongly consider protons, heavy ions, or SRS if skull base location
Chordoma or chondrosarcoma, oligometastatic	Resection of all lesions or SRS/SBRT to unresectable sites; trial enrollment
Chordoma or chondrosarcoma, widely metastatic	Surgery or RT for symptomatic sites; systemic therapy for selected histologies; trial enrollment

EPIDEMIOLOGY: Chondrosarcoma is the third most common primary bone tumor (after myeloma and osteosarcoma).[1] It is the most common primary bone tumor in older populations, with most patients older than age 50 at diagnosis.[2] Incidence is 0.5 in 100,000 per year, with slight male predominance.[2,3] Chordomas are exceedingly rare, with an incidence of 0.08 in 100,000 per year.[4] Similarly to chondrosarcoma, chordoma is more common in older populations, with a median age at diagnosis of 60, and a male predominance.[5]

RISK FACTORS: There are no known environmental risk factors for chordoma or chondrosarcoma, and no known predisposing conditions for chordoma. Most chondrosarcomas are sporadic and de novo. However, some can arise from the malignant transformation of osteochondromas and enchondromas, the latter of which can be solitary or multiple in the context of enchondromatosis. Osteochondromas are cartilage-capped projections from bony surfaces, of which 5% transform to chondrosarcoma. Solitary enchondromas are benign cartilaginous tumors within bone marrow, in whom transformation is extremely rare. Enchondromatosis is associated with Ollier disease, Maffucci syndrome, or multiple hereditary exostoses; 25% to 30% transform to chondrosarcoma.[1,6]

ANATOMY: Chondrosarcomas: Can arise in any bone with equal incidence in axial and appendicular skeleton. Proximal femur most common site, followed by proximal humerus, distal femur, ribs.[3] Can also involve spine, scapula, sternum; can rarely involve facial bones, neck, forearm, clavicle, small tubular bones.[3] Further subdivided into conventional and rare types based on a combination of anatomical location within bone, and pathologic features.

Conventional chondrosarcomas include the following:

- Central (75%): Arise within medullary cavity of any bone; up to 40% arise from enchondroma; typically an older male patient.
- Peripheral (10%): Arise within cartilage cap of preexisting osteochondroma.
- Periosteal (<1%): Arise on surface of bone; patients typically younger (20s to 30s).[3]

Rare chondrosarcoma subtypes are based on histology rather than anatomy, and include dedifferentiated, mesenchymal, clear cell, and myxoid. See Pathology.

Chordomas: As these malignancies arise from remnants of the notochord (see Pathology), they are most commonly found in the midline, although they can also arise in the clinoid process or temporal bone because the notochord projects into these areas. Historically, chordomas were thought to occur most commonly in the sacrum, but newer series demonstrate an approximately equal incidence in the skull base, mobile spine, and sacrum.[7]

PATHOLOGY: *Chondrosarcomas:* Conventional chondrosarcomas are classified as grade 1, 2, or 3 based on cellularity, abundance of hyaline matrix, nuclear size, and frequency of mitoses. Grade 1 chondrosarcomas are often difficult to distinguish from benign enchondroma, even to experienced pathologists. Rare, "nonconventional" subtypes represent <15% of chondrosarcomas and include dedifferentiated, mesenchymal (the only radiosensitive histology), clear cell, and myxoid. Grade is the single most important prognostic factor for chondrosarcomas, as demonstrated by worsening OS with increasing grade: grade 1, 10-year OS 83% to 95%; grade 2, 10-year OS 64% to 86%; grade 3, 10-year OS 29% to 55%. Risk of distant metastasis is 1% in grade 1 chondrosarcoma, 10% to 15% in grade 2, and up to 70% in grade 3.[8–10]

Chordomas: Arise from remnants of the embryonic notochord. Three histologic subtypes: classical (conventional), chondroid, and dedifferentiated. Classical chordomas appear as soft, gray–white, lobulated tumors composed of groups of cells separated by fibrous septa. These cells have round nuclei and an abundant vacuolated cytoplasm and are termed *physaliferous* cells. The chondroid subtype has a better prognosis and has a predilection for skull base location. Chordomas stain positive for S-100, cytokeratins, and brachyury; expression of brachyury is helpful in differentiating chordoma from chondrosarcoma (see Genetics).[7,11]

GENETICS: Chondrosarcoma: About 90% of patients with multiple osteochondromas have inherited germline mutation in tumor suppressors EXT1 or EXT2; however, presence or absence of mutation is not associated with malignant transformation. Ollier disease and Maffucci syndrome are both caused by somatic mosaic mutations in IDH1 or IDH26. However, there are no known genes associated with sporadic chondrosarcoma.[12]

Chordoma: The vast majority are sporadic, and as discussed earlier, there are no known syndromes associated with chordoma. However, the transcription factor brachyury, which is involved in notochord development, is overexpressed in >95% of chordomas. Brachyury is not expressed in chondrosarcomas.[13,14]

CLINICAL PRESENTATION: Dependent on site and histology. Patients with chondrosarcomas usually have a long, indolent course; 80% present with bony pain, which is often insidious, slowly progressive, and worse at night.[3] About 27% present with associated pathologic fracture.[3] Soft tissue swelling is also common. Symptoms may persist for months or years before diagnosis. Similarly, chordomas are often indolent and slow-growing, and patients are often asymptomatic until late stages. Chordoma of the mobile spine and sacrum can present with pain and neurologic deficits at the corresponding spinal nerve root level. Skull base chordoma presentation varies with location (see Table 10.2).[15]

Table 10.2: Skull Base Tumor Locations and Their Associated Presentations	
Middle fossa	Sensory deficits in the first, second, or third branches of CN V; masseter weakness; diplopia; dysarthria and dysphagia; headache
Jugular foramen	Occipital headache that worsens with movement; CN IX–XII dysfunction (dysarthria, dysphagia, reduced tongue/palate sensation, sternocleidomastoid and shrug weakness, deviation of the tongue on protrusion); glossopharyngeal neuralgia (shooting pain in the throat)
Clivus	Headache most severe at the vertex that worsens with neck flexion; possible dysfunction of CN IV–XII
Orbital or parasellar	Frontal or orbital headache, diplopia, visual deficits, restricted extraocular movements, proptosis
Sphenoid sinus	Frontal headache with or without orbital pain, nasal congestion, diplopia, restricted extraocular movements (especially abduction)
Occipital condyle	Occipital headache and deviation of the tongue on protrusion due to CN XII dysfunction

WORKUP: H&P including careful musculoskeletal and complete neurologic exam.

Labs: For skull base tumors, consider endocrine and ophthalmologic evaluation.

Imaging: Plain radiograph of affected bone, CT, MRI. Chondrosarcomas have high water content, which leads to low attenuation on CT and high signal intensity on T2 MRI. Classic descriptions of central chondrosarcomas on XR: fusiform expansion in metaphysis or diaphysis, mixed radiolucent and sclerotic appearance, punctate or ring-and-arc pattern of calcifications. Periosteal chondrosarcomas appear as round soft tissue mass on bone surface. Chordomas often demonstrate an origin in the bone and an extensive and destructive adjacent soft tissue component; calcifications and expansion of the involved bone are common. They are typically iso- or hypointense on T1 MRI, hyperintense on T2 MRI, and hetereogeneously enhancing with gadolinium contrast due to intratumoral necrosis, which leads to a "honeycomb" appearance.[16] If grade 2 to 3 chondrosarcoma, obtain CT chest to evaluate for lung metastases.

Biopsy: For non–skull base bony locations, core biopsy preferred to establish the diagnosis. May start with percutaneous approach, but may not reflect grade accurately due to lesion heterogeneity; biopsy should be aimed at most aggressive-looking part of lesion (soft tissue or enhancing components).[17] For skull base, open, endoscopic, or fine needle biopsy as anatomically feasible.

PROGNOSTIC FACTORS: Extent of resection is the most important treatment-related prognostic factor for both of these histologies. Grade for chondrosarcomas and histologic subtype for chordomas are most important tumor-related prognostic factors; 10-year OS for chondrosarcoma above 90% for grade 1 disease, as low as 30% for grade 3 disease, or even poorer for nonconventional subtypes. For chordoma, SEER data suggest MS of ~7.5 years.[18]

STAGING: Chondrosarcoma: MSTS system most commonly used. AJCC 8 staging also exists for bone tumors of appendicular skeleton/trunk/skull/facial bones, spine, and pelvis; however, no AJCC prognostic stage groupings exist for spine and pelvis. In MSTS, "extracompartmental" is defined as extension of tumor through cortex of involved bone.

Table 10.3: MSTS Staging for Sarcomas	
Stage IA	Low grade, intracompartmental
Stage IB	Low grade, extracompartmental
Stage IIA	High grade, intracompartmental
Stage IIB	High grade, extracompartmental
Stage III	Systemic or regional metastases

Table 10.4: AJCC 8th Edition (2017): Staging for Bony Tumors of Appendicular Skeleton, Trunk, Skull, and Facial Bones

Tumor*		Node		Distant Metastasis		Grade	
T1	≤8 cm	N0	No regional LNs	M0	No distant metastasis	G1	Well differentiated, low grade
T2	>8 cm	N1	Regional LNs	M1a	Distant metastasis to lung	G2	Moderately differentiated, high grade
T3	Discontinuous tumors in primary bone site			M1b	Distant metastasis to nonlung site	G3	Poorly differentiated, high grade

Note: There is no T4 designation for these sites.

TNM	Grade	Group Stage
T1N0M0	G1	IA
T2–3N0M0	G1	IB
T1N0M0	G2 to G3	IIA
T2N0M0	G2 to G3	IIB
T3N0M0	G2 to G3	III
Any T, N0, M1a	Any G	IVA
Any T, N1; any M	Any G	IVB

TREATMENT PARADIGM

Surgery: *Chondrosarcoma:* Complete resection is considered the only curative option. Surgical approach depends on stage, grade, and location. For grade 1 lesions, goal is to minimize functional disability. For small grade 1 lesions in extremity, manage with intralesional curettage followed by phenolization or cryotherapy and then cementation or bone grafting of cavity; this approach has fewer complications than wide local excision, and offers excellent outcomes, with LC and OS >90% at 10 years.[19–23] For large grade 1 lesion in extremity, or any size axial/pelvis: wide local excision, due to difficulty of complete curettage and therefore higher local recurrence rate. LC and OS >90% at 5 years.[24] For grade 2 to 3 disease, wide en bloc local excision is required for all nonmetastatic cases; this may entail an extensive reconstruction; 10-year OS 70%.[25] For peripheral chondrosarcomas, cartilage cap with its pseudocapsule must be completely resected. 10-year LC 82%, 10-year OS 95%.[26] For recurrent disease, preferred management is repeat resection based on grade, as in the preceding discussion.

Chordoma: Similarly to chondrosarcoma, surgery is the mainstay of treatment.[27–29] However, complete resection is often impossible due to anatomic location; in these cases, postoperative RT is recommended. Surgical approach and technique is dependent on anatomic location. For sacral lesions lower than S3, en bloc resection is often feasible with a posterior or transperineal approach with low morbidity. Sacral lesions above S3 often require both an anterior and a posterior approach, with open laparotomy and dissection of tumor away from viscera, significantly increasing morbidity.[30] All approaches are associated with a significant risk of bowel and bladder incontinence. For skull base lesions, a variety of approaches can be employed depending on specific patient and tumor anatomy, including open transsphenoidal, transmaxillary, transnasal, transoral, or endoscopic approaches.

Chemotherapy: Essentially no role in most cases of chondrosarcoma and chordoma. Chondrosarcomas have poor vascularity, large amounts of extracellular matrix, and expression of the efflux pump MDR1, rendering them particularly chemoresistant; CHT response rates are as low as 0%.[31–35] Per NCCN guidelines, dasatinib can be attempted for widely metastatic chondrosarcoma, with an 18% response rate in one phase II study.[36] Traditional chemotherapeutic agents are similarly ineffective in chordomas. Very small series have suggested some efficacy of imatinib or sunitinib.[5,37]

Radiation

Chondrosarcoma: Indications: Generally radioresistant due to the low proportion of actively dividing cells, and therefore no major role for RT, with the following few specific indications: Post-op after incomplete resection of high-grade, dedifferentiated, or mesenchymal; locally recurrent cases; definitive management of unresectable lesions. May also be employed in the palliative setting for symptomatic metastatic lesions. No guidelines exist for target delineation. Dose: Postoperative doses of ≥60 Gy commonly used in historical series. Cases of true definitive RT (i.e., without any degree of preceding resection) are rare in the literature. Optimal dose unknown, but probably >60 to 70 Gy.

Chordoma: Indications: Similarly to chondrosarcoma, radioresistant. Dose: Treatment to <70 Gy associated with dismal local control. Treatment to doses higher than 70 Gy with photons to certain anatomical sites, particularly the skull base or sacrococcygeal region, may not be feasible and may require consideration of proton or carbon ion therapy. Japanese series of definitive carbon ion RT for unresectable sacral chordomas, with most patients treated to 67 to 70 GyE, have suggested good outcomes, with acceptable safety and with 5-year LC of ≥80%.[38,39]

Toxicity: All sites: Fatigue, CNS necrosis. Skull base: Hearing loss, trismus, osteoradionecrosis, brain necrosis, cranial nerve dysfunction. Spine: Pain flare, vertebral compression fracture, nausea/vomiting/diarrhea, radiation myelopathy.

■ EVIDENCE-BASED Q&A

▦ Is there a role for postoperative RT in chondrosarcoma and chordoma?

For completely resected lesions, no survival or local control benefit has been seen with adjuvant RT. In patients with less than completely resected disease, evidence for the utility of postoperative RT is mixed.

York et al (*J Neurosurg* 1999, PMID 10413129): Single-institution RR of 28 patients with chondrosarcoma of the spine treated with surgery with or without postoperative RT over 43 years; 18 patients underwent 28 surgeries; 75% STR; 10 patients had postoperative RT; doses ranged from 40 to 70 Gy. DFS (16 months vs. 44 months) between surgery alone and surgery + RT groups was not statistically significant. However, STR was associated with a statistically significantly lower DFS compared to GTR. **Conclusion: For spine chondrosarcomas, no clear benefit to post-op RT. Complete resection associated with better DFS.**

Sahgal (*Neuro Oncol* 2015, PMID 25543126): RR of 18 patients with skull base chondrosarcoma and 24 with skull base chordoma treated with surgery and post-op IMRT. 36% had GTR. Chondrosarcomas treated to median 70 Gy; 5-year LC 88%, 5-year OS 87%. GTR and age were only predictors of LC. **Conclusion: Good LC and OS with surgery + post-op RT compared to other series. Complete resection associated with better LC and OS.**

Goda (*Cancer* 2011, PMID 21246520): RR of 60 patients with extracranial chondrosarcoma who had surgery with pre-op (40%) or post-op (60%) RT; 50% had R0 resection. RT dose ranged from 40 to 70 Gy; 10-year LC for R0, R1, R2 resection was 100%, 94%, and 42%, respectively. Only grade and younger age were associated with poorer outcomes. **Conclusion: In a population with a significant proportion of patients with incomplete resection, surgery with pre-op or post-op RT offers good long-term LC.**

▦ Is there a role for SRS in chondrosarcoma and chordoma?

SRS offers good outcomes in the skull base and spine, as demonstrated by the following studies. For a discussion of the role of SRS in the management of spine metastases, see Chapter 67.

Kano, North American Gamma Knife Consortium (*J Neurosurg* 2011, PMID 21135744): RR of 71 patients who underwent definitive, postoperative, or salvage SRS for skull base chordomas. Median dose 15 Gy (range 9–25 Gy); 5-year LC 66%, 5-year OS 80% for the cohort. On subset analysis based on receipt of prior RT, LC was similar, but OS significantly higher for patients who did not receive prior RT (93% vs. 43%). On MVA, older age, prior RT, and larger tumor were associated with poorer LC. **Conclusion: SRS offers modest LC for skull base chordomas. Poor prognostic factors include age, prior RT, and larger tumor size.**

Kano, North American Gamma Knife Consortium (*J Neurosurg* 2015, PMID 26115468): RR of 46 patients who underwent definitive or postoperative SRS for skull base chondrosarcoma. Median dose 15 Gy (range 10.5–20 Gy); 5-year PFS 85%, 10-year PFS 70%, 5-year OS 86%, 10-year OS 76%; 13% of patients had cranial nerve toxicities attributable to RT. **Conclusion: SRS offers excellent LC, with modest toxicity outcomes.**

- **What are the roles of proton and heavy particle therapy in the treatment of chordoma and chondrosarcoma?**

Given that many of these lesions occur in anatomically critical locations (skull base, sacrococcygeus), there has been interest in particle therapy for potential ability to dose-escalate while relatively sparing OARs. Institutional series and a meta-analysis suggest that particle therapy may offer good local control outcomes, with acceptable toxicity.

Rosenberg, MGH (*Am J Surg Pathol* 1999, PMID 10555005): RR of 200 patients with grade 1 or 2 skull base chondrosarcoma treated with surgery and photon + proton RT; 95% had STR. RT was combination of photon 3D-CRT and 180 MeV proton; median dose 72.1 GyE. 5-year LC 99%, 10-year LC 98%. **Conclusion: Surgery and proton + photon RT offers excellent long-term LC for skull base chondrosarcoma.**

Imai, Japan (*IJROBP* 2016, PMID 27084649): RR of 188 patients with unresectable sacral chordoma treated with definitive carbon ion RT. All but one patient treated to 67.2 GyE or higher (maximum 73.6 GyE); 5-year LC 77%, 5-year OS 81%; 97% of patients retained ability to walk; worst toxicities were grade 3 neuropathy in 6 patients and grade 4 skin toxicity in 2 patients. **Conclusion: Carbon ion RT offers good local control outcomes with acceptable toxicity and ability to preserve ambulation.**

Guan, China (*Radiat Oncol* 2019, PMID 31752953): RR of 91 patients with skull base or C-spine chordoma or chondrosarcoma treated with protons, carbon ions, or both; 50% definitive, 50% re-RT. Proton-only therapy was 70 GyE/35 fx; combination or carbon ion therapy was to a total dose of 63 to 71 GyE in 2 to 3 Gy/fx; 2-year LC 86%, 2-year PFS 77%, and 2-year OS 87%; 21% of patients had late grade 1 to 2 toxicities (most commonly hearing loss); no grade 3 + late toxicities. On MVA, tumor volume >60 mL was associated with poorer PFS and OS. Re-RT was also associated with poorer OS. **Conclusion: For chordomas and chondrosarcomas of the skull base and cervical spine, particle therapy offers good local control outcomes with acceptable toxicity.**

Zhou, Meta-Analysis (*World Neurosurg* 2018, PMID 29879512): Meta-analysis of 25 studies of a total of 996 patients with chordoma s/p resection who underwent post-op RT via conventionally fractionated photons, SRS, protons, or carbon ions; 3-year OS was comparable for SRS, protons, and carbon ions (92%, 89%, and 93%, respectively, NS), which were superior to conventional RT (70%). Similarly, 5-year OS was favorable for SRS, protons, and carbon ions (81%, 79%, and 87%, respectively) compared to conventional RT (46%). Long-term data were limited, but at 10 years, protons appeared to be associated with the most favorable OS (60%) compared to conventional RT (21%), SRS (40%), and carbon ions (45%). **Conclusion: For patients s/p surgery who go on to RT, SRS and particle therapy may offer favorable survival outcomes compared to conventionally fractionated RT.**

- **Are there any society guidelines regarding the management of chordoma?**

In 2017, the Chordoma Global Consensus Group defined consensus recommendations for the management of recurrent chordoma.

Stacchiotti, CGCG Position Paper (*Ann Oncol* 2017, PMID 28184416): Defined recommendations for the management of recurrent chordoma. For skull base recurrence, high-dose (re)RT preferred over resection. For mobile spine/sacrum recurrence, high-dose (re)RT preferred in most cases, except those with surgically accessible tumor without history of prior piecemeal resection or surgical rupture, in which case maximal safe resection preferred. For any site, if neither high-dose RT nor GTR feasible, palliative management (which may include palliative RT or surgical debulking). **Conclusion: Re-RT to high doses generally preferred for recurrent chordoma when feasible.**

REFERENCES

1. Gelderblom H, Hogendoorn PC, Dijkstra SD, et al. The clinical approach towards chondrosarcoma. *Oncologist.* 2008;13(3):320–329. doi:10.1634/theoncologist.2007-0237

2. van Praag Veroniek VM, Rueten-Budde AJ, Ho V, et al. Incidence, outcomes and prognostic factors during 25 years of treatment of chondrosarcomas. *Surg Oncol.* 2018;27(3):402–408. doi:10.1016/j.suronc.2018.05.009

3. Kim MJ, Cho KJ, Ayala AG, Ro JY. Chondrosarcoma: with updates on molecular genetics. *Sarcoma.* 2011;2011:405437. doi:10.1155/2011/405437

4. Frezza AM, Botta L, Trama A, et al. Chordoma: update on disease, epidemiology, biology and medical therapies. *Curr Opin Oncol.* 2019;31(2):114–120. doi:10.1097/CCO.0000000000000502

5. Alan O, Akin Telli T, Ercelep O, et al. Chordoma: a case series and review of the literature. *J Med Case Rep.* 2018;12(1):239. doi:10.1186/s13256-018-1784-y

6. Silve C, Juppner H. Ollier disease. *Orphanet J Rare Dis.* 2006;1:37. doi:10.1186/1750-1172-1-37

7. George B, Bresson D, Herman P, Froelich S. Chordomas: a review. *Neurosurg Clin N Am.* 2015;26(3):437–452. doi:10.1016/j.nec.2015.03.012

8. Angelini A, Guerra G, Mavrogenis AF, et al. Clinical outcome of central conventional chondrosarcoma. *J Surg Oncol.* 2012;106(8):929–937. doi:10.1002/jso.23173

9. Bjornsson J, McLeod RA, Unni KK, et al. Primary chondrosarcoma of long bones and limb girdles. *Cancer.* 1998;83(10):2105–2119. doi:10.1002/(SICI)1097-0142(19981115)83:10<2105::AID-CNCR9>3.0.CO;2-U

10. Evans HL, Ayala AG, Romsdahl MM. Prognostic factors in chondrosarcoma of bone: a clinicopathologic analysis with emphasis on histologic grading. *Cancer.* 1977;40(2):818–831. doi:10.1002/1097-0142(197708)40:2<818::AID-CNCR2820400234>3.0.CO;2-B

11. Shen J, Shi Q, Lu J, et al. Histological study of chordoma origin from fetal notochordal cell rests. *Spine (Phila Pa 1976).* 2013;38(25):2165–2170. doi:10.1097/BRS.0000000000000010

12. Pedrini E, Jennes I, Tremosini M, et al. Genotype-phenotype correlation study in 529 patients with multiple hereditary exostoses: identification of "protective" and "risk" factors. *J Bone Joint Surg Am.* 2011;93(24):2294–2302. doi:10.2106/JBJS.J.00949

13. Vujovic S, Henderson S, Presneau N, et al. Brachyury, a crucial regulator of notochordal development, is a novel biomarker for chordomas. *J Pathol.* 2006;209(2):157–165. doi:10.1002/path.1969

14. Kitamura Y, Sasaki H, Yoshida K. Genetic aberrations and molecular biology of skull base chordoma and chondrosarcoma. *Brain Tumor Pathol.* 2017;34(2):78–90. doi:10.1007/s10014-017-0283-y

15. Jacox A., Carr, D. B., Payne, R., et al. (1994). *Management of Cancer Plan. Clinical Practice Guideline No. 9* (AHCPR Pub. No. 94–0592). Rockville, MD: Agency for Health Care Policy and Research, U.S. Department of Health and Human Services, Public Health Service; 1994: 31–32.

16. Youssef C, Aoun SG, Moreno JR, Bagley CA. Recent advances in understanding and managing chordomas. *F1000Res.* 2016;5:2902. doi:10.12688/f1000research.9499.1

17. Normand AN, Cannon CP, Lewis VO, et al. Curettage of biopsy-diagnosed grade 1 periacetabular chondrosarcoma. *Clin Orthop Relat Res.* 2007;459:146–149. doi:10.1097/BLO.0b013e3180619554

18. Smoll NR, Gautschi OP, Radovanovic I, et al. Incidence and relative survival of chordomas: the standardized mortality ratio and the impact of chordomas on a population. *Cancer.* 2013;119(11):2029–2037. doi:10.1002/cncr.28032

19. Bauer HC, Brosjo O, Kreicbergs A, Lindholm J. Low risk of recurrence of enchondroma and low-grade chondrosarcoma in extremities. 80 patients followed for 2–25 years. *Acta Orthop Scand.* 1995;66(3):283–288. doi:10.3109/17453679508995543

20. Donati D, Colangeli S, Colangeli M, et al. Surgical treatment of grade I central chondrosarcoma. *Clin Orthop Relat Res.* 2010;468(2):581–589. doi:10.1007/s11999-009-1056-7

21. Hickey M, Farrokhyar F, Deheshi B, et al. A systematic review and meta-analysis of intralesional versus wide resection for intramedullary grade I chondrosarcoma of the extremities. *Ann Surg Oncol.* 2011;18(6):1705–1709. doi:10.1245/s10434-010-1532-z

22. van der Geest IC, de Valk MH, de Rooy JW, et al. Oncological and functional results of cryosurgical therapy of enchondromas and chondrosarcomas grade 1. *J Surg Oncol.* 2008;98(6):421–426. doi:10.1002/jso.21122

23. Leerapun T, Hugate RR, Inwards CY, et al. Surgical management of conventional grade I chondrosarcoma of long bones. *Clin Orthop Relat Res.* 2007;463:166–172. doi:10.1097/BLO.0b013e318146830f

24. Streitburger A, Ahrens H, Balke M, et al. Grade I chondrosarcoma of bone: the munster experience. *J Cancer Res Clin Oncol.* 2009;135(4):543–550. doi:10.1007/s00432-008-0486-z

25. Fiorenza F, Abudu A, Grimer RJ, et al. Risk factors for survival and local control in chondrosarcoma of bone. *J Bone Joint Surg Br.* 2002;84(1):93–99. doi:10.1302/0301-620X.84B1.0840093

26. Ahmed AR, Tan TS, Unni KK, et al. Secondary chondrosarcoma in osteochondroma: report of 107 patients. *Clin Orthop Relat Res.* 2003(411):193–206. doi:10.1097/01.blo.0000069888.31220.2b

27. Stacchiotti S, Casali PG, Lo Vullo S, et al. Chordoma of the mobile spine and sacrum: a retrospective analysis of a series of patients surgically treated at two referral centers. *Ann Surg Oncol.* 2010;17(1):211–219. doi:10.1245/s10434-009-0740-x

28. Osaka S, Kodoh O, Sugita H, et al. Clinical significance of a wide excision policy for sacrococcygeal chordoma. *J Cancer Res Clin Oncol.* 2006;132(4):213–218. doi:10.1007/s00432-005-0067-3

29. York JE, Kaczaraj A, Abi-Said D, et al. Sacral chordoma: 40-year experience at a major cancer center. *Neurosurgery*. 1999;44(1):74–79: discussion 79–80. doi:10.1097/00006123-199901000-00041

30. Yin X, Fan WL, Liu F, et al. Technique and surgical outcome of total resection of lower sacral tumor. *Int J Clin Exp Med*. 2015;8(2):2284–2288.

31. Wyman JJ, Hornstein AM, Meitner PA, et al. Multidrug resistance-1 and p-glycoprotein in human chondrosarcoma cell lines: expression correlates with decreased intracellular doxorubicin and in vitro chemoresistance. *J Orthop Res*. 1999;17(6):935–940. doi:10.1002/jor.1100170619

32. van Oosterwijk JG, Herpers B, Meijer D, et al. Restoration of chemosensitivity for doxorubicin and cisplatin in chondrosarcoma in vitro: BCL-2 family members cause chemoresistance. *Ann Oncol*. 2012;23(6):1617–1626. doi:10.1093/annonc/mdr512

33. van Oosterwijk JG, Meijer D, van Ruler MA, et al. Screening for potential targets for therapy in mesenchymal, clear cell, and dedifferentiated chondrosarcoma reveals Bcl-2 family members and TGFbeta as potential targets. *Am J Pathol*. 2013;182(4):1347–1356. doi:10.1016/j.ajpath.2012.12.036

34. Terek RM, Schwartz GK, Devaney K, et al. Chemotherapy and P-glycoprotein expression in chondrosarcoma. *J Orthop Res*. 1998;16(5):585–590. doi:10.1002/jor.1100160510

35. Italiano A, Mir O, Cioffi A, et al. Advanced chondrosarcomas: role of chemotherapy and survival. *Ann Oncol*. 2013;24(11):2916–2922. doi:10.1093/annonc/mdt374

36. Schuetze SM, Bolejack V, Choy E, et al. Phase 2 study of dasatinib in patients with alveolar soft part sarcoma, chondrosarcoma, chordoma, epithelioid sarcoma, or solitary fibrous tumor. *Cancer*. 2017;123(1):90–97. doi:10.1002/cncr.30379

37. Casali PG, Messina A, Stacchiotti S, et al. Imatinib mesylate in chordoma. *Cancer*. 2004;101(9):2086–2097. doi:10.1002/cncr.20618

38. Imai R, Kamada T, Araki N, Working Group for B, Soft Tissue S. Carbon Ion Radiation Therapy for Unresectable Sacral Chordoma: an analysis of 188 cases. *Int J Radiat Oncol Biol Phys*. 2016;95(1):322–327. doi:10.1016/j.ijrobp.2016.02.012

39. Nishida Y, Kamada T, Imai R, et al. Clinical outcome of sacral chordoma with carbon ion radiotherapy compared with surgery. *Int J Radiat Oncol Biol Phys*. 2011;79(1):110–116. doi:10.1016/j.ijrobp.2009.10.051

II ■ HEAD AND NECK

11 ■ OROPHARYNX CANCER

Shireen Parsai, Aditya Juloori, Nikhil P. Joshi, and Shlomo A. Koyfman

QUICK HIT ■ SCC of the oropharynx is currently the most common H&N cancer in the United States. Its incidence continues to rise with increasing prevalence of HPV. There are two etiologies: those associated with tobacco and alcohol, which are often HPV negative, and those associated with HPV infection. These are classified as two distinct diseases per the AJCC 8th edition staging system. Both are currently treated with the same approach, but treatment paradigms are evolving to account for differences in outcome.

Table 11.1 General Treatment Paradigm for Oropharynx Cancer	
	Treatment Options
T1–2N0–1	Definitive IMRT Or TORS (or other function-preserving surgery), neck dissection, and risk-adapted adjuvant therapy (Chapter 17)
T3–4 and/or N1–3	Definitive chemoRT Or Surgery (select patients) with risk-adapted PORT ± CHT

EPIDEMIOLOGY: Estimated 35,610 tongue and pharynx cases in 2020 with 6,470 deaths.[1] Male-to-female ratio approximately 4:1.[2] In the United States, incidence of HPV-associated OPC increased by 225% from 1988 to 2004 and HPV-negative cancer declined by 50% in the same time frame.[3] Prevalence of HPV was 39.5% on RTOG 9003, which increased to 68% on RTOG 0129 and further to 73% on RTOG 0522.[4-6] Peak prevalence of oral HPV DNA is bimodal: 7% for ages 30 to 34 and 11% for ages 60 to 64.[4]

RISK FACTORS: Age, high-risk sexual behavior (HPV+), tobacco, alcohol (HPV−).[4,7]

ANATOMY: Oropharynx consists of base of tongue (lingual tonsil), vallecula, palatine tonsil, soft palate, and posterior oropharyngeal wall. The superior border of the OPX is the soft palate and the inferior border is the hyoid–lingual surface of the epiglottis. The base of tongue is separated from the oral tongue by the circumvallate papillae. The base of tongue is the posterior one third of the tongue and composed of lingual lymphatic tissue. The palatine tonsils sit between an arch formed by the anterior and posterior tonsillar pillars.

Table 11.2 Oropharynx Borders	
Site	**Boundaries**
BOT	Anteriorly by circumvallate papillae, laterally by glossopalatine sulci, and inferiorly by vallecula. Includes pharyngoepiglottic and glossoepiglottic fold.
Tonsillar complex	Composed of anterior and posterior tonsillar pillars, true palatine tonsil, and tonsillar fossa. Tonsillar pillars are mucosal folds over glossopalatine and pharyngopalatine muscles. Tonsillar fossa is a triangular region bounded by pillars, inferiorly by glossotonsillar sulcus and pharyngoepiglottic fold and laterally by pharyngeal constrictor muscles.
Soft palate	Defined anteriorly by hard palate, laterally by palatopharyngeal and superior pharyngeal constrictor muscles and posteriorly by palatopharyngeal arch/uvula. Forms roof of oropharynx and floor of nasopharynx.
PPW	Spans area defined by soft palate, epiglottis, posterior edge of tonsillar complexes, and lateral aspects of pyriform sinuses inferiorly. Inferior to oropharyngeal PPW is PPW of hypopharynx, one of the three subsites of hypopharynx.

PATHOLOGY: Approximately 95% of OPC are SCCs.[8] Remaining 5% of cases consist of lymphoma, minor salivary cancers (e.g., mucoepidermoid, adenoid cystic; see Chapter 15), and rare sarcomas. HPV-positive and -negative cancers appear different pathologically. HPV-positive tumors often originate from the lymphoid tissue of tonsil or BOT and are more likely to be poorly differentiated/nonkeratinizing and basaloid in appearance. HPV-negative tumors have no predilection for location and are often keratinizing. *HPV 16* serotype accounts for ~90% of HPV-associated cases. HPV viral proteins E6 and E7 bind p53 and Rb respectively with subsequent loss of tumor suppression. When E7 binds to Rb, transcription factor E2F is released and allows cyclin to bypass G1/S checkpoint. Reflexive expression of p16 protein inhibits cyclin D-CDK4 complex in an effort to prevent uncontrolled cell cycling. Overexpression of p16 protein serves as a surrogate marker of HPV integration into DNA. p16 protein can be detected by IHC. HPV DNA is detected by FISH. p16 is more sensitive but less specific than HPV16 DNA. On RTOG 0129, 19% of HPV-negative patients were p16+ but only 3% of p16– were HPV16–. In HPV-endemic areas such as the United States, PPV of p16 status in OPC is high (~90%), but in HPV-uncommon disease sites or in the developing world, PPV of p16 status is poor (<40%). EGFR is more commonly amplified in HPV-negative tumors and is associated with poor prognosis.[2,9]

Table 11.3 Factors Associated With HPV Status in OPC	
HPV+	**HPV–**
- Younger	- Older
- Non/light smoker	- Heavy smoking/drinking
- Caucasian	- Non-Caucasian
- High-risk sexual behavior	- Not related to sexual behavior
- More likely tonsil/base of tongue	- No tissue preference
- Nonkeratinizing	- Keratinizing
- Basaloid	- p53 mutation
- p16 upregulated	- EGFR amplified
- Poorly differentiated	

CLINICAL PRESENTATION: Most common presentation of OPC is painless neck mass. Other symptoms related to local invasion include dysphagia, odynophagia, or otalgia referred from cranial nerve IX via tympanic nerve of Jacobson. Oral tongue fixation (unable to protrude tongue) suggests deep musculature involvement. Trismus suggests medial pterygoid invasion.[2]

WORKUP: H&P with careful attention to H&N including palpation of BOT, dental exam, neurologic exam, mirror exam, and/or flexible laryngoscopy.

Labs: CBC and BMP with attention to renal function. Measurement of HPV-circulating tumor DNA, obtained at baseline and posttreatment, is an evolving strategy for surveillance.[10]

Imaging: CT of neck with contrast is most helpful for primary tumor delineation; PET/CT is also recommended for staging and evaluation of lymphadenopathy. Consider MRI if concerns exist for perineural or skull base invasion.[2,11] After chemoRT, it is more cost effective to perform PET/CT at 12 weeks and proceed to neck dissection if positive than to perform planned neck dissection.[12]

Procedures: Initial biopsy via FNA of lymphadenopathy acceptable although confirmatory biopsy of primary via tonsillectomy or BOT biopsy with detailed exam under anesthesia is recommended. Tumor HPV testing recommended per NCCN.

Other: Nutrition, speech and swallowing evaluation/therapy, and audiogram as clinically indicated. EUA with endoscopy as clinically indicated. Smoking cessation counseling should also be advised as appropriate.

PROGNOSTIC FACTORS: Age, smoking (both 10 and 20 pack-year cutoffs have been used for stratification, may be less relevant than current/former smoking status[13]), comorbidities, performance status, stage, HPV status, PET SUV.[14–16] Staging and prognostic stratification of HPV-positive patients is rapidly evolving (see Tables 11.4 and 11.5).

NATURAL HISTORY: Nodal involvement is common and initial site of drainage from oropharynx is to neck level II and subsequently down jugular chain to levels III to IV. Levels IB, V and retropharyngeal nodes can be involved but are less common.[8] Historically, locoregional recurrence was responsible for the majority of cancer-related morbidity and mortality.[17] While this remains true for HPV-negative disease, locoregional recurrence of HPV-positive disease is generally uncommon. Distant metastases, however, develop in both subgroups at similar rates. Most common sites of distant metastases are lung and bone.[14,18]

Table 11.4 AJCC 8th Edition (2017): Staging for Oropharynx (p16−)		cN0	cN1	cN2a	cN2b	cN2c	cN3a	cN3b
T/M ＼ N								
T1	• ≤2 cm	I						
T2	• 2.1 to 4 cm	II	III	IVA				
T3	• >4 cm • Extension							
T4a	• Invasion[1]							
T4b	• Invasion[2]			IVB				
M1	• Distant metastasis			IVC				

Notes: Extension = extension to lingual surface of epiglottis. Invasion[1] = invasion into larynx, extrinsic musculature of tongue, medial pterygoid muscle, hard palate, or mandible. Invasion[2] = invasion into lateral pterygoid, pterygoid plates, lateral nasopharynx, skull base or encases carotid artery.
cN1, single ipsilateral LN (≤3 cm) and −ENE; cN2a, single ipsilateral LN (3.1–6 cm) and −ENE; cN2b, multiple ipsilateral LN (≤6 cm) and −ENE; cN2c, bilateral or contralateral LN (≤6 cm) and −ENE; cN3a, LN (>6 cm) and no ENE; cN3b, clinically overt ENE.
pN1, single LN (≤3 cm) and −ENE; pN2a, single ipsilateral or contralateral LN (≤3 cm) and −ENE or single ipsilateral LN (3.1–6 cm) and −ENE; pN2b, multiple ipsilateral LN (≤6 cm) and −ENE; pN2c, bilateral or contralateral LN (≤6 cm) and −ENE; pN3a, LN (>6 cm) and −ENE; pN3b, LN (>3 cm) and + ENE.

Table 11.5 AJCC 8th Edition (2017): Staging for HPV-Mediated (p16+) Oropharyngeal Cancer		cN0	cN1	cN2	cN3
T/M ＼ N					
T1	• ≤2 cm	I		II	III
T2	• 2.1 to 4 cm				
T3	• >4 cm • Extension				
T4	• Invasion				
M1	• Distant metastases			IV	

Notes: Extension = Extension to lingual surface of epiglottis. Invasion = invasion into larynx, extrinsic muscles of tongue, medial pterygoid, hard palate, or beyond.
cN1, one or more ipsilateral LN (≤6 cm); cN2, contralateral or bilateral LN (≤6 cm); cN3, LN (>6 cm).
pN1, ≤4 LNs; pN2, >4 LNs.

TREATMENT PARADIGM

Surgery: Classic oncologic surgery for OPC consists of radical tonsillectomy (simple tonsillectomy performed for biopsy is generally not sufficient for oncologic control), glossectomy (often requiring mandibulotomy), palatectomy, or pharyngectomy with ipsilateral or bilateral neck dissection depending on nodal status and laterality of primary tumor. Because of functional deficits left by these procedures, nonoperative approaches became standard in the 1970s and beyond. Over the past decade, however, minimally invasive procedures such as TLM and TORS have reduced morbidity of surgery and are now standard options for T1–2 and select T3 lesions (see Evidence-Based Q&A).[11] Only one historical trial has compared surgery with RT to definitive RT (RTOG 7303) and with small numbers found similar OS for both approaches; this is the same with the modern ORATOR trial (see following).[19] See Chapter 17 for details on adjuvant RT. Radical neck dissection: levels IB to V with sacrifice of internal and external jugular veins, SCM, omohyoid, CN XI, and submandibular gland. Modified radical neck dissection: levels IB to V but leaves one or more of jugular veins, SCM, omohyoid, or CN XI. Selective neck dissection: modified radical but leaves one or more of levels IB to V. Supraomohyoid neck dissection: resection of levels I to III. Recently, SLNB (followed by neck dissection if positive) has been found to be oncologically equivalent to neck lymph node dissections for patients with operable oral and oropharyngeal cT1–T2N0 cancer. There is also lower morbidity associated with SLNB during the first 6 months after surgery.[20]

Chemotherapy: Concurrent cisplatin is standard for eligible patients receiving definitive RT with stage III to IV disease. Cisplatin can be given concurrently with RT as 100 mg/m^2 weeks 1, 4, and 7 (NCCN Category 1) or 40 mg/m^2 weekly (NCCN Category 2B).[11] Carboplatin/infusional 5-FU is also considered an NCCN category 1 recommended regimen to be administered concurrently with RT. Cetuximab given concurrent with RT for nonplatinum candidates can be considered, though it has inferior outcomes without overall decreased toxicity for patients who are eligible to receive cisplatin (NCCN category 2B; see Evidence-Based Q&A).[21] Cetuximab starts 1 week prior to RT as loading dose of 400 mg/m^2 followed by 250 mg/m^2 weekly during RT.[22] Other less common concurrent regimens include carboplatin/paclitaxel, cisplatin/5-FU, and 5-FU/hydroxyurea. Induction CHT consists of cisplatin, 5-FU, and docetaxel (TPF) every 3 weeks for 4 cycles completing 4 to 7 weeks prior to RT alone or with cetuximab or carboplatin (see Evidence-Based Q&A).[11,23] Cisplatin-based induction CHT has not been proven to increase overall survival as compared to proceeding directly to concurrent chemoradiation regimens.

Radiation

Indications: RT is indicated for definitive treatment of OPC or in postoperative setting (see Chapter 17).

Dose: In a definitive setting, standard dose is 70 Gy/35 fx. Various elective nodal doses have been used including 56 Gy/35 fx (simultaneous boost) and 50 Gy/25 (sequential boost to 70 Gy). RTOG 1016 used a third lower dose to "low-risk" neck to 50 to 52.5 Gy/35 fx. For cT1-2N0-1 OPC, 66 Gy/30 fx RT alone with elective dose of 54 Gy/30 fx (simultaneous) is reasonable based on RTOG 0022 (see Evidence-Based Q&A). Dose reduction for HPV+ patients is the subject of clinical trials.

Toxicity: Acute: Fatigue, mucositis, dysphagia, odynophagia, xerostomia, dermatitis, aspiration. Chronic: Dysphagia, neck fibrosis, xerostomia, trismus, osteoradionecrosis, hypothyroidism, brachial plexopathy (rare but take care with gross disease in low neck).

Procedure: See *Handbook of Treatment Planning in Radiation Oncology*, Chapter 4.[24]

▪ EVIDENCE-BASED Q&A

▪ Can definitive RT lead to similar control and survival compared to radical surgeries?

This was a key question in the 1970s, when surgery was the definitive treatment of choice, often requiring mandibulotomy for BOT access and subsequent functional deficits. RTOG 7303 is the only historical PRT addressing this question; definitive RT has subsequently become the standard option to preserve functional outcomes.

Kramer, RTOG 7303 (*Head Neck Surg* 1987, PMID 3449477): Advanced SCC of oropharynx or oral cavity randomly assigned to preoperative RT, PORT, or definitive RT (65–70 Gy). Larynx or hypopharynx cancers randomized to either preoperative (50 Gy) or PORT (60 Gy). For oral cavity or OPC patients, 4-year OS was similar between all groups: 30% preoperative, 36% postoperative, 33% definitive. 4-year LRC was 43% preoperative, 52% postoperative, and 38% definitive. **Conclusion: Definitive RT is an ethically justified alternative compared to radical surgery.**

▪ Can the efficacy of RT be improved by altering fractionation?

SCC is known to undergo accelerated repopulation and is sensitive to reoxygenation, so fractionation was thought to play an important role in outcomes with definitive RT. Multiple trials and meta-analysis demonstrated improved LRC and OS with AF for treating locoregionally advanced patients.

Horiot, EORTC 22791 (*Radiother Oncol* 1992, PMID 1480768): PRT of 356 patients randomized to 70 Gy/35 to 40 fx or hyperfractionation of 80.5 Gy/70 fx. T2–3 oropharynx (excluding BOT) cancers,

N0–1 were included from 1980 to 1987. Hyperfractionation demonstrated LRC benefit and trend toward OS in T3N0–1 patients but not T2.

Fu, RTOG 9003 (*IJROBP* 2000, PMID 10924966; Update Beitler *IJROBP* 2014, PMID 24613816): PRT 1,073 patients with stage III to stage IV SCC of oral cavity, oropharynx, supraglottic larynx or stage II to stage IV of BOT or hypopharynx randomized to one of four arms: (a) standard fractionation to 70 Gy/35 fx, (b) hyperfractionation to 81.6 Gy/68 fx at 1.2 Gy/fx BID with 6-hour interfraction interval, (c) split-course accelerated hyperfractionation to 67.2 Gy/42 fx given 1.6 Gy/fx BID with 6-hour interfraction interval and 2-week rest after 38.4 Gy, or (d) accelerated hyperfractionation with concomitant boost to 72 Gy/42 fx given at 1.8 Gy/fx 5 days a week with 1.5 Gy/fraction to boost field as second daily treatment given 6 hours apart for last 12 treatment days. Primary end point was 2-year LRC. Results at initial report: At MFU of 23 months, both hyperfractionation (2) and concomitant boost (4) arms showed improved LRC but no significant difference in OS. All 3 AF arms showed increased acute effects but only concomitant boost arm showed increased late effects. In final update, hyperfractionation (2) and concomitant boost (4) decreased 5-year LRR compared to standard fractionation, but hyperfractionation did not increase late effects. When using only 5-year follow-up, hyperfractionation improved OS (HR: 0.81, $p = .05$) but not when all follow-up data were included. **Conclusion: AF improves disease control in locoregionally advanced squamous carcinoma of H&N.**

Table 11.6 Results of RTOG 9003			
	Regimen	2-Yr LRC	2-Yr OS
1. Standard	70 Gy/35 fx daily	46%	46%
2. Hyperfractionation	81.6 Gy/68 fx BID	54%*	54.5%[†]
3. Split course	67.2 Gy/42 fx BID with 2-week break	47.5%	46.2%
4. Concomitant boost	72 Gy/42 fx (BID final 12 days)	54.5%[‡]	50.9%

*Statistically significant difference in original and final reports.
[†]Statistically significant difference (only when limited to 5-year follow-up).
[‡]Statistically significant difference compared to standard arm in original report.

Overgaard, DAHANCA 6 and 7 Combined Analysis (*Lancet* 2003, PMID 14511925): Combined analysis of two trials performed from 1992 to 1999 including 1,485 patients with stage I to stage IV SCC; DAHANCA 6 of glottis carcinoma testing fractionation and DAHANCA 7 of supraglottic, pharynx, and oral cavity cancers testing fractionation and radiosensitizer nimorazole. RT given to 62 to 68 Gy at 2 Gy/fx and randomized to either 5 or 6 fractions per week. Overall 5-year LRC was improved with acceleration (70% vs. 60%, $p = .0005$). Disease-specific survival but not OS was also improved by acceleration. **Conclusion: Six fractions weekly became standard in Denmark. This result was independent of p16 status.**[25]

Bourhis, MARCH Meta-Analysis (*Lancet* 2006, PMID 16950362; Update Lacas, *Lancet Oncol* 2017, PMID 28757375): Patient-level meta-analysis of 11,969 patients from 34 trials with MFU 6 years, 75% oropharynx and larynx cancers and 75% stage III to stage IV. AF was associated with a significant OS benefit of 3.1% at 5 years ($p = .003$). The significant survival benefit was attributed to hyperfractionation alone, which had the most OS benefit (8.1%). OS was significantly worse (5.8% decrement at 5 years) with AF RT alone compared with concurrent chemoRT (HR: 1.22, $p = .01$). **Conclusion: AF, specifically hyperfractionation, improves OS in H&N cancer. The comparison between hyperfractionated RT and concurrent chemoRT remains to be specifically tested.**

■ **Does CHT add benefit to conventionally fractionated RT?**

Adelstein, H&N Intergroup (*JCO* 2003, PMID 12506176): PRT of 271 of planned 362 patients between 1992 and 1999 with stage III to stage IV unresectable SCC (all sites except sinus, nasopharynx, or salivary) randomized to (a) RT alone (70 Gy/35 fx); (b) cisplatin with RT (100 mg/m² weeks 1, 4, and 7); or (c) split-course chemoRT (cisplatin 75 mg/m² with 5-FU 1,000 mg/m² every 4 weeks with 30 Gy/15 fx 1st course followed by surgical evaluation and if CR or unresectable, another 30–40 Gy given with 3rd cycle of CHT). Trial closed early due to slow accrual; 3-year OS for chemoRT (arm B) was superior to that of arm A or arm C; 89% of patients in arm B experienced grades 3 to 5 toxicity. **Conclusion: High-dose cisplatin when added to conventionally fractionated RT improves OS.**

Table 11.7 Results of H&N Intergroup			
	CR	3-Yr OS	Grades 3 to 5 Toxicity
Arm A: RT	27.4%	23%	52%
Arm B: CRT	40.2%	37%*	89%*
Arm C: split-course CRT	49.4%*	27%	77%*

Statistically significant relative to arm A.

Calais, GORTEC 94-01 (*JNCI* 1999, PMID 10601378; Denis *JCO* 2004 PMID 14657228): PRT of 226 patients with stage III to stage IV SCC of oropharynx randomized to RT alone (70 Gy/35 fx) with or without concurrent carboplatin and 5-FU for 3 cycles. OS (22% vs. 16%), DFS (27% vs. 15%), and LRC (48% vs. 25%) were all improved by statistically significant amount. Grade 3 or higher late effects occurred in 30% vs. 56% ($p = .12$). **Conclusion: CHT improved survival without increasing late toxicity.**

◼ Does CHT add benefit to hyperfractionated RT?

Although hyperfractionated RT adds benefit over conventional fractionation, CHT remains beneficial.

Brizel, Duke (*NEJM* 1998, PMID 9632446): PRT of 116 patients with T3–4 N0–3 SCC of H&N (and T2N0 BOT) treated to 75 Gy/60 fx BID and randomized to either no concurrent therapy or concurrent cisplatin (60 mg/m^2) and 5-FU (600 mg/m^2) weeks 1 and 6. At MFU of 41 months, 3-year OS 55% in CHT arm vs. 34% in hyperfractionated group ($p = .07$). LRC was also improved (44% vs. 70%, $p = .01$). Toxicity was comparable. **Conclusion: CHT adds benefit to hyperfractionated RT with similar toxicity.**

Bourhis, GORTEC 99-02 (*Lancet Oncol* 2012, PMID 22261362): Three-arm PRT of stage III to stage IV SCC of H&N randomized to standard chemoRT (70 Gy/35 fx with carboplatin and 5-FU), accelerated chemoRT (70 Gy in 6 weeks with carboplatin and 5-FU), or very accelerated RT alone (64.8 Gy/36 fx BID in 3.5 weeks). Standard chemoRT and accelerated chemoRT were similar in terms of PFS ($p = .88$). Conventional chemoRT improved PFS compared with very accelerated RT ($p = .04$). **Conclusion: Acceleration alone cannot completely compensate for absence of CHT.**

◼ Does hyperfractionated RT add benefit to chemoRT?

This question is the inverse of the previous question and was partially addressed by GORTEC 99-02 earlier, but was also addressed by the RTOG (although this was not the most significant finding from RTOG 0129; see HPV section later).

Nguyen-Tan, RTOG 0129 (*JCO* 2014, PMID 25366680): PRT of 721 patients with SCC of oral cavity, oropharynx, larynx, or hypopharynx to either 70 Gy/35 fx or 72 Gy/42 fx over 6 weeks with concomitant boost schedule (see RTOG 9003 earlier). Both arms received cisplatin 100 mg/m^2 every 3 weeks (2 cycles for accelerated arm, 3 for standard arm). After MFU 7.9 years, no differences were observed in any end point (OS, PFS, LRC, or DM). **Conclusion: No benefit to acceleration in presence of concurrent CHT.**

◼ What is the overall summary of chemoRT trials?

Pignon, MACH-NC Meta-analysis (*Lancet* 2000, PMID 10768432; Update Pignon *Radiother Oncol* 2009, PMID 19446902; By Disease Site: Blanchard *Radiother Oncol* 2011, PMID 21684027): Patient-level meta-analysis of over 17,000 patients from 93 trials demonstrated OS benefit to addition of CHT of 4.5% at 5 years. Concurrent chemoRT showed absolute benefit of 6.5% at 5 years (SS); induction 2.4% at 5 years (NS). Patients above 70 years of age did not benefit in terms of OS. Both concurrent and induction CHT improved distant control (update: HR 0.73 and 0.88, $p = .0001$ and .04 but not different when compared to each other).

◼ Is cetuximab of benefit compared to RT alone?

An EGFR inhibitor, cetuximab is active against H&N cancer and improved OS compared to RT alone.

Bonner (*NEJM* 2006, PMID 16467544; Update *Lancet Oncol* 2010, PMID 19897418): PRT of 424 patients from 1999 to 2002 with stage III to stage IV SCC of oropharynx, hypopharynx, or larynx randomized to either RT alone (3 regimens permitted: daily, BID, and concomitant boost) or RT with cetuximab given 400 mg/m² loading dose 1 week before RT and 250 mg/m² weekly during RT. Primary end point was LRC. Cetuximab improved LRC and OS (MS 29 vs. 49 months, $p = .03$). Toxicity was not different with exception of infusion reactions and acneiform rash. Subsequent analyses did not show interaction with HPV status.[26] Survival was improved in cetuximab patients who developed grade 2 or higher acneiform rash compared to those without rash. **Conclusion: Cetuximab improves OS compared to RT alone.**

■ **Does cetuximab improve survival when added to cisplatin?**

Ang, RTOG 0522 (*JCO* 2014, PMID 25154822): PRT of 891 patients with stages III to IV H&N cancer randomized to RT with cisplatin with or without cetuximab. Addition of cetuximab did not improve OS, DFS, LRC, or DM but did increase toxicity. EGFR expression did not predict outcome. **Conclusion: No benefit to addition of cetuximab to cisplatin.**

■ **Is concurrent cetuximab directly comparable and less toxic than concurrent cisplatin?**

It was hypothesized that concurrent cetuximab may provide similar oncologic outcomes to cisplatin but with reduced toxicity. Three phase III RCTs directly compared RT with concurrent cetuximab vs. concurrent cisplatin among patients with HPV+ oropharyngeal cancer; each demonstrated reduced survival with cetuximab without dramatic reductions in toxicity.

Gillison, RTOG 1016 (*Lancet* 2019, PMID 30449625): PRT of HPV+ oropharyngeal cancer (AJCC 7th edition: T1–2, N2a–N3 or T3–4, N0–3) treated with accelerated IMRT (70 Gy/35 fx, 6 fx/week) with either concurrent cisplatin (100 mg/m² days 1 and 22) or concurrent cetuximab. Primary end point OS. Of 805 patients with 4.5-year MFU, OS with cetuximab was not non-inferior to cisplatin (HR: 1.45, $p = .5$). Furthermore, cetuximab was associated with significantly inferior OS, PFS, and LRF, but not DM; 5-year OS was 84.6% with cetuximab vs. 77.9% with cetuximab ($p = .016$); 5-year LRF was 9.9% with cisplatin vs. 17.3% with cetuximab ($p = .0005$). Moderate to severe acute and late toxicities were similar. **Conclusion: For HPV + oropharyngeal cancer, concurrent cetuximab has inferior OS compared to concurrent cisplatin without a dramatic reduction in toxicity.**

Mehanna, De-ESCALATE (*Lancet* 2019, PMID 30449623): PRT with HPV+ low-risk (p16+ and <10 smoking pack-years) oropharyngeal cancer treated with RT (70 Gy/35 fx) with either concurrent cisplatin (100 mg/m² days 1, 22, and 43) or concurrent cetuximab. Primary end point was overall G3–5 toxicity at 2 years, and of 334 patients, it was not significantly different ($p = .98$); 2-year OS worse with cetuximab vs. cisplatin (89.4% vs. 97.5%; $p = .001$), as was 2-year any-recurrence (16.1% vs. 6%, $p = .0007$). Giving cetuximab instead of cisplatin was estimated to lead to 1 extra death at 2 years for every 12 patients treated. **Conclusion: For low-risk HPV + oropharyngeal cancer, concurrent cetuximab showed no benefit in terms of reduced toxicity, but instead showed inferior OS and disease control compared to cisplatin.**

Gebre-Medhin, ARTSCAN III (*JCO* 2021, PMID 33052757): Swedish PRT of 291 patients; about 15% were non-OPC and 10% p16-negative. Randomized to weekly cisplatin 40 mg/m² vs. cetuximab. Second randomization for cT3–4 tumors to 68 Gy vs. 73.1 Gy. Stopped early due to inferiority of cetuximab; 3-year OS was 88% for cisplatin and 78% for cetuximab ($p = .086$). LRC and EFS inferior in cetuximab arm, DM not different. Escalation to 73.1 Gy not clearly beneficial. **Conclusion: Cetuximab is clearly inferior to cisplatin.**

■ **Can induction CHT improve survival by reducing rate of distant metastases?**

This subject has been extensively studied and is controversial. In summary, TPF is the preferred induction regimen but superiority of induction CHT has not been established compared to concurrent chemoRT.

Vermorken, TAX 323 (*NEJM* 2007, PMID 17960012): PRT randomized 358 stage III to stage IV H&N cancer to 4 cycles of induction cisplatin/5-FU (PF) with or without docetaxel (TPF) followed by RT alone. TPF demonstrated OS benefit (MS 14.5 vs. 18.8 months). **Conclusion: TPF is induction CHT regimen of choice.**

Posner, TAX 324 (*NEJM* 2007, PMID 17960013; Update Lorch *Lancet Oncol* 2011, PMID 21233014): PRT randomized 501 stage III to stage IV H&N cancer to 3 cycles of induction cisplatin/5-FU

(PF) with or without docetaxel (TPF) followed by RT with concurrent carboplatin. Updated results continued to show survival benefit (MS 34.8 vs. 70.6 months). **Conclusion: TPF is induction CHT regimen of choice.**

Haddad, PARADIGM (*Lancet Oncol* 2013, PMID 23414589): PRT of patients with T3–4 or N2–3 SCC comparing 3 cycles of TPF followed by chemoRT with either docetaxel or carboplatin vs. chemoRT with 2 cycles of cisplatin 100 mg/m^2. Trial closed early after 145 patients were enrolled. No differences observed in terms of OS or PFS. Induction patients experienced more febrile neutropenia. **Conclusion: No clear benefit to induction CHT compared to concurrent cisplatin.**

Cohen, DeCIDE (*JCO* 2014, PMID 25049329): PRT of patients with N2–3 H&N cancer treated with either concurrent CHT (docetaxel, 5-FU, and hydroxyurea) or 2 cycles of TPF induction CHT with same concurrent chemoRT. RT was 74 to 75 Gy given BID. Trial closed early due to slow accrual; 285 patients included. MFU 30 months. No difference in OS, RFS, or distant failure-free survival. **Conclusion: TPF cannot be routinely recommended for N2–3 patients.**

■ **Which tonsil tumors can be treated with unilateral neck RT?**

O'Sullivan published the classic series defining unilateral RT to be safe for T1–2N0 lateralized tonsil tumors with ≤1 cm of soft palate or superficial base of tongue invasion. Subsequent series have expanded indications to well-lateralized node-positive patients, although this is more controversial.[27–29] Modern trials (NRG HN-002) recommend unilateral RT for cT1–3 tonsil tumors, well lateralized (<1 cm soft palate, base of tongue invasion) with minimal nodal disease (N0–2a, no ECE) with unilateral RT optional for N2b patients confined to level II without ECE. Guidelines exist on this topic for clarity.[30]

O'Sullivan, PMH (*IJROBP* 2001, PMID 11567806): RR of 228 patients with carcinoma of tonsillar region treated with unilateral RT between 1970 and 1991; 84% were T1–2, 58% N0. Crude rate of contralateral failure was 3.5%: T1 0% (0/67), T2 1.5% (2/118), T3 10% (3/30), T4 0% (0/7). Risk was >10% if involving medial one-third of soft palate or base of tongue involved. **Conclusion: Unilateral RT is safe in select tonsil cancers >1 cm from midline. Extension to BOT is considered relative contraindication to ipsilateral RT.**

Huang, PMH (*IJROBP* 2017, PMID 28258895): RR of 379 patients treated with unilateral RT. T1–T2N0–N2b tonsil cancer treated between 1999 and 2014 stratified by HPV status. MFU 5.03 years. Regional control was not statistically different compared between HPV+ or HPV– patients. Overall, 5-year contralateral neck failures were 2%. **Conclusion: Ipsilateral RT to selected T1–T2N0–N2b tonsil patients results in equally excellent outcomes regardless of tumor HPV status. When considering ipsilateral RT, ≤1 cm superficial involvement of soft palate or BOT is safe, but suspicion of deeper invasion should be approached cautiously.**

■ **When is it necessary to irradiate levels IB and V?**

With modern imaging, it is likely safe to spare levels IB and V for T1–2 OPC if not involved on imaging.

Sanguineti, Johns Hopkins (*IJROBP* 2009, PMID 19131181): RR of 103 patients with T1–2, clinically node-positive OPC staged with CT imaging who underwent initial neck dissection. Overall, if CT was negative, levels IB, IV, and V were involved in 3%, 6%, and 1%, respectively. Levels IB and V were <4% regardless of pathologic involvement of II to IV. Level IV was 5% if level III was not involved but 11% if level III was involved. **Conclusion: Levels IB and V are low risk and can be spared in cT1–2 OPC.**

Sanguineti, Johns Hopkins (*Acta Oncol* 2014, PMID 24274389): RR of 91 patients with HPV+ OPC and clinically positive neck nodes who underwent ipsilateral neck dissection between 1998 and 2010. Pathology was reviewed to determine risk of subclinical disease at each neck level (not evident on CT). Risk of subclinical disease in both levels IB and V is <5%, while it is 6.5% (95% CI: 3.1–9.9) for level IV. Level IB subclinical involvement >5% when 2+ ipsilateral levels besides IB are involved. Risk of occult disease in level IV is <5% when level III is not involved. Low number of events in level V did not allow analysis of predictors of involvement. **Conclusion: Consider electively covering level IB if 2+ other levels are involved. Level IV may be spared when level III is negative.**

■ **What prospective data guided the adoption of IMRT for OPC in the United States?**

Although IMRT is now standard in the treatment of H&N cancer, RTOG 0022 is one of the few prospective trials investigating safety and efficacy in cooperative group setting. It is also a trial that demonstrates good outcomes for T1–2N0–1 OPC treated with RT alone.

Eisbruch, RTOG 0022 (*IJROBP* 2010, PMID 19540060): Initial RTOG multi-institutional trial demonstrating safety and efficacy of IMRT. Prospective phase II trial of 69 T1–2 N0–1 OPC treated with RT alone to 66 Gy/30 fx with IMRT; 2-year LRF was 9%. LRF was increased in those with major deviations: 2/4 patients with deviations (50%) vs. 3/49 without (6%, $p = .04$). **Conclusion: IMRT is feasible with encouraging acute and late toxicity. Quality of IMRT is important to avoid LRF.**

■ **What are expected outcomes with TORS? Who are ideal candidates?**

TORS (and TLM) has transformed morbidity associated with surgical resection of OPC. FDA approval was obtained for DaVinci robot in resection of T1–2 OPC in 2009 and NCCN guidelines allow for TORS as option for select patients.[10] Series from multiple institutions have established the safety and efficacy of TORS.[31–38] For now, TORS remains institution- and surgeon-dependent and comparative data are limited to QOL, as shown in ORATOR trial in the following.

Nichols, ORATOR (*Lancet Oncol* 2019, PMID 31416685): Multicenter phase II PRT of 68 patients with T1–2N0–2 (≤4 cm) OPX SCC comparing TORS + neck LND vs. RT (70 Gy/35 fx). CHT added to RT if N1–2; PORT with 60 Gy/30 fx (<2 mm margin, pT3/4, N+, LVSI) or CRT with 64 Gy/30 fx and concurrent CHT (positive margins or ECE) added to TORS based on pathology. Primary end point was swallowing-related QOL at 1 year using MDADI score, powered to detect "clinically meaningful" improvement in TORS group compared to RT group. MDADI scores at 1 year for TORS vs. RT did not meet clinically meaningful thresholds, although patients treated with RT demonstrated statistically significant improvement in swallowing-related QOL scores. Of the TORS patients, 47% received PORT and 24% received adjuvant CRT. Worse hearing loss, tinnitus, and neutropenia in the RT group, whereas worse trismus in the TORS group. One death was recorded due to bleeding after TORS. **Conclusion: Patients treated with RT did not have a clinically meaningful change in swallowing compared to those who underwent TORS. Discussion of toxicity profiles of TORS and RT/CRT should take place with patients considering options.**

■ **Do HPV-positive tumors behave differently than HPV-negative tumors?**

HPV+ OPC is now classified as distinct disease.

Ang, RTOG 0129 (*NEJM* 2010, PMID 20530316): Retrospective analysis of RTOG 0129 (see Nguyen-Tan 2014 in the preceding) investigating role of HPV. HPV status was determined by both FISH for HPV DNA and IHC for p16; 64% of patients had HPV-positive tumors and 3-year OS was markedly improved for these patients (82% vs. 57%, $p < .001$); 3-year rate of local–regional disease lower for patients with HPV+ tumors vs. HPV– tumors: 13.6% vs. 35.1% ($p < .001$). Smoking and nodal stage were prognostic. RPA for OS divided patients into 3 classes based on HPV status, smoking, T and N stages: low risk (HPV-positive and ≤10 pack-years or HPV-positive, >10 pack-years, and N0–2a), intermediate risk (HPV-positive, >10 pack-years, and N2b–3 or HPV-negative, ≤10 pack-years, and T2–3), or high risk (HPV-negative, ≤10 pack-years, and T4 or >10 pack-years). **Conclusion: This trial defined impact of HPV status on prognosis for oropharynx patients.**

Fakhry, RTOG 2nd Analysis (*JCO* 2014, PMID 24958820): Second analysis of RTOG 0129 and 0522 including patients with initially locally advanced oropharyngeal SCC (206 HPV+, 117 HPV–) who developed recurrent disease after primary treatment. Investigated effect of HPV status on survival after disease progression. Median time to progression 8.2 months for p16+ vs. 7.3 months for p16– (NS); 55% of patients had LRR only, 40% had DM only, 5% had both. MFU time after first event of disease progression was 4 years. p16+ patients had significantly improved OS after disease progression when compared to p16– patients (2.6 years vs. 0.8 years). Salvage surgery reduced risk of death after disease progression. **Conclusion: Patterns of failure do not differ based on p16 status (similar time to disease progression and anatomic site involvement), but p16+ patients have improved survival after first recurrence.**

O'Sullivan, PMH (*JCO* 2013, PMID 23295795): RR of 505 OPC patients; 382 HPV-positive. Although OS, LC (94% vs. 80%), and regional control (95% vs. 82%) were improved in HPV+ patients, distant control was similar (90% vs. 86%). RPA for distant control divided patients into 4 classes: HPV+ low (N0–N2c and T1–3) or high risk (N0–2c and T4 or N3) and HPV– low (N0–2c and T1–2) or high risk (N0–2c and T3–4 or N3). CHT seemed to reduce distant metastases for HPV+ low-risk category patients with N2b–N2c disease. **Conclusion: HPV+ patients with low risk of distant metastases (T1–3N0–2a) may be candidates for treatment de-intensification.**

■ **Are there opportunities to de-intensify treatment for HPV-positive patients?**

No standard regimen has been identified to date, but multiple trials are ongoing investigating de-intensification for low-risk HPV-positive patients. Given the inferior results of the three preceding cetuximab trials, de-escalation should be reserved for patients treated on protocol until phase III data is available.

Chera, UNC/UF/Rex Trial (*JCO* 2019, PMID 31411949): Prospective phase II trial of HPV-positive patients with T0–3N0–2c and ≤10 pack-years or 10 to 30 pack-years but abstinent for >5 years. This was a FU trial to initial phase II where pCR was the end point;[39] in this study, the primary end point was 2-year PFS and PET/CT guided surgery. Patients received 60 Gy/30 fx with weekly cisplatin 30 mg/m^2 (no CHT for cT0–2N0–1). Results: 114 enrolled, MFU 31.8 months. Clinical CR on PET was 93% at primary; 6 were observed without recurrence, 2 biopsied, and 1 had persistence who died. CR in the neck was 80%, neck dissection positive in 4 of 11. PFS was 86% at 2 years, LRC 95%, DMFS 91%. **Conclusion: De-intensification is likely safe for low-risk HPV-positive patients. Further trials are ongoing.**

Marur, ECOG 1308 (*JCO* 2017, PMID 28029303): Phase II trial of 80 patients evaluating whether cCR to induction CHT could select patients with HPV+ OPC who could receive de-intensified therapy with goal of sparing late sequelae. Eligibility criteria: Stage III to stage IV, T1–3N0–N2b OPC, p16+ or HPV+, ≤10 pack-year smoking history. Treated with 3 cycles of induction CHT with cisplatin, paclitaxel, and cetuximab. If cCR of primary site, went on to receive IMRT to 54 Gy with weekly cetuximab. If PR at primary site or nodes, patients went on to receive 69.3 Gy to involved site and cetuximab. Primary end point was 2-year PFS; 70% had primary site cCR and received low-dose arm; these patients had 2-year PFS 80%. At 12 months, patients treated with RT ≤54 Gy had less difficulty swallowing solids (40% vs. 89%, $p = .011$) or impaired nutrition (10% vs. 44%, $p = .025$); 8 of 9 failures in reduced-dose arm were locoregional. **Conclusion: For patients who respond to induction CHT, reduced-dose IMRT with concurrent cetuximab for favorable HPV-associated patients may have improved swallowing and nutritional status.**

Chen, UCLA (*Lancet Oncol* 2017, PMID 28434660): Single-arm phase II trial with biopsy-proven stage III to stage IV (AJCC 7th edition) HPV+ OPC received carboplatin/paclitaxel x2 cycles. CR or PR received 54 Gy/27 fx, less than PR received 60 Gy/30 fx, both concurrent with paclitaxel. Primary end point PFS; 45 patients, MFU 30 months; 3 LRF, 1 DM; 2-year PFS 92% (95% CI: 77–97); 39% grade 3 toxicity (mostly during induction CHT); 2% feeding tube dependence at 3 months, 0% at 6 months. **Conclusion: Reduced-dose chemoRT is associated with high PFS.**

Yom, NRG HN002 (*JCO* 2021, PMID 33507809): Phase II PRT of 306 patients with T1–2N1–2b or T3N0–2b (AJCC 7th edition) OPC with ≤10 pack-year smoking history, randomized to 60 Gy/30 fx + weekly cisplatin (IMRT + C) vs. modestly accelerated IMRT alone 60 Gy/30 fx with 6 fx/week. Powered to detect acceptable prespecified 2-year PFS of ≥85% without worse swallowing QOL at 1 year per MDADI as coprimary end point. MFU 2.6 years, 2-year PFS for IMRT + C was 90.5% (84.5–94.7, $p = .04$), which met prespecified PFS end point, while it was 87.6% (81.1–92.5, $p = .228$) for IMRT-alone arm, which failed to meet prespecified PFS end point. Both arms passed MDADI dysphagia threshold. Similar rates of mucositis, but higher rates of acute dysphagia and hematologic toxicity in IMRT + C arm. No difference in late toxicity or 2-year OS. **Conclusion: De-intensification of chemoradiotherapy for HPV+ OPC with 60 Gy/30 fx and weekly cisplatin warrants phase III comparison with 70 Gy, which is currently ongoing in NRG HN-005.**

REFERENCES

1. Siegel RL, Miller KD, Jemal A. Cancer statistics, 2020. *CA Cancer J Clin.* 2020;70(1):7–30. doi:10.3322/caac.21387
2. Salama JK, Gillison ML, Brizel DM. Oropharynx. In: Halperin EC, Wazer DE, Perez CA, Brady LW, eds. *Principles and Practice of Radiation Oncology.* 6th ed. Lippincott Williams & Wilkins; 2013:817–832.

3. Chaturvedi AK, Engels EA, Pfeiffer RM, et al. Human papillomavirus and rising oropharyngeal cancer incidence in the United States. *J Clin Oncol.* 2011;29(32):42944301. doi:10.1200/JCO.2011.36.4596

4. Gillison ML, Broutian T, Pickard RK, et al. Prevalence of oral HPV infection in the United States, 2009–2010. *JAMA.* 2012;307(7):693–703. doi:10.1001/jama.2012.101

5. Gillison ML, Zhang Q, Jordan R, et al. Tobacco smoking and increased risk of death and progression for patients with p16-positive and p16-negative oropharyngeal cancer. *J Clin Oncol.* 2012;30(17):2102–2111. doi:10.1200/JCO.2011.38.4099

6. Ang KK, Trotti A, Brown BW, et al. Randomized trial addressing risk features and time factors of surgery plus radiotherapy in advanced head-and-neck cancer. *Int J Radiat Oncol Biol Phys.* 2001;51(3):571–578. doi:10.1016/S0360-3016(01)01690-X

7. Bagnardi V, Rota M, Botteri E, et al. Light alcohol drinking and cancer: a meta-analysis. *Ann Oncol.* 2013;24(2):301–308. doi:10.1093/annonc/mds337

8. Cannon GM, Harari PM, Gentry LR, et al. Oropharyngeal cancer. In: Gunderson L, Tepper J, eds. *Clinical Radiation Oncology.* 3rd ed. Elsevier; 2012:585–617. doi:10.1016/B978-1-4377-1637-5.00031-6

9. Chung CH, Gillison ML. Human papillomavirus in head and neck cancer: its role in pathogenesis and clinical implications. *Clin Cancer Res.* 2009;15(22):6758–6762. doi:10.1158/1078-0432.CCR-09-0784

10. Chera BS, Kumar S, Shen C, et al. Plasma circulating tumor HPV DNA for the surveillance of cancer recurrence in HPV-associated oropharyngeal cancer. *J Clin Oncol.* 2020;38(10):1050–1058. doi:10.1200/JCO.19.02444

11. NCCN Clinical Practice Guidelines in Oncology: Head and Neck Cancers. 2017. https://www.nccn.org

12. Mehanna H, Wong WL, McConkey CC, et al. PET-CT surveillance versus neck dissection in advanced head and neck cancer. *N Engl J Med.* 2016;374(15):1444–1454. doi:10.1056/NEJMoa1514493

13. Broughman JR, Xiong DD, Moeller BJ, et al. Rethinking the 10-pack-year rule for favorable human papilloma-virus-associated oropharynx carcinoma: a multi-institution analysis. *Cancer.* 2020;126(12):2784–2790. doi:10.1002/cncr.32849

14. Ang KK, Harris J, Wheeler R, et al. Human papillomavirus and survival of patients with oropharyngeal cancer. *N Engl J Med.* 2010;363(1):24–35. doi:10.1056/NEJMoa0912217

15. Schwartz DL, Harris J, Yao M, et al. Metabolic tumor volume as a prognostic imaging-based biomarker for head-and-neck cancer: pilot results from radiation therapy oncology group protocol 0522. *Int J Radiat Oncol Biol Phys.* 2015;91(4):721–729. doi:10.1016/j.ijrobp.2014.12.023

16. Huang SH, Xu W, Waldron J, et al. Refining american joint committee on cancer/union for international cancer control TNM stage and prognostic groups for human papillomavirus-related oropharyngeal carcinomas. *J Clin Oncol.* 2015;33(8):836–845. doi:10.1200/JCO.2014.58.6412

17. Beitler JJ, Muller S, Grist WJ, et al. Prognostic accuracy of computed tomography findings for patients with laryn-geal cancer undergoing laryngectomy. *J Clin Oncol.* 2010;28(14):2318–2322. doi:10.1200/JCO.2009.24.7544

18. O'Sullivan B, Huang SH, Siu LL, et al. Deintensification candidate subgroups in human papillomavirus-related oropharyngeal cancer according to minimal risk of distant metastasis. *J Clin Oncol.* 2013;31(5):543–550. doi:10.1200/JCO.2012.44.0164

19. Kramer S, Gelber RD, Snow JB, et al. Combined radiation therapy and surgery in the management of advanced head and neck cancer: final report of study 73-03 of the radiation therapy oncology group. *Head Neck Surg.* 1987;10(1):19–30. doi:10.1002/hed.2890100105

20. Garrel R, Poissonnet G, Moyà Plana A, et al. Equivalence randomized trial to compare treatment on the basis of sentinel node biopsy versus neck node dissection in operable T1-T2N0 oral and oropharyngeal cancer. *J Clin Oncol.* 2020;38(34):4010–4018. doi:10.1200/JCO.20.01661

21. Gillison ML, Trotti AM, Harris J, et al. Radiotherapy plus cetuximab or cisplatin in human papillomavirus-posi-tive oropharyngeal cancer (NRG Oncology RTOG 1016): a randomised, multicentre, non-inferiority trial. *Lancet.* 2019;393(10166):40–50. doi:10.1016/S0140-6736(18)32779-X

22. Bonner JA, Harari PM, Giralt J, et al. Radiotherapy plus cetuximab for squamous-cell carcinoma of the head and neck. *N Engl J Med.* 2006;354(6):567–578. doi:10.1056/NEJMoa053422

23. Vermorken JB, Remenar E, van Herpen C, et al. Cisplatin, fluorouracil, and docetaxel in unresectable head and neck cancer. *N Engl J Med.* 2007;357(17):1695–1704. doi:10.1056/NEJMoa071028

24. Videtic GMM, Woody N, Vassil AD. *Handbook of Treatment Planning in Radiation Oncology.* 3rd ed. Demos Medical; 2020. doi:10.1891/9780826168429

25. Lassen P, Eriksen JG, Krogdahl A, et al. The influence of HPV-associated p16-expression on accelerated fraction-ated radiotherapy in head and neck cancer: evaluation of the randomised DAHANCA 6&7 trial. *Radiother Oncol.* 2011;100(1):49–55. doi:10.1016/j.radonc.2011.02.010

26. Rosenthal DI, Harari PM, Giralt J, et al. Association of human papillomavirus and p16 status with outcomes in the IMCL-9815 Phase III registration trial for patients with locoregionally advanced oropharyngeal squamous cell car-cinoma of the head and neck treated with radiotherapy with or without cetuximab. *J Clin Oncol.* 2016;34(12):1300–1308. doi:10.1200/JCO.2015.62.5970

27. Chronowski GM, Garden AS, Morrison WH, et al. Unilateral radiotherapy for the treatment of tonsil cancer. *Int J Radiat Oncol Biol Phys.* 2012;83(1):204–209. doi:10.1016/j.ijrobp.2011.06.1975

28. Al-Mamgani A, van Rooij P, Fransen D, Levendag P. Unilateral neck irradiation for well-lateralized oropharyngeal cancer. *Radiother Oncol.* 2013;106(1):69–73. doi:10.1016/j.radonc.2012.12.006

29. Liu C, Dutu G, Peters LJ, et al. Tonsillar cancer: the peter maccallum experience with unilateral and bilateral irradi-ation. *Head Neck.* 2014;36(3):317–322. doi:10.1002/hed.23297

30. Tsai CJ, Galloway TJ, Margalit DN, et al. Ipsilateral radiation for squamous cell carcinoma of the tonsil: american radium society appropriate use criteria executive summary. *Head Neck.* 2021;43(1):392–406. doi:10.1002/hed.26492

31. de Almeida JR, Li R, Magnuson JS, et al. Oncologic outcomes after transoral robotic surgery: a multi-institutional study. *JAMA Otolaryngol Head Neck Surg.* 2015;141(12):1043–1051. doi:10.1001/jamaoto.2015.1508

32. Hutcheson KA, Holsinger FC, Kupferman ME, Lewin JS. Functional outcomes after TORS for oropharyngeal cancer: a systematic review. *Eur Arch Otorhinolaryngol.* 2015;272(2):463–471. doi:10.1007/s00405-014-2985-7

33. Leonhardt FD, Quon H, Abrahão M, et al. Transoral robotic surgery for oropharyngeal carcinoma and its impact on patient-reported quality of life and function. *Head Neck.* 2012;34(2):146–154. doi:10.1002/hed.21688

34. Park YM, Kim WS, Byeon HK, et al. Oncological and functional outcomes of transoral robotic surgery for oropharyngeal cancer. *Br J Oral Maxillofac Surg.* 2013;51(5):408–412. doi:10.1016/j.bjoms.2012.08.015

35. Weinstein GS, O'Malley BW Jr, Snyder W, et al. Transoral robotic surgery: radical tonsillectomy. *Arch Otolaryngol Head Neck Surg.* 2007;133(12):1220–1226. doi:10.1001/archotol.133.12.1220

36. Weinstein GS, Quon H, O'Malley BW, et al. Selective neck dissection and deintensified postoperative radiation and chemotherapy for oropharyngeal cancer: a subset analysis of the university of pennsylvania transoral robotic surgery trial. *Laryngoscope.* 2010;120(9):1749–1755. doi:10.1002/lary.21021

37. Weinstein GS, O'Malley BW Jr, Magnuson JS, et al. Transoral robotic surgery: a multicenter study to assess feasibility, safety, and surgical margins. *Laryngoscope.* 2012;122(8):1701–1707. doi:10.1002/lary.23294

38. Desai SC, Sung CK, Jang DW, Genden EM. Transoral robotic surgery using a carbon dioxide flexible laser for tumors of the upper aerodigestive tract. *Laryngoscope.* 2008;118(12):2187–2189. doi:10.1097/MLG.0b013e31818379e4

39. Chera BS, Amdur RJ, Tepper J, et al. Phase 2 trial of de-intensified chemoradiation therapy for favorable-risk human papillomavirus-associated oropharyngeal squamous cell carcinoma. *Int J Radiat Oncol Biol Phys.* 2015;93(5):976–985. doi:10.1016/j.ijrobp.2015.08.033

12 ■ ORAL CAVITY CANCER

Kailin Yang, Bindu V. Manyam, and Neil M. Woody

> **QUICK HIT** ■ Unlike oropharyngeal SCC, HPV infection is not associated with oral cavity SCC (OC-SCC). Primary management of oral cavity cancers is generally surgical resection with selective neck dissection (levels IB–III, others as indicated by primary site location and stage), followed by risk-adapted postoperative RT with or without concurrent CHT. Early-stage lesions (particularly lip) may be treated with definitive RT using brachytherapy. DOI is important for decision-making in oral cavity cancers.

EPIDEMIOLOGY: Estimated incidence of 35,000 and 7,000 deaths in the United States in 2020 and comprises 30% of all H&N malignancies. Male-to-female ratio is approximately 3:2.[1] Most common sites for oral cavity cancer in the United States are lip and tongue. Incidence is markedly higher internationally (20-fold increase in South Asia).[2]

RISK FACTORS: Smoking and alcohol are primary risk factors for OC-SCC. Other risk factors include chewing tobacco, poor oral hygiene, periodontal disease, chronic irritation from ill-fitting dentures, betel nut, chronic sun exposure (for lip cancer), and immune suppression (HIV or solid organ transplant). Unlike OPC, majority of OC-SCC are negative for HPV, unless near circumvallate papillae.[3] Genetic syndromes associated with OC-SCC include Fanconi anemia and dyskeratosis congenita.[4,5]

ANATOMY: Oral cavity boundaries: anterior border junction of skin and vermilion border of lip; posterior border: junction of hard and soft palate; posterior–inferior border: circumvallate papillae of tongue; lateral border: anterior tonsillar pillars/buccal mucosa (Anatomic definition of oral cavity is listed in Table 12.1.). Atlases are available for neck nodal level definition.[6]

Table 12.1 Oral Cavity Anatomic Definition

Site	Key Features	Pattern of Drainage
Mucosal lip	Bordered by upper and lower lip vermillion. Upper lip innervated by infraorbital nerve (V2) and lower lip innervated by mental nerve (V3).	IA (lower lip), IB, II, III, facial lymphatics (upper lip)
Buccal mucosa	Mucosa of inner cheek and lips to attachment of mucosa of alveolar ridge and pterygomandibular raphe.	IB, II to IV
Alveolar ridges	Mucosa overlying alveolar process of maxilla (upper) and mandible (lower). Posterior margin of upper alveolar ridge is pterygopalatine arch and posterior margin of lower alveolar ridge is ascending ramus of mandible.	IB, II to IV
Retromolar trigone	Mucosa overlying ascending ramus of mandible, from posterior surface of last molar tooth to tuberosity of maxilla.	IB, II to IV
Floor of mouth	Mucosa overlying mylohyoid and hyoglossus muscles, extending from inner surface of lower alveolar ridge to dorsal surface of tongue.	IA, IB, II to IV

(continued)

Table 12.1 Oral Cavity Anatomic Definition (continued).		
Site	Key Features	Pattern of Drainage
Hard palate	Mucosa extending from inner surface of superior alveolar ridge to posterior edge of palatine bone of maxillae.	II to IV
Oral tongue (anterior two-thirds of tongue)	Mobile portion of tongue from circumvallate papillae to dorsal surface of tongue at junction of floor of mouth. Sensation is from lingual nerve (V3), taste is from chorda tympani (CN VII), and motor function is from hypoglossal nerve (CN XII).	Three routes of drainage: Tip of tongue–submental nodes Lateral tongue–IB Medial tongue–deep cervical LN II to IV 15% drain to levels III to IV skipping II

PATHOLOGY: SCC comprises 95% of oral cavity cancers.[7] Less common histologies include minor salivary gland carcinomas, mucosal melanoma, lymphoma, and sarcoma. Basal cell carcinomas can arise from vermillion border of lip. Routine HPV testing is not recommended and p16 is not specific to HPV infection in oral cavity.

GENETICS: Mutation in p53, CDKN2A, Rb loss of function, and increased expression of EGFR are associated with worse prognosis.[4,5] Next-generation sequencing has identified subgroups of oral cavity tumors genetically distinct from other HPV-negative H&N cancers.[8]

SCREENING: There is no effective screening program routinely used in the United States. One study of 4,611 tobacco users older than 40 were screened with systematic inspection of oral mucosa, in which abnormal findings were seen in over 70% of patients, but cancer diagnosed in only 3% of patients.[9] One study in India suggested 27% relative reduction in risk of oral cancer death with screening by physical examination and identified subsets of patients with highest risks who derive the greatest absolute benefit.[10]

CLINICAL PRESENTATION: Symptoms include pain, nonhealing ulcer, bleeding, dysphagia, ill-fitting dentures, and halitosis. Advanced lesions can present with symptoms of facial numbness, difficulty with protrusion of tongue, and trismus. On examination, may present as visible or palpable mass or ulceration in oral cavity or palpable cervical lymphadenopathy.

WORKUP: H&P including visual inspection of tumor, size and location, palpation of tumor borders, cranial nerve examination, and cervical lymph node examination. Exam should include flexible nasopharyngolaryngoscopy to rule out second primary neoplasm. Dental evaluation is important to identify need for extraction and risk of osteoradionecrosis. Speech and nutrition evaluation as indicated.

Imaging: CT neck with contrast. PET/CT is challenging to interpret in oral cavity, but remains useful for nodal and distant staging. MRI if concern for perineural spread.

Biopsy: In-office biopsy is common if safe but EUA with biopsy may be required.

PROGNOSTIC FACTORS: Age, smoking, tumor location, stage (Table 12.2), and pathologic features (histologic grade, DOI, PNI, margin status, number and size of lymph nodes, extracapsular extension) have been associated with prognosis. Lymph node involvement was shown to be the most important prognostic factor for OC-SCC.[11] One study determined oral tongue to be associated with higher rate of local failure, distant metastases, and lower OS compared to other oral cavity subsites, while other studies have suggested no significant difference in prognosis.[12,13]

NATURAL HISTORY: Premalignant changes (white plaques known as "leukoplakia") are often present before development of invasive carcinoma. Risk of development of leukoplakia into invasive carcinoma is estimated to be 1% to 20% in 10 years.[14] Patients with stage I to stage II OC-SCC have been shown to have 5-year OS about 83% and patients with stage III to stage IVa disease have 5-year OS of 55%.[15,16] Compared with other H&N sites, OC-SCCs have higher rate of local recurrence after definitive therapy. Most frequent sites of distant metastasis are lung and bone.

STAGING

	N	cN0	cN1	cN2a	cN2b	cN2c	cN3a	cN3b
T/M								
T1	• ≤2 cm • DOI ≤5 mm	I	III	IVA				
T2	• ≤2 cm and DOI (5.1–10 mm) • 2.1 to 4 cm and DOI ≤10 mm	II						
T3	• >4 cm • DOI >10 mm							
T4a lip	• Invasion[1]							
T4a oral cavity	• Invasion[2]							
T4b oral cavity	• Invasion[3]	IVB						
M1	• Distant metastasis	IVC						

Table 12.2 AJCC 8th Edition (2017): Staging for Oral Cavity

Notes: Invasion[1] = invasion into cortical bone or involves inferior alveolar nerve, floor of mouth, or skin of face. Invasion[2] = invasion through cortical bone or mandible/maxilla, into maxillary sinus, or skin of face. Invasion[3] = invasion into masticator space, pterygoid plates, or skull base, and/or encases internal carotid artery.

cN1, single ipsilateral LN (≤3 cm) and −ENE; cN2a, single ipsilateral LN (3.1–6 cm) and −ENE; cN2b, multiple ipsilateral LN (≤6 cm) and −ENE; cN2c, bilateral or contralateral LN (≤6 cm) and −ENE; cN3a, LN (>6 cm) and − ENE; cN3b, clinically overt ENE.

pN1, single LN (≤3 cm) and −ENE; pN2a, single ipsilateral or contralateral LN (≤3 cm) and +ENE or single ipsilateral LN (3.1–6 cm) and −ENE; pN2b, multiple ipsilateral LN (≤6 cm) and −ENE; pN2c, bilateral or contralateral LN (≤6 cm) and −ENE; pN3a, LN (>6 cm) and −ENE; pN3b, LN (>3 cm) and +ENE or multiple LN any with +ENE or a single contralateral node with +ENE.

TREATMENT PARADIGM

Surgery: Initial surgical resection is standard of care. Randomized trials comparing upfront surgery vs. RT demonstrated significantly worse OS with RT alone.[17,18] Achieving negative surgical margins is critical, and if feasible, repeat resection of positive margin is preferred. Close surgical margin has historically been defined as within 5 mm; however, retrospective review demonstrated local recurrence–free survival was significantly higher with margins ≤2.2 mm, suggesting new definition for close margin to stratify patients for local recurrence.[19]

Early-stage OC-SCC can be resected without significant functional or cosmetic deficits, though hemiglossectomy, maxillectomy, and mandibulotomy for locally advanced disease can lead to significant speech and swallowing deficits, which can be managed with reconstruction. Standard transoral or open approaches are used, and minimally invasive surgery with transoral laser or robotic surgery has not been shown to provide relative benefit in this setting.[20]

For T1 lip, upper alveolar ridge, and hard palate cancer, lymph node dissection may be able to be omitted, as risk of metastasis is low. For T1 or T2 oral tongue cancer, elective lymph node dissection of levels I to IV is typically recommended for all tumors ≥2 mm DOI. Recent Senti-MERORL trial demonstrated oncologic equivalence of SLNB compared to LND for operable T1–T2 N0 patients.[21] Lower alveolar ridge, floor of mouth, buccal, and retromolar trigone cancers with clinically node-negative neck should undergo level I to level III lymph node dissection due to high incidence of occult nodal metastases. Patients with primary tumors near or involving midline should be managed with bilateral neck dissection.

Chemotherapy: Combined analysis of two prospective randomized trials demonstrated significant LRC, DFS, and OS benefit with addition of concurrent CHT to PORT in patients with ECE and positive margin (see Chapter 17 for details).[22] Two PRTs examining role of preoperative CHT demonstrated no improvement in OS with cisplatin and 5-FU or docetaxel, cisplatin, and 5-FU (TPF).[23,24]

Radiation

Indications: Typical indications include pT3–T4a; pN2–3; pT1–2N0–1 *and* one or more of the following: PNI, LVSI, margin <5 mm, or T2 oral cavity cancer with ≥5 mm DOI (can consider 4 mm based on Ganly data).[25] MSKCC and PMH nomograms can be used to assess potential benefits of PORT.[26,27] PORT should start 4 to 6 weeks after surgery. PORT can be omitted for pathologic N0 neck given excellent control rate.[28] For nonoperative cases, definitive chemoRT is a feasible and viable approach based on University of Chicago experience.[29]

Intraoral cone RT: Classic technique for small tumor size (<3 cm) of floor of mouth. Preserves salivary gland function and decreases risk of osteoradionecrosis. Intraoral cone RT uses 100 to 250 kVp x-rays or 6 MeV electrons. Local control rate around 85%.[30]

Brachytherapy: Interstitial implant can be used alone or in combination with EBRT for treatment of oral tongue, floor of mouth, or buccal mucosa. Isotopes used include Ir-192, Ra-226, Cs-137, Au-198, tantalum-182. For tumor thickness <1 cm, single-plane implant is adequate; otherwise, double-plane or volumetric implant is used. Surface mold brachytherapy can be used for select superficial (<1 cm depth) or recurrent superficial lesions of hard palate, lower gingiva, and floor of mouth. Impression is made of surface to be irradiated with HDR catheters inserted into predrilled holes or grooves in mold and sealed with dental plaster.[31]

Dose: See Chapter 17 for details. For T1–T2N0 lesions, interstitial LDR brachytherapy dose is 60 to 70 Gy delivered over 6 to 7 days, with minimum tumor dose rate at 30 to 60 cGy/hr. When brachytherapy is used in combination with EBRT, implant dose should be at least 40 Gy.

Toxicity: Acute complications include mucositis, loss of taste, xerostomia, thrush, dermatitis, dysphagia, odynophagia. Chronic toxicity includes xerostomia, lifelong need for fluoride prophylaxis, risk for dental caries and osteoradionecrosis.

Procedure: See *Handbook of Treatment Planning in Radiation Oncology*, Chapter 4 for details.[32]

■ EVIDENCE-BASED Q&A

▓ Why is initial surgical resection preferred over definitive RT for initial management of OC-SCC?

Two PRTs, as well as several retrospective studies, suggest LRC and OS benefit for surgical resection compared to definitive RT.[17,18]

Robertson, Glasgow (*Clin Oncol* 1998, PMID 9704176): PRT of 35 patients with T2–4N0–2 OC-SCC and oropharynx randomized to surgery followed by PORT (60 Gy/30 fx) vs. RT alone (66 Gy/33 fx). Trial designed to recruit 350 patients, but was closed after only 35 patients due to significantly worse OS with RT alone. MFU 23 months. OS significantly better with surgery and PORT (relative death rate 0.24, *p* = .001). Duration of LC was significantly decreased with RT alone (*p* = .037). **Conclusion: Definitive RT is suboptimal for oral cavity cancer.**

Iyer, Singapore (*Cancer* 2015, PMID 25639864): PRT of 119 patients with stage III to stage IV H&N SCC randomized to surgery followed by PORT vs. concurrent CHT and RT. MFU 13 years. No significant difference in OS for entire cohort (45% vs. 35%; *p* = .262) and DSS (56% vs. 46%; *p* = .637) at 5 years for surgery vs. RT alone, respectively. For patients with OC-SCC, surgery up front significantly improved 5-year OS (68% vs. 12%; *p* = .038). **Conclusion: OS and DSS are significantly improved with surgery and PORT compared to RT alone for OC-SCC, but not for other sites of H&N.**

■ Is there benefit for elective neck dissection compared to neck dissection at nodal relapse?

Randomized data suggest survival benefit to up-front neck dissection compared to neck dissection at time of nodal relapse, though stage, pathologic features, and location of primary should be considered.

D'Cruz, India (*NEJM* 2015, PMID 26027881): PRT of 596 patients with lateralized T1–2 OC-SCC randomized to elective ipsilateral neck dissection vs. therapeutic neck dissection (at time of nodal relapse). MFU 39 months. At 3 years, elective neck dissection demonstrated significantly improved OS (80% vs. 67.5%; p = .01) and DFS (69.5% vs. 45.9%; p < .001) compared to therapeutic neck dissection. Overall rate of pathologic nodal positivity in clinically node-negative neck was 30%. Rates of adverse events were 6.6% and 3.6% in elective neck dissection and therapeutic neck dissection arms, respectively. **Conclusion: Ipsilateral elective neck dissection provides OS and DFS benefit in patients with early-stage, well-lateralized OC-SCC, compared to therapeutic neck dissection.** *Comment: Note that nodal positivity (including pN1) guided RT decision leading to imbalance, possibly explaining survival difference.*

■ At what DOI should neck dissection be performed in early-stage (cT1–2N0) oral tongue cancer?

Several retrospective studies have demonstrated DOI as a significant predictor for locoregional recurrence. DOI ≥4 to 5 mm has been suggested as threshold for neck dissection.

Huang, PMH Meta-Analysis (*Cancer* 2009, PMID: 19197973): Meta-analysis of 16 studies investigated negative predictive value of DOI from 3 to 6 mm for cT1–2N0 oral tongue cancer. Probability of lymph node positivity at time of dissection or nodal relapse after ≥2 years follow-up increased ≥5 mm DOI (Table 12.3). There was significant increase in nodal positivity between 4 and 5 mm DOI (p = .007). **Conclusion: DOI strongly predicts for cervical lymph node involvement. Elective neck dissection should be considered in patients with cN0 disease with DOI >4 mm.**

Table 12.3 PMH Meta-Analysis	
DOI (mm)	False Negative Rate (%)
3	5.3
4	4.5
5	16.6
6	13

Ganly, MSKCC & PMH Combined Analysis (*Cancer* 2013, PMID 23184439): Combined analysis of 164 patients from MSKCC and PMH with pT1–2N0 oral tongue cancer treated with surgery alone (ipsilateral neck dissection, no PORT). MFU 66 months. Locoregional recurrence-free survival at 5 years was 79.9%. Regional recurrence was ipsilateral in 61% of cases and contralateral in 39% of cases. Regional recurrence was 5.7% for tumors with <4 mm DOI and 24% for ≥4 mm DOI. MVA demonstrated that tumor thickness ≥4 mm was significantly associated with regional recurrence free survival (p = .02). Patients with regional recurrence had significantly worse DSS (33% vs. 97%; p < .0001). **Conclusion: Neck recurrence was significantly higher with DOI ≥4 mm, with contralateral failures accounting for 40% of recurrences.**

■ What are indications and benefits for postoperative RT for OC-SCC?

Typical indications include pT3–T4a; pN2–3; pT1–2N0–1 and one or more of the following: PNI, LVSI, close margin <5 mm, or T2 oral cavity cancer with ≥5 mm DOI (can consider 4 mm based on the preceding Ganly data).[25] These are inclusion criteria for RTOG 0920, investigating the role of postoperative RT with or without cetuximab. These features have also been identified in various retrospective studies as significantly associated with inferior LRC, increased DM, and inferior OS.[33,34] Many historical H&N studies included patients with OC-SCC (though lip subsite was often excluded).[22,34–36]

■ **What are indications and benefits for addition of CHT to postoperative RT?**

The combined analysis of Bernier and Cooper (EORTC 22931 and RTOG 9501) suggests that ECE and positive margins are indications for postoperative concurrent chemoRT (see Chapter 17 for details). One recent trial at Tata Memorial in India also addressed this question.

Laskar (*ASCO* 2016, Abstract 6004): PRT of 900 patients with resectable OC-SCC who underwent surgery randomized to PORT alone (56–60 Gy in 5 fx/week; Arm A), PORT with concurrent weekly cisplatin (30 mg/m^2; Arm B), or accelerated PORT (6 fx/week; Arm C). MFU was 58 months. LRC at 5 years was 59.9% and 65.1% for Arm A vs. Arm B ($p = .203$) and 58.2% for Arm C (p = NS). Unplanned subset analysis demonstrated significantly improved LRC, DFS, and OS for patients with high-risk features (T3–T4, N2–3, and ECE) and for patients treated with standard fractionation RT and concurrent chemoRT compared to accelerated RT. **Conclusion: Intensification of therapy with concurrent CHT or accelerated RT did not improve outcomes in these patients with OC-SCC.** *Comment: Final manuscript is pending, and oral cavity cancer may have different biology in India than in the United States.*

■ **Is there benefit to preoperative CHT, RT, or chemoRT prior to surgical resection in OC-SCC?**

Several PRTs have investigated the role of induction CHT with cisplatin/5-FU or TPF with no improvement in OS. Retrospective evidence suggests benefit to downstaging for patients with unresectable disease.

Zhong, China (*JCO* 2013, PMID 23129742): PRT of 256 patients with stage III to IVA resectable OC-SCC randomized to 2 cycles of induction TPF (docetaxel 75 mg/m^2 on day 1, cisplatin 75 mg/m^2 on day 1, and 5-FU 750 mg/m^2 on days 1–5) followed by surgery and PORT (54–66 Gy) vs. surgery followed by PORT. MFU 30 months. Clinical response rate to induction CHT was 80.6%. No significant difference in OS (HR: 0.977, $p = .918$) or DFS (HR: 0.974, $p = .897$) with induction TPF. Patients with clinical response or favorable pathologic response (≤10% viable tumor cells) had superior OS, LRC, and distant control with induction TPF. **Conclusion: There was no significant survival benefit with induction TPF.**

Licitra, Italy (*JCO* 2003, PMID 12525526): PRT of 195 patients with T2–4 (>3 cm) N0–2 resectable OC-SCC randomized to 3 cycles of cisplatin and 5-FU followed by surgery vs. surgery alone. PORT was included for positive margin, soft tissue invasion of face, >3 lymph nodes, and/or ECE. No significant difference in 5-year OS between induction CHT and surgery alone (55% vs. 55%). Fewer patients required PORT in CHT arm (33% vs. 46%). Patients who had pCR had significantly improved 10-year OS (76% vs. 41%). **Conclusion: Induction CHT does not provide survival benefit and may decrease need for PORT.**

Mohr, Germany (*Int J Oral Maxillofac Surg* 1994, PMID 7930766): PRT of 268 patients with T2–4N0–3 OC-SCC and oropharyngeal cancer randomized to preoperative chemoRT (36 Gy/18 fx with concurrent cisplatin) followed by surgery vs. surgery alone. Surgery was completed 10 to 14 days after preoperative chemoRT. Locoregional recurrence was higher with surgery alone compared to preoperative chemoRT (31% vs. 15.6%). OS for preoperative chemoRT vs. surgery alone was 19% vs. 28%, respectively. **Conclusion: Induction chemoRT may provide LRC and OS benefit compared to surgery alone.**

■ **What are the patterns of failure after PORT?**

Retrospective series have demonstrated that contralateral neck failure is common after ipsilateral neck RT and majority of failures are local, within high-dose RT field.

Chan, PMH (*Oral Oncol* 2013, PMID 23079695): RR of 180 patients treated with PORT for stage I to stage IV OC-SCC (46% oral tongue, 23% floor of mouth, 12% hard palate, 9% buccal). MFU 34 months. LC, LRC, and OS at 2 years were 87%, 78%, and 65%, respectively. Of 38 locoregional failures, 26 were in-field. Contralateral failure occurred in 3 of 12 patients treated to ipsilateral neck only and more common in patients with N2b disease. **Conclusion: Bilateral neck RT may be beneficial in patients with N2b disease.**

Yao, University of Iowa (*IJROBP* 2007, PMID 17276613): RR of 55 patients treated with IMRT for OC-SCC (49 patients received PORT, 5 received definitive RT, and 1 received preoperative RT). OS and LRC at 2 years were 68% and 85%, respectively. All failures were in high-dose RT field, except for 1 patient who failed in lower contralateral neck. Median time to LRR was 4.1 months and LRC was significantly lower in patients with ECE. **Conclusion: Most failures after PORT are in-field.**

REFERENCES

1. Siegel RL, Miller KD, Jemal A. Cancer statistics, 2020. *CA Cancer J Clin.* 2020;70(1):7–30. doi:10.3322/caac.21387
2. Warnakulasuriya S. Global epidemiology of oral and oropharyngeal cancer. *Oral Oncol.* 2009;45(4–5):309–316. doi:10.1016/j.oraloncology.2008.06.002
3. Castellsague X, Alemany L, Quer M, et al. HPV involvement in head and neck cancers: comprehensive assessment of biomarkers in 3680 patients. *J Natl Cancer Inst.* 2016;108(6):djv403.
4. Kiaris H, Spandidos DA, Jones AS, et al. Mutations, expression and genomic instability of the H-ras proto-oncogene in squamous cell carcinomas of the head and neck. *Br J Cancer.* 1995;72(1):123–128. doi:10.1038/bjc.1995.287
5. Zhu X, Zhang F, Zhang W, et al. Prognostic role of epidermal growth factor receptor in head and neck cancer: a meta-analysis. *J Surg Oncol.* 2013;108(6):387–397. doi:10.1002/jso.23406
6. Grégoire V, Ang K, Budach W, et al. Delineation of the neck node levels for head and neck tumors: a 2013 update. DAHANCA, EORTC, HKNPCSG, NCIC CTG, NCRI, RTOG, TROG consensus guidelines. *Radiother Oncol.* 2014;110(1):172–181. doi:10.1016/j.radonc.2013.10.010
7. Wolff KD, Follmann M, Nast A. The diagnosis and treatment of oral cavity cancer. *Dtsch Arztebl Int.* 2012;109(48):829–835. doi:10.3238/arztebl.2012.0829
8. Cancer Genome Atlas Network. Comprehensive genomic characterization of head and neck squamous cell carcinomas. *Nature.* 2015;517(7536):576–582. doi:10.1038/nature14129
9. Prout MN, Sidari JN, Witzburg RA, et al. Head and neck cancer screening among 4611 tobacco users older than forty years. *Otolaryngol Head Neck Surg.* 1997;116(2):201–208. doi:10.1016/S0194-5998(97)70326-7
10. Cheung LC, Ramadas K, Muwonge R, et al. Risk-based selection of individuals for oral cancer screening. *J Clin Oncol.* 2021;39(6):663–674. doi:10.1200/JCO.20.02855
11. Shah JP, Cendon RA, Farr HW, Strong EW. Carcinoma of the oral cavity: factors affecting treatment failure at the primary site and neck. *Am J Surg.* 1976;132(4):504–507. doi:10.1016/0002-9610(76)90328-7
12. Zelefsky MJ, Harrison LB, Fass DE, et al. Postoperative radiotherapy for oral cavity cancers: impact of anatomic subsite on treatment outcome. *Head Neck.* 1990;12(6):470–475. doi:10.1002/hed.2880120604
13. Bell RB, Kademani D, Homer L, et al. Tongue cancer: is there a difference in survival compared with other subsites in the oral cavity? *J Oral Maxillofac Surg.* 2007;65(2):229–236. doi:10.1016/j.joms.2005.11.094
14. Lee JJ, Hong WK, Hittelman WN, et al. Predicting cancer development in oral leukoplakia: ten years of translational research. *Clin Cancer Res.* 2000;6(5):1702–1710.
15. Luryi AL, Chen MM, Mehra S, et al. Treatment factors associated with survival in early-stage oral cavity cancer: analysis of 6830 cases from the national cancer data base. *JAMA Otolaryngol Head Neck Surg.* 2015;141(7):593–598. doi:10.1001/jamaoto.2015.0719
16. Liao CT, Chang JT, Wang HM, et al. Survival in squamous cell carcinoma of the oral cavity: differences between pT4 N0 and other stage IVA categories. *Cancer.* 2007;110(3):564–571. doi:10.1002/cncr.22814
17. Robertson AG, Soutar DS, Paul J, et al. Early closure of a randomized trial: surgery and postoperative radiotherapy versus radiotherapy in the management of intra-oral tumours. *Clin Oncol (R Coll Radiol).* 1998;10(3):155–160. doi:10.1016/S0936-6555(98)80055-1
18. Iyer NG, Tan DS, Tan VK, et al. Randomized trial comparing surgery and adjuvant radiotherapy versus concurrent chemoradiotherapy in patients with advanced, nonmetastatic squamous cell carcinoma of the head and neck: 10-year update and subset analysis. *Cancer.* 2015;121(10):1599–1607. doi:10.1002/cncr.29251
19. Zanoni DK, Migliacci JC, Xu B, et al. A proposal to redefine close surgical margins in squamous cell carcinoma of the oral tongue. *JAMA Otolaryngol Head Neck Surg.* 2017;143(6):555–560. doi:10.1001/jamaoto.2016.4238
20. Boudreaux BA, Rosenthal EL, Magnuson JS, et al. Robot-assisted surgery for upper aerodigestive tract neoplasms. *Arch Otolaryngol Head Neck Surg.* 2009;135(4):397–401. doi:10.1001/archoto.2009.24
21. Garrel R, Poissonnet G, Moya Plana A, et al. Equivalence randomized trial to compare treatment on the basis of sentinel node biopsy versus neck node dissection in operable T1-T2N0 oral and oropharyngeal cancer. *J Clin Oncol.* 2020;38(34):4010–4018. doi:10.1200/JCO.20.01661
22. Bernier J, Cooper JS, Pajak TF, et al. Defining risk levels in locally advanced head and neck cancers: a comparative analysis of concurrent postoperative radiation plus chemotherapy trials of the EORTC (#22931) and RTOG (#9501). *Head Neck.* 2005;27(10):843–850. doi:10.1002/hed.20279
23. Bossi P, Lo Vullo S, Guzzo M, et al. Preoperative chemotherapy in advanced resectable OCSCC: long-term results of a randomized phase III trial. *Ann Oncol.* 2014;25(2):462–466. doi:10.1093/annonc/mdt555

24. Zhong LP, Zhang CP, Ren GX, et al. Randomized phase III trial of induction chemotherapy with docetaxel, cisplatin, and fluorouracil followed by surgery versus up-front surgery in locally advanced resectable oral squamous cell carcinoma. *J Clin Oncol*. 2013;31(6):744–751. doi:10.1200/JCO.2012.43.8820

25. Ganly I, Goldstein D, Carlson DL, et al. Long-term regional control and survival in patients with "low-risk," early stage oral tongue cancer managed by partial glossectomy and neck dissection without postoperative radiation: the importance of tumor thickness. *Cancer*. 2013;119(6):1168–1176. doi:10.1002/cncr.27872

26. Gross ND, Patel SG, Carvalho AL, et al. Nomogram for deciding adjuvant treatment after surgery for oral cavity squamous cell carcinoma. *Head Neck*. 2008;30(10):1352–1360. doi:10.1002/hed.20879

27. Wang SJ, Patel SG, Shah JP, et al. An oral cavity carcinoma nomogram to predict benefit of adjuvant radiotherapy. *JAMA Otolaryngol Head Neck Surg*. 2013;139(6):554–559.

28. Contreras JA, Spencer C, DeWees T, et al. Eliminating postoperative radiation to the pathologically node-negative neck: long-term results of a prospective phase II study. *J Clin Oncol*. 2019;37(28):2548–2555. doi:10.1200/JCO.19.00186

29. Foster CC, Melotek JM, Brisson RJ, et al. Definitive chemoradiation for locally-advanced oral cavity cancer: a 20-year experience. *Oral Oncol*. 2018;80:16–22. doi:10.1016/j.oraloncology.2018.03.008

30. Wang CC, Doppke KP, Biggs PJ. Intra-oral cone radiation therapy for selected carcinomas of the oral cavity. *Int J Radiat Oncol, Biol, Phys*. 1983;9(8):1185–1189. doi:10.1016/0360-3016(83)90178-5

31. Mazeron JJ, Ardiet JM, Haie-Meder C, et al. GEC-ESTRO recommendations for brachytherapy for head and neck squamous cell carcinomas. *Radiother Oncol*. 2009;91(2):150–156. doi:10.1016/j.radonc.2009.01.005

32. Videtic GMM WN, Vassil AD. *Handbook of Treatment Planning in Radiation Oncology*. 2nd ed. Demos Medical; 2015. doi:10.1891/9781617051975

33. Ang KK, Trotti A, Brown BW, et al. Randomized trial addressing risk features and time factors of surgery plus radiotherapy in advanced head-and-neck cancer. *Int J Radiat Oncol, Biol, Phys*. 2001;51(3):571–578. doi:10.1016/S0360-3016(01)01690-X

34. Peters LJ, Goepfert H, Ang KK, et al. Evaluation of the dose for postoperative radiation therapy of head and neck cancer: first report of a prospective randomized trial. *Int J Radiat Oncol Biol Phys*. 1993;26(1):3–11. doi:10.1016/0360-3016(93)90167-T

35. Bernier J, Domenge C, Ozsahin M, et al. Postoperative irradiation with or without concomitant chemotherapy for locally advanced head and neck cancer. *N Engl J Med*. 2004;350(19):1945–1952. doi:10.1056/NEJMoa032641

36. Cooper JS, Pajak TF, Forastiere AA, et al. Postoperative concurrent radiotherapy and chemotherapy for high-risk squamous-cell carcinoma of the head and neck. *N Engl J Med*. 2004;350(19):1937–1944. doi:10.1056/NEJMoa032646

13 ■ NASOPHARYNGEAL CANCER

Christopher W. Fleming, Shireen Parsai, and Nikhil P. Joshi

QUICK HIT ■ Nasopharyngeal Cancer (NPC) is rare in the United States, with high prevalence in endemic regions (South China, Southeast Asia, North Africa). The majority of U.S. cases (and nearly all cases in endemic areas) are related to EBV, and use of EBV DNA as a biomarker to guide therapy is under active investigation. Treatment is typically non-operative (Table 13.1).

Table 13.1 General Treatment Paradigm for Nasopharyngeal Cancer[1]	
	Treatment Options
T1N0M0	Definitive IMRT (70 Gy/35 fx) + elective neck irradiation*
T1N1–3 and T2–4N0-3	Definitive concurrent chemoRT with adjuvant or induction CHT
M1	CHT ± locoregional RT (70 Gy) based on response

*If N0, treat RPNs and bilateral levels II to V; if node +, treat IB as well.
Source: From NCCN Clinical Practice Guidelines in Oncology: Head and Neck Cancers (Version 1). 2021. https://www.nccn.org/professionals/physician_gls/pdf/head-and-neck.pdf

EPIDEMIOLOGY: A total of 3,200 cases per year in the United States (0.5–2 per 100,000). Endemic in South China, Hong Kong, Southeast Asia, and North Africa (rates as high as 25 per 100,000). Estimated 51,000 deaths worldwide. More common in males (2.3:1 ratio).[2] In endemic areas, incidence peaks at 50 to 59 years of age; otherwise, in low-risk populations incidence appears to increase with age.[3]

RISK FACTORS: EBV, salt-preserved fish, preserved foods, low fruit/vegetable diet, tobacco smoke, family history, HPV.[3]

ANATOMY: The nasopharynx is a cuboidal space bordered anteriorly by the choanae, posteriorly by the clivus and cervical vertebrae (C1–2), superiorly by the skull base (sphenoid sinus), and inferiorly by the soft palate. The lateral walls consist of the Eustachian tube orifice bounded by the torus tubarius, with the fossa of Rosenmüller located further posteriorly. Most NPCs arise from fossa of Rosenmüller.[4]

PATHOLOGY: WHO classification is divided into three groups: *keratinizing* squamous cell carcinoma, *nonkeratinizing* carcinoma (further subdivided into differentiated and undifferentiated subgroups), and *basaloid* squamous cell carcinoma (see Table 13.2).

Table 13.2 WHO Classification for Nasopharyngeal Cancer			
WHO Classification[5]	**U.S. Incidence**	**Endemic Incidence[6]**	**Notes[7]**
Keratinizing	25%	1%	WHO type I (squamous cell carcinoma), associated with smoking and occasionally HPV
Nonkeratinizing • Differentiated	12%	3%	WHO type II (transitional cell carcinoma)
• Undifferentiated	63%	95%	WHO type III (lymphoepithelial carcinoma), endemic, associated with EBV, most favorable prognosis
Basaloid	–	<0.2%	Aggressive clinical course, poor survival

SCREENING: Screening methods have been studied in endemic areas (e.g., IgA to EBV viral capsid antigen, circulating plasma EBV DNA), though currently no established screening protocols exist.[8]

CLINICAL PRESENTATION: Most common presentations are painless neck mass, nasal or ear symptoms, headache, diplopia, or facial numbness.[1] Diplopia occurs due to local invasion, with CN VI often compressed first. Jacod's triad of vision loss, ophthalmoplegia, and trigeminal neuralgia result from cavernous sinus invasion. Dysphagia, hoarseness, Horner's syndrome, and CN XI deficits can occur from lateral RPN compression on CNs IX to XII (Villaret's syndrome) or from invasion into jugular foramen (Vernet's syndrome). LN involvement is extremely common at diagnosis (75%–90%, bilateral in 50%). Five percent to 11% of patients have metastatic disease at the time of diagnosis. Most common sites for DM are bone, lung, and liver.[9–11]

WORKUP: H&P with attention to cranial nerves and neck adenopathy, nasopharyngoscopy. Dental, nutritional, speech and swallowing, and audiology exam as clinically indicated. Ophthalmologic and endocrine evaluation as clinically indicated. Smoking cessation should be advised.

Labs: Routine CBC, CMP, as well as EBV DNA testing. Pretreatment plasma EBV DNA levels are prognostic.[1]

Imaging: MRI and CT with contrast evaluating base of skull and regional node involvement. PET/CT for distant disease, especially for T3–4 or node-positive patients, as well as those with high EBV viral load.

PROGNOSTIC FACTORS: Performance status, stage, WHO classification (keratinizing worse, EBV-associated better), post-RT EBV DNA.[6]

STAGING (SEE TABLE 13.3):

Table 13.3 AJCC 8th ed. (2017): Staging for Nasopharynx Cancer		cN0	cN1	cN2	cN3
T0	• No primary tumor, but EBV-positive cervical node (unknown primary)				
T1	• Confined to nasopharynx or extension to oropharynx/nasal cavity	I	II	III	IVA
T2	• Extension to parapharyngeal space and/or medial pterygoid, lateral pterygoid, prevertebral muscles				
T3	• Infiltration of bony structures[1]				
T4	• Extension[2]				
M1	• Distant metastasis		IVB		

Notes: Infiltration of bony structures[1] = Skull base, cervical vertebrae, pterygoid plates, paranasal sinuses. Extension[2] = Intracranial extension and/or involvement of cranial nerves, hypopharynx, orbit, parotid gland, soft tissue beyond lateral surface of lateral pterygoid muscle.
cN1, unilateral LNs and/or unilateral or bilateral metastasis in RPNs (≤6 cm), above caudal border of cricoid; cN2, bilateral LNs (≤6 cm), above caudal border of cricoid; cN3, unilateral or bilateral LNs (>6 cm) and/or LNs below caudal border of cricoid cartilage.

TREATMENT PARADIGM

Surgery: Surgery is not routine in up-front setting but rather reserved as salvage option in select patients. Persistent nodal disease after primary therapy or nodal recurrence may be treated with neck dissection.

Chemotherapy: Concurrent chemoradiation (chemoRT) with adjuvant CHT has historically been the standard treatment regimen in the United States for patients with stage II to stage IVB disease. However, induction CHT is a reasonable alternative to adjuvant (see Q&A section), with the advantage of potentially reducing RT volumes. Cisplatin is given concurrently with RT as 100 mg/m² bolus at weeks 1, 4, and 7 or 40 mg/m² weekly. Adjuvant CHT consists of cisplatin (80 mg/m²) and 5-FU (1,000 mg/m² continuous infusion for 4 days) every 4 weeks for 3 cycles beginning 4 weeks after completion of RT. Induction CHT consists of cisplatin (80 mg/m² day 1) and gemcitabine (1 gm/m² days 1 and 8) q3 weeks x 3 cycles; other induction regimens include TPF (docetaxel, cisplatin, and 5-FU) and cisplatin with 5-FU. Results from NPC 0501 suggest that it may be feasible to replace 5-FU with capecitabine.[12]

Radiation

Indications: Stage I disease (T1N0M0) is generally treated with RT alone. Stage II to stage IVB NPC are treated with concurrent chemoRT followed by adjuvant CHT, or induction CHT followed by concurrent chemoradiation.

Dose: Treat primary site to 70 Gy/35 fx or 69.96 Gy/33 fx. Elective nodal RT (bilateral in all) to RPNs, levels II to V. Treat level IB in node-positive patients or those with primary tumor extension to nasal cavity, hard palate or maxillary sinus. The following at-risk sites are also included in the elective volume: entirety of the nasopharynx, anterior one third of the clivus (the entire clivus if involved), foramen ovale, foramen rotundum, pterygoid fossae, parapharyngeal space, inferior sphenoid sinus (entire sphenoid sinus if T3–4), posterior fourth of the nasal cavity and maxillary sinuses. Cavernous sinus can also be considered for T3–4 tumors.

Toxicity: Acute: xerostomia, dysphagia, odynophagia, nausea, weight loss. *Late:* Hearing loss, dental carries, trismus, brainstem necrosis, optic neuritis, endocrinopathy, cranial nerve palsies, stroke.

Procedure: See *Handbook of Treatment Planning in Radiation Oncology*, Chapter 4.[13]

■ EVIDENCE-BASED Q&A

▓ What is the role of CHT in treatment of nasopharyngeal cancer?

Concurrent chemoRT followed by adjuvant CHT has been the standard of care in the United States. Historically, most patients were treated with RT alone, until the Intergroup Al-Sarraf trial demonstrated OS benefit to concurrent and adjuvant CHT compared to definitive RT alone in patients with stage III to stage IV NPC (AJCC, 4th edition). These results were initially controversial, particularly in Asia. Critics argued outcomes of definitive RT alone arm were worse than historical standards. In addition, high proportion of WHO type I patients (22%) may account for poor outcomes and need for CHT. WHO type I histology is more common in the United States compared to endemic regions. Since then, multiple randomized trials have defined benefit of concurrent CHT, and the MAC-NPC meta-analysis demonstrated absolute survival benefit of 6.3% at 5 years with concomitant CHT.[14] Recently, induction CHT followed by concurrent chemoRT has emerged as a new standard of care for select patients.

Al-Sarraf, Intergroup 0099 (*JCO* 1998, PMID 9552031): PRT of 193 patients with biopsy proven stage III to IV (M0) NPC. Note that *AJCC* 4th edition included N1 patients in stage III (now stage II). Randomized to RT alone vs. RT with concurrent cisplatin and adjuvant CHT with cisplatin and 5-FU (see Chemotherapy section). Study was closed early after interim analysis of 147 patients demonstrated OS benefit in experimental arm (see Table 13.4). Sixty-three percent completed all concurrent CHT, 55% completed all cycles of adjuvant. **Conclusion: Concurrent and adjuvant CHT with RT improves OS for stage III to stage IV (and N1, 7/8th edition stage II) nasopharyngeal cancer.**

Table 13.4 Results of Al-Sarraf INT 0099 Nasopharynx Trial		
	5-Yr PFS*	**5-Yr OS***
RT	29%	37%
ChemoRT + Adjuvant CHT	58%	67%
*p < .001		

Blanchard, MAC-NPC Meta-analysis (*IJROBP* 2006, PMID 16377415; Update *Lancet Oncol* 2015, PMID 25957714): Update with 4,806 patients. MFU 7.7 years; addition of CHT to RT improved OS with absolute benefit of 6.3% at 5 years (*p* < .0001). Addition of CHT also improved PFS, LRC, distant control, and cancer mortality. Increase in OS was statistically significant for concomitant CHT (with and without adjuvant CHT), but not adjuvant CHT alone or induction CHT alone. **Conclusion: Concurrent CHT improves OS in locally advanced NPC.**

■ Is adjuvant CHT necessary?

This is an area of controversy (see Table 13.5). There has been one trial to directly address this question, detailed as follows. Although the trial was negative, it was heavily criticized (see the following comment). 2020 NCCN guidelines report concurrent chemoRT followed by adjuvant CHT a category 2A recommendation and concurrent chemoRT alone category a 2B recommendation.

Chen, Sun Yat-sen China (*Lancet Oncol* 2012, PMID 22154591): Multi-institution PRT involving institutions in China; 508 patients with stage III/IV (T3–4N0 excluded) randomized to concurrent chemoRT ± adjuvant CHT (cisplatin 80 mg/m² and 5-FU 800 mg/m² for 120 hours q4 weeks x3 cycles). Primary endpoint was FFS. Two-year FFS rate was 84% in concurrent-only arm and 86% in concurrent + adjuvant arm (*p* = .13). **Conclusion: Adjuvant CHT did not improve FFS.** *Comment: Did not use noninferiority design, 18% randomized to adjuvant CHT did not receive it, nearly 60% did not complete concurrent CHT, 50% required RT dose reduction, and 70% had treatment delays.*

Table 13.5 Pros and Cons of Adjuvant CHT for NPC	
Rationale for Eliminating Adjuvant CHT	**Rationale for Employing Adjuvant CHT**
• Historical trials investigating use of adjuvant CHT after definitive RT have been negative. • PRTs evaluating RT alone vs. chemoRT (w/o adjuvant) show survival benefit to concurrent CHT (Taiwan, Hong Kong, China). • Two meta-analyses investigating impact of CHT on outcomes have suggested that major driver of benefit is concurrent phase. The analysis of Baujat et al. found 18% reduction in HR of death with CHT overall, with 40% risk reduction with concurrent and 3% risk reduction with adjuvant.[15] The analysis of Langendijk et al. suggested 20% survival benefit at 5 years with concurrent CHT and no benefit to adjuvant.[16] • PRT from China randomized patients to chemoRT with weekly cisplatin ± 3 cycles adjuvant cisplatin/5-FU. While there were more failures in the arm without adjuvant CHT, they were not statistically different (*p* = .13).[17] • Compliance is poor; generally, only 50% to 60% of patients complete full course of adjuvant therapy on PRTs.	• Data from Taiwan suggest that for patients at high risk of distant failure, concurrent chemoRT is insufficient.[18] • Analysis of phase III Hong Kong data showed that concurrent cisplatin plus adjuvant cisplatin/5-FU was associated with improved distant control. In patients who received 0 to 1 cycles, 5-yr distant FFR was 68% vs. 78% for 2 to 3 cycles.[18] • Chinese PRT did not use noninferiority design; therefore, premature to suggest it should change practice. Additionally, 18% of patients in adjuvant arm did not receive it, 50% required RT dose reduction, and 70% had treatment delays. • In modern series using IMRT, LRC is excellent, and major pattern of failure is now distant.

■ Which patients benefit from CHT?

Patients with stage I NPC can be treated with definitive RT alone. Majority of clinical trials demonstrating benefit with addition of CHT to RT (including INT 0099) included patients with stage III to stage IV disease. Patients with stage II disease have been found to have worse outcomes compared to stage I with distant failure rates as high as 10% to 15% with N1 disease. RR from Taiwan suggested that addition of CHT in stage II patients resulted in similar outcomes to those found in stage I patients treated with RT alone.[19] This led to the following phase III trial in China.

Chen, Sun Yat-sen China (*JNCI* 2011, PMID 22056739): PRT of 230 patients with stage II NPC randomized to concurrent chemoRT with weekly cisplatin (30 mg/m²) vs. RT alone. See Table 13.6. Concurrent CHT significantly improved OS (*p* = .007), PFS (*p* = .017), and DMFS (*p* = .007), at expense of worse acute toxicity (*p* = .001). OS advantage driven by improvement in DMFS; LRC unchanged. MVA showed that the number of CHT cycles delivered was the only factor associated with improved OS, PFS, and distant control. **Conclusion: Concurrent CHT improved survival for patients with stage II NPC.**

Table 13.6 Sun Yat-sen Trial (China) Investigating Concurrent ChemoRT for NPC						
	5-Yr LRC	**5-Yr PFS**	**5-Yr DMFS**	**5-Yr OS**	**Acute G3–4**	**Late G3–4**
RT	91%	79%	84%	86%	40%	10%
ChemoRT	93%	88%	95%	95%	64%	14%

■ What is the role of induction CHT?

There has been significant interest in adding induction CHT to chemoRT due to the potential benefits of improved compliance (relative to adjuvant CHT) and downstaging to allow for reduced RT volumes. Note that RT volume reduction is particularly helpful for NPC due to proximity to serial structures such as optic structures and brainstem, in comparison to other H&N sites away from serial structures. Phase IIR trial from Hong Kong demonstrated 26.5% absolute improvement in 3-year OS by adding induction cisplatin and docetaxel to chemoRT with no compromise in ability to deliver full course of chemoRT afterward.[20] However, phase IIR trial from Europe was negative.[21] NPC 0501 (six-arm trial investigating induction–concurrent sequence, use of capecitabine, and accelerated fractionation) found no difference in outcomes based on CHT sequence or RT acceleration; however, secondary analyses suggested improved efficacy of induction regimen.[12]

Sun, China (*Lancet Oncol* 2016, PMID 27686945): Multicenter PRT involving 10 institutions in China, 480 patients, evaluating addition of induction CHT (TPF: cisplatin, 5-FU, docetaxel q3 weeks x 3 cycles) to concurrent chemoRT in locally advanced NPC. Eligibility criteria included stage III to IVB (except T3-4N0). Concurrent CHT was high-dose cisplatin. Primary endpoint FFS. MFU 45 months, 3-year FFS increased from 72% to 80% (*p* = .034) in favor of induction CHT. Induction CHT was associated with increased grade 3/4 toxicity: 42% vs. 17% neutropenia, 41% vs. 17% leukopenia, 41% vs. 35% stomatitis. **Conclusion: Induction CHT significantly improved 3-year FFS compared to concurrent chemoRT alone.**

Zhang, China (*NEJM* 2019, PMID 31150573): Multicenter PRT of 480 patients with stage III to stage IVB NPC with involved lymph nodes, randomized to induction cisplatin/gemcitabine followed by chemoRT vs. chemoRT alone. Induction CHT was cisplatin (80 mg/m^2 day 1) and gemcitabine (1 gm/m^2 days 1 and 8) q3 weeks x 3 cycles. Concurrent CHT was high-dose cisplatin. Induction CHT improved 3-year RFS (85.3% vs. 76.5%, HR 0.51, CI 0.34–0.77) and 3-year OS (94.6% vs. 90.3%, HR 0.43, CI 0.24–0.77). Vast majority of induction patients completed CHT (96.7%). G3 or higher acute toxicity increased with induction, 75.7% vs. 55.7%. Late G3 or higher toxicity was similar, 9.2% induction vs. 11.4% chemoRT alone. **Conclusion: Induction CHT with cisplatin and gemcitabine significantly improved RFS and OS over chemoRT alone. Comment: no adjuvant CHT used in comparison arm.**

■ What is the role of adaptive replanning?

Adaptive replanning should be strongly considered. NPC is radiosensitive tumor, and large anatomic changes are possible during treatment. Dosimetric studies have shown that replanning can improve coverage as well as reduce dose to surrounding critical structures. In a prospective study from China, 129 patients with M0 NPC were enrolled, 86 of whom were replanned before 25th fraction. Patients who were replanned were found to have superior 2-year LRC (97% vs. 92%) and reported improved global QOL, functional QOL, and symptoms (dyspnea, appetite loss, speech problems, dry mouth, etc.).[22]

■ What is the role of serum EBV DNA levels?

EBV is the primary etiologic agent in pathogenesis of NPC, and EBV levels both pre- and posttreatment are prognostic for survival. Patients with pre-treatment values ranging from <1,500 copies/mL to <4,000 copies/ mL tend to have improved survival. Multiple studies have shown that detectable EBV after definitive RT is a poor prognostic marker.[23,24] NRG HN001 is an ongoing phase II/III study of individualized treatment for NPC based on posttreatment EBV DNA. Undetectable patients are randomized to adjuvant CHT vs. observation, while detectable patients are randomized between cisplatin/5-FU and gemcitabine/paclitaxel.[25]

■ Do metastatic patients benefit from locoregional RT?

A phase III trial showed an improvement in OS with the addition of locoregional RT in patients with metastatic nasopharyngeal cancer and initial response to CHT.[26] See Chapter 71 for details.

■ How is pediatric NPC treated?

In the United States, induction CHT is the standard treatment paradigm, illustrated by the following COG protocol, investigating dose-adapting RT based on response to CHT.

Rodriguez-Galindo, COG ARAR0331 (JCO 2019, PMID 31553639): Single-arm prospective study of 111 patients, median age 15, stage IIb to stage IV. Patients received 3 cycles induction cisplatin (80 mg/m² day 1) and 5-FU (1,000 mg/m²/d continuous infusion days 1–4), every 3 weeks, followed by chemoRT with high-dose cisplatin. Dose was adapted from 61.2 Gy to 71.2 Gy based on response to induction CHT. After feasibility analysis, study was amended to reduce cisplatin from 3 to 2 cycles. Five-year EFS and OS were 84.3% and 89.2%, respectively. Five-year EFS for stage IV patients was 82.7%. Five-year local and distant failure were 3.7% and 8.7%, respectively. Patients treated with 3 cycles concurrent cisplatin had numerically higher 5-year EFS compared to those receiving 2 cycles (90.7% vs. 81.2%, $p = .14$). **Conclusion: Treatment with induction CHT resulted in excellent outcomes. Dose reduction is possible for patients with response to induction CHT. Three cycles of concurrent cisplatin may improve EFS compared to two cycles.**

REFERENCES

1. NCCN Clinical Practice Guidelines in Oncology: Head and Neck Cancers (Version 1). 2021. https://www.nccn.org/professionals/physician_gls/pdf/head-and-neck.pdf
2. Ferlay J, Soerjomataram I, Dikshit R, et al. Cancer incidence and mortality worldwide: sources, methods and major patterns in GLOBOCAN 2012. *Int J Cancer.* 2015;136(5):E359–E386. doi:10.1002/ijc.29210
3. Chang ET, Adami HO. The enigmatic epidemiology of nasopharyngeal carcinoma. *Cancer Epidemiol Biomarkers Prev.* 2006;15(10):1765–1777. doi:10.1158/1055-9965.EPI-06-0353
4. Halperin E, Perez C, Brady L. *Principles and Practice of Radiation Oncology.* 6th ed. Lippincott Williams & Wilkins; 2013.
5. Stelow EB, Wenig BM. Update from the 4th edition of the world health organization classification of head and neck tumours: nasopharynx. *Head Neck Pathol.* 2017;11(1):16–22. doi:10.1007/s12105-017-0787-0
6. Wei WI, Sham JS. Nasopharyngeal carcinoma. *Lancet.* 2005;365(9476):2041–2054. doi:10.1016/S0140-6736(05)66698-6
7. Amin MB, Edge S, Greene F, et al., eds. *AJCC Cancer Staging Manual.* 8th ed. Springer International Publishing: American Joint Commission on Cancer; 2017.
8. Tabuchi K, Nakayama M, Nishimura B, et al. Early detection of nasopharyngeal carcinoma. *Int J Otolaryngol.* 2011;2011:638058. doi:10.1155/2011/638058
9. Vokes EE, Liebowitz DN, Weichselbaum RR. Nasopharyngeal carcinoma. *Lancet.* 1997;350(9084):1087–1091. doi:10.1016/S0140-6736(97)07269-3
10. Hsu MM, Tu SM. Nasopharyngeal carcinoma in Taiwan: clinical manifestations and results of therapy. *Cancer.* 1983;52(2):362–368. doi:10.1002/1097-0142(19830715)52:2<362::AID-CNCR2820520230>3.0.CO;2-V
11. Altun M, Fandi A, Dupuis O, et al. Undifferentiated nasopharyngeal cancer (UCNT): current diagnostic and therapeutic aspects. *Int J Radiat Oncol Biol Phys.* 1995;32(3):859–877. doi:10.1016/0360-3016(95)00516-2
12. Lee AWM, Ngan RKC, Ng WT, et al. NPC-0501 trial on the value of changing chemoradiotherapy sequence, replacing 5-fluorouracil with capecitabine, and altering fractionation for patients with advanced nasopharyngeal carcinoma. *Cancer.* 2020;126(16):3674–3688. doi:10.1002/cncr.32972
13. Videtic GMM, Vassil AD. *Handbook of Treatment Planning in Radiation Oncology,* 3rd ed. Demos Medical; 2020. doi:10.1891/9780826168429
14. Blanchard P, Lee A, Marguet S, et al. Chemotherapy and radiotherapy in nasopharyngeal carcinoma: an update of the MAC-NPC meta-analysis. *Lancet Oncol.* 2015;16(6):645–655. doi:10.1016/S1470-2045(15)70126-9
15. Baujat B, Audry H, Bourhis J, et al. Chemotherapy in locally advanced nasopharyngeal carcinoma: an individual patient data meta-analysis of eight randomized trials and 1753 patients. *Int J Radiat Oncol Biol Phys.* 2006;64(1):47–56. doi:10.1016/j.ijrobp.2005.06.037
16. Langendijk JA, Leemans CR, Buter J, et al. The additional value of chemotherapy to radiotherapy in locally advanced nasopharyngeal carcinoma: a meta-analysis of the published literature. *J Clin Oncol.* 2004;22(22):4604–4612. doi:10.1200/JCO.2004.10.074
17. Chen L, Hu CS, Chen XZ, et al. Concurrent chemoradiotherapy plus adjuvant chemotherapy versus concurrent chemoradiotherapy alone in patients with locoregionally advanced nasopharyngeal carcinoma: a phase 3 multicentre randomised controlled trial. *Lancet Oncol.* 2012;13(2):163–171. doi:10.1016/S1470-2045(11)70320-5
18. Lin JC, Liang WM, Jan JS, et al. Another way to estimate outcome of advanced nasopharyngeal carcinoma: is concurrent chemoradiotherapy adequate? *Int J Radiat Oncol Biol Phys.* 2004;60(1):156–164. doi:10.1016/j.ijrobp.2004.03.002
19. Cheng SH, Tsai SY, Yen KL, et al. Concomitant radiotherapy and chemotherapy for early-stage nasopharyngeal carcinoma. *J Clin Oncol.* 2000;18(10):2040–2045. doi:10.1200/JCO.2000.18.10.2040
20. Hui EP, Ma BB, Leung SF, et al. Randomized phase II trial of concurrent cisplatin-radiotherapy with or without neoadjuvant docetaxel and cisplatin in advanced nasopharyngeal carcinoma. *J Clin Oncol.* 2009;27(2):242–249. doi:10.1200/JCO.2008.18.1545
21. Fountzilas G, Ciuleanu E, Bobos M, et al. Induction chemotherapy followed by concomitant radiotherapy and weekly cisplatin versus the same concomitant chemoradiotherapy in patients with nasopharyngeal carcinoma: a

randomized phase II study conducted by the hellenic cooperative oncology group (HeCOG) with biomarker evaluation. *Ann Oncol*. 2012;23(2):427–435. doi:10.1093/annonc/mdr116

22. Yang H, Hu W, Wang W, et al. Replanning during intensity modulated radiation therapy improved quality of life in patients with nasopharyngeal carcinoma. *Int J Radiat Oncol Biol Phys*. 2013;85(1):e47–e54. doi:10.1016/j.ijrobp.2012.09.033

23. Lin JC, Wang WY, Chen KY, et al. Quantification of plasma epstein-barr virus DNA in patients with advanced nasopharyngeal carcinoma. *N Engl J Med*. 2004;350(24):2461–2470. doi:10.1056/NEJMoa032260

24. Leung SF, Zee B, Ma BB, et al. Plasma Epstein-Barr viral deoxyribonucleic acid quantitation complements tumor-node-metastasis staging prognostication in nasopharyngeal carcinoma. *J Clin Oncol*. 2006;24(34):5414–5418. doi:10.1200/JCO.2006.07.7982

25. Individualized Treatment in Treating Patients With Stage II-IVB Nasopharyngeal Cancer Based on EBV DNA. NRG Oncology. https://ClinicalTrials.gov/show/NCT02135042. Accessed June 9, 2021.

26. You R, Liu YP, Huang PY, et al. Efficacy and safety of locoregional radiotherapy with chemotherapy vs chemotherapy alone in de novo metastatic nasopharyngeal carcinoma: a multicenter phase 3 randomized clinical trial. *JAMA Oncol*. 2020;6(9):1345–1352. doi:10.1001/jamaoncol.2020.1808

14 ■ LARYNGEAL CANCER

Aditya Juloori, Shauna R. Campbell, and Shlomo A. Koyfman

QUICK HIT ■ Laryngeal cancer includes squamous carcinoma originating from the supraglottis, glottis, or rarely the subglottis. Goal of treatment is to achieve disease control while maintaining organ function, defined as functional voice with intact swallowing. Early-stage glottic cancers can be managed with RT alone or microsurgery. Locoregionally advanced disease, defined as T3–4 or node-positive, frequently requires either total laryngectomy (with adjuvant RT as indicated) or definitive chemoRT to attempt voice preservation. For patients with T4a disease with extralaryngeal spread, total laryngectomy with PORT is preferred over definitive chemoRT (Table 14.1).

Table 14.1 General Treatment Paradigm for Larynx Cancer

	Supraglottic	Glottic
Tis	Endoscopic Surgery	
T1N0	Larynx-sparing surgery OR Definitive RT (66–70 Gy) to primary tumor + elective LN levels II to IV	Definitive RT (63 Gy/28 fx at 2.25 Gy/fx) OR larynx-sparing surgery
T2N0		Definitive RT (65.25 Gy/29 fx at 2.25 Gy/fx) OR larynx-sparing surgery
T3 or node-positive	Larynx-sparing surgery w/ PORT OR definitive chemoRT (70 Gy/35 fx) to tumor + elective LN II to IV (V if LN +) w/ cisplatin	
T4a	Total laryngectomy (preferred for thyroid cartilage penetration or significant soft-tissue extension) with adjuvant RT ± concurrent cisplatin as indicated OR Larynx preservation with concurrent chemoRT to 70 Gy/35 fx with cisplatin	

EPIDEMIOLOGY: A total of 12,400 new diagnoses of laryngeal cancer in the United States with estimated 3,750 deaths in 2020. More common in men than women; incidence increases with age.[1]

RISK FACTORS: Smoking, alcohol, environmental exposures (asbestos, cement, wood dust, perchlorethylene).

ANATOMY: Major functions of larynx are voice production, airway patency during breathing, and airway occlusion during swallowing. It spans from C3 to C6 vertebral bodies and is bordered superiorly by hyoepiglottic ligament, inferiorly by cricoid, anteriorly by thyrohyoid membrane/thyroid cartilage, and posteriorly by arytenoid cartilage. Preepiglottic and paraglottic spaces are one continuous space anterosuperiorly. Laryngeal muscles (with exception of cricothyroid) are innervated by recurrent laryngeal nerve (branch of vagus nerve). Damage to this nerve results in a fixed, midline cord. Cricothyroid muscle is innervated by superior laryngeal nerve. Damage to this nerve results in mobile, "bowed" cords.

The larynx is divided into three segments:

1. *Supraglottis* (one third of all laryngeal cancers,[1] mnemonic FAVEA: false vocal cords, arytenoids, ventricles, epiglottis, aryepiglottic folds): Bordered superiorly by epiglottis, posteriorly by arytenoids, anteriorly by posterior edge of vallecula and anterior false cord, and inferiorly by epithelium of true vocal cord as it turns upward to form apex of ventricle. More than 50% of patients with supraglottic primaries present with node-positive disease due to presence of extensive lymphatics in this part of larynx. Levels II to IV are primary drainage sites for supraglottis.
2. *Glottis* (two thirds of all laryngeal cancers[2]): Consists of true vocal cords and anterior and posterior commissures. Due to sparse lymphatics, early-stage disease rarely involves regional nodes. True

vocal cord is made up of the following layers: epithelial mucosa, basement membrane, superficial layer of lamina propria, and thyroarytenoid muscle.

3. *Subglottis* (1%–2% of all laryngeal cancers[3]): Starts 5 mm inferior to margin of vocal cords to inferior aspect of cricoid cartilage. Subglottic tumors can drain to pretracheal (Delphian) nodes.

PATHOLOGY: Ninety-five percent of tumors are SCC. Carcinoma in situ occurs in vocal cords but is rare in supraglottis. Rare malignancies: malignant minor salivary gland, small cell, lymphoma, plasmacytoma, carcinoid, soft-tissue sarcoma, chondrosarcoma, osteosarcoma, malignant melanoma. HPV positivity has not been shown to be prognostic or predictive in laryngeal cancer.

CLINICAL PRESENTATION: Presenting clinical symptoms are classically related to site of origin. Glottic cancers often present at early stage with hoarseness but as disease progresses, patients develop otalgia, dysphagia, cough, hemoptysis, stridor. In supraglottis, cancers are often detected later and commonly present with dysphagia, globus sensation, airway obstruction, and lymphadenopathy. Otalgia is due to referred pain to auricular branch of Arnold (from vagus nerve).

WORKUP: H&P including flexible nasopharyngolaryngoscopy. Videostroboscopy can be used to evaluate mucosal wave of true cords. Pain with palpation of thyroid cartilage can be reflective of cartilage invasion.

Labs: Routine CBC and CMP. Pre-CHT audiology exam.

Imaging: CT neck with contrast and PET/CT for stage III/IV disease. CT scan has high positive-predictive value for thyroid cartilage penetration (74%) and extralaryngeal spread (81%).[4]

Procedure: EUA with triple endoscopy (~4% incidence of second primary) and biopsy. Dental, nutrition, speech and swallow evaluation as indicated.

STAGING

Table 14.2 AJCC 8th ed. (2017): Staging for Larynx Cancer									
SUPRAGLOTTIS									
T/M	N	cN0	cN1	cN2a	cN2b	cN2c	cN3a	cN3b
T1	Limited to 1 subsite of supraglottis with normal vocal cord mobility	I						
T2	Invades mucosa of >1 adjacent subsite of supraglottis or glottis, or region outside supraglottis without fixation of larynx[1]	II	III	IVA			IVB	
T3	• Limited to larynx with vocal cord fixation • Invasion[2]							
T4	a. Moderately advanced local disease[3]							
	b. Very advanced local disease[4]							
M1	Distant metastasis	IVC						

Notes: Larynx[1] = Regions include mucosa of BOT, vallecula, medial wall of pyriform sinus. Invades[2] = Postcricoid area, preepiglottic space, paraglottic space, and/or inner cortex of thyroid cartilage. Disease[3] = invades through thyroid cartilage outer cortex, trachea, soft tissues of neck, deep extrinsic muscles of tongue, strap muscles, thyroid, or esophagus. Disease[4] = Invades prevertebral space, encases carotid artery, or invades mediastinal structures.
cN1, single ipsilateral LN (≤3 cm) and ENE; cN2a, single ipsilateral LN (3.1–6 cm) and –ENE; cN2b, multiple ipsilateral LN (≤6 cm) and –ENE; cN2c, bilateral or contralateral LN (≤6 cm) and –ENE; cN3a, LN (>6 cm) and –ENE; cN3b, clinically overt ENE.
pN1, single LN (≤3 cm) and –ENE; pN2a, single ipsilateral or contralateral LN (≤3 cm) and +ENE or single ipsilateral LN (3.1–6 cm) and –ENE; pN2b, multiple ipsilateral LN (≤6 cm) and –ENE; pN2c, bilateral or contralateral LN (≤6 cm) and –ENE; pN3a, LN (>6 cm) and –ENE; pN3b, LN (>3 cm) and +ENE.

GLOTTIS									
T/M	**N**	cN0	cN1	cN2a	cN2b	cN2c	cN3a	cN3b
T1	a. Limited to 1 vocal cord with normal mobility	I						
	b. Involves 2 vocal cords with normal mobility							
T2	Extends to supraglottis and/or subglottis and/or with impaired vocal cord mobility[1]	II	III		IVA			IVB
T3	• Limited to larynx with vocal cord fixation • Invades[2]							
T4	a. Moderately advanced local disease[3]							
	b. Very advanced local disease[4]							
M1	Distant metastasis				IVC			

Notes: Mobility[1] = Unofficially, T2 can be divided into T2a (mobile cord) and T2b (impaired cord mobility). Invades[2] = Paraglottic space and/or inner cortex of thyroid cartilage. Disease[3] = invades through thyroid cartilage outer cortex, trachea, soft tissues of neck, deep extrinsic muscles of tongue, strap muscles, thyroid, or esophagus. Disease[4] = Invades prevertebral space, encases carotid artery, or invades mediastinal structures.
Refer to supraglottic larynx for nodal staging.

SUBGLOTTIS									
T/M	**N**	cN0	cN1	cN2a	cN2b	cN2c	cN3a	cN3b
T1	Limited to subglottis	I						
T2	Extends to vocal cords with normal or impaired mobility	II	III		IVA			IVB
T3	• Limited to larynx with vocal cord fixation • Invades[1]							
T4	a. Moderately advanced local disease[2]							
	b. Very advanced local disease[3]							
M1	Distant metastasis				IVC			

Notes: Invades[1] = Invasion of paraglottic space and/or inner cortex of thyroid cartilage. Disease[2] = invades through thyroid cartilage outer cortex, trachea, soft tissues of neck, deep extrinsic muscles of tongue, strap muscles, thyroid, or esophagus. Disease[3] = Invades prevertebral space, encases carotid artery, or invades mediastinal structures.

TREATMENT PARADIGM

Surgery

Glottis: Modern surgical options for early glottic tumors focus on endoscopic resection with aim of preserving laryngeal function and have largely replaced external approaches. Note that at least one mobile arytenoid complex must be preserved to maintain adequate function of larynx. Endoscopic techniques can include mucosal stripping (for in situ disease), microdissection (including TORS), electrocautery, CO_2 laser (TLM or TOLM), among others. Other voice-conserving options are as follows:

Vertical hemilaryngectomy: Removes up to one true vocal cord as well as one-third of contralateral true cord. Appropriate for lesions with up to 1 cm anterior subglottic extension and 5 mm posterior subglottic extension.[5]

SCPL–CHEP: Resection of true and false cords, paraglottic spaces, and entire thyroid cartilage. Arytenoids and cricoid cartilage are preserved. CHEP is performed, which involves reconstruction by suturing cricoid to hyoid and epiglottis.

Supraglottis: Voice-preserving options include the following:

SGL: Swallow- and voice-preserving surgery that may be used for tumors of epiglottis, single arytenoid, aryepiglottic fold, or false cord. Included in resection are hyoid bone, epiglottis, superior half of thyroid cartilage, AE folds, and false cords to arytenoids.

SCPL–CHEP: Resection of both true and false cords, paraglottic space, preepiglottic space, epiglottis, and thyroid cartilage. Reconstruction includes suturing of cricoid to hyoid, cricohyoidopexy. Total laryngectomy includes removal of larynx, pharynx is reconstructed (often with free flap), and permanent tracheostomy is required. For patients treated with primary surgical approach, elective neck dissection of bilateral levels II to IV is warranted for most patients with supraglottic cancer and for locally advanced glottic disease.

Chemotherapy: Concurrent CHT is not routinely given for early-stage disease, but is considered by some for unfavorable T2 disease (impaired mobility). In definitive chemoRT for T2b or stage III to stage IVB disease, concurrent cisplatin is the standard of care, given as 100 mg/m² bolus weeks 1, 4, 7 (NCCN Category 1) OR 40 mg/m² weekly (NCCN category 2B). Cetuximab can be used for nonplatinum candidates, with loading dose of 400 mg/m² 1 week prior to RT followed by 250 mg/m² weekly during RT. Use of induction CHT is controversial but has been used to select patients for laryngectomy versus preservation and consists of docetaxel, cisplatin, 5-fluorouracil (TPF) q3 weeks × 4 cycles completed 4 to 7 weeks prior to RT.

Radiation

Indications: Early-stage disease (cT1–T2N0) is typically treated with RT alone. Locally advanced disease is treated definitively (larynx preservation) or postoperatively (see Chapter 17). Nodal basins are typically not electively included in RT volumes in early-stage glottic patients unless supraglottic involvement is suspected, making risk of occult nodal metastasis higher. Cervical LN levels II to IV are targeted bilaterally and level V is included for node-positive hemineck or with primary tumor extension to base of tongue. Consider inclusion of level VIa for anterior soft-tissue extension or emergency tracheostomy with tumor cut-through. Consider level VIb with subglottic extension of primary tumor.

Dose: For T1N0 glottic cancers, accelerated hypofractionation has been shown to improve LC compared to standard fractionation. Recommended dose is 63 Gy/28 fx (2.25 Gy/fx). For T2aN0 disease, common dose is 65.25 Gy/29 fx. For patients with T2bN0 disease, LC is inferior with RT alone and thus alternative approaches including addition of concurrent CHT or hyperfractionation are considered. For locally advanced disease, 70 Gy/35 fx with CHT is common.

Toxicity: Acute: Fatigue, dysphagia, mucositis, hoarseness, xerostomia, odynophagia, RT dermatitis, dysgeusia, aspiration. Late: Dysphagia, esophageal stricture, aspiration, hoarseness, hearing loss, renal insufficiency, neck fibrosis, stroke, hypothyroidism.

Procedure: See *Handbook of Treatment Planning in Radiation Oncology*, Chapter 4.[6]

■ EVIDENCE-BASED Q&A

EARLY-STAGE DISEASE

■ What is the general treatment paradigm for early-stage disease?

Both RT and laryngeal preservation surgery provide excellent outcomes for early-stage disease.

Retrospective evidence demonstrates 5-year DFS above 90% for stage I disease and around 80% for stage II disease with either definitive RT or surgery.[7] Randomized data are sparse, however. Small randomized trial published in 2014[8] did show less patient-reported hoarseness in those treated with RT compared to those treated with transoral laser surgery, but overall voice quality was similar. In general, voice quality is related to amount of vocal cord resected.

■ What is the impact of larger fraction size for early-stage disease?

Mild hypofractionation and acceleration has shown consistent improvement in local control for early disease.

Le, UCSF (*IJROBP* 1997, PMID 9300746): RR of 398 patients with T1 to T2 glottic cancer (315 T1, 83 T2) treated with definitive RT to median dose of 63 Gy. Overall, 5-yr LC was 85% for T1 patients and 70% for T2 patients. Anterior commissure involvement and earlier treatment era predicted for worse LC in T1 patients. In T2 patients (but NOT T1), poor prognostic factors for LC included overall treatment time (>43 days), smaller fraction size (<1.8 Gy/fx), lower total dose (≤65 Gy) impaired VC mobility, and subglottic extension.

Table 14.3 UCSF Experience in Early Larynx Cancer (cT2 patients)				5-Yr LC		5-Yr LC
	5-Yr LC					
Treatment time ≤43 days	100%	Fx ≥ 2.25 Gy/day	100%		>65 Gy	78%
Treatment time >43 days	84%	Fx < 1.8 Gy/day	44%		≤65 Gy	60%
p value	.003	p value	.003		p value	.01
No VC mobility impaired	79%	No subglottic extension	77%			
VC mobility impaired	45%	Subglottic extension	58%			
p value	.02	p value	.04			

Yamazaki, Japan (*IJROBP* 2006, PMID 16169681): PRT of 180 patients with T1N0 SCC of glottis (80% T1a) treated with definitive RT and randomized to 2 Gy/fx or 2.25 Gy/fx. For standard fractionation arm, patients treated to 60 Gy for tumor length <⅔ of glottis and to 66 Gy for ≥⅔ of glottis. In 2.25 Gy/fx arm, total dose was 56.25 and 63 Gy respectively for tumor length <⅔ and ≥⅔ of glottis respectively; 5-yr LC was 92% in hypofractionation arm compared to 77% in standard fractionation arm. Fraction size was independent predictor for LC. Acute and late toxicities were equivalent. **Conclusion: Decreasing overall treatment time with larger fraction sizes improved LC without causing increased acute or late toxicity in patients with T1N0 glottic cancer.**

■ What is impact of hyperfractionation for early-stage disease?

RTOG 95-12 demonstrated modest, but not statistically significant, benefit in local control with use of hyperfractionated RT in patients with T2N0 glottic cancer. T2b was a negative prognostic factor.

Trotti, RTOG 9512 (*IJROBP* 2014 PMID 25035199): PRT of 250 patients with T2N0 SCC of glottis treated with definitive RT randomized to hyperfractionation (79.2 Gy/66 fx at 1.2 Gy BID) or standard fractionation (70 Gy/35 fx). Primary end point was LC. While there were trends toward improved outcomes with HFRT, there were no significant differences in 5-yr LC (78% vs. 70%, $p = .14$), 5-yr DFS (49% vs. 40%, $p = .13$), or 5-yr OS (72% vs. 63%, $p = .29$). LC in T2b patients was relatively lower (70% T2b vs. 76% T2a, $p = .1$). No difference in rates of grade 3 to grade 4 late toxicity between treatment arms. Of note, the trial was powered to detect 15% absolute difference in 5-yr LC. **Conclusion: Hyperfractionation modestly improves LC, as seen in other disease sites of head and neck, though not statistically significant in this study.**

■ How should T2B patients be treated?

T2b glottic cancer has not been adopted by the AJCC but has been described as presence of hypomobile cord. Patients with T2b disease had worse control in RTOG 9512 (LC 70 vs. 76% $p = .10$ and LRC 63% vs. 74%, $p = .03$) and in other large retrospective series[9,10] and thus may benefit from alteration from standard treatment. Options to improve local control in this unfavorable subset include hyperfractionation, hypofractionation (e.g., 65.25 Gy/29 fx), or addition of concurrent CHT.[11]

■ **Is there any role for IMRT in early-stage population?**

There is no routine role, and IMRT should be considered investigational. Proposed rationale is late toxicity avoidance, particularly vascular toxicity with carotid sparing. Early series have shown that carotid sparing is feasible without detriment in local control,[12,13] but results are still immature at this time.

LOCALLY ADVANCED DISEASE

■ **What is the basis for larynx preservation for locally advanced disease?**

While definitive surgery followed by PORT had been the traditional paradigm, the VA Larynx Study prospectively demonstrated equivalent survival rates with nonoperative approach and RTOG 91-11 demonstrated superior rates of larynx preservation with concurrent chemoRT compared to patients treated with either induction CHT or RT, or RT alone. T4 patients had higher rate of needing salvage laryngectomy in VA Larynx study and thus a large volume of T4 patients were excluded in RTOG 91-11. However, an NCDB analysis demonstrated that majority of patients with T4a disease still undergo organ preservation paradigm in clinical practice, despite general guidelines, with inferior overall survival compared to those who had TL (median survival 61 mos vs. 39 mos).[14] Multiple individual retrospective series have also identified tumor volume as prognostic for outcomes in addition to T stage.

Wolf, VA Larynx Study (*NEJM* 1991, PMID 2034244): PRT of 332 patients with stage III to stage IV locally advanced SCC of larynx (63% supraglottis, 57% vocal cord fixation) randomized to induction CHT followed by RT or total laryngectomy followed by post-op RT. Patients in larynx preservation arm received cisplatin 100 mg/m^2 and 5-FU 1,000 mg/m^2/d × 5 days on days 1 and 22. Tumor response was assessed by exam and indirect laryngoscopy 18 to 21 days after 2nd cycle. Patients w/o at least PR in larynx and those w/ any evidence of disease progression (including neck disease) underwent salvage laryngectomy. Patients w/ at least PR at primary tumor site and no progression of any neck lymphadenopathy received 3rd cycle of CHT on day 43. This was followed by definitive RT consisting of 66 to 76 Gy delivered at 1.8 to 2 Gy/fx to primary tumor site and 50 to 75 Gy to LNs. Twelve weeks after completion of RT, tumor response was reassessed; patients w/ persistent disease in larynx underwent salvage laryngectomy. Patients w/ persistent neck disease alone underwent neck dissection only. All laryngectomy patients underwent post-op RT consisting of 50 to 50.4 Gy for microscopic disease, 60 to 60.4 Gy for areas felt to be at high risk for local recurrence and 65 to 74.2 Gy for areas of residual disease. MFU 33 mos. Thirty-one percent had CR and 54% had PR after 2 cycles of CHT. Lack of response to induction CHT, however, was not associated with reduced OS. Rate of laryngeal preservation was 64%. Fifty-six percent of patients with T4 primary tumors required salvage laryngectomy (vs. 29% in remainder of study population). Rate of DM was lower in CHT arm, but LC was inferior. **Conclusion: Induction CHT followed by definitive RT can be effective in preserving larynx in high percentage of patients, w/o compromising OS.**

Table 14.4 Results of VA Larynx Study				
	2-Yr OS	2-Yr LC	Recurrence at Site of Primary	DM
Induction CHT + Definitive RT	68%	80%	12%	11%
TL + PORT	68%	93%	2%	17%
p value	.9846	.001	.001	.001

Forastiere, RTOG 91-11 (*NEJM* 2003, PMID 14645636; Update *JCO* 2013, PMID 23182993): PRT of 518 patients with SCC of supraglottic/glottic larynx, stage III to stage IV (T1 or T4 with tumor extending through thyroid cartilage into neck of soft tissue or >1 cm of BOT involvement were excluded) randomized to 1 of 3 arms: Arm 1 (Induction, from VA Larynx): cisplatin 100 mg/m^2 day 1 + 5-FU 1,000 mg/m^2/day for 5 days for 2 cycles on day 1 and day 22 followed by response evaluation. Those with less than PR or progression proceeded to laryngectomy with PORT. Those with CR or PR continued to additional cycle of cisplatin/5-FU followed by 70 Gy/35 fx RT alone. Arm 2 (chemoRT): cisplatin 100 mg/m^2 days 1, 22, 43 concurrent with 70 Gy/35 fx. Arm 3 (RT alone): 70 Gy/35 fx. Patients with single LN >3 cm or multiple LNs underwent neck dissection 8 weeks after completion of therapy. Seven end points were reported but primary end point was LFS. Standard arm was induction. Update published with MFU of 10.8 yrs. In an update, compared to induction, chemoRT improved larynx preservation, LC, and LRC but not LFS (primary end point) and trended to worse OS ($P = .08$) potentially suggestive of unexplained late effects. See Table 14.5. **Conclusion: Concurrent chemoRT declared "winner" due to LRC and LP benefit although LFS was similar.**

Table 14.5 Ten-Year Results of the RTOG 9111 Larynx Preservation Trial							
Arm	LFS (1°)	LP	LC	LRC	DC	DFS	OS
1. Induction	28.9%*	67.5%	53.7%	48.9%	83.4%	20.4%	38.8%
2. ChemoRT	23.5%*	81.7%*†	69.2%*†	65.3%*†	83.9%	21.6%*	27.5%
3. RT alone	17.2%†	63.8%	50.1%	47.2%	76.0%	14.8%	31.5%

*Significant relative to RT alone.
†Significant relative to induction (standard arm).

■ What is role of cetuximab for locally advanced laryngeal cancer?

The Bonner trial[14] established survival benefit with addition of cetuximab to RT in patients with locally advanced SCCHN.

Bonner, Cetuximab Secondary Analysis (*JAMA Otolaryngol Head Neck Surg* 2016, PMID 27389475): Secondary analysis of original Bonner trial investigating role of cetuximab in larynx preservation. Arms included RT alone vs. RT with concurrent cetuximab; 168 patients with larynx or hypopharynx cancers were included in this subset (90 in cetuximab, 78 in RT alone). Two-year rates of larynx preservation were 87.9% for cetuximab and 85.7% for RT alone (HR: 0.57, 95% CI: 0.23–1.42, $p = .22$). HR for laryngectomy-free survival was 0.78 ($p = .17$). No difference in OS. **Conclusion: There was statistically nonsignificant benefit to cetuximab with regard to larynx preservation and laryngectomy-free survival.** *Comment: Conclusions are limited by lack of power and retrospective nature of subset analysis.*

REFERENCES

1. Siegel RL, Miller KD, Jemal A. Cancer statistics, 2020. *CA Cancer J Clin.* 2020;70(1):7–30. doi:10.3322/caac.21590
2. Hoffman HT, Porter K, Karnell LH, et al. Laryngeal cancer in united states: changes in demographics, patterns of care, and survival. *Laryngoscope.* 2006;116(9, Pt 2, Suppl 111):1–13. doi:10.1097/01.mlg.0000236095.97947.26
3. Dahm JD, Sessions DG, Paniello RC, Harvey J. Primary subglottic cancer. *Laryngoscope.* 1998;108(5):741–746. doi:10.1097/00005537-199805000-00022
4. Beitler JJ, Muller S, Grist WJ, et al. Prognostic accuracy of computed tomography findings for patients with laryngeal cancer undergoing laryngectomy. *J Clin Oncol.* 2010;28(14):2318–2322. doi:10.1200/JCO.2009.24.7544
5. Fein DA, Mendenhall WM, Parsons JT, Million RR. T1-T2 squamous cell carcinoma of glottic larynx treated with RT: multivariate analysis of variables potentially influencing local control. *Int J Radiat Oncol Biol Phys.* 1993;25(4):605–611. doi:10.1016/0360-3016(93)90005-G
6. Videtic GMM, Woody N, Vassil AD. *Handbook of Treatment Planning in RT Oncology.* 3rd ed. Demos Medical; 2020. doi:10.1891/9780826168429
7. Tamura Y, Tanaka S, Asato R, et al. Therapeutic outcomes of laryngeal cancer at kyoto university hospital for 10 years. *Acta Otolaryngol Suppl.* 2007(557):62–65. doi:10.1080/00016480601067990
8. Aaltonen LM, Rautiainen N, Sellman J, et al. Voice quality after treatment of early vocal cord cancer: randomized trial comparing laser surgery with RT therapy. *Int J Radiat Oncol Biol Phys.* 2014;90(2):255–260. doi:10.1016/j.ijrobp.2014.06.032
9. Mendenhall WM, Amdur RJ, Morris CG, Hinerman RW. T1-T2N0 squamous cell carcinoma of glottic larynx treated with RT therapy. *J Clin Oncol.* 2001;19(20):4029–4036. doi:10.1200/JCO.2001.19.20.4029
10. Le QT, Fu KK, Kroll S, et al. Influence of fraction size, total dose, and overall time on local control of T1-T2 glottic carcinoma. *Int J Radiat Oncol Biol Phys.* 1997;39(1):115–126. doi:10.1016/S0360-3016(97)00284-8
11. Bhateja P, Ward MC, Hunter GH, et al. Impaired vocal cord mobility in T2N0 glottic carcinoma: suboptimal local control with RT alone. *Head Neck.* 2016;38(12):1832–1836. doi:10.1002/hed.24520
12. Zumsteg ZS, Riaz N, Jaffery S, et al. Carotid sparing intensity-modulated RT therapy achieves comparable locoregional control to conventional RT in T1-2N0 laryngeal carcinoma. *Oral Oncol.* 2015;51(7):716–723. doi:10.1016/j.oraloncology.2015.02.003
13. Ward MC, Pham YD, Kotecha R, et al. Clinical and dosimetric implications of intensity-modulated RT for early-stage glottic carcinoma. *Med Dosim.* 2016;41(1):64–69. doi:10.1016/j.meddos.2015.08.004
14. Grover S, Swisher-McClure S, Mitra N, et al. Total laryngectomy versus larynx preservation for T4a larynx cancer: patterns of care and survival outcomes. *Int J Radiat Oncol Biol Phys.* 2015;92(3):594–601. doi:10.1016/j.ijrobp.2015.03.004

15 ■ SALIVARY GLAND TUMORS

Sarah S. Kilic, Martin C. Tom, Shlomo A. Koyfman, and Nikhil P. Joshi

QUICK HIT: ■ Salivary gland tumors are an uncommon group of benign and malignant neoplasms with natural histories that vary by histology. The most common benign histology is pleomorphic adenoma. The most common malignant histology depends on location: parotid gland, mucoepidermoid carcinoma; submandibular and minor salivary glands, adenoid cystic carcinoma. Surgery is the standard of care for all histologies; the facial nerve should be preserved if possible. Postoperative RT should be considered for those at high risk of recurrence (Table 15.1). No benefit to CHT has been demonstrated prospectively.

Table 15.1 General Treatment Paradigm for Malignant Salivary Cancer				
Surgical Resection With Consideration of Adjuvant RT as Follows				
Primary Site			**Ipsilateral Neck**	
Stage I to stage II and no risk factors	Observation		cN0 or pN0 and low risk	Observation
T3–4, PNI, deep lobe involvement, bone involvement, high grade or recurrent disease	60 Gy		Pathologic node-negative with risk factors (*see Terhaard and RTOG 1008*): T3–4, high grade, facial nerve deficit, recurrent disease	50 to 54 Gy levels II to IV
			Node-positive, resected	60 Gy levels Ib to V
Margin-positive or close margins (<1 mm)	66 Gy		ECE	66 Gy
Gross disease	70 Gy		Gross nodal disease	70 Gy

EPIDEMIOLOGY: Salivary gland tumors are rare neoplasms that represent approximately 6% of H&N cancers[1], with roughly 2,500 cases in the United States annually.[2] Benign histologies are more common in young females (median age 46).[3,4] Malignant histologies are more common with older age (median age 54) and have an increasing male predilection with increasing age.[2,4] Histology is classified according to the WHO 2005 system, with over 40 different histologies defined.[2] The parotid gland is the most common site (70% of all tumors, 75% of which are benign), with 22% in minor glands and 8% in submandibular glands.[4]

RISK FACTORS: Risk factors are not clearly defined. Strongest evidence is for RT exposure, as shown among Hiroshima/Nagasaki survivors.[5] Smoking is not a risk factor (except in Warthin's tumor; see Table 15.2). EBV has been implicated in lymphoepithelial carcinomas,[6] and other viruses are under investigation.

ANATOMY: Major salivary glands consist of parotid, submandibular, and sublingual gland (between mylohyoid and floor of mouth mucosa). Borders of parotid are second maxillary molar (anterior), zygomatic arch (superior), internal jugular vein (deep), mastoid tip (posterior), and posterior digastric muscle (inferior). Parotid contributes primarily to stimulated serous saliva production, and submandibular to unstimulated mucous/serous saliva (and, therefore, RT-induced xerostomia).[7] Parotid lies behind ramus of mandible and is separated into superficial and deep lobes by facial nerve. Retromandibular vein is common radiographic landmark for facial nerve. Stensen's duct drains to buccal mucosa. Facial nerve (CN VII) courses through parotid after exiting stylomastoid foramen. There are five branches of CN VII: temporal, zygomatic, buccal, marginal mandibular, and cervical. CN VII controls facial muscles and taste to oral tongue. Auriculotemporal nerve originates from V3, innervates parotid (salivation/parasympathetic), and can be route of perineural spread; if damaged during surgery, this can aberrantly regenerate to innervate skin, causing auriculotemporal syndrome (preauricular sweating and flushing), also called Frey's syndrome after Dr. Lucie Frey, one of the first female European neurologists, who characterized it in 1923.[7] Submandibular is innervated by chorda tympani, and perineural spread can be to CN XII, to CN V via lingual nerve, or to CN VII via chorda tympani. Minor salivary glands are distributed throughout aerodigestive epithelium. Multiple contouring guides are available to aid in anatomy of cranial nerves when PNI is present.[8,9]

Table 15.2 Characteristics of Salivary Tumors

	Parotid	Submandibular	Sublingual	Minor Glands
Pathology[4,10]	75% benign, 25% malignant	50% benign, 50% malignant	75% malignant	
Frequency[4]	70%	8%	22%	
Salivary fluid[3,10]	Serous	Mixed	Mucous	
Associated nerves	CN VII (facial) with spread to V3 via chorda tympani	V3 (lingual) and XII (hypoglossal)	V3 (lingual)	Location dependent

PATHOLOGY: Most common histologies listed in Tables 15.3 and 15.4, in order of decreasing incidence. Grade is prognostic for mucoepidermoid carcinoma, adenocarcinoma, salivary duct carcinoma, and acinic cell carcinoma.[2] Adenoid cystic carcinoma is graded by percentage of solid component (high grade if >30% solid).

Table 15.3 Benign Salivary Tumor Histologies

Pleomorphic adenoma	Most common salivary gland tumor, two thirds of parotid tumors, two thirds are females in their 40s. Treatment is surgery, with <5% risk of recurrence, but beware of tumor spillage, in which case recurrence can be up to 45%. Risk of second recurrence is 46%. Can transform into carcinoma *ex* pleomorphic adenoma (CExP). Rate of transformation is <1% in patients without recurrence; 4% with recurrence.[3] Consider RT to 50 to 60 Gy for multiple recurrences, deep involvement, or large tumors.[11]
Warthin's tumor	Often of parotid, often bilateral (6%).[12] Associated with smoking, more common in men.[13] Can be highly PET-avid and is often an incidental finding on PET. Malignant degeneration is rare (<1%)[10]; observation is reasonable.
Basal cell adenoma	Approximately 2% of salivary tumors.[10] May be confused with basal cell of skin metastatic to parotid lymph nodes.
Oncocytoma	1% of salivary tumors. Slowly progressive parotid tumor in older patients.

Table 15.4 Malignant Salivary Tumor Histologies

Mucoepidermoid	Most common parotid malignancy. Grade is prognostic. Most are curable with surgery alone.
Adenoid cystic carcinoma	Almost always demonstrates PNI and can track along cranial nerves. Tubular pattern is most favorable, cribriform is intermediate, and solid is least favorable. Greater than 30% solid pattern is considered high-grade. Long natural history. Risk of nodal involvement classically thought to be <5%, but recent data as high as 37% in oral cavity and 19% in major glands.[14,15] Indolent distant metastases to lungs in up to 50%.[10] Late recurrences (>20 years) can be seen. Most benefit from adjuvant RT.[16]
Adenocarcinoma, NOS	Grade is prognostic, nodal metastases seen in 50% to 60% of high-grade lesions.[15]
Acinic cell carcinoma	Low-grade, slowly progressive tumors, 80% within parotid. Submandibular tumors are uncommon and most aggressive.[10]
Carcinoma *ex* pleomorphic adenoma	4% of salivary tumors, 12% of malignancies. Degenerated pleomorphic adenoma. More than 80% of patients do not have history of known pleomorphic adenoma.[10]

(continued)

Table 15.4 Malignant Salivary Tumor Histologies (*continued*)

Salivary duct carcinoma	9% of salivary malignancies. Males more common (4:1). Aggressive, high grade, similar to high-grade breast ductal carcinoma.[10] Androgen receptor and HER2 amplification common.
Metastasis to salivary gland	5% of salivary malignancies,[10] incidence varies by region based on frequency of skin cancer. Mostly squamous cell carcinoma of skin followed by melanoma.
Epithelial–myoepithelial	Only 1% of salivary tumors, twice as common in women, 60% parotid, typically slow growing.

GENETICS: EGFR, c-kit, HER2, NTRK fusion, and androgen receptor positivity have all been described, most commonly in salivary duct carcinomas,[17] but no standard role for targeted agents in the non-metastatic setting.

CLINICAL PRESENTATION: Most present initially as slowly progressive painless mass. Adenoid cystic carcinoma may present initially as neuropathic pain (misdiagnosis as trigeminal neuralgia) and progress to facial nerve motor deficit.

WORKUP: H&P, including H&N exam with cranial nerve exam. Ultrasound can be helpful to differentiate between benign vs. malignant prior to biopsy. FNA sensitivity and specificity are 80% and >95%, respectively.[11] Contrast-enhanced MRI is critical for evaluation of perineural spread in malignant histologies. CT chest for malignant histologies. PET is not standard. Dental, nutrition, speech, and swallow evaluation as indicated.

PROGNOSTIC FACTORS: Stage, grade, histology, recurrence, positive margins, bone invasion, positive lymph nodes, facial nerve palsy.[11,18,19]

TREATMENT PARADIGM

Observation: Observation can be appropriate for benign histologies other than pleomorphic adenoma. Pleomorphic adenoma should be treated upfront in healthy patients due to risk of malignant transformation. Malignant histologies should always be treated.

Surgery: Surgical resection of the primary tumor is the standard of care for all technically resectable salivary gland tumors warranting treatment. Care should be taken to minimize risk of tumor spillage; enucleation should not be performed. Preservation of functional cranial nerves should be attempted. Microscopic margins preferred over facial nerve sacrifice, although not at the expense of residual gross disease.[20] Consider nerve grafting for reconstruction of sacrificed cranial nerve. For all locations and histologies, clinically node-positive neck should be dissected. For parotid tumors, elective nodal dissection of levels II to III, and possibly IV, may be recommended, and is surgeon dependent based on risk factors (size, stage, grade, histology, location). For submandibular tumors, elective dissection of levels I to III, again surgeon dependent. For parotid tumors, levels I and V may be at risk only if levels II to IV are involved.[11]

Table 15.5 AJCC 8th ed. (2017): Staging for Salivary Gland Cancer (Note that minor salivary cancers are staged according to their site of origin)

T/M \ N		cN0	cN1	cN2a	cN2b	cN2c	cN3a	cN3b
T1	• ≤2 cm	I						
T2	• 2.1 to 4 cm	II	III		IVA			
T3	• >4 cm and/or extraparenchymal extension							
T4a	• Invasion[1]							
T4b	• Invasion[2]				IVB			
M1	• Distant metastasis				IVC			

Notes: Invasion[1] = Invasion of skin, mandible, ear canal, or facial nerve. Invasion[2] = Invasion of skull base, pterygoid plates and/or encasing carotid artery. Nodal category definition is similar to other non-HPV-associated head and neck cancers; see Table 11.4 for clinical and pathologic nodal categories.

Chemotherapy: Addition of CHT for high-risk lesions is investigational and retrospective data are inconsistent.[21-23] *RTOG 1008 is an ongoing phase II/III study of adjuvant RT 60–66 Gy vs. adjuvant RT 60–66 Gy with concurrent cisplatin 40 mg/m² weekly. Included are patients with resected intermediate- or high-grade adenocarcinoma, intermediate- or high-grade mucoepidermoid carcinoma, high-grade salivary duct carcinoma, high-grade acinic cell carcinoma, and high-grade (>30% solid component) adenoid cystic carcinoma with any of the following risk factors: T3–T4, or N+, or T1–T2 AND positive/close (≤1 mm) margins.* Regarding targeted therapies, many early studies (imatinib,[24] lapatinib,[25] and dasatinib[26]) for salivary tumors have had disappointing results. Notably, the tyrosine kinase inhibitors larotrectinib and entrectinib have shown encouraging response rates (>75%) for NTRK fusion-positive tumors across various primary sites, including salivary gland.[27] Phase I/II studies of combined androgen blockade (for androgen receptor-positive salivary duct carcinomas),[28] lenvatinib (for adenoid cystic carcinoma),[29] and pembrolizumab (for any PD-L1-positive histology)[30] have shown some promise.

Radiation

Indications and dose: Consider RT for pT3–4 disease, close or positive margins, high-grade, recurrent disease, positive lymph nodes, PNI, LVSI, or bone invasion. Adenoid cystic carcinomas typically display significant PNI and are treated with RT. Role of RT for T1 lesions with risk factors is unclear (NCCN category 2B):[20] 60 Gy to primary site and 54 Gy to elective neck (if included) is recommended. Dose should be escalated to 66 Gy for positive margins or extracapsular extension, and to 70 Gy for gross disease.[11,20] Treatment of ipsilateral neck for pathologically node-positive disease is required, and elective nodal coverage should be considered for pT3–4, high-grade, facial nerve deficits, or recurrent disease.

Procedure: See *Handbook of Treatment Planning in Radiation Oncology*, Chapter 4.[31]

Complications: Oral mucositis, odynophagia, skin erythema, altered taste, partial xerostomia, trismus, hypothyroidism, and ear complications (secretory otitis media or partial hearing loss). Limit contralateral parotid to mean 26 Gy if possible. TD 5/5 of parotid is 32 Gy.

Neutrons: Higher LC, but more late effects than photons. RBE is >2.6. Neutrons lack skin sparing, are less affected by hypoxia, and are less cell cycle dependent than photons. Consider for unresectable or recurrent tumors, particularly adenoid cystic. In one small series of tumors involving base of skull, 3-year LC doubled (39%–82%) with SRS boost following neutron treatment, without increased toxicity.[32] Complications include osteoradionecrosis, fibrosis, cervical myelopathy, CNS necrosis, optic neuritis, palatal fistula, retinopathy, and glaucoma.

■ EVIDENCE-BASED Q&A

▨ What are the indications for postoperative RT?

Because salivary cancer is relatively rare, no prospective trials have been performed. Therefore, indications for postoperative RT are based on retrospective evidence. In general, adjuvant RT indications include pT3–4 disease, close or positive margins, high-grade, recurrent disease, positive lymph nodes, PNI, LVSI, or bone invasion.

Terhaard, Netherlands (*Head & Neck* 2005, PMID 15629600): RR of 498 patients treated for salivary cancers between 1984 and 1995; 386 patients received RT to median dose of 62 Gy (60.7 Gy for negative margins, 62.4 Gy for close, and 64 Gy for positive). Forty percent received elective nodal RT. Ten-year LC improved for those with T3–4 tumors, close (<5 mm) and positive margins, PNI, and bone invasion. Unresectable patients showed dose response, with 5-year LC of 0% for <66 Gy, and 50% for ≥66 Gy. **Conclusion: Postoperative RT indicated for T3–4 disease, close or positive margins, bone invasion, and PNI. Risk of nodal disease was defined using T-stage and histology.**

Armstrong, Memorial Sloan Kettering (*Arch Otolaryngol Head Neck Surg* 1990, PMID 2306346): Matched-pair analysis of 46 patients treated with postoperative RT after 1966 matched to those treated with surgery alone prior to 1966. Median RT dose was 56.64 Gy. For entire cohort, 5-yr CSS and LC were not statistically significantly different between surgery alone and surgery plus RT groups. However, RT did improve CSS (51% vs. 10%, $p = .015$) and LC (73% vs. 66%, $p = $ NS) for stages III–IV patients. Node-positive patients also had CSS (49% vs. 19%, $p = .015$) and local control (69% vs. 40%, $p = .05$) benefits. **Conclusion: Stages III to IV and node positivity are indications for postoperative radiotherapy.**

Table 15.6 Results of Terhaard et al, 2005

10-Year Local Control	No RT	RT		Risk of Positive Neck Nodes (%) by Score and Primary Location				
				T Score + Histology Score*	Parotid	Submandibular	Oral Cavity	Other
T3–4 tumor	18%	84%		2	4%	0%	4%	0%

10-Year Local Control	No RT	RT		Risk of Positive Neck Nodes (%) by Score and Primary Location				
				T Score + Histology Score*	Parotid	Submandibular	Oral Cavity	Other
Close margins	55%	95%		3	12%	33%	13%	29%
Positive margins	44%	82%		4	25%	57%	19%	56%
Bone invasion	54%	86%		5	33%	60%	–	–
PNI	60%	88%		6	38%	50%	–	–
All results statistically significant.				*Scoring: T1 = 1, T2 = 2, T3-4 = 3. Acinic/adenoid cystic/CExP = 1, MucoEp = 2, Squamous/Undifferentiated = 3.				

North, Johns Hopkins (*IJROBP* 1990, PMID 2115032): RR of 87 patients with major salivary gland tumors treated from 1975 to 1987 with surgery with or without RT. Thirty-four percent had neck dissection. Seventy-four percent received RT (60 Gy for negative margins, 66 Gy for close or positive margins, and 72 Gy for gross disease). Postoperative RT improved local recurrence for untreated and recurrent patients and improved 5-yr OS (75% vs. 59%, $p = .014$). Negative prognostic factors included facial nerve palsy, undifferentiated histology, male gender, skin involvement, and no RT. **Conclusion: RT should only be omitted for patients with low-grade T1–2 tumors with negative margins.**

Cho, Korea (*Ann Surg Oncol* 2016, PMID 27342828): RR of 179 patients with low-grade salivary gland cancers (LGSGC). Ten-year OS was 96.6% and RFS was 89.6%. Adjuvant RT improved RFS for patients with node positivity, PNI, LVSI, extraparenchymal extension, positive margin, or T3–4. Close margins (<5 mm) did not increase risk of recurrence. T1–2 patients without risk factors had low risk of recurrence after surgery alone. **Conclusion: Adjuvant RT improves RFS for high-risk LGSGC. Low-risk LGSGC (T1–2 without risk factors) have good outcomes after surgery alone.**

■ **Which patients are at higher risk of nodal metastasis?**

High-grade, vascular invasion, facial nerve palsy, histology, and higher T stage appear to predict risk for nodal metastases.

Xiao, NCDB Analysis (*Otolaryngol Head Neck Surg* 2016, PMID 26419838): NCDB analysis of 22,653 cases of primary parotid cancer with pathologic LN evaluation. N0 patients had improved 5-yr OS compared to N+ (79% vs. 40%, $p < .001$). Patients with low-grade tumors had improved 5-yr OS vs. high grade (88% vs. 69%, $p < .001$). Incidence of N+ independently predicted by high grade (50.9% vs. 9.3% in low grade) and high T stage. **Conclusion: Incidence of occult nodal disease varies by histology. High T stage and grade predict nodal disease in most histologies.**

Table 15.7 Incidence of Nodal Metastases in Parotid Malignancies

Primary Parotid Cancer Histology	cN+ (%)	Occult N+ (%)	Occult N+ (High Grade % N+ /T4 % N+)
Salivary ductal carcinoma	53.5	23.6	36/40
Adenocarcinoma NOS	45.2	19.9	31.6/31.6
Carcinoma ex-pleomorphic adenoma	23.9	11.8	19.2/35.5

(continued)

Table 15.7 Incidence of Nodal Metastases in Parotid Malignancies (*continued*)			
Primary Parotid Cancer Histology	cN+ (%)	Occult N+ (%)	Occult N+ (High Grade % N + /T4 % N+)
Mucoepidermoid carcinoma	20.2	9.3	21.8/21.6
Adenoid cystic carcinoma	14.2	7.0	9.6/13
Acinar cell carcinoma	10	4.4	24.5/11.5
Basal cell adenocarcinoma	9.4	6.3	6.7/22.2
Epithelial–myoepithelial carcinoma	4.8	1.5	0/0
Average	24.4	10.2	

■ **Can salivary cancer be treated with RT alone?**

Based on retrospective evidence, surgery is essential for local control and is the accepted standard of care for medically operable and technically resectable patients.

Mendenhall, University of Florida (*Cancer* 2005, PMID 15880750): RR of 224 patients treated between 1964 and 2003 with RT alone (*n* = 64) or surgery with RT (*n* = 160). Median dose was 74 Gy for RT alone and 66 Gy for postoperative. LRC was significantly worse with RT alone (stages I–III 89% vs. 70%, *p* = .01; stage IV 66% vs. 24%, *p* = .002; overall 81% vs. 40%, *p* < .0001). In patients with technically unresectable disease treated with RT alone, 10-yr LRC was 20%. **Conclusion: RT alone is inferior to surgery combined with RT in terms of LRC.**

■ **Does neutron therapy offer improved control or survival outcomes?**

Local control is improved without survival benefit. Cost and toxicity are significant.

Laramore, RTOG 8001-MRC Trial (*IJROBP* 1993, PMID 8407397): PRT in England and the United States of 25 patients with inoperable or unresectable salivary cancer randomized to photon/electron therapy or neutron therapy. CR was more frequent in neutron arm. LC was significantly improved in neutron arm (56% vs. 17%, *p* = .009), leading to early closure of trial. No difference in OS (15% vs. 25%, *p* = NS). However, severe late complications were seen in 69% of neutron patients vs. 15% of photon patients (*p* = .07). **Conclusion: Neutron RT improves local control, but does not improve survival, and has a much higher rate of long-term toxicity.**

Douglas, University of Washington (*Arch Otolaryngol Head Neck Surg* 2003, PMID 12975266): RR of 279 patients treated with fast neutrons for salivary gland cancers, 263 of whom had evidence of gross disease at time of treatment. MFU of 36 months. Total dose delivered was between 17.4 and 20.7 nGy, with fractions given 3 to 4 times per week. CSS and LRC were 67% and 59% at 6 years, respectively. Grades 3–4 RTOG toxicity at 6 years was 10%. **Conclusion: For gross residual disease, neutrons offer modest local control and good survival outcomes.**

■ **Is modern RT as effective as neutron therapy with less toxicity?**

This was suggested by a small RR from MSKCC, though data are limited.

Spratt, MSKCC (*Radiol Oncol* 2014, PMID 24587780): RR of 27 patients with unresectable salivary cancer treated with photons to median dose of 70 Gy with IMRT or 3D-CRT. Eighteen patients also received CHT. At MFU 52 months, 5-yr LRC was 47%, which compared favorably to neutron arm of RTOG 8001. **Conclusion: Modern photon therapy with or without CHT may be a reasonable alternative to neutrons with less toxicity.**

■ **Is there a role for carbon ion therapy in the treatment of salivary gland tumors?**

Jensen, COSMIC Trial (IJROBP 2015, PMID 26279022): *German prospective phase II trial of 53 patients with malignant salivary gland tumors. All patients treated with 24 Gy (RBE) C12 followed by IMRT 50 Gy. MFU 42 months. At 3 years, LC 82%, PFS 58%, and OS 78%. High rates of long-term hearing impairment*

(25%) and "adverse events of the eye" (20%). **Conclusion: Carbon ion + IMRT treatment offered good control outcomes, but with significant late toxicities.**

■ **Does the addition of adjuvant chemoRT improve outcomes compared to adjuvant RT alone?**

Several small retrospective analyses have demonstrated promising control rates.[21–23] Conversely, an NCDB analysis actually revealed inferior survival with adjuvant chemoRT compared to RT alone.[33] RTOG 1008 is a phase II/III RCT that aims to answer this question in high-risk salivary gland cancer.

Amini, NCDB (*JAMA Otolaryngol Head Neck Surg*** 2016, PMID: 27541166):** NCDB analysis of 2,210 patients with salivary gland cancer s/p resection comparing adjuvant chemoRT to adjuvant RT alone. Included grade 2 or 3 with ≥1 adverse feature (T3–4, N+, or margin 83% received RT, 17% received chemoRT). At MFU of 39 months, 5-yr OS was inferior with chemoRT compared to RT alone (39% vs. 54%, $p < .001$). OS with chemoRT was inferior on MVA (HR: 1.22, $p = .02$) and trended to inferiority on propensity score matched analysis (HR: 1.20, $p = .08$). **Conclusion: In high-risk salivary gland cancer, adjuvant chemoRT was not associated with improved OS compared to adjuvant RT alone, and may actually worsen outcomes.**

REFERENCES

1. Boukheris H, Curtis RE, Land CE, Dores GM. Incidence of carcinoma of the major salivary glands according to the WHO classification, 1992 to 2006: a population-based study in the United States. *Cancer Epidemiol Biomarkers Prev.* 2009;18(11):2899–2906. doi:10.1158/1055-9965.EPI-09-0638

2. Guzzo M, Locati LD, Prott FJ, et al. Major and minor salivary gland tumors. *Crit Rev Oncol Hematol.* 2010;74(2):134–148. doi:10.1016/j.critrevonc.2009.10.004

3. Andreasen S, Therkildsen MH, Bjorndal K, Homoe P. Pleomorphic adenoma of the parotid gland 1985–2010: a danish nationwide study of incidence, recurrence rate, and malignant transformation. *Head Neck.* 2016;38 Suppl 1:E1364–E1369. doi:10.1002/hed.24228

4. Spiro RH. Salivary neoplasms: overview of a 35-year experience with 2,807 patients. *Head Neck Surg.* 1986;8(3):177–184. doi:10.1002/hed.2890080309

5. Saku T, Hayashi Y, Takahara O, et al. Salivary gland tumors among atomic bomb survivors, 1950–1987. *Cancer.* 1997;79(8):1465–1475. doi:10.1002/(SICI)1097-0142(19970415)79:8<1465::AID-CNCR4>3.0.CO;2-A

6. Leung SY, Chung LP, Yuen ST, et al. Lymphoepithelial carcinoma of the salivary gland: in situ detection of epstein-barr virus. *J Clin Pathol.* 1995;48(11):1022–1027. doi:10.1136/jcp.48.11.1022

7. Motz KM, Kim YJ. Auriculotemporal syndrome (Frey Syndrome). *Otolaryngol Clin North Am.* 2016;49(2):501–509. doi:10.1016/j.otc.2015.10.010

8. Gluck I, Ibrahim M, Popovtzer A, et al. Skin cancer of the head and neck with perineural invasion: defining the clinical target volumes based on the pattern of failure. *Int J Radiat Oncol Biol Phys.* 2009;74(1):38–46. doi:10.1016/j.ijrobp.2008.06.1943

9. Ko HC, Gupta V, Mourad WF, et al. A contouring guide for head and neck cancers with perineural invasion. *Pract Radiat Oncol.* 2014;4(6):e247–e258. doi:10.1016/j.prro.2014.02.001

10. Fang P. Internal mammary misfortune. *Int J Radiat Oncol Biol Phys.* 2017;97(3):447. doi:10.1016/j.ijrobp.2016.10.032

11. Halperin EC, Brady LW, Perez CA, Wazer DE. *Perez & Brady's Principles and Practice of Radiation Oncology.* LWW; 2013.

12. Maiorano E, Lo Muzio L, Favia G, Piattelli A. Warthin's tumour: a study of 78 cases with emphasis on bilaterality, multifocality and association with other malignancies. *Oral Oncol.* 2002;38(1):35–40. doi:10.1016/S1368-8375(01)00019-7

13. Pinkston JA, Cole P. Cigarette smoking and warthin's tumor. *Am J Epidemiol.* 1996;144(2):183–187. doi:10.1093/oxfordjournals.aje.a008906

14. Amit M, Binenbaum Y, Sharma K, et al. Incidence of cervical lymph node metastasis and its association with outcomes in patients with adenoid cystic carcinoma. An International Collaborative Study. *Head Neck.* 2015;37(7):1032–1037. doi:10.1002/hed.23711

15. Xiao CC, Zhan KY, White-Gilbertson SJ, Day TA. Predictors of nodal metastasis in parotid malignancies: a national cancer data base study of 22,653 patients. *Otolaryngol Head Neck Surg.* 2016;154(1):121–130. doi:10.1177/0194599815607449

16. Lee A, Givi B, Osborn VW, et al. Patterns of care and survival of adjuvant radiation for major salivary adenoid cystic carcinoma. *Laryngoscope.* 2017;127(9):2057–2062. doi:10.1002/lary.26516

17. Can NT, Lingen MW, Mashek H, et al. Expression of hormone receptors and her-2 in benign and malignant salivary gland tumors. *Head Neck Pathol.* 2018;12(1):95–104. doi:10.1007/s12105-017-0833-y

18. Carrillo JF, Vazquez R, Ramirez-Ortega MC, et al. Multivariate prediction of the probability of recurrence in patients with carcinoma of the parotid gland. *Cancer.* 2007;109(10):2043–2051. doi:10.1002/cncr.22647

19. Storey MR, Garden AS, Morrison WH, et al. Postoperative radiotherapy for malignant tumors of the submandibular gland. *Int J Radiat Oncol, Biol, Phys.* 2001;51(4):952–958. doi:10.1016/S0360-3016(01)01724-2

20. Douglas JG, Koh WJ, Austin-Seymour M, Laramore GE. Treatment of salivary gland neoplasms with fast neutron radiotherapy. *Arch Otolaryngol Head Neck Surg.* 2003;129(9):944–948. doi:10.1001/archotol.129.9.944

21. Pederson AW, Salama JK, Haraf DJ, et al. Adjuvant chemoradiotherapy for locoregionally advanced and high-risk salivary gland malignancies. *Head Neck Oncol.* 2011;3:31. doi:10.1186/1758-3284-3-31

22. Schoenfeld JD, Sher DJ, Norris CM Jr, et al. Salivary gland tumors treated with adjuvant intensity-modulated radiotherapy with or without concurrent chemotherapy. *Int J Radiat Oncol Biol Phys.* 2012;82(1):308–314. doi:10.1016/j.ijrobp.2010.09.042

23. Tanvetyanon T, Qin D, Padhya T, et al. Outcomes of postoperative concurrent chemoradiotherapy for locally advanced major salivary gland carcinoma. *Arch Otolaryngol Head Neck Surg.* 2009;135(7):687–692. doi:10.1001/archoto.2009.70

24. Hotte SJ, Winquist EW, Lamont E, et al. Imatinib mesylate in patients with adenoid cystic cancers of the salivary glands expressing c-kit: a princess margaret hospital phase II consortium study. *J Clin Oncol.* 2005;23(3):585–590. doi:10.1200/JCO.2005.06.125

25. Agulnik M, Cohen EW, Cohen RB, et al. Phase II study of lapatinib in recurrent or metastatic epidermal growth factor receptor and/or erbB2 expressing adenoid cystic carcinoma and non adenoid cystic carcinoma malignant tumors of the salivary glands. *J Clin Oncol.* 2007;25(25):3978–3984. doi:10.1200/JCO.2007.11.8612

26. Wong SJ, Karrison T, Hayes DN, et al. Phase II trial of dasatinib for recurrent or metastatic c-KIT expressing adenoid cystic carcinoma and for nonadenoid cystic malignant salivary tumors. *Ann Oncol.* 2016;27(2):318–323. doi:10.1093/annonc/mdv537

27. Cocco E, Scaltriti M, Drilon A. NTRK fusion-positive cancers and TRK inhibitor therapy. *Nat Rev Clin Oncol.* 2018;15(12):731–747. doi:10.1038/s41571-018-0113-0

28. Fushimi C, Tada Y, Takahashi H, et al. A prospective phase II study of combined androgen blockade in patients with androgen receptor-positive metastatic or locally advanced unresectable salivary gland carcinoma. *Ann Oncol.* 2018;29(4):979–984. doi:10.1093/annonc/mdx771

29. Tchekmedyian V, Sherman EJ, Dunn L, et al. Phase II study of lenvatinib in patients with progressive, recurrent or metastatic adenoid cystic carcinoma. *J Clin Oncol.* 2019;37(18):1529–1537. doi:10.1200/JCO.18.01859

30. Cohen RB, Delord JP, Doi T, et al. Pembrolizumab for the treatment of advanced salivary gland carcinoma: findings of the phase 1b KEYNOTE-028 study. *Am J Clin Oncol.* 2018;41(11):1083–1088.

31. Videtic GMM WN, Vassil AD. *Handbook of Treatment Planning in Radiation Oncology.* 2nd ed. Demos Medical; 2015. doi:10.1891/9781617051975

32. Douglas JG, Goodkin R, Laramore GE. Gamma knife stereotactic radiosurgery for salivary gland neoplasms with base of skull invasion following neutron radiotherapy. *Head Neck.* 2008;30(4):492–496. doi:10.1002/hed.20729

33. Amini A, Waxweiler TV, Brower JV, et al. Association of adjuvant chemoradiotherapy vs radiotherapy alone with survival in patients with resected major salivary gland carcinoma: data from the national cancer data base. *JAMA Otolaryngol Head Neck Surg.* 2016;142(11):1100–1110. doi:10.1001/jamaoto.2016.2168

16 ■ CARCINOMA OF UNKNOWN PRIMARY OF THE HEAD AND NECK

Monica E. Shukla and Jeffrey A. Kittel

QUICK HIT ■ Head and neck CUP represents ~3% of H&N cancers. Detailed diagnostic workup is required to identify a primary source for malignancy (must include): comprehensive H&P, analysis of the histology and anatomic disease distribution (nodal levels), presence/absence of biomarkers (p16, HPV DNA, EBV DNA) advanced imaging (e.g., contrast-enhanced CT and PET/CT), diagnostic surgical procedures (e.g., palatine tonsillectomy), with further therapy guided by findings. Biopsy showing adenocarcinoma in the low neck should prompt evaluation for a salivary gland tumor, thoracic, gynecologic, or gastrointestinal primary. SCCUPs despite thorough workup are assumed to arise from H&N sites (mucosal or skin) and treated based on the probability of the primary site given anatomic location of nodal involvement and presence/absence of biomarkers. Two broad treatment approaches exist: primary surgery (with risk-adapted adjuvant RT ± chemotherapy) and definitive RT (± chemotherapy) (Table 16.1).

Table 16.1 General Treatment Paradigm for Unknown Primary Presenting as Squamous Carcinoma of H&N Lymph Nodes	
	Treatment Options
cT0N1	Option 1: Neck dissection (at least levels II–IV with or without TORS lingual tonsillectomy) • Observation with no additional adverse features • Add postoperative RT (PORT) for pN2/3 (see Chapter 17) • Add chemoRT for extranodal extension (ENE+) Option 2: RT alone
cT0N2-3	Option 1: Definitive chemoRT (favored for bilateral/bulky presentation or radiographic concern for ENE to avoid tri-modality therapy) Option 2: Neck dissection (with or without TORS lingual tonsillectomy) • Add PORT for pN2/3 (see Chapter 17) • Add chemoRT for ENE+

Dose: In 2 Gy/fx, treat gross disease to 66 to 70 Gy, low-risk neck to 54 to 56 Gy, and potential primary sites to 50 to 60 Gy (or a biologically equivalent dose scheme)

EPIDEMIOLOGY: CUP represents 2% to 3% of all newly diagnosed H&N carcinomas. Median age at diagnosis is 50 to 70 years with male predominance (M:F of 4:1). The majority of HNSCCUP in the United States are now HPV associated.[1]

RISK FACTORS: Standard risk factors for H&N cancer apply, as do those of other primaries that spread to cervical lymph nodes.

General: Alcohol, tobacco, betel and areca nuts, Plummer–Vinson syndrome. Oropharyngeal: HPV infection.

Nasopharyngeal: EBV infection, salt-cured foods, occupational smoke/dust exposure. Sinonasal: Nickel, wood dust, leather tanning agents. Cutaneous: UV exposure

ANATOMY: Pattern of nodal involvement on physical exam helps direct further workup toward potential sites of the occult primary.

Table 16.2 Lymph Node Levels* and Correlation With Possible Primary Site		
Level	Anatomic Correlation	Possible Primary Site
Ia	Submental	Anterior oral cavity/lower lip
Ib	Submandibular	Oral cavity (upper and lower lip, cheek, nose) and skin (lip, nose, medial canthus)
II	Upper jugular	Oropharynx, hypopharynx, oral cavity, larynx
III	Middle jugular	Oropharynx, larynx, hypopharynx, thyroid
IV	Lower jugular	Larynx, hypopharynx, thyroid, cervical esophagus, trachea
V	Posterior cervical triangle	Nasopharynx, skin of posterior neck, scalp, hypopharynx
VI	Anterior cervical (prelaryngeal (Delphian), pre/paratracheal, tracheoesophageal)	Larynx, thyroid
VII	Lateral retropharyngeal and retrostyloid	Nasopharynx, oropharyngeal wall or soft palate, hypopharynx, paranasal sinuses
Supraclavicular	Medial SCV (IVa) and lateral SCV (Vc)	Thyroid, cervical esophagus, infraclavicular primary (e.g., lung, gastrointestinal or gynecologic)
VIII	Intra/periparotid	Skin

*Cervical LN levels as per Robbins et al.[2]

PATHOLOGY: Most common pathology of HNCUP is SCC. Adenocarcinoma and neuroendocrine carcinomas are less common. Lymphoma, sarcoma, thyroid, melanoma, and germ cell tumors may also be encountered.

CLINICAL PRESENTATION: Classic presentation is unilateral painless neck mass in level II (~50%) ± level III. N1 presentation occurs in ~25%. With the rise of HPV-related cancers, some centers have noted a higher incidence of HNSCCUP,[3] with the hypothesis that HPV-related disease often presents with a small primary tumor,[4] which can be difficult to identify against a background of often irregular-appearing lymphoid tissue.

WORKUP:

Comprehensive H&P: Attention to past history of malignancy (including skin cancers) and risk factors. Exam should include direct inspection of the mucosal surfaces of the upper aerodigestive tract (including flexible nasopharyngolaryngoscopy to visualize surfaces not able to be evaluated on standard exam, that is, nasal cavity, nasopharynx, posterior/inferior oropharynx, larynx, and hypopharynx); digital exam of high-risk sites to evaluate for palpable abnormalities (without a visual correlate) and thorough exam of the skin of the head and neck. Anatomic location of the pathologic lymph node and histology will provide clues as to the primary site (Table 16.2).

Labs: CBC, CMP (thyroglobulin and calcitonin if adenocarcinoma).

Biopsy: FNA of pathologic LN for initial sampling (unless suspicious for lymphoma). If FNA is nondiagnostic, proceed to core needle biopsy. Excisional biopsy is a less favored alternative; if done, ideally with planned neck dissection to follow. Excisional biopsy alone is not recommended due to disruption of tissue planes, which can alter lymphatic drainage (non-oncologic resection). In the current era, testing of viral and other biomarkers from the biopsy specimen is essential in directing the search for a primary tumor (Table 16.3). IHC for p16 protein or another HPV-specific test should be performed on every SCCUP with levels II–III LN involvement ± with other levels as clinically indicated. If p16 is negative, other markers (e.g., EBV) should be performed.

Table 16.3 Pathologic Markers and Correlation With Possible Primary Site

Marker	Possible Primary Site
EBV	Nasopharynx
p16+, HPV ISH+	Oropharynx
p16+, HPV ISH-	Skin[5]
Adenocarcinoma, TTF+	Thyroid, lung

Imaging: CECT is the primary imaging modality for evaluation of cervical lymphadenopathy. PET/CT is the next test of choice if CECT and clinical exam (including scope) are unrevealing for a primary site. MRI not clearly superior to CECT; although it could help guide biopsies if substantial metal artifact, iodine contrast allergy, or if nasopharynx primary is suspected.[6] Imaging should be performed prior to panendoscopy to guide selection of biopsy sites and to avoid uncertainties of interpretation due to false-positive FDG avidity at sites manipulated during endoscopy. PET detection rate of primary tumor is approximately 30% in patients with HNCUP after standard workup.[7]

Procedures: Following PET/CT, next step is EUA w/panendoscopy with directed biopsies of any suspicious areas. With panendoscopy, the primary site is identified in 50% to 65% of patients with suspicious radiographic or physical findings, but only in 15% to 29% of those without.[8,9] Utility of random biopsies in absence of PET/CT or clinical suspicion is very low and no longer recommended.[10] If LN levels I–III are involved, ipsilateral palatine tonsillectomy is still recommended, and increases detection of the primary tumor by about 10-fold as compared to tonsillar biopsy (3% vs. 30%).[11,12] Particularly in the p16+ setting, consider lingual tonsillectomy if palatine tonsillectomy is negative. Meta-analyses of lingual tonsillectomy a.k.a. "tongue base mucosectomy" with transoral approach (via TORS or TLM) demonstrated 78% of patients had a primary site in the BOT after negative comprehensive workup.[13] Palatine and/or lingual tonsillectomies can be unilateral if there is only unilateral lymph node involvement.[10] If bilateral lymph nodes are involved, the primary site is more likely to be in the BOT than the palatine tonsil. Consider unilateral lingual tonsillectomy on the side with greatest nodal burden and contralateral lingual tonsillectomy if frozen sections are negative. Consider unilateral palatine tonsillectomy if lingual tonsillectomy is negative but avoid bilateral palatine tonsillectomy and bilateral lingual tonsillectomy due to morbidity.[10] Tissue specimens taken during diagnostic evaluation ideally are anatomically oriented and margin evaluation performed.

PROGNOSTIC FACTORS: Histology, number of LNs, LN level (upper vs. lower/SCV), KPS, extracapsular extension, and grade among others.

NATURAL HISTORY: Mucosal emergence rates, historically, are low after comprehensive RT. One series suggested rates of 25% after neck dissection alone and rates from 8% to 14% with RT. These rates may be lower in the modern era with improved imaging. Regional failure in neck and distant metastases are more common at 20% to 35%.[14]

STAGING: T-classification for cancer of unknown primary is T0 (not TX, which implies incomplete workup). LN staging for squamous cancers is per standard H&N staging (see Chapter 11 for details). EBV-associated unknown primary follows nasopharyngeal LN staging.

TREATMENT PARADIGM: Initial treatment can follow a paradigm of primary surgery (with risk-adapted adjuvant RT ± CHT as indicated) or primary RT (± CHT as indicated). Results have generally been comparable with either approach, and institutional preference often determines treatment algorithm.[15–17] Treatment strategy should take into account analysis of toxicities of each therapy.[18]

Surgery: For HNSCCUP, NCCN guidelines recommend surgery/neck dissection (preferred) or radiation therapy as primary therapy for N1 disease.[11] With modern staging, outcomes after surgery alone for N1 disease are excellent with 90% control above clavicles.[19] Typically, selective dissection is performed with levels IIA–IV routinely dissected ± other levels based on anatomic location of involved nodes, nodal burden, and suspected primary site.[10] Potential complications of neck dissection include hematoma, seroma, chyle leak, lymphedema, wound infection/dehiscence, fistula, cranial nerve damage (e.g., CN XI), and carotid rupture. The major potential complication of lingual tonsillectomy is hemorrhage, occurring in 4.9% of patients.[13] After surgery, adjuvant RT ± CHT should be offered based on standard recommendations for HN cancer (see Chapter 17 for details).

Chemotherapy: Concurrent CHT with radiation therapy is recommended for patients with either (a) ENE or residual disease after a neck dissection or (b) cN2–3 disease treated nonoperatively. These concepts are largely extrapolated from major definitive and post-op studies in setting of known H&N primaries (see Chapters 11–15 and 17). There have been small observational studies in setting of unknown primary that have shown good outcomes with chemoRT for patients with N2–N3 nodal disease.[18,20–22] If delivered, CHT dosing strategy is similar to that of other H&N sites, commonly high-dose cisplatin 100 mg/m^2 on days 1, 22, and 43 or cisplatin 40 mg/m^2 weekly. CHT may not be recommended concurrently with adjuvant radiation after resection of LN metastases with high suspicion for a skin primary due to lack of benefit seen on TROG 05.01,[23] though some may still consider concurrently for treatment in the definitive setting.

Radiation

Indications: RT can be employed in either the (a) high-risk postoperative setting or the (b) definitive setting. Following neck dissection, RT indications mimic standard indications for PORT in the head and neck: more than one involved node (N2–3), ENE, or positive margin. In the definitive setting, RT can be delivered alone or with concurrent CHT (e.g., cN2–3; see the preceding text).

Fields: Most commonly, RT is delivered to putative mucosal sites along with bilateral neck, unless skin primary is suspected.

- Primary: Classically, comprehensive RT for likely mucosal primaries included the nasopharynx, oropharynx, and hypopharynx with exclusion of oral cavity and larynx (sites that can be easily visualized). Potential gain w/ comprehensive RT in controlling primary should be weighed against its effects on QOL/toxicity. Target volumes have evolved and are often modified by HPV/EBV status and diagnostic interventions (e.g., palatine or lingual tonsillectomy). Guidelines recommend targeting only oropharynx for HPV+ disease (ipsilateral tonsil ± soft palate and bilateral BOT, modified by prior surgical diagnostic interventions).[10] Consider treating only nasopharynx for EBV+ disease. For HPV– disease in levels II–III, we consider the ipsilateral tonsil, entire base of tongue, ipsilateral Fossa of Rosenmüller, and ipsilateral pyriform sinus to be at risk.
- Neck/lymphatics: Most treat bilateral neck levels II to IV with RP, though other levels (IB, V, RP) should be included as indicated by presumed primary location (e.g., include V and RP with EBV+ presumed nasopharyngeal primary). Unilateral nodal treatment for suspected mucosal primaries is controversial and should be considered only with involvement of a single node (unless concerned for nasopharyngeal primary, in which bilateral coverage is recommended).[10] In the adjuvant setting, putative primary sites are treated as in definitive setting.[10] Omitting putative mucosal sites after comprehensive surgical diagnostics (at least ipsilateral palatine tonsillectomy and high-quality bilateral lingual tonsillectomy) is investigational. Pathologic N1 disease (small, single LN involved without ENE) can be observed.[10]

Dose: As in target delineation, dosing is heterogeneous. An acceptable dose scheme in the definitive setting is 70 Gy/35 fx to gross disease, 56 to 63 Gy/35 fx to mucosal sites at risk, and 56 Gy/35 fx to the uninvolved neck (or a radiobiologic equivalent scheme). Postoperatively, an acceptable dose regimen is 66 Gy in 30 to 33 fx to areas harboring ENE (or gross residual disease), 60 Gy in 30 fx to the postoperative bed and pathologically involved nodal levels, and 54 Gy in 30 fx to the uninvolved neck (or a radiobiologic equivalent scheme).

Toxicity:

- Acute: Mucositis, skin erythema/desquamation, odynophagia, dysphagia, fatigue, aspiration, xerostomia/thickened secretions, taste alterations.
- Late: Xerostomia, taste alteration, fibrosis, trismus, decreased hearing, hypothyroidism, submental lymphedema, dysphagia, esophageal strictures, bone/soft tissue necrosis, secondary malignancy.

■ EVIDENCE-BASED Q&A

■ Does association with HPV carry same implications in HNCUP as it does in oropharyngeal cancer?

Yes. HPV-associated HNCUPs have a better prognosis relative to their p16-negative counterparts, independent of nodal status.[24] In one study, 5-year OS was 92% if p16+ vs. 30% if p16–.[1] HPV positivity also leads practitioners to target only likely primary sites (i.e., oropharynx), which may decrease toxicity of treatment.

■ What is role of transoral lingual tonsillectomy in workup of HNCUP?

Recently, TORS has been used to perform lingual tonsillectomy in search of occult primary and appears to increase the likelihood of detecting a primary site when added to the standard diagnostic algorithm.

Mehta, Pittsburgh (*Laryngoscope* 2013, PMID 23154813): Ten patients with SCCUP underwent transoral robotic base-of-tongue resection (lingual tonsillectomy). In 9 of 10 patients (90%), primary was detected with mean diameter of 0.9 cm.

Patel, Multi-Institution (*JAMA Otolaryngol Head Neck Surg* 2013, PMID 24136446): Retrospective multi-institution series of patients treated with TORS to identify primary site in patients with SCCUP of head and neck. Six institutions enrolled a total of 47 patients. Primary site was found in 72%. Primary was in BOT in 59% and in tonsil in 38%. In 18 patients without suspicious radiographic or examination findings, 72% of primaries were identified with TORS.

Farooq, Meta-analysis (*Oral Oncol* 2019, PMID 30926070): Meta-analysis including 21 studies. In patients with negative exam, conventional imaging, and PET/CT, tongue base mucosectomy identified the primary in 64% of cases, which rose to 78% in patients who also had a negative EUA and tonsillectomy.

■ Does bilateral neck RT improve outcomes as compared to unilateral treatment?

Unilateral treatment is controversial considering that occult primary tumors presumed to be arising from the oropharynx often reside in the base of tongue, which is a midline structure. Table 16.4 provides a summary of various series investigating unilateral treatment. Although failure rates appear low (approximately 10%), this remains controversial. Of note, many of the historical papers compared ipsilateral RT without mucosal coverage to comprehensive RT. Less controversy exists in the setting of a single LN without clinical or radiologic evidence of ENE, in which case, it is reasonable to consider unilateral neck RT with coverage of putative mucosal sites.[10]

Table 16.4 Studies Investigating Unilateral Neck Treatment

Author	Institution	Year	Ipsilateral LN Treated, N	Contralateral Failure, N (%)	Comment
Carlson et al.[25]	MDACC	1986	13	2 (15.6%)	2D fields, no CT imaging
Colletier et al.[26]	MDACC	1998	14	1 (7.1%)	May overlap with Carlson; unclear if one contralateral failure was in ipsilateral-only-treated patient
Reddy et al.[27]	U Chicago	1997	16	9 (56%)	All nodes treated ipsilaterally with electron beam only; 5 of 9 recurrences were primary and contralateral nodes synchronously

(continued)

Table 16.4 Studies Investigating Unilateral Neck Treatment (*continued*)					
Author	Institution	Year	Ipsilateral LN Treated, N	Contralateral Failure, N (%)	Comment
Grau et al.[28]	Denmark	2000	26	1 (4%)	Patients treated with bilateral RT on study had 2% contralateral failure
Beldi et al.[29]	Milan	2007	33	Not reported	Report worse survival in unilateral patients but many were treated palliatively
Ligey et al.[30]	Dijon	2009	59	6 (10.2%)	Seven primary tumors emerged in unilateral group
Fakhrian et al.[31]	Munich	2012	17	1 (5.9%)	Comprehensive RT not associated with OS/RFS.
Cuaron et al.[32]	MSKCC	2015	6	0 (0%)	Small, but all CT imaging
Perkins et al.[33]	Wash U	2012	21	1 (5%)	All treated post neck dissection
Overall approximate crude rate			172	21 (12.2%)	Excluding Reddy: 12/156 = 7.7%

REFERENCES

1. Keller LM, Galloway TJ, Holdbrook T, et al. p16 status, pathologic and clinical characteristics, biomolecular signature, and long-term outcomes in head and neck squamous cell carcinomas of unknown primary. *Head Neck.* 2014;36(12):1677–1684. doi:10.1002/hed.23514
2. Robbins KT, Clayman G, Levine PA, et al. Neck dissection classification update: revisions proposed by the american head and neck society and the american academy of otolaryngology-head and neck surgery. *Arch Otolaryngol Head Neck Surg.* 2002;128(7):751–758. doi:10.1001/archotol.128.7.751
3. Motz K, Qualliotine JR, Rettig E, et al. Changes in unknown primary squamous cell carcinoma of the head and neck at initial presentation in the era of human papillomavirus. *JAMA Otolaryngol Head Neck Surg.* 2016;142(3):223–228. doi:10.1001/jamaoto.2015.3228
4. Huang SH, Perez-Ordonez B, Liu FF, et al. Atypical clinical behavior of p16-confirmed HPV-related oropharyngeal squamous cell carcinoma treated with radical radiotherapy. *Int J Radiat Oncol Biol Phys.* 2012;82(1):276–283. doi:10.1016/j.ijrobp.2010.08.031
5. McDowell LJ, Young RJ, Johnston ML, et al. p16-positive lymph node metastases from cutaneous head and neck squamous cell carcinoma: no association with high-risk human papillomavirus or prognosis and implications for the workup of the unknown primary. *Cancer.* 2016;122(8):1201–1208. doi:10.1002/cncr.29901
6. Ruhlmann V, Ruhlmann M, Bellendorf A, et al. Hybrid imaging for detection of carcinoma of unknown primary: a preliminary comparison trial of whole body PET/MRI versus PET/CT. *Eur J Radio.* 2016;85(11):1941–1947. doi:10.1016/j.ejrad.2016.08.020
7. Johansen J, Buus S, Loft A, et al. Prospective study of 18FDG-PET in the detection and management of patients with lymph node metastases to the neck from an unknown primary tumor. Results from the DAHANCA-13 study. *Head Neck.* 2008;30(4):471–478. doi:10.1002/hed.20734
8. Cianchetti M, Mancuso AA, Amdur RJ, et al. Diagnostic evaluation of squamous cell carcinoma metastatic to cervical lymph nodes from an unknown head and neck primary site. *Laryngoscope.* 2009;119(12):2348–2354. doi:10.1002/lary.20638
9. Mendenhall WM, Mancuso AA, Parsons JT, et al. Diagnostic evaluation of squamous cell carcinoma metastatic to cervical lymph nodes from an unknown head and neck primary site. *Head Neck.* 1998;20(8):739–744. doi:10.1002/(SICI)1097-0347(199812)20:8<739::AID-HED13>3.0.CO;2-0
10. Maghami E, Ismaila N, Alvarez A, et al. Diagnosis and management of squamous cell carcinoma of unknown primary in the head and neck: ASCO guideline. *J Clin Oncol.* 2020;38(22):2570–2596. doi:10.1200/JCO.20.00275
11. Head and Neck Cancers. NCCN Clinical Practice Guidelines in Oncology. 2020; Version 2.2020 — June 9, 2020.
12. Waltonen JD, Ozer E, Schuller DE, Agrawal A. Tonsillectomy vs. deep tonsil biopsies in detecting occult tonsil tumors. *Laryngoscope.* 2009;119(1):102–106. doi:10.1002/lary.20017

13. Farooq S, Khandavilli S, Dretzke J, et al. Transoral tongue base mucosectomy for the identification of the primary site in the work-up of cancers of unknown origin: systematic review and meta-analysis. *Oral Oncol.* 2019;91:97–106. doi:10.1016/j.oraloncology.2019.02.018

14. Nieder C, Ang KK. Cervical lymph node metastases from occult squamous cell carcinoma. *Curr Treat Options Oncol.* 2002;3(1):33–40. doi:10.1007/s11864-002-0039-7

15. Demiroz C, Vainshtein JM, Koukourakis GV, et al. Head and neck squamous cell carcinoma of unknown primary: neck dissection and radiotherapy or definitive radiotherapy. *Head Neck.* 2014;36(11):1589–1595. doi:10.1002/hed.23479

16. Christiansen H, Hermann RM, Martin A, et al. Neck lymph node metastases from an unknown primary tumor retrospective study and review of literature. *Strahlenther Onkol.* 2005;181(6):355–362. doi:10.1007/s00066-005-1338-2

17. Balaker AE, Abemayor E, Elashoff D, St John MA. Cancer of unknown primary: does treatment modality make a difference? *Laryngoscope.* 2012;122(6):1279–1282. doi:10.1002/lary.22424

18. Chen AM, Farwell DG, Lau DH, et al. Radiation therapy in the management of head-and-neck cancer of unknown primary origin: how does the addition of concurrent chemotherapy affect the therapeutic ratio? *Int J Radiat Oncol Biol Phys.* 2011;81(2):346–352. doi:10.1016/j.ijrobp.2010.06.031

19. Galloway TJ, Ridge JA. Management of squamous cancer metastatic to cervical nodes with an unknown primary site. *J Clin Oncol.* 2015;33(29):3328–3337. doi:10.1200/JCO.2015.61.0063

20. Sher DJ, Balboni TA, Haddad RI, et al. Efficacy and toxicity of chemoradiotherapy using intensity-modulated radiotherapy for unknown primary of head and neck. *Int J Radiat Oncol Biol Phys.* 2011;80(5):1405–1411. doi:10.1016/j.ijrobp.2010.04.029

21. Argiris A, Smith SM, Stenson K, et al. Concurrent chemoradiotherapy for N2 or N3 squamous cell carcinoma of the head and neck from an occult primary. *Ann Oncol.* 2003;14(8):1306–1311. doi:10.1093/annonc/mdg330

22. Shehadeh NJ, Ensley JF, Kucuk O, et al. Benefit of postoperative chemoradiotherapy for patients with unknown primary squamous cell carcinoma of the head and neck. *Head Neck.* 2006;28(12):1090–1098. doi:10.1002/hed.20470

23. Porceddu SV, Bressel M, Poulsen MG, et al. Postoperative concurrent chemoradiotherapy versus postoperative radiotherapy in high-risk cutaneous squamous cell carcinoma of the head and neck: the Randomized Phase III TROG 05.01 Trial. *J Clin Oncol.* 2018;36(13):1275–1283. doi:10.1200/JCO.2017.77.0941

24. Dixon JG, Bognar BA, Keyserling TC, et al. Teaching women's health skills: confidence, attitudes and practice patterns of academic generalist physician. *J Gen Intern Med.* 2003;18(6):411–418. doi:10.1046/j.1525-1497.2003.10511.x

25. Carlson LS, Fletcher GH, Oswald MJ. Guidelines for radiotherapeutic techniques for cervical metastases from an unknown primary. *Int J Radiat Oncol Biol Phys.* 1986;12(12):2101–2110. doi:10.1016/0360-3016(86)90008-8

26. Colletier PJ, Garden AS, Morrison WH, et al. Postoperative radiation for squamous cell carcinoma metastatic to cervical lymph nodes from an unknown primary site: outcomes and patterns of failure. *Head Neck.* 1998;20(8):674–681. doi:10.1002/(SICI)1097-0347(199812)20:8<674::AID-HED3>3.0.CO;2-H

27. Reddy SP, Marks JE. Metastatic carcinoma in the cervical lymph nodes from an unknown primary site: results of bilateral neck plus mucosal irradiation vs. ipsilateral neck irradiation. *Int J Radiat Oncol Biol Phys.* 1997;37(4):797–802. doi:10.1016/S0360-3016(97)00025-4

28. Grau C, Johansen LV, Jakobsen J, et al. Cervical lymph node metastases from unknown primary tumours: results from a national survey by the Danish Society for Head and Neck Oncology. *Radiother Oncol.* 2000;55(2):121–129. doi:10.1016/S0167-8140(00)00172-9

29. Beldi D, Jereczek-Fossa BA, D'Onofrio A, et al. Role of radiotherapy in the treatment of cervical lymph node metastases from an unknown primary site: retrospective analysis of 113 patients. *Int J Radiat Oncol Biol Phys.* 2007;69(4):1051–1058. doi:10.1016/j.ijrobp.2007.04.039

30. Ligey A, Gentil J, Crehange G, et al. Impact of target volumes and radiation technique on loco-regional control and survival for patients with unilateral cervical lymph node metastases from an unknown primary. *Radiother Oncol.* 2009;93(3):483–487. doi:10.1016/j.radonc.2009.08.027

31. Fakhrian K, Thamm R, Knapp S, et al. Radio(chemo)therapy in the management of squamous cell carcinoma of cervical lymph nodes from an unknown primary site: a retrospective analysis. *Strahlenther Onkol.* 2012;188(1):56–61. doi:10.1007/s00066-011-0017-8

32. Cuaron J, Rao S, Wolden S, et al. Patterns of failure in patients with head and neck carcinoma of unknown primary treated with radiation therapy. *Head Neck.* 2016;38 Suppl 1:E426–E431. doi:10.1002/hed.24013

33. Perkins SM, Spencer CR, Chernock RD, et al. Radiotherapeutic management of cervical lymph node metastases from an unknown primary site. *Arch Otolaryngol Head Neck Surg.* 2012;138(7):656–661. doi:10.1001/archoto.2012.1110

17 ■ POSTOPERATIVE RADIATION FOR HEAD AND NECK CANCER

Timothy D. Smile and Carryn M. Anderson

QUICK HIT ■ Surgery is the preferred initial management of resectable H&N cancers of oral cavity, salivary gland, nasal cavity/paranasal sinuses, thyroid, and some oropharynx and larynx cancers. Oncologic surgery alone is often sufficient treatment for T1-T2N0-1 tumors when resected with negative margins. Adjuvant RT (PORT) is recommended for specific pathologic risk factors with concurrent CHT given for positive margins and ECE in mucosal HNSCC.

Table 17.1 PORT Indications and Dosing Summary

Risk Group	Treatment	Patient Characteristics
Low risk	Observation	pT1–T2, pN0-1, –PNI, –LVSI, –margins, –ECE
Intermediate risk	60 Gy	pT3–T4, pN2–3 disease, PNI, LVSI, close margins (<5 mm), pT1-2N0-1 with multiple minor risk factors or depth of invasion >4 mm in oral tongue[1]
	66 Gy	Multiple of above risk factors
High risk	66 Gy + CHT	+ECE, microscopic positive margins[2]
	70 Gy + CHT	Residual gross disease

EPIDEMIOLOGY: Worldwide incidence of >550,000 (fifth most common cancer), male-to-female ratio 3:1, 2020 estimated U.S. incidence of 53,260 cases and 9,570 deaths.[3]

RISK FACTORS: Tobacco (cigarettes and chew, 5–25× increased risk), alcohol (dose dependent and synergistic with tobacco), HPV infection (oropharyngeal), HIV, immunosuppressed from transplant drugs or autoimmune diseases, betel nut chewing (oral cavity), sun exposure (skin), previous radiation, occupational/environmental exposures.

ANATOMY: See Chapters 11 to 15 for site-specific anatomy. For maxillary sinus tumors, one important landmark is Ohngren's line: extends from medial canthus of eye to angle of mandible. Anteroinferior/infrastructures have good prognosis, whereas superoposterior/suprastructures have poor prognosis and have early extension into eye, skull base, pterygoids, and infratemporal fossa.

PATHOLOGY: Most common histology is SCC: "keratin pearls" are seen in well-differentiated SCC, often associated with classic HNSCC related to smoking/alcohol abuse; nonkeratinizing poorly differentiated "basaloid" squamous cancers often associated with HPV-associated p16+ oropharyngeal SCC. Other histologies include mucoepidermoid carcinoma, adenoid cystic carcinoma, adenosquamous, adenocarcinoma, acinic cell, lymphoma, lymphoepithelial carcinoma, and melanoma.

GENETICS: Mutation of p53, CDKN2A, Rb loss of function, and increased expression of EGFR are associated with worse prognosis in oral cavity cancers.[4,5]

SCREENING: No established role for screening in H&N cancers managed with surgical resection. See Chapters 13 and 14 for further discussion of screening investigations.

CLINICAL PRESENTATION: Dependent on primary site. Paranasal sinus/nasal cavity/nasopharynx: nasal obstruction, epistaxis, lateral gaze palsy, unilateral hearing loss, epiphora. Oropharynx: dysphagia, trismus, otalgia, odynophagia. Oral cavity: nonhealing ulceration, dysarthria, loose teeth. Larynx: hoarseness, stridor, dysphagia, odynophagia, otalgia. Hypopharynx: dysphagia, hoarseness, weight loss. Many patients are asymptomatic from their primary disease and present with adenopathy, most commonly level II jugulodigastric node.

WORKUP: H&P including flexible nasopharyngolaryngoscopy or mirror examination.

Labs: Routine labs including CBC, CMP, audiology if platinum CHT.

Imaging: CT neck with contrast, PET/CT for stage III/IV patients, CT chest to screen if PET/CT not obtained. If unknown primary by office exam and imaging, obtain PET/CT prior to panendoscopy/exam under anesthesia.[6]

Pathology: FNA biopsy of neck node and/or biopsy of primary site. See Chapters 11 to 15 for site-specific workup. Optimally, multidisciplinary consult should be performed prior to resection.

PROGNOSTIC FACTORS: Positive margins and ECE are most important pathologic prognostic factors. Other negative pathologic factors include close margins, PNI, LVSI, tumor size, depth of invasion (oral tongue in particular). HPV-associated oropharynx cancers have better prognosis overall, and ECE and advanced nodal stage do not have same negative impact on survival, as reflected in AJCC's 8th edition of the Staging Manual. *Extracapsular extension* ranges from microscopic (small break in capsule, desmoplastic stromal reaction) to macroscopic (visible to eye at surgery) to gross soft tissue deposits (no evidence of LN architecture, which likely represents complete LN replacement).[7] Recurrence rates double when ECE is present. CT can predict ECE with frequent false negatives but uncommon false positives (Sens/Spec/PPV/NPV 43%, 97%, 82%, and 87%).[6] Nodes <2.5 cm on CT imaging have approximately 6% rate of pathologic ECE as compared to larger nodes with 32% rate.[8]

NATURAL HISTORY: Majority of disease-related recurrences will be locoregional and occur within first 2 years of treatment completion. Most common site of distant metastasis is lung, with bone second most common. HPV-associated cancers have been known to spread to less common sites such as liver, skin, soft tissues, brain, and leptomeninges.[9]

STAGING: See Chapters 11 to 16 and 18 to 19 for staging details.

TREATMENT PARADIGM

Observation: Observation is appropriate following surgery for low-risk patients, loosely defined as pT1-2N0-1 without LVSI, PNI, ECE, shallow depth of invasion (especially oral tongue, <4 mm) and with negative margins (>5 mm ideally).

Surgery: Resection of primary should be performed with least morbidity possible. Free flap reconstruction may be necessary for larger tumors (hemiglossectomy, total glossectomy, mandibular reconstruction, laryngopharyngectomy, etc.). Free flaps typically include radial forearm, anterolateral thigh or fibula (when bone is required). Minimally invasive techniques such as TORS and TLM are available at expert centers. TORS is performed using robotic platform, suggested for oropharynx and possibly larynx/hypopharynx primaries. TORS is FDA approved for cT1–2 tumors.[10] TLM is piecemeal removal of tumor through laryngoscope using CO_2 laser aimed via micromanipulator attached to microscope (only available at few specialized centers). Both are suggested as a possible method to improve toxicity through lower RT doses (70 Gy+cisplatin needed for definitive vs. 60–66 Gy±CHT post-op) and as a way to intensify treatment for advanced disease (see terminated RTOG 1221). See review for issues specific to TORS/TLM.[11,12] For sinonasal tumors, endoscopic surgery is preferred, performed in piecemeal way. Neck dissection typically performed at time of surgery (see Table 17.2).

Chemotherapy: CHT can be added concurrently with RT in postoperative setting to escalate treatment for high-risk cancers. High-dose cisplatin is most common, given at 100 mg/m² at days 1, 22, 43. Weekly cisplatin 40 mg/m² is an acceptable alternative. Ongoing trials are investigating role of cetuximab (RTOG 0920) for intermediate risk and alternative multiagent regimens for high-risk patients (RTOG 1216).

Table 17.2 Neck Dissection Types for H&N Cancer	
Radical neck dissection	All LN groups I–V, CN XI, IJ vein, SCM
Modified radical neck dissection	All LN groups I–V, preserves ≥1 of CN XI, IJ, SCM
Selective neck dissection (SND)	Preservation of ≥1 LN group
Supraomohyoid	SND of only I–III, considered for oral cavity cases
Lateral neck dissection (thyroid cancer)	SND II–IV (oropharynx, hypopharynx, larynx)
Central neck dissection (thyroid cancer)	SND VI

Radiation

Indications: Risk-adapted approach to RT is used to escalate therapy in postoperative setting. Indications for PORT are described (Table 17.1) by loosely defined risk groups of low (observation), intermediate (RT alone, defined by RTOG 0920), and high (chemoRT, defined by RTOG 1216). For sinonasal tumors, PORT is almost always recommended (except for T1 ethmoid). RT should be initiated within 6 weeks of surgery for optimal LRC and OS.[13]

Dose: In era of IMRT SIB technique, doses of 66 Gy, 59.4 Gy, and 56.1 Gy in 33 fx to areas of high risk (microscopic margin positive, ECE, or multiple primary site risk factors), intermediate risk (post-op bed or undissected neck at risk), and low risk (elective lower risk nodal areas), respectively, are commonly used. In cases without high-risk features, 60 Gy/30 fx is delivered to post-op bed simultaneously with 54 Gy to high-risk undissected/low-risk neck.

■ EVIDENCE-BASED Q&A

■ What evidence suggests that PORT is effective?

Most evidence is retrospective although there are two older randomized trials demonstrating improved LRF with PORT compared to observation.[14,15]

■ Historically, what evidence suggests postoperative RT is superior to preoperative radiation?

Tupchong, RTOG 7303 (*IJROBP* 1991, PMID 1993628): Phase III PRT of preoperative RT vs. PORT for supraglottic larynx and hypopharynx cancer. Preoperative RT was 50 Gy, PORT was 60 Gy; 277 patients, follow-up from 9 to 15 years. LRC improved in PORT group compared to preoperative (70% vs. 58%, $p = .04$). No difference in OS ($p = .15$). **Conclusion: PORT improves LRC compared to preoperative RT. Because of this trial, PORT has become standard in patients managed with primary surgery.**

■ What data support current standard dosing for PORT?

All patients require minimum dose of 57.6 Gy at 1.8 Gy/fx to whole operative bed. High-risk areas of ≥2 adverse factors or ECE requires 63 Gy at 1.8 Gy/fx.

Peters, MD Anderson (*IJROBP* 1993, PMID 8482629): PRT of stage III/IV SCC of oral cavity, oropharynx, hypopharynx, and larynx stratified by risk factors. Lower-risk patients randomized to 52.2 to 57.6 Gy vs. 63 Gy and higher-risk patients randomized to 63 Gy vs. 68.4 Gy, all in 1.8 Gy fractions. On interim analysis, patients who received dose of ≤54 Gy had significantly higher primary failure rate and dose group was increased to 57.6 Gy, improving LRF ($p = .02$). Overall, no dose response was demonstrated. However, if ECE was present, recurrence was significantly higher at 57.6 Gy than at ≥63 Gy. ECE was the only independent variable prognostic of LRR. Having two or more of following were progressively prognostic: oral cavity primary, mucosal margins close or positive, nerve invasion, ≥2 positive lymph nodes, largest node 3 cm, treatment delay greater than 6 weeks, and Zubrod performance status ≥2. **Conclusion: Minimum dose of 57.6 Gy to whole operative bed should be delivered with boost of 63 Gy to sites of increased risk (e.g., ECE). Treatment should be started as soon as possible after surgery. Dose escalation above 63 Gy does not appear to improve therapeutic ratio. This trial defined most common dosing regimens used today (60–66 Gy).**

■ **What data support risk-adapted approach to PORT?**

Ang, MD Anderson (*IJROBP* 2001, PMID 11597795): Multi-institutional PRT of 213 patients with advanced HNSCC of oral cavity, oropharynx, larynx, and hypopharynx assessing role of risk stratification and PORT scheduling (concomitant boost vs. standard). Patients received therapy predicated on set of pathologic risk features: oral cavity site, mucosal margin status, nerve invasion, 1 positive node, >1 positive nodal group, largest node >3 cm, ECE, and treatment delay of >6 weeks. See Table 17.3. **Conclusion: Dosing based on risk stratification is legitimate approach to PORT for H&N cancer.** (*See altered fractionation in the following for the second conclusion.*)

Table 17.3 Results of MD Anderson Risk-Adapted PORT for H&N Cancer			
Risk Group	PORT	5-Yr LRC (%)	5-Yr OS (%)
Low Risk: no adverse factors	None	90	83
Intermediate risk: one adverse factor other than ECE	57.6 Gy/6.5 weeks	94	66
High risk: ≥2 adverse factors or ECE	63 Gy/5 or 7 weeks (±conc. boost)	68	42

■ **With definitive RT, altered fractionation improves control (RTOG 9003), so should we accelerate patients receiving PORT?**

No benefit for most patients; however, acceleration may compensate for delay in PORT after surgery beyond 6 weeks.

Sanguineti, Italy (*IJROBP* 2005, PMID 15708255): Phase III trial of PORT 60 Gy/6 weeks (CF) or AF with "biphasic concomitant boost" schedule, with boost delivered during first and last weeks of treatment (64 Gy/5 weeks); 2-yr LRC CF 80% vs. AF 78% ($p = .52$), trend to benefit for patients with RT delay >7 weeks; 2-yr OS 67% vs. 64% ($p = .84$). Toxicity: Confluent mucositis CF 27% vs. AF 50% ($p = .006$), duration same. Late toxicity 18% vs. 27% (NS). **Conclusion: Accelerated fractionation not beneficial overall, might be option for patients who delay starting RT.**

Ang, MD Anderson (*IJROBP* 2001, PMID 11597795): Same trial as detailed earlier. Regarding hyperfractionation, only "trend" to benefit when comparing 5 weeks vs. 7 weeks in high-risk patients (LRC $p = .11$, OS $p = .08$). However, when looking at interval from surgery to PORT initiation for high-risk patients, acceleration seemed to make up for delay. **Conclusion: Hyperfractionation may be beneficial, particularly in patients with treatment delay >6 weeks from surgery.**

CHEMOTHERAPY

■ **Which patients benefit from treatment escalation with concurrent chemoRT?**

In high-risk patients, those with ECE or positive margins seem to benefit based on combined RTOG 9501/ EORTC 22931 analyses.

Bernier, EORTC 22931 (*NEJM* 2004, PMID 15128894): PRT of 334 patients w/ HNSCC (oral cavity, oropharynx, hypopharynx, or larynx) s/p primary surgical resection w/ high-risk features comparing postop RT alone (66 Gy/33 fx) vs. chemoRT (cisplatin 100 mg/m² on days 1, 22, 43 w/ same RT). Eligible patients included pT3–4 and N_{any} (except pT3N0 of larynx w/ negative margins), or T1–2 and N2–3, or T1-2N0-1 w/ unfavorable pathologic findings (ENE, + margins, PNI or vascular tumor embolism), or oral cavity/oropharynx tumors w/ levels IV–V LNs. Overall, 67% had pT3–4, 57% had pN2–3, 28% had +margins, 54% had ≥2 positive LNs. MFU 60 mos. See Table 17.4. Acute Gr 3–4 mucosal adverse effects were worse w/ chemoRT (41% vs. 21%, $p = .001$), while cumulative incidence of late effects was not. **Conclusion: Post-op chemoRT improves survival over RT alone for patients w/ locally advanced HNSCC (and w/ unfavorable clinical + pathologic factors) w/o high incidence of late effects.**

Table 17.4 Results of Bernier EORTC CHT Trial

	Median PFS	5-Yr PFS	MS	5-Yr OS	5-Yr LRR	5-Yr DM
Post-op RT	23 mos	36%	32 mos	40%	31%	25%
Post-op chemoRT	55 mos	47%	72 mos	53%	18%	21%
p value	.04		.02		.007	.61

Cooper, RTOG 9501 (*NEJM* 2004, PMID 15128893, Update Cooper *IJROBP* 2012, PMID 2274963): PRT of 416 patients (update 410 patients) w/ HNSCC (oral cavity, oropharynx, hypopharynx, or larynx) s/p macroscopic complete resection w/ high-risk features (any or all of: histologic invasion of ≥2 LNs, ECE or +margins) comparing RT alone (60–66 Gy/30–33 fx) vs. chemoRT (cisplatin 100 mg/m² on days 1, 22, 43). Overall, 18% had positive margins, 82% had ≥2 LNs or ECE. MFU 6.1 yrs, update 9.4 yrs for survivors. See Table 17.5. Incidence of acute adverse effects ≥ grade 3 was 34% and 77% in RT and chemoRT arms, respectively (*p* < .001). In the first report, CHT improved LRF and DFS but not OS. With long-term follow-up CHT improved LRF in patients with ECE or +margins. **Conclusion: ECE and +margins remain indications for concurrent CHT and PORT.**

Table 17.5 Results of RTOG 9501 Postoperative CHT Trial

	Original Report (2004)			Long-Term Update (2012)		
	2-Yr LRC (2004)	2-Yr DFS (2004)	2-Yr OS (2004)	10-Yr LRF, All (2012)	10-Yr LRF, ECE or +margins (2012)	10-Yr OS, ECE or +margins (2012)
PORT	72%	HR 0.78	HR 0.84	28.8%	33.1%	19.6
Postop chemoRT	82%			22.3%	21.0%	27.1
p value	.01	.04	.19	.10	.02	.07

Bernier, Pooled Analysis EORTC and RTOG (*Head Neck* 2005, PMID 16161069): Data from EORTC 22931 and RTOG 95-01 were pooled for comparative analysis. ECE and/or microscopically +margins were only risk factors with significant impact of chemoRT in both trials. **Conclusion: +margins and ECE are most significant prognostic factors for poor outcomes, and postop chemoRT improves outcomes in patients w/ one or both of these risk factors.**

■ **Does the schedule of cisplatin (q3 weekly vs. weekly) influence outcomes?**

Noronha, India (*JCO* 2018, PMID 22920295): PRT of 300 patients w/ stages III–IV SCC of oral cavity, oropharynx, hypopharynx, larynx, or unknown primary, randomized to weekly cisplatin (30 mg/m²) vs. high-dose cisplatin (100 mg/m² q3 weeks). High-dose cisplatin arm resulted in higher 2-yr LRC (58.5% vs. 73.1%, *p* = .014) and higher G3+ toxicity (71.6% vs. 84.6%, *p* = .006). OS 39.5 months in weekly arm vs. not reached in high-dose arm (HR, 1.14 [95% CI, 0.79 to 1.65]; *p* = .48). **Conclusion: High-dose cisplatin should remain preferred CHT regimen.**

■ **How much ECE should trigger the addition of CHT?**

Randomized data included any ECE. Recent data show survival detriment proportional to amount of ECE.[16,17] There does not appear to be a level of ECE low enough to omit CHT and levels with gross ECE have inferior survival even with chemotherapy. In HPV era, this is evolving with multiple trials investigating omission of CHT for those with minor ECE ≤1 mm.

MANAGEMENT OF LOW-RISK PATIENTS

■ Is PORT necessary in N1 patients?

A microscopic single node without other risk factors was not sufficient to receive PORT in the preceding Ang trial. However, any node positivity was an indication for PORT in the Tata Memorial study of oral cavity patients, which may have contributed to the difference in OS (see Chapter 12).[18] It is likely that carefully selected pN1 non-oral cavity patients, in absence of other risk factors and after adequate neck dissection, can be observed.[19,20]

■ Can the treatment volumes be decreased in PORT?

A small phase II study (mixture of primary sites, selected group) of omitting the pathologically node-negative neck demonstrated favorable local control. This is only the beginning of such investigations and should be approached with caution off-study.

Contreras (*JCO* 2019, PMID 31246526): Phase II study with 72 patients who underwent resection of the primary and bilateral neck dissection (6 patients were unable to undergo contralateral neck dissection), with high-risk features warranting PORT. The pN0 neck was not irradiated (if patient had bilateral pN0, only the primary was irradiated). Primary end point was rate of recurrence in unirradiated pN0 neck (aimed to demonstrate <10% failure). Sites included oral cavity (20%), oropharynx (51%), hypopharynx (6%), larynx (22%), and unknown primary (1%). No patients were treated to contralateral neck; 24% of patients received RT to the primary only. No failures were observed in the unirradiated pN0 neck. Distant failure occurred in 26% of patients; 5-yr OS was 64%. **Conclusion: In this small study, eliminating PORT to the pN0 neck had favorable control rates without long-term adverse effects on global QOL.**

Swisher-McClure, AVOID trial (*IJROBP* 2020, PMID 31785337): Single-arm phase 2 prospective trial of 60 patients with stage pT1–2 N1–3 HPV-associated OPSCC treated with TORS and selective neck dissection at a single institution. Patients had favorable features at the primary site (negative surgical margins ≥2 mm, no PNI, and no LVSI) but required adjuvant therapy based on LN involvement. PORT to at-risk areas in the involved neck (60–66 Gy) and uninvolved neck (54 Gy). The resected primary site was treated as an active avoidance structure. Concurrent CHT was given for ECE. Median follow-up was 2.4 yrs. A single patient recurred at the primary site, for 2-yr local control of 98.3%. One patient (1.7%) developed a regional neck recurrence, and 2 patients (3.3%) developed distant metastases; 2-yr LRFS was 97.9%. OS was 100% at the time of analysis. The mean RT dose to the primary site was 36.9 Gy. **Conclusion: Deintensified PORT that avoids the resected primary tumor site for selected patients with HPV-associated OPSCC appears safe and is worthy of further study.**

■ Can PORT dose be deintensified after surgery for HPV+ patients?

There are select patients for whom reduced dose PORT without chemotherapy seems sufficient based on the ECOG/ACRIN 3311 randomized trial presented in abstract form at ASCO in 2020 and 2021.[21] For post-TORS patients with negative margins, <5 involved nodes, and minimal ENE (<1 mm), reduced-dose PORT with 50 Gy had similar 2-yr PFS to 60 Gy (95% vs. 98.6%, respectively). Phase II data from Mayo Clinic suggests comparable LRC rates to historical controls using 30–36 Gy PORT after transoral surgery with good QOL and swallowing function. TORS with de-escalated PORT should be evaluated in a phase III trial.

Ma, Mayo MC1273 (*JCO* 2019, PMID 31163012): Single-arm phase II trial of RT de-escalation after transoral surgery. Included patients with p16-positive oropharyngeal SCC, smoking history of <10 pack-years, and negative margins. Cohort A (intermediate risk) received 30 Gy (1.5-Gy/fx given BID) with 15 mg/m^2 docetaxel weekly. Cohort B included patients with ECE who received the same treatment plus a simultaneous integrated boost to nodal levels with ECE to 36 Gy in 1.8 Gy fx, given BID. Median follow-up was 36 months. The 2-yr LRC rate was 96.2%, with PFS of 91.1% and OS of 98.7%. Grade 3 or worse toxicity at pre-RT and 1 and 2 yrs post-RT were 2.5%, 0%, and 0%. Swallowing function improved slightly between pre-RT and 12 months post-RT, with one patient requiring temporary feeding tube. **Conclusion: Aggressive RT de-escalation resulted in locoregional tumor control rates comparable to those of historical controls, low toxicity, and little decrement in swallowing function or QOL.**

REFERENCES

1. Ganly I, Goldstein D, Carlson DL, et al. Long-term regional control and survival in patients with "low-risk," early stage oral tongue cancer managed by partial glossectomy and neck dissection without postoperative radiation: the importance of tumor thickness. *Cancer.* 2013;119(6):1168–1176. doi:10.1002/cncr.27872

2. Bernier J, Cooper JS, Pajak TF, et al. Defining risk levels in locally advanced head and neck cancers: a comparative analysis of concurrent postoperative radiation plus chemotherapy trials of the EORTC (#22931) and RTOG (# 9501). *Head Neck.* 2005;27(10):843–850. doi:10.1002/hed.20279

3. Siegel RL, Miller KD, Jemal A. Cancer statistics, 2020. *CA Cancer J Clin.* 2020;70(1):7–30. doi:10.3322/caac.21590

4. Kiaris H, Spandidos DA, Jones AS, et al. Mutations, expression and genomic instability of the H-ras proto-oncogene in squamous cell carcinomas of the head and neck. *Br J Cancer.* 1995;72(1):123–128. doi:10.1038/bjc.1995.287

5. Zhu X, Zhang F, Zhang W, et al. Prognostic role of epidermal growth factor receptor in head and neck cancer: a meta-analysis. *J Surg Oncol.* 2013;108(6):387–397. doi:10.1002/jso.23406

6. Mani N, George MM, Nash L, et al. Role of 18-Fludeoxyglucose positron emission tomography-computed tomography and subsequent panendoscopy in head and neck squamous cell carcinoma of unknown primary. *Laryngoscope.* 2016;126(6):1354–1358. doi:10.1002/lary.25783

7. Lewis JS Jr, Carpenter DH, Thorstad WL, et al. Extracapsular extension is a poor predictor of disease recurrence in surgically treated oropharyngeal squamous cell carcinoma. *Mod Pathol.* 2011;24(11):1413–1420. doi:10.1038/modpathol.2011.105

8. Prabhu RS, Magliocca KR, Hanasoge S, et al. Accuracy of computed tomography for predicting pathologic nodal extracapsular extension in patients with head-and-neck cancer undergoing initial surgical resection. *Int J Radiat Oncol, Biol Phy.* 2014;88(1):122–129. doi:10.1016/j.ijrobp.2013.10.002

9. Trosman SJ, Koyfman SA, Ward MC, et al. Effect of human papillomavirus on patterns of distant metastatic failure in oropharyngeal squamous cell carcinoma treated with chemoradiotherapy. *JAMA Otolaryngol Head Neck Surg.* 2015;141(5):457–462. doi:10.1001/jamaoto.2015.136

10. FDA510(k) summary. 2009. http://www.accessdata.fda.gov/cdrh_docs/pdf9/K090993.pdf

11. Ward MC, Koyfman SA. Transoral robotic surgery: The radiation oncologist's perspective. *Oral Oncol.* 2016;60:96–102. doi:10.1016/j.oraloncology.2016.07.008

12. Huang SH, Hansen A, Rathod S, O'Sullivan B. Primary surgery versus (chemo)radiotherapy in oropharyngeal cancer: the radiation oncologist's and medical oncologist's perspectives. *Curr Opin Otolaryngol Head Neck Surg.* 2015;23(2):139–147. doi:10.1097/MOO.0000000000000141

13. Tribius S, Donner J, Pazdyka H, et al. Survival and overall treatment time after postoperative radio(chemo)therapy in patients with head and neck cancer. *Head Neck.* 2016;38(7):1058–1065. doi:10.1002/hed.24407

14. Kokal WA, Neifeld JP, Eisert D, et al. Postoperative radiation as adjuvant treatment for carcinoma of the oral cavity, larynx, and pharynx: preliminary report of a prospective randomized trial. *J Surg oncol.* 1988;38(2):71–76. doi:10.1002/hed.24407

15. Mishra RC, Singh DN, Mishra TK. Post-operative radiotherapy in carcinoma of buccal mucosa, a prospective randomized trial. *European Journal Surg oncol.* 1996;22(5):502–504. doi:10.1016/S0748-7983(96)92969-8

16. Prabhu RS, Hanasoge S, Magliocca KR, et al. Extent of pathologic extracapsular extension and outcomes in patients with nonoropharyngeal head and neck cancer treated with initial surgical resection. *Cancer.* 2014;120(10):1499–1506. doi:10.1002/cncr.28596

17. Greenberg JS, Fowler R, Gomez J, et al. Extent of extracapsular spread: a critical prognosticator in oral tongue cancer. *Cancer.* 2003;97(6):1464–1470. doi:10.1002/cncr.11202

18. D'Cruz AK, Vaish R, Kapre N, et al. Elective versus Therapeutic Neck Dissection in Node-Negative Oral Cancer. *N Engl J Med.* 2015;373(6):521–529. doi:10.1056/NEJMoa1506007

19. Schmitz S, Machiels JP, Weynand B, et al. Results of selective neck dissection in the primary management of head and neck squamous cell carcinoma. *Eur Arch Otorhinolaryngol.* 2009;266(3):437–443. doi:10.1007/s00405-008-0767-9

20. Jäckel MC, Ambrosch P, Christiansen H, et al. Value of postoperative radiotherapy in patients with pathologic N1 neck disease. *Head Neck.* 2008;30(7):875–882. doi:10.1002/hed.20794

21. Ferris RL, Flamand Y, Weinstein GS, et al. Updated report of a phase II randomized trial of transoral surgical resection followed by low-dose or standard postoperative therapy in resectable p16+ locally advanced oropharynx cancer: A trial of the ECOG-ACRIN cancer research group (E3311). *J Clin Oncol.* 2021;39(15). https://ascopubs.org/doi/abs/10.1200/JCO.2021.39.15_suppl.6010. Accessed Jun 11, 2021.

18 ■ THYROID CANCER

James R. Broughman and Nikhil P. Joshi

QUICK HIT ■ PTC and FTC are forms of differentiated thyroid cancer that are treated with surgical resection (thyroid lobectomy and isthmusectomy vs. total thyroidectomy) followed by adjuvant therapy dependent upon ATA risk group. RAI is delivered to ablate residual thyroid tissue and microscopic disease. MTC is a neuroendocrine thyroid tumor that produces calcitonin and CEA and is associated with the MEN2 syndrome. Adjuvant EBRT is used infrequently for differentiated/medullary thyroid cancers, but may be indicated after resection of recurrent disease at high risk for additional unresectable recurrence (positive margins, gross extrathyroidal extension, gross and extensive extracapsular nodal extension, insular or poorly differentiated, tall cell, hobnail or other high-risk histology).

ATC is an aggressive disease managed with resection followed by chemoRT vs. definitive chemoRT vs. palliative RT and targeted therapy as applicable. RAI is not effective for MTC or ATC.

EPIDEMIOLOGY: There were an estimated 53,000 new cases (PTC 60%, FTC 25%, MTC 5%, ATC <5%) and 2,200 deaths in the United States in 2020.[1]

RISK FACTORS: Previous radiation exposure particularly during childhood.[2] Approximately 85% of RT-induced thyroid cancers are well-differentiated PTC. Other factors include iodine deficiency, family history of thyroid cancer, and female gender.

GENETICS: MEN2 is a rare, autosomal-dominant syndrome in which nearly all patients develop MTC due to mutations in the RET proto-oncogene.

ANATOMY: Bilobed gland joined near lower pole by the isthmus, crossing the trachea anteriorly just below the cricoid cartilage. Thyroid gland is composed of follicles or acini, each with a basement membrane lined with a single layer of follicular cells responsible for thyroid hormone synthesis. Each contains a central space with thyroglobulin (Tg), the molecule upon which the thyroid hormones are synthesized and stored prior to release by TSH stimulation. *Lymphatics:* LN spread has more prognostic significance in MTC than for the well-differentiated subtypes. The 1st echelon is paratracheal, paralaryngeal, and prelaryngeal (Delphian) nodes of level VI. Secondary spread is to mid/lower jugular (levels III–IV) and supraclavicular LNs. *Physiology:* Hypothalamus secretes thyrotropin-releasing hormone, which stimulates anterior pituitary to secrete TSH, which stimulates thyroid to make T3 (triiodothyronine) and T4 (thyroxine), which control cellular metabolic activity in all cellular tissues and exert negative feedback on hypothalamus and pituitary. Tg is a storage form of T3 and T4. Nearly 90% of well-differentiated thyroid cancers secrete Tg, and 60% take up radioiodine detectable on imaging. Thus, radioiodine is used in diagnosis/treatment of differentiated thyroid cancers, under maximal TSH stimulation. T3 half-life ~2.5 days. T4 half-life ~6.5 days.

PATHOLOGY: Four major subtypes (see Table 18.1); rare histologies include lymphoma or metastasis (usually breast, colon, renal, or melanoma).

CLINICAL PRESENTATION: Commonly presents as palpable nodule or hoarseness if recurrent laryngeal nerve is involved. ATC presents as rapidly enlarging neck mass. Differential diagnosis includes thyroid lymphoma, metastasis, benign thyroid nodule, thyroiditis.

Table 18.1 Thyroid Cancer Subtypes	
Subtype	Description
Papillary	• Accounts for 60% of thyroid cancer cases. • Well-differentiated. Arise from follicular cells. Produce and secrete T3, T4 (RAI effective). • Associated with psammoma bodies; slow growing, indolent; multifocal in 75%; metastasizes locally to LNs, less commonly DM. Better long-term prognosis than follicular. • Good prognostic variants: papillary microcarcinoma (<1 cm), encapsulated, solid, and follicular. • Poor prognostic variants: tall-cell, hobnail, columnar-cell, and diffuse sclerosing. These variants often do not concentrate ^{131}I to a degree that is curative.
Follicular	• Accounts for 25% of thyroid cancer cases. • Well-differentiated. Arise from follicular cells. Produce and secrete T3, T4 (RAI effective). • Metastasizes hematogenously to lung and bone. Compared to PTC, has lower predilection for LN spread and occurs in older population. • Hurthle cell variant has a worse prognosis and is less likely to uptake [131]I. Need ≥75% Hurthle cells present (characterized by abundant eosinophilic granular content).
Medullary	• Accounts for 5% of thyroid cancer cases. • Arise from the parafollicular or C cells (neural crest, i.e., neuroendocrine). • Produce and secrete calcitonin and CEA. • RAI ineffective.
Anaplastic	• Accounts for <5% of thyroid cancer cases, but 40% of all thyroid cancer deaths.[3] • Extremely aggressive. Always classified as stage IV regardless of size, invasion, nodal status, or DM. • RAI ineffective. • 20% have history of differentiated thyroid cancer. • Variants include spindle cell, squamoid, and pleomorphic giant cell. • 45% have DM at diagnosis, most often to lung and bone.

WORKUP: H&P. US and/or MRI (preferred over CT to avoid iodine contamination from contrast for PTC/FTC, but neither is reliable at distinguishing malignant nodules). Laryngoscopy for VC movement. If nodule present with TSH normal or elevated, proceed to FNA. If TSH low, ^{131}I scan performed to see if the thyroid nodule is functioning/hot (97% benign) or non-functioning/cold (10% malignant). If cold, proceed to FNA.[4] Hurthle cell cancers have poor ^{131}I uptake and are better seen by Tc-99m sestamibi scan. PET may be used for poorly differentiated tumors with elevated Tg level and a negative ^{131}I scan. For MTC, check calcitonin and CEA levels pre-op and post-op. Obtain US of neck and CT C/A/P. Consider serum calcium and urinary excretion of metanephrines and catecholamines to evaluate for possible MEN syndrome. For ATC, get US neck, CT neck, PET/CT, and CT or MRI brain.

PROGNOSTIC FACTORS: Tumor size (>1.5 cm), age (<20 or >55 years is worse), male sex (worse), extent of local and distant spread, stage, extent of surgery, response to RAI, and histology.[5] Unilateral LN spread does not impact OS, but bilateral or mediastinal LN involvement has poor prognosis. Elevated serum Tg correlates with recurrence post-op (most sensitive when hypothyroid with high TSH).

STAGING:

Table 18.2 AJCC 8th ed. (2017): Staging for Papillary, Follicular, Poorly Differentiated, Hurthle cell, and Anaplastic Thyroid Carcinoma						
T/M	N	N0a	N0b	N1a	N1b
T1	a. ≤1 cm, limited to the thyroid		I (see note*)		II (see note*)	
	b. 1.1–2 cm, limited to the thyroid					
T2	2.1–4 cm, limited to the thyroid					
T3	a. >4 cm, limited to the thyroid					
	b. Gross extension[1]					

(continued)

Table 18.2 AJCC 8th ed. (2017): Staging for Papillary, Follicular, Poorly Differentiated, Hurthle Cell, and Anaplastic Thyroid Carcinoma (*continued*)

T/M		N	N0a	N0b	N1a	N1b
T4	a. Gross extension[2]		III (see note*)			
	b. Gross extension[3]		IVA (see note*)			
M1	Distant metastasis		IVB (see note*)			

Notes: Extension[1] = extension invading only strap muscles (sternohyoid, sternothyroid, thyrohyoid, or omohyoid muscles). Extension[2] = extension invading subcutaneous soft tissue, larynx, trachea, esophagus, or recurrent laryngeal nerve. Extension[3] = extension invading prevertebral fascia or encasing the carotid artery or mediastinal vessels. Solitary tumor (s) or multifocal tumor (m) identifiers may be used.
N0a, >1 pathologically confirmed benign LNs; N0b, no radiologic or clinical evidence of LNs; N1a, unilateral or bilateral metastasis to level VI or VII LNs; N1b, Unilateral, bilateral, or contralateral metastasis to levels I–V or RP LNs.
*Only for patients >55 y/o. In patients <55 y/o, M0 disease is stage I and M1 disease is stage II, regardless of T and N staging. **Anaplastic thyroid carcinoma uses same TNM stage, but separate group staging with T1-3aN0 Stage IVA and all T3b-T4 or N+ as IVB and metastatic as IVC.**

TREATMENT PARADIGM

Well-Differentiated Thyroid Cancer (PTC or FTC)

Surgery: Surgery is the primary treatment for well-differentiated thyroid cancer. Options include thyroid lobectomy plus isthmusectomy vs. total thyroidectomy. Thyroid hormone (T4, levothyroxine) replacement therapy is required following total thyroidectomy to prevent hypothyroidism and to minimize potential TSH stimulation of tumor growth. Lobectomy plus isthmusectomy is an option for select patients unable or unwilling to undergo lifelong thyroid hormone replacement. Total thyroidectomy is recommended for patients with tumors ≥4 cm, extrathyroidal extension, cervical node involvement, distant metastases, or poorly differentiated histology. Consider regional nodal dissection for clinically involved nodes, tumor >4 cm, or extrathyroidal invasion.[6]

Table 18.3 American Thyroid Association (ATA) 2016 risk of recurrence for differentiated thyroid cancer	
Low Risk	• PTC histology and all of the following: no local or DM, all macroscopic tumor resected, no invasion of locoregional tissues, no aggressive histology (tall cell, insular, columnar cell carcinoma, Hurthle cell carcinoma, follicular thyroid cancer, hobnail variant), no vascular invasion, no ^{131}I uptake outside the thyroid bed on the post-treatment scan (if done), clinical N0 or ≤5 pathologic N1 micrometastases (<0.2 cm in largest dimension) • Intrathyroidal, encapsulated follicular variant of PTC • Intrathyroidal, well-differentiated follicular thyroid cancer with capsular invasion and no or minimal (<4 foci) vascular invasion • Intrathyroidal, papillary microcarcinoma, unifocal or multifocal, including BRAF V600E mutated (if known)
Intermediate Risk	*Any are present:* • Microscopic invasion into the perithyroidal soft tissues • Cervical lymph node metastases or ^{131}I avid metastatic foci in the neck on the post treatment scan done after thyroid remnant ablation • Tumor with aggressive histology or vascular invasion (aggressive histologies include tall cell, insular, columnar cell carcinoma, Hurthle cell carcinoma, follicular thyroid cancer, hobnail variant) • Clinical N1 or >5 pathologic N1 with all involved lymph nodes <3 cm in largest dimension • Multifocal papillary thyroid microcarcinoma with extrathyroidal extension and BRAF V600E mutated (if known)
High Risk	*Any are present:* • Macroscopic tumor invasion • Incomplete tumor resection with gross residual disease • Distant metastases • Postoperative serum thyroglobulin suggestive of distant metastases • Pathologic N1 with any metastatic lymph node ≥3 cm in largest dimension • Follicular thyroid cancer with extensive vascular invasion (>4 foci of vascular invasion)

Radioiodine: TSH stimulates radioiodine uptake into follicular cells through sodium-iodide transporters. This leads to acute thyroid-cell death by emission of short path-length (1–2 mm) β particles. [131]I must be taken up by thyroid tissue to be effective and is of no value to thyroid cancers that do not concentrate iodide (i.e., MTC, ATC). A radioactive uptake study using ^{123}I is typically performed prior to ^{131}I administration to ensure adequate iodine uptake. [123]I is a γ emitter used for imaging only. Patients are instructed to follow a low-iodine diet, avoid IV iodinated contrast, and temporarily stop thyroid hormone replacement prior to administration to ensure adequate uptake. The entire body is imaged ~1 week after ^{131}I administration to document the quality of treatment.

Indications: Postoperatively for ATA intermediate and high-risk patients, and select low risk patients.

Table 18.4 Indications for [131]I Ablation Based on ATA Risk Group[6]			
Surgical Resection	ATA Risk Group	[131]I ablation (RAI)	Initial Goal TSH (mU/L) via T4 replacement
	Low	Do not routinely give [131]I	0.5 to 2.0 (if Tg undetectable); 0.1 to 0.5 (if Tg detectable)
	Intermediate	Give [131]I	0.1–0.5
	High	Give [131]I	<0.1

Source: From Haugen BR, Alexander EK, Bible KC, et al. 2015 American thyroid association management guidelines for adult patients with thyroid nodules and differentiated thyroid cancer: the American thyroid association guidelines task force on thyroid nodules and differentiated thyroid cancer. *Thyroid.* 2016;26(1):1–133. doi:10.1089/thy.2015.0020.

Radiation: There is no consensus for the role of adjuvant EBRT, though it may be considered for patients with residual disease unlikely to respond to RAI (absent or inadequate radioiodine avidity), unresectable residual disease, at high risk for residual disease (age >55, positive margins, gross extrathyroidal extension, insular or poorly differentiated histology), or recurrent disease. Consider omitting EBRT in patients under age 45 who may not benefit from treatment and may be at risk for 2nd malignancies. Dose is 60 to 66 Gy in 30 to 33 fx.

MTC

Surgery: All should undergo total thyroidectomy if possible. Completeness of surgical removal is the most important prognostic factor for long-term survival.[7] Central compartment neck dissection is indicated, with sampling of cervical and mediastinal nodes. Consider modified neck or mediastinal dissection if positive. Radical neck dissection does not improve prognosis and is not indicated. Serum calcitonin and CEA should be measured 2 to 3 months after surgery to detect the presence of residual disease. Patients with normal calcitonin and CEA are considered biochemically cured and continue surveillance. Patients with postop calcitonin levels detectable but <150 pg/mL (2–6 mo after surgery) should have neck imaging (US ± CT or MRI) to identify persistent locoregional disease. Patients with postop calcitonin levels ≥150 pg/mL (2–6 mo after surgery) should undergo additional imaging (CT or MRI neck, C/A/P, bone scan or bone MRI in patients suspected of having skeletal metastases) to identify possible DM.[8]

Radioiodine: Not indicated, because the tumor cells do not concentrate iodine.

Thyroid Hormone Replacement: Thyroxine (T4, levothyroxine) replacement therapy should be started immediately after surgery. The goal of T4 therapy is to restore and maintain euthyroidism. Suppression of serum TSH is not indicated with MTC because C cells are not TSH-responsive.

Radiation: Indications are similar to those of well-differentiated thyroid tumors. Some consider EBRT for persistently elevated calcitonin/CEA levels following surgery without evidence of gross disease or DM, though not routine. Dose is 63 Gy and 56 Gy in 35 fx or 66 Gy and 59.4 Gy in 33 fx and can be delivered similar to RTOG 0912.

Systemic Therapy: Reserved for patients with DM. Patients with asymptomatic small and slow-growing DM can be observed. Otherwise, initial treatment is with an oral TKI, such as cabozantinib or vandetanib, followed by sorafenib, sunitinib, or lenvatinib. Cytotoxic CHT for patients who fail TKIs includes dacarbazine-based regimens such as cyclophosphamide-vincristine-dacarbazine.

Anaplastic Thyroid Cancer (ATC)

Typically presents with a rapidly enlarging neck mass and cause of death is often asphyxiation. DM at presentation is common. Surgery is recommended for resectable disease, which is followed by adjuvant chemoRT. Many patients present with unresectable disease, and those with good KPS can receive definitive chemoRT. Patients with DM and good KPS can be considered for definitive chemoRT to the primary for locoregional control. Many follow RTOG 0912, which delivers 66 Gy and 59.4 Gy in 33 fx with concurrent paclitaxel.[9] Other strategies include hyperfractionation with 60 Gy/40 fx BID with weekly doxorubicin. For DM, dabrafenib and trametinib have demonstrated 1-yr OS of 80% in BRAF V600 mutant anaplastic thyroid cancer in a 16-patient phase II study.[10]

Radioiodine: RAI is not indicated, because the tumor cells do not concentrate iodine.

■ **EVIDENCE-BASED Q&A**

■ **What are the indications for EBRT in differentiated thyroid cancer?**

The role of adjuvant EBRT in patients with well-differentiated thyroid cancer has been studied only retrospectively, and many of the studies included patients at low risk of recurrence who were unlikely to benefit from the therapy. Those who are most likely to benefit are probably patients with evidence of extrathyroidal extension at the time of surgery. The addition of EBRT to patients with recurrent or high-risk differentiated thyroid cancer can lead to LC and OS outcomes comparable to historical controls. EBRT can improve outcomes in patients with gross residual disease[11] but may need to be given in partnership with RAI[12] and outcomes overall may be worse.[13] EBRT seems to be well tolerated.[14]

Tam, MDACC Matched Pair Analysis (*JAMA Otolaryngol* 2017, PMID 29098272): Matched pair analysis of 88 patients with surgically resected T4a-differentiated thyroid cancer comparing RAI vs. RAI plus EBRT; 5-yr DFS was 43% in RAI alone group compared with 57% in RAI plus EBRT (effect size = 14%; 95% CI, −7% to 33%). RAI alone had increased LRF (effect size -32%). Age and esophageal invasion predicted worse DFS. **Conclusion: Addition of EBRT to RAI results in good disease control for locally advanced differentiated thyroid cancer.**

ATA 2015 Guidelines (*Thyroid* 2016, PMID 26462967): Recommend EBRT (in combination with surgery and RAI) for patients with aerodigestive invasive disease. Recommend against routine adjuvant EBRT in patients who have had initial complete surgical resection. However, the use of EBRT in this latter setting is controversial. Selective use of EBRT may be considered in patients with initial complete surgical resection who have locally advanced disease and in patients >60 years with extrathyroidal extension. It is unknown whether EBRT reduces the risk of recurrence in patients with aggressive histologic subtypes who have adequate initial surgery and/or RAI.

■ **How should thyroid cancer follow-up be done?**

Most recurrences occur within first 5 years, but recurrences can happen even decades after PTC diagnosis. US has been particularly useful at identifying malignant cervical lymph nodes, the most common site of recurrent PTC. Serum thyroglobulin is a useful marker of persistent or recurrent tumor in patients after thyroidectomy and ablation of residual normal thyroid tissue. If initial surgery and thyroid-remnant ablation are successful, the serum thyroglobulin concentration should be very low, both during thyroxine therapy and after it is discontinued or stimulated by recombinant human TSH. A stimulated thyroglobulin value of ≥ 2 ng/mL suggests disease is present and more extensive evaluation is indicated. Antithyroglobulin antibodies, present initially in ~25% of patients with thyroid cancer, may interfere with assays for thyroglobulin, and antithyroglobulin antibodies should be tested for prior to measuring serum thyroglobulin.

■ **What is the standard treatment regimen for patients with anaplastic thyroid cancer?**

There are no randomized data to guide treatment given the rare nature of the disease. Most retrospective series utilize surgery (if possible) and concurrent chemoRT for all who can tolerate. Concurrent low-dose doxorubicin is common, although targeted agents are being investigated. Palliative treatment is appropriate for urgent airway compromise, and tracheostomy should be considered if possible.

Sherman, MSKCC (*Radiother Oncol* 2011, PMID 21981877): RR of 37 patients treated with weekly doxorubicin (10 mg/m^2) and RT to median of 57.6 Gy; 1-yr OS was 28%. **Conclusion: Weekly doxorubicin is feasible although outcomes remain poor.**

REFERENCES

1. Siegel RL, Miller KD, Jemal A. Cancer statistics, 2020. *CA Cancer J Clin.* 2020;70(1):7–30. doi:10.3322/caac.21590
2. Schneider AB, Sarne DH. Long-term risks for thyroid cancer and other neoplasms after exposure to radiation. *Nat Clin Pract Endo Metab.* 2005;1(2):82–91. doi:10.1038/ncpendmet0022
3. Are C, Shaha AR. Anaplastic thyroid carcinoma: biology, pathogenesis, prognostic factors, and treatment approaches. *Ann Surg oncol.* 2006;13(4):453–464. doi:10.1245/ASO.2006.05.042
4. Cabanillas ME, McFadden DG, Durante C. Thyroid cancer. *Lancet (London, England).* 2016;388(10061):2783–2795. doi:10.1016/S0140-6736(16)30172-6
5. Duntas L, Grab-Duntas BM. Risk and prognostic factors for differentiated thyroid cancer. *Hell J Nucl Med.* 2006;9(3):156–162.
6. Haugen BR, Alexander EK, Bible KC, et al. 2015 American thyroid association management guidelines for adult patients with thyroid nodules and differentiated thyroid cancer: the American thyroid association guidelines task force on thyroid nodules and differentiated thyroid cancer. *Thyroid.* 2016;26(1):1–133. doi:10.1089/thy.2015.0020
7. Momin S, Chute D, Burkey B, Scharpf J. Prognostic variables affecting primary treatment outcome for medullary thyroid cancer. *Endoc Pratc.* 2017;23(9):1053–1058. doi:10.4158/EP161684.OR
8. Wells SA, Jr., Asa SL, Dralle H, et al. Revised American Thyroid Association guidelines for the management of medullary thyroid carcinoma. *Thyroid : official journal of the American Thyroid Association.* 2015;25(6):567–610. doi:10.1089/thy.2014.0335
9. Sherman EJ, Harris J, Bible KC, et al. 1914MO Randomized phase II study of radiation therapy and paclitaxel with pazopanib or placebo: NRG-RTOG 0912. *Ann Oncol.* 2020;31:S10–S85. doi:10.1016/j.annonc.2020.08.1402
10. Subbiah V, Kreitman RJ, Wainberg ZA, et al. Dabrafenib and Trametinib Treatment in Patients With Locally Advanced or Metastatic BRAF V600-Mutant Anaplastic Thyroid Cancer. *J Clin Oncol.* 2018;36(1):7–13. doi:10.1200/JCO.2017.73.6785
11. Chow SM, Law SC, Mendenhall WM, et al. Papillary thyroid carcinoma: prognostic factors and the role of radioiodine and external radiotherapy. *Int J Radiat Oncol Biol Phsy.* 2002;52(3):784–795. doi:10.1016/S0360-3016(01)02686-4
12. Tsang RW, Brierley JD, Simpson WJ, et al. The effects of surgery, radioiodine, and external radiation therapy on the clinical outcome of patients with differentiated thyroid carcinoma. *Cancer.* 1998;82(2):375–388. doi:10.1002/(SICI)1097-0142(19980115)82:2<389::AID-CNCR19>3.0.CO;2-V
13. Schwartz DL, Lobo MJ, Ang KK, et al. Postoperative external beam radiotherapy for differentiated thyroid cancer: outcomes and morbidity with conformal treatment. *Int J Radiat Oncol Biol Phsy.* 2009;74(4):1083–1091. doi:10.1016/j.ijrobp.2008.09.023
14. Kwon J, Wu HG, Youn YK, et al. Role of adjuvant postoperative external beam radiotherapy for well differentiated thyroid cancer. *Radiat Oncol J.* 2013;31(3):162–170. doi:10.3857/roj.2013.31.3.162

19 ■ SINONASAL TUMORS

Timothy D. Smile and Neil M. Woody

QUICK HIT ■ Sinonasal tumors include a range of malignancies that can develop in the maxillary, ethmoid, sphenoid, or frontal sinuses and in the nasal cavity. Squamous cell carcinoma and adenocarcinoma of the maxillary sinus, nasal cavity, and the ethmoid sinus are the most common.

Table 19.1 General Treatment Paradigm for Sinonasal Tumors	
Stage	**Treatment Options**
Stage I/II	Surgical resection (preferred) and observation (only T1 ethmoid), RT, or chemoRT based on postoperative risk factors OR definitive RT
Stage III/IVA	Surgical resection (preferred) followed by RT or chemoRT based on postoperative risk factors OR definitive chemoRT
Stage IVB	ChemoRT or RT alone

EPIDEMIOLOGY: Sinonasal cancers cover a range of rare malignancies and account for ~3% of all head and neck cancers, with an annual incidence of 1 case per 100,000 people worldwide (~2000 cases).[1] M:F ratio of 1.8:1. Tumors generally develop after age 40 and usually between the ages of 60 and 70. The maxillary sinus is the most common paranasal sinus cancer (60%–70%), followed by nasal cavity (20%–30%), ethmoid sinus (10%–15%), and frontal and sphenoid sinuses (1%–2%). Prevalence is higher in Asia and Africa.

RISK FACTORS: Occupational exposure (including leather tanners, textile, wood dust ACA, and formaldehyde), air pollution, and tobacco smoke. There is some recent evidence that HPV infection can be associated with malignant degeneration of an inverted papilloma.[2] There is also evidence of a connection between EBV virus infection and subsequent development of a sinonasal tract lymphoma.[3] Chronic sinusitis is not causative.

ANATOMY: The paranasal sinuses are air-filled spaces that are located within the bones of the skull and face. They are centered on the nasal cavity and consist of four sets of paired sinuses: maxillary, frontal, sphenoid, and ethmoid.

Maxillary Sinus: Largest paranasal sinus in the shape of a pyramid with the base along the nasal wall and the apex pointing laterally toward the zygoma. The anterior maxillary sinus wall houses the infraorbital nerve, which runs through the infraorbital canal along the roof of the sinus and sends branches to the soft tissues of the cheek. The roof of the maxillary sinus is the floor of the orbit. The posteromedial wall of the maxillary sinus is adjacent to the pterygopalatine fossa, and the posterolateral wall is adjacent to the infratemporal fossa. The maxillary sinus is innervated by branches of V2 (infraorbital nerve and the greater palatine nerves).

Frontal Sinus: Located in the frontal bone superior to the orbits in the forehead. The posterior wall of the frontal sinus separates the sinus from the anterior cranial fossa (much thinner than anterior wall). It is innervated by the supraorbital and supratrochlear nerves of V1.

Sphenoid Sinus: Located in the center of the head in the sphenoid bone and may extend posteriorly as far as the foramen magnum. Innervation of the sphenoid sinus is from V1 and V2 branches.

Ethmoid Sinus: Air cells between the orbits in the ethmoid bone. The ethmoid cells are shaped like pyramids and are divided by thin septa. Lamina papyracea paper-thin bone separate ethmoid cells from orbit.

PATHOLOGY: The most common histology of sinonasal tract tumors is squamous cell carcinoma (~80% of cases). Other common histologies include adenocarcinoma, adenoid cystic carcinoma, and mucoepidermoid carcinoma. Other rarer histologies include SNUC, HMPC, angiosarcoma, rhabdomyosarcoma, lymphoma, olfactory neuroblastoma (esthesioneuroblastoma), mucosal melanoma, NUT-midline carcinoma, teratocarcinosarcoma, meningioma, plasmacytoma, and metastasis. Benign etiologies to consider include sinonasal polyposis, choanal polyps, and juvenile angiofibromas.

CLINICAL PRESENTATION: Most patients are asymptomatic or have nonspecific sinonasal symptoms that mimic benign tissue until they invade an adjacent structure and cause more urgent medical attention or more detailed evaluation. Therefore, most patients have locally advanced disease at presentation (a triad of facial asymmetry, palpable or visible tumor in the oral cavity, and visible intranasal disease occurs in ~50% of patients). Common initial symptoms include facial or dental pain, nasal obstruction, and epistaxis. Less common symptoms include cranial neuropathy (extraocular movements or trigeminal nerve symptomatology), chronic sinusitis, facial edema, vision loss, headaches, rhinorrhea, and hyposmia.

WORKUP: History and physical exam with particular attention to cranial nerves and evidence of local invasion. Nasal endoscopy as clinically indicated. Dental consult.

Labs: CBC and BMP.

Imaging: CT sinuses and MRI are both performed to evaluate disease extent and distinguish from benign causes (infection, retained secretions, granulation of scar tissue). CT chest for earlier stage disease and PET/CT for stage III/IV patients. CT provides information about bone invasion and MRI about the involvement of soft tissues, nerves, skull base, and brain, and better differentiation of fluid from solid tumor.

Biopsy: Endoscopic biopsy is typically performed unless tumor is protruding through nasal cavity or oral cavity. Maxillary sinus lesions biopsied intranasally or through gingivobuccal sulcus if tumor extends through the anterior maxilla. Ethmoid sinus lesions are biopsied through endoscopic or transnasal approach in exam under anesthesia. Frontal sinus lesions are biopsied through endoscopic approach or via the frontal recess in the OR as well.

PROGNOSTIC FACTORS: The 5-year OS for patients is 50% for those with local disease, 30% with regional disease, and 15% for those with distant metastatic disease. Favorable prognostic factors: lower T stage (T1/T2 vs. T3/T4), N status (N0 vs. N+), histology (adenocarcinoma vs. squamous cell or undifferentiated), sinus location (maxillary sinus vs. ethmoid sinus). Poor prognostic factors: intracranial extension, infiltration into the pterygopalatine fossa, skull base, dura, cribriform plate, or orbits.

Table 19.2 AJCC 8th Edition (2017): Staging for Maxillary Sinus Tumors									
T/M	N	cN0	cN1	cN2a	cN2b	cN2c	cN3a	cN3b	
T1	Tumor limited to maxillary sinus mucosa with no erosion or destruction of bone	I							
T2	Extension	II	III	IVA					
T3	Invasion[1]								
T4a	Invasion[2]								
T4b	Invasion[3]	IVB							
M1	Distant metastasis	IVC							

Notes: Extension = extension into the hard palate and/or middle nasal meatus, except extension to posterior wall of maxillary sinus and pterygoid plates, or bone erosion. Invasion[1] = Invasion of posterior wall of maxillary sinus, subcutaneous tissues, floor or medial wall of orbit, pterygoid fossa, or ethmoid sinuses. Invasion[2] = Invasion of anterior orbital contents, skin of cheek, pterygoid plates, infratemporal fossa, cribriform plate, sphenoid or frontal sinuses. Invasion[3] = Invasion of orbital apex, dura, brain, middle cranial fossa, cranial nerves other than V2, nasopharynx, or clivus.

N1 = single ipsilateral LN ≤ 3 cm without extranodal extension (ENE), N2a = single ipsilateral LN 3–6 cm without ENE, N2b = multiple ipsilateral LNs ≤ 6 cm without ENE, N2c = bilateral or contralateral LN ≤ 6 cm without ENE, N3a = LN > 6 cm without ENE, N3b = any node with clinically overt ENE.

T/M \ N		cN0	cN1	cN2a	cN2b	cN2c	cN3a	cN3b
Table 19.3 AJCC 8th Edition (2017): Staging for Nasal Cavity and Ethmoid Sinus Tumors								
T1	Tumor limited to any one subsite, with or without bony invasion	I						
T2	Invasion[1]	II	III			IVA		
T3	Extension							
T4a	Invasion[2]							
T4b	Invasion[3]				IVB			
M1	Distant metastasis				IVC			

Notes: Invasion[1] = invasion of two subsites in a single region or extending to involve an adjacent region within the nasoethmoidal complex, with or without bony invasion. Extension = extension to invade the medial wall or floor of the orbit, maxillary sinus, palate, or cribriform plate. Invasion[2] = Invasion of anterior orbital contents, skin of nose or cheek, minimal extension to anterior cranial fossa, pterygoid plates, sphenoid or frontal sinuses. Invasion[3] = Invasion of orbital apex, dura, brain, middle cranial fossa, cranial nerves other than V2, nasopharynx, or clivus.

TREATMENT PARADIGM

In general, there are no randomized trials to define optimal treatment paradigms due to the rarity, heterogeneity in histology, and variability in site of origin.

Surgery: Resection with either open or endoscopic surgery with the goal of a gross-total resection of involved bone and soft tissue is standard of care. Imaged-guided endoscopic techniques are becoming increasingly popular and are performed by both ENT and neurosurgeons with lower frequencies of surgical complications and decreased morbidity. The endoscopic method was historically criticized because it involves piecemeal resection of tumor (vs. en-bloc resection). However, negative margin status is now known to be the most important factor for local control, and this is equivalent between approaches. Advantages of endoscopic approach over open surgery include no facial incision, no craniotomy, no facial bone osteotomy, shorter hospital stay, and faster recovery time. Endoscopic sinus surgery alone can be used for early-stage lesions or in combination with open craniofacial surgery for locally advanced cases. Contraindications to endoscopic surgery include extensive dural involvement or extension into facial or orbital soft tissues. Prior to surgery, it is important to evaluate the extent of disease with regard to orbital involvement. There are three grades of orbital invasion:

■ Grade I—destruction of medial orbital wall.
■ Grade II—invasion of the periorbital fat, extraconal.
■ Grade III—invasion of the medial rectus, optic nerve bulb, or eyelid skin, which implies breaching of the periorbita/periosteum.

Orbital exenteration should be performed for those with grade III invasion (gross transgression of the periorbita with orbital invasion) since orbital preservation with periosteal resection in cases of incomplete periosteal invasion yields comparable survivals and allows for functional eye preservation. After resection, most patients undergo surgical and/or prosthetic reconstruction to improve cosmesis, function, and quality of life. Complications of surgery include meningitis, hemorrhage, wound infection, abscess, CSF leak, pneumocephalus, trismus, and blindness. Regarding management of the neck, cervical lymph node metastases are typically uncommon for patients with sinonasal cancers (see following). Neck management (RT or neck dissection) should be performed in patients who have documented cervical lymph node involvement or locally advanced disease (T3/T4).

Chemotherapy: Although no prospective randomized trials have been performed in sinonasal cancer specifically regarding CHT recommendations, typically, management is similar to other H&N squamous cell carcinomas. Cisplatin-based CHT given concurrently with RT is recommended in cases of unresectable disease or postoperatively in patients with positive margins and extracapsular spread and can be considered for multiple intermediate risk factors (appropriate for SCC or ACA, but benefit is unclear for other histologies). For patients with borderline resectable disease, preoperative CHT or chemoRT can decrease tumor size to facilitate surgery. A small prospective series of cisplatin-based induction CHT for patients with T3 or T4 tumors followed by surgery and postoperative RT demonstrated favorable 3-year EFS of 69%[4] and OS of 57%.[4]

Radiation: Typically, postoperative RT (started within 6 weeks of surgery) is used after maximum surgical resection and reconstruction. Definitive RT is recommended for patients with unresectable disease or for medically inoperable patients. Extrapolating from other H&N sites: 60 Gy for completely resected disease, 66 Gy for positive margins, and 70 Gy for unresectable or gross residual disease. In the paranasal sinus area, 1.8 Gy/fraction can be considered if multiple neural structures are treated or if escalating dose to >70 Gy. Refer to PORT Chapter 17 for more detailed information.

■ **EVIDENCE-BASED Q&A**

SINONASAL TUMORS

▧ **What is the risk of lymph node involvement?**

In general, LN involvement is rare (<15% to 20%) at the time of diagnosis for patients with sinonasal tumors. However, in patients with SCC or poorly differentiated histology, this could be as high as 30%. The risk of lymph node involvement correlates with advanced T classification and inferior involvement of the alveolar ridge, gingivobuccal sulcus, and palate. In retrospective series, adjuvant elective nodal RT is associated with improved LC and RFS in these subgroups.[5-7] Nasal, ethmoidal, sphenoid, and frontal sinus cancers rarely metastasize regionally. The most commonly involved LNs levels are ipsilateral Ib and II, but consider RP and parotid for cancers of the mid-face or with lateral extension; contralateral involvement is rare.

▧ **What are the toxicities of RT in the current era?**

Previous reports had high risks of toxicities to surrounding structures when treating patients with sinonasal cancer including visual complications (chronic pain and vision loss), pituitary dysfunction, osteoradionecrosis, and frontal/temporal lobe necrosis. IMRT has resulted in a decline in these complications without sacrificing LC or OS.[8]

▧ **Is there a role for proton beam therapy for patients with sinonasal cancer?**

PBT has been observed to be safe and efficacious in multiple retrospective series, but prospective validation has yet to be published.

Yu, Multi-Institutional (*Adv Radiat Oncol* 2019, PMID 31673662): RR of 69 patients who underwent curative-intent PBT for sinonasal tumors from 2010 to 2016. Forty-two patients received de novo RT and 27 received re-RT; most common histology was SCC, and median dose was 58.5 GyE. With MFU 26 months, de novo patients experienced 3-yr OS, FFDP, and FFLR rates of 100%, 84%, and 77%, respectively. Re-RT patients experienced 3-yr OS, FFDP, and FFLR rates of 76.2%, 32.1%, and 33.8%, respectively, and also experienced freedom from distant metastasis rate of 47.4%. Late toxicity observed in 15% of patients with no grade >3 toxicities and no incidence of vision loss or symptomatic brain necrosis. **Conclusion: PBT appears safe and efficacious for patients with sinonasal tumors.**

▧ **Is there a role for charged-particle therapy for patients with sinonasal cancer?**

Potentially, to spare the retina and uninvolved brain, but requires prospective investigation.

Patel, Mayo Arizona (*Lancet Oncol* 2014, PMID 24980873): Meta-analysis of 41 studies of nasal cavity and paranasal sinus tumors including 43 cohorts of treatment-naive patients (primary and adjuvant RT) and those with recurrent disease who were treated with CPT and photon therapy. Overall, higher 5-yr OS (RR 1.51, $p = .0038$) and DFS (RR 1.93, $p = .0003$) but no difference in 5-yr LRC (RR 1.06, $p = .79$) but was higher in CPT cohort at long-term follow-up (RR 1.18, $p = .031$). Subgroup analysis compared IMRT to CPT showed higher DFS (RR 1.44, $p = .045$) and LRC (RR 1.26, $p = .011$). **Conclusion: CPT may lead to improvements in LRC, DFS, and OS but prospective studies are necessary.**

SNUC

SNUC is a rare, poorly differentiated, rapidly growing malignancy that arises from the mucosa of the nasal cavity or paranasal sinuses. SNUC historically accounted for 3% to 5% of sinonasal carcinomas, but retrospective pathology review in light of recent new histologic classifications (see following) has changed SNUC to a diagnosis of exclusion.[9,10] SNUC is associated with a poor prognosis, generally presenting with locally advanced disease (80% are T4 at presentation) and a high frequency of distant metastases, even when local disease control can be achieved. There are no prospective randomized clinical trials to guide treatment; however, a prospective series from MD Anderson evaluating induction CHT followed by response-adapted local therapy is described in the following. Otherwise, treatment involves surgery with adjuvant chemoRT or definitive chemoRT.

■ What are the outcomes with multimodality therapy in SNUC?

An NCDB analysis suggests combined modality therapy; either chemoRT alone or surgery combined with chemoRT yields the best survival rates.

Kuo, NCDB (*Otol Head Neck Surg* 2017, PMID 27703092): Retrospective NCDB analysis of 435 patients treated from 2004 to 2012. Multivariate cox regression evaluated OS based on treatment when adjusting for other prognostic factors (age, primary site, sex, race, comorbidity, insurance, and TNM stage). Results: OS was 41.5%. On MVA, surgery + chemoRT was associated with significantly higher OS compared to surgery + RT and RT alone. Surgery + chemoRT was not significantly different than chemoRT alone. **Conclusion: Combined modality therapy (chemoRT or surgery + chemoRT) is associated with improved OS vs. other treatment modalities in patients with SNUC.**

■ Is there a benefit to induction CHT in SNUC?

The following study from MD Anderson in the only prospective study to guide therapy for patients with SNUC.

Amit, MDACC (*JCO* 2019, PMID 30615549): Prospective cohort study of 95 patients with treatment-naive SNUC undergoing induction CHT prior to definitive locoregional therapy with either definitive chemoRT or surgery followed by RT or chemoRT; 5-yr DSS was 59% for the entire cohort. For patients with PR or CR after induction CHT, 5-yr DSS estimates for patients treated with chemoRT vs. surgery with post-op RT or chemoRT (not randomized) were 81% and 54%, respectively (log-rank *p* = .001). For patients without at least PR after induction CHT, 5-yr DSS estimates for chemoRT vs. surgery with post-op RT or chemoRT were 0% and 39%, respectively (adjusted HR 5.68, 95% CI 2.89–9.36). **Conclusion: For patients with favorable response after induction CHT, chemoRT was associated with improved OS compared to surgery. However, for patients without favorable response to induction CHT, surgery was associated with improved disease control and OS.**

■ How should the neck be managed in SNUC?

While prospective data are lacking, a meta-analysis of 12 studies demonstrated fewer regional recurrences with elective neck treatment in patients with clinically node negative necks, specifically showing regional failures in 3.7% of patients undergoing elective neck therapy vs. 26.4% in those without (OR 0.2, 95% CI 0.08–0.49, p = .0004).[11]

RARE SINONASAL CANCER SUBTYPES

■ What are the recently classified histological subtypes of sinonasal malignancies?

There are several emerging rare histologies of sinonasal malignancy recently characterized in the pathology literature[12] some of them have not been distinctly classified by the World Health Organization.

HMSC: Rare entity characterized by indolent clinical course despite aggressive appearing histologic morphology with high rates of local recurrence. Mediated by HPV subtype 33 rather than 16, which is common in oropharyngeal HPV-related SCC. Commonly locally invasive at presentation. A retrospective case series of 57 patients demonstrated LR rate of 36.4% among all patients, with LR rates of 40% if PNI+ and 60% if bone invasion.[13] Despite these high rates of LR, there were no nodal recurrences and no cases of disease-specific mortality.

NUT-midline carcinoma: Arises from translocation of the nuclear protein on the testis called *NUTM1* on chromosome 15q14.6. These tumors represent ~2% of sinonasal carcinomas and are observed more in teens and young adults. These are aggressive tumors, with half of patients presenting with locoregional or distant metastases. Treatment involves surgery with adjuvant cisplatin-based chemoRT as previously noted. Prognosis is poor for this almost uniformly fatal disease with MS of 9 months.

SMARCB1 (INI-1)-deficient sinonasal carcinoma: Locally aggressive tumor usually presenting as T4 disease. The name is derived from the deletion of the tumor-suppressor gene *SMARCB1* found on chromosome 22. These tumors often arise in the ethmoid sinus and can demonstrate local invasion into the orbit or anterior cranial fossa. Imaging can demonstrate calcifications and "hair on end" phenomenon suggestive of aggressive periosteal reaction.

Olfactory neuroblastoma (Esthesioneuroblastoma): Small round blue-cell tumor arising from the olfactory epithelium. General treatment paradigm includes aggressive locoregional therapy with endoscopic resection followed by adjuvant RT for Kadish stage B through D patients (Table 19.5). Kadish stage A patients may be observed postoperatively. Standard post-op RT dosing recommended with minimum dose of 54 Gy. The risk of cervical nodal metastasis at diagnosis is 5%, but delayed cervical LN metastasis is common. Prophylactic vs. salvage management of the neck is controversial, but patients with Kadish stage C or Hyams grade III or IV disease are thought to be at higher risk of LN relapse. NCDB analysis demonstrated that prognosis is good for Kadish A–C patients (5-yr OS 80%, 88%, and 77% for stage A, B, and C, respectively) but worse for stage D (5-yr OS 50%).[14] However, a meta-analysis and SEER data demonstrate higher risk of DM and worse OS correlating with higher Hyams grade, suggesting grade is more prognostic than stage.[15,16] Concurrent CHT with cisplatin/etoposide added to adjuvant RT is indicated for positive margins or extranodal extension.

TABLE 19.4 Hyams Histologic Grading System: Esthesioneuroblastoma	
Grade I	Prominent fibrillary matrix, tumor cells with uniform nuclei, absent mitotic activity, and no necrosis
Grade II	Some fibrillary matrix, moderate nuclear pleomorphism with some mitotic activity, and no necrosis
Grade III	Minimal fibrillary matrix, Flexner-type rosettes present, more prominent mitotic activity and nuclear pleomorphism, and some necrosis possible
Grade IV	No fibrillary matrix or rosettes, marked nuclear pleomorphism, increased mitotic activity, and frequent necrosis

TABLE 19.5 Kadish Staging System: Esthesioneuroblastoma	
Stage	**Definition**
A	Confined to the nasal cavity
B	Involves the nasal cavity and one or more paranasal sinuses
C	Extending beyond the nasal cavity or paranasal sinuses
D	Regional lymph node or distant metastasis

REFERENCES

1. Siegel RL, Miller KD, Jemal A. Cancer statistics, 2020. *CA Cancer J Clin.* 2020;70(1):7–30. doi:10.3322/caac.21387
2. Re M, Gioacchini FM, Bajraktari A, et al. Malignant transformation of sinonasal inverted papilloma and related genetic alterations: a systematic review. *Eur Arch Otorhinolaryngol.* 2017;274(8):2991–3000. doi:10.1007/s00405-017-4571-2
3. Mitarnun W, Suwiwat S, Pradutkanchana J. Epstein-Barr virus-associated extranodal non-Hodgkin's lymphoma of the sinonasal tract and nasopharynx in Thailand. *Asian Pac J Cancer Prev.* 2006;7(1):91–94.
4. Licitra L, Locati LD, Cavina R, et al. Primary chemotherapy followed by anterior craniofacial resection and radiotherapy for paranasal cancer. *Ann Oncol.* 2003;14(3):367–372. doi:10.1093/annonc/mdg113
5. Jiang GL, Ang KK, Peters LJ, et al. Maxillary sinus carcinomas: natural history and results of postoperative radiotherapy. *Radiother Oncol.* 1991;21(3):193–200. doi:10.1016/0167-8140(91)90037-H

6. Bristol IJ, Ahamad A, Garden AS, et al. Postoperative radiotherapy for maxillary sinus cancer: long-term outcomes and toxicities of treatment. *Int J Radiat Oncol Biol Phys.* 2007;68(3):719–730. doi:10.1016/j.ijrobp.2007.01.032
7. Le QT, Fu KK, Kaplan MJ, et al. Lymph node metastasis in maxillary sinus carcinoma. *Int J Radiat Oncol Biol Phys.* 2000;46(3):541–549. doi:10.1016/S0360-3016(99)00453-8
8. Madani I, Bonte K, Vakaet L, et al. Intensity-modulated radiotherapy for sinonasal tumors: Ghent University Hospital update. *Int J Radiat Oncol Biol Phys.* 2009;73(2):424–432. doi:10.1016/j.ijrobp.2008.04.037
9. Llorente JL, López F, Suárez C, Hermsen MA. Sinonasal carcinoma: clinical, pathological, genetic and therapeutic advances. *Nat Rev Clin Oncol.* 2014;11(8):460–472. doi:10.1038/nrclinonc.2014.97
10. Frierson HF, Jr., Mills SE, Fechner RE, Taxy JB, Levine PA. Sinonasal undifferentiated carcinoma: an aggressive neoplasm derived from schneiderian epithelium and distinct from olfactory neuroblastoma. *Am J Surg Pathol.* 1986;10(11):771–779. doi:10.1097/00000478-198611000-00004
11. Faisal M, Seemann R, Lill C, et al. Elective neck treatment in sinonasal undifferentiated carcinoma: systematic review and meta-analysis. *Head Neck.* 2020;42(5):1057–1066. doi:10.1002/hed.26077
12. Contrera KJ, Woody NM, Rahman M, et al. Clinical management of emerging sinonasal malignancies. *Head Neck.* 2020. doi:10.1002/hed.26150
13. Ward ML, Kernig M, Willson TJ. HPV-related multiphenotypic sinonasal carcinoma: a case report and literature review. *Laryngoscope.* 2020. doi:10.1002/lary.28598
14. Konuthula N, Iloreta AM, Miles B, et al. Prognostic significance of Kadish staging in esthesioneuroblastoma: an analysis of the National Cancer Database. *Head Neck.* 2017;39(10):1962-1968. doi:10.1002/hed.24770
15. Dulguerov P, Allal AS, Calcaterra TC. Esthesioneuroblastoma: a meta-analysis and review. *Lancet Oncol.* 2001;2(11):683–690. doi:10.1016/S1470-2045(01)00558-7
16. Tajudeen BA, Arshi A, Suh JD, St etal. Importance of tumor grade in esthesioneuroblastoma survival: a population-based analysis. *JAMA Otolaryngol Head Neck Surg.* 2014;140(12):1124–1129. doi:10.1001/jamaoto.2014.2541

III ■ SKIN

20 ■ NONMELANOMA SKIN CANCER

Ian W. Winter, Neil M. Woody, and Shlomo A. Koyfman

> **QUICK HIT** ■ Nonmelanomatous skin cancer is the most common cancer. BCC and SCC represent the majority of cases. The vast majority of patients are classified as low risk and effectively treated with surgical excision or other focal therapy. Infrequently, lesions may act aggressively and require aggressive surgical resection with adjuvant RT or definitive RT. MCC is a rare primary neuroendocrine malignancy of skin that can be aggressive with rapid regional, in transit, marginal, and distant recurrence. Management is primarily surgical with WLE + SLNB standard (depending on site and nodal drainage) followed by wide-field adjuvant RT. Definitive RT is an option for unresectable lesions (Table 20.1).

Table 20.1: General Treatment Paradigm for Nonmelanoma Skin Cancer		
SCC or BCC	Low risk	Surgical resection (Mohs, WLE for noncosmetic areas), electrodissection, curettage, definitive RT (nonsurgical)
	High risk	Surgery (WLE or Mohs) + adjuvant RT (indications: +extensive PNI, vascular invasion, +margins, deep tissue invasion, multiple recurrences, node-positive) Or Definitive RT (nonsurgical candidates)
	Node positive	Nodal dissection followed by adjuvant RT (pN2 or greater, pN1 controversial). Rare for BCC
	Very locally advanced/ Metastatic	Cemiplimab or pembrolizumab (SCC) Agree with change (BCC, although mets are rare)
MCC	Localized disease	WLE + SLNB followed by wide-field adjuvant RT to primary site, with inclusion of regional nodes in cases of nodal involvement (can consider observation if SLNB negative or single node microscopically positive after full dissection)
	Very locally advanced/ Metastatic	Immunotherapy (pembrolizumab, avelumab, nivolumab), can consider CHT if checkpoint inhibitors contraindicated

EPIDEMIOLOGY: Nonmelanomatous skin cancer includes cutaneous SCC, BCC, and MCC. Prevalence in the United States was estimated to be 5.4 million cases in 2012. BCC accounts for 65% to 70% of cases while SCC accounts for 30%, with MCC representing small percentage of cases.[1] MCC incidence estimated at 0.7 per 100,000[2]; occurs mostly in older adults (average age 74 to 76), with fair skin; male-to-female ratio approximately 2:1.

RISK FACTORS: Older age, higher UV exposure (UV-B 290–320 nm is higher risk than UV-A), fair complexion, prior RT exposure (e.g., uranium miners, prior RT, tinea capitis, acne, enlarged thymus, childhood cancer survivors), chemical exposure (arsenic, coal tar), prior phototherapy, steroid use, and chronic ulcers/scars/inflammation. Of note, chronic inflammation increases risk of SCC significantly more than risk of BCC. SCC is a major contributor to morbidity and mortality in immune-suppressed patients (65× risk,[3] organ-transplant patients on calcineurin inhibitors have higher risk than mTOR inhibitor sirolimus; see the following for details). Risk factors for MCC include light skin, older age, UV exposure, immune suppression, organ transplant (×24 risk),[4] CLL, melanoma, and myeloma.[5] Merkel cell polyomavirus is ubiquitous and can be detected in normal skin flora as well as other tumors, but clonal integration of viral DNA provides evidence of causal relationship.[6]

ANATOMY: Skin is the largest organ in the body and composed of two primary layers: epidermis superficially (devoid of lymphatics) and dermis, which contains superficial lymphatic plexus. Dermis is composed of papillary region superficially connecting with epidermis and reticular region below. Beneath the dermis is the subdermis (or hypodermis), composed primarily of fat and connective tissue. Basement membrane separates epidermis from dermis. Tumors of skin may be characterized by Clark's levels—level 1: tumor confined to epidermis (in situ); level 2: invasion into papillary dermis; level 3: invasion into junction of papillary and reticular dermis; level 4: invasion into reticular dermis; and level 5: invasion into subcutaneous fat. Normal Merkel cells exist in basal epidermis and around hair follicles and act as mechanoreceptors. MCC is most common in sun-exposed areas (42.6% H&N, 23.6% upper limb, 15.3% lower limb as per NCDB).[7]

PATHOLOGY

BCC: Arises from basal layer of epidermis and has three presentations. Nodular subtype accounts for 60% of cases and presents with pink- or flesh-colored papule. These may become ulcerated and hence the term "noduloulcerative" ("rodent ulcer"). Superficial subtype accounts for 30% of cases and demonstrates red, scaly macule. Morpheaform subtype accounts for 5% to 10% of cases and presents as light-colored macules, or shiny, atrophic lesions with indistinct margins; morpheaform subtype is more likely to have infiltrating growth. Rare subtypes include infiltrative and basosquamous subtypes, which are more aggressive with basosquamous behaving similarly to SCC.

SCC: Clinically, often begin as round to irregular, plaque-like or nodular, and overlaid with warty keratotic scale or conical keratinized protrusion ("cutaneous horn"). May also see as ulcer or induration and propensity to bleed. Histology demonstrates pleomorphism, numerous and atypical mitoses, dyskeratosis, and "horn pearl" formation. Bowen's disease: SCC in situ; red-brown epidermal plaque is in sun-exposed sites. Known as "erythroplasia of Queyrat" if on glans penis.

MCC: Small round blue cell tumor of uncertain origin. Merkel cell polyomavirus detected in >80% of MCC.[8,9] Theories of origin include sensory cells in skin mechanoreceptors or skin stem cells that undergo malignant differentiation.[10,11] Three subtypes exist (small cell type, trabecular type, and intermediate type), but these are not thought to be prognostic. Immunostaining includes CK20 and cytokeratin (typically positive) as well as TTF1 and CK7 (negative in MCC, positive in SCLC).

GENETICS: Basal cell nevus syndrome (Gorlin syndrome) is disorder of PTCH, which results in macrocephaly, frontal bossing, bifid ribs, palmar and plantar pitting, medulloblastoma, and bone cysts. PTCH is in SHH signaling pathway. BCC is also associated with Bazex–Dupré–Christol syndrome, which is an X-linked dominant syndrome characterized by multiple BCC and pitting or "ice pick" scars of skin (follicular atrophoderma). Others: XP with 57% lifetime incidence of skin cancer (AR disorder associated with mutations in 7 identified genes [XPA to XPG] resulting in impaired ability to correct UV-related DNA damage due to nucleotide excision repair), albinism with 35% lifetime incidence of skin cancer, Bloom's syndrome, epidermolysis bullosa, Fanconi anemia, and Muir–Torre syndrome (AD disorder characterized by sebaceous skin tumors [eyelid] ± keratoacanthoma and internal malignancies [GI/GU]). Associated with germline mutation of DNA mismatch repair genes: MSH-1 and MLH-1 exhibiting microsatellite instability.

SCREENING: Patients with prior diagnosis of BCC or SCC should be screened by dermatologists at regular intervals to detect new skin cancers. The American Academy of Dermatology provides guidelines for patient self-surveillance while USPSTF suggests there is insufficient evidence to recommend routine screening of asymptomatic patients. Two PRTs confirm that application of sunscreen reduces incidence of AK, BCC, and SCC.[12,13]

CLINICAL PRESENTATION: Appearance of primary BCC and SCC described earlier under pathology. MCCs typically present as firm, painless, rapidly growing, single red or purple cutaneous dome-shaped nodule. Sixty-five percent present with localized disease.[7]

WORKUP: H&P including history of prior operations, procedures, or prior RT to involved area or other history of skin cancers or premalignant lesions. Complete skin examination with investigation for skip lesions, and regional nodal examination. Review for any neurologic symptoms suggestive of PNI. Biopsy confirmation of nonmelanoma skin cancer is recommended.

Biopsy approaches include punch, shave, or excisional biopsy. Sentinel node biopsy is generally recommended for MCC.

Imaging: CT/MRI should be considered for lesions involving medial/lateral canthi, positive PNI or suspicious symptoms, lymphadenopathy, or fixed lesion to underlying muscle, bone, or fascia. For MCC, PET/CT recommended for regional and distant staging, MRI with contrast of primary tumor as clinically indicated to assess for deep/adjacent structure invasion, MRI brain recommended for clinical suspicion.

PROGNOSTIC FACTORS: Include tumor size, depth of invasion, immunosuppression, location, chronic inflammation, prior RT, neurologic symptoms, recurrent tumor, and poor differentiation. NCCN defines high-risk factors, which can be used to stratify patients.

Table 20.2: NCCN Definition of High Risk for Nonmelanoma Skin Cancers[14,15]		
	SCC	**BCC**
Location/size	• Trunk or extremities and size ≥20 mm • Cheeks, forehead, scalp, neck, and pretibia and ≥10 mm • "Mask" area (central face, eyelids, eyebrows, periorbital, nose, lips, chin, mandible, pre/postauricular, temple, ear), genitalia, hands and feet, and ≥ 6 mm	
Borders	Poorly defined	
Recurrent	Yes	
Immunosuppression	Present	
Subtype	Adenoid, adenosquamous, desmoplastic, or metaplastic	Aggressive growth pattern (morpheaform, basosquamous, sclerosing, mixed infiltrative, or micronodular features)
Perineural, lymphatic, or vascular involvement	Yes	Yes
Prior RT to site	Yes, or site of chronic inflammation	Yes
Differentiation	Poorly differentiated	
Depth	Clark's levels IV–V or depth ≥2mm	
Symptoms	Neurologic symptoms, rapid growth	

Source: From NCCN Clinical Practice Guidelines in Oncology: Basal Cell Skin Cancer. 2020;1.2020; NCCN. NCCN Clinical Practice Guidelines in Oncology: Squamous Cell Skin Cancer. 2020.

MCC: Presence of nodal disease is the most important prognostic factor. Merkel cell virus antigen expression and presence of tumor-infiltrating lymphocytes[16] are associated with favorable prognosis. LVSI, large tumor size, infiltrating pattern, deep invasion, extracapsular extension, and older age are associated with unfavorable prognosis.[17] Anti-VP1 (Merkel polyomavirus) antibody titer >10,000 copies are associated with favorable prognosis.[18] Local and nodal failure is common. Recurrences can occur early (start RT early if concerned), with median time to recurrence of 9 months. Nodal failure is the most common site of first failure (55% of failures), followed by distant (29% of failures), local (15% of failures), and in transit (9% of failures).[19]

STAGING: BCC and SCC of the H&N are staged according to AJCC 8th edition staging system (Tables 20.3 and 20.4), with the exception of SCC of eyelid, which is staged separately.[3] MCC is also staged separately (Table 20.5).

Table 20.3: AJCC 8th Edition (2017): Staging System for Cutaneous Squamous Cell Carcinoma of H&N (BCC and SCC)

T/M \ N		cN0	cN1	cN2a	cN2b	cN2c	cN3a	cN3b
T1	• <2 cm	I						
T2	• 2.1 to 4 cm	II	III		IVA			
T3	• >4 cm • 1 high-risk feature[1]							
T4a	• Gross cortical bone							
T4b	• Invasion into skull base			IVB				
M1	• Distant metastasis		IVC					

Notes: 1 high risk feature[1] = minor bone erosion, PNI (nerve measuring ≥0.1 mm), or deep invasion (beyond subcutaneous fat or >6 mm depth). Nodal category definition is similar to other non–HPV-associated H&N cancers; see Chapter 11 for clinical and pathologic nodal categories.

Prognostic Stage Groups	
Stage 0	TisN0M0
Stage I	T1N0M0
Stage II	T2N0M0
Stage III	T3N0M0, T1–T3N1M0
Stage IV	T4, any N; T1–3N2; any T, N3; any TN w/ M1

A second Brigham and Women's Hospital staging system has been proposed for SCC. This T-staging system was found to better discriminate prognosis of patients in an internal cohort than the AJCC staging system.[20]

Table 20.4: Brigham and Women's Hospital Staging System for Cutaneous SCC

		10-Yr LR	High-Risk Factors
T1	0 high-risk factor	0.6%	Tumor ≥2 cm
T2a	1 high-risk factor	5%	Poor differentiation
T2b	2–3 high-risk factors	21%	PNI ≥0.1 mm
T3	≥4 high-risk factors	67%	Tumor beyond fat (bone invasion automatically T3)

TREATMENT PARADIGM: General treatment paradigm for early-stage low-risk SCC and BCC lesions is surgical excision or alternative focal therapy. For high-risk lesions, or LN involvement, resection followed by adjuvant therapy where indicated. Paradigm for nonmetastatic MCC is surgical resection followed by adjuvant RT.

Surgery: Surgical resection has two forms: wide local excision and Mohs surgery. Wide local excision is appropriate for small BCC and SCC in noncritical areas, and is the mainstay of treatment in MCC. SM should be 3 to 5 mm w/ BCC, 4 to 6 mm w/ SCC, and 1 to 2 cm with MCC. Alternatively, Mohs surgery provides on-site *comprehensive* margin assessment and is preferred for lesions located in critical areas for which larger surgery would be disfiguring. During Mohs, horizontal layers of tissue are serially excised at an oblique angle and systematically mapped w/ particular attention to peripheral and deep margins. Map of resection is typically created to guide this process, and location of positive margins during excision process is generated and can help inform planning of adjuvant RT. Goal of Mohs resection is to obtain negative margins with maximal sparing of normal tissue. It involves comprehensive margin assessment, where 100% of the margin is pathologically

T/M \ N		cN0	cN1	pN1a(sn)	pN1a	pN1b	c/pN2	c/pN3
Table 20.5: AJCC 8th Edition (2017): Staging for MCC[3]								
T1	• ≤2 cm	I						
T2	• 2.1–5 cm	IIA	IIIA		IIIB			
T3	• >5 cm							
T4	• Invasion[1]	IIB						
M1a	• Distant skin • Subcutaneous tissue • Distant LN	IV						
M1b	• Lung							
M1c	• Any other visceral sites							

Notes: Invasion[1] = invasion into fascia, cartilage, bone, or muscle.
cN1, metastasis in regional LN(s); pN1a(sn), clinically occult regional LN identified by sentinel lymph node biopsy only; pN1a, clinically occult regional LN following lymph node dissection; pN1b, clinically and/or radiologically detected regional LN with microscopic confirmation; c/pN2, in-transit metastasis (discontinuous from primary tumor, located between primary tumor and draining lymph node basin), without LN metastasis; c/pN3, in-transit metastasis with LN metastasis.

Prognostic Stage Groups			
Clinical		**Pathologic**	
Stage 0	TisN0M0	Stage 0	TisN0M0
Stage I	T1N0M0	Stage I	T1N0M0
Stage IIA	T2–3N0M0	Stage IIA	T2–3N0M0
Stage IIB	T4N0M0	Stage IIB	T4N0M0
Stage III	T0–4N1–3M0	Stage IIIA	T0N1bM0, T1–3N1aM0
		Stage IIIB	T1–4, N1b–N3, M0
Stage IV	Any T, any N, M1	Stage IV	Any T, any N, M1

assessed. Standard pathologic assessment using "bread loafing" technique typically examines 3% to 5% of tissue. Mohs surgery is associated with cure rates for BCC around 99% for primary and 95% for recurrent tumors.

MCC: For clinically node-negative patients, SLNB should be performed (SLNB controversial in H&N locations). If lymph nodes are clinically positive, either regional lymph node dissection should be performed or biopsy should be obtained (FNA appropriate) with subsequent regional nodal RT. If surgery to primary would be disfiguring or otherwise morbid, definitive RT may be appropriate.

Other Local Therapies: Local therapies are appropriate for small low-risk BCC and SCC lesions: Cryotherapy with liquid nitrogen for two to three applications can be employed for low-risk lesions with cell kill resulting from hypertonic damage. Cryotherapy is both convenient and inexpensive but provides no histologic diagnosis, no margin assessment, and is associated with subsequent hypopigmentation. Curettage and electrodessication is similar to cryotherapy, where tumor is scraped with curette and base electrodessicated. Procedure is guided by "feel" of tumor vs. dermis with the goal of achieving 3 to 4 mm margin on curetting. It may have superior cosmetic outcomes to cryotherapy, but is contraindicated in patients with pacemakers or other electronic implants and is not recommended in hair-bearing areas where feel of tumor vs. normal tissue is more difficult due to hair follicles. Topical CHT: Active agents include 5-FU and cisplatin. Topical therapy is applied twice daily for 5 to 6, or sometimes up to 10, weeks depending on clinical response. Topical 5-FU is often employed for preinvasive lesions including Bowen's disease, AKs, and cases of Gorlin syndrome. Imiquimod is immune response modifier thought to promote apoptosis and/or stimulate release of tumoricidal mediated immunity factors from monocytes/macrophages. Cure rates are as high as 90% for low-risk BCC, but only 75% for nodular BCC.

Systemic Therapy: For SCC, immunotherapy with cemiplimab or pembrolizumab is recommended for DM or locally advanced or recurrent disease not amenable to curative surgery or RT.[15,21,22] For patients not eligible for checkpoint inhibitors or clinical trials, consider cisplatin ± 5-FU, EGFR inhibitors (e.g., cetuximab), or carboplatin.[15]

For BCC, disruption of SHH pathway with vismodegib or sonidegib is systemic therapy of choice, with response rates of 48.5% to 66.7%.[23–25] Many patients have AEs leading to discontinuation. After discontinuation, median RFS is 18.4 months, with a rechallenge response rate of 85% in the event of progression.[26] Itraconazole (anti-SHH signaling activity) has also been employed in BCC.

For MCC, there is no clear role for concurrent or adjuvant CHT for locoregionally confined disease, although phase II data do exist with concurrent cisplatin/etoposide.[27] In metastatic setting, phase II data suggest response rates of >50% to PD-1 or PD-L1 inhibition.[28–31]

Radiation

Indications: RT is indicated as definitive therapy for unresectable, inoperable, or cosmetically unacceptable cases (Table 20.6).[32] For lesions of eyelid, external ear, or nose, RT is often preferred.

Table 20.6: Indications for PORT[14,15,33]		
SCC	**BCC**	**MCC**
Gross perineural spread that is clinically or radiologically apparent, close or positive margins not amenable to further surgery, recurrence after prior margin-negative resection		Indicated for primary site (can consider observation for small <1 cm tumors widely excised with no risk factors), may omit nodal basin if full node dissection performed and negative, or if SLNB negative without high-risk features for false-negative SLNB
BWH T2b or higher, especially in setting of chronic immunosuppression. Multiple nodes positive	Locally advanced or neglected tumors involving bone or infiltrating muscle	

Source: From NCCN Clinical Practice Guidelines in Oncology: Basal Cell Skin Cancer. 2020;1.2020; NCCN. NCCN Clinical Practice Guidelines in Oncology: Squamous Cell Skin Cancer. 2020; NCCN. NCCN Clinical Practice Guidelines: Merkel-Cell Carcinoma. 2020;1.2020.

In cases of PNI (particularly clinically symptomatic PNI), multiply recurrent tumor, or bone/cartilage invasion, consider treating entire nerves up to BOS and certainly if major named nerves are clinically/radiographically involved. Ipsilateral LNs should be treated in cases of parotid LN involvement, or N2/3 disease.[34] RT has advantages of being noninvasive and cosmetically favorable. RT cosmesis outcomes worsen with time and are increased with use of larger fx sizes. For MCC, there is limited evidence suggesting that RT reduces LRR. Risk factors include LVSI, immune suppression, positive margins (further resection not possible).[33,35] PORT for MCC should be initiated without delay (~4 weeks) as rapid recurrences can occur.

Dose: ACR appropriateness criteria[36] recommend the following as curative regimens for nonmelanomatous skin cancer: 60 to 70 Gy/30 to 35 fx, 50 to 55 Gy/17 to 20 fx, 40 to 44 Gy/10 fx, 40 Gy/5 fx (twice weekly), 30 Gy/3 fx (once weekly), or 20 to 25 Gy/1 fx. In areas where target volumes exist in close proximity to critical structures or cosmetically sensitive areas (overlying cartilage), more protracted RT courses are recommended. For adjuvant therapy to primary site, NCCN guidelines recommend 64 to 66 Gy/32 to 33 fx, 55 Gy/20 fx, or others. For adjuvant therapy to lymph nodes, consider standard H&N dosing schemes at 2 Gy/fx. For MCC, adjuvant dosing varies by margin status and nodal involvement.

Table 20.7: Adjuvant RT Dosing for Postoperative Treatment of MCC[33]		Regional Lymph Nodes	
Negative margins	50–56 Gy/25–28 fx	Negative SLNB	Observe (*unless accuracy of SLNB is in question, such as in H&N*)
Microscopic margins	56–60 Gy/28–30 fx	Microscopic node-positive	50–56 Gy (*or observation after full dissection with only 1 positive node*)
Gross residual or definitive RT	60–66 Gy/30–33 fx	Extracapsular extension	56–60 Gy

Source: From NCCN. NCCN Clinical Practice Guidelines: Merkel Cell Carcinoma. 2020;1.2020.

Toxicity: Acute: Fatigue, erythema, RT dermatitis, hypo/hyperpigmentation, alopecia/epilation, others location-dependent. Late: Hypo/hyperpigmentation, fibrosis, ulceration, alopecia/epilation, lymphedema, others location-dependent.

■ **EVIDENCE-BASED Q&A**

SCC AND BCC

■ **What are outcomes of definitive RT for BCC and SCC?**

Several retrospective series have reported outcomes of definitive RT for BCC and SCC with excellent LC (~90%–95%) and reasonable cosmesis.[37,38] Large tumors and those with cartilage or bone invasion have worse LC (~65%–75%) and more commonly have subsequent nodal failure.[38,39] A variety of dose and fractionation schemes have been used in reported series with no consensus, though one series that reported fraction sizes >2 Gy may have better LC in those with BCC between 1 and 5 cm in size.[38,40]

■ **How does definitive RT compare with surgical resection?**

Avril, Institut Gustave Roussy (*Br J Cancer* 1997, PMID 9218740): PRT of 347 patients with primary BCC of face <4 cm in maximal diameter randomized to Mohs resection vs. definitive RT. RT techniques included ^{192}Ir brachytherapy to 65 to 70 Gy over 5 to 7 days (55%), contact therapy with 2 fractions of 18 to 20 Gy spaced 2 weeks apart (33%), and orthovoltage RT with 2 to 4 Gy per day to total dose of up to 60 Gy (12%). Mohs surgery was associated with significantly improved 4-year failure rate of 0.7% vs. 7.5%. Cosmetic results were good for 87% of surgical patients and 69% of RT patients. **Conclusion: Mohs surgery offers improved control and cosmesis of facial BCC compared to RT although comparison is not with electron or modern photon RT.**

■ **What are the advantages of Mohs surgery over conventional excision?**

Smeets, Netherlands (*Lancet* 2004, PMID 15541449): PRT of 612 BCCs (408 primary, 204 recurrent) of Mohs vs. WLE. Mohs trended to better 2-year LC at 2% vs. 3% for primary and 2% vs. 8% for recurrent. WLE with worse cosmesis and more likely to have +margins (in 18% of primary and 32% of recurrent), especially with aggressive histology, high-risk location (except lips and preauricular), and recurrent tumor. **Conclusion: Mohs surgery may permit better cosmesis and reduce +margin rate for tumors in difficult locations or recurrent tumors.**

■ **What studies have defined worse prognosis of immunosuppressed SCC patients?**

Manyam, Multi-Institution (*Cancer* 2017, PMID 28171708): Multi-institutional RR of 205 patients from 3 institutions investigating effect of immune status on disease outcomes in patients with primary or recurrent stages I–IV SCC of H&N who underwent surgery and received post-op RT between 1995 and 2015; 138 patients (67.3%) were immunocompetent and 67 (32.7%) were immunosuppressed (chronic hematologic malignancy, HIV/AIDS, or had received immunosuppressive therapy for organ transplantation ≥6 months before diagnosis). Locoregional RFS (47.3% vs. 86.1%; p < .0001) and PFS (38.7% vs. 71.6%; p = .002) were significantly lower in immunosuppressed patients at 2 years; 2-year OS rate in immunosuppressed patients demonstrated similar trend (60.9% vs. 78.1%; p = .135) but did not meet significance. On MVA, immunosuppressed status (HR: 3.79, p < .0001), recurrent disease (HR: 2.67, p = .001), poor differentiation (HR: 2.08, p = .006), and PNI (HR: 2.05, p = .009) were significantly associated with LRR. **Conclusion: Immunosuppression led to dramatically inferior outcomes compared with immunocompetent status, despite receiving bimodality therapy.**

■ **Can alteration of specific immunosuppressive agents prevent recurrent SCC?**

mTOR inhibitors (sirolimus) improve outcomes in immunosuppressed patients compared to calcineurin inhibitors (tacrolimus, cyclosporine).

Euvrard, TUMORAPA (*NEJM* 2012, PMID 22830463): Multicenter PRT in kidney-transplant patients with hx of at least one SCC while on calcineurin inhibitors randomized to either same therapy (56 patients) vs. switching to sirolimus (64 patients). Primary end point was survival free of SCC at 2 years. Secondary end points included time until onset of new SCC, occurrence of other skin tumors, graft function, and problems with sirolimus. Survival free of SCC was significantly longer in sirolimus group than in calcineurin inhibitor group. Overall, new SCC developed in 14 patients (22%) in sirolimus group (6 after withdrawal of sirolimus) and in 22 (39%) in calcineurin inhibitor group (median time until onset, 15 vs. 7 months, p = .02), with relative risk reduction in sirolimus group of 0.56 (95% CI: 0.32–0.98); 60 serious adverse events in sirolimus group, as compared with 14 events in calcineurin inhibitor group (average, 0.938 vs. 0.250). **Conclusion: Switching from calcineurin inhibitors to sirolimus had antitumoral effect among kidney-transplant patients with previous SCC. These observations may have implications concerning immunosuppressive treatment of patients with SCC.**

■ **What data guides treatment of patients with node-positive SCC or those at risk of node-positive disease?**

Veness, Australia (*Laryngoscope* 2005, PMID 15867656): RR of 167 patients with SCC with parotid or LN metastasis (50% parotid only) with 87% receiving adjuvant RT to median dose 60 Gy/30 fx to dissected necks and 50 Gy to sites of subclinical disease. LF was 20% for treated vs. 43% for untreated necks; 73% of patients who experienced LF died of disease.

Moore, MDACC (*Laryngoscope* 2005, PMID 16148695): Prospective cohort evaluation of 193 patients with SCC in H&N. Forty patients (21%) found to have LN or parotid metastases at presentation. Thirty-seven of these patients received adjuvant RT to median dose of 60 Gy. Recurrent tumor, poorly differentiated histology, LVSI, inflammation and invasion beyond subcutaneous fat were all associated with nodal metastases. Thirty-seven percent of lesions >4 cm and 31% of lesions invading >8 mm were LN positive. **Conclusion: Patients with ipsilateral neck or parotid LN metastasis from SCC should receive adjuvant RT regardless of clinical nodal status.** *Exception may be single node <3 cm without ECE/PNI. Patients with direct invasion of parotid, tumor >2 cm, PNI, or recurrence in tissue adjacent to parotid or immune compromised state should be considered for LN dissection and may also benefit from adjuvant RT.*

■ **Which patients with cutaneous nonmelanoma skin cancer of the H&N are most likely to benefit from adjuvant RT?**

Harris (*JAMA Otol HNS* 2019, PMID 30570645): RR of 349 H&N cSCC patients at 2 tertiary care centers treated with primary resection with or without RT. A subset analysis was conducted for tumors with PNI and for patients with regional disease (N2 or greater nodal disease). In tumors with PNI, adjuvant RT was associated with improved OS (HR: 0.44, 95% CI: 0.24–0.86). In patients with regional disease, adjuvant RT was associated with improved OS (HR: 0.30, 95% CI: 0.15–0.61). **Conclusion: Adjuvant RT was associated with improved OS in those with PNI and regional disease.**

■ **What is the importance of clinical and microscopic PNI in SCC?**

Garcia-Serra, University of Florida (*Head Neck* 2003, PMID 14648861): RR of 135 patients with PNI (microscopic in 59, clinical in 76) treated with surgery and RT or RT alone; 5-year LC was 87% in cases of microscopic PNI and 55% in cases of clinical PNI. Positive SM on initial resection was present in 88% of cases experiencing LF.

Jackson, Australia (*Head Neck* 2009, PMID 19132719): RR of 118 patients with cutaneous H&N cancer with PNI treated with surgery and post-op RT (median dose 55 Gy). At MFU of 84 months, 5-year LC was 90% for microscopic PNI compared to 57% for patients with clinical/symptomatic PNI ($p <$ .0001). DFS and OS was inferior for clinical PNI. **Conclusion: It is important to identify clinical PNI to determine risk of recurrence with treatment.**

Gluck, Michigan (*IJROBP* 2009, PMID 18938044): Patterns of failure study of 11 patients with cPNI tx with 3D-CRT or IMRT who recurred. Most patients had single nerve involved initially, while all patients recurred with involvement of multiple nerves, indicating substantial cross communication between nerve branches of cranial nerves V and VII. **Conclusion: In cases of PNI, it is crucial to cover involved nerve proximally to cavernous sinus.** *For CN VII, cover nerve to brainstem and distally, skin innervated by nerve, major communicating branches, and compartment in which it is embedded/innervates (e.g., orbit for V1 or V2 involvement; masticator space for V3 involvement; parotid gland for VII involvement).*

■ **Is there a role for concurrent chemoRT for the treatment of high-risk cutaneous SCC?**

Porceddu, TROG 05.01 (*JCO* 2018, PMID 29537906): PRT of 321 patients with high-risk (T3–T4, in-transit metastases, intraparotid metastases, or cervical nodal metastases either $\geq$3 cm or $\geq$2 involved nodes or with ECE) cutaneous SCC of the H&N randomized to adjuvant RT (60 or 66 Gy) ± CHT (carboplatin AUC 2 × 6c). Primary end point was LC and secondary end points were DFS and OS. Results: 238 patients (77%) had high-risk nodal disease, 59 patients (19%) had high-risk primary or in-transit disease, and 13 patients (4%) had both; 84% completed all 6 cycles of CHT. The 2- and 5-year LRC rates were 88% and 83%, respectively, for RT and 89% and 87% ($p =$ .58), respectively, for chemoRT. No differences in DFS or OS. Locoregional failure was the most common site of failure and distant-only failure occurred in 7% of patients in both arms. **Conclusion: No benefit of addition of carboplatin to RT for the adjuvant management of high-risk cutaneous SCC.**

■ **Is immunotherapy effective in the management of cutaneous SCC?**

Recent phase I and phase II studies have shown safety and efficacy of cemiplimab and pembrolizumab for patients with locally advanced or metastatic cutaneous SCC.[21,22,41] Overall response rate with cemiplimab was 50% for metastatic disease and 44% in locally advanced disease. Pembrolizumab had a 34% response rate overall. Both drugs had acceptable safety profiles. Further studies investigating the role of immunotherapy are ongoing.

■ **Is there any role for RT in the management of early-stage nonmelanoma skin cancer?**

There have been several single-center short-term studies demonstrating the effectiveness of electronic brachytherapy in the treatment of early-stage disease. Typical fractionation schemes range from 36 Gy/3 fx to 40–42 Gy/7–8 fx delivered by specialized HDR electronic brachytherapy surface applicators. While there is a lack of long-term outcomes, local control is good with rates of 98% at 1 year, with 85% to 94% of patients achieving excellent cosmesis.[42,43]

MCC

■ **Does RT improve survival for early-stage MCC?**

Mojica, SEER (*JCO* 2007, PMID 17369567): SEER analysis of 1,665 patients investigating the role of adjuvant RT; 89% were treated with surgery and 40% of these with adjuvant RT. Adjuvant RT was associated with improved OS (MS 63 vs. 45 months, $p =$ .0002). This association was true for all primary tumor sizes, but particularly those >2 cm.

Kim, SEER (*JAMA Dermatol*** 2013, PMID 23864085):** SEER analysis of 747 patients (eliminated patients with survival <4 months arguing this biased the Mojica analysis). Performed propensity-matched analysis comparing surgery alone to surgery with adjuvant RT. Age and stage correlated with OS and MCC-specific survival. Matched analysis demonstrated improved OS but not MCC-specific survival in group receiving adjuvant RT. **Conclusion: Survival differences observed in adjuvant RT group are related to selection bias.** *Comment: Analysis may be underpowered.*

Bhatia, NCDB (*JNCI*** 2016, PMID 2725173):** NCDB analysis of 6,908 patients with stages I–III MCC investigating role of adjuvant RT. After adjustment, adjuvant RT was associated with improved OS in stages I–II MCC but not in stage III patients (stage I HR: 0.71, $p < .001$; stage II HR: 0.77, $p < .001$; stage III HR: 0.98, $p = .80$). Less than 5% of stage I, ~10% of stage II, and 29% of stage III patients received CHT. CHT was not associated with improved OS in any stage. **Conclusion: Adjuvant RT is associated with improved OS in stage I–II MCC.**

Vargo, NCDB Reanalysis (*JNCI*** 2016, PMID 28423400):** Extended Bhatia NCDB analysis to include variables previously omitted including type of primary surgery. Also performed propensity matching, which confirmed association with RT and improved OS (HR: 0.76, $p < .001$). Best OS was demonstrated in WLE plus RT group. **Conclusion: Adjuvant RT remains associated with improved OS.**

■ Is RT to lymph nodes indicated in stage I patients?

In pre-SLNB and pre-PET/CT era, RT improved nodal recurrence rates. In the modern era, omission of nodal RT is recommended for patients with negative SLNB. For patients with positive SLNB but no nodal dissection, RT is recommended. For patients with complete nodal dissection, RT is recommended for multiple positive nodes or ECE.[33]

Jouary, France (*Ann Oncol*** 2012, PMID 21750118):** PRT from 1993 to 2005 including patients with stage I MCC treated with WLE and RT to primary tumor bed, then randomized to observation of regional nodes vs. prophylactic RT. Notably excluded patients with unclear nodal drainage (median head and trunk), immune suppression, and for delay in RT initiation over 6 weeks. RT consisted of 50 Gy to primary bed and nodal region (if randomized to nodal RT) with 3 cm margin. Powered to detect 20% gain in OS (n = 105). Study stopped early after 83 patients accrued as SLNB became common in France and this was not permitted per protocol. No difference in OS. Regional recurrence 16.7% vs. 0% favoring nodal RT ($p = .007$). PFS 89.7% vs. 81.2% favoring nodal RT ($p = .4$). **Conclusion: In pre-SLNB, pre-PET/CT era, nodal RT improved rate of nodal recurrence, but trial did not accrue sufficiently to detect impact on OS.**

■ What is the optimal dose for definitive treatment of MCC?

Retrospective evidence suggests that doses >50 Gy are necessary to achieve locoregional control.[44] *NCDB supports doses ranging from 50 to 55 Gy, although selection bias may factor into doses above 55 Gy.*[45] *Furthermore, impressive results have been observed in metastatic setting from 8 Gy/1 fx, with complete response rates of up to 45%.*[46] *This suggests that there may be immune–system interaction. Further work is ongoing.*

■ What treatment margins should be used around tumor bed?

Given proclivity for in-transit recurrences and lymphovascular spread, wide margins of 3 to 4 cm are generally recommended.[44] *Treat regional lymphatics in continuity (same field) with primary lesion if tolerable (the TROG 9607 trial defined "tolerable" as less than 20 cm with cone down).*[27]

■ Is there benefit to addition of concurrent CHT with RT?

Concurrent chemoRT has been studied but is not standard given good responses seen with RT alone and unclear benefit with CHT.

Poulsen, TROG 9607 (*JCO*** 2003, PMID 14645427):** Single-arm phase II of 53 nonmetastatic MCC patients with either high-risk postoperative (gross residual, tumor >1 cm, involved nodes) occult primary with positive nodes or recurrent disease. Twenty-eight percent treated definitively, 72% adjuvantly. Patients treated to 50 Gy/25 fx; 45 Gy with boost to 50 Gy (shrinking field) was possible for large fields and 45 Gy alone recommended if 50 Gy was felt to be intolerable. Four cycles of concurrent and adjuvant carboplatin AUC 4.5 and etoposide (80 mg/m^2/day for 3 days) were delivered on weeks 1, 4, 7, and 10; 3-year OS, LRC, and DC were 76%, 75%, and 76%, respectively. Tumor location and presence of nodes were associated with LC and OS. **Conclusion: High levels of LC and OS were achieved compared to historical controls; further study is warranted.**

■ **Is there a role for immunotherapy in the treatment of MCC?**

A phase II study of patients with metastatic or recurrent MCC treated with pembrolizumab showed a 56% response rate with 24% having a complete response. Durable antitumor activity was sustained with MS and median duration of response not reached after MFU of 15 months.[29,31]

REFERENCES

1. Rogers HW, Weinstock MA, Feldman SR, Coldiron BM. Incidence estimate of nonmelanoma skin cancer (Keratinocyte Carcinomas) in the U.S. population, 2012. *JAMA Dermatol.* 2015;151(10):1081–1086. doi:10.1001/jamadermatol.2015.1187
2. Paulson KG, Park SY, Vandeven NA, et al. Merkel cell carcinoma: current US incidence and projected increases based on changing demographics. *J Am Acad Dermatol.* 2018;78(3):457–463 e452. doi:10.1016/j.jaad.2017.10.028
3. *AJCC Cancer Staging Manual, Eighth Edition.* 8th ed: Springer Publishing Company; 2017.
4. Clarke CA, Robbins HA, Tatalovich Z, et al. Risk of merkel cell carcinoma after solid organ transplantation. *J Natl Cancer Inst.* 2015;107(2):dju382. doi:10.1093/jnci/dju382
5. Howard RA, Dores GM, Curtis RE, et al. Merkel cell carcinoma and multiple primary cancers. *Cancer Epidemiol Biomarkers Prev.* 2006;15(8):1545–1549. doi:10.1158/1055-9965.EPI-05-0895
6. Feng H, Shuda M, Chang Y, Moore PS. Clonal integration of a polyomavirus in human Merkel cell carcinoma. *Science.* 2008;319(5866):1096–1100. doi:10.1126/science.1152586
7. Harms KL, Healy MA, Nghiem P, et al. Analysis of prognostic factors from 9387 Merkel cell carcinoma cases forms the basis for the new 8th edition AJCC staging system. *Ann Surg Oncol.* 2016;23(11):3564–3571. doi:10.1245/s10434-016-5266-4
8. Santos-Juanes J, Fernández-Vega I, Fuentes N, et al. Merkel cell carcinoma and Merkel cell polyomavirus: a systematic review and meta-analysis. *Br J Dermatol.* 2015;173(1):42–49. doi:10.1111/bjd.13870
9. Rodig SJ, Cheng J, Wardzala J, et al. Improved detection suggests all Merkel cell carcinomas harbor Merkel polyomavirus. *J Clin Invest.* 2012;122(12):4645–4653. doi:10.1172/JCI64116
10. Tilling T, Moll I. Which are the cells of origin in Merkel cell carcinoma? *J Skin Cancer.* 2012;2012:680410. doi:10.1155/2012/680410
11. Ratner D, Nelson BR, Brown MD, Johnson TM. Merkel cell carcinoma. *J Am Acad Dermatol.* 1993;29(2 Pt 1):143–156. doi:10.1016/0190-9622(93)70159-Q
12. Thompson SC, Jolley D, Marks R. Reduction of solar keratoses by regular sunscreen use. *N Engl J Med.* 1993;329(16):1147–1151. doi:10.1056/NEJM199310143291602
13. Green A, Williams G, Neale R, et al. Daily sunscreen application and betacarotene supplementation in prevention of basal-cell and squamous-cell carcinomas of the skin: a randomised controlled trial. *Lancet.* 1999;354(9180):723–729. doi:10.1016/S0140-6736(98)12168-2
14. NCCN Clinical Practice Guidelines in Oncology: Basal Cell Skin Cancer. 2020;1.2020.
15. NCCN. NCCN Clinical Practice Guidelines in Oncology: Squamous Cell Skin Cancer. 2020.
16. Paulson KG, Iyer JG, Tegeder AR, et al. Transcriptome-wide studies of Merkel cell carcinoma and validation of intratumoral CD8+ lymphocyte invasion as an independent predictor of survival. *J Clin Oncol.* 2011;29(12):1539–1546. doi:10.1200/JCO.2010.30.6308
17. Sihto H, Kukko H, Koljonen V, et al. Merkel cell polyomavirus infection, large T antigen, retinoblastoma protein and outcome in Merkel cell carcinoma. *Clin Cancer Res.* 2011;17(14):4806–4813. doi:10.1158/1078-0432.CCR-10-3363
18. Touzé A, Le Bidre E, Laude H, et al. High levels of antibodies against Merkel cell polyomavirus identify a subset of patients with Merkel cell carcinoma with better clinical outcome. *J Clin Oncol.* 2011;29(12):1612–1619. doi:10.1200/JCO.2010.31.1704
19. Allen PJ, Bowne WB, Jaques DP, et al. Merkel cell carcinoma: prognosis and treatment of patients from a single institution. *J Clin Oncol.* 2005;23(10):2300–2309. doi:10.1200/JCO.2005.02.329
20. Karia PS, Jambusaria-Pahlajani A, Harrington DP, et al. Evaluation of American Joint Committee on Cancer, International Union Against Cancer, and Brigham and Women's Hospital tumor staging for cutaneous squamous cell carcinoma. *J Clin Oncol.* 2014;32(4):327–334. doi:10.1200/JCO.2012.48.5326
21. Migden MR, Rischin D, Schmults CD, et al. PD-1 blockade with cemiplimab in advanced cutaneous squamous-cell carcinoma. *N Engl J Med.* 2018;379(4):341–351. doi:10.1056/NEJMoa1805131

22. Grob JJ, Gonzalez R, Basset-Seguin N, et al. Pembrolizumab monotherapy for recurrent or metastatic cutaneous squamous cell carcinoma: a single-arm phase II trial (KEYNOTE-629). *J Clin Oncol.* 2020;38(25):2916–2925. doi:10.1200/JCO.19.03054

23. Sekulic A, Migden MR, Basset-Seguin N, et al. Long-term safety and efficacy of vismodegib in patients with advanced basal cell carcinoma: final update of the pivotal ERIVANCE BCC study. *BMC Cancer.* 2017;17(1):332. doi:10.1186/s12885-017-3286-5

24. Basset-Seguin N, Hauschild A, Kunstfeld R, et al. Vismodegib in patients with advanced basal cell carcinoma: primary analysis of STEVIE, an international, open-label trial. *Eur J Cancer.* 2017;86:334–348. doi:10.1016/j.ejca.2017.08.022

25. Dummer R, Guminski A, Gutzmer R, et al. The 12-month analysis from Basal Cell Carcinoma Outcomes with LDE225 Treatment (BOLT): a phase II, randomized, double-blind study of sonidegib in patients with advanced basal cell carcinoma. *J Am Acad Dermatol.* 2016;75(1):113–125.e115. doi:10.1016/j.jaad.2016.02.1226

26. Herms F, Lambert J, Grob JJ, et al. Follow-up of patients with complete remission of locally advanced basal cell carcinoma after vismodegib discontinuation: a multicenter french study of 116 patients. *J Clin Oncol.* 2019;37(34):3275–3282. doi:10.1200/JCO.18.00794

27. Poulsen M, Rischin D, Walpole E, et al. High-risk Merkel cell carcinoma of the skin treated with synchronous carboplatin/etoposide and radiation: a Trans-Tasman Radiation Oncology Group Study--TROG 96:07. *J Clin Oncol.* 2003;21(23):4371–4376. doi:10.1200/JCO.2003.03.154

28. Winkler JK, Bender C, Kratochwil C, et al. PD-1 blockade: a therapeutic option for treatment of metastatic Merkel cell carcinoma. *Br J Dermatol.* 2017;176(1):216–219. doi:10.1111/bjd.14632

29. Nghiem PT, Bhatia S, Lipson EJ, et al. PD-1 Blockade with Pembrolizumab in Advanced Merkel-Cell Carcinoma. *N Engl J Med.* 2016;374(26):2542–2552. doi:10.1056/NEJMoa1603702

30. Kaufman HL, Russell J, Hamid O, et al. Avelumab in patients with chemotherapy-refractory metastatic Merkel cell carcinoma: a multicentre, single-group, open-label, phase 2 trial. *Lancet Oncol.* 2016;17(10):1374–1385. doi:10.1016/S1470-2045(16)30364-3

31. Nghiem P, Bhatia S, Lipson EJ, et al. Durable tumor regression and overall survival in patients with advanced Merkel cell carcinoma receiving pembrolizumab as first-line therapy. *J Clin Oncol.* 2019;37(9):693–702. doi:10.1200/JCO.18.01896

32. Mendenhall WM, Amdur RJ, Hinerman RW, et al. Radiotherapy for cutaneous squamous and basal cell carcinomas of the head and neck. *Laryngoscope.* 2009;119(10):1994–1999. doi:10.1002/lary.20608

33. NCCN. NCCN Clinical Practice Guidelines: Merkel Cell Carcinoma. 2020;1.2020.

34. Veness MJ, Morgan GJ, Palme CE, Gebski V. Surgery and adjuvant radiotherapy in patients with cutaneous head and neck squamous cell carcinoma metastatic to lymph nodes: combined treatment should be considered best practice. *Laryngoscope.* 2005;115(5):870–875. doi:10.1097/01.MLG.0000158349.64337.ED

35. Decker RH, Wilson LD. Role of radiotherapy in the management of Merkel cell carcinoma of the skin. *J Natl Compr Canc Netw.* 2006;4(7):713–718. doi:10.6004/jnccn.2006.0061

36. Koyfman SA, Cooper JS, Beitler JJ, et al. ACR Appropriateness Criteria(®) Aggressive Nonmelanomatous Skin Cancer of the Head and Neck. *Head Neck.* 2016;38(2):175–182. doi:10.1002/hed.24171

37. Schulte KW, Lippold A, Auras C, et al. Soft x-ray therapy for cutaneous basal cell and squamous cell carcinomas. *J Am Acad Dermatol.* 2005;53(6):993–1001. doi:10.1016/j.jaad.2005.07.045

38. Locke J, Karimpour S, Young G, et al. Radiotherapy for epithelial skin cancer. *Int J Radiat Oncol Biol Phys.* 2001;51(3):748–755. doi:10.1016/S0360-3016(01)01656-X

39. Kwan W, Wilson D, Moravan V. Radiotherapy for locally advanced basal cell and squamous cell carcinomas of the skin. *Int J Radiat Oncol Biol Phys.* 2004;60(2):406–411. doi:10.1016/j.ijrobp.2004.03.006

40. National Comprehensive Cancer Network. Breast Cancer (version 2.2016). 2016. https://www.nccn.org/professionals/physician_gls/pdf/breast.pdf

41. Migden MR, Khushalani NI, Chang ALS, et al. Cemiplimab in locally advanced cutaneous squamous cell carcinoma: results from an open-label, phase 2, single-arm trial. *Lancet Oncol.* 2020;21(2):294–305. doi:10.1016/S1470-2045(19)30728-4

42. Paravati AJ, Hawkins PG, Martin AN, et al. Clinical and cosmetic outcomes in patients treated with high-dose-rate electronic brachytherapy for nonmelanoma skin cancer. *Pract Radiat Oncol.* 2015;5(6):e659-664. doi:10.1016/j.prro.2015.07.002

43. Gauden R, Pracy M, Avery AM, et al. HDR brachytherapy for superficial non-melanoma skin cancers. *J Med Imaging Radiat Oncol.* 2013;57(2):212–217. doi:10.1111/j.1754-9485.2012.02466.x

44. Veness M, Foote M, Gebski V, Poulsen M. The role of radiotherapy alone in patients with merkel cell carcinoma: reporting the Australian experience of 43 patients. *Int J Radiat Oncol Biol Phys.* 2010;78(3):703–709. doi:10.1016/j.ijrobp.2009.08.011

45. Patel SA, Qureshi MM, Mak KS, et al. Impact of total radiotherapy dose on survival for head and neck Merkel cell carcinoma after resection. *Head Neck.* 2017;39(7):1371–1377. doi:10.1002/hed.24776

46. Iyer JG, Parvathaneni U, Gooley T, et al. Single-fraction radiation therapy in patients with metastatic Merkel cell carcinoma. *Cancer Med.* 2015;4(8):1161–1170. doi:10.1002/cam4.458

Sarah S. Kilic, Aditya Juloori, and Nikhil P. Joshi

QUICK HIT ■ Melanoma is increasing in incidence. Primary treatment is surgical excision with lymph node evaluation (SLNB vs. complete dissection). Immunotherapies and targeted therapies are the mainstay of systemic treatment in the adjuvant, unresectable, and metastatic settings. The role of adjuvant RT is controversial, though it may be considered in patients with multiple risk factors to improve local and/or regional control. Definitive RT can be used for lentigo maligna melanoma when surgery would be disfiguring (Table 21.1).

Table 21.1: General Indications for Adjuvant RT of Malignant Melanoma After Resection	
Primary site	Desmoplastic neurotropic histology Ulceration Satellitosis Breslow depth >4 mm Positive margins Locally recurrent disease
Regional lymph nodes	Gross ECE Multiple positive LNs (see Burmeister et al.; criteria vary by site) Size ≥3 to 4 cm

EPIDEMIOLOGY: Rising incidence over the past 30 years; 100,350 new diagnoses and 6,850 deaths in the United States expected per year.[1] Incidence increases with age (median age at diagnosis 63). In patients younger than 45, melanoma is more commonly diagnosed in females, but by age 65, the incidence is twice as high in men as in women; 20 times more common in Caucasians than Blacks.[2] Roughly 84% present with localized disease, 9% with regional disease, and 4% with distant metastatic disease.[3]

RISK FACTORS: Fair skin (particularly Fitzpatrick skin types I and II), red/blond hair, high-density freckling, light eyes (green/hazel/blue), increased lifetime exposure to sunlight (natural or artificial), family history of melanoma or dysplastic nevi, immunosuppression (congenital or acquired).[4] UVB (intermittent exposure, sunburn during early ages) is higher risk than UVA (tanning beds, PUVA therapy); 10% of cases are familial with mutations in *CDKN2A, CDK4, XP,* or *BRCA2* genes.[5]

ANATOMY: Human skin is composed of, from superficial to deep, epidermis, dermis, and hypodermis (subcutis). The hypodermis contains collagen and fat cells. The dermis consists of a superficial papillary layer and a deep reticular layer and contains sweat glands, vessels, lymphatics, pain and touch receptors, and follicles, and is highly collagenized. The epidermis is subdivided into five layers, which are, from superficial to deep, stratum corneum (dead, fully keratinized anucleate keratinocytes), stratum lucidum (highly keratinized), stratum granulosum (cells contain keratin precursors), stratum spinosum (contains dendritic cells), stratum basale (contains melanocytes and mitotically active keratinocyte progenitors that contribute to constant regeneration of the overlying layers). Malignant melanoma originates from the neoplastic proliferation of melanocytes, the melanin pigment–producing cells of the skin that arise from the neural crest during embryonic development and migrate to the stratum basale. Melanocytes are present in skin, eye, sinonasal tract, upper respiratory, GI, and GU tracts, and thus, malignant melanoma can arise in cutaneous, conjunctival/uveal, and mucosal sites.

PATHOLOGY: The most common subtype is superficial spreading, comprising 70% of melanoma.[6] These usually occur in trunk and extremities and are commonly related to sun exposure. The nodular melanoma subtype makes up 15% to 30% of cases.[6] The lentigo maligna subtype commonly occurs in older patients in sun-damaged areas of skin, and often presents as a mildly pigmented macule.[7] The least common subtype is acral lentiginous melanoma, which comprises less than 5% of cases.[6] Acral lentiginous melanoma is the most common subtype in patients of Asian origin and in those with dark skin; most commonly arises in palms of hand and soles of feet. Mucosal melanoma is rare, and makes up approximately 1% of all melanoma cases. These most commonly occur in head and neck, anorectum, vagina, and vulva.[8] *BRAF* mutation status can help guide systemic therapy; targetable mutations include V600E and V600K (see Table 21.4).

SCREENING: Clinician skin exams may reduce the risk of advanced melanoma, but no prospective randomized evidence exists to suggest decreased mortality/morbidity with clinical exams. Per USPSTF recommendations, there is insufficient evidence to recommend either for or against routine screening for the general population. The AAD recommends that those at high risk (strong family history of melanoma or personal history of multiple clinically atypical moles) undergo frequent self-examination with at least annual physician exam. The ABCDE system is useful for screening: **a**symmetry, **b**order irregularities, **c**olor variegation (different colors in same region), **d**iameter >6 mm, **e**nlargement or evolution of color change, shape, or symptoms. Genetic counseling should be considered for those with a strong family history.[5]

WORKUP: H&P with full-body skin exam and thorough lymph node evaluation; 20% of clinically node-negative patients have metastatic involvement, while 20% of clinically node-positive patients are pathologically negative.

Pathology: Excisional biopsy of lesion with at least 1 to 3 mm margins. Alternatively, clinician can consider full-thickness punch or incisional biopsy depending on location (palm/sole, digit, face, ear) or for larger tumors. If clinical suspicion is low, shave biopsy may be used, but this may complicate depth assessment if malignancy is identified. Per NCCN guidelines, SLNB is routinely recommended for patients with any of the following: lesion <0.8 mm thick with ulceration, lesion >0.8 mm thick regardless of ulceration, any lesion with LVSI or high mitotic index (>2 mitoses per mm^2), microscopic satellites in biopsy, or wide excision specimen.[9] SLNB may be less accurate after a prior wide excision, rotation flap, or skin graft closure, but these are not contraindications to attempting the procedure. Historically important features on pathology include Breslow depth (thickness of the lesion, measured to the tenth of a millimeter) and Clark level (scored 1 through 5 based on deepest involved layer of skin, with 1 being confined to the epidermis and 5 invading into the hypodermis).

Imaging: Cross-sectional imaging (CT, PET, and MRI brain) can be considered for patients with a single clinically occult positive node identified on SLNB alone (pathologic stage IIIA), should be performed for all patients with any clinically positive node or more extensive nodal disease (pIIIB–D), and should be performed for any patient with symptoms suspicious for locoregional or distant metastatic disease.[9]

PROGNOSTIC FACTORS: SLNB status is the most important predictor for local recurrence and DSS. ECE, number of lymph nodes, lymph node size, anatomic region, pathologic factures, and margins are used to determine benefit to adjuvant primary or nodal RT. Historically important pathologic features were Breslow thickness and Clark level; Breslow is more prognostic than Clark, but both have been supplanted by AJCC 8th staging.

TREATMENT PARADIGM

Surgery: Surgical excision is the primary treatment for melanoma. Wide local excision is recommended, with margin requirement based on thickness of tumor. NCCN 2020 guidelines outline the following margin requirements (Table 21.3) based on findings from multiple randomized surgical trials, though these can be modified for individual anatomic or functional needs.[9]

Table 21.2: AJCC 8th Edition: Clinical Staging for Cutaneous Malignant Melanoma

T/N		cN0	cN1a	cN1b	cN1c	cN2a	cN2b	cN2c	cN3a	cN3b	cN3c
T1a		IA									
T1b	<0.8 mm thick with ulceration 0.8 to 1.0 mm thick	IB									
T2a	1 to 2 mm with no ulceration										
T2b	1 to 2 mm with ulceration	IIA					III				
T3a	2 to 4 mm with no ulceration										
T3b	2 to 4 mm with ulceration	IIB									
T4a	>4 mm with no ulceration										
T4b	>4 mm with ulceration	IIC									
M1a	Skin, muscle, nonregional LNs										
M1b	Lung						IV				
M1c	Non-CNS visceral										
M1d	CNS										

cN1a, 1 clinically occult LN (detected by SLN biopsy); cN1b, 1 clinically detected LN; cN1c, negative regional LN, with in-transit, satellite, or microsatellite metastasis; cN2a, 2–3 clinically occult LN; cN2b, 2–3 LN, at least one of which clinically detected; cN2c, 1 clinically occult or clinically detected LN with in-transit, satellite, or microsatellite metastasis; cN3a, ≥4 clinically occult LN; cN3b, ≥4 LN, at least one of which was clinically detected or presence of any number of matted nodes without in-transit, satellite, or microsatellite metastasis; cN3c, ≥2 clinically occult or clinically detected LN and/or presence of any number of matted nodes with presence of in-transit, satellite, or microsatellite metastasis.

Table 21.3: NCCN-Recommended Clinical Margins for Malignant Melanoma	
Tumor Thickness	**NCCN-Recommended Clinical Margins**
In situ	0.5 to 1.0 cm
≤1.0 mm	1.0 cm
1 to 2 mm	1 to 2 cm
2.01 to 4 mm	2.0 cm
>4 mm	2.0 cm

SLNB is recommended for patients based on lesion thickness and other pathologic features, as discussed earlier. Completion lymphadenectomy is recommended if positive SLNB, as ~18% of those with +SLN will have additional regional LN.[10,11] The MSLT-II trial randomized patients with positive SLNB to immediate completion dissection or nodal observation with ultrasound and found that patients who underwent completion dissection had favorable regional disease control, though there was no improvement in melanoma-specific survival.[12] Complete dissection is required for any clinically node-positive patient. Adequate dissections require >10 LNs in groin, >15 LNs in axilla and neck.

Systemic Therapy: Previously, adjuvant high-dose interferon for at least 1 year was standard of care after multiple randomized trials demonstrated improved DFS with this intervention. However, targeted therapies and modern immunotherapy have replaced interferon as the systemic treatment of choice in the adjuvant, unresectable, and metastatic setting. The 2020 NCCN guidelines provide recommendations for targeted therapies and immune checkpoint inhibitors in the unresectable/metastatic and adjuvant settings, as detailed in Table 21.4.[9]

Table 21.4: Immunotherapeutic and Targeted Therapies for Cutaneous Melanoma			
Drug	**Indications in Unresectable/ Metastatic Setting**	**Indications in Adjuvant Setting**	**Notable Study**
Immunotherapy agents			
Ipilimumab (CTLA-4 inhibitor)	Unresectable or metastatic	Pathologically positive regional nodes >1 mm s/p complete resection and total lymphadenectomy	EORTC 18071: ipi improves RFS, DMFS, and OS vs. placebo after resection[13]
Nivolumab (PD-1 inhibitor)	Unresectable or metastatic	S/p complete resection with nodal involvement or metastases	CheckMate 238: nivo improves RFS and DMFS vs. ipi after resection and in metastatic setting[14]
Pembrolizumab (PD-1 inhibitor)	Unresectable or metastatic	S/p complete resection with nodal involvement	KEYNOTE-054: pembro improves RFS and DM vs. placebo after resection[15]
Ipilimumab + nivolumab	Unresectable or metastatic	Not FDA approved	CheckMate 067: ipi + nivo improves OS vs. ipi or nivo alone in previously untreated stages III–IV[16]
BRAF inhibitors			
Dabrafenib	Unresectable or metastatic with BRAF V600E mutation	Not FDA approved	
Vemurafenib	Unresectable or metastatic with BRAF V600E mutation	Not FDA approved	BRIM8: vem improves DFS vs. placebo after resection[17]

(continued)

Table 21.4: Immunotherapeutic and Targeted Therapies for Cutaneous Melanoma (*continued*)			
Drug	Indications in Unresectable/ Metastatic Setting	Indications in Adjuvant Setting	Notable Study
BRAF inhibitor/MEK inhibitor combinations			
Dabrafenib + trametinib	Unresectable or metastatic with BRAF V600E or V600K mutation	BRAF V600E or BRAF V600K mutation, s/p complete resection with nodal involvement	COMBI-AD: dab + tri improves RFS vs. placebo after resection[18]
Vemurafenib + cobimetinib	Unresectable or metastatic with BRAF V600E mutation	Not FDA approved	
Encorafenib + binimetinib	Unresectable or metastatic with BRAF V600E or V600K mutation	Not FDA approved	

Source: Adapted from April 2020 NCCN Guidelines.

Radiation

Definitive: For lentigo maligna melanoma, definitive RT is used when surgery would be disfiguring. There is no standard dose, but 50 Gy/20 fx with electrons is a commonly used regimen.[19]

Adjuvant: Per NCCN guidelines, indications for treating primary tumor include desmoplastic or neurotropic features, and thick lesions (>4 mm), particularly if ulcerated or associated with satellitosis. For positive margins, re-resection is preferred, but adjuvant RT can be employed if resection to a negative margin is not feasible. Potential indications for treating regional LNs include multiple positive LNs, ECE, lymph node size ≥3 to 4 cm, SLN involvement but without complete or inadequate lymph node dissection, and recurrent disease.[9] Indications for RT are stronger if multiple risk factors are present.

Dose: Most common dose/fx regimens include 48 Gy/20 fx over 4 weeks (see Burmeister) or 30 Gy/5 fx over 2.5 weeks (see Ang).

Toxicity: Acute: Fatigue, RT dermatitis, others location dependent. Late: Fibrosis, hypo/hyperpigmentation, lymphedema, others location dependent.

■ EVIDENCE-BASED Q&A

■ Which patients benefit from adjuvant RT to regional nodal basin?

Even with adequate lymphadenectomy, recurrence in nodal basin is relatively common and quite morbid, negatively impacting quality of life. This led to multiple prospective studies evaluating nodal RT (as summarized in the following), which were generally completed before the era of modern immunotherapy/targeted therapy. Given that regional failure is low (10%–20%) with modern adjuvant systemic therapy, the role of adjuvant RT has become even more controversial in the modern era.[15,18,20] The decision regarding adjuvant RT should be undertaken in a comprehensive multidisciplinary manner to ensure selection of patients who are most likely to benefit from treatment. Patients who present with locoregional recurrence after adjuvant systemic treatment are likely to benefit from adjuvant RT after salvage surgery.

Ang, MDACC (*IJROBP* 1994, PMID 7960981; Update *Cancer* 2003, PMID 12655537): Phase II study of 160 patients managed with one of the following: (a) elective RT after WLE of lesions >1.5 mm thick/Clark level IV/V, (b) adjuvant RT after WLE/LND with pN+ (stage II/III), or (c) RT for nodal only relapse s/p nodal dissection. RT was 30 Gy/5 fx over 2.5 weeks. MFU 78 months; 10-year local and locoregional control of 94% and 91%. Authors recommended adjuvant RT for ECE, LN ≥3 cm (in axilla or inguinal region), LN ≥2 cm (cervical), involvement of multiple lymph nodes (≥4 nodes in axilla or inguinal region, 2 or more if cervical), recurrent disease, or selective LND (rather than modified radical or radical LND). **Conclusion: Hypofractionated RT (30 Gy/5 fx) is safe and effective for adjuvant treatment of melanoma with excellent 10-year LRC and rare toxicity.**

Burmeister, ANZMTG 01.02/TROG 02.01 (*Lancet* 2012, PMID 22575589; **Update** *Lancet* 2015, **PMID 26206146**): PRT of 250 patients with clinically node-positive melanoma after LND with specific high-risk features: ≥1 parotid, ≥2 cervical or axillary, or ≥3 groin nodes, ENE, maximum metastatic node diameter ≥3 cm in neck or ≥4 cm in groin/axilla randomized to adjuvant RT (48 Gy/20 fx over 4 weeks) or observation. For margin-positive patients, dose was escalated to 50 Gy/21 fx. Previous phase II study described the regional fields used in detail.[21] Patients in observation group who recurred received resection and RT at that time. At 6 years, lymph node field relapse significantly improved with RT (21% vs. 36%). OS and RFS similar between groups; 22% of patients experienced grade 3 to 4 toxicity, mostly skin/subcutaneous. **Conclusion: Adjuvant nodal RT reduces nodal recurrence in select patients with high-risk features after nodal dissection.** *Comment: Trial was performed prior to systemic therapy/immunotherapy era (<5% received interferon); 23 of 26 patients in observation group with regional failure underwent salvage surgery with similar 5-year OS to overall cohort.*

◼ What should the field extent be for patients treated with axillary nodal RT?

In patients with axillary metastasis, limiting RT field to axilla rather than extending it to supraclavicular region provided equivalent local control rates, and extended field RT was associated with significantly higher rate of treatment-related complications.

Beadle, MDACC (*Cancer* 2009, PMID 18774657): RR of 200 patients with melanoma metastatic to axillary lymph node region who had high-risk features and received postoperative RT. High risk was defined as LN ≥3 cm in size, ≥4 positive lymph nodes, presence of ECE, or recurrent disease after initial resection; 48% of patients were treated to axilla only and 52% were treated to axilla and supraclavicular fossa. Dose was 30 Gy/5 fx. MFU 59 months; 5-year axillary control was 89% for axilla only vs. 84% for axilla and supraclavicular fossa (NS). OS, DSS, and DMFS were not significantly different. On MVA, extended field RT was associated with increased risk of complications. **Conclusion: Limiting RT field to axilla rather than extending to adjacent SCV nodal area provides equivalent control with decreased toxicity.**

◼ Which patients benefit from adjuvant RT to primary site?

The data for primary site RT are sparse. Risk factors associated with a higher risk of local recurrence that have been demonstrated in surgical series include increased tumor thickness, ulceration, head and neck location, and desmoplastic/neurotropic features, and therefore, adjuvant RT to the primary site is sometimes considered for patients with one or more of these features. Desmoplastic melanoma is a rare subtype that tends to be locally aggressive, with increased incidence of LR rather than nodal or distant metastasis. It has a neurotropic predilection and tends to spread along large named nerves, especially in the head and neck, where wide surgical margins are difficult to achieve. Retrospective evidence from MDACC suggests that the use of postoperative RT significantly reduces local recurrence in patients with desmoplastic melanoma.[22] TROG (TROG 08.09)/ANZ Melanoma Trials Group (ANZMTG 01.09) is an ongoing randomized trial that prospectively evaluates the impact of adjuvant RT in this population.

◼ What is the role of sentinel lymph node biopsy in the surgical management of melanoma?

The MSLT trials investigated this question and found that SLNB is useful for prognostication but does not improve disease-specific survival in most patients; additionally, in patients with a positive SLNB, completion dissection does not improve disease-specific survival.

Morton, MSLT-I (*NEJM* 2014, PMID 24521106): PRT of 1,661 patients with clinically node-negative cutaneous melanoma s/p wide excision, then randomized to up-front SLNB (followed by immediate lymphadenectomy if positive SLNB) or observation (with lymphadenectomy at nodal recurrence); 16% of patients in SLNB arm had positive lymph node; 17% of patients in observation arm had eventual nodal recurrence. For the entire cohort, no difference in 10-year DSS between SLNB compared to observation. However, in patients with intermediate-thickness tumors, those with positive SLNB had improved melanoma-specific survival compared to those initially observed who later developed nodal metastases. In patients with intermediate (1.2–3.5 mm) or thick (>3.5 mm) tumors, 10-year melanoma-specific survival was significantly lower in patients with a positive

SLNB (intermediate: 62% vs. 85%; thick: 48% vs. 66%) compared to those who had negative biopsy **Conclusion: SLNB is useful for staging and prognostication. However, SLNB does not improve melanoma-specific survival.**

Faries, MSLT-II (*NEJM* 2017, PMID 28591523): PRT of 1,934 patients with cutaneous melanoma s/p wide local excision and positive SLNB randomized to completion dissection or nodal observation. No difference in 3-year melanoma-specific survival between groups. At 3 years, regional nodal control (92% vs. 77%) and nodal recurrence (hazard ratio 0.31) were improved in the completion dissection group. Significantly more lymphedema in the completion dissection group (24% vs. 6%). **Conclusion: Completion dissection improves nodal disease control, but does not improve melanoma-specific survival, and is associated with a higher rate of lymphedema.** *Comment: Most patients had a low disease burden (70% had only one positive sentinel node; 12% had only PCR evidence of nodal disease); some feel results may not apply to higher disease burdens.*

▪ Can RT replace neck dissection?

Single-institution retrospective data from MDACC suggest that patients with stage I/II cutaneous melanoma who did not have SLNB or LND and had subsequent adjuvant treatment with hypofractionated regional nodal RT had good outcomes (89% 5- and 10-year actuarial regional controls and 10-year symptomatic complication rate of 6%).[23] This is not standard of care and is limited by retrospective analysis and selection bias. If the sentinel node does not map, a multidisciplinary decision between observation, adjuvant immunotherapy and nodal dissection will be required—elective RT is not common.

▪ When is definitive RT considered?

Definitive RT is not preferred for most cases. RT alone is considered in patients with superficial lentigo maligna (confined to epidermis) and lentigo maligna melanoma (invasive into dermis). These patients are often older adults and can present with large superficial lesions on the face; therefore, nonsurgical options can offer better function and cosmesis. In this setting, dose fractionation schedules vary widely, but generally, good local control outcomes have been observed (70%–90%).[24] The currently ongoing RADICAL trial randomizes patients with lentigo maligna who are not surgical candidates or who refuse surgery to definitive radiation or imiquimod and will offer some of the first prospective data regarding this question.

REFERENCES

1. Siegel RL MK, Jemal A. Cancer Statistics, 2020. *CA Cancer J Clin.* 2020;70(1):7–30. doi:10.3322/caac.21590
2. Bradford PT. Skin cancer in skin of color. *Dermatol Nurs.* 2009;21(4):170–177,206.
3. Harlan LC, Lynch CF, Ballard-Barbash R, Zeruto C. Trends in the treatment and survival for local and regional cutaneous melanoma in a US population-based study. *Melanoma Res.* 2011;21(6):547–554. doi:10.1097/CMR.0b013e32834b58e4
4. Rastrelli M, Tropea S, Rossi CR, Alaibac M. Melanoma: epidemiology, risk factors, pathogenesis, diagnosis and classification. *In Vivo.* 2014;28(6):1005–1011.
5. Leachman SA, Lucero OM, Sampson JE, et al. Identification, genetic testing, and management of hereditary melanoma. *Cancer Metastasis Rev.* 2017;36(1):77–90. doi:10.1007/s10555-017-9661-5
6. Fitzpatrick TB, Wolff K. *Fitzpatrick's Dermatology in General Medicine.* 7th ed. McGraw-Hill Medical; 2008.
7. Star P, Guitera P. Lentigo maligna, macules of the face, and lesions on sun-damaged skin: confocal makes the difference. *Dermatol Clin.* 2016;34(4):421–429. doi:10.1016/j.det.2016.05.005
8. Chang AE, Karnell LH, Menck HR. The national cancer data base report on cutaneous and noncutaneous melanoma: a summary of 84,836 cases from the past decade. The American college of surgeons commission on cancer and the American cancer society. *Cancer.* 1998;83(8):1664–1678. doi:10.1002/(SICI)1097-0142(19981015)83:8<1664::AID-CNCR23>3.0.CO;2-G
9. Swetter SM, Thompson JA, Albertini MR, et al. NCCN Guidelines Version 4.2020 Cutaneous Melanoma. 2020.
10. Cascinelli N, Bombardieri E, Bufalino R, et al. Sentinel and nonsentinel node status in stage IB and II melanoma patients: two-step prognostic indicators of survival. *J Clin Oncol.* 2006;24(27):4464–4471. doi:10.1200/JCO.2006.06.3198
11. Lee JH, Essner R, Torisu-Itakura H, et al. Factors predictive of tumor-positive nonsentinel lymph nodes after tumor-positive sentinel lymph node dissection for melanoma. *J Clin Oncol.* 2004;22(18):3677–3684. doi:10.1200/JCO.2004.01.012
12. Faries MB, Thompson JF, Cochran AJ, et al. Completion dissection or observation for sentinel-node metastasis in melanoma. *N Engl J Med.* 2017;376(23):2211–2222.

13. Eggermont AM, Chiarion-Sileni V, Grob JJ, et al. Adjuvant ipilimumab versus placebo after complete resection of high-risk stage III melanoma (EORTC 18071): a randomised, double-blind, phase 3 trial. *Lancet Oncol.* 2015;16(5):522–530. doi:10.1016/S1470-2045(15)70122-1

14. Weber J, Mandala M, Del Vecchio M, et al. Adjuvant nivolumab versus ipilimumab in resected stage III or IV melanoma. *N Engl J Med.* 2017;377(19):1824–1835. doi:10.1056/NEJMoa1709030

15. Eggermont AMM, Blank CU, Mandala M, et al. Adjuvant pembrolizumab versus placebo in resected stage III melanoma. *N Engl J Med.* 2018;378(19):1789–1801. doi:10.1056/NEJMoa1802357

16. Wolchok JD, Chiarion-Sileni V, Gonzalez R, et al. Overall survival with combined nivolumab and ipilimumab in advanced melanoma. *N Engl J Med.* 2017;377(14):1345–1356.

17. Maio M, Lewis K, Demidov L, et al. Adjuvant vemurafenib in resected, BRAF(V600) mutation-positive melanoma (BRIM8): a randomised, double-blind, placebo-controlled, multicentre, phase 3 trial. *Lancet Oncol.* 2018;19(4):510–520.

18. Long GV, Hauschild A, Santinami M, et al. Adjuvant dabrafenib plus trametinib in stage III BRAF-mutated melanoma. *N Engl J Med.* 2017;377(19):1813–1823. doi:10.1056/NEJMoa1708539

19. Fogarty GB, Hong A, Economides A, Guitera P. Experience with treating lentigo maligna with definitive radiotherapy. *Dermatol Res Pract.* 2018;2018:7439807. doi:10.1155/2018/7439807

20. Eggermont AM, Chiarion-Sileni V, Grob JJ, et al. Prolonged survival in stage III melanoma with ipilimumab adjuvant therapy. *N Engl J Med.* 2016;375(19):1845–1855. doi:10.1056/NEJMoa1611299

21. Burmeister BH, Mark Smithers B, Burmeister E, et al. A prospective phase II study of adjuvant postoperative radiation therapy following nodal surgery in malignant melanoma-Trans Tasman Radiation Oncology Group (TROG) Study 96.06. *Radiother Oncol.* 2006;81(2):136–142. doi:10.1016/j.radonc.2006.10.001

22. Guadagnolo BA, Prieto V, Weber R, et al. The role of adjuvant radiotherapy in the local management of desmoplastic melanoma. *Cancer.* 2014;120(9):1361–1368. doi:10.1002/cncr.28415

23. Bonnen MD, Ballo MT, Myers JN, et al. Elective radiotherapy provides regional control for patients with cutaneous melanoma of the head and neck. *Cancer.* 2004;100(2):383–389. doi:10.1002/cncr.11921

24. Hendrickx A, Cozzio A, Plasswilm L, Panje CM. Radiotherapy for lentigo maligna and lentigo maligna melanoma: a systematic review. *Radiat Oncol.* 2020;15(1):174. doi:10.1002/cncr.11921

22 ■ MYCOSIS FUNGOIDES

Vamsi Varra, Matthew C. Ward, and Gregory M. M. Videtic

QUICK HIT ■ MF is the most common cutaneous lymphoma in the United States and originates from the T-cell. The final diagnosis is often revealed by skin biopsies since it is often confused with other entities. Appropriate imaging and lymph node biopsies are utilized to evaluate for extracutaneous disease. Treatments tend to be localized (skin-directed therapy, phototherapy, and localized superficial irradiation) for early stages of disease and systemic for more advanced or refractory disease (Table 22.1).

Table 22.1: General Treatment Paradigm for Mycosis Fungoides[1]	
Stage I	Observation, skin-directed therapy, phototherapy, TSEBT
Stage II	Observation, skin-directed therapy, phototherapy, TSEBT, interferon alpha
Stage III	TSEBT, photophoresis, interferon alpha, phototherapy, methotrexate
Stage IV	CHT, TSEBT, oral bexarotene, interferon alpha, vorinostat, romidepsin, low-dose methotrexate, clinical trials

Source: From Trautinger F, Eder J, Assaf C, et al. European Organisation for Research and Treatment of Cancer consensus recommendations for the treatment of mycosis fungoides/Sezary syndrome: update 2017. *Eur J Cancer.* 2017;77:57–74. doi:10.1016/j.ejca.2017.02.027

EPIDEMIOLOGY: In America and Europe, six cases of mycosis fungoides are diagnosed annually per million people. Disease accounts for approximately 4% of all non-Hodgkin's lymphoma diagnoses. It affects men almost twice as often as women and has higher prevalence in the Black population.[2] Median age at diagnosis is 55 to 60.[3]

RISK FACTORS: Risk factors for MF are unclear. Although HTLV1 has been found in skin lesions of patients with mycosis fungoides, there are also studies providing evidence against role of HTLV1 as risk factor.[4]

ANATOMY: Lesions can present anywhere on the body, but are most commonly seen in a truncal distribution.[5] In rare cases, malignant T-cells can be found in peripheral blood and in advanced stages, disease may present in regional or distant lymph nodes, or other organ systems, most commonly including lungs, oral cavity, pharynx, or central nervous system.[3,6]

PATHOLOGY: Pathogenesis of MF is currently unclear. On histology, skin biopsies show Pautrier's abscesses (pathognomonic, present in 38% of cases), haloed lymphocytes, exocytosis, disproportionate epidermotropism, epidermal lymphocytes larger than dermal lymphocytes, hyperconvoluted intraepidermal lymphocytes, and lymphocytes aligned within basal layer.[7] Disease can also present with circulating malignant T-cells (Sézary cells) that usually possess CD4+/CD7– or CD4+/CD26– immunophenotype.[8]

CLINICAL PRESENTATION: Typical clinical presentation is preceded by a premycotic period, defined by nonspecific, slightly scaling lesions, accompanied by nondiagnostic skin biopsies. As deposition of malignant T-cells becomes more persistent, disease presents with heterogeneous patches that may evolve into plaques, and then finally cutaneous tumors. MF commonly presents with debilitating pruritus.[9]

WORKUP: H&P including percentage of body surface area affected by patches, plaques, or tumor lesions. Laboratory studies should include CBC, CMP, LFTs, and serum LDH, as well as evaluation for Sézary cells (PCR/flow cytometry). Skin biopsies should be taken from at least two sites, and should be assessed with H&E staining, immunostaining for surface marker expression profiles, and PCR for clonal TCR rearrangement. If only one biopsy can be obtained, lesion with greatest induration should be chosen.[8] Chest x-ray or nodal ultrasound is sufficient for patients with early-stage disease. However, CT scan of chest, abdomen, and pelvis, or whole-body integrated PET/CT should be performed for patients with T2b disease or greater in order to rule out any lymphadenopathy or visceral involvement.[10]

PROGNOSTIC FACTORS: Advanced clinical stage, large cell histology, folliculotropic disease, age >60, increased LDH, and extracutaneous involvement have worse prognosis.[11]

STAGING: Current standard for staging MF utilizes TNMB system proposed by ISCL/EORTC. Patients with limited patches, papules, and/or plaques that cover <10% of the skin are classified as T1. Patients with lesions covering ≥10% of the skin surface are classified as T2. If ≥1 tumor ≥1 cm in diameter, then they are classified as T3. Erythema covering ≥80% of the body surface is classified as T4.[8]

Disease with clinically abnormal peripheral lymph nodes with a histopathology Dutch grade of 1 or NCI LN0–2 is N1. Nodal disease with a histopathology Dutch grade of 2 or NCI LN3 is N2. Nodal disease with a histopathology Dutch grade of 3 to 4 or NCI LN4 is N3. Clinically abnormal peripheral lymph nodes without histologic confirmation are NX.[8] Patients with visceral organ involvement are M1.

A peripheral blood involvement classification of B0 is defined by absence of significant blood involvement (≤5% of peripheral blood lymphocytes as atypical Sézary cells). B1 disease is defined by a low blood-tumor burden: >5% of peripheral blood lymphocytes as Sézary cells, but still less than the B2 criterion, which is greater than 1,000 Sézary cells/μL with positive clone.[8]

Note that N1a/b, N2a/b, B0a/b, B1a/b subclassifications are defined but not included here for brevity and can be found in the original definition by Olsen et al.[8] Grouped stage is provided in Table 22.2.

Table 22.2: TNMB Clinical Staging System				
N T/B/M	N0	N1	N2	N3
T1	IA	IIA		IVA2
T2	IB			
T3	IIB			
T4	IIIA (if B0) or IIIB (if B1)			
B2	IVA1			
M1	IVB			

Source: From Olsen E, Vonderheid E, Pimpinelli N, et al. Revisions to the staging and classification of mycosis fungoides and Sezary syndrome: a proposal of the International Society for Cutaneous Lymphomas (ISCL) and the cutaneous lymphoma task force of the European Organization of Research and Treatment of Cancer (EORTC). *Blood.* 2007;110(6):1713–1722. doi:10.1182/blood-2007-03-055749

TREATMENT PARADIGM

Observation: Expectant observation is recommended for informed patients with stage IA disease but requires attentive monitoring and proper patient education.[1]

Medical: Various skin-directed therapies should be considered as first-line treatment in early disease and supplemental treatment in more advanced disease. Preferred initial skin-directed therapies are topical corticosteroids, topical nitrogen mustard (e.g., carmustine), and topical retinoids.[1] Pruritus is highly prevalent and should be treated according to general guidelines for managing pruritus.

Surgery: There is no clear role for surgical resection in MF.

Chemotherapy: Although skin-directed therapies should be attempted initially in patients with early disease, CHT should be considered early in patients with extensive, advanced, or refractory disease. Common CHT regimens include low-dose methotrexate, pegylated liposomal doxorubicin, gemcitabine, pralatrexate, fludarabine with cyclophosphamides, fludarabine with interferon alpha, CHOP (cyclophosphamide, doxorubicin, vincristine, and prednisolone), and EPOCH (etoposide, vincristine, doxorubicin, cyclophosphamide, and prednisolone).[12] Other systemic therapies include retinoids, histone deacetylase inhibitors, brentuximab vedotin, mogamulizumab (anti-CCR4), pembrolizumab, and bortezimib.[1,13,14]

Radiation: Localized RT is indicated for patients with stage IA disease presenting with one to three lesions that are in close enough proximity to be targeted by single or abutting RT fields.[15] It is also indicated as palliative treatment for patients with advanced disease. Photons as well as electron beam may be used. Local superficial irradiation for curative treatment of unilesional stage IA disease should be dosed at least 20 to 30 Gy at 2 Gy per fraction with 5 fractions per week, and palliative treatment for advanced disease can be dosed at 8 to 20 Gy given in 1 to 5 fractions.[16,17] Adverse effects include mild dermatitis, local alopecia, and pigmentation changes.[15]

TSEBT: In TSEBT, electrons are calibrated to penetrate skin to limited depth, targeting epidermis, adnexal structures, and dermis. It can be considered in all stages of disease. Historically treatment dosed to 26–36 Gy to 4- to 6-mm depth (surface dose 31–36 Gy), given in 30 to 36 treatments (2 days per fraction) over 9 weeks, 4 days per week. Recent evidence suggests shorter course of 12 Gy may be effective, with shorter duration of control. During treatment, some symptoms, such as pruritus and cutaneous erythema, may be exacerbated. In addition, alopecia, temporary nail stasis, peripheral edema, epistaxis, blisters of fingers and feet, anhidrosis, parotitis, gynecomastia, corneal tears, chronic nail dystrophy, chronic xerosis, and fingertip dysesthesias may occur.[18] For technical details regarding both local superficial irradiation and TSEBT, see *Handbook of Treatment Planning in Radiation Oncology*, Chapter 10.[19]

Other Modalities: Phototherapy may be used in treatment of MF, including UVB and PUVA. More recently, treatments also include UVA1 and excimer laser.[20] In cases refractory to other modalities, allogenic hematopoietic stem cell transplant may be considered.[21]

■ **EVIDENCE-BASED Q&A**

▓ **Do patients benefit from early aggressive therapy?**

While CR is higher in those undergoing aggressive therapy with TSEBT and CHT, there is no benefit in DFS or OS with significantly increased toxicity rate.

Kaye (*NEJM* 1989, PMID 2594037): RCT of 103 patients w/ MF randomized to 30 Gy TSEBT w/ CHT (cyclophosphamide, doxorubicin, etoposide, and vincristine) or sequential topical treatment. Higher rate of CR in patients treated w/ combination therapy (38% vs. 18%, $p = .032$) but no difference in DFS or OS after 75 months of FU. Increased toxicity in combination therapy group including hospitalization for fever/neutropenia, and CHF. **Conclusion: Early aggressive therapy with RT and CHT does not improve prognosis for patients with MF as compared with conservative treatment beginning with sequential topical therapies.**

▓ **What dose should be used for localized disease?**

When using standard fractionation, doses of 20 to 30 Gy are necessary for durable response. However, recently, doses as low as 7 Gy have been shown to be effective.

Cotter (*IJROBP* 1983, PMID 6195138): RR of 110 lesions from 14 patients with MF who underwent RT with Co-60 or electrons. Doses ranged from 6 to 40 Gy; 53% of lesions were plaques, 20% were tumors ≤3 cm in diameter, 27% were tumors >3 cm in diameter. CR in 95% of plaques, 95% of tumors ≤3 cm, and 93% in tumors >3 cm in diameter. CR in all tumors receiving >20 Gy. In lesions having CR, 42% had in-field recurrence if they received <10 Gy, 32% for 10 to 20 Gy, 21% for 20 to 30 Gy, and 0% for >30 Gy with mean time to first recurrence of 5 months, 10 months, and 16 months, respectively, for each dose range. Eighty-three percent of 30 recurrences were within 1 year while 100% were within

2 years of treatment. **Conclusion: Tumor doses equivalent to at least 30 Gy at 2 Gy per fraction, 5 fractions per week are suggested for adequate local control of cutaneous MF lesions.**

Thomas, Northwestern University (*IJROBP* 2013, PMID 22818412): RR of 270 patients treated with single-fraction RT dose of ≥7 Gy or more. MFU 41.3 months. CR in 94.4% of patients, PR in 3.7%, conversion to CR after second treatment in 1.5%, and no response in 0.4%. **Conclusion: Single fraction of 7 to 8 Gy is sufficient to provide palliation for CTCL lesions. New lesions can develop outside the treated field.**

Wilson, Yale (*IJROBP* 1998, PMID 9422565): RR of 21 patients with 32 lesions receiving curative LSRT for stage IA MF; 9 patients received prior focal therapy (steroids, PUVA, BCNU, UVB) and 6 received adjuvant therapy after local RT (PUVA, steroids). Median FU was 36 months. Median surface dose was 20 Gy (6–40 Gy) with median 5 fractions. For fields receiving >20 Gy, median fraction number was 10. CR was 97% overall with one patient having PR, treated with 6 Gy. Three patients had LR at 52 months (8 Gy), 16 months (20 Gy), and 4 months (20 Gy); 10-year DFS of 91% for those receiving ≥20 Gy with 91% LC. **Conclusion: Patients should be offered choice of LSRT alone, without adjuvant therapies, to dose of 20 Gy or greater with minimum margin of 1 to 2 cm around target.**

■ **What dose should be used for TSEBT?**

TSEBT is conventionally dosed to at least 30 Gy, yielding greater CR rates and lower rates of disease recurrence. However, recent phase II studies suggest 12 Gy can provide rapid reduction of disease burden for a sustained period of time and reduce toxicity.

Hoppe, Stanford (*IJROBP* 1977, PMID 591404): A total of 176 patients with MF treated with TSEBT from 1958 to 1975 with varying doses. CR rates increased with decreased skin involvement, ranging from 86% in limited plaques to 44% in tumors. Survival also related to extent of disease with 10-year OS of 76%, 44%, and 6% in those with limited plaques, generalized plaques, and tumors, respectively. Stage also correlated with survival, exemplified by 5-year OS of 80% and 51% for stage I and stage II patients respectively, along with lack of stage III/IV long-term survivors. CR was directly related to initial dose of TSEBT with 18% CR for 8 to 9.9 Gy, 55% for 10 to 19.9 Gy, 66% for 20 to 24.9 Gy, 75% for 25 to 29.9 Gy, and 94% for 30 to 36 Gy. Thirty-nine percent (20 patients) who had CR after TSEBT >30 Gy remained without disease 3 to 14 years after completion. **Conclusion: Patients receiving TSEBT dose of at least 30 Gy experienced greatest rates of CR and had lower rates of disease recurrence.**

Hoppe, Stanford (*J Am Acad Dermatol* 2015, PMID 25476993): Pooled data from three clinical trials using low-dose (12 Gy) TSEBT. All trials involved TSEBT-naive patients with stage IB to IIIA MF. Treatment was 12 Gy, 1 Gy per fraction over 3 weeks. Primary end point was clinical response rate; 33 patients enrolled; 18 males. Stages were 22 IB, 2 IIA, 7 IIB, and 2 IIIA. Overall response rate was 88% (29/33), including nine patients with complete response. Median time to response was 7.6 weeks (3–12.4 weeks). Median duration of clinical benefit was 70.7 weeks (95% CI: 41.8–133.8). **Conclusion: Low-dose TSEBT provides reliable and rapid reduction of MF, can be administered safely multiple times during the course of a patient's disease, and has acceptable toxicity profile.**

Morris (*IJROBP* 2017, PMID 28843374): Prospective cohort study of 103 patients with MF treated with low-dose TSEBT (12 Gy/8 fx). Stages were 54 IB, 33 IIB, 12 III, and 4 IV. CR in 18% and PR in 69%. Eight percent of patients had stable disease and 5% progressed on treatment. In patients with CR, median time to relapse was 7.3 months and median response duration was 11.8 months. Median PFS for the whole cohort was 13.2 months. **Conclusion: Low-dose TSEBT of 12 Gy in 8 fractions is effective and well tolerated.**

REFERENCES

1. Trautinger F, Eder J, Assaf C, et al. European organisation for research and treatment of cancer consensus recommendations for the treatment of mycosis fungoides/Sezary syndrome: update 2017. *Eur J Cancer.* 2017;77:57–74. doi:10.1016/j.ejca.2017.02.027
2. Criscione VD, Weinstock MA. Incidence of cutaneous T-cell lymphoma in the United States, 1973–2002. *Arch Dermatol.* 2007;143(7):854–859. doi:10.1001/archderm.143.7.854

3. Willemze R, Jaffe ES, Burg G, et al. WHO-EORTC classification for cutaneous lymphomas. *Blood.* 2005;105(10):3768–3785. doi:10.1182/blood-2004-09-3502

4. Wood GS, Salvekar A, Schaffer J, et al. Evidence against a role for human T-cell lymphotrophic virus type I (HTLV-I) in the pathogenesis of American cutaneous T-cell lymphoma. *J Invest Dermatol.* 1996;107(3):301–307. doi:10.1111/1523-1747.ep12363010

5. Pimpinelli N, Olsen EA, Santucci M, et al. Defining early mycosis fungoides. *J Am Acad Dermatol.* 2005;53(6):1053–1063. doi:10.1016/j.jaad.2005.08.057

6. Kim YH, Liu HL, Mraz-Gernhard S, et al. Long-term outcome of 525 patients with mycosis fungoides and Sezary syndrome: clinical prognostic factors and risk for disease progression. *Arch Dermatol.* 2003;139(7):857–866. doi:10.1001/archderm.139.7.857

7. Smoller BR, Bishop K, Glusac E, et al. Reassessment of histologic parameters in the diagnosis of mycosis fungoides. *Am J Surg Pathol.* 1995;19(12):1423–1430. doi:10.1097/00000478-199512000-00009

8. Olsen E, Vonderheid E, Pimpinelli N, et al. Revisions to the staging and classification of mycosis fungoides and Sezary syndrome: a proposal of the International Society for Cutaneous Lymphomas (ISCL) and the cutaneous lymphoma task force of the European Organization of Research and Treatment of Cancer (EORTC). *Blood.* 2007;110(6):1713–1722. doi:10.1182/blood-2007-03-055749

9. Olsen EA, Whittaker S, Kim YH, et al. Clinical end points and response criteria in mycosis fungoides and Sezary syndrome: a consensus statement of the International Society for Cutaneous Lymphomas, the United States Cutaneous Lymphoma Consortium, and the Cutaneous Lymphoma Task Force of the European Organisation for Research and Treatment of Cancer. *J Clin Oncol.* 2011;29(18):2598–2607. doi:10.1200/JCO.2010.32.0630

10. Tsai EY, Taur A, Espinosa L, et al. Staging accuracy in mycosis fungoides and sezary syndrome using integrated positron emission tomography and computed tomography. *Arch Dermatol.* 2006;142(5):577–584. doi:10.1001/archderm.142.5.577

11. Scarisbrick JJ, Prince HM, Vermeer MH, et al. Cutaneous Lymphoma International Consortium study of outcome in advanced stages of mycosis fungoides and Sézary syndrome: effect of specific prognostic markers on survival and development of a prognostic model. *J Clin Oncol.* 2015;33(32):3766–3773. doi:10.1200/JCO.2015.61.7142.

12. Hughes CF, Khot A, McCormack C, et al. Lack of durable disease control with chemotherapy for mycosis fungoides and Sezary syndrome: a comparative study of systemic therapy. *Blood.* 2015;125(1):71–81. doi:10.1182/blood-2014-07-588236

13. Larocca C, Kupper T. Mycosis fungoides and Sézary syndrome: an update. *Hematol. Oncol Clin North Am.* 2019;33(1):103–120. doi:10.1016/j.hoc.2018.09.001

14. Kim YH, Bagot M, Pinter-Brown L, et al. Mogamulizumab versus vorinostat in previously treated cutaneous T-cell lymphoma (MAVORIC): an international, open-label, randomised, controlled phase 3 trial. *Lancet Oncol.* 2018;19(9):1192–1204. doi:10.1016/S1470-2045(18)30379-6.

15. Wilson LD, Kacinski BM, Jones GW. Local superficial radiotherapy in the management of minimal stage IA cutaneous T-cell lymphoma (mycosis fungoides). *Int J Radiat Oncol Biol Phys.* 1998;40(1):109–115. doi:10.1016/S0360-3016(97)00553-1

16. Cotter GW, Baglan RJ, Wasserman TH, Mill W. Palliative radiation treatment of cutaneous mycosis fungoides: a dose response. *Int J Radiat Oncol Biol Phys.* 1983;9(10):1477–1480. doi:10.1016/0360-3016(83)90321-8

17. Neelis KJ, Schimmel EC, Vermeer MH, et al. Low-dose palliative radiotherapy for cutaneous B-and T-cell lymphomas. *Int J Radiat Oncol Biol Phys.* 2009;74(1):154–158. doi:10.1016/j.ijrobp.2008.06.1918

18. Jones GW, Kacinski BM, Wilson LD, et al. Total skin electron radiation in the management of mycosis fungoides: consensus of the European Organization for Research and Treatment of Cancer (EORTC) Cutaneous Lymphoma Project Group. *J Am Acad Dermatol.* 2002;47(3):364–370. doi:10.1067/mjd.2002.123482

19. Videtic GMM, Woody N, Vassil AD. *Handbook of Treatment Planning in Radiation Oncology.* 3rd ed. Demos Medical; 2020. doi:10.1891/9780826168429

20. Olsen EA, Hodak E, Anderson T, et al. Guidelines for phototherapy of mycosis fungoides and Sezary syndrome: a consensus statement of the United States Cutaneous Lymphoma Consortium. *J Am Acad Dermatol.* 2016;74(1):27–58. doi:10.1016/j.jaad.2015.09.033

21. Duarte RF, Boumendil A, Onida F, et al. Long-term outcome of allogeneic hematopoietic cell transplantation for patients with mycosis fungoides and Sezary syndrome: a European society for blood and marrow transplantation lymphoma working party extended analysis. *J Clin Oncol.* 2014;32(29):3347–3348. doi:10.1200/JCO.2014.57.5597

IV ■ BREAST

23 ■ EARLY-STAGE BREAST CANCER

Kailin Yang, Rahul D. Tendulkar, and Chirag Shah

QUICK HIT ■ For early-stage breast cancer, treatment typically involves surgical resection followed by adjuvant therapy (CHT, RT, and/or endocrine therapy) depending on pathologic features. BCS + adjuvant RT is an equivalent alternative (LC and OS) to mastectomy for most patients with unifocal cancers who desire organ preservation. WBI after BCS improves LR rates (from 26% to 7% at 5 years) and OS by 5% at 15 years.[1] Conventional WBI dose is 45 to 50 Gy, followed by a tumor bed boost of 10 to 16 Gy in some patients. Hypofractionated WBI regimens (40–42.5 Gy/15–16 fx or 26-28.5 Gy/5 fx) have replaced conventional WBI for most patients, particularly in those not requiring elective nodal irradiation. In patients with limited axillary nodal involvement on SLNB, a completion ALND is not necessary, provided the patient undergoes WBI ± RNI. Lower risk patients (e.g., older age, T1N0, ER+, negative margins) may be eligible for PBI, intraoperative RT, or endocrine therapy alone after lumpectomy.

EPIDEMIOLOGY: Worldwide, breast cancer is the most frequently diagnosed and leading cause of cancer death in women. In the United States, >250,000 new diagnoses in 2020 and >40,000 deaths were reported.[2] Lifetime risk is 1 in 8 women (~1 in 50 by age 50). Median age at diagnosis is 61. About two-thirds of new diagnoses have no significant risk factors. Males account for 1% (a/w Klinefelter syndrome and BRCA2; 90% are ER+).

RISK FACTORS

Estrogen Exposure: Female gender, older age, early menarche, nulliparity, older age at first birth (>30 years), lack of breastfeeding, late menopause (>55 years), hormone replacement therapy.

Family History: Risk increases with more first-degree relatives.

Genetics (5%–10% hereditary): BRCA1—AD (17q21), 60% to 80% lifetime risk of breast cancer, 30% to 50% lifetime risk of ovarian cancer, higher risk of triple negative (ER–/PR–/HER2–); BRCA2—AD (13q12), 50% to 60% lifetime risk of breast cancer, 10% to 20% lifetime risk of ovarian cancer, male breast cancer, prostate, bladder, endometrial, and pancreatic cancers; Li–Fraumeni—AD (17p), p53, a/w sarcoma, leukemia, brain, adrenocortical carcinoma; Cowden syndrome—AD (10q23), PTEN, a/w hamartomas of skin and oral cavity; ataxia–telangiectasia—AR (11q22), ATM; Peutz–Jeghers.

Personal History of Breast Disease: Prior breast cancer, DCIS, LCIS, atypical ductal hyperplasia, dense breast tissue, history of RT during youth (age <30 years).

Lifestyle/Exposure: High-fat diet, postmenopausal obesity, sedentary lifestyle.

ANATOMY: The breast overlies the pectoralis major muscle, extends from approximately the second to the sixth rib and from the lateral sternum to anterior axillary fold. The axillary tail of Spence extends laterally into the low axilla. Glandular tissue is arranged in 15 to 20 lobes with a system of lactiferous ducts that open at the nipple. UOQ contains the greatest volume of glandular tissue (most common location of breast cancers). The least common location is the lower inner quadrant. Breast is supported by Cooper's ligaments, which are fibrous septae joining the superficial fascia (skin) and deep fascia covering the pectoralis major muscle. Lymphatic drainage is primarily to the axilla. ALN levels I, II, and III are respectively located inferolateral, deep, and superomedial to pectoralis minor, which inserts on coracoid process of the scapula. Rotter's nodes are located between pectoralis major and minor (anterior to level II). IMNs are situated along IM vessels adjacent to sternum in the first three intercostal spaces, about 2 to 3 cm lateral to midline, and 2 to 3 cm deep. Approximately 30% of medial tumors and 15% of lateral tumors drain to the IMN.

PATHOLOGY: Breast carcinomas arise from epithelial elements and comprise a diverse group of lesions with differing biologic behavior, although often discussed as a single disease with similar management guidelines. ER and/or PR are expressed in 70% of tumors (more common in postmenopausal patients). HER2/neu (c-ERbB-2 or human epidermal growth factor receptor 2) is a receptor tyrosine kinase, with HER2 amplification seen in 25% to 30% of invasive cancers. TNBC is an aggressive entity in which tumors do not express ER, PR, or HER2, accounting for ~15% of cases and more commonly found in BRCA mutation carriers.

Invasive Ductal Carcinoma: Eighty percent of cases, firm mass with desmoplastic reaction, solid cords of cells.

Invasive Lobular Carcinoma: Five percent to 10% of cases, rubbery texture, less visible on mammogram (better imaged with MRI), "Indian filing" histology, often bilateral/multicentric, >80% ER+, spreads to unusual locations such as meninges, serosal surfaces, BM, ovary, and RP.

Rarer Subtypes (Need >90% Predominant Pattern): *Tubular*—small, well-differentiated variant of IDC, >75% tubules, usually ER+/PR+. *Medullary*—a/w BRCA1, presents at younger age (<50 years), LNs are large/hyperplastic, most are triple negative. *Mucinous/colloid*—older patients, favorable. *Papillary*—older patients, often multifocal/diffuse, often LN+ even when small size. *Cribriform*—ER+/PR+. *Other uncommon variants* include metaplastic (poor prognosis), squamous cell, invasive micropapillary, adenoid cystic, mucoepidermoid, secretory, apocrine, spindle cell, lymphoma, neuroendocrine small cell, and clear cell. Mammary carcinoma is a mixture of invasive ductal and lobular carcinoma.

EIC: Defined as ≥25% DCIS within the invasive carcinoma specimen and extending beyond edges of tumor. Originally identified as a risk factor for LR after BCT, but no longer considered the case provided margins are negative.[3]

Paget's Disease: Chronic eczematous changes of the nipple–areolar complex, with an underlying intraepidermal adenocarcinoma of the nipple (in 95%). About 50% have a palpable mass (>90% are invasive cancer) and 50% have no mass (typically DCIS). Low risk of axillary nodal mets.

Cystosarcoma Phyllodes: Fibroepithelial, "leaf-like," large, encapsulated tumors, usually benign w/o invasion. Can grow slowly and then have sudden rapid increase in size. Uncommonly malignant and nodal mets are rare.

GENETICS: A number of gene expression profiling models exist, including the Amsterdam 70-gene good-versus-poor outcome model (low signature vs. high signature),[4] the 21-gene recurrence score model,[5] and the intrinsic subtype model.[6] The 21-gene recurrence score (Oncotype DX) was developed for patients w/ LN-negative, ER+ breast cancers, receiving tamoxifen ± CHT on NSABP B-14, and is stratified into low risk (<18 score), intermediate risk (18–30), and high risk (>30) of recurrence in order to estimate the relative benefit of CHT in addition to hormonal therapy.[5] Rates of distant recurrence in the low-risk, intermediate-risk, and high-risk groups were 6.8%, 14.3%, and 30.5% at 10 years. The TAILORx study showed noninferiority of endocrine therapy alone over endocrine + CHT in women with intermediate risk (revised score of 11–25).[7] There are four main intrinsic subtypes: luminal A (best prognosis), luminal B, HER2 enriched (HER2+), and basal-like (worst prognosis).[6] Note that the luminal A and B clinicopathologic surrogate definitions have been updated: *luminal A–like*: ER+/HER2– with either low Ki-67 (<14%) or combination of PR+ (≤20%) and intermediate Ki-67 (14%–19%); *luminal B–like*: ER+/HER2– with either high Ki-67 (≤20%) or combination of intermediate Ki-67 (14%–19%) with PR– or low (<20%), or ER+/PR+ with HER2+; *basal-like*: usually triple negative (~70%–80% correlation), high prevalence in young Black women and BRCA mutation carriers; *HER2 enriched*: usually ER–/PR–, HER2+, high Ki-67.[8] The luminal subtypes, while usually HER2–, can be HER2+. Higher response rates to neoadjuvant CHT are seen with basal-like and HER2 enriched cancers.[9]

SCREENING: Screening mammograms (90% sensitive/specific) reduce mortality by 35% (relative risk) in women 50 to 74 years of age; 40% of breast lesions are detected by mammogram only, but 10% have palpable tumors that are not visualized.

- *ACR Appropriateness Guidelines*:[10] Begin annual screening at 40 y/o; screen at 25 to 30 y/o for BRCA mutation carriers and untested first-degree relatives of carriers; screen at 25 to 30 y/o or 10 years earlier than first-degree relatives (whichever is later) with lifetime risk for breast cancer ≤20%.

Screen 8 years after or at 25 y/o (whichever is later) for women who received mantle RT/thoracic RT between 10 and 30 y/o. Screen annually for women with biopsy-proven lobular neoplasia, atypical ductal hyperplasia, or personal history of breast cancer beginning at diagnosis, but not when <30 y/o. Supplemental screening may be necessary in women with genetic predisposition to disease and/or dense breasts. Clinical breast examination not recommended in average risk women.

- *USPSTF:*[11] Recommends biennial screening for ages 50 to 74, no routine screening for 40 to 49 (self-exams controversial). High-risk women should begin screening 10 years before age of youngest first-degree relative diagnosed. Insufficient evidence for benefit/harm of clinical exam; however, recommended against teaching breast self-examination.

ACS guidelines recommend screening MRI for women with 20% to 25% or greater lifetime risk of breast cancer, including women with hereditary mutations (BRCA, Li–Fraumeni, Cowden), strong family history of breast/ovarian cancer, and women who received prior thoracic RT for Hodgkin's disease before 30 years of age.[12,13]

CLINICAL PRESENTATION: Typically detected by screening mammogram (~90%), self-breast exam, and/or clinical exam (~10%).[14] Most common presentation is a painless mass, but can occasionally present with pain (~5%), nipple discharge (though usually benign), nipple retraction or axillary lymphadenopathy with occult primary. A mass is less concerning for malignancy if associated with changes in menstrual cycle. Most common location is UOQ (40%), followed by central area (30%), UIQ (15%), LOQ (10%), and LIQ (5%). Bilateral disease in 1% to 3% of cases. Risk of developing contralateral cancer after primary diagnosis is 0.75% per year. *Multifocal* defined as ≥2 cancer foci in same quadrant (typically eligible for breast conservation). *Multicentric:* ≥2 foci in different quadrants or >5 cm apart (typically not eligible for breast conservation). *Differential Diagnosis:* Fibroadenoma (solitary mass, well defined, mobile); cysts (more diffuse and less firm, suspicious if blood in aspirate or contents reaccumulate quickly); infection (mastitis or abscess); Mondor's cord (thrombophlebitis of superficial breast veins); fat necrosis; intraductal papilloma (common cause of bloody discharge); sclerosing adenosis (nodular benign condition consisting of hyperplastic lobules of acinar tissue); lactocele.

TABLE 23.1: Breast Imaging and Reporting Data System Classification

BI-RADS	Description	Malignancy %	Follow-Up
0	Incomplete	1%	Completion of imaging or review of previous imaging not previously available
1	Negative	<1%	Routine annual screening
2	Benign lesion	<1%	Routine annual screening
3	Probably benign	<2%	Short interval f/u (6 months)
4a	Low suspicion for malignancy	2%–10%	Biopsy
4b	Moderate suspicion for malignancy	10%–50%	Biopsy
4c	High suspicion for malignancy	50%–95%	Biopsy
5	Highly suggestive of malignancy	>95%	Biopsy
6	Biopsy-proven malignancy	100%	Appropriate treatment per stage

Source: From Vanel D. The American College of Radiology (ACR) Breast Imaging and Reporting Data System (BI-RADS): a step towards a universal radiological language? *Eur J Radiol.* 2007;61(2):183. doi:10.1016/j.ejrad.2006.08.030

WORKUP

H&P: Full H&P with attention to breast and LN exam (axilla and SCV)

Imaging: Mammogram (Table 23.1) and ultrasound are typical first steps.[15] Systemic staging workup is not routinely indicated per NCCN for anatomic stages I to II in the absence of suspicious symptoms, physical exam findings, or lab abnormalities (e.g., elevated alk phos or LFTs). If suspicious, studies may include PET/CT or CT chest/abdomen/pelvis and bone scan, ± MRI brain.

- *Mammography*: On CC view, the lateral edge of the film is typically marked by "CC" marker. On MLO view, assess for image quality by ensuring pectoralis muscle is included. Concerning mammographic findings: calcifications 100 to 300 microns, >10 clustered linear calcifications, spiculated lesions. Spot compression views are useful for suspicious masses (vs. disappearance of dense breast tissue on compression), and magnification views are used for evaluation of calcifications.
- *Ultrasound*: Helps distinguish solid from cystic masses (but not useful for calcifications) and to evaluate nonpalpable masses identified on mammogram.
- *MRI*: Higher sensitivity (>90%) than mammography, but lower specificity (39%–95%) due to false positives. Suspicious features for malignancy: strong, rapid contrast enhancement, spiculated margins, rim enhancement, heterogeneous appearance. Potential indications for MRI include an obscured breast (silicone implants), suspicious masses with negative mammogram and ultrasound, evaluation of poorly imaged tumors such as ILC or DCIS without microcalcifications, or patients presenting with positive axillary nodes of unknown primary (MRI detects primary tumor 80%–90% of the time). MRI can change surgical management in 25% of cases but does not reduce positive margins, re-excision rates, or LR rates.[16–18]

Procedures: Core biopsy, needle aspirate (if cystic on ultrasound). FNA may detect abnormal cells, but cannot distinguish DCIS from IDC and cannot identify ER/PR/HER2 status; thus core biopsy is preferred. US core biopsy for palpable masses. Stereotactic core biopsy or needle localization if nonpalpable lesion with suspicious calcifications. MRI-guided biopsy if only visible on MRI. Punch biopsy for Paget's or if suspicious of dermal involvement (e.g., suspected inflammatory breast cancer).

PROGNOSTIC FACTORS: Poor prognostic factors include LN+ (strongest factor), young age, ER/PR negativity, HER2/neu amplification (in the absence of HER2-directed therapy), high grade, LVSI+, basal-like subtype.[19]

STAGING (TABLE 23.2):

TABLE 23.2: AJCC 8th Edition (2017): Staging for Breast Cancer					
cT/pT		cN		pN	
Tis	• Carcinoma in situ	N0	• No palpable LNs	N0	(i–) negative IHC
					(i+) positive IHC (≤0.2 mm)
					(mol–) negative RT-PCR
					(mol+) positive RT-PCR
T1mic	• ≤0.1 cm	N1	• Mobile ipsilateral level I/II axillary LNs	N1	mi >0.2 mm and/or >200 cells, but ≤2 mm
					a. 1–3 axillary LNs
					b. IM LN+ pathologically, but not clinically
					c. pN1a + pN1b

(continued)

TABLE 23.2: AJCC 8th Edition (2017): Staging for Breast Cancer (*continued*)

cT/pT		cN		pN	
T1	a. >0.1 cm and ≤0.5 cm	**N2a**	• Fixed/matted ipsilateral axillary LNs	**N2**	a. 4–9 axillary LNs
	b. >0.5 cm and ≤1 cm				
	c. >1 cm and ≤2 cm				b. IM LNs+ pathologically and clinically, but with negative axillary LNs
T2	• >2 cm and ≤5 cm	**N2b**	• Clinically detected ipsilateral IM LNs, without axillary LNs	**N3**	a. ≤10 axillary LNs or + infraclavicular LNs
					b. Pathologically and clinically + IM LNs with + axillary LNs; or pathologically, but not clinically + IM LNs with >3 axillary LNs
					c. Ipsilateral SCV LNs
T3	• >5 cm	**N3a**	• Ipsilateral infraclavicular LNs	**Group Staging**	
T4	a. Extension to chest wall (except pectoralis major)	**N3b**	• Ipsilateral IM and axillary LNs	**0**	Tis
				. **IA**	T1N0M0
	b. Peau d'orange, ulcer, or satellite skin nodules			**IB**	T0–1N1miM0
				IIA	T0–1N1M0, T2N0M0
	c. Both T4a and T4b			**IIB**	T2N1M0, T3N0M0
	d. Inflammatory carcinoma			**IIIA**	T0–3N2M0, T3N1M0
cT/pT		**cN**		**pN**	
M0(i+)	• Circulating tumor cells in bone marrow	**N3c**	• Ipsilateral supraclavicular LNs	**IIIB**	T4N0-2M0
				IIIC	Any T, N3M0
M1	• Distant metastasis			**IV**	M0(i+), M1

Note: In addition to the preceding anatomic staging, prognostic group staging was developed in the AJCC 8th edition, which includes grade and ER/PR/HER2 status and is preferred over the historic anatomic group staging.

TREATMENT PARADIGM: Local therapy options include MRM or BCT composed of lumpectomy ± RT (see Table 23.3 for surgical options). There are no significant differences in LR (with negative margins), distant DFS, or OS between MRM and BCT at extended follow-up in at least six prospective trials. CHT, if needed, is delivered either neoadjuvantly or postoperatively, but generally before RT (the Recht trial initially demonstrated reduced recurrence rates in patients treated with CHT prior to RT, although the curves converged at later follow-up).[20,21] Hormonal therapy is indicated for hormone receptor–positive cancers, and usually follows all other therapies. Breast cancer is both a local and a distant disease. Halsted theorized that breast cancer spreads with orderly anatomic progression of disease, such that aggressive local treatment should improve survival. Fisher theorized that intrinsic tumor factors dictate patterns of spread, such that systemic therapy should improve outcomes. Hellman merged the two theories, recognizing that breast cancers fall under a heterogeneous spectrum, and that optimizing both LC and systemic therapy can provide the best outcomes.[22]

Prevention: Tamoxifen as chemoprevention reduces the risk of noninvasive and invasive cancers in high-risk women by up to 50% (NSABP P-1).[23] Raloxifene is as effective as tamoxifen and with lower rate of thromboembolic events (NSABP P-2 "STAR").[24] Prophylactic mastectomy reduces breast cancer risk by >90% in those with a strong family history and may improve survival in BRCA carriers.[25] Prophylactic oophorectomy decreases risk in BRCA carriers by 50% if before 40 years of age.[26] No conclusive evidence of a benefit from special dietary changes; however, alcohol/obesity is associated with increased risk of developing breast cancer.

Surgery

TABLE 23.3: Surgical Options for Breast Cancer	
Radical mastectomy	Popularized by Halsted starting in 1894. Involves en bloc removal of the breast, overlying skin, pectoralis major, pectoralis minor, and level I, II, and III lymph nodes; there are currently no absolute indications for this procedure.
Modified radical mastectomy	Complete removal of breast tissue, pectoralis fascia, and level I and II lymph nodes (preserves pectoralis major, lateral pectoral nerve, and level III nodes).
Total mastectomy	Removal of breast tissue only (preservation of both pectoralis muscles and axillary lymph nodes).
Skin-sparing mastectomy	Resection of biopsy scar and/or skin immediately overlying the tumor, and removal of breast parenchyma. Preservation of majority of breast skin for reconstruction.
Nipple-sparing mastectomy	Skin-sparing mastectomy with preservation of the nipple–areolar complex.
Lumpectomy or partial mastectomy	Removal of only part of the breast containing the cancer (i.e., BCS). Margins are considered negative if there is "no tumor on ink."[27]
Axillary lymph node dissection	A typical level I and II ALND yields ~15 nodes. A complete ALND with removal of level III nodes is generally unnecessary unless grossly positive. Incidence of skip metastases to level III nodes without involved level I nodes is <3%.
Sentinel lymph node biopsy	Tc-99m sulfur colloid and/or isosulfan blue dye are injected at tumor site for 3–7 minutes, and gamma camera identifies SLNs. False negative rate is 8%–10% after negative SLNB.[28] Results in less lymphedema, less pain, and better arm mobility compared to ALND.

Chemotherapy: Typically given pre- or post-op to LN+ patients, ER−, HER2+, and women with multiple adverse features (e.g., young age or high Oncotype DX scores). Neoadjuvant CHT has equivalent survival as adjuvant (NSABP B-18) but may allow for less extensive surgery. For patients with ER+ and N0-N1, gene expression assays such as Oncotype DX and MammaPrint can be considered for addition of adjuvant CHT to endocrine therapy.[7,29] Virtually all subgroups of women have a benefit in DFS from adjuvant CHT, though benefit is more pronounced in younger women, LN+, and ER− patients. Note: Role of CHT is unclear in women >70 y/o because this age group was excluded from early clinical trials. *Trastuzumab* has OS advantage for HER2+ patients in addition to cytotoxic CHT.[30] Trastuzumab is not given concurrently with Adriamycin because of cardiotoxicity concerns, but is safe to give with RT. Trastuzumab-related cardiac effects are reversible, so obtain cardiac echo q3 months to monitor. Pertuzumab has been added to trastuzumab to provide dual anti-HER2 therapy, which results in pCR rates of 50% to 60% in the neoadjuvant setting. Common CHT regimens include the following:

- AC: Adriamycin 60 mg/m^2 + cyclophosphamide 600 mg/m^2 q3weeks × 4 cycles.
- AC→T: Adriamycin 60 mg/m^2 + cyclophosphamide 600 mg/m^2 q3weeks × 4 cycles followed by paclitaxel 175 mg/m^2 q3weeks × 4 cycles or 80 mg/m^2 q1week × 12 weeks (dose-dense regimen is q2weeks w/ filgrastim or pegfilgrastim for support).
- AC→TH: same as AC→T, with the addition of trastuzumab 4 mg/kg loading dose followed by 2 mg/kg per week concurrently with paclitaxel, then trastuzumab monotherapy (6 mg/kg q3weeks) for 1 year.
- TC: docetaxel 75 mg/m^2 and cyclophosphamide 600 mg/m^2.
- TCHP: nonanthracycline regimen consisting of docetaxel 75 mg/m^2 + carboplatin (AUC 6 mg/mL/min) q3weeks × 6 cycles + trastuzumab (8 mg/kg loading dose followed by 6 mg/kg q3weeks for 1 year) + pertuzumab (840 mg loading dose followed by 420 mg q3weeks).

Anthracycline-based CHT is superior to nonanthracycline-based regimens, and may especially benefit HER2+ patients. The addition of a taxane has OS benefit for LN+ patients compared to AC alone.[31,32] Dose-dense regimens (q2weeks instead of q3weeks) offer OS advantage for high-risk patients as well.[33] TC provides OS benefit compared to AC.[34] Other CHT regimens include the following: TAC: docetaxel, Adriamycin, and cyclophosphamide; CMF: cyclophosphamide, methotrexate, fluorouracil; FAC: fluorouracil, doxorubicin, cyclophosphamide; FEC: fluorouracil, epirubicin, cyclophosphamide.

Hormone Therapy: Indicated for essentially all ER+ or PR+ patients, unless a specific contraindication exists. *Tamoxifen* is a partial estrogen agonist that functions as a competitive inhibitor. Premenopausal women are typically treated with tamoxifen 20 mg daily for 5 years, though 10 years of therapy was recently found to further reduce recurrence and breast cancer mortality by approximately one-third in the first 10 years following diagnosis and by approximately half subsequently.[35] Side effects include hot flashes, vaginal discharge/bleeding, cataracts, retinopathy, thromboembolic events (1%), endometrial cancer (RR 2–7), and uterine sarcomas. AIs such as anastrozole or letrozole block conversion of androgens to estrogen in fat, liver, and muscle and are ineffective in premenopausal women (due to ovarian production of estrogen). Postmenopausal women are typically treated with anastrozole 1 mg daily for 5 years. Compared to tamoxifen in postmenopausal women, AIs improve DFS and have higher rates of myalgias, arthralgias, and osteoporosis, but less risk of endometrial cancer and DVTs.[36,37]

Radiation: WBI after lumpectomy significantly lowers risk of LRR when compared to lumpectomy alone, and improves 15-year OS by reducing BCM.[1]

Indications: WBI is indicated in most patients following BCS. Favorable subgroups (e.g., older patients with T1N0 ER+ breast cancers) may be treated with APBI, IORT, or adjuvant endocrine therapy alone.

Absolute contraindications to BCS: Persistently positive resection margins after re-excision attempts, multicentric tumors, diffuse malignant-appearing mammographic microcalcifications, prior RT to the breast or chest wall, inflammatory breast cancer.

Relative contraindications to BCS: Pregnancy (can perform BCS in third trimester and defer RT until after delivery), active lupus/scleroderma, large tumor in a small breast (cosmetic outcome may not be satisfactory). BRCA mutation carriers are not contraindicated to receive RT; however, their risk of developing new primary cancers remains high after BCT, so bilateral mastectomies are commonly performed.

Dose: Conventional WBI (45–50.4 Gy in 1.8–2 Gy/fx, typically with boost of 10–16 Gy) is no longer necessary in most cases of early breast cancer. Hypofractionated regimens (typically 40–42.5 Gy at 2.66 Gy/fx with consideration of boost) are the current standard for most early-stage breast cancer.[38] Other hypofractionated WBI regimens include 28.5 Gy / 5 fx once weekly or 26 Gy / 5 fx once daily. Regimens for APBI include 30 Gy in 5 fx QOD and 38.5 Gy in 10 fx BID.[39]

Timing: RT usually starts within 4 to 6 weeks of completion of surgery or CHT; delaying RT for longer than 16 weeks after surgery is a/w higher breast relapse rates.[40]

Procedure: See *Handbook of Treatment Planning in Radiation Oncology*, Chapter 5.[41]

Toxicity: Acute effects: erythema, pruritus, tenderness, desquamation. Late effects: hyperpigmentation, volume loss, fibrosis, rib fracture, lymphedema, pulmonary fibrosis, secondary malignancies (<1% at 10 years, with angiosarcoma being most common) and cardiac effects.[42]

- **EVIDENCE-BASED Q&A**

- **Is there a role for radical mastectomy in the modern era?**

NSABP B-04 established there is no advantage to radical mastectomy vs. total mastectomy with or without RT.

Fisher, NSABP B-04 (*NEJM* 2002, PMID 12192016): PRT of nonfixed, operable tumors confined to breast/axilla (n = 1079 LN– and n = 586 LN+). Randomization of cN0 patients to RM vs. TM + RT (50 Gy/25 fx tangents + PAB; 45 Gy/25 fx IM + SCV; boost if LN+) vs. TM alone; cN+ patients randomized to RM vs. TM + RT. No significant differences between the three arms of LN– patients or between the two arms of LN+ patients for DFS, RFS, or OS (Table 23.4). Among cN0 patients, no difference in OS between RM vs. TM ± RT, and no survival benefit to RT (after TM in cN0). ALN status is a strong prognostic indicator, but no survival advantage to removing occult positive nodes at surgery. Forty percent of cN0 women had pathologically positive nodes in RM arm; 17.8% of TM alone patients needed delayed ALND for axillary failure, usually within first 2 years. **Conclusion: RM not necessary for operable breast cancer.**

TABLE 23.4: NSABP B-04 Results

	25-Yr DFS		25-Yr RFS		25-Yr Distant DFS		25-Yr OS		25-Yr LR	
	LN–	LN+	LN–	LN+	LN–	LN+	LN–	LN+	LN–	LN+
RM	19%	11%	53%	36%	46%	32%	25%	14%	5%	8%
TM + RT	13%	10%	52%	33%	38%	29%	19%	14%	1%	3%
TM	19%	–	50%	–	43%	–	26%		7%	

- **How does mastectomy compare with breast conservation?**

At least six randomized trials have demonstrated no significant differences in OS between BCT and mastectomy (Table 23.5). Two trials, which did not require negative margin lumpectomies (e.g., 48% in the EORTC trial had positive margins), found higher LR rates with BCT, likely due to inadequate surgery.[43,44] At 20-year follow-up in the Milan trial, there were higher rates of LR in the BCT arm (8.8% after quadrantectomy vs. 2.3% after RM), likely due to new primary tumors (two thirds of recurrences were in other quadrants and only one third occurred in the index quadrant scar).[45] A 1992 NCI consensus statement declared both mastectomy and BCT to be acceptable standards of care for operable breast cancer.

TABLE 23.5: Prospective Randomized Trials of Breast Conservation Therapy vs. MRM

Trial	Years	N	Stage	Surgery	Adjuvant	F/U	OS % (p)	DFS % (p)	LR % (p)
Milan[45]	1973–1980	701	I	Q/RM	CMF	20 yrs	58/59 (NS)		9/2 (<.001)
Gustave-Roussy[46]	1972–1980	179	I	WE/MRM	None	15 yrs	73/65 (.19)		9/14 (NS)
NSABP B-06[47]	1976–1984	1,851	I–II	WE/MRM	MF	20 yrs	46/47 (.74)	35/36 (.95)	2.7/10.2
NCI[48]	1979–1987	237	I–II	WE/MRM	AC	25 yrs	38/44 (.38)	56/29 (.0017)	22/1.0 (<.001)
EORTC 10801[49]	1980–1986	868	I–II	LE/MRM	CMF	22 yrs	39/45 (NS)		20/12 (.01)
Danish[50]	1983–1989	904	I–III	Q, WE/MRM	CMF, Tam	6 yrs	79/82 (NS)	70/66 (NS)	3/4 (NS)

■ What is the role of adjuvant WBI after breast-conserving surgery?

Up to 40% of women after surgical resection of gross tumor will have residual microscopic disease that can develop into recurrence. The Holland study demonstrated that 43% of unifocal cancers in mastectomy specimens had tumor foci >2 cm from the index lesion.[51] NSABP B-06 showed that 20-year LR rates were reduced from 39% to 14% with the addition of RT.[47] The EBCTCG meta-analysis was the first study large enough to demonstrate that adjuvant WBI improves survival—the individual trials were not sufficiently powered. RT decreased 15-year risk of death from breast cancer from 31% to 26% for LN– patients and 55% to 48% for LN+.[1] The EBCTCG meta-analysis suggested a "4:1 ratio"—one breast cancer death was avoided by year 15 for every four local recurrences prevented by year 5 and for every four overall recurrences prevented by year 10.[52] There has been no subgroup (age, grade, size, hormone status), which has not been shown to benefit from RT.

Fisher, NSABP B-06 (*NEJM* 2002, PMID 12393820): PRT of 1,851 patients from 1976 to 1984 with stage I to II, mobile tumor ≤4 cm, mobile axillary LNs, and negative margins randomized to MRM vs. lumpectomy vs. lumpectomy + WBI 50 Gy/25 fx. ALND was levels I to II. Patients with +LNs received CHT (5-FU and melphalan). Similar DFS and OS observed between MRM and BCT (Table 23.6). The 20-year IBTR rate was 39% after lumpectomy alone and 14% after lumpectomy + RT, with significant benefit to RT in both LN+ and LN–. **Conclusion: Mastectomy and BCT have similar long-term outcomes. Adjuvant WBI after lumpectomy reduces IBTR by ~2/3.**

TABLE 23.6: Results of NSABP B-06						
NSABP B-06	**5-Yr IBTR**	**5-Yr DFS**	**5-Yr OS**	**20-Yr IBTR**	**20-Yr DFS**	**20-Yr OS**
MRM (TM + ALND)		67%	82%		36%	47%
Lumpectomy	28%	64%	83%	39%	35%	46%
Lumpectomy + RT	8%	71%	84%	14%	35%	46%

EBCTCG 2005 Meta-Analysis (*Lancet* 2005, PMID 15894097): Meta-analysis of 42,080 women with breast cancer treated on 78 randomized trials that began by 1995. Studies included RT vs. no RT (N ~23,500), more vs. less surgery (N ~9,300), and more surgery vs. RT (N ~9,300). In 10 trials, 7,311 patients were treated with BCS + RT vs. BCS alone. Overall, RT reduces the RR of 5-year LR by 70% (Table 23.7). The absolute 19% reduction in LR at 5 years translated to a 5% reduction in BCM at 15 years; hence for every four LR prevented, one death was avoided.

TABLE 23.7: 2005 EBCTCG Meta-Analysis							
	All patients (N = 7,311)			**LN– (N = 6,097)**		**LN+ (N = 1,214)**	
	5-yr LR	**15-yr BCM**	**15-yr OS**	**5-yr LR**	**15-yr BCM**	**5-yr LR**	**15-yr BCM**
BCS + RT	7%	31%	65%	7%	26%	11%	48%
BCS alone	26%	36%	60%	23%	31%	41%	55%
p value	<.00001	.0002	.005	sig	.006	sig	.01

EBCTCG 2011 Meta-analysis (*Lancet* 2011, PMID 22019144): Meta-analysis of 10,801 early-stage breast cancer patients s/p BCS from 17 PRTs, 77% pN0. RT reduced the 10-year risk of any recurrence by approximately half (Table 23.8). With addition of RT to BCS, about one breast cancer death was avoided by year 15 for every four overall recurrences avoided at 10 years, another 4:1 ratio.

TABLE 23.8: 2011 EBCTCG Meta-Analysis						
	10-Yr Recurrence (Any)			15-Yr BCM		
	All	pN0	pN+	All	pN0	pN+
BCS + RT	19%	16%	43%	21%	17%	43%
BCS alone	35%	31%	64%	25%	21%	51%

■ **Does completion ALND after a positive SLNB benefit cN0 patients? Can RT replace ALND in select cN0 patients?**

NSABP B-04 demonstrated that not all undissected nodal disease results in clinical recurrence. Several randomized trials have since shown similar rates of axillary recurrence and DFS between SLNB and ALND among clinically node-negative patients, most of whom received adjuvant RT. ACOSOG Z0011 and IBCSG 23-01 showed that completion ALND after SLNB offered no improvement over SLNB alone in SLN+ patients receiving BCS and WBI, for both macrometastases and micrometastases. The AMAROS trial evaluated ALND vs. axillary RT after a positive SLNB, and found no difference in recurrence rates, but ALND had twice the rate of lymphedema (28% vs. 14%). Patients undergoing mastectomy were not well represented in AMAROS, and so completion ALND remains appropriate for SLN+ patients after mastectomy. Select patients in whom PMRT is already planned may be spared ALND, provided there are no grossly enlarged LNs on exam or imaging.

Guiliano, ACOSOG Z0011 (*JAMA* 2011, PMID 21304082; **Lucci** *JCO* 2007, PMID 17485711; **Jagsi** *JCO* 2014 PMID 25135994; **Update** *Ann Surg* 2016, PMID 27513155; **Update** *JAMA* 2017, **PMID: 28898379**): PRT of 891 patients with cT1–T2 N0 who underwent lumpectomy and SLNB with 1 to 2 LN+, randomized to completion ALND or not. All patients received WBI, without node-directed RT (per protocol). Patients were excluded for >2 LN+, matted LNs, gross ENE, received neoadjuvant CHT, or underwent mastectomy. Target enrollment was 1,900 but closed early due to very low event rate. Primary end point of OS was similar in both arms; 96% to 97% received systemic therapy. Median 17 ALNs removed in ALND arm and 2 in SLNB arm ($p < .001$). In ALND arm, 27% had additional metastases in dissected LNs, and 14% had ≤4 LN+. ALND arm had higher rates of subjective lymphedema (13% vs. 2% at 1 year, $p < .0001$), wound infections, axillary seromas, and paresthesias than SLNB alone. While standard tangent fields were specified by protocol, ~50% utilized high tangents (defined as ≤2 cm from humeral head), and 19% received RNI to include at least SCV nodes. At 10-year update, nodal recurrences were 0.5% in ALND arm vs. 1.5% in SLNB arm, and 10-year IBTR were 6.2% vs. 5.3% (p = NS) (Table 23.9). **Conclusion: Completion ALND is not necessary in patients with 1 to 2 SLN metastases who receive WBI and systemic therapy.**

TABLE 23.9: ACOSOG Z0011 Results					
	10-Yr IBTR	Nodal Recurrence	Lymphedema	10-Yr DFS	10-Yr OS
BCS + ALND + RT	6.2%	0.5%	13%	78%	84%
BCS + SLNB + RT	5.3%	1.5%	2%	80%	86%

Galimberti, IBCSG 23-01 (*Lancet Oncol* 2013, PMID 23491275; **Update** *Lancet* Oncol 2018, **PMID 30196031**): PRT of 931 patients with cT1-2N0 who underwent SLNB and had ≤1 micrometastatic (≤2 mm) SLN w/o ECE, randomized to completion ALND or not (noninferiority design). Ninety-one percent underwent BCT, 9% had mastectomy. Median 21 LNs removed at ALND, and 13% had additional nodal metastases; 10-year DFS, 76.8% in SLNB arm vs. 74.9% in ALND arm (p = .24); 10-year OS also similar (90.8% in SLNB arm and 88.2% in ALND arm). **Conclusion: Supports ACOSOG Z-11 trial in omission of completion ALND for low-volume SLN metastases.**

Donker, AMAROS/EORTC 10981/22023 (*Lancet* 2014, PMID 25439688; **SABCS 2018, Abstract GS4-01**): A total of 4,806 patients with cT1-2N0 breast cancer registered and randomized preoperatively prior to SLNB; 1,425 patients (30% of initial cohort) with SLN+ received axillary RT (n = 681) vs. completion ALND (n = 744) in a noninferiority design. Axillary RT to levels I–III and SCV fossa to 50

Gy/25 fx. 82% underwent BCT and 18% mastectomy; 33% of those undergoing ALND had additional LN+. Primary end point was 5-year axillary recurrence rate, which was 0.43% after ALND vs. 1.19% with axillary RT (NS). In comparison, nonrandomized patients with negative SLNB had similar axillary recurrence rate of 0.8%. OS and DFS rates similar between ALND and RT; however, lymphedema more frequent after ALND (28% vs. 14%) (Table 23.10). **Conclusion: For SLN+ patients, axillary RT provides similar control with less risk of lymphedema compared to ALND.**

TABLE 23.10: AMAROS Trial Results

	Lymphedema	10-Yr DFS	10-Yr OS
BCT + ALND	28%	82%	85%
BCT + RT	14%	78%	81%
p value	<.001	.18	.34

Wong, Harvard (*IJROBP* 2008, PMID 18394815): Prospective, single-arm trial of 74 patients >55 y/o with stage I/II, cN0, ER+ breast cancer treated with lumpectomy (negative margins) without ALND or SLNB and WBI with high tangents (blocked humeral head) + tumor bed boost + 5 years hormonal therapy. Median age 74.5, median tumor size 1.2 cm. MFU 52 months. No patient had local or axillary recurrence. **Conclusion: High tangential RT and hormonal therapy w/o ALND is a reasonable option in older patients with early-stage ER/PR+ cN0 breast cancer.**

■ **What is the role of regional nodal irradiation in breast conservation patients undergoing axillary dissection?**

After lumpectomy, RNI is indicated for certain high-risk patients, such as those with LN+ and/or ER-negative disease. The NCIC MA.20 and EORTC 22922/10925 trials showed an improvement in LRR, DM, DFS and a trend toward OS with the use of comprehensive nodal radiation.[53,54] It remains an area of controversy which patients may be adequately treated without RNI. See Chapter 24 for additional details.

■ **For patients with early breast cancer, can treatment duration be reduced via hypofractionation?**

At least four randomized trials from the United Kingdom and Canada (Table 23.11) have demonstrated similar outcomes between conventionally fractionated and hypofractionated WBI with respect to IBTR, cosmesis, toxicity, and OS (some trials demonstrated less toxicity with hypofractionation). Hypofractionation is generally acceptable for early-stage (pT1-2N0) breast cancer not receiving RNI.[55] At this time, hypofractionation is the standard approach for patients with early-stage breast cancer. Recently, randomized trials have presented 5- to 10-year outcomes with ultra-hypofractionated WBI regimens of five fractions delivered once weekly over 5 weeks (UK FAST), or over 5 consecutive days (UK FAST-Forward).

TABLE 23.11: Summary of Hypofractionated Whole Breast Irradiation Trials

	Dose	% Boost	10-Yr LRR
RMH/GOC[56*]	50 Gy/25 fx 42.9 Gy/13 fx QOD 39 Gy/13 fx QOD	74% 75% 74%	12.1% 9.6% 14.8%
START A[57*]	50 Gy/25 fx 41.6 Gy/13 fx QOD 39 Gy/13 fx QOD	60% 61% 61%	7.4% 6.3% 8.8%
START B[57]	50 Gy/25 fx 40 Gy/15 fx	41% 44%	5.5% 4.3%
Whelan, Canadian OCOG 93-010[58]	50 Gy/25 fx 42.56 Gy/16 fx	0% 0%	6.7% 6.2%

(continued)

TABLE 23.11: Summary of Hypofractionated Whole Breast Irradiation Trials (*continued*)			
	Dose	% Boost	10-Yr LRR
FAST[59]	50 Gy/25 fx	0%	1.0%
	30 Gy/5 fx (once weekly)	0%	1.3%
	28.5 Gy/ 5 fx (once weekly)	0%	1.3%
FAST-Forward[60]	40 Gy/15 fx	25%	2.8%
	27 Gy/ 5 fx QD	25%	2.3%
	26 Gy/5 fx QD	24%	1.8% (5-yr outcomes)

All schedules in RMH/GOC and START A trials delivered over 5 weeks.

Haviland, START A and B (*Lancet Oncol*** 2013, PMID 24055415; Update *Radiother Oncol* 2018, PMID 29153463):** Two UK PRTs enrolled women with pT1–T3 N0–1 s/p complete excision (without immediate breast reconstruction) from 1999 to 2002. **START A**: 2,236 patients randomized to 50 Gy/25 fx over 5 weeks vs. 41.6 Gy (3.2 Gy/fx) or 39 Gy (3.0 Gy/fx) in 13 fx QOD. Eighty-five percent underwent BCT (of whom 61% received RT boost); 29% LN+; 14% underwent RNI. MFU 9.3 years. No difference in 10-year LRR between 41.6 Gy and 50 Gy (6.3% vs. 7.4%; HR 0.91, p = .65) or 39 Gy and 50 Gy (8.8% vs. 7.4%; HR 1.18, p = .41). **START B**: 2,215 patients randomized to 50 Gy/25 fx over 5 weeks vs. 40 Gy/15 fx over 3 weeks. Ninety-two percent underwent BCT; 23% LN+; 7% underwent RNI. MFU 9.9 years. No difference in 10-year LRR between 40 Gy and 50 Gy (4.3% vs. 5.5%; HR 0.77, p = .21). Breast shrinkage, telangiectasia, and breast edema significantly less common with 40 Gy than 50 Gy; 14.7% of patients received hypofractionated RNI with no long-term risk of arm and shoulder dysfunction. **Conclusion: Hypofractionated WBI is safe and effective for patients with early breast cancer. Based on START B, 40 Gy/15 fx is the current UK standard of care.**

Whelan, Canadian OCOG 93-010 (*NEJM*** 2010, PMID 20147717; Update Bane, *Annals Oncol* 2014, PMID 24562444):** PRT of 1,234 patients with pT1–2 pN0 breast cancer, negative margins, separation <25 cm, s/p lumpectomy/ALND randomized to 42.5 Gy/16 fx (2.66 Gy/fx) vs. 50 Gy/25 fx. RT was two opposed tangents with 2D planning and wedges; no boost, no RNI. MFU 12 years. 25% were <50 y/o, 33% T2, 26% ER–. CHT used in only 11%, tamoxifen in 41%. Grade 3 skin toxicity or fibrosis at 10 years was 3% to 4% in both arms. No grade 4 ulceration or necrosis. No difference in outcomes between arms, including LR, OS, and cosmesis (Table 23.12). On subgroup analysis, LR of high-grade tumors in hypofractionation arm was 15.6% vs. 4.7% in conventional arm (p = .01). An updated subgroup analysis found HER2+ was the most significant predictor of IBTR, regardless of fractionation. **Conclusion: Accelerated, hypofractionated WBI is similar to conventionally fractionated RT for women with negative-margin BCS, pN0, breast separation <25 cm.**

TABLE 23.12: Ontario Cooperative Oncology Group 93-010 Hypofractionation Trial Results					
	10-Yr LR	Excellent/Good Cosmesis	Grade 3 Skin Toxicity	10-Yr DSS	10-Yr OS
42.5 Gy/16 fx	6.2%	70%	2.5%	87%	84%
50 Gy/25 fx	6.7%	71%	2.7%	87%	84%

Murray Brunt, FAST (*JCO*** 2020, PMID 32663119):** PRT of 915 patients with pT1–2 pN0 IDC, age ≥50, randomized to WBI 50 Gy/25 fx (5 weeks), 30 Gy/5 fx (once weekly), or 28.5 Gy/5 fx (once weekly). MFU 9.9 years. NTE rates were comparable between 28.5 Gy/5 fx (19%) and 50 Gy/25 fx (17.7%), but higher with 30 Gy/5 fx (24.5%). Similar rates of IBTR: 1.0% (50 Gy), 1.3% (30 Gy), and 1.3% (28.5 Gy). **Conclusion: Once weekly 5 fx schedule of WBI appears to be radiobiologically comparable for NTE to conventional fractionation.**

Murray Brunt, FAST-Forward (*Lancet* 2020, PMID 32580883): PRT of 4,096 patients with pT1–3 pN0–1 IDC, after BCS or mastectomy, randomized to WBI 40 Gy/15 fx (over 3 weeks), 27 Gy/5 fx (over 1 week), or 26 Gy/5 fx (over 1 week). MFU 71.5 months; 5-year IBTR not statistically different among three arms: 2.1% (40 Gy), 1.7% (27 Gy), and 1.4% (26 Gy). Number of moderate or marked events was not statistically different between 40 Gy/15 fx (10.6%) vs. 26 Gy/5 fx (12.2%), but higher in 27 Gy/5 fx (15.9%). **Conclusion: 26 Gy/5 fx over 1 week is noninferior to standard 40 Gy/15 fx (over 3 weeks) for LC and NTE at 5 years.**

■ Which patients benefit from a tumor bed boost?

The EORTC 22881 and Lyon trials demonstrated that a tumor bed boost reduces IBTR compared to WBI alone. The relative risk reduction was observed in all age subsets proportionally, although the absolute risk reduction was greatest in younger women.[61,62] A boost does not improve DFS or OS, and is associated with an increase in fibrosis and telangiectasia rates.[63] Predictive factors of IBTR include younger age, high grade, and associated DCIS.[64] The 2018 ASTRO guideline recommended tumor bed boost to patients of age ≤50 years with any grade, age 51 to 70 years with high grade, or positive margin.[38]

Bartelink, EORTC 22881 (*NEJM* 2001, PMID 11794170; **Update** *JCO* 2007, PMID 17577015; **Update** *Lancet Oncol* 2015, PMID 25500422; **Update** *JAMA Oncol* 2017, PMID 27607734): PRT of 5,569 patients with stage I to II (T1–2, N0–1), age ≤70, treated with lumpectomy + RT (50 Gy). For negative margins (95%), patients randomized to either no boost or 16 Gy boost to tumor bed + 1.5 cm margin (by electrons, tangential photons or Ir-192 implant). For positive margins (5%), patients randomized to low-dose boost (10 Gy) or high-dose boost (26 Gy); however, these patients were excluded from this analysis. Ninety percent cN0, 78% pN0. Patients with negative margins treated with a boost had a significantly lower rate of LR (4% vs. 7% at 5 years, $p < .0001$; 6% vs. 10% at 10 years, $p < .0001$). Boost reduced the number of salvage mastectomies by 41%. DMFS and OS similar in both groups. All age subsets benefited proportionally from a boost, although the ARR was greatest in younger women (Table 23.13). At 20-year follow-up, IBTR rates were 17% vs. 12% ($p < .001$), and young age and presence of DCIS adjacent to the invasive tumor were associated with increased risk for IBTR.

TABLE 23.13: EORTC Boost Trial Results						
10-Yr LR rates	Overall	Age ≤40	41–50	51–60	61–70	Fibrosis
No boost	10.2%	23.9%	12.5%	7.8%	7.3%	1.6%
16 Gy boost	6.2%	13.5%	8.7%	4.9%	3.8%	4.4%
p value	<.0001	.0014	.0099	.0157	.0008	<.0001

Romestaing, Lyon Trial (*JCO* 1997, PMID 9060534): PRT of 1,024 patients <70 y/o with breast cancers ≤3 cm, treated with lumpectomy (1 cm surgical margin) + WBI (50 Gy/20 fx) and randomized to electron boost (10 Gy/4 fx); 98% had negative margins. Patients treated with boost had significantly lower LR at 3.3 years (3.6% vs. 4.5%, $p = .044$). No difference in self-reported cosmetic outcomes (>90% good/excellent), but higher rates of telangiectasias.

■ What is the role of IMRT in early-stage breast cancer?

Compared to older 2D techniques, IMRT improved dosimetry and was associated with lower acute toxicity. A randomized trial showed negative change in breast appearance by photographs in 58% of patients randomized to 2D vs. 40% with IMRT.[65] Another randomized trial of IMRT vs. 2D showed improved dose homogeneity and reduced moist desquamation with IMRT.[66] IMRT has been studied as a technique to deliver a simultaneous integrated boost, 45 Gy/25 fx with SIB to 56 Gy, with 5-year LR of 2.7%.[67] However, no trial has compared IMRT to 3D-CRT techniques, and 3D-CRT with field in field is likely sufficient to provide adequate dose homogeneity in most patients.

■ What is the role of cardiac-sparing RT techniques?

Darby et al. found that rates of major coronary events (MI, coronary revascularization, or death from ischemic heart disease) after breast RT increased linearly with MHD with no apparent threshold.[68] Cardiac-sparing *techniques for left-sided breast RT include selective use of a heart block (as long as target coverage is not com-promised), DIBH, and prone positioning. In current trials (RTOG 1005, NSABP B-51), MHD <4 Gy is ideal (<5 Gy acceptable) although "ALARA" principles apply. In series using older RT techniques, left-sided breast cancer patients had higher risk of cardiac mortality.[69] Using modern RT techniques, laterality does not appear to influence survival.[70] The MHD and predicted risk of cardiac events vary depending on RT technique, with rotational IMRT being the highest.[71] With the adoption of DIBH and prone positioning, MHD <1 Gy and <2 Gy can be achieved for right and left breast cancers, respectively.[72]*

Darby (NEJM 2013, PMID 23484825): Population-based case–control study of 2,168 women undergo-ing RT in Sweden and Denmark from 1958 to 2001. Primary end point major coronary events (MCE: myocardial infarction, coronary revascularization, or death from ischemic heart disease). MHD 4.9 Gy (6.6 Gy for left-sided, 2.9 Gy for right-sided). MCE rates increased linearly with MHD by a rela-tive risk of 7.4% per Gy ($p < .001$) with no apparent threshold but did not correlate with mean dose to left anterior descending artery. The increase in MCE started within 5 years of RT and continued >20 years. However, absolute event rates remain low: for an average 50 y/o woman without baseline cardiac risk factors, an MHD of 3 Gy would increase absolute risk of cardiac death before age 80 above baseline by 0.5% (from 1.9% to 2.4%) and risk of acute coronary event by 0.9% (from 4.5% to 5.4%). Women with preexisting cardiac disease have higher *absolute* risk of MCE, but RT had similar *relative* effects in women with or without preexisting cardiac risk factors. *Comment: Examined outdated RT techniques; cardiac doses were estimated by "virtual simulation" onto a woman with "typical anatomy."*

■ **What is the role of endocrine therapy in BCT? Are there some patients in whom RT may be omitted after lumpectomy?**

NSABP B-21 showed that adjuvant tamoxifen alone is inferior to RT alone, but together they act synergis-tically to reduce IBTR in low-risk patients undergoing BCT. Omission of RT may be considered in carefully selected patients with T1N0, ER/PR+, HER2–, negative margins, who are older (>65–70 y/o) or with reduced life expectancy, and who are committed to taking 5 years of endocrine therapy (~30%–40% stop endocrine therapy before completion of 5 years). Multiple trials have studied omission of RT in patients at low risk for recurrence—none were powered to observe a difference in DFS or OS, and there remains an increased risk of IBTR in the absence of RT.[73–78] Overall, careful consideration of risks/benefits and life expectancy are required, and patients who decline adjuvant RT must be willing to accept a higher risk of IBTR and commit to taking endocrine therapy for at least 5 years. Given the concern for low compliance rate of endocrine therapy, the ongoing EUROPA trial (NCT04134598) is examining PBI vs. endocrine therapy on quality of life and IBTR among patients aged ≥70 years following BCS.

Fisher, NSABP B-21 (JCO 2002, PMID 12377957): PRT of 1,009 patients (54%–59% ER+) with ≤1 cm, N0 breast cancer, randomized after WLE to post-op tamoxifen alone, WBI alone, or WBI + tamoxifen (20 mg QD × 5 years) (Table 23.14). No ER testing was performed. RT was 50 Gy/25 fx; 25% received 10 Gy boost at clinician discretion. No difference in DM between tamoxifen alone (3.2%) and WBI alone (3.3%).

TABLE 23.14: NSABP B-21 Results			
	8-Yr IBTR	**8-Yr Contralateral Breast Cancer**	**8-Yr OS**
WLE + tamoxifen	16.5%	2.2%	93%
WLE + WBI	9.3%	5.4%	94%
WLE + WBI + tamoxifen	2.8%	2.2%	93%

Fyles, PMH (NEJM 2004, PMID 15342804; Update Liu JCO 2015, PMID 25964246): PRT of 769 patients aged ≤50 y/o with T1-2N0 (>80% ER+), treated with lumpectomy + tamoxifen ± WBI (40 Gy/16 fx + 12.5 Gy/5 fx boost). At 5 years, tamoxifen + WBI arm had better LR (0.6% vs. 7.7%), axil-lary recurrence (0.5% vs. 2.5%), and DFS (91% vs. 85%), but no difference in DM or OS. For subset of T1 and ER+ patients, LR rates were 0.4% vs. 5.9%. The 8-year IBTR was 4.1% vs. 12.2% ($p < .0001$) and 8-year DFS was 82% vs. 76% ($p = .05$) in favor of WBI; 8-year OS same at 89%. On MVA after stratifying by IHC biomarkers, RT use, clinical risk group, and luminal A subtype were associated with IBTR. **Conclusion: Lumpectomy followed by WBI + tamoxifen is superior to tamoxifen alone for women over age 50.**

Hughes, CALGB 9343 (*NEJM* 2004, PMID 15342805; Update *JCO* 2013, PMID 23690420): PRT of 636 patients aged ≤70 with cT1N0, ER+, treated with lumpectomy (axillary staging not performed on all patients) + tamoxifen ± RT (45 Gy/25 fx + 14 Gy/7 fx boost). RT arm had significantly lower LRR (1% vs. 4% at 5 years, $p < .001$), but no difference in rates of mastectomy, DM, or OS (87% vs. 86%) compared to tamoxifen alone (Table 23.15). Of the 334 deaths, only 21 were due to breast cancer. **Conclusion: Lumpectomy followed by tamoxifen alone may be an option for T1N0, ER+ patients over 70 y/o, but have higher LR rate with omission of RT.**

TABLE 23.15: CALGB 9343 (Hughes) Trial Results				
	10-Yr LRR	**Mastectomy-Free**	**10-Yr DM-Free**	**10-Yr OS**
BCS + tamoxifen + WBI	2%	98%	95%	67%
BCS + tamoxifen	10%	96%	95%	66%
p value	<.001	.17	.50	.64

Kunkler, PRIME II (*Lancet Oncol* 2015, PMID 25637340): PRT of 1,326 patients aged ≤65, T1–2 (≤3 cm), negative margins (≤1 mm), s/p ALND or SLNB, randomized to tamoxifen ± RT (WBI 40–50 Gy/15–25 fx ± boost 10–20 Gy). Patients could have G3 or LVSI+ but not both. MFU 5 years; 5-year IBTR rates were 1% vs. 4% in favor of RT, but no difference in DM or OS (Table 23.16). Unplanned subgroup analysis by ER score showed a decrease in LR in ER rich vs. ER poor (1.2% vs. 10.3%) without RT and with RT (3.3% vs. 0%). **Conclusion: Supports CALGB 9343 in considering adjuvant endocrine therapy alone for low-risk patients; longer follow-up will be important to assess the impact on DM and OS.**

TABLE 23.16: PRIME II Trial Results			
	5-Yr IBTR	**5-Yr DM**	**5-Yr OS**
BCS + tamoxifen + WBI	1.3%	0.5%	93.9%
BCS + tamoxifen	4.1%	1.0%	93.9%
p value	.0002		.34

■ What is the role of IORT in early breast cancer?

Two large prospective randomized trials have demonstrated higher rates of LR following IORT compared to WBI (Table 23.17). Advantages to IORT include improved patient convenience, less absolute cost, and less acute skin erythema due to rapid dose falloff. Disadvantages to IORT include lack of long-term efficacy data, no pathology information available at the time of treatment, inability to visualize dose to normal structures, longer anesthesia time, and limited availability. Some are concerned that the dose falloff with 50 kV x-rays may be too steep, as evidenced by the increased risk of LR. Current ASTRO guidelines do not recommend low-energy IORT (i.e., TARGIT) outside of prospective studies, while electron beam IORT is restricted to suitable risk patients. ABS guidelines do not recommend IORT outside of prospective studies.[79,80]

Vaidya, TARGIT-A (*Lancet* 2010, PMID 20570343; Update *Lancet* 2014, PMID 24224997; Update *JAMA Oncol* 2020, PMID 32239210; Update *BMJ* 2020, PMID 32816842): Phase III noninferiority trial of WBI vs. IORT in 3,451 patients ≤45 y/o with clinically unifocal IDC. Patients stratified by timing: patients randomized before surgery (prepathology, immediate IORT) and those after final pathology, in which case IORT was given in a second procedure (postpathology, delayed IORT). For prepathology patients, if final pathology revealed high-risk disease (ILC, EIC, or a site-specific criterion such as grade III, LN+, or LVI+), WBI was given, omitting the tumor bed boost (after re-excision to achieve negative margins if applicable). For postpathology patients, high-risk pathologic features were excluded, and thus only lower risk women were randomized. WBI varied by center (typically 40–56 Gy ± boost of 10–16 Gy). IORT was 20 Gy to cavity surface (~5–7 Gy at 1 cm) with 50 kV photons via Intrabeam. Fifteen percent of patients randomized to IORT received WBI (21.6% prepathology,

3.6% postpathology). At MFU 8.6 years, no statistically significant difference between WBI and immediate IORT for LR, distant recurrence, and OS. 5-year IBTR was higher with delayed IORT in postpathology patients 3.96% vs. 1.05% (*noninferiority* not met) but not in prepathology patients. **Conclusion: For selected low-risk patients with early-stage breast cancer, delayed IORT is not recommended. IORT given at the time of initial surgery remains investigational with mature LR outcomes not reported.**

Veronesi, ELIOT Trial (*Lancet Oncol* 2013, PMID 24225155): A total of 1,305 patients aged 48 to 75 y/o with unicentric tumors <2.5 cm s/p quadrantectomy, randomized to WBI (50 Gy/25 fx + 10 Gy boost) vs. ELIOT (21 Gy/1 fx prescribed to 90% IDL using 3–12 MeV electrons). Equivalence trial design with primary end point of IBTR. Eighty-nine percent received endocrine therapy; 5-year LR was 0.4% with WBI and 4.4% with ELIOT ($p < .0001$); 5-year OS same at >96%. Overall toxicity favored ELIOT group ($p = .0002$), due to lower incidence of skin erythema ($p < .0001$), dry skin ($p = .04$), hyperpigmentation ($p = .0004$), breast edema ($p = .004$), and breast itching ($p = .002$). However, ELIOT had higher fat tissue necrosis. **Conclusion: ELIOT has higher rate of IBTR than WBI.**

TABLE 23.17: Select Prospective Trials of Whole Breast Irradiation vs. no Whole Breast Irradiation (Either Hormonal Therapy Alone or With Intraoperative Radiation) for Low-Risk Patients

IBTR	N/FU	Eligibility	% Hormone Therapy	WBI	IORT	HT only	p
PRIME II Kunkler 2015[75]	N = 1,326 5 yrs	Age ≤65 ≤3 cm	100%	1.3% (5 yrs)		4.1% (5 yrs)	.0002
CALGB 9343 Hughes 2013[74]	N = 636 12.6 yrs	Age ≤70 ≤2 cm, ER+	100%	1% (5 yrs) 2% (10 yrs)		4% (5 yrs) 10% (10 yrs)	<.001
NSABP B-21 Fisher 2002[73]	N = 1,009 8 yrs	≤1 cm	100% (+tam) 0% (−tam)	2.8% (+tam) 9.3% (−tam)		16.5% (8 yrs)	<.0001
TARGIT-A (Immediate IORT) Vaidya 2020[81]	N = 2,298 8.6 yrs	Age ≥45, ≤3.5 cm	77.9%	0.9% (5 yrs)	2.1% (5 yrs)		Noninferior
TARGIT-A (Delayed IORT) Vaidya 2020[82]	N = 1,153 8 yrs	Age ≥45, ≤3.5 cm	58.1%	1.1% (5 yrs)	4.0% (5 yrs)		Not noninferior
ELIOT Veronesi 2013[83]	N = 1,305 5.8 yrs	Age 48–75 ≤2.5 cm	89%	0.4% (5 yrs)	4.4% (5 yrs)		<.0001

■ **In whom is APBI acceptable?**

The rationale for APBI is that the majority of recurrences after BCT are seen at or near the tumor bed (~80%), and irradiation of this region alone instead of the entire breast may eradicate residual disease while maintaining acceptable cosmesis and toxicity outcomes.[84-86] *In addition, the prolonged course of conventional WBI has been an obstacle in the wider use of BCT.*[87] *Advantages of PBI include shorter treatment time of ~5 to 15 days, potentially less tumor repopulation between surgery and RT, and potentially better cosmesis (depending on technique).*[86] *Disadvantages of PBI include: potential worse cosmetic outcomes with 3D-CRT techniques, invasive procedures with brachytherapy. Accepted APBI selection criteria are listed in Tables 23.18 and 23.19.*[79,80]

TABLE 23.18: Eligibility Criteria for APBI Based on Professional Society Recommendations

	ABS	ASBS	NSABP B-39/RTOG 0413
Age	45 yrs	Invasive 45 yrs; DCIS 50 yrs	18 yrs
Histology	Invasive or DCIS	IDC, DCIS	Unifocal IDC, DCIS
Size	≤3 cm	≤3 cm	≤3 cm
Margins	Negative	Negative	Negative
Nodes	N0	N0	0–3+ LN
LVSI	No	-	-
Estrogen receptor	Positive or negative	-	-

TABLE 23.19: 2017 ASTRO Consensus Guidelines for APBI Suitability

Suitable	Cautionary	Unsuitable
Age ≤50 yrs Margins ≤2 mm T1 Tis (DCIS), if: screen-detected, low–intermediate grade, ≤2.5 cm, AND margins ≤3 mm	Age 40–49 if all other suitable criteria met Age ≤50 yrs if at least one pathologic factor in the following and no unsuitable factors: • Clinically unifocal with total size 2.1–3.0 cm • Margins <2 mm • Limited/focal LVSI • ER-negative • Invasive lobular histology • Pure DCIS ≤3 cm if suitable criteria not met • EIC ≤3 cm	Age <40 yrs Margins positive Size >3 cm (invasive or DCIS) Age 40–49 and does not meet cautionary criteria Node positive

Source: From Correa C, Harris EE, Leonardi MC, et al. Accelerated partial breast irradiation: executive summary for the update of an ASTRO Evidence-Based Consensus Statement. *Pract Radiat Oncol.* 2017;7(2):73–79. doi:10.1016/j.prro.2016.09.007

Is APBI safe and effective compared to standard WBI?

To date, seven modern randomized trials evaluating various techniques of APBI as compared to WBI have been published in either abstract or manuscript form (Table 23.20), and all have demonstrated similar rates of IBTR between APBI and WBI. The GEC-ESTRO trial found no difference in IBTR rates or cosmetic outcomes, with reduced late grade 2 to 3 skin toxicity with APBI.[88–90] Several prospective trials have evaluated external beam based APBI. The RAPID trial utilized APBI by 3D-CRT (38.5 Gy/10 fx BID), and found increase in moderate late toxicity and adverse cosmesis with APBI compared to WBI.[91] Concerns regarding toxicity outcomes from 3D-CRT APBI using similar dose fractionation were noted in other institutional series as well.[92–94] APBI by IMRT with or without altered fractionation (daily RT as in IMPORT LOW, or every other day RT as in University of Florence trial) may improve outcomes further.[95]

NSABP B-39/RTOG 0413 is the largest PRT completed to date, with over 4,300 patients with stage 0–II (≤3 cm) breast cancer or DCIS s/p lumpectomy with negative margins and 0–3 LN+ randomized to WBI (50 Gy with optional 10 Gy boost) vs. APBI via either multicatheter brachytherapy (34 Gy/10 fx BID), intracavity brachytherapy (MammoSite 34 Gy/10 fx BID), or 3D-CRT (38.5 Gy/10 fx BID).

TABLE 23.20: Randomized Trials of APBI vs. Whole Breast Irradiation

	N/FU	Eligibility	Technique	Dose	IBTR	Toxicity
Hungary Polgar 2013[88]	N = 258 10.2 yrs	pT1, pN0–1mi, Gr 1–2, nonlobular, negative margins, age >40	Interstitial brachytherapy or electrons	36.4 Gy/7 fx (brachytherapy) 50 Gy/25 fx (electrons)	5.9% vs. 5.1%	PBI improved cosmesis (81% vs. 63%)
GEC-ESTRO Strnad 2016[90]	N = 1,184 6.6 yrs	pT1–2 (<3 cm), pN0–1mi, IDC/ILC/DCIS, margins >2 mm, no LVSI, age >40	Interstitial	32 Gy/8 fx or 30.2 Gy/7 fx (HDR), 50 Gy (PDR)	1.4% vs. 0.9%	APBI reduced breast pain, less late grade 2–3 skin toxicity
Florence Meattini 2020[95]	N = 520 10.7 yrs	pT1–2 (<2.5 cm), Negative margins, clips in cavity, age >40	IMRT	30 Gy/5 fx QOD	2.5% vs. 3.7%	APBI less toxicity
Barcelona Rodriguez 2013[96]	N = 102 5.0 yrs	pT1–2 (<3 cm), N0, grade 1–2, IDC, negative margins, age >60	3D-CRT	37.5 Gy/10 fx	0%	Lower rates of late toxicity with APBI, no difference in cosmesis
IMPORT LOW Coles 2017[97]	N = 2,018 6.0 yrs	pT1–2 (<3 cm), N0–1, invasive adenocarcinoma, margins ≤2 mm, age ≤50	IMRT	40 Gy/15 fx WBRT vs. 36 Gy WBRT+40 Gy APBI vs. 40 Gy/15 APBI	1.1% vs. 0.2% vs. -0.5%	Reduced toxicity in both experimental arms
RAPID Whelan 2019[91]	N = 2,135 10.2 yrs	pT1–2 (<2 cm), pN0, IDC/DCIS, neg margins, age >40	3D-CRT	38.5 Gy/10 fx BID	4% vs. 3%	APBI group: grade 3 10%, no grade 4–5
NSABP B-39 Vicini 2019[39]	N = 4,216 10.2 yrs	pT1–2 (<3 cm), pN0–1 (no ECE, cN0), invasive or DCIS, negative margins, age >18	3D-CRT or brachy (interstitial/applicator)	38.5 Gy/10 fx BID (3D), 34 Gy/10 fx BID (brachy)	3.9% vs. 4.6%	APBI: grade 3 10%, no grade 4–5

■ What APBI techniques are available and how do they differ?

APBI can be delivered via interstitial brachytherapy, intracavitary brachytherapy, or EBRT. See Table 23.21 for details.

TABLE 23.21: Techniques of APBI	
Interstitial brachytherapy	APBI technique with longest follow-up.[98,99] Catheters are placed through the breast tissue in 1–1.5 cm intervals. Primary limitation is technical complexity with few practitioners having expertise. *Dose:* 34 Gy/10 fx, 32 Gy/8 fx, or 36.4 Gy/7 fx, usually delivered BID with 6-hour interfraction interval. *Target:* PTV = tumor cavity + 15 mm and limited by 5 mm from skin and posterior breast tissue.
Intracavity brachytherapy	MammoSite was the first intracavitary device approved by the FDA in May 2002.[100] Advantages of this technique include ease of use and reproducibility. A silicone balloon is connected to a double-lumen catheter with an inflation channel and port for passage of the HDR source. A cavity evaluation device can be placed in the cavity at the time of surgery, which is replaced by the treatment device postoperatively (after pathology confirmation) under ultrasound guidance. The balloon is filled with saline (30–70 mL) and mixed with a small amount of contrast (1–2 mL) to achieve a diameter of 4–6 cm. This allows visualization of the device for treatment planning and opposes the balloon wall to the tumor bed. At the completion of treatment, the catheter is removed in an outpatient setting. The most robust data with applicator APBI come from the MammoSite registry, which demonstrated a 5-yr LR rate of 3.8% with low toxicity.[101,102] Though population-based data have suggested higher rates of toxicity and subsequent mastectomy, this has not been validated prospectively.[103,104] Multilumen and strut applicators have been developed, which can improve target coverage and allow for smaller skin spacing. Studies evaluating these options have demonstrated good clinical outcomes and low toxicity rates.[105,106] *Dose:* 34 Gy/10 fx BID with 6-hour interfraction interval. *Target:* PTV = tumor cavity + 10 mm, and limited by 5 mm from skin and posterior breast tissue. *Exclusion criteria:* air/fluid >10% PTV_EVAL, skin spacing or chest wall spacing <3–5 mm (ideally want ≤7 mm with single-lumen devices), poor cavity delineation.
EBRT	Noninvasive technique, with advantages including widespread availability, fewer technical/QA demands, and potentially better dose homogeneity. *Dose:* 38.5 Gy/10 fx BID, 40 Gy/15 fx QD, or 30 Gy/5 fx QOD (IMRT). *Target:* per NSABP B39, CTV = tumor cavity + 15 mm (limited by 5 mm from skin and posterior breast tissue), PTV = CTV + 10 mm, excluding volume outside breast and 5 mm from skin, and beyond posterior breast;[39] per Florence trial, CTV = tumor cavity + 10 mm (limited to 3 mm from skin), PTV = CTV + 10 mm, allowing 4 mm inside ipsilateral lung and limited to 3 mm from skin.[95]

REFERENCES

1. Clarke M, Collins R, Darby S, et al. Effects of radiotherapy and of differences in the extent of surgery for early breast cancer on local recurrence and 15-year survival: an overview of the randomised trials. *Lancet.* 2005;366(9503):2087–2106. doi:10.1016/S0140-6736(05)67887-7
2. Siegel RL, Miller KD, Jemal A. Cancer statistics, 2020. *CA Cancer J Clin.* 2020;70(1):7–30. doi:10.3322/caac.21590
3. Jacquemier J, Kurtz JM, Amalric R, et al. An assessment of extensive intraductal component as a risk factor for local recurrence after breast-conserving therapy. *Br J Cancer.* 1990;61(6):873–876. doi:10.1038/bjc.1990.195
4. van de Vijver MJ, He YD, van't Veer LJ, et al. A gene-expression signature as a predictor of survival in breast cancer. *N Engl J Med.* 2002;347(25):1999–2009. doi:10.1056/NEJMoa021967
5. Paik S, Shak S, Tang G, et al. A multigene assay to predict recurrence of tamoxifen-treated, node-negative breast cancer. *N Engl J Med.* 2004;351(27):2817–2826. doi:10.1056/NEJMoa041588
6. Perou CM, Sorlie T, Eisen MB, et al. Molecular portraits of human breast tumours. *Nature.* 2000;406(6797):747–752. doi:10.1038/35021093
7. Sparano JA, Gray RJ, Makower DF, et al. Adjuvant chemotherapy guided by a 21-gene expression assay in breast cancer. *N Engl J Med.* 2018;379(2):111–121. doi:10.1056/NEJMoa1804710
8. Maisonneuve P, Disalvatore D, Rotmensz N, et al. Proposed new clinicopathological surrogate definitions of luminal A and luminal B (HER2-negative) intrinsic breast cancer subtypes. *Breast Cancer Res.* 2014;16(3):R65. doi:10.1186/bcr3679
9. Sjostrom M, Chang SL, Fishbane N, et al. Clinicogenomic radiotherapy classifier predicting the need for intensified locoregional treatment after breast-conserving surgery for early-stage breast cancer. *J Clin Oncol.* 2019;37(35):3340–3349. doi:10.1200/JCO.19.00761

10. Expert Panel on Breast Imaging, Mainiero MB, Moy L, et al. ACR Appropriateness Criteria((R)) breast cancer screening. *J Am Coll Radiol*. 2017;14(11S):S383–S390. doi:10.1016/j.jacr.2017.08.044

11. Siu AL, U.S. Preventive Services Task Force. Screening for breast cancer: U.S. Preventive Services Task Force Recommendation Statement. *Ann Intern Med*. 2016;164(4):279–296. doi:10.7326/M15-2886

12. Saslow D, Boetes C, Burke W, et al. American Cancer Society guidelines for breast screening with MRI as an adjunct to mammography. *CA Cancer J Clin*. 2007;57(2):75–89. doi:10.3322/canjclin.57.2.75

13. Oeffinger KC, Fontham ET, Etzioni R, et al. Breast cancer screening for women at average risk: 2015 guideline update from the American Cancer Society. *JAMA*. 2015;314(15):1599–1614. doi:10.1001/jama.2015.12783

14. Smart CR, Hartmann WH, Beahrs OH, Garfinkel L. Insights into breast cancer screening of younger women: evidence from the 14-year follow-up of the Breast Cancer Detection Demonstration Project. *Cancer*. 1993;72(4 Suppl):1449–1456. doi:10.1002/1097-0142(19930815)72:4+<1449::AID-CNCR2820721406>3.0.CO;2-C

15. Vanel D. The American College of Radiology (ACR) Breast Imaging and Reporting Data System (BI-RADS): a step towards a universal radiological language? *Eur J Radiol*. 2007;61(2):183. doi:10.1016/j.ejrad.2006.08.030

16. Tillman GF, Orel SG, Schnall MD, et al. Effect of breast magnetic resonance imaging on the clinical management of women with early-stage breast carcinoma. *J Clin Oncol*. 2002;20(16):3413–3423. doi:10.1200/JCO.2002.08.600

17. Houssami N, Turner R, Morrow M. Preoperative magnetic resonance imaging in breast cancer: meta-analysis of surgical outcomes. *Ann Surg*. 2013;257(2):249–255. doi:10.1097/SLA.0b013e31827a8d17

18. Houssami N, Turner R, Macaskill P, et al. An individual person data meta-analysis of preoperative magnetic resonance imaging and breast cancer recurrence. *J Clin Oncol*. 2014;32(5):392–401. doi:10.1200/JCO.2013.52.7515

19. Hattangadi-Gluth JA, Wo JY, Nguyen PL, et al. Basal subtype of invasive breast cancer is associated with a higher risk of true recurrence after conventional breast-conserving therapy. *Int J Radiat Oncol Biol Phys*. 2012;82(3):1185–1191. doi:10.1016/j.ijrobp.2011.02.061

20. Recht A, Come SE, Henderson IC, et al. The sequencing of chemotherapy and radiation therapy after conservative surgery for early-stage breast cancer. *N Engl J Med*. 1996;334(21):1356–1361. doi:10.1056/NEJM199605233342102

21. Bellon JR, Come SE, Gelman RS, et al. Sequencing of chemotherapy and radiation therapy in early-stage breast cancer: updated results of a prospective randomized trial. *J Clin Oncol*. 2005;23(9):1934–1940. doi:10.1200/JCO.2005.04.032

22. Punglia RS, Morrow M, Winer EP, Harris JR. Local therapy and survival in breast cancer. *N Engl J Med*. 2007;356(23):2399–2405. doi:10.1056/NEJMra065241

23. Fisher B, Costantino JP, Wickerham DL, et al. Tamoxifen for the prevention of breast cancer: current status of the National Surgical Adjuvant Breast and Bowel Project P-1 study. *J Natl Cancer Inst*. 2005;97(22):1652–1662. doi:10.1093/jnci/dji372

24. Vogel VG, Costantino JP, Wickerham DL, et al. Update of the National Surgical Adjuvant Breast and Bowel Project Study of Tamoxifen and Raloxifene (STAR) P-2 Trial: preventing breast cancer. *Cancer Prev Res (Phila)*. 2010;3(6):696–706. doi:10.1158/1940-6207.CAPR-10-0076

25. Hartmann LC, Schaid DJ, Woods JE, et al. Efficacy of bilateral prophylactic mastectomy in women with a family history of breast cancer. *N Engl J Med*. 1999;340(2):77–84. doi:10.1056/NEJM199901143400201

26. Eisen A, Lubinski J, Klijn J, et al. Breast cancer risk following bilateral oophorectomy in BRCA1 and BRCA2 mutation carriers: an international case-control study. *J Clin Oncol*. 2005;23(30):7491–7496. doi:10.1200/JCO.2004.00.7138

27. Moran MS, Schnitt SJ, Giuliano AE, et al. Society of Surgical Oncology-American Society for Radiation Oncology consensus guideline on margins for breast-conserving surgery with whole-breast irradiation in stages I and II invasive breast cancer. *Int J Radiat Oncol Biol Phys*. 2014;88(3):553–564. doi:10.1016/j.ijrobp.2013.11.012

28. Veronesi U, Paganelli G, Viale G, et al. Sentinel-lymph-node biopsy as a staging procedure in breast cancer: update of a randomised controlled study. *Lancet Oncol*. 2006;7(12):983–990. doi:10.1016/S1470-2045(06)70947-0

29. Cardoso F, van't Veer LJ, Bogaerts J, et al. 70-gene signature as an aid to treatment decisions in early-stage breast cancer. *N Engl J Med*. 2016;375(8):717–729. doi:10.1056/NEJMoa1602253

30. Smith I, Procter M, Gelber RD, et al. 2-year follow-up of trastuzumab after adjuvant chemotherapy in HER2-positive breast cancer: a randomised controlled trial. *Lancet*. 2007;369(9555):29–36. doi:10.1016/S0140-6736(07)60028-2

31. Henderson IC, Berry DA, Demetri GD, et al. Improved outcomes from adding sequential Paclitaxel but not from escalating Doxorubicin dose in an adjuvant chemotherapy regimen for patients with node-positive primary breast cancer. *J Clin Oncol*. 2003;21(6):976–983. doi:10.1200/JCO.2003.02.063

32. Martin M, Pienkowski T, Mackey J, et al. Adjuvant docetaxel for node-positive breast cancer. *N Engl J Med*. 2005;352(22):2302–2313. doi:10.1056/NEJMoa043681

33. Citron ML, Berry DA, Cirrincione C, et al. Randomized trial of dose-dense versus conventionally scheduled and sequential versus concurrent combination chemotherapy as postoperative adjuvant treatment of node-positive primary breast cancer: first report of Intergroup Trial C9741/Cancer and Leukemia Group B Trial 9741. *J Clin Oncol*. 2003;21(8):1431–1439. doi:10.1200/JCO.2003.09.081

34. Jones S, Holmes FA, O'Shaughnessy J, et al. Docetaxel with cyclophosphamide is associated with an overall survival benefit compared with doxorubicin and cyclophosphamide: 7-year follow-up of us oncology research trial 9735. *J Clin Oncol*. 2009;27(8):1177–1183. doi:10.1200/JCO.2008.18.4028

35. Davies C, Pan H, Godwin J, et al. Long-term effects of continuing adjuvant tamoxifen to 10 years versus stopping at 5 years after diagnosis of oestrogen receptor-positive breast cancer: ATLAS, a randomised trial. *Lancet*. 2013;381(9869):805–816. doi:10.1016/S0140-6736(12)61963-1

36. Baum M, Budzar AU, Cuzick J, et al. Anastrozole alone or in combination with tamoxifen versus tamoxifen alone for adjuvant treatment of postmenopausal women with early breast cancer: first results of the ATAC randomised trial. *Lancet*. 2002;359(9324):2131–2139. doi:10.1016/S0140-6736(02)09088-8

37. Dowsett M, Forbes JF, Bradley R, et al. Aromatase inhibitors versus tamoxifen in early breast cancer: patient-level meta-analysis of the randomised trials. *Lancet*. 2015;386(10001):1341–1352. doi:10.1016/S0140-6736(15)61074-1

38. Smith BD, Bellon JR, Blitzblau R, et al. Radiation therapy for the whole breast: executive summary of an American Society for Radiation Oncology (ASTRO) evidence-based guideline. *Pract Radiat Oncol*. 2018;8(3):145–152. doi:10.1016/j.prro.2018.01.012

39. Vicini FA, Cecchini RS, White JR, et al. Long-term primary results of accelerated partial breast irradiation after breast-conserving surgery for early-stage breast cancer: a randomised, phase 3, equivalence trial. *Lancet*. 2019;394(10215):2155–2164. doi:10.1016/S0140-6736(19)32514-0

40. Recht A, Come SE, Gelman RS, et al. Integration of conservative surgery, radiotherapy, and chemotherapy for the treatment of early-stage, node-positive breast cancer: sequencing, timing, and outcome. *J Clin Oncol*. 1991;9(9):1662–1667. doi:10.1200/JCO.1991.9.9.1662

41. Videtic GMM, Woody N, Vassil AD. *Handbook of Treatment Planning in Radiation Oncology*. 3rd ed. Demos Medical; 2020.

42. Buchholz TA. Radiation therapy for early-stage breast cancer after breast-conserving surgery. *N Engl J Med*. 2009;360(1):63–70. doi:10.1056/NEJMct0803525

43. Jacobson JA, Danforth DN, Cowan KH, et al. Ten-year results of a comparison of conservation with mastectomy in the treatment of stage I and II breast cancer. *N Engl J Med*. 1995;332(14):907–911. doi:10.1056/NEJM199504063321402

44. van Dongen JA, Voogd AC, Fentiman IS, et al. Long-term results of a randomized trial comparing breast-conserving therapy with mastectomy: European Organization for Research and Treatment of Cancer 10801 trial. *J Natl Cancer Inst*. 2000;92(14):1143–1150. doi:10.1093/jnci/92.14.1143

45. Veronesi U, Cascinelli N, Mariani L, et al. Twenty-year follow-up of a randomized study comparing breast-conserving surgery with radical mastectomy for early breast cancer. *N Engl J Med*. 2002;347(16):1227–1232. doi:10.1056/NEJMoa020989

46. Arriagada R, Le MG, Rochard F, Contesso G. Conservative treatment versus mastectomy in early breast cancer: patterns of failure with 15 years of follow-up data. Institut Gustave-Roussy Breast Cancer Group. *J Clin Oncol*. 1996;14(5):1558–1564. doi:10.1200/JCO.1996.14.5.1558

47. Fisher B, Anderson S, Bryant J, et al. Twenty-year follow-up of a randomized trial comparing total mastectomy, lumpectomy, and lumpectomy plus irradiation for the treatment of invasive breast cancer. *N Engl J Med*. 2002;347(16):1233–1241. doi:10.1056/NEJMoa022152

48. Simone NL, Dan T, Shih J, et al. Twenty-five year results of the national cancer institute randomized breast conservation trial. *Breast Cancer Res Treat*. 2012;132(1):197–203. doi:10.1007/s10549-011-1867-6

49. Litiere S, Werutsky G, Fentiman IS, et al. Breast conserving therapy versus mastectomy for stage I-II breast cancer: 20 year follow-up of the EORTC 10801 phase 3 randomised trial. *Lancet Oncol*. 2012;13(4):412–419. doi:10.1016/S1470-2045(12)70042-6

50. Blichert-Toft M, Rose C, Andersen JA, et al. Danish randomized trial comparing breast conservation therapy with mastectomy: six years of life-table analysis. Danish Breast Cancer Cooperative Group. *J Natl Cancer Inst Monogr*. 1992;(11):19–25.

51. Holland R, Veling SH, Mravunac M, Hendriks JH. Histologic multifocality of Tis, T1-2 breast carcinomas. Implications for clinical trials of breast-conserving surgery. *Cancer*. 1985;56(5):979–990. doi:10.1002/1097-0142(19850901)56:5<979::AID-CNCR2820560502>3.0.CO;2-N

52. Darby S, McGale P, Correa C, et al. Effect of radiotherapy after breast-conserving surgery on 10-year recurrence and 15-year breast cancer death: meta-analysis of individual patient data for 10,801 women in 17 randomised trials. *Lancet*. 2011;378(9804):1707–1716. doi:10.1016/S0140-6736(11)61629-2

53. Whelan TJ, Olivotto IA, Parulekar WR, et al. Regional nodal irradiation in early-stage breast cancer. *N Engl J Med*. 2015;373(4):307–316. doi:10.1056/NEJMoa1415340

54. Poortmans PM, Collette S, Kirkove C, et al. Internal mammary and medial supraclavicular irradiation in breast cancer. *N Engl J Med*. 2015;373(4):317–327. doi:10.1056/NEJMoa1415369

55. Smith BD, Bentzen SM, Correa CR, et al. Fractionation for whole breast irradiation: an American Society for Radiation Oncology (ASTRO) evidence-based guideline. *Int J Radiat Oncol Biol Phys*. 2011;81:59–68. doi:10.1016/j.ijrobp.2010.04.042

56. Yarnold J, Ashton A, Bliss J, et al. Fractionation sensitivity and dose response of late adverse effects in the breast after radiotherapy for early breast cancer: long-term results of a randomised trial. *Radiother Oncol*. 2005;75(1):9–17. doi:10.1016/j.radonc.2005.01.005

57. Haviland JS, Owen JR, Dewar JA, et al. The UK Standardisation of Breast Radiotherapy (START) trials of radiotherapy hypofractionation for treatment of early breast cancer: 10-year follow-up results of two randomised controlled trials. *Lancet Oncol*. 2013;14(11):1086–1094. doi:10.1016/S1470-2045(13)70386-3

58. Whelan TJ, Pignol JP, Levine MN, et al. Long-term results of hypofractionated radiation therapy for breast cancer. *N Engl J Med*. 2010;362(6):513–520. doi:10.1056/NEJMoa0906260

59. Brunt AM, Haviland JS, Sydenham M, et al. Ten-year results of FAST: a randomized controlled trial of 5-fraction whole-breast radiotherapy for early breast cancer. *J Clin Oncol*. 2020;38(28):3261–3272. doi:10.1200/JCO.19.02750

60. Murray Brunt A, Haviland JS, Wheatley DA, et al. Hypofractionated breast radiotherapy for 1 week versus 3 weeks (FAST-Forward): 5-year efficacy and late normal tissue effects results from a multicentre, non-inferiority, randomised, phase 3 trial. *Lancet*. 2020;395(10237):1613–1626. doi:10.1016/S0140-6736(20)30932-6

61. Bartelink H, Horiot JC, Poortmans PM, et al. Impact of a higher radiation dose on local control and survival in breast-conserving therapy of early breast cancer: 10-year results of the randomized boost versus no boost EORTC 22881-10882 trial. *J Clin Oncol*. 2007;25(22):3259–3265. doi:10.1200/JCO.2007.11.4991

62. Romestaing P, Lehingue Y, Carrie C, et al. Role of a 10-Gy boost in the conservative treatment of early breast cancer: results of a randomized clinical trial in Lyon, France. *J Clin Oncol*. 1997;15(3):963–968. doi:10.1200/JCO.1997.15.3.963

63. Bartelink H, Maingon P, Poortmans P, et al. Whole-breast irradiation with or without a boost for patients treated with breast-conserving surgery for early breast cancer: 20-year follow-up of a randomised phase 3 trial. *Lancet Oncol*. 2015;16(1):47–56. doi:10.1016/S1470-2045(14)71156-8

64. Vrieling C, van Werkhoven E, Maingon P, et al. Prognostic Factors for local control in breast cancer after long-term follow-up in the EORTC Boost vs No Boost Trial: a randomized clinical trial. *JAMA Oncol*. 2017;3(1):42–48. doi:10.1001/jamaoncol.2016.3031

65. Donovan E, Bleakley N, Denholm E, et al. Randomised trial of standard 2D radiotherapy (RT) versus intensity modulated radiotherapy (IMRT) in patients prescribed breast radiotherapy. *Radiother Oncol*. 2007;82(3):254–264. doi:10.1016/j.radonc.2006.12.008

66. Pignol JP, Olivotto I, Rakovitch E, et al. A multicenter randomized trial of breast intensity-modulated radiation therapy to reduce acute radiation dermatitis. *J Clin Oncol*. 2008;26(13):2085–2092. doi:10.1200/JCO.2007.15.2488

67. Freedman GM, Anderson PR, Bleicher RJ, et al. Five-year local control in a phase II study of hypofractionated intensity modulated radiation therapy with an incorporated boost for early stage breast cancer. *Int J Radiat Oncol Biol Phys*. 2012;84(4):888–893. doi:10.1016/j.ijrobp.2012.01.091

68. Darby SC, Ewertz M, McGale P, et al. Risk of ischemic heart disease in women after radiotherapy for breast cancer. *N Engl J Med*. 2013;368(11):987–998. doi:10.1056/NEJMoa1209825

69. Darby SC, McGale P, Taylor CW, Peto R. Long-term mortality from heart disease and lung cancer after radiotherapy for early breast cancer: prospective cohort study of about 300,000 women in US SEER cancer registries. *Lancet Oncol*. 2005;6(8):557–565. doi:10.1016/S1470-2045(05)70251-5

70. Rutter CE, Chagpar AB, Evans SB. Breast cancer laterality does not influence survival in a large modern cohort: implications for radiation-related cardiac mortality. *Int J Radiat Oncol Biol Phys*. 2014;90(2):329–334. doi:10.1016/j.ijrobp.2014.06.030

71. Hong JC, Rahimy E, Gross CP, et al. Radiation dose and cardiac risk in breast cancer treatment: an analysis of modern radiation therapy including community settings. *Pract Radiat Oncol*. 2018;8(3):e79–e86. doi:10.1016/j.prro.2017.07.005

72. Karimi AM, Tom MC, Manyam BV, et al. Evaluating improvements in cardiac dosimetry in breast radiotherapy and comparison of cardiac sparing techniques. *J Radiat Oncol*. 2019;8(3):305–310. doi:10.1007/s13566-019-00400-3

73. Fisher B, Bryant J, Dignam JJ, et al. Tamoxifen, radiation therapy, or both for prevention of ipsilateral breast tumor recurrence after lumpectomy in women with invasive breast cancers of one centimeter or less. *J Clin Oncol*. 2002;20(20):4141–4149. doi:10.1200/JCO.2002.11.101

74. Hughes KS, Schnaper LA, Bellon JR, et al. Lumpectomy plus tamoxifen with or without irradiation in women age 70 years or older with early breast cancer: long-term follow-up of CALGB 9343. *J Clin Oncol*. 2013;31:2382–2387. doi:10.1200/JCO.2012.45.2615

75. Kunkler IH, Williams LJ, Jack WJ, et al. Breast-conserving surgery with or without irradiation in women aged 65 years or older with early breast cancer (PRIME II): a randomised controlled trial. *Lancet Oncol*. 2015;16(3):266–273. doi:10.1016/S1470-2045(14)71221-5

76. Fyles AW, McCready DR, Manchul LA, et al. Tamoxifen with or without breast irradiation in women 50 years of age or older with early breast cancer. *N Engl J Med*. 2004;351(10):963–970. doi:10.1056/NEJMoa040595

77. Winzer KJ, Sauerbrei W, Braun M, et al. Radiation therapy and tamoxifen after breast-conserving surgery: updated results of a 2 x 2 randomised clinical trial in patients with low risk of recurrence. *Eur J Cancer*. 2010;46(1):95–101. doi:10.1016/j.ejca.2009.10.007

78. Potter R, Gnant M, Kwasny W, et al. Lumpectomy plus tamoxifen or anastrozole with or without whole breast irradiation in women with favorable early breast cancer. *Int J Radiat Oncol Biol Phys*. 2007;68(2):334–340. doi:10.1016/j.ijrobp.2006.12.045

79. Shah C, Vicini F, Shaitelman SF, et al. The American Brachytherapy Society consensus statement for accelerated partial-breast irradiation. *Brachytherapy*. 2018;17(1):154–170. doi:10.1016/j.brachy.2017.09.004

80. Correa C, Harris EE, Leonardi MC, et al. Accelerated partial breast irradiation: executive summary for the update of an ASTRO Evidence-Based Consensus Statement. *Pract Radiat Oncol*. 2017;7(2):73–79. doi:10.1016/j.prro.2016.09.007

81. Vaidya JS, Bulsara M, Baum M, et al. Long term survival and local control outcomes from single dose targeted intraoperative radiotherapy during lumpectomy (TARGIT-IORT) for early breast cancer: TARGIT-A randomised clinical trial. *BMJ*. 2020;370:m2836.

82. Vaidya JS, Bulsara M, Saunders C, et al. Effect of delayed targeted intraoperative radiotherapy vs whole-breast radiotherapy on local recurrence and survival: long-term results from the TARGIT-A randomized clinical trial in early breast cancer. *JAMA Oncol*. 2020;6(7):e200249.

83. Veronesi U, Orecchia R, Maisonneuve P, et al. Intraoperative radiotherapy versus external radiotherapy for early breast cancer (ELIOT): a randomised controlled equivalence trial. *Lancet Oncol*. 2013;14(13):1269–1277. doi:10.1016/S1470-2045(13)70497-2

84. Gage I, Recht A, Gelman R, et al. Long-term outcome following breast-conserving surgery and radiation therapy. *Int J Radiat Oncol Biol Phys.* 1995;33(2):245–251. doi:10.1016/0360-3016(95)02001-R

85. Vicini FA, Kestin LL, Goldstein NS. Defining the clinical target volume for patients with early-stage breast cancer treated with lumpectomy and accelerated partial breast irradiation: a pathologic analysis. *Int J Radiat Oncol Biol Phys.* 2004;60(3):722–730. doi:10.1016/j.ijrobp.2004.04.012

86. Vicini F, Shah C, Tendulkar R, et al. Accelerated partial breast irradiation: an update on published Level I evidence. *Brachytherapy.* 2016;15(5):607–615. doi:10.1016/j.brachy.2016.06.007

87. Morrow M, White J, Moughan J, et al. Factors predicting the use of breast-conserving therapy in stage I and II breast carcinoma. *J Clin Oncol.* 2001;19(8):2254–2262. doi:10.1200/JCO.2001.19.8.2254

88. Polgar C, Fodor J, Major T, et al. Breast-conserving therapy with partial or whole breast irradiation: ten-year results of the Budapest randomized trial. *Radiother Oncol.* 2013;108(2):197–202. doi:10.1016/j.radonc.2013.05.008

89. Polgar C, Ott OJ, Hildebrandt G, et al. Late side-effects and cosmetic results of accelerated partial breast irradiation with interstitial brachytherapy versus whole-breast irradiation after breast-conserving surgery for low-risk invasive and in-situ carcinoma of the female breast: 5-year results of a randomised, controlled, phase 3 trial. *Lancet Oncol.* 2017;18(2):259–268. doi:10.1016/S1470-2045(17)30011-6

90. Strnad V, Ott OJ, Hildebrandt G, et al. 5-year results of accelerated partial breast irradiation using sole interstitial multicatheter brachytherapy versus whole-breast irradiation with boost after breast-conserving surgery for low-risk invasive and in-situ carcinoma of the female breast: a randomised, phase 3, non-inferiority trial. *Lancet.* 2016;387(10015):229–238. doi:10.1016/S0140-6736(15)00471-7

91. Whelan TJ, Julian JA, Berrang TS, et al. External beam accelerated partial breast irradiation versus whole breast irradiation after breast conserving surgery in women with ductal carcinoma in situ and node-negative breast cancer (RAPID): a randomised controlled trial. *Lancet.* 2019;394(10215):2165–2172. doi:10.1016/S0140-6736(19)32515-2

92. Liss AL, Ben-David MA, Jagsi R, et al. Decline of cosmetic outcomes following accelerated partial breast irradiation using intensity modulated radiation therapy: results of a single-institution prospective clinical trial. *Int J Radiat Oncol Biol Phys.* 2014;89(1):96–102. doi:10.1016/j.ijrobp.2014.01.005

93. Hepel JT, Tokita M, MacAusland SG, et al. Toxicity of three-dimensional conformal radiotherapy for accelerated partial breast irradiation. *Int J Radiat Oncol Biol Phys.* 2009;75(5):1290–1296. doi:10.1016/j.ijrobp.2009.01.009

94. Chafe S, Moughan J, McCormick B, et al. Late toxicity and patient self-assessment of breast appearance/satisfaction on RTOG 0319: a phase 2 trial of 3-dimensional conformal radiation therapy-accelerated partial breast irradiation following lumpectomy for stages I and II breast cancer. *Int J Radiat Oncol Biol Phys.* 2013;86(5):854–859. doi:10.1016/j.ijrobp.2013.04.005

95. Meattini I, Marrazzo L, Saieva C, et al. Accelerated partial-breast irradiation compared with whole-breast irradiation for early breast cancer: long-term results of the randomized phase III APBI-IMRT-florence trial. *J Clin Oncol.* 2020;38(35):4175–4183. doi:10.1200/JCO.20.00650

96. Rodriguez N, Sanz X, Dengra J, et al. Five-year outcomes, cosmesis, and toxicity with 3-dimensional conformal external beam radiation therapy to deliver accelerated partial breast irradiation. *Int J Radiat Oncol Biol Phys.* 2013;87(5):1051–1057. doi:10.1016/j.ijrobp.2013.08.046

97. Coles CE, Griffin CL, Kirby AM, et al. Partial-breast radiotherapy after breast conservation surgery for patients with early breast cancer (UK IMPORT LOW trial): 5-year results from a multicentre, randomised, controlled, phase 3, non-inferiority trial. *Lancet.* 2017;390(10099):1048–1060. doi:10.1016/S0140-6736(17)31145-5

98. Polgar C, Major T, Fodor J, et al. Accelerated partial-breast irradiation using high-dose-rate interstitial brachytherapy: 12-year update of a prospective clinical study. *Radiother Oncol.* 2010;94(3):274–279. doi:10.1016/j.radonc.2010.01.019

99. Shah C, Antonucci JV, Wilkinson JB, et al. Twelve-year clinical outcomes and patterns of failure with accelerated partial breast irradiation versus whole-breast irradiation: results of a matched-pair analysis. *Radiother Oncol.* 2011;100(2):210–214. doi:10.1016/j.radonc.2011.03.011

100. Benitez PR, Keisch ME, Vicini F, et al. Five-year results: the initial clinical trial of MammoSite balloon brachytherapy for partial breast irradiation in early-stage breast cancer. *Am J Surg.* 2007;194(4):456–462. doi:10.1016/j.amjsurg.2007.06.010

101. Shah C, Badiyan S, Ben Wilkinson J, et al. Treatment efficacy with accelerated partial breast irradiation (APBI): final analysis of the American Society of Breast Surgeons MammoSite((R)) breast brachytherapy registry trial. *Ann Surg Oncol.* 2013;20(10):3279–3285. doi:10.1245/s10434-013-3158-4

102. Shah C, Khwaja S, Badiyan S, et al. Brachytherapy-based partial breast irradiation is associated with low rates of complications and excellent cosmesis. *Brachytherapy.* 2013;12(4):278–284. doi:10.1016/j.brachy.2013.04.005

103. Smith GL, Xu Y, Buchholz TA, et al. Association between treatment with brachytherapy vs whole-breast irradiation and subsequent mastectomy, complications, and survival among older women with invasive breast cancer. *JAMA.* 2012;307(17):1827–1837. doi:10.1001/jama.2012.3481

104. Presley CJ, Soulos PR, Herrin J, et al. Patterns of use and short-term complications of breast brachytherapy in the national medicare population from 2008-2009. *J Clin Oncol.* 2012;30(35):4302–4307. doi:10.1200/JCO.2012.43.5297

105. Cuttino LW, Arthur DW, Vicini F, et al. Long-term results from the Contura multilumen balloon breast brachytherapy catheter phase 4 registry trial. *Int J Radiat Oncol Biol Phys.* 2014;90(5):1025–1029. doi:10.1016/j.ijrobp.2014.08.341

106. Yashar C, Attai D, Butler E, et al. Strut-based accelerated partial breast irradiation: report of treatment results for 250 consecutive patients at 5 years from a multicenter retrospective study. *Brachytherapy.* 2016;15(6):780–787. doi:10.1016/j.brachy.2016.07.002

24 ■ LOCALLY ADVANCED BREAST CANCER

Christopher W. Fleming, Yvonne D. Pham, and Rahul D. Tendulkar

QUICK HIT ■ LABC is characterized by advanced tumor (T3 or T4) or nodal stage (N2 or N3), generally including clinical stage IIB (T3N0) to stage III. Patients are generally treated with neoadjuvant CHT, followed by surgery and adjuvant RT (Table 24.1). IBC represents an aggressive subset of LABC.

Table 24.1: General Treatment Paradigm	
NACT	Associated with high rates (up to 60%) of pCR and allows for cosmetically acceptable surgery, but has similar DFS and OS compared to adjuvant CHT. For HER2+ disease, add trastuzumab and pertuzumab to CHT. Response to neoadjuvant therapy may direct need for adjuvant treatment.
Surgery	Performed 3 to 6 weeks after completing NACT. Usually MRM w/ ALND, although LABC is not a contraindication to BCT.
RT	Initiated about 4 weeks following surgery (or CHT if given adjuvantly). Indications for PMRT are generally based on initial clinical stage as well as response to neoadjuvant CHT. PMRT is indicated for clinical or pathologic stage III (T3N1 or T4 or N2), and is controversial for stage II (T1-T2N1 or T3N0).

EPIDEMIOLOGY: Approximately one-quarter of new breast cancer diagnoses are locally advanced at presentation. From 2012 to 2016, the incidence of LABC declined by 0.8% per year, which may reflect a shift toward earlier stage at diagnosis.[1] LABC represents a heterogeneous class of tumors. Some cases present between routine screening mammograms and represent disease with a rapid growth rate. This is particularly true for IBC, which accounts for ~2% of all new breast malignancies.[2] LABC also includes patients with slow-growing, neglected tumors that have become extensive over time. There are no clear risk factors unique to patients presenting with advanced disease; however, young/premenopausal women are more likely to present with LABC.[3]

RISK FACTORS, ANATOMY, PATHOLOGY, GENETICS, SCREENING: See Chapter 23 for details.

CLINICAL PRESENTATION: Breast masses are typically found by self-breast exam, mammogram, or clinical exam, and are rarely painful (~5%). Lesions present late (T3/T4) usually as a result of lack of screening, delay due to patient neglect or misdiagnosis, or aggressive tumor biology. Other LABC signs may include axillary adenopathy, skin erythema, dimpling, nipple retraction, bloody discharge, or change in size or shape of the breast. IBC is a clinical diagnosis that requires erythema and dermal edema (peau d'orange) of ≥1/3 of the breast, which develops in ≤6 months and includes rapid enlargement of the breast, generalized induration in the presence or absence of a distinct breast mass, and a biopsy-proven carcinoma. The pathologic hallmark for IBC is tumor emboli within the dermal lymphatics (present in 50%–75% of cases), but this is neither sufficient nor required for diagnosis of IBC. Occult dermal lymphatic invasion w/o clinical signs of IBC is unusual (<2% of cases).[4] Patients with IBC are more frequently hormone receptor–negative and HER2+ than other breast cancers; most are LN positive and ~30% present with distant metastases.

WORKUP: H&P with attention to extent of disease, especially the extent of skin involvement if IBC (photo documentation); assess mobility/fixation of the tumor and LNs. As many patients will receive NACT, it is important to assess and document extent of disease prior to therapy.

Labs: CBC, CMP, alkaline phosphatase.

Imaging: Bilateral mammograms and ultrasound as necessary. For clinical stage IIIA and higher (T3N1, T4, or N2), CT chest/abdomen/pelvis and bone scan or PET/CT for identifying unsuspected regional nodal disease and/or distant metastases.[5] Additional imaging may include MRI brain if neurologic symptoms are present, and plain films of areas of increased uptake on bone scan.

Procedures: Core needle biopsy (full thickness of skin for IBC) rather than FNA for determination of ER/PR and HER2 status.

Other: Echocardiography to evaluate left ventricular ejection fraction prior to anthracycline CHT (Adriamycin contraindicated w/ LVEF <30% to 35%; cardiotoxicity seen after cumulative dose of 450–500 mg/m^2) and trastuzumab-containing regimens.[5]

PROGNOSTIC FACTORS: Adverse prognostic factors include LN involvement (most important), young age, smoking, presentation in pregnancy, palpable mass, extensive erythema, IBC, high grade, LVSI, positive margins, high Oncotype DX 21-gene Recurrence Score, ER-negative, incomplete response to NACT.

STAGING: See Chapter 23 for AJCC staging system.

TREATMENT PARADIGM

In general, CHT and RT are indicated for almost all LABC. CHT is commonly delivered neoadjuvantly, while RT is reserved for the adjuvant setting.

Chemotherapy: Node positivity is generally an indication for cytotoxic CHT. However, Oncotype DX 21-gene Recurrence Score has shown to be predictive of benefit of CHT for hormone-positive, HER2-negative patients, even for node-positive women, prompting some practitioners to withhold CHT for node-positive patients with low Oncotype scores.[6] RxPONDER and SWOG S1007 are ongoing trials evaluating the omission of CHT in this group. There is no difference in DFS or OS between NACT and adjuvant CHT,[7,8] but NACT may help make up-front inoperable disease more amenable to surgery, improve cosmetic outcomes following surgery, and direct adjuvant therapy based on response to neoadjuvant therapy. Patients diagnosed during pregnancy and unable to have surgery may also benefit from NACT. The choice of a specific NACT regimen should be based on tumor biology and the cancer subset type. Common regimens are detailed in Chapter 23. TNBC and HER2+ subtypes have the highest likelihood of pCR, generally 50% to 60%,[9,10] while ER-positive tumors have pCR rates closer to 15% to 25%.[11] Patients with pCR have significant improvements in DFS (HR 0.48) and OS (HR 0.48) compared to those with residual disease.[12,13] Patients without pCR to NACT may undergo additional adjuvant systemic therapy. The CREATE-X trial found OS benefit to 6 to 8 cycles adjuvant capecitabine in HER2-negative breast cancer without pCR to NACT.[14] Similarly, the KATHERINE trial found adjuvant T-DM1 improved invasive DFS for HER2+ breast cancer with residual disease.[15]

Surgery: Prior to NACT, evaluation of the tumor and lymph nodes should be performed. Radio-opaque clips should be placed in the tumor to aid in planning of locoregional treatment and subsequent pathologic assessment (facilitates locoregional treatment should a CR to CHT occur). Tumor size should be documented for staging (using ultrasound or breast MRI). For suspicion of an involved axilla, perform FNA and/or core needle biopsy with placement of a radio-opaque clip in the suspicious lymph node. If the axilla is clinically benign, can consider pre-NACT SLNB (institutional preference) or wait until the time of surgery; if negative, no further evaluation.

Surgery is typically performed 3 to 6 weeks after completing NACT and usually consists of MRM w/ ALND. ALND involves levels I and II axillary dissections; level III may be dissected if disease is apparent in level I or II. LABC is not a contraindication to BCT but must be undertaken with caution; at least one trial found that after NACT, IBTR was higher in patients who required downstaging to be eligible for BCT.[16] For the initially clinically node-negative axilla, a negative SLNB is generally sufficient.[17] Clinically N1 women with CR to NACT may be considered for SLNB alone to avoid ALND, assuming SLNB shows no residual nodal disease.[18] If SLNB is positive after NACT, ALND should be performed.

Radiation

Indications: Indications for PMRT generally include clinical stage III (regardless of response to NACT), residual LN-positive after NACT, or pathologic stage III, but is controversial for T3N0 or T1–2N1 patients.[19] PMRT generally includes RT of the chest wall, as well as comprehensive nodal RT to the axilla, supraclavicular lymph nodes, and internal mammary (IM) nodes. Historical indications for treating the full axilla with a PAB are based on historical risk factors for subsequent axillary recurrence: gross extranodal extension, ≥10 +LNs, >50% +LN nodal ratio, or undissected axilla. IM nodal RT has been controversial over the rarity of documented IM nodal failures and concerns about cardiotoxicity, but was performed in all the classic PMRT trials. Indications for IM nodal RT may include clinically positive IM nodes, central/medial tumor location, or axillary LN-positive disease. RT usually initiated 4 to 6 weeks following surgery or CHT (whichever is last) provided adequate healing has taken place. In the KATHERINE trial, patients receiving adjuvant T-DM1 received concurrent RT, while CREATE-X allowed for RT delivered either before or after capecitabine. Both allowed concurrent use of endocrine therapy with RT.

Dose: Conventional dose to chest wall and regional lymph nodes is 50 Gy/25 fx; however, a Chinese randomized trial found noninferiority of hypofractionated PMRT (43.5 Gy/15 fx) in patients without breast reconstruction.[20] The ongoing Alliance A221505: RT CHARM trial is evaluating the tolerability of hypofractionated PMRT in the reconstruction setting. There is insufficient evidence per PMRT guidelines to recommend a total dose, fraction size, use of scar boosts or bolus.[21] If margins are close or positive, consider boost to 60 Gy (conventional fractionation) and boost gross residual (unresectable) disease to ≥66 Gy. For IBC, treat with trimodality including NACT, mastectomy, and PMRT (regardless of response to NACT).

Procedure: See *Handbook of Treatment Planning in Radiation Oncology*, Chapter 5.[22]

■ EVIDENCE-BASED Q&A

■ What are the classic data on recurrence patterns after mastectomy and adjuvant CHT?

Fowble, ECOG Pooled Analysis (*JCO* 1988, PMID 3292711): RR of 627 women treated on ECOG adjuvant CHT trials from 1978 to 1982 without RT. Pre- and postmenopausal patients undergoing mastectomy included. Eligibility criteria: age <66, primary tumor confined to breast and ipsilateral axilla w/o fixation, arm edema, inflammatory changes, ulceration, satellite skin nodules, peau d'orange >1/3 of the breast, or skin infiltration >2 cm. All patients had positive LNs. MFU 4.5 years. On MVA, the following factors were significant for LRR within 3 years: tumor size >5 cm, ≥4 LN+, ER-negative, tumor necrosis, and pectoral fascia involvement (Table 24.2). **Conclusion: Consider PMRT for LN+ patients with high-risk features.**

Table 24.2: Factors Associated With LRR in ECOG Trials									
	LRR	*p Value*		LRR	*p Value*			LRR	*p Value*
Tumor Size		.004	ER status		.02	Pectoral fascia involvement			.007
≤2 cm	9%		Positive	8%					
2–5 cm	9%								
>5 cm	19%		Negative	14%		Absent		10%	
LNs		.006	Tumor necrosis		.002	Present		29%	
1–3+	7%		Absent	8%					
4–7+	15%		Present	17%					
≥8+	15%								

Taghian, NSABP Pooled Analysis (*JCO* 2004, PMID 15452182): Pooled analysis from multiple NSABP trials (B-15, B-16, B-18, B-22, and B-25) of LN+ patients treated with mastectomy and adjuvant CHT (90% received doxorubicin-based CHT) ± tamoxifen and without PMRT. At 10 years, 12.2% had isolated LRF, 19.8% had LRF with or without DF, and 43.3% had DF alone as a first event. LRF (± DF) as a first event was 13% for 1 to 3 +LN, 24.4% for 4 to 9 +LN, and 31.9% for ≥10 +LN ($p < .0001$). LRF was 14.9% for tumors ≤2 cm, 21.3% for 2.1 to 5 cm, and 24.6% for >5 cm ($p < .0001$). The majority of recurrences occurred in the chest wall and around the mastectomy scar (56.9%), followed by supra-clavicular LN (22.6% of all LRF) and axillary LN (11.7%). Parasternal and subclavicular failures were <1% of the total LRF. Age, tumor size, premenopausal status, number of +LN, and number of dissected LN were significant predictors on MVA for LRF as first event. **Conclusion: LRF as first event is high for patients with large tumors and ≥4 positive LNs, and therefore, recommend PMRT to those groups. Axillary LN status is the most important predictor for LRR, of which the majority occur in the chest wall.**

■ **What is the benefit of RT after mastectomy?**

At least three randomized trials have demonstrated a survival benefit to PMRT for high-risk patients, particularly those with LN+ disease. In the modern era, the risk of LRR in pT1–2N1 patients without PMRT is less (<10%) compared to historical series (20%–30%), and so this remains a controversial subgroup.

Ragaz, British Columbia (*NEJM* 1997, PMID 9309100; Update *JNCI* 2005, PMID 15657341): PRT of 318 premenopausal women with stages I–II breast cancer, enrolled if pathologically node-positive after MRM + ALND (levels I and II) comparing adjuvant CHT with CMF + PMRT vs. CMF alone. Median 11 LNs removed. CMF given for 6 to 12 months. PMRT delivered between the 4th and 5th cycles of CHT. Chest wall was treated to 37.5 Gy/16 fx w/ opposed tangents and midaxilla received 35 Gy/16 fx through an AP SCV field and PAB. A direct IM field treating both IM chains received 37.5 Gy/16 fx. All fields treated w/ Co-60. MFU 150 months. **Conclusion: PMRT improves long-term LRC, DFS, and OS (Table 24.3).**

Table 24.3: Results of British Columbia PMRT Trial						
	15-Yr LRC	15-Yr DFS	15-Yr OS	20-Yr LRC	20-Yr DFS	20-Yr OS
CMF + PMRT	87%	50%	54%	90%	48%	47%
CMF alone	67%	33%	46%	74%	30%	37%
p value	.003	.007	.07	.002	.001	.03

Overgaard, Danish Breast Cancer Cooperative Group 82b (*NEJM* 1997, PMID 9395428): PRT of 1,708 premenopausal high-risk women who had TM w/ ALND for stage II or III breast cancer, comparing adjuvant CHT with CMF + PMRT vs. CMF alone. "High risk" defined as +axillary LNs, tumor >5 cm, and/or invasion of the skin or pectoral fascia. Premenopausal defined as amenorrhea for <5 years or hysterectomy before the age of 55. Median 7 LNs removed. CHT consisted of 8 cycles of CMF in patients receiving RT and 9 cycles in those treated w/ CHT alone. RT given after 1st cycle of CHT. CHT then resumed 1 to 2 weeks after RT. RT delivered in five-field arrangement to a median dose of 50 Gy/25 fx in 35 days or 48 Gy/22 fx in 38 days to axilla, SCV, ICV, chest wall, and IM nodes (upper four intercostal spaces). Posterior axillary fields recommended if AP diameter too large to limit maximum dose to 55 Gy/25 fx or 52.8 Gy/22 fx. Most were treated w/ linac. MFU 114 months. **Conclusion: Statistically significant survival benefit with PMRT for all T stages, N stages (even N0), and histopathologic grades (Table 24.4).** *Comment: Median of 7 LNs dissected was low for this era, likely understaging many patients.*

Table 24.4: Results of Danish 82b PMRT Trial			
	10-Yr LRC	10-Yr DFS	10-Yr OS
CMF + RT	91%	48%	54%
CMF alone	68%	34%	45%
p value	<.001	<.001	<.001

Overgaard, Danish Breast Cancer Cooperative Group 82c (*Lancet* 1999, PMID 10335782): PRT of 1,375 postmenopausal high-risk women <70 years s/p TM w/ ALND for stage II or III breast cancer randomized to PMRT + tamoxifen vs. tamoxifen alone vs. CMF + tamoxifen (arm not reported). "High risk" defined as in 82b trial. Postmenopausal defined as ≥5 years of amenorrhea, or hysterectomy after the age of 55; 58% of patients had 1 to 3 LN+. All patients received tamoxifen 30 mg/day for 1 year. Median 7 LNs removed. PMRT same as 82b. All but 69 patients were treated with linacs. MFU 123 months. **Conclusion: The addition of PMRT to adjuvant tamoxifen reduces LRR and prolongs OS in high-risk postmenopausal women with breast cancer (Table 24.5).** *Comment: Only 1 year of tamoxifen is insufficient systemic therapy.*

Table 24.5: Results of Danish 82b PMRT Trial					
	LRR as First Site of Recurrence	DM First Recurrence	10-Yr DFS	5-Yr OS	10-Yr OS
Tam + PMRT	8%	39%	36%	63%	45%
Tam alone	35%	25%	24%	62%	36%
p value	<.001		<.001		.03

Overgaard, 82b and 82c Combined Analysis (*Radiother Oncol* 2007, PMID 17306393): Because many women on 82b and 82c had limited ALNDs, a subgroup analysis was done for 1,152 patients with ≥8 LNs removed, which showed that PMRT significantly improved LRC and OS in all LN+ patients, with the magnitude of improvement similar in 1 to 3 vs. ≥4 LN+ patients (Table 24.6). Overall, this indicated that PMRT is beneficial and unrelated to the absolute number of positive LNs.

Table 24.6: Combined 82b and 82c Analysis in Patients With ≥8 LNs Removed					
	15-Yr OS All Patients	15-Yr LRF 1 to 3 LN+	15-Yr OS 1 to 3 LN+	15-Yr LRF 4+ LN+	15-Yr OS 4+ LN+
No PMRT	29%	27%	48%	51%	12%
PMRT	39%	4%	57%	10%	21%
p value	.015	<.001	.03	<.001	.03

Clarke, EBCTCG Meta-Analysis (*Lancet* 2005, PMID 16360786; Update *Lancet* 2014, PMID 24656685): Meta-analysis of individual data for 8,135 women in 22 RCTs from 1964 to 1986 who underwent mastectomy and ALND ± PMRT; 3,786 women had ALND of levels I and II; median of 10 LNs removed. All patients enrolled into trials in which RT included the chest wall, SCV or axilla fossa (or both), and IM chain. For 3,131 pN+ patients, PMRT improved 10-year risk of LRR and AR as well as 20-year risk of BCM. There was no benefit to PMRT for patients who were node negative (Table 24.7). For 1,772 women with ≥4 LN+, PMRT significantly improved outcomes. For subset of 1,314 patients with 1 to 3 LN+, PMRT significantly reduced LRR, AR, and BCM (Table 24.8).

Table 24.7: Early Breast Cancer Trialists' Collaborative Group Meta-Analysis (2014 Update)			
	10-Yr LRR	10-Yr Any Recurrence	20-Yr BCM
pN0 (700)			
RT	3.0%	22.4%	28.8%
No RT	1.6%	21.1%	26.6%
p value	p > .1	RR 1.06, p > .1	RR 1.18, p > .1
pN+ (3,131)			

(continued)

Table 24.7: Early Breast Cancer Trialists' Collaborative Group Meta-Analysis (2014 Update) (continued)			
	10-Yr LRR	10-Yr AR	20-Yr BCM
RT	8.1%	51.9%	58.3%
No RT	26.0%	62.5%	66.4%
p value	p < .00001	p < .00001	p = .001
pN1 (1314)			
RT	3.8%	34.2%	42.3%
No RT	20.3%	45.7%	50.2%
p value	p < .00001	p = .00006	p = .01
pN2–3 (1772)			
RT	13.0%	66.3%	70.7%
No RT	32.1%	75.1%	80.0%
p value	p < .00001	p = .0003	p = .04

Table 24.8: EBCTCG Subset of 1,133 Patients With 1 to 3 LN+ Who Received Systemic Therapy			
pN1 (1,133)	10-Yr LRR	10-Yr AR	20-Yr BCM
RT	4.3%	33.8%	41.5%
No RT	21.0%	45.5%	49.4%
p value	p = .00001	p = .00009	p = .01

■ **Are T3N0 tumors at high risk for recurrence?**

The utility of PMRT for pT3N0 patients is controversial. At least two large RRs show low LF rates <10% for mastectomy + systemic therapy alone for pT3N0. Conversely, a 2014 SEER analysis and single-institution data suggest a benefit with PMRT for pT3N0 patients. Notably, cT3N0 are often understaged in terms of nodal involvement, and thus have a different prognosis than pT3N0.

Taghian, NSABP Pooled Analysis (*JCO* 2006, PMID 16921044): RR of 313 patients from 5 NSABP PRTs (B-13, B-14, B-19, B-20, B-23) for pT3N0 breast cancers treated with mastectomy without PMRT. MFU 15 years; 34% received adjuvant CHT, 21% adjuvant tamoxifen, 19% both, and 26% no systemic tx; 28 patients experienced LRF. Only 7% of patients with tumors = 5 cm and 7.2% of patients with >5 cm had LRF. The overall 10-year cumulative incidences of isolated LRF, LRF with and w/o DM, and DF alone at first event were 7.1%, 10.0%, and 23.6%, respectively; 24 of 28 failures occurred on chest wall. Patients with >10 LNs removed had 7.3% LRF vs. 1–5 LNs removed had 16.7% LRF (p = .21). For patients who underwent no systemic treatment, CHT alone, tamoxifen alone, or CHT plus tamoxifen, the LRF incidences were 12.6%, 5.6%, 4.6%, and 5.3%, respectively (p = .2). **Conclusion: Patients who are pT3N0, treated by mastectomy w/ adjuvant systemic therapy and no PMRT have low rates of LRF. PMRT is not routinely indicated for these patients.**

Johnson, SEER Analysis (*Cancer* 2014, PMID 24985911): RR of 2,525 T3N0 patients from 2000 to 2010 who underwent MRM, 1,063 received PMRT. On UVA at 8 years, PMRT was associated with improved OS (76.5% vs. 61.8%, p < .01) and CSS (85.0% vs. 82.4%, p < .01). Use of PMRT remained significant on MVA for OS (HR: 0.63, p < .001) and CSS (HR: 0.77, p = .045). **Conclusion: PMRT should be considered in T3N0M0 patients, and is associated with improvement in OS and CSS, although selection bias remains a potential confounder.**

Jagsi, MGH (*IJROBP* 2005, PMID 15990006): RR of 877 pN0 patients who received mastectomy alone. 10-year LRR 6.0%. Negative prognostic factors included (a) size >2 cm, (b) margin <2 mm, (c) premenopausal status, and (d) LVI; 10-year LRR was 1.2% with 0 risk factors, 10.0% with 1 risk factor, 17.9% with 2 risk factors, and 40.6% for those with 3 risk factors. Chest wall was the site of failure in

80% of patients. **Conclusion: Node-negative patients with multiple adverse risk factors may benefit from PMRT.**

Nagar, MDACC (*IJROBP* 2011, PMID 21885207): RR of 162 patients with cT3N0 who received NACT and underwent mastectomy. Median number of LNs dissected was 15; 45% of patients were ypN+ after NACT; 119 patients (73%) received PMRT and 43 patients did not. MFU 75 months. For all patients, 5-year LRR rate was 9%; 5-year LRR rate after PMRT was 4% vs. 24% for those who did not receive PMRT ($p < .001$). CW was most common site of LR, then axilla and SCV (equally). A significantly higher proportion of irradiated patients had ypLN+ and were ≤40 years of age. **Conclusion: Consider PMRT for patients with cT3N0 as LRR risk remains high without PMRT.** *Comment: Clinical understaging of axillary lymph nodes is common, as 45% of cT3N0 patients were found to have residual ypN+ disease even after NACT.*

■ What is the role of PMRT for patients with a TNBC molecular subtype?

Women with TNBC have an aggressive clinical course (early relapse, higher incidence of visceral and brain metastases, and relatively poor prognosis compared to other subtypes), so some consider PMRT in these patients even with earlier stage disease.

Wang, China (*Radiother Oncol* 2011, PMID 21852010): Multicenter PRT of 681 women with TNBC stage I–II (82% LN-negative) s/p mastectomy, randomized to CHT ± PMRT (50 Gy/25 fx +/– RNI as clinically indicated). At an MFU 7.2 years, PMRT improved 5-year RFS (74.6%–88.3%, $p = .02$) and 5-year OS (78.7% vs. 90.4%, $p = .03$). **Conclusion: Adjuvant CHT plus RT was more effective than CHT alone in women with triple-negative early-stage breast cancer after mastectomy.** *Comment: Independent confirmation would be valuable to confirm the role of PMRT in LN-negative TNBC.*

■ What is the preferred sequencing of CHT, neoadjuvant or adjuvant?

There is no difference in DFS or OS between neoadjuvant or adjuvant CHT. NACT is associated with high rates of pathologic response and a higher likelihood for allowing a cosmetically acceptable surgery. With NACT, there is downstaging of the tumor and involved axillary LNs with an increased opportunity for BCT.

Fisher, NSABP B-18 (*JCO* 1997, PMID 9215816; Update *JCO* 1998, PMID 9704717; Wolmark *J Natl Cancer Inst Monogr* 2001, PMID 11773300; Rastogi *JCO* 2008, PMID 18258986): PRT of 1,523 patients with operable breast cancer (T1–3N0–1M0) randomized to pre-op AC × 4 vs. post-op AC × 4. CHT was q21 days, doxorubicin 60 mg/m^2, and cyclophosphamide 600 mg/m^2. Tamoxifen (10 mg BID × 5 years) was given to all patients ≥50 y/o regardless of ER status (status unknown for many patients). All patients who had a lumpectomy received RT to 50 Gy. Breast tumor size decreased by ≥50% in 80% of patients. Patients in preoperative AC group had 36% cCR, 43% cPR, and 13% pCR. Patients with pCR had significantly improved DFS (HR: 0.47, $p < .0001$) and OS (HR: 0.32, $p < .0001$) vs. patients who did not have a pCR. MVA showed that posttreatment pathologic nodal status was also a strong predictor of OS and DFS ($p < .0001$). IBTR was greater in the pre-op group who had BCT due to downstaging vs. patients who were planned to have BCT (14.5% vs. 6.9%, $p = .04$).[18] **Conclusion: Preoperative CHT is equivalent to adjuvant CHT in regard to OS and DFS (Table 24.9).**

Table 24.9: NSABP B-18 Results (16-Yr Data)					
	pN+	BCS Rate	IBTR	DFS	OS
Pre-op CHT	42%	68%	13%	42%	55%
Post-op CHT	58%	60%	10%	39%	55%
p value	.001	.001	.21	.27	.90

Van Der Hage, EORTC 10902 (*JCO* 2001, PMID 11709566; Update Van Nes, *Breast Cancer Res Treat* 2009, PMID 18484198): PRT of 698 patients with operable breast cancer (T1c-3,T4b, N0–1M0) comparing pre-op FEC (5-FU, epirubicin, cyclophosphamide) × 4 vs. post-op FEC. All patients who had BCT received RT to 50 Gy to breast and 45 Gy to IM nodes and SCV. Tamoxifen 20 mg QD given to all patients ≥50 regardless of ER status. Tumors were assessed by clinical and mammographic evaluation. MFU 10 years. No difference in OS, DFS, or LRR between groups. NACT improves the rate of BCT compared to adjuvant CHT (35% vs. 22%, respectively). Patients who received BCT due to tumor downsizing did not have an increase in LRR or worse OS compared to patients who had BCT without downsizing of the tumor. **Conclusion: NACT does not lead to a detriment in OS or DFS compared to adjuvant CHT.**

- **Which patients are at increased risk for LRR after NACT alone (and therefore should consider additional therapy)?**

Mamounas, Combined NSABP B-18 and B-27 (*JCO* 2012, PMID 23032615): Combined analysis of NSABP B-18 and B-27, included 3,088 patients with cT1–3, N0–N1 patients. NACT was either AC alone or AC followed by neoadjuvant/adjuvant docetaxel. Lumpectomy patients received breast RT alone while mastectomy patients did not undergo PMRT. The 10-year cumulative LRR rate in mastectomy patients was 12.3% (8.9% local; 3.4% regional); predictors of LRR on MVA included clinical tumor size >5 cm (before NACT), clinical N+ (before NACT), and incomplete pathologic response in the breast or axillary LNs. For lumpectomy patients, the LRR was 10.3% (8.1% local; 2.2% regional); predictors of LRR included age <50, clinical N+ (before NACT), and incomplete pathologic response in the breast or axillary LNs. **Conclusion: The 10-year risk of LRR is significant after NACT (>10%). Tumor size >5 cm, positive axillary lymph nodes, younger age, and incomplete response to NACT portend a higher risk of LRR.**

- **In those groups with an increased risk for LRR after NACT, which studies show a benefit to adding RT?**

Huang, MDACC (*JCO* 2004, PMID 15570071): RR of 542 patients treated on 6 consecutive prospective trials with NACT followed by mastectomy and PMRT compared to 134 patients on same trials who did not receive PMRT. PMRT reduced 10-year LRR from 22% to 11%, $p = .0001$. On MVA, PMRT improved 10-year LRR in the following groups: cT3–4, clinical stage IIB or higher, pT2–4, and pN2–3. For patients with pCR to NACT, PMRT improved LRR for clinical stage III or higher (33% vs. 3%, $p = .006$). PMRT improved CSS in the following groups: cT4, pN2–3, clinical stage IIIB or higher. **Conclusion: PMRT improves LRC and CSS in high-risk groups after NACT.**

Krug, Meta-Analysis of Gepar Trials (*Ann Surg Oncol* 2019): Pooled analysis of the randomized NACT trials GeparTrio, GeparQuattro, and GeparQuinto; included 817 patients who underwent mastectomy after NACT; 83% received RT; 5-year cumulative incidence of LRR was 15.2% (95% CI: 9.0%–22.8%) in patients treated without RT and 11.3% in patients treated with RT (95% CI: 8.7%–14.3%). On MVA, RT was associated with a lower risk of LRR (HR: 0.51, $p = .05$). This effect was shown especially in patients with cT3–4 tumors, as well as in patients who were cN+ before neoadjuvant therapy, including those with pCR. **Conclusion: RT reduces LRR rates in breast cancer patients who undergo mastectomy after NACT, including high-risk patients with pCR to NACT.**

- **What are the current indications for PMRT?**

Recht, ASCO/ASTRO/SSO Guidelines (*JCO* 2016, 27646947): PMRT for patients with T1–2N1 reduces LRF, AR, and BCM, but PMRT should be used only if expected benefits outweigh potential toxicity risks. PMRT indicated for patients who are ypN+ (any T) after NACT. For patients who are cN0 before NACT or have a complete pathologic response in the axilla, there is insufficient evidence to recommend for or against PMRT, and it is recommended to enroll these patients into clinical trials (such as NSABP B-51). When PMRT is used, it should routinely include the chest wall/reconstructed breast, supraclavicular–axillary apical nodes, and internal mammary nodes, although there are subgroups that may not derive benefit from treating all nodal regions.

- **For patients with incomplete response to NACT, is there benefit to further systemic therapy?**

Masuda, CREATE-X (*NEJM* 2017, PMID 28564564): PRT of 910 patients with HER2-negative breast cancer with residual disease after NACT randomized to standard adjuvant therapy with or without capecitabine, 1,250 mg/m^2 BID on days 1 to 14 every 3 weeks for 6 to 8 cycles. RT was delivered as needed, either before or after capecitabine; 68% hormone positive, 32% TNBC. Capecitabine improved 5-year DFS (74.1% vs. 67.6%, $p = .01$) and 5-year OS (89.2% vs. 83.6%, $p = .01$). For TNBC patients, DFS 69.8% vs. 56.1% (HR: 0.58, 95% CI: 0.39–0.87) and OS 78.8% vs. 70.3% (HR: 0.52, 95% CI:

0.30–0.90). For hormone-positive patients, DFS 76.4% vs. 73.4% (HR: 0.81, 95% CI: 0.55–1.17) and OS 93.4% vs. 90.0% (HR: 0.73, 95% CI: 0.38–1.40). **Conclusion: Adjuvant capecitabine prolongs DFS and OS in HER2-negative patients with residual disease after NACT.**

Von Minckwitz, KATHERINE (*NEJM* 2019, PMID 30516102): PRT of 1,486 HER2+ patients with residual disease after NACT containing a taxane and trastuzumab, randomized to adjuvant T-DM1 or trastuzumab for 14 cycles. If indicated, PMRT was delivered concurrently. T-DM1 improved 3-year DFS (88.3% vs. 77.0%, *p* < .001). **Conclusion: Adjuvant T-DM1 prolongs DFS in HER2+ patients with residual disease after NACT.**

■ Can hypofractionated RT be delivered to the chest wall and regional nodes?

Though Ragaz's British Columbia randomized study evaluating the role of PMRT utilized a hypofractionated regimen (37.5 Gy in 16 fractions), the majority of PMRT studies have used regimens of either 1.8 or 2 Gy per day. A study from the Chinese Academy of Medical Sciences evaluated the efficacy and tolerance of hypofractionated RT in the modern era; none of these patients had reconstruction. Additionally, long-term toxicity results from the minority of patients (~15%) on the START A/B trials who received hypofractionated lymph node irradiation were reported in 2017.

Wang, China (*Lancet Oncol* 2019, PMID 30711522): Noninferiority trial comparing 50 Gy/25 fx to 43.5 Gy/15 fx (all 2D planning) in pT3–4 or pN2+ patients s/p mastectomy. RT delivered to chest wall and regional nodes. Results: 820 patients enrolled between 2008 and 2016. For both arms, 5-year LRR was 8%. No significant difference in acute and late toxicities other than fewer patients in the hypofractionated group experienced grade 3 acute skin toxicity (3% vs. 8%, *p* < .0001). **Conclusion: Hypofractionated PMRT was noninferior to conventional PMRT in both efficacy and toxicity.**

Haviland, START A/B Late Effects (*Radiother Oncol* 2017, PMID 29153463): 14.7% of the patients enrolled in the START trials received comprehensive chest wall and nodal RT. With 10 years of follow-up, no significant differences between the hypofractionated and conventionally fractionated arms. **Conclusion: Hypofractionated RNI is safe.**

■ How does PMRT impact implant-related complications?

PMRT increases complication rates after breast reconstruction. Though the previously mentioned trials support the safety of hypofractionated PMRT, it is unknown if hypofractionation remains safe for reconstructed patients. This question is being tested in the Alliance A221505: RT CHARM trial.

Naoum, Harvard (*IJROBP* 2019, PMID 31756414): RR of 1,286 patients who underwent 1,814 breast reconstructions with or without PMRT. Evaluated rates of reconstruction complications in those who underwent TE/I, SSPI, and autologous tissue reconstructions; 5-year cumulative incidence of any reconstruction complications with and without PMRT: autologous 15.1% vs. 11.1%, SSPI 18.2% vs. 12.6%, TE/I 36.8% vs. 19.5%. **Conclusion: Complication rates after TE/I are high with PMRT. SSPI and autologous reconstructions have significantly lower complications rates than TE/I.**

■ Should the SCV and/or IM nodes be included in the radiation field?

IMNs were included in the three randomized PMRT trials (British Columbia, DBCCG 82b/82c), although isolated recurrence in the IMN is low (~1% or less). The incidence of IMN involvement in extended radical mastectomy series was based on the location and size of the primary tumor along with the extent of axillary involvement. Hennequin et al. showed no OS benefit (though underpowered), while a Danish prospective nonrandomized cohort study suggested an OS benefit. The EORTC 22922 trial demonstrated a DFS benefit to including IMN-SCV fields over omitting them, although it remains unclear whether the benefit was achieved by inclusion of the IMN or SCV fields (or both).

Hennequin, French Trial (*IJROBP* 2013, PMID 23664327): PRT of 1,334 patients w/ axillary LN+ or central/medial tumors (irrespective of axillary involvement). All patients underwent MRM with ALND of levels I and II. No IMN dissection allowed. PMRT delivered to chest wall + SCV. For pN+ cases, levels I + II covered, mainly 50 Gy/25 fx. Randomized between ± IMNI (included first 5 intercostal spaces) to a dose of 45 Gy/18 fx (2.5 Gy/fx) using mixed photon and electron fields. MFU 11.3 years; 10-year OS 59.3% without IMNI vs. 62.6% with IMNI (*p* = .8). IMNI did not significantly improve OS for any subgroup. **Conclusion: No benefit to IMNI.** *Comment: Included node-negative patients (25%) who have lower risk for IMN involvement; used 2D planning, which may have underestimated the coverage of IMNs; study was powered for a 10% survival benefit, which is likely optimistic given that the British Columbia/Danish trials of PMRT vs. no RT showed a ~10% OS benefit.*

Poortmans, EORTC 22922–10925 (*NEJM* 2015, PMID 26200978, Update *Lancet Oncol* 2020, PMID 33152277): PRT of 4,004 patients with axillary LN+ and/or a medially located primary tumor (irrespective of axillary involvement), randomized between ± IM and medial SCV irradiation (IM-MS); 7.4% of control vs. 8.3% in IM-MS group received axillary RT. BCT in 76%; mastectomy in 24%. After mastectomy, chest wall RT was given to 73% in both arms; 44% were node negative. Updated MFU 15.7 years, any breast cancer recurrence and BCM were reduced with IM-MS RT, though OS, DFS, and DMFS were not. **Conclusion: IM-MS RT significantly reduced BCM and any breast cancer recurrence (Table 24.10). However, an OS difference was not statistically significant.**

Table 24.10: EORTC 22922 Results						
15-Yr Results	DFS	Any Breast Recurrence	BCM	OS	Pulmonary Fibrosis	Cardiac Disease
Surgery + IM-MS RT	60.8%	24.5%	16.0%	73.1%	4.4%	6.5%
Surgery	59.9%	27.1%	19.8%	70.9%	1.7%	5.6%
p value	*p* = .18	*p* = .024	*p* = .0055	*p* = .36	NR	NR

Whelan, MA.20/NCIC-CTG (*NEJM* 2015, PMID 26200977): PRT of 1,832 patients who underwent BCT and SLNB or ALND found to be pN+ or pN0 with high-risk features (tumor ≥5 cm, or tumor ≥2 cm with <10 ALNs removed and at least one of the following: grade 3, ER–, LVSI). All patients received adjuvant systemic therapy with CHT, endocrine therapy, or both. Exclusion: T4, cN2–3, M1. Patients randomized to WBI only (50 Gy/25 fx +/– boost) ± RNI. RNI included IM nodes in first three intercostal spaces + SCV + axilla (covered levels I + II if <10 axillary nodes removed or >3 LN+) with optional PAB. Primary end point was OS. MFU 9.5 years; 85% had 1 to 3 positive LNs, 5% had ≥4 positive LNs, and 10% were LN–. Absolute magnitude of benefit is variable across the population and suggests need for risk-stratified approach to these patients (Table 24.11). In subgroup of ER-negative patients, DFS was significantly improved with RNI (82% vs. 71%, *p* = .04) and OS approached significance (81.3% vs. 73.9%, HR: 0.69, 95% CI: 0.47–1.00, *p* = .05). **Conclusion: RNI improved DFS, locoregional DFS, and distant DFS in high-risk patients after BCT, but no OS benefit was observed.**

Table 24.11: NCIC MA.20 Results							
10-Yr Results	DFS	Locoregional DFS	Distant DFS	BCM	OS	Pneumonitis	Lymphedema
BCS + CHT + WBI + RNI	82%	95.2%	86.3%	10.3%	82.8%	1.2%	8.4%
BCS + CHT + WBI	77%	92.2%	82.4%	12.3%	81.8%	0.2%	4.5%
p value	*p* = .01	*p* = .009	*p* = .03	*p* = .11	*p* = .38	*p* < .001	*p* < .001

Thorsen, DBCG-IMN (*JCO* 2015, PMID 26598752): Prospective population-based cohort study of 3,089 patients with unilateral LN+ breast cancer underwent mastectomy or BCS with ALND (levels I–II). Included pT1–T3 and pN1–3. Patients with right-sided disease received IMNI while left-sided disease did not receive IMNI (due to concerns of RT-induced heart disease). RT to breast/chest wall, scar, SCV, infraclavicular (level III), and axillary levels I–II to 48 Gy/24 fx. IMNI in right-sided cancer included intercostal spaces 1 to 4 treated with anterior electron field or included in tangential photon fields. Primary end point was OS. MFU 8.9 years; 3% OS benefit with IMNI (75.9% vs. 72.2%, *p* = .005); 3% of right-sided did not receive IMNI, while 10% of left-sided received IMNI. Equal number of cardiac deaths in two groups. Subgroup analysis showed lateral tumors with ≥4 LNs had OS benefit with IMNI (HR: 0.71, 95% CI: 0.57–0.89). **Conclusion: IMNI may improve OS in LN+ breast cancer.** *Comment: Not a randomized trial and excluded patients unfit for standard RT, which may potentially lead to overestimation of IMNI effect.*

Table 24.12: DBCG-IMN Results

DBCG-IMN 8-Yr Results	OS	BCM	DM
With IMNI	75.9%	20.9%	27.4%
Without IMNI	72.2%	23.4%	29.7%
p value	*p* = .005	*p* = .03	*p* = .07

REFERENCES

1. American Cancer Society. *Breast cancer facts & figures 2019–2020.* American Cancer Society, Inc; 2019.

2. Levine PH, Steinhorn SC, Ries LG, Aron JL. Inflammatory breast cancer: the experience of the surveillance, epidemiology, and end results (SEER) program. *J Natl Cancer Inst.* 1985;74(2):291–297.

3. Li CI, Malone KE, Daling JR. Differences in breast cancer hormone receptor status and histology by race and ethnicity among women 50 years of age and older. *Cancer Epidemiol Biomarkers Prev.* 2002;11(7):601–607.

4. Gruber G, Ciriolo M, Altermatt HJ, et al. Prognosis of dermal lymphatic invasion with or without clinical signs of inflammatory breast cancer. *Int J Cancer.* 2004;109(1):144–148. doi:10.1002/ijc.11684

5. Fisher B, Anderson S, Bryant J, et al. Twenty-year follow-up of a randomized trial comparing total mastectomy, lumpectomy, and lumpectomy plus irradiation for the treatment of invasive breast cancer. *N Eng J Med.* 2002;347:1233–1241. doi:10.1056/NEJMoa022152

6. Mamounas EP, Russell CA, Lau A, et al. Clinical relevance of the 21-gene Recurrence Score((R)) assay in treatment decisions for patients with node-positive breast cancer in the genomic era. *NPJ Breast Cancer.* 2018;4:27. doi:10.1038/s41523-018-0082-6

7. Fisher B, Brown A, Mamounas E, et al. Effect of preoperative chemotherapy on local-regional disease in women with operable breast cancer: findings from National Surgical Adjuvant Breast and Bowel Project B-18. *J Clin Oncol.* 1997;15(7):2483–2493. doi:10.1200/JCO.1997.15.7.2483

8. van der Hage JA, van de Velde CJ, Julien JP, et al. Preoperative chemotherapy in primary operable breast cancer: results from the European Organization for Research and Treatment of Cancer trial 10902. *J Clin Oncol.* 2001;19(22):4224–4237. doi:10.1200/JCO.2001.19.22.4224

9. Gianni L, Pienkowski T, Im YH, et al. Efficacy and safety of neoadjuvant pertuzumab and trastuzumab in women with locally advanced, inflammatory, or early HER2-positive breast cancer (NeoSphere): a randomised multicentre, open-label, phase 2 trial. *Lancet Oncol.* 2012;13(1):25–32. doi:10.1016/S1470-2045(11)70336-9

10. Schneeweiss A, Chia S, Hickish T, et al. Pertuzumab plus trastuzumab in combination with standard neoadjuvant anthracycline-containing and anthracycline-free chemotherapy regimens in patients with HER2-positive early breast cancer: a randomized phase II cardiac safety study (TRYPHAENA). *Ann Oncol.* 2013;24(9):2278–2284. doi:10.1093/annonc/mdt182

11. Bear HD, Anderson S, Brown A, et al. The effect on tumor response of adding sequential preoperative docetaxel to preoperative doxorubicin and cyclophosphamide: preliminary results from National Surgical Adjuvant Breast and Bowel Project Protocol B-27. *J Clin Oncol* 2003;21(22):4165–4174. doi:10.1200/JCO.2003.12.005

12. Mieog JS, van der Hage JA, van de Velde CJ. Preoperative chemotherapy for women with operable breast cancer. *Cochrane Database Syst Rev.* 2007;(2):CD005002. doi:10.1002/14651858.CD005002.pub2

13. Untch M, Fasching PA, Konecny GE, et al. Pathologic complete response after neoadjuvant chemotherapy plus trastuzumab predicts favorable survival in human epidermal growth factor receptor 2-overexpressing breast cancer: results from the TECHNO trial of the AGO and GBG study groups. *J Clin Oncol.* 2011;29(25):3351–3357. doi:10.1200/JCO.2010.31.4930

14. Masuda N, Lee SJ, Ohtani S, et al. Adjuvant capecitabine for breast cancer after preoperative chemotherapy. *N Engl J Med.* 2017;376(22):2147–2159. doi:10.1056/NEJMoa1612645

15. von Minckwitz G, Huang CS, Mano MS, et al. Trastuzumab Emtansine for Residual Invasive HER2-Positive Breast Cancer. *N Engl J Med.* 2019;380(7):617–628. doi:10.1056/NEJMoa1814017

16. Fisher B, Bryant J, Wolmark N, et al. Effect of preoperative chemotherapy on the outcome of women with operable breast cancer. *J Clin Oncol.* 1998;16(8):2672–2685. doi:10.1200/JCO.1998.16.8.2672

17. Geng C, Chen X, Pan X, Li J. The feasibility and accuracy of sentinel lymph node biopsy in initially clinically node-negative breast cancer after neoadjuvant chemotherapy: a systematic review and meta-analysis. *PLoS One.* 2016;11(9):e0162605. doi:10.1371/journal.pone.0162605

18. El Hage Chehade H, Headon H, et al. Is sentinel lymph node biopsy a viable alternative to complete axillary dissection following neoadjuvant chemotherapy in women with node-positive breast cancer at diagnosis? An updated meta-analysis involving 3,398 patients. *Am J Surg.* 2016;212(5):969–981. doi:10.1016/j.amjsurg.2016.07.018

19. Recht A, Comen EA, Fine RE, et al. Postmastectomy radiotherapy: an american society of clinical oncology, american society for radiation oncology, and society of surgical oncology focused guideline update. *Ann Surg Oncol*. 2017;24(1):38–51. doi:10.1245/s10434-016-5558-8

20. Wang SL, Fang H, Song YW, et al. Hypofractionated versus conventional fractionated postmastectomy radiotherapy for patients with high-risk breast cancer: a randomised, non-inferiority, open-label, phase 3 trial. *Lancet Oncol*. 2019;20(3):352–360. doi:10.1016/S1470-2045(18)30813-1

21. Recht A, Edge SB, Solin LJ, et al. Postmastectomy radiotherapy: clinical practice guidelines of the american society of clinical oncology. *J Clin Oncol*. 2001;19(5):1539–1569. doi:10.1200/JCO.2001.19.5.1539

22. Videtic GMM, Woody N, Vassil AD. *Handbook of treatment planning in radiation oncology*. 2nd ed. Demos Medical; 2015. doi:10.1891/9781617051975

25 ■ DUCTAL CARCINOMA IN SITU

Timothy D. Smile, Rahul D. Tendulkar, and Chirag Shah

QUICK HIT ■ Ductal carcinoma in situ (also known as intraductal carcinoma) represents ~20% of all BCs. Without treatment, up to 25% to 30% of DCIS cases can progress to invasive BC over 30 years. Standard treatment involves either breast conservation therapy (lumpectomy plus adjuvant RT) or mastectomy. After lumpectomy, adjuvant RT results in 50% relative RR in LR (with approximately half of recurrences being invasive cancers) but no improvement in overall survival. Absolute risk of IBTR depends on grade, histologic subtype, size, ER status, and margin status. LCIS is a distinct entity from DCIS, which is mammographically undetectable and does not require a negative margin excision (except possibly pleomorphic subtype) or adjuvant RT.

EPIDEMIOLOGY: Over 60,000 cases of in situ BCs are diagnosed in the United States annually, of which roughly 80% are DCIS and 20% are LCIS.[1] Incidence increased fivefold with the introduction of mammography. DCIS is less common than invasive BC (~200,000 per year). Left untreated, ~25% to 30% of patients with DCIS develop invasive cancer over 30 years.[2–4]

RISK FACTORS: Similar to invasive BC: female gender, older age, BRCA status, family history (first-degree relative), unopposed estrogen (includes early menarche, late menopause, nulliparity, late age at first birth), obesity, alcohol (dose-dependent), prior RT, atypical ductal hyperplasia.

PATHOLOGY: DCIS implies that the basement membrane is preserved despite carcinoma in situ cells arising from the ductal epithelium. Typically grows toward nipple. Five histologic subtypes (mnemonic: C²PMS): cribriform, comedo (worst prognosis), papillary, micropapillary, solid (second worst prognosis). Overall three main categories of grading:

■ *Grade 1 (low grade):* Monomorphous nuclei with inconspicuous nucleoli and diffuse chromatin. Typically ER- and PR-positive, have a low proliferative rate and rarely (if ever) show abnormalities of the HER2/neu or p53 oncogenes.
■ *Grade 2 (intermediate grade):* Nuclei are neither grade 1 nor 3.
■ *Grade 3 (high grade):* Nuclei are large and pleomorphic, >1 nucleolus per cell, irregular chromatin. Typically exhibit aneuploidy, ER- and PR-negative and have a high proliferative rate, overexpression of the HER2 oncogene, mutations of the p53 tumor suppressor, and angiogenesis in the surrounding stroma.

LCIS can be commonly associated with or without atypical ductal hyperplasia or atypical lobular hyperplasia and is not considered a malignancy. However, pleomorphic LCIS is considered to have similar biologic behavior as DCIS, and clinicians may consider complete excision with negative margins, albeit data are lacking. Furthermore, multifocal/extensive LCIS involving >4 terminal ductal lobular units on core biopsy is thought to increase chances of finding invasive cancer on surgical excision.

Seventy-five percent to 80% of DCIS cases are ER-positive. Up to 35% are HER2/neu amplified, and the clinical significance is under investigation.[5]

GENETICS: The Oncotype Dx DCIS Score multigene expression assay may have utility as a prognostic biomarker for recurrence.[6,7] However, the test's cost-effectiveness is uncertain.[8]

SCREENING: Mammographic screening reduces BC mortality by 20% (relative risk).[9] ACS, ACR, AMA, NCI, and NCCN recommend routine screening initiated at age 40. See Chapter 23 for additional details. Risk-prediction models may help with patient-specific decisions. MRI screening is recommended by the NCI/ACS for patients with a 20% to 25% lifetime risk of BC (BRCA mutation, first-degree relative with BRCA mutation, history of thoracic RT, Li–Fraumeni/Cowden syndrome, or based on family history calculator).[10,11] MRI screening is not recommended for <15% risk (prior BC, atypical ductal hyperplasia, DCIS, ALH, LCIS, dense breasts).

CLINICAL PRESENTATION: In situ breast disease is generally asymptomatic and usually detected mammographically. On occasion, DCIS may be palpable. It may also be discovered incidentally during investigation of a nearby breast mass (benign or malignant).

WORKUP: H&P with breast and lymph node exam.

Imaging: Bilateral diagnostic mammograms with spot compression views (to evaluate masses) and magnification (to evaluate calcifications) as necessary. Concerning findings on mammography: 100 to 300 μm clustered or linear calcifications, spiculated or new lesions. Linear/branching calcifications are associated with high-grade DCIS and necrosis whereas fine/granular calcifications are associated with low-grade DCIS.[12] Ninety percent of DCIS present with calcifications, and 80% of lesions with calcifications contain DCIS.[12,13] The BI-RADS is the standard mammographic terminology. MRI may be superior to mammography for detecting DCIS (especially high-grade or multicentric disease) but has a high rate of false positives.[14] Concerning MRI findings include non–mass-like enhancement with segmental or ductal distribution and granular internal enhancement (BI-RADS 5), or enhancement in late postcontrast phase, or enhancement not following milk ducts, or asymmetric (BI-RADS 4).

Biopsy Technique: FNA is inadequate to distinguish DCIS from invasive cancer, and therefore stereotactic core or excisional biopsy is recommended. Stereotactic guided "bracketing" of the suspicious areas to help facilitate excision. Use ultrasound guidance for masses. Atypical ductal hyperplasia on core biopsy requires complete excision as 20% of patients are upstaged.[15]

PROGNOSTIC FACTORS: Higher risk of recurrence for young age, high grade, comedonecrosis, multifocality, large tumor size, positive surgical margins, ER-negativity, HER2/neu amplification.[16] The VNPI quantifies prognostic factors for LR in patients with DCIS (low score 4–6, intermediate 7–9, and high 10–12) (see Table 25.1).[17,18] Note that VNPI has not been prospectively validated.[19,20]

Table 25.1: Updated VNPI			
Score	1	2	3
Size	≤15 mm	16 to 40 mm	>40 mm
Margin	≥10 mm	1 to 9 mm	<1 mm
Grade	Grade 1/2 without necrosis	Grade 1/2 with necrosis	Grade 3
Age	>60	40 to 60	<40

STAGING: T classification is Tis and stage is 0 for all DCIS/LCIS.

TREATMENT PARADIGM: Options include observation if short life expectancy due to comorbidities, lumpectomy alone, lumpectomy with adjuvant RT ± tamoxifen/anastrozole (based on menopausal status and if ER-positive) or mastectomy. A risk-based patient-specific assessment is necessary.

Prevention: Tamoxifen and raloxifene both reduce the risk of BC (invasive and noninvasive) by ~50% in high-risk populations. ER-positive tumors are reduced by ~70% but no difference in ER-negative tumors.

Surgery: Either lumpectomy (LR reduced by adjuvant RT)[16] or simple mastectomy (LR 1%–2% without RT).[21] No trials have compared breast-conserving therapy (lumpectomy + RT; BCT) to mastectomy. Data from the Netherlands show only 8% of DCIS is present beyond 1 cm from the initial focus.[22] According to NCCN guidelines, sentinel node dissection should not be performed in the absence of invasive cancer but may be considered for microinvasion or for large tumors >4 cm.[23]

SLNB should be considered in those undergoing mastectomy given the limitation of future sampling if invasion is demonstrated on final pathology. Ten percent to 20% of patients diagnosed with DCIS only on biopsy will have invasive cancer identified at surgery.[24,25] Follow-up specimen radiograph prior to RT useful to confirm complete excision of the suspicious calcifications.

Chemotherapy: No indication in DCIS/LCIS. The NSABP B-43/RTOG 0974 trial is investigating the role of trastuzumab for HER2/neu amplified cases.

Hormonal Therapy: Consider adjuvant tamoxifen given 20 mg/day or anastrozole 1 mg/day for 5 years after excision of ER-positive DCIS. Low-dose tamoxifen (5 mg/day) for 3 years is also an option based on the TAM01 trial discussed in the following.[26] NCCN recommends tamoxifen for patients with ER-positive tumors treated with excision alone or lumpectomy and RT.[23]

Radiation

Indications: RT after surgery is indicated for most patients choosing BCT. Five randomized controlled trials have demonstrated a LC benefit to RT, although CSS and OS are similar to lumpectomy alone. NCCN guidelines suggest either mastectomy or BCT as level 1 treatment options, and lumpectomy alone as 2B.[23]

WBI: Treat whole breast using opposed tangents to 40.05 to 42.5 Gy/15–16 fx. Prospective and retrospective series have demonstrated similar outcomes between hypofractionation and standard fractionation.[27,28] While a boost of 10 to 16 Gy in 5 to 8 fractions can be considered, ASTRO consensus guidelines do not recommend boost given the lack of prospective randomized evidence showing benefit in DCIS population.[29]

APBI: Rationale: Approximately 80% to 90% of LR occur at/near lumpectomy site, underutilization of BCT due to treatment duration, transportation. Modalities: applicator brachytherapy, multicatheter interstitial, EBRT.

IORT: Higher rates of LR in two randomized trials for invasive BC; however, limited data in DCIS. IORT not recommended for DCIS off protocol.

BCT contraindications: Absolute: persistently positive surgical margins despite maximal re-excision, multicentric tumors (unless resected as single specimen), diffuse malignant-appearing calcifications, inability to receive post-op RT (prior chest/breast irradiation, pregnancy). *Relative:* active connective tissue disease (scleroderma, active lupus), ataxia telangiectasia, poor cosmesis (large tumor [>4–5 cm] in small breast).

Toxicity: Acute effects: erythema, pruritus, tenderness, desquamation. Late effects: altered pigmentation, volume loss, fibrosis, rib fracture, lymphedema, pulmonary fibrosis, secondary malignancies, and cardiac toxicity.

■ **EVIDENCE-BASED Q&A**

▓ **Can RT reduce the risk of recurrence after lumpectomy?**

Yes, RT has consistently demonstrated an approximately 50% relative reduction in the risk of recurrence of both DCIS and invasive recurrence across all trials and in a meta-analysis.

EBCTCG Meta-analysis (*JNCI Monographs* 2010, PMID 20956824): Individual patient data from four PRTs of lumpectomy with or without RT; 3,729 patients. RT reduced 10-year risk of IBTR by 54% relative RR and 15% absolute RR (NNT 6.7), with a greater proportional reduction in older women. No difference by subgroup when divided by age, extent of resection, tamoxifen, method of detection, margins, focality, grade, necrosis, architecture, or size. Even in small, low-grade tumors resected with negative margins, RT still reduced 10-year IBTR risk by 18% absolute and 52% relative risk. There was no effect on mortality (BCSM, non-BC, or all cause); 10-year BCSM was 4.1% vs. 3.7% with and without RT, respectively. **Conclusion: RT reduced 10-year risk of invasive and noninvasive IBTR after lumpectomy irrespective of risk factors, but no effect was seen on mortality.**

Fisher, NSABP B-17 (*NEJM* 1993, PMID 8292119; *JCO* 1998, PMID 9469327; *Semin Oncol* 2001, PMID 11498833; *JNCI* 2011, PMID 21398619): PRT of 818 DCIS patients randomized to excision with or without WBI. Stratified by age (≤49 or >49 years), tumor type (DCIS or DCIS + LCIS), detection (mammography, clinical exam, or both), or axillary dissection (performed or not). All margins were tumor free and RT was initiated within 8 weeks of lumpectomy to a dose of 50 Gy/25 fx. Nine percent of patients received a tumor bed boost. RT reduced the risk of recurrence by 58%. Comedonecrosis was an independent predictor of IBTR. **Conclusion: Lumpectomy with RT reduces LR over lumpectomy alone.**

Holmberg, SweDCIS (*JCO* 2008, PMID 18250350; *JCO* 2014, PMID 25311220): PRT of 1,067 patients with DCIS treated with lumpectomy and randomized to RT or observation. RT was WBI 50 Gy/25 fx with no boost. Stratified by age, size, focality, detection mode, and margins; 20-year absolute RR of IBE of 12% and a 37% relative RR with the addition of RT; 59.4% and 45.4% of IBE were invasive in the RT and control arms, respectively. No effect on survival. Increasing effect of RT with age (8-year IBTR rates: 24% vs. 8% in >60 years of age and 31% vs. 20% in <50 years of age). No group was identified with an acceptably low risk of recurrence without RT. All women had at least a 1% per year incidence of recurrence in absence of RT. **Conclusion: All women benefit from RT and "further search for clinical variables predictive of a low-risk group that does not need RT does not seem fruitful."** *Comment: No formal histopathologic protocol, ~10% margin status unknown.*

Julien, EORTC 10853 (*Lancet* 2000, PMID 10683002; *JCO* 2006, PMID 16801628; *JCO* 2013, PMID 24043739): PRT of 1,002 patients (<70 y/o, DCIS ≤5 cm) treated with lumpectomy and randomized to observation or WBI. Margins must have no DCIS at the sample margin. Post-op mammograms or specimen radiographs were not required. RT given <12 weeks post-op, using opposed tangents 50 Gy/25 fx with no boost recommended (although 5% received a tumor bed boost with median 10 Gy). LR-free rate at 15 years was 69% vs. 82% in favor of RT. **Conclusion: RT after local excision of DCIS reduced overall number of invasive and noninvasive recurrences in ipsilateral breast.**

Wapnir, NSABP-B17/24 Long-Term Outcomes (*JNCI* 2011, PMID 21398619): Long-term outcomes of invasive IBTR after lumpectomy for DCIS. RT reduced invasive IBTR by 52%. Invasive IBTR was associated with increased mortality risk (HR of death 1.75, 95% CI: 1.45–2.96, p < .001). After invasive IBTR, 22/39 deaths were attributed to BC.

Table 25.2: Summary of DCIS Trials Evaluating RT Vs. No RT									
	EBCTG 10-Yr		NSABP-B17 15-Yr		SweDCIS 20-Yr		EORTC 10853 15-Yr		UK/ANZ RT Arm 12.7-Yr	
	RT	No RT	RT	No RT	RT	No RT	RT	No RT	RT	No RT
IBTR	12.9*	28.1	19.8*	35	20.0*	32.0	18*	31	7.1*	19.4
Invasive recurrence	NR	NR	10.7*	19.6	15.1	20.1	10*	16	3.3*	9.1
CSS	95.9	96.3	95.3	96.9	95.9	95.8	96	95	NR	NR
OS	91.6	91.8	82.9	84.2	77.2	73.0	88	90	NR	NR

*Statistically significant difference.

■ **Is there a subset of patients at a low enough absolute risk of recurrence that RT can be omitted?**

Although there are women with a low risk of recurrence, this subset has not been clearly defined and remains a patient-specific decision based on life expectancy and patient wishes. See the preceding VNPI and the following prospective data.

Wong, Dana Farber/Harvard (*JCO* 2006, PMID 16461781; *BCRT* 2014, PMID 24346130): Prospective single-arm study enrolling "low-risk" women with DCIS defined as predominantly grades 1 to 2, ≤2.5 cm mammographically with margins ≥1 cm or re-excision without residual DCIS and no tamoxifen. Accrued 158/200 patients (stopped early). At 8 years, the incidence of LR was 13%, and 32% of recurrences were invasive. **Conclusion: Despite margins of ≥1 cm, LR is substantial in patients with small low-grade DCIS treated by excision alone. The estimated annual risk of LR in this group of patients is 1.9% per year.**

Solin, ECOG 5194 (*JCO* 2009, PMID 19826126; *JCO* 2015, PMID 26371148): Single-arm trial of 711 DCIS patients (grades 1 to 2 and ≤2.5 cm or grade 3 and ≤1 cm) treated with local excision only (margins ≥3 mm; 30% received tamoxifen). Median tumor sizes were 7 and 6 mm, respectively. The 12-year IBE was 14.4% for grades 1 to 2 and 24.6% for grade 3. The 12-year IBR was 7.5% for grades 1 to 2 and 13.4% for grade 3. **Conclusion: Rate of recurrence increases without plateau (~1% per year for grades 1 to 2 and 2% per year for grade 3).**

McCormick, RTOG 9804 (*JCO* 2015, PMID 25605856): PRT of "low-risk" DCIS (grades 1 to 2, size <2.5 cm, mammographically detected with margins ≥3 mm) randomized to WBI 50 Gy/25 fx vs. observation; 636 patients enrolled of a planned 1,790. MFU 7.2 years; 62% received tamoxifen (optional). Primary end point was ipsilateral LR. At 7 years, LR was 0.9% RT vs. 6.7% observation ($p < .001$). **Conclusion: RT reduces LR even in a very low-risk cohort.**

■ **Is adjuvant tamoxifen beneficial? Who should receive it? What is the optimal dose?**

Tamoxifen lowers the incidence of any breast event (B24 and UK/ANZ) and contralateral breast events but does not affect ipsilateral invasive recurrences and therefore is not a substitute for RT (UK/ANZ). Tamoxifen benefits only ER-positive patients (B-24).

Fisher, NSABP B-24 (*Lancet* 1999, PMID 10376613; *JNCI* 2011, PMID 21398619): PRT of 1,798 DCIS patients comparing BCS with RT with or without tamoxifen. Stratified by age (≤49 or >49 years), tumor type (DCIS or DCIS + LCIS), and detection method (mammography, clinical exam, or both). Patients with a positive margin or residual scattered calcifications were eligible. RT given within 8 weeks of lumpectomy with tangents to 50 Gy/25 fx. Placebo or tamoxifen 10 mg BID given within 56 days of lumpectomy for 5 years. Thirty-one percent stopped tamoxifen due to side effects, personal reasons, or unspecified reasons. Any BC event was decreased with tamoxifen (13% vs. 8% at 5 years, $p = .0009$), as did the rate of invasive BC (7% vs. 4%, $p = .004$). *Note that ER status was initially unknown (see Allred).*

Allred, NSABP B-24 subgroup (*JCO* 2012, PMID 22393101): A total of 732 patients evaluated from B-24 for ER status; 76% were ER+ and in these patients, tamoxifen decreased the 10-year incidence of BC (HR: 0.49, $p < .001$) but showed no benefit with ER-negative patients.

Houghton, UK/ANZ Trial (*Lancet* 2003, PMID 12867108; *Lancet Oncol* 2011, PMID 21145284): Four-arm PRT of 1,694 DCIS patients after lumpectomy randomized using a 2 × 2 design: ± RT and ± tamoxifen. Surgery was a resection with specimen radiograph and negative margins; microinvasion was allowed. RT was 50 Gy/25 fx without a boost. Tamoxifen: 20 mg QD for 5 years. Patients could choose the four-way randomization or one of the two-way randomizations. Only patients randomized to a treatment were analyzed for that arm. At 10 years, risk of any breast event was no adjuvant treatment (32%), tamoxifen alone (24%), RT alone (13%), RT and tamoxifen (10%). Both tamoxifen and RT significantly decreased the risk of IBTR. Tamoxifen did not affect invasive recurrences and therefore is not a substitute for RT.

Table 25.3: Summary of DCIS Trials Evaluating Tamoxifen Vs. No Tamoxifen						
	NSABP B24 10 Yrs			**UK/ANZ Tamoxifen Randomization 12.7 Yrs**		
	Tam	No Tam	HR	Tam	No Tam	HR
IBTR	13.2	16.6	0.68*	15.7	19.6	0.78*
Invasive recurrence	6.6	9	NR	6.8	6.9	0.95
CBTR	4.9	8.1	0.68*	1.9	4.2	0.44*
OS	82.9	85.6	NR	NR	NR	NR

*Statistically significant difference.

DeCensi, TAM01 (*JCO* 2019, PMID 30973790): PRT of 500 patients ≤75 y/o with ER+ DCIS randomized to low-dose tamoxifen (5 mg/day) or placebo for 3 years. MFU 5.1 years, the low-dose tamoxifen arm had fewer cumulative breast events (6% vs. 11%; $p = .02$) and contralateral breast events (1.2% vs. 4.8%; $p = .02$). No difference in patient-reported outcomes except for slight increase in daily hot flashes with tamoxifen ($p = .02$). Conclusion: Low-dose tamoxifen decreased contralateral breast events by 75% with limited toxicity.

■ **Since tamoxifen prevents contralateral recurrences in the preceding trials, can we use it to prevent BC in high-risk patients?**

Yes, although often the side effects make this less frequently used.

Fisher, NSABP P-1 (*JNCI* 1998, PMID 9747868): A total of 13,388 women with risk factors ($\geq$60 y/o or with risk $\geq$1.66% or with a history of LCIS) randomized to placebo or tamoxifen for 5 years. Tamoxifen reduced the risk of invasive BC by 49% with older women benefiting more. All subgroups benefited. ER-positive tumors were reduced by 69%, but no difference was seen in ER-negative.

Vogel, NSABP P-2 "STAR" (*JAMA* 2006, PMID 16754727): PRT comparing tamoxifen to raloxifene with the goal of reducing side effects of tamoxifen and testing efficacy of raloxifene. Overall raloxifene appeared similar in efficacy with a lower rate of thromboembolic events.

■ **Is anastrozole superior to tamoxifen for DCIS?**

Margolese, NSABP B-35 (*Lancet* 2016, PMID 26686957): Phase III PRT of 3,104 postmenopausal women with ER- or PR-positive DCIS comparing 1 mg/day anastrozole to 20 mg/day tamoxifen for 5 years. The primary end point was BCFI, defined as the time from randomization to any BCE including local, regional, distant recurrence or contralateral disease, invasive or DCIS. MFU 8.6 years. BCFI at 10 years was 89% vs. 93% (HR 0.73) in favor of anastrozole ($p = .03$). Benefit was primarily in women <60 years of age. There was a NS trend for a reduction in second primary breast cancers with anastrozole (HR: 0.68, $p = .07$); 10-year estimates for OS were 92.1% for tamoxifen, 92.5% for anastrozole (NS).

■ **What is the optimal dose and fractionation for DCIS? Is hypofractionation appropriate?**

Most prospective DCIS trials used 50 Gy/25 fx with or without a boost. Hypofractionation has been studied prospectively (DBCG and MD Anderson trials) with oncologic outcomes pending.[27,30] However, given the established efficacy and safety in invasive BC, most consider hypofractionation to be appropriate for DCIS.

Lalani, Ontario Series (*IJROBP* 2014, PMID 25220719): RR of 1,609 patients treated from 1994 to 2003. Sixty percent treated with conventional RT, 40% with hypofractionation (42.4 Gy/16 fx). Fifteen percent of conventional patients received a boost whereas 54% of the hypofractionated patients received a boost. MFU 9.2 years; 10-year LRFS 86% vs. 89% for hypofractionated ($p = .03$). Hypofractionation was not associated with recurrence on multivariate analysis. **Conclusion: Hypofractionation was of similar efficacy to conventional schedules.**

Offersen, DBCG HYPO Trial (*JCO* 2020, PMID 32910709): PRT of 1,842 women with node-negative BC or DCIS s/p BCS randomized to WBI with either 50 Gy/25 fx or 40 Gy/15 fx. 246 women had DCIS. Primary end point was grade 2 to 3 breast induration at 3 years. The rates of induration at 3 years were 11.8% vs. 9.0% in the 50 Gy and 40 Gy arms, respectively ($p = .07$). Systemic therapy and RT boost did not increase risk of induration; 9-year LRR 3.3% vs. 3.0% in the 50 Gy and 40 Gy arms, respectively (NS). OS was comparable. **Conclusion: Hypofractionation was of similar efficacy to conventional schedules.**

■ **Is it necessary to boost the tumor bed for DCIS patients?**

This is controversial as there is no prospective randomized evidence directly comparing oncologic outcomes (trials ongoing). Cosmesis and arm/shoulder function were negatively affected by the addition of tumor bed boost in conventionally fractionated and hypofractionated WBI regimens in the BIG 3–07/TROG 07.01 trial, while LR outcomes are still pending.[28] Note that a boost was performed in a small minority of patients on prospective trials (5%–9% NSABP B-17/EORTC, not recommended on SweDCIS/UK/ANZ/RTOG 9804). Retrospective series are noted in the following. ASTRO guidelines do not recommend boost given the lack of evidence to support it.

Omlin, Switzerland (*Lancet Oncol* 2006, PMID 16887482): RR of 373 patients from 18 institutions, all ≤45 years of age. Fifteen percent had no RT after surgery, 45% had RT without boost, 40% had RT with a 10 Gy boost. LRFS at 10 years improved for those given a boost (no RT 46%, RT no boost 72%, RT with boost 86%). **Conclusion: Boost should be considered in young patients.**

Wai, British Columbia (*Cancer* 2011, PMID 20803608): RR of 957 patients between 1985 and 1999 with MFU 9.3 years; 50% had no RT, 35% had RT without boost, and 15% had RT with a boost. While RT was associated with improved LC, no difference between those with or without a boost.

Moran, Multi-Institutional (*JAMA Oncol* 2017, PMID 28358936): RR of pooled patient-level data from 10 institutions including 4,131 patients treated between 1980 and 2010. Boost associated with significantly lower rate of ipsilateral breast tumor recurrence with benefit of 0.8% at 5 years, 1.6% at 10 years, and 3.6% at 15 years. **Conclusion: Boost reduced rate of ipsilateral breast tumor recurrence across all age groups, similar to findings with invasive BCs.**

■ **What factors predict for recurrence?**

Beyond the VNPI, other studies have discussed predictive factors that can aid in patient selection. A combined analysis of B-17 and B-24 demonstrated younger age, clinically detected DCIS, comedonecrosis, and positive margins to be associated with a higher risk of recurrence.[31] On SweDCIS trial, grade III histology and necrosis were predictors for recurrence.[32] Additional retrospective reviews have shown that younger age and multifocality may also be associated with higher rates of recurrence.[33,34]

■ **What surgical margins are necessary?**

Dunne, Ireland (*JCO* 2009, PMID 19255332). Study-level meta-analysis of 4,660 patients on 22 trials of BCT in DCIS looking at IBTR and margin status. Median time to IBTR 5 years. Negative margins had lower IBTR than positive (64% less), close or unknown margins after RT. No significant difference in IBTR with 2 mm vs. >5 mm margins. **Conclusion: Margins of ≥2 mm are sufficient when RT is used.**

Morrow, SSO/ASTRO/ASCO Consensus Guideline (*JCO* 2016, PMID 2758719): No prior consensus regarding the optimal margin width for DCIS treated with BCT. Multidisciplinary consensus panel used a meta-analysis of margin width and IBTR rates from a systematic review of 20 studies including 7,883 patients and other published literature to obtain guidelines. Negative margins (no DCIS on ink) halve the risk of IBTR compared with positive margins. When WBI is given, a 2-mm margin minimizes the risk of IBTR compared with smaller negative margins with statistically significant OR of 0.51. Margins ≥2 mm and up to 10 mm do not significantly decrease IBTR compared with 2 mm margins (with WBI). Clinical judgment should be used in determining the need for further surgery in patients with negative margins <2 mm.

■ **Are there any patients who require radiation after a mastectomy for DCIS?**

Childs, Harvard (*IJROBP* 2012, PMID 22975615): RR of 142 patients with mastectomy without post-op RT with pure DCIS (no microinvasion). Fifteen percent with positive margin, 16% with margin ≤2 mm. One patient with positive margin and one patient with close margins experienced chest wall recurrence. **Conclusion: PMRT not routinely warranted even with positive margins.**

Chan, UCSF (*IJROBP* 2010, PMID 20646871): RR of 193 patients with mastectomy: 55 with close margin, 4 with positive margin. Risk of chest wall recurrence 1.7% for all, and 3.4% for high-grade patients.

Carlson, Emory (*JACS* 2007, PMID 17481544): RR of 223 patients with skin-sparing mastectomy and reconstruction without RT. LR 3.3%, regional recurrence 0.9%, distant recurrence 0.9%. If margin <1 mm, LR 10%.

■ **Can genomic assays be used to guide prognosis and treatment for DCIS patients?**

Genomic assays may have utility as independent prognostic tools for estimating the risk of recurrence.[6,7] However, the test may not be cost effective[8] as the low-risk subset has a risk of 10%, and many women may choose RT anyway in this situation.

Solin, ECOG E5194 (*JNCI* 2013, PMID 23641039): Molecular profiling of patients with negative margins treated without RT on the ECOG E5194 study. Oncotype DX performed on subset of 327 patients. Identified three groups (70% low risk, 16% intermediate, and 14% high) with IBTR risks of 10.6%, 26.7%, and 25.9% at 10 years, respectively. Invasive recurrence risks were 3.7%, 12.3%, and 19.2% for low, intermediate, and high risk, respectively. Prognostic value persisted on multivariate analysis.

Rakovitch, DCIS Oncotype (*Breast Cancer Res Treat* 2015, PMID 26119102): Validated Oncotype DX in a retrospective population-based cohort of 718 cases treated with surgery alone with negative margins. MFU 9.6 years. Oncotype DX independently predicted the risk of recurrence on MVA. The 10-year LR risks for low-, intermediate-, and high-risk groups were 12.7%, 33%, and 27.8%, respectively. **Conclusion: Oncotype for DCIS adds independent value in an external subset; however, even in the low-risk group, the LR risk may be high enough to offer RT.**

■ **Is APBI feasible in DCIS?**

Multiple studies support the use of APBI in appropriately selected patients. Current ASTRO,[29] ABS[35], and ASBS[36] guidelines support the use of APBI for selected patients with DCIS.

Shah, MammoSite Registry (*Ann Surg Oncol* 2013, PMID 23975302): A total of 194 patients with DCIS who underwent APBI with MammoSite (34 Gy/10 fx). MFU 63 months; 5-year actuarial IBTR rate 4.1%. Tumor size (OR = 1.1, $p = .03$) and ER-negativity (OR = 3.0, $p = .0009$) were associated with IBTR, while a trend noted for positive margins (OR = 2.0, $p = .06$) and cautionary/unsuitable status compared with suitable status (OR = 1.8, $p = .07$).

Vicini, ASBS/WBH Pooled Analysis (*Ann Surg Oncol* 2013, PMID 23054123): Pooled analysis from ASBS MammoSite Registry Trial and William Beaumont Hospital of 300 women with DCIS who underwent APBI over 17-year period. Rate of IBTR was 2.6% at 5 years with no regional recurrences, CSS 99.5% and OS 99.5%. When comparing cautionary DCIS group to invasive suitable/cautionary group, no difference in IBTR noted (2.6% vs. 3.1%, $p = .90$) with significant improvements in DM (0% vs. 2.5%, $p = .05$), DFS (98.5% vs. 94.4%, $p = .05$), and OS (95.7% vs. 90.8%, $p = .03$) noted for DCIS patients. When comparing cautionary DCIS patients to invasive suitable patients, no difference in IBTR noted (2.6% vs. 2.4%, $p = .76$), while improved OS for DCIS patients was noted (95.7% vs. 90.9%, $p = .02$).

Strnad, GEC-ESTRO Multicatheter Trial (*Lancet* 2015, PMID 26494415): PRT of 1,184 women randomized to multicatheter brachytherapy vs. WBI (50 Gy + 10 Gy boost). Included women with stage 0–IIA tumors ≤3 cm, pN0/Nmi, no LVSI, and clear margins ≥2 mm (≥5 mm for DCIS). For DCIS, only VNPI low or intermediate scores (<8) included ($n = 60$; 5%). APBI performed to the tumor bed with ≥2 cm margins to 32 Gy in 8 fx or 30.3 Gy in 7 fx BID or pulsed-dose brachytherapy to 50 Gy. APBI was considered noninferior if the 5-year LR rate in APBI arm did not exceed 3% more than the WBI arm; 5-year LR rate was 0.92% in the WBI arm vs. 1.44% in the APBI arm.

■ **Is there a role for IORT in the treatment of DCIS?**

IORT has been shown to have higher rates of LR in two randomized trials (TARGIT and ELIOT). Limited data are available for patients with DCIS and thus IORT is not recommended off protocol at this time.

Rivera, IORT for DCIS (*Breast* 2016, PMID 26534876): Prospective nonrandomized trial of 30 women with pure DCIS considered eligible for IORT based on preoperative mammography and CE-MRI. Inclusion: lesion ≤4 cm in maximal diameter on both digital mammography and CE-MRI, pure DCIS on biopsy or wide local excision, and considered resectable with clear surgical margins (2 mm) using BCS. Median age was 57 years (range 42–79 years) and median lesion size was 15.6 mm (2–40 mm). A total of 14.3% (5/35) of patients required some form of additional therapy. At 36 months MFU (range of 2–83 months), only 2 patients experienced LR of cancer (DCIS only), yielding a 5.7% LR rate. No deaths or DM were observed.

■ Is there a survival benefit to radiation after DCIS?

None of the prospective trials or the meta-analysis mentioned earlier demonstrated a survival benefit (although women on NSABP B-24 who developed an invasive recurrence demonstrated inferior survival).

Narod, SEER (*JAMA Oncol* 2015, PMID 26291673): SEER analysis of 108,196 DCIS patients with MFU of 7.5 years; 20-year BCSM 3.3% and was higher in women <35 years of age and Black women. RT reduced the risk of invasive recurrence at 10 years (2.5% vs. 4.9%) but did not improve BCSM. **Conclusion: Prevention of IBTR did not alter BC mortality at 10 years.**

■ With long-term follow-up, do the outcomes for DCIS change?

Solin, Multi-Institutional (*Cancer* 2005, PMID 15674853): A total of 1,003 women treated at 10 North American centers with BCT; 15-year rate of any LF was 19%. Older patients (≥50) and negative margins experienced fewer failures. CSS was 98%.

■ What is LCIS and how does it differ from DCIS?

LCIS is asymptomatic and is not considered a premalignant condition but rather a risk factor for developing invasive BC.[1] The exception is pleomorphic LCIS, which may be treated surgically with excellent outcomes if negative margins are obtained.[37] The risk of developing BC is approximately 7% at 10 years with an equal chance of developing a malignancy in either breast.[38] If a suspicious lesion is detected on mammography and only LCIS is discovered on biopsy, it is important to repeat imaging/excision to ensure the entire suspicious area was removed and no underlying DCIS or malignancy is present. There is no role for RT in the treatment of LCIS.

REFERENCES

1. Siegel RL, Miller KD, Jemal A. Cancer statistics, 2020. *CA Cancer J Clin.* 2020;70(1):7–30. doi:10.3322/caac.21590
2. Collins LC, Tamimi RM, Baer HJ, et al. Outcome of patients with ductal carcinoma in situ untreated after diagnostic biopsy: results from the Nurses' Health Study. *Cancer.* 2005;103(9):1778–1784. doi:10.1002/cncr.20979
3. Eusebi V, Feudale E, Foschini MP, et al. Long-term follow-up of in situ carcinoma of the breast. *Semin Diagn Pathol.* 1994;11(3):223–235.
4. Sanders ME, Schuyler PA, Dupont WD, Page DL. The natural history of low-grade ductal carcinoma in situ of the breast in women treated by biopsy only revealed over 30 years of long-term follow-up. *Cancer.* 2005;103(12):2481–2484. doi:10.1007/s10549-013-2755-z
5. Siziopikou KP, Anderson SJ, Cobleigh MA, et al. Preliminary results of centralized HER2 testing in ductal carcinoma in situ (DCIS): NSABP B-43. *Breast Cancer Res Treat.* 2013;142(2):415–421. doi:10.1007/s10549-013-2755-z
6. Rakovitch E, Nofech-Mozes S, Hanna W, et al. A population-based validation study of the DCIS Score predicting recurrence risk in individuals treated by breast-conserving surgery alone. *Breast Cancer Res Treat.* 2015;152(2):389–398. doi:10.1007/s10549-015-3464-6
7. Solin LJ, Gray R, Baehner FL, et al. A multigene expression assay to predict local recurrence risk for ductal carcinoma in situ of the breast. *J Natl Cancer Inst.* 2013;105(10):701–710. doi:10.1093/jnci/djt067
8. Raldow AC, Sher D, Chen AB, et al. Cost effectiveness of the oncotype DX DCIS score for guiding treatment of patients with ductal carcinoma in situ. *J Clin Oncol.* 2016;34(33):3963–3968. doi:10.1200/JCO.2016.67.8532
9. The benefits and harms of breast cancer screening: an independent review. *Lancet (London, England).* 2012;380(9855):1778–1786. doi:10.1016/S0140-6736(12)61611-0
10. Bevers TB, Helvie M, Bonaccio E, et al. Breast cancer screening and diagnosis, version 3.2018, NCCN clinical practice guidelines in oncology. *J Natl Compr Canc Netw.* 2018;16(11):1362–1389. doi:10.6004/jnccn.2018.0083.
11. Saslow D, Boetes C, Burke W, et al. American Cancer Society guidelines for breast screening with MRI as an adjunct to mammography. *CA Cancer J Clin.* 2007;57(2):75–89. doi:10.3322/canjclin.57.2.75
12. Holland R, Hendriks JH, Vebeek AL, et al. Extent, distribution, and mammographic/histological correlations of breast ductal carcinoma in situ. *Lancet (London, England).* 1990;335(8688):519–522. doi:10.1016/0140-6736(90)90747-S
13. Dershaw DD, Abramson A, Kinne DW. Ductal carcinoma in situ: mammographic findings and clinical implications. *Radiology.* 1989;170(2):411–415. doi:10.1148/radiology.170.2.2536185
14. Kuhl CK, Schrading S, Bieling HB, et al. MRI for diagnosis of pure ductal carcinoma in situ: a prospective observational study. *Lancet (London, England).* 2007;370(9586):485–492. doi:10.1016/S0140-6736(07)61232-X
15. McGhan LJ, Pockaj BA, Wasif N, et al. Atypical ductal hyperplasia on core biopsy: an automatic trigger for excisional biopsy? *Ann Surg Oncol.* 2012;19(10):3264–3269. doi:10.1245/s10434-012-2575-0
16. Correa C, McGale P, Taylor C, et al. Overview of the randomized trials of radiotherapy in ductal carcinoma in situ of the breast. *J Natl Cancer Inst Monogr.* 2010;2010(41):162–177. doi:10.1093/jncimonographs/lgq039

17. Silverstein MJ. An argument against routine use of radiotherapy for ductal carcinoma in situ. *Oncology.* 2003;17(11):1511–1533; discussion 1533–1514, 1539, 1542 passim.

18. Silverstein MJ, Lagios MD. Choosing treatment for patients with ductal carcinoma in situ: fine tuning the University of Southern California/Van Nuys Prognostic Index. *J Natl Cancer Inst Monogr.* 2010;2010(41):193–196. doi:10.1093/jncimonographs/lgq040

19. Whitfield R, Kollias J, de Silva P, et al. Management of ductal carcinoma in situ according to Van Nuys Prognostic Index in Australia and New Zealand. *ANZ J Surg.* 2012;82(7–8):518–523. doi:10.1111/j.1445-2197.2012.06133.x

20. MacAusland SG, Hepel JT, Chong FK, et al. An attempt to independently verify the utility of the Van Nuys Prognostic Index for ductal carcinoma in situ. *Cancer.* 2007;110(12):2648–2653. doi:10.1002/cncr.23089

21. Hwang ES. The impact of surgery on ductal carcinoma in situ outcomes: the use of mastectomy. *J Natl Cancer Inst Monogr.* 2010;2010(41):197–199. doi:10.1093/jncimonographs/lgq032

22. Faverly DR, Burgers L, Bult P, Holland R. Three dimensional imaging of mammary ductal carcinoma in situ: clinical implications. *Semin Diagn Pathol.* 1994;11(3):193–198.

23. Gradishar WJ, Anderson BO, Abraham J, et al. Breast cancer, version 3.2020, NCCN clinical practice guidelines in oncology. *J Natl Compr Canc Netw.* 2020;18(4):452–478.

24. Kurniawan ED, Rose A, Mou A, et al. Risk factors for invasive breast cancer when core needle biopsy shows ductal carcinoma in situ. *Arch Surg.* 2010;145(11):1098–1104. doi:10.1001/archsurg.2010.243

25. Yen TW, Hunt KK, Ross MI, et al. Predictors of invasive breast cancer in patients with an initial diagnosis of ductal carcinoma in situ: a guide to selective use of sentinel lymph node biopsy in management of ductal carcinoma in situ. *J Am Coll Surg.* 2005;200(4):516–526. doi:10.1016/j.jamcollsurg.2004.11.012

26. DeCensi A, Puntoni M, Guerrieri-Gonzaga A, et al. Randomized placebo controlled trial of low-dose tamoxifen to prevent local and contralateral recurrence in breast intraepithelial neoplasia. *J Clin Oncol.* 2019;37(19):1629–1637. doi:10.1200/JCO.18.01779

27. Offersen BV, Alsner J, Nielsen HM, et al. Hypofractionated versus standard fractionated radiotherapy in patients with early breast cancer or ductal carcinoma in situ in a randomized Phase III Trial: the DBCG HYPO Trial. *J Clin Oncol.* 2020;38(31):3615–3625. doi:10.1200/JCO.18.01779

28. King MT, Link EK, Whelan TJ, et al. Quality of life after breast-conserving therapy and adjuvant radiotherapy for non-low-risk ductal carcinoma in situ (BIG 3–07/TROG 07.01): 2-year results of a randomised, controlled, phase 3 trial. *Lancet Oncol.* 2020;21(5):685–698.

29. Morrow M, Van Zee KJ, Solin LJ, et al. Society of surgical oncology-american society for radiation oncology-american society of clinical oncology consensus guideline on margins for breast-conserving surgery with whole-breast irradiation in ductal carcinoma in situ. *J Clin Oncol.* 2016;34(33):4040–4046. doi:10.1200/JCO.2016.68.3573

30. Shaitelman SF, Schlembach PJ, Arzu I, et al. Acute and short-term toxic effects of conventionally fractionated vs hypofractionated whole-breast irradiation: a randomized clinical trial. *JAMA Oncol.* 2015;1(7):931–941. doi:10.1001/jamaoncol.2015.2666

31. Wapnir IL, Dignam JJ, Fisher B, et al. Long-term outcomes of invasive ipsilateral breast tumor recurrences after lumpectomy in NSABP B-17 and B-24 randomized clinical trials for DCIS. *J Natl Cancer Inst.* 2011;103(6):478–488. doi:10.1093/jnci/djr027

32. Ringberg A, Nordgren H, Thorstensson S, et al. Histopathological risk factors for ipsilateral breast events after breast conserving treatment for ductal carcinoma in situ of the breast-results from the swedish randomised trial. *Eur J Cancer.* 2007;43(2):291–298. doi:10.1016/j.ejca.2006.09.018

33. Vicini FA, Recht A. Age at diagnosis and outcome for women with ductal carcinoma-in-situ of the breast: a critical review of the literature. *J Clin Oncol.* 2002;20(11):2736–2744. doi:10.1200/JCO.2002.07.137

34. Meijnen P, Bartelink H. Multifocal ductal carcinoma in situ of the breast: a contraindication for breast-conserving treatment? *J Clin Oncol.* 2007;25(35):5548–5549. doi:10.1200/JCO.2007.13.9121

35. Shah C, Vicini F, Shaitelman SF, et al. The American brachytherapy society consensus statement for accelerated partial-breast irradiation. *Brachytherapy.* 2018;17(1):154–170. doi:10.1016/j.brachy.2017.09.004

36. Consensus Guideline on Accelerated Partial Breast Irradiation. 2018; https://www.breastsurgeons.org/docs/statements/Consensus-Statement-for-Accelerated-Partial-Breast-Irradiation.pdf

37. Flanagan MR, Rendi MH, Calhoun KE, et al. Pleomorphic lobular carcinoma in situ: radiologic-pathologic features and clinical management. *Ann Surg Oncol.* 2015;22(13):4263–4269. doi:10.1245/s10434-015-4552-x

38. Chuba PJ, Hamre MR, Yap J, et al. Bilateral risk for subsequent breast cancer after lobular carcinoma-in-situ: analysis of surveillance, epidemiology, and end results data. *J Clin Oncol.* 2005;23(24):5534–5541. doi:10.1200/JCO.2005.04.038

26 ■ RECURRENT BREAST CANCER

Ian W. Winter, Camille A. Berriochoa, and Chirag Shah

QUICK HIT ■ LRR of breast cancer is associated with an increased risk of distant metastases and mortality. The majority of recurrences occur in the ipsilateral breast or chest wall within 5 years of initial treatment. Treatment is dependent upon initial management and the location of recurrence, with consideration for surgery, RT/re-irradiation, CHT, and/or endocrine therapy (Table 26.1). RT may also be given with concurrent hyperthermia or CHT.

Table 26.1: General Treatment Paradigm for Locoregionally Recurrent Breast Cancer

Local recurrence only	Initial BCS + RT	Total mastectomy + ALND (if level I/II dissection not previously done), then consider CHT (based on receptor status); if mastectomy refused can consider repeat breast conservation
	Initial mastectomy only	Surgery if possible + RT, then consider CHT either pre-op or post-op (based on receptor status)
	Initial mastectomy + ALN I/II dissection + RT	Consider CHT (based on receptor status), surgery if possible, then consider re-irradiation
Regional ± local recurrence	ALN recurrence	CHT, then surgery + RT if possible (consider re-irradiation)
	SCV or IMN recurrence	CHT, then RT/re-irradiation if possible

EPIDEMIOLOGY: There are ~3.9 million breast cancer survivors in the United States.[1] LRR occurs in approximately 5% to 15%, with decreasing rates in modern studies.[2-5] Most LRR occurs within 5 years of diagnosis, with recurrences after mastectomy occurring earlier than after BCT (~1.2 years earlier).[6] Following LRR, 5-year OS varies widely, ranging from 25% to 75%.[6-9]

RISK FACTORS: Younger age, premenopausal status, larger tumor size, higher BMI, increasing number of LN+, decreased number of dissected LN, ER-negative, HER2+ not treated with trastuzumab, high grade, lymphovascular invasion, not receiving endocrine therapy, margin positivity, BCS without RT, and mastectomy without RT when indicated.[10-15] Genetic susceptibility (BRCA1 or BRCA2) increases the risk of a new primary cancer.

ANATOMY: Following BCT, LRR occurs most commonly in the ipsilateral breast. Following mastectomy, LRR occurs on the CW (~60%) > SCV (~20%) > ALN (~10%).[10]

CLINICAL PRESENTATION: Usually detected via mammography (following BCT), physical exam, or other imaging. Symptoms can include palpable mass, skin changes, new-onset lymphedema, palpable LN, skin changes, or brachial plexopathy.[16-18]

WORKUP:

Labs: CBC, LFT, alkaline phosphatase, and creatinine to evaluate renal function in anticipation of contrast-enhanced imaging.

Imaging: CT chest, CT abdomen/pelvis, MRI brain if symptomatic, bone scan, PET/CT, x-rays of symptomatic bones or suspicious areas noted on bone scan, biopsy with comparison to original pathology, receptor status evaluation, genetic counseling (if high risk).[19] Consider breast MRI for those with intact breast and MRI of the brachial plexus for those with brachial plexopathy symptoms.

PROGNOSTIC FACTORS: Prognosis is better if LRR is isolated in the CW/axilla/IM nodes only (5-yr OS 44%–49%) vs. SCV/multiple sites (5-yr OS 21%–24%).[20] Worse prognosis if LRR within 2 years of initial treatment, following mastectomy (vs. following BCT), skin involvement, larger primary tumor, initial multiple LN+, older age, or higher BMI.[8,13,20,21]

STAGING: Assign a recurrent TNM (rTNM) stage per AJCC (see Chapter 23 for staging).

TREATMENT PARADIGM

Surgery: Surgical options are dependent on the location of the recurrence, previous surgery performed, and feasibility of resection. In general, in-breast recurrences after previous lumpectomy may be salvaged with mastectomy; repeat breast conservation can be considered in select patients not wishing to undergo mastectomy. CW recurrences and nodal recurrences should be excised if feasible, sometimes after cytoreductive systemic therapy.

Chemotherapy: Choices of systemic therapy are determined by the tumor receptor status (ER, PR, HER2) and previous therapy received. CHT concurrent with RT may be considered in select patients typically with gross residual disease. Consider CHT after maximum local control achieved for ER-negative cancers (per the CALOR trial).[22]

Radiation: In the radiation-naive patient, adjuvant RT to the CW with doses of 50 to 60 Gy are appropriate; for positive margins, doses of 60 to 66 Gy or higher are recommended; for gross disease, doses of 66 to 70 Gy are recommended, with consideration of concurrent CHT (capecitabine). Many different regimens have been used for re-irradiation. One option for repeat breast conservation includes 45 Gy at 1.5 Gy/fx given BID to the partial breast (RTOG 1014).[23] For re-irradiation of gross disease, consider concurrent hyperthermia to improve LC. Sequelae can include fatigue, radiation dermatitis, fibrosis, lymphedema, brachial plexopathy, chest wall pain, rib fracture, pneumonitis, and cardiotoxicity.

Hyperthermia (HT): Typically given to superficial CW recurrences concurrent with re-irradiation to temperatures of 43°C. When used in conjunction with RT, HT impairs the cell's ability to repair RT-induced DNA damage, resulting in more effective tumor cell kill. At 43°C there is a dramatic decrease in the cell survival slope (Arrhenius plot). HT dosing is frequently described in terms of CEM43°C T90, which represents the number of cumulative equivalent minutes at 43°C exceeded by 90% of the monitored points within the tumor. HT-related damage is cell cycle nonspecific (as opposed to RT, which is most damaging during G2/M and least effective in S). However, cells may develop thermotolerance[24] (resistance to subsequent HT), which is a phenomenon thought to be due to the production of heat shock proteins; therefore, HT is not delivered daily. A commonly used treatment RT dosing regimen is 32 Gy in 8 fx delivered twice weekly with concurrent HT per the ESHO trial published in 1996,[25] with more recent data using this regimen published by Dutch investigators in 2015.[26] HT techniques include microwave heating, regional perfusional HT, ultrasound, and wrapping.

■ EVIDENCE-BASED Q&A

■ **How are true recurrences (TR) and new primaries (NP) differentiated? How does this change prognosis?**

Characteristics of a NP include different histology, change in receptor status, different location, LOH, and change from aneuploid to diploid compared to the original tumor. NP and TR occur at a similar rate until 8 years; subsequently NP occurs more frequently. An NP has a more favorable prognosis compared to a TR (10-yr OS 75% vs. 55%).[27–29]

■ **Can a sentinel lymph node biopsy be repeated for LRR breast cancer?**

Yes. A 2018 meta-analysis found repeat SLNB was feasible, accurate, spared patients from unnecessary ALND, and provided information that can alter management. It included 1,761 patients who had prior SLNB or ALND who underwent repeat SLNB. There was successful SLN identification in 64.3% (more successful if no prior ALND) with 18.2% node positive. Aberrant drainage was seen more frequently in those with prior ALND.

The negative predictive value was 96.5%. There was no statistical difference between those with previous RT vs. those without.[30]

LOCAL RECURRENCE AFTER BCT

■ What is the preferred treatment for LRR after initial BCT?

Mastectomy is typically preferred; ~80% to 95% of patients with LRR after BCT are suitable mastectomy candidates.[31,32] After salvage mastectomy, second LRR ranges from 4% to 25%, with 5-year OS ranging from 57% to 100%, and 10-year OS ~66% (see Table 26.2).[33]

■ After initial BCT, is salvage BCS an option?

Many clinicians prefer salvage mastectomy given the higher observed LR rates following salvage BCS (4%–25% vs. 7%–49%, respectively).[33] However, no prospective trials have compared the two strategies. Retrospective studies showed that following primary BCT with a subsequent IBTR, salvage mastectomy vs. salvage BCS had no difference in OS, with the caveat that the Milan study showed worse LR with repeat BCS (Table 26.3). RTOG 1014 is a phase II study that provides a framework for repeat BCS with re-irradiation.

Alpert, Yale (*IJROBP* 2005, PMID 16199315): RR of 146 patients s/p BCT with IBTR. Thirty had salvage BCS, 116 underwent salvage mastectomy. MFU 13.8 years. OS similar (salvage BCS 58.0% vs. salvage mastectomy 65.7%, *p* = NS). LR and DM rate similar between groups, both ~7%. **Conclusion: Salvage BCS is feasible with comparable outcomes to salvage mastectomy, but patients remain at risk for further IBTR.**

Table 26.2: Outcomes After Salvage Mastectomy for IBTR After BCT				
Series	N	MFU (mos)	LR (%)	5-Yr OS (%)
Alpert et al.[32]	116	166	6.9	
Shah et al.[33]	18	49	10	100
Dalberg et al.[34]	65	156	12	
Kurtz et al.[35]	43	53	12	
Jacobson et al.[36]	18	120	17	
Voogd et al.[37]	208	52	25	
Salvadori et al.[38]	134	60	4	70
Ofuchi et al.[39]	51	53	11	57–100
Kurtz et al.[40]	66	84	12.1	68
Chen et al.[41]	568			78

Table 26.3: Outcomes After Excision Alone for IBTR After BCT				
Series	N	MFU (mos)	LR (%)	5-Yr OS (%)
Alpert et al.[32]	30	116	6.7	
Shah et al.[33]	18	49	0	100
Dalberg et al.[34]	14	13	33	
Kurtz et al.[35]	46	53	36	
Voogd et al.[37]	16	52	38	
Salvadori et al.[38]	57	60	14	85
Ofuchi et al.[39]	73	53	49	89–94
Kurtz et al.[40]	52	84	23	79
Chen et al.[41]	179			67

■ **After initial BCT, is re-irradiation safe and feasible?**

Yes. RTOG 1014 (repeat BCT with 3D partial breast re-irradiation) evaluated repeat breast conservation. Five-year data demonstrated low rates of toxicity and promising control rates; however, one must consider its stringent entrance criteria.

Arthur, RTOG 1014 (*JAMA Oncol* 2019, PMID 31750868): Phase II, 3D conformal partial breast re-irradiation (PBrI) following repeat lumpectomy for IBTR after previous BCT. Included unifocal IBTR >1 year following BCT, <3 cm, negative margins, ≤3 LN+ without ECE. PBrI to surgical cavity + 1.5 cm CTV, + 1 cm PTV. Dose was 45 Gy in 30 fx delivered at 1.5 Gy BID with 3DCRT; 58 patients (35 invasive, 23 DCIS, mean age 65 years). MFU 5.5 years; 7% late grade 3 AE, no grade 4; 5-year IBTR 5%, ipsilateral mastectomy 10%, DMFS 95%, and OS 95%. **Conclusion: PBrI may be a reasonable alternative to mastectomy, with second breast conservation achievable in 90% of patients with low risk of second recurrence at 5 years.**

Wahl, Multi-institutional (*IJROBP* 2008, PMID 17869019): RR of 81 patients with LRR who underwent repeat RT to breast or chest wall. Median first course RT was 60 Gy and second course was 48 Gy, with median total dose 106 Gy. Twenty percent received BID RT, 54% received concurrent HT, and 54% concurrent CHT. MFU from second RT was 1 year. Four patients had late grade 3/4 toxicity. CR in 57%, with trend to improved CR with HT (67% vs. 39%, $p = .08$); 1-year local DFS 100% if no gross disease vs. 53% with gross disease. No treatment-related mortality. **Conclusion: Repeat RT is feasible with acceptable toxicity.**

■ **Is interstitial brachytherapy after LRR safe and feasible?**

Yes, though data are limited. The largest retrospective study suggests outcomes are comparable to those of mastectomy with promising cosmetic results and limited toxicity.

Hannoun-Levi, GEC-ESTRO (*Radiother Oncol* 2013, PMID 23647758): RR of 217 patients with IBTR following primary BCT (surgery + whole breast with or without regional nodes) re-treated with lumpectomy followed by interstitial multi-catheter brachytherapy (MCB; LDR, PDR, or HDR). MFU 3.9 yrs; 10-year rates of second LR, DM, and OS were 7%, 19%, and 76%, respectively. Excellent/good cosmetic result achieved in 85%. **Conclusion: With IBTR, lumpectomy plus MCB is feasible and effective in preventing second LR with an OS rate at least equivalent to those achieved with salvage mastectomy.**

LOCAL RECURRENCE AFTER MASTECTOMY

■ **How should local/CW recurrences after mastectomy be treated?**

Excision (rather than incisional biopsy) improves outcomes. If possible, aggressive RT after resection is preferred (see Halverson) with consideration of CHT afterward per the CALOR study for receptor negative cancers.

Halverson, Washington U. (*IJROBP* 1990, PMID 2211253): RR of 244 patients with LRR following mastectomy alone. Based on findings, the authors had four recommendations: (a) large-field RT (i.e., entire CW) improved control compared to localized RT (i.e., lesion +1 to 2-cm margin); 10-yr control 63% vs. 18%, $p < .01$. (b) Elective RT to SCV nodes 46 to 50 Gy reduced SCV failure from 16% to 6%, $p = .049$. (c) Elective RT to uninvolved CW to >50 Gy. Patients with SCV or ALN disease failed in CW 29% and 21%, respectively. RT to uninvolved CW decreased recurrence from 27% vs 17%, $p = .32$. (d) Treatment to >50 Gy for completely excised recurrences and >60 Gy for incompletely excised <3 cm recurrences (tumors <3 cm control with ≥60 Gy vs. <60 Gy was 100% vs. 76%). Tumor control for >3 cm lesions was only 50% despite doses of 70 Gy.

■ **Is re-irradiation in the postmastectomy setting safe and feasible?**

The Wahl study (described earlier) included 31 patients s/p mastectomy and demonstrated that re-irradiation to the CW appears safe. Acute/late toxicity occurred at acceptable rates and were most commonly skin related (e.g., dermatitis, fibrosis, skin infection) or the development of lymphedema. The risk of pneumonitis is low with modern techniques.[42] However, one must account for the risk of brachial plexopathy, which has been shown to increase significantly with cumulative doses above 95 Gy and with re-irradiation intervals less than 1 year.[43]

Regional Recurrence to Axillary Lymph Nodes or Supraclavicular Lymph Nodes

Following mastectomy, LRR occurs in the chest wall (~60%) > SCV (~20%) > ALN (~10%).[11] Prognosis is better if LRR is isolated to CW/ALNs/IMNs alone (5-year OS 44%–49%) vs. SCV/multiple sites (5-year OS 21%–24%).[20]

■ **What are outcomes after treatment for supraclavicular recurrence?**

SCV recurrence (SCVr) is associated with a poor prognosis. However, long-term survival is possible with SCVr and aggressive treatment may benefit these patients.

Reddy, MD Anderson (*IJROBP* 2011, PMID 21168284): RR of 140 patients with LRR following initial MRM and CHT, 47 patients involving SCV (23 isolated SCVr). Patients with SCVr had worse DMFS and OS than those without SCV involvement. However, those with isolated SCVr did similar to those with isolated CW LRR with 5-year OS of 25%. **Conclusion: SCVr carries a poor prognosis, but those with isolated SCVr can achieve long-term OS.**

■ **How should isolated internal mammary nodal recurrences be managed?**

There are few data available to guide management of internal mammary recurrences. Options include surgery, SBRT, and fractionated radiotherapy, often preceded by chemotherapy depending on receptor status and resectability.[44–47]

■ **Are there any techniques to reduce the incidence of lymphedema in patients with recurrent breast cancer?**

Lymphovenous bypass surgery can be considered in selected patients to reduce the risk of lymphedema.[48]

■ **What is the role of chemotherapy for locoregional recurrence?**

Especially for ER negative recurrences, consider CHT after maximum local control achieved (as per CALOR trial), or preoperatively to facilitate a gross total resection.

Aebi, CALOR Trial (*Lancet Oncol* 2014, PMID 24439313; Wapnir *JCO* 2018 PMID: 29443653): PRT of 162 patients with isolated LRR s/p radical resection (R0 or R1) randomized to adjuvant multiagent CHT or observation. All could receive hormone/HER2 therapy or RT. Excluded SCVr. The CHT used was not standardized and left to clinician discretion. MFU 9 years. For ER-negative patients, 10-year DFS 70% vs. 34% for CHT vs. no CHT, with HR 0.29 (95% CI 0.13–0.67). In ER-positive patients, 10-year DFS 50% vs. 59% for CHT vs. no CHT, with HR 1.07 (95% CI 0.32–1.55). OS was not significantly different between groups regardless of ER status. **Conclusion: Following complete resection for isolated LRR, adjuvant CHT should be recommended for those who are ER negative.**

■ **Does RT with hyperthermia (HT) improve complete response (CR) rates compared to RT alone?**

Yes. Two prospective studies and a meta-analysis show significantly improved CR rates with RT and HT compared to RT alone (~40% vs. ~60%), and favorable CR rates (~66%) for re-irradiation with HT.

Datta, Meta-analysis (*IJROBP* 2016, PMID 26899950): Meta-analysis of RT+HT in locally recurrent breast cancers treated without surgery or CHT; 34 studies (8 two-arm, 26 single-arm). Treatment was median of seven HT sessions at an average of 42.5°C, mean RT dose 38.2 Gy (26–60 Gy). In the two-arm studies (627 patients) RT+HT had CR in 60% vs. RT alone 38% (SS). In the single-arm studies, RT+HT had CR rate of 63%. Among the 779 patients with previous RT, RT+HT had CR of 67%. Mean acute and late grade 3/4 toxicities with RT+HT were 14% and 5%, respectively. **Conclusion: In LRBC, RT+HT improves CR rates compared to RT alone. For reirradiation + HT, CR was achieved in 67% of patients.**

Linthorst (*Radiother Oncol* 2015, PMID 26002305): RR of 248 patients with breast cancer recurrence treated with re-irradiation (32 Gy/8 fx, twice weekly) and HT (once weekly after RT). MFU 32 months. CR 70%. LC and OS at 1, 3, and 5 years was 53%, 40%, and 39%, and 66%, 32%, and 18% respectively; 10-year OS was 10%. Thermal burns in 23%, but healed with conservative tx; 5-year late G3 toxicity 1%. **Conclusion: Re-irradiation has high rate of LC with acceptable late toxicity. Many patients achieved LC during survival period.**

Jones, Duke (*JCO* 2005, PMID 15860867): PRT of 109 patients with superficial tumors (≤3 cm depth) comparing RT ± HT. In the RT + HT arm, 66% had CR vs. 42% in RT alone arm. Patients with prior RT had most benefit (68% vs. 23%, SS). No OS benefit was seen. Toxicity well tolerated, one grade III thermal burn. **Conclusion: Adjuvant HT with a thermal dose >10 CEM 43°C T(90) significantly improves LC in patients with superficial tumors receiving RT.**

Vernon, International Collaborative Hyperthermia Group (*IJROBP* 1996, PMID 8690639): Merged five PRTs (including the ESHO 5–88 PRT from the Netherlands) due to slow accrual. A total of 306 patients with advanced primary or recurrent breast cancer. Target 43°C with RT given in various fractionations. Primary endpoint was local CR. Overall CR for RT alone 41% vs. RT+HT 59% (*p* = SS). Greatest effect of HT in recurrent lesions after previous RT, where re-irradiation dose was low; 2-year OS ~40% (*p* = NS), 74% patients progressed outside HT area during follow-up. **Conclusion: There seems to be a benefit to HT, but well-designed, prospective trials with appropriate criteria are warranted.**

REFERENCES

1. Miller KD, Nogueira L, Mariotto AB, et al. Cancer treatment and survivorship statistics, 2019. *CA Cancer J Clin.* 2019;69(5):363–385. doi:10.3322/caac.21565

2. Fisher B, Anderson S, Bryant J, et al. Twenty-year follow-up of a randomized trial comparing total mastectomy, lumpectomy, and lumpectomy plus irradiation for the treatment of invasive breast cancer. *N Engl J Med.* 2002;347(16):1233–1241. doi:10.1056/NEJMoa022152

3. Ragaz J, Jackson SM, Le N, et al. Adjuvant radiotherapy and chemotherapy in node-positive premenopausal women with breast cancer. *N Engl J Med.* 1997;337(14):956–962. doi:10.1056/NEJM199710023371402

4. Overgaard M, Nielsen HM, Overgaard J. Is the benefit of postmastectomy irradiation limited to patients with four or more positive nodes, as recommended in international consensus reports? A subgroup analysis of the DBCG 82 b&c randomized trials. *Radiother Oncol.* 2007;82(3):247–253. doi:10.1016/j.radonc.2007.02.001

5. Overgaard M, Jensen MB, Overgaard J, et al. Postoperative radiotherapy in high-risk postmenopausal breast-cancer patients given adjuvant tamoxifen: danish breast cancer cooperative group DBCG 82c randomised trial. *Lancet.* 1999;353(9165):16411648. doi:10.1016/S0140-6736(98)09201-0

6. van Tienhoven G, Voogd AC, Peterse JL, et al. Prognosis after treatment for loco-regional recurrence after mastectomy or breast conserving therapy in two randomised trials (EORTC 10801 and DBCG-82TM). EORTC breast cancer cooperative group and the danish breast cancer cooperative group. *Eur J Cancer.* 1999;35(1):32–38. doi:10.1016/S0140-6736(98)09201-0

7. Wapnir IL, Anderson SJ, Mamounas EP, et al. Prognosis after ipsilateral breast tumor recurrence and locoregional recurrences in five national surgical adjuvant breast and bowel project node-positive adjuvant breast cancer trials. *J Clin Oncol.* 2006;24(13):2028–2037. doi:10.1200/JCO.2005.04.3273

8. Anderson SJ, Wapnir I, Dignam JJ, et al. Prognosis after ipsilateral breast tumor recurrence and locoregional recurrences in patients treated by breast-conserving therapy in five national surgical adjuvant breast and bowel project protocols of node-negative breast cancer. *J Clin Oncol.* 2009;27(15):2466–2473. doi:10.1200/JCO.2008.19.8424

9. Reddy JP, Levy L, Oh JL, et al. Long-term outcomes in patients with isolated supraclavicular nodal recurrence after mastectomy and doxorubicin-based chemotherapy for breast cancer. *Int J Radiat Oncol Biol Phys.* 2011;80(5):1453–1457. doi:10.1016/j.ijrobp.2010.04.015

10. Taghian A, Jeong JH, Mamounas E, et al. Patterns of locoregional failure in patients with operable breast cancer treated by mastectomy and adjuvant chemotherapy with or without tamoxifen and without radiotherapy: results from five national surgical adjuvant breast and bowel project randomized clinical trials. *J Clin Oncol.* 2004;22(21):4247–4254. doi:10.1200/JCO.2004.01.042

11. Recht A, Gray R, Davidson NE, et al. Locoregional failure 10 years after mastectomy and adjuvant chemotherapy with or without tamoxifen without irradiation: experience of the eastern cooperative oncology group. *J Clin Oncol.* 1999;17(6):1689–1700. doi:10.1200/JCO.1999.17.6.1689

12. Cheng SH, Horng CF, Clarke JL, et al. Prognostic index score and clinical prediction model of local regional recurrence after mastectomy in breast cancer patients. *Int J Radiat Oncol Biol Phys.* 2006;64(5):1401–1409. doi:10.1016/j.ijrobp.2005.11.015

13. Nielsen HM, Overgaard M, Grau C, et al. Loco-regional recurrence after mastectomy in high-risk breast cancer--risk and prognosis: an analysis of patients from the DBCG 82 b&c randomization trials. *Radiother Oncol.* 2006;79(2):147–155. doi:10.1016/j.radonc.2006.04.006

14. Wo JY, Taghian AG, Nguyen PL, et al. The association between biological subtype and isolated regional nodal failure after breast-conserving therapy. *Int J Radiat Oncol Biol Phys.* 2010;77(1):188–196. doi:10.1016/j.ijrobp.2009.04.059

15. Warren LE, Ligibel JA, Chen YH, et al. Body mass index and locoregional recurrence in women with early-stage breast cancer. *Ann Surg Oncol.* 2016;23(12):3870–3879. doi:10.1245/s10434-016-5437-3

16. Dershaw DD, McCormick B, Osborne MP. Detection of local recurrence after conservative therapy for breast carcinoma. *Cancer.* 1992;70(2):493–496. doi:10.1002/1097-0142(19920715)70:2<493::AID-CNCR2820700219>3.0.CO;2-3

17. Montgomery DA, Krupa K, Jack WJ, et al. Changing pattern of the detection of locoregional relapse in breast cancer: the Edinburgh experience. *Br J Cancer*. 2007;96(12):1802–1807. doi:10.1038/sj.bjc.6603815

18. Montgomery DA, Krupa K, Cooke TG. Follow-up in breast cancer: does routine clinical examination improve outcome? A systematic review of the literature. *Br J Cancer*. 2007;97(12):1632–1641. doi:10.1038/sj.bjc.6604065

19. National Comprehensive Cancer Network. NCCN clinical practice guidelines in oncology: breast cancer. 2015(5.2020).

20. Halverson KJ, Perez CA, Kuske RR, et al. Survival following locoregional recurrence of breast cancer: univariate and multivariate analysis. *Int J Radiat Oncol Biol Phys*. 1992;23(2):285–291. doi:10.1016/0360-3016(92)90743-2

21. Gage I, Schnitt SJ, Recht A, et al. Skin recurrences after breast-conserving therapy for early-stage breast cancer. *J Clin Oncol*. 1998;16(2):480–486. doi:10.1200/JCO.1998.16.2.480

22. Wapnir IL, Price KN, Anderson SJ, et al. Efficacy of chemotherapy for ER-negative and ER-positive isolated locoregional recurrence of breast cancer: final analysis of the CALOR trial. *J Clin Oncol*. 2018;36(11):1073–1079. doi:10.1200/JCO.2017.76.5719

23. Arthur DW, Winter KA, Kuerer HM, et al. Effectiveness of breast-conserving surgery and 3-dimensional conformal partial breast reirradiation for recurrence of breast cancer in the ipsilateral breast: The NRG oncology/RTOG 1014 Phase 2 Clinical Trial. *JAMA Oncol*. 2019;6(1):75–82. doi:10.1001/jamaoncol.2019.4320

24. Hall EJ, Giaccia AJ. *Radiobiology for the Radiologist*. 8th ed. Wolters Kluwer; 2019.

25. Vernon CC, Hand JW, Field SB, et al. Radiotherapy with or without hyperthermia in the treatment of superficial localized breast cancer: results from five randomized controlled trials. International collaborative hyperthermia group. *Int J Radiat Oncol Biol Phys*. 1996;35(4):731–744. doi:10.1016/0360-3016(96)00154-X

26. Linthorst M, Baaijens M, Wiggenraad R, et al. Local control rate after the combination of re-irradiation and hyperthermia for irresectable recurrent breast cancer: results in 248 patients. *Radiother Oncol*. 2015;117(2):217–222. doi:10.1016/j.radonc.2015.04.019

27. Smith TE, Lee D, Turner BC, et al. True recurrence vs. new primary ipsilateral breast tumor relapse: an analysis of clinical and pathologic differences and their implications in natural history, prognoses, and therapeutic management. *Int J Radiat Oncol Biol Phys*. 2000;48(5):1281–1289. doi:10.1016/S0360-3016(00)01378-X

28. Huang E, Buchholz TA, Meric F, et al. Classifying local disease recurrences after breast conservation therapy based on location and histology: new primary tumors have more favorable outcomes than true local disease recurrences. *Cancer*. 2002;95(10):2059–2067. doi:10.1002/cncr.10952

29. McGrath S, Antonucci J, Goldstein N, et al. Long-term patterns of in-breast failure in patients with early stage breast cancer treated with breast-conserving therapy: a molecular based clonality evaluation. *Am J Clin Oncol*. 2010;33(1):17–22. doi:10.1097/COC.0b013e31819cccc3

30. Poodt IGM, Vugts G, Schipper RJ, Nieuwenhuijzen GAP. Repeat sentinel lymph node biopsy for ipsilateral breast tumor recurrence: a systematic review of the results and impact on prognosis. *Ann Surg Oncol*. 2018;25(5):1329–1339. doi:10.1245/s10434-018-6358-0

31. Kurtz JM, Jacquemier J, Amalric R, et al. Is breast conservation after local recurrence feasible? *Eur J Cancer*. 1991;27(3):240–244. doi:10.1016/0277-5379(91)90505-8

32. Alpert TE, Kuerer HM, Arthur DW, et al. Ipsilateral breast tumor recurrence after breast conservation therapy: outcomes of salvage mastectomy vs. salvage breast-conserving surgery and prognostic factors for salvage breast preservation. *Int J Radiat Oncol Biol Phys*. 2005;63(3):845–851. doi:10.1016/j.ijrobp.2005.02.035

33. Shah C, Wilkinson JB, Jawad M, et al. Outcome after ipsilateral breast tumor recurrence in patients with early-stage breast cancer treated with accelerated partial breast irradiation. *Clin Breast Cancer*. 2012;12(6):392–397. doi:10.1016/j.clbc.2012.09.006

34. Dalberg K, Mattsson A, Sandelin K, Rutqvist LE. Outcome of treatment for ipsilateral breast tumor recurrence in early-stage breast cancer. *Breast Cancer Res Treat*. 1998;49(1):69–78. doi:10.1023/A:1005934513072

35. Kurtz JM, Amalric R, Brandone H, et al. Local recurrence after breast-conserving surgery and radiotherapy: frequency, time course, and prognosis. *Cancer*. 1989;63(10):1912–1917. doi:10.1002/1097-0142(19890515)63:10<1912::AID-CNCR2820631007>3.0.CO;2-Y

36. Jacobson JA, Danforth DN, Cowan KH, et al. Ten-year results of a comparison of conservation with mastectomy in the treatment of stage I and II breast cancer. *N Engl J Med*. 1995;332(14):907–911. doi:10.1056/NEJM199504063321402

37. Voogd AC, van Tienhoven G, Peterse HL, et al. Local recurrence after breast conservation therapy for early stage breast carcinoma: detection, treatment, and outcome in 266 patients. Dutch study group on local recurrence after breast conservation (BORST). *Cancer*. 1999;85(2):437–446. doi:10.1002/(SICI)1097-0142(19990115)85:2<437::AID-CNCR23>3.0.CO;2-1

38. Salvadori B, Marubini E, Miceli R, et al. Reoperation for locally recurrent breast cancer in patients previously treated with conservative surgery. *Br J Surg*. 1999;86(1):84–87. doi:10.1046/j.1365-2168.1999.00961.x

39. Ofuchi T, Amemiya A, Hatayama J. Salvage surgery for patients with ipsilateral breast tumor recurrence after breast-conserving treatment. *Nihon Rinsho*. 2007;65 Suppl 6:439–444.

40. Kurtz JM, Amalric R, Brandone H, et al. Results of salvage surgery for mammary recurrence following breast-conserving therapy. *Ann Surg*. 1988;207(3):347–351. doi:10.1097/00000658-198803000-00021

41. Chen SL, Martinez SR. The survival impact of the choice of surgical procedure after ipsilateral breast cancer recurrence. *Am J Surg*. 2008;196(4):495–499. doi:10.1016/j.amjsurg.2008.06.018

42. Wahl AO, Rademaker A, Kiel KD, et al. Multi-institutional review of repeat irradiation of chest wall and breast for recurrent breast cancer. *Int J Radiat Oncol Biol Phys.* 2008;70(2):477–484. doi:10.1016/j.ijrobp.2007.06.035

43. Chen AM, Yoshizaki T, Velez MA, et al. Tolerance of the brachial plexus to high-dose reirradiation. *Int J Radiat Oncol Biol Phys.* 2017;98(1):83–90. doi:10.1016/j.ijrobp.2017.01.244

44. Fang P. Internal mammary misfortune. *Int J Radiat Oncol Biol Phys.* 2017;97(3):447. doi:10.1016/j.ijrobp.2016.10.032

45. Melotek JM, Chmura SJ. Oligometastasis-directed ablative therapy: a clinical trial question. *Int J Radiat Oncol Biol Phys.* 2017;97(3):448. doi:10.1016/j.ijrobp.2016.10.023

46. Rahimi A, Timmerman R. Ablative therapy: a reasonable approach. *Int J Radiat Oncol Biol Phys.* 2017;97(3):448–449. doi:10.1016/j.ijrobp.2016.10.028

47. Angervall L, Enzinger FM. Extraskeletal neoplasm resembling ewing's sarcoma. *Cancer.* 1975;36:240–251. doi:10.1002/1097-0142(197507)36:1<240::AID-CNCR2820360127>3.0.CO;2-H

48. Schwarz GS, Grobmyer SR, Djohan RS, et al. Axillary reverse mapping and lymphaticovenous bypass: lymphedema prevention through enhanced lymphatic visualization and restoration of flow. *J Surg Oncol.* 2019;120(2):160–167. doi:10.1002/jso.25513

V ■ THORACIC

Sarah S. Kilic, Gaurav Marwaha, Kevin L. Stephans, and Gregory M. M. Videtic

QUICK HIT ■ Surgical resection is the standard of care for operable early-stage NSCLC. For medically inoperable patients, SBRT is the standard of care. For high-risk operable patients, given the absence of completed randomized trials, there is controversy regarding whether surgery or SBRT is the preferred option with regard to the endpoint of overall survival (see Table 27.1).

Table 27.1: General Treatment Paradigm for Early-Stage NSCLC

	Operable			Medically Inoperable (FEV1 <40%, DLCO <40%)
	Surgery	CHT	RT	
Stage IA (cT1a-bN0)	Lobectomy + mediastinal LND	No (unless in Japan)	No PORT (except for positive margins or pN2*)	SBRT *Peripheral: 60 Gy/3 fx (54 Gy with heterogeneity correction), 50 Gy/5 fx, 48 Gy/4 fx, 34 Gy/1 fx, 30 Gy/1 fx (without heterogeneity correction)*
Stage IB (cT2aN0)		Debatable (LACE meta-analysis)		
IIA and select IIB (cT2bN0, cT3N0)		Yes (LACE meta-analysis)		*Central: 50 (-60) Gy/5 fx (RTOG 0813)*

*Controversial given preliminary results of LungART; see Chapter 28.

EPIDEMIOLOGY: Lung cancer is the most common noncutaneous cancer worldwide, the second most common in the United States, and the leading cause of cancer mortality in the United States with an estimated 228,820 new cases and 135,720 deaths annually.[1] NSCLC comprises ~80% of all lung cancers, and 15% to 20% of NSCLC patients present with early-stage disease.

RISK FACTORS: Smoking, radon, asbestos, family history, pulmonary fibrosis, occupational exposures (silica, cadmium, arsenic, beryllium, diesel exhaust, coal soot).

ANATOMY: Lobes in both lungs separated by the oblique fissure, right lung also separated by the horizontal fissure. Trachea starts at C3/4, carina at T5. Nodal stations range from 1 to 14; see atlas by Lynch.[2]

PATHOLOGY

- *Adenocarcinoma*: Most common histology, 38% of all lung cancers. Majority are peripheral. Bronchioloalveolar carcinoma (subtype of adenocarcinoma) arises from type II pneumocytes, grows along alveolar septa, and has a long natural history.
- *Squamous*: ~20% of all lung cancers. Majority are central.
- *SCC*: Thirteen percent of all lung cancers, almost always associated with smoking (see Chapter 29).
- *Other*: Consists of other rare histologies and other neuroendocrine carcinomas such as large cell or carcinoid.

GENETICS: Greater than 95% of clinically-relevant mutations are found in adenocarcinomas. EGFR is a transmembrane tyrosine kinase mutated in ~17% of NSCLC. These mutants are targetable with TKIs such as osimertinib, erlotinib, gefitinib, and afatinib. ALK rearrangements are found in ~5% of NSCLC. These mutants are associated with younger age and never smokers; these respond to TKIs like crizotinib, alectinib, and ceritinib. *ROS-1* mutations are seen in 1% to 2% of NSCLC and can respond to crizotinib.[3] *BRAF V600E, MET, RET, and KRAS* are emerging driver mutations that are thought to respond to vemurafenib, crizotinib, cabozantinib, and sotorasib, respectively.

SCREENING: USPSTF criteria: screen with low-dose CT for patients ages 50 to 80 and ≥20 pack-year smoker and cessation <15 years ago. Of note, the recent International Lung Screening Trial, currently reported as abstract only, suggests that additional screening criteria based on clinical features such as age, race, education, and BMI may be more sensitive than current USPSTF criteria.[4]

CLINICAL PRESENTATION: Cough, dyspnea, wheeze, stridor, hemoptysis, anorexia, weight loss, decline in performance status, paraneoplastic syndromes such as hypercalcemia from PTHrP (SCC) or hypertrophic osteoarthropathy.

WORKUP: H&P. PFT: See ACCP guidelines for details.[5] Medical inoperability used on trials to define criteria for SBRT (Indiana University criteria): baseline FEV1 <40% predicted, predicted post-op FEV1 <30% predicted, DLCO <40% predicted, pO_2 <70 mmHg, pCO_2 >50 mmHg, exercise oxygen consumption <50% predicted. Preoperative cardiac workup if necessary.

Labs: CBC, CMP.

Imaging: CT chest (with contrast if evaluating nodes), consider CT abdomen for metastatic workup but at least review liver and adrenal on CT chest, PET scan. "Pathologic" lymph nodes defined as short-axis diameter >1.0 cm and "bulky" lymphadenopathy as short axis >3.0 cm, multiple matted nodes, radiographic ECE or ≥3 stations involved. MRI of thoracic inlet for superior sulcus tumors and octreotide scan for carcinoid. MRI brain for stage II or higher (NCCN 2017); consider MRI brain for central stage IB (NCCN optional recommendation); otherwise, brain imaging unnecessary unless neurological symptoms are present. CT brain with contrast sufficient if MRI is not feasible.[6]

Procedures: Biopsy indicated (EBUS, CT-guided, or thoracentesis depending on location/presence of effusion; sputum pathology is unreliable but at least 3 needed to be negative). EBUS/mediastinoscopy to confirm positive nodes on CT or PET and for all T3 or central T1–2 tumors (see Table 27.2). EBUS allows sampling of stations 2, 4, 7, and 10. Mediastinoscopy allows sampling of 2, 4, and 7. Chamberlain procedure or VATS are required to reach stations 5 and 6. EUS required for stations 8 and 9.

PROGNOSTIC FACTORS: Stage, weight loss >5% in 3 months, KPS <90, age >70, +LVSI, marital status.

STAGING

Table 27.2: AJCC 8th Edition (2017): Staging for Lung Cancer						
T/M	N		cN0	cN1	cN2	cN3
T1	≤1 cm[1]		IA1	IIB	IIIA	IIIB
	1.1–2 cm		IA2			
	2.1–3 cm		IA3			
T2[2]	3.1–4 cm		IB			
	4.1–5 cm		IIA			
T3	5.1–7 cm Invasion[3] Same lobe nodules		IIB	IIIA	IIIB	IIIC
T4	>7 cm Invasion[4] Separate lobe nodules					
M1a	• Separate nodules in contralateral lobe • Pleural nodules • Malignant pleural/pericardial effusion		IVA			
M1b	• Single extrathoracic metastasis in single organ • Single non-regional lymph node					
M1c	• Multiple extrathoracic metastases		IVB			

Notes: ≤1 cm[1]: or rare superficial spreading tumor with invasive component limited to bronchial wall. T2[2]: or involves main bronchus, but not carina, invades visceral pleura, or atelectasis or obstructive pneumonitis extending to hilar region. Invasion[3]: Invasion of parietal pleura, chest wall, phrenic nerve, or parietal pericardium. Invasion[4]: Invasion of diaphragm, mediastinum, great vessels, trachea, carina, recurrent laryngeal nerve, esophagus, or vertebral body.
cN1, Ipsilateral peribronchial and/or ipsilateral hilar LNs (stations 10–14); cN2, ipsilateral mediastinal and/or subcarinal LNs (stations 2–9); cN3, contralateral mediastinal, hilar, or any scalene or supraclavicular LNs (station 1).

TREATMENT PARADIGM

Observation: "Active surveillance" is not an established option for NSCLC because even in medically-inoperable patients, lung cancer–specific mortality is 53%.[7] Therefore, postponement of treatment is generally inappropriate unless the lesion is too small to diagnose (see following).

Solitary Pulmonary Nodule: Discrete opacity in lung parenchyma ≤3 cm (>3 cm is "mass," and malignancy until proven otherwise). Differential includes granuloma, abscess, fungal infection, hamartoma, tuberculosis, metastasis, lymphoma, and carcinoid. Factors associated with malignancy: faster growth rate, lack of calcifications, greater size, spiculated (vs. smooth or lobulated) margins, air bronchograms, solid appearance (vs. ground glass), contrast enhancement, high SUV. If ≥8 mm, consider PET/CT or biopsy, see NCCN for additional size-specific follow-up guidelines. Lung-RADS is evolving standardization system for follow-up of indeterminate nodules on lung cancer screening CT reporting.

Surgery: Standard treatment for medically-operable patients. Lobectomy superior to wedge/segmentectomy. VATS lobectomy comparable to open lobectomy.[8] For accurate staging, mediastinal LN dissection should be performed. Preoperative medical workup including PFTs (see Workup) and cardiac clearance necessary.

Chemotherapy: See LACE pooled analysis in the following. Generally no role for stage I. Note also that uracil–tegafur has been shown to be beneficial in the Japanese population, but is not used in the United States due to nonreproducible results.[9]

RFA: Placement of electrode in tumor with ablative heating. Retrospective series have reported complete radiographic responses from 38% to 93% with relapse rates from 8% to 43%. Factors associated with CR include smaller tumors, metastases, and ablation zone 4× tumor diameter. Pneumothorax is a risk associated with the procedure.

Radiation

Indications: Historically, fractionated RT was standard treatment for medically-inoperable patients, with results inferior to surgery. SBRT, however, may be comparable to surgery, and is now the treatment of choice (rather than wedge or RFA) for medically-inoperable patients. Adjuvant RT is not indicated in completely resected stage I/II patients (although Italian trial by Trodella et al. does show benefit; other trials have not).

Dose: Common fractionation schemes for SBRT include 54 Gy/3 fx with heterogeneity correction or 60 Gy/3 fx without heterogeneity correction, given with an interfraction interval of 40 hours to 7 days, with an overall treatment time of 8 to 14 days. 50 Gy/5 daily fx is the Japanese standard, and is standard for central tumors; 50Gy/5 every-other-day fractions is also utilized for central tumors, 60Gy/5fx and 60Gy/8fx have also been used.[10] Post-op dose is 54 to 60 Gy for microscopically (R1) positive margins and ≥60 Gy for macroscopically (R2) positive margins.[9]

Toxicity: Acute: Fatigue. Rarely, cough, pneumonitis, esophagitis, subacute chest wall pain. Late: Radiation pneumonitis, chest wall pain. On average, PFTs remain stable (some improve, some decrease, often related to baseline comorbidity).

Procedure: See *Handbook of Treatment Planning in Radiation Oncology*, Chapter 6.[11]

■ EVIDENCE-BASED Q&A

SCREENING AND STAGING

■ **Is there benefit to routine radiographic screening for lung cancer? Which patients should be screened?**

Previously, routine screening with CXR or sputum cytology had not been shown to reduce mortality. The National Lung Screening Trial was paradigm-changing and led to the revision of NCCN and USPSTF guidelines.

National Lung Screening Trial (*NEJM* **2011, PMID 21714641**): PRT of 54,454 patients at high risk for lung cancer randomized to three annual screenings with either low dose CT or single-view PA CXR.

Results: There were 247 vs. 309 deaths from lung cancer per 100,000 person-years in low dose CT group vs. CXR group, representing relative reduction in mortality from lung cancer of 20% ($p = .004$). Rate of death from any cause was also reduced by 6.7% ($p = .02$) in low-dose CT group compared to CXR group. Notably, false positive rate was 96.4% in low-dose CT group and 94.5% in CXR group, but majority of false positives (>90%) were observed with serial imaging and did not result in unnecessary procedures. Number needed to screen with low-dose CT to prevent 1 lung cancer death was 320. **Conclusion: CT screening reduces mortality from lung cancer.**

■ **What defines "early-stage" lung cancer? Why is it important to investigate the mediastinum?**

Early stage is typically defined as stage I or II, but treatment decision-making is based on presence or absence of nodal involvement. Therefore, careful staging of mediastinum is necessary. PET/CT has sensitivity of 79% (CT staging 60%),[11] but investigation of the mediastinum via either mediastinoscopy or EBUS can improve this.

■ **What is the difference between mediastinoscopy and EBUS? What is the sensitivity and specificity of either approach or a combination?**

Mediastinoscopy is the historical standard for evaluation of regional lymph nodes, but EBUS has advantages of being less invasive and providing access to station 10 (hilar nodes). Accurate clinical staging is important to avoid unnecessary thoracotomies: that is, those who will need CHT and/or RT anyway and would not benefit from surgery. Historically, 25% to 30% of thoracotomies were unnecessary due to incomplete clinical staging.

Annema, ASTER Trial (*JAMA* 2010, PMID 21098770): PRT of 241 patients with resectable NSCLC randomized to mediastinoscopy or EUS-FNA/EBUS followed by mediastinoscopy if no nodes found. All patients without evidence of mediastinal tumor spread then underwent thoracotomy with lymph node dissection. Primary outcome was sensitivity for N2/N3 metastases. All patients received PET/CT up-front, and known N2-3 patients excluded. Results: Sensitivity of mediastinoscopy: 79%, EBUS: 85%, EUS-FNA/EBUS followed by mediastinoscopy: 94%. Unnecessary thoracotomies: 18% (mediastinoscopy) vs. 7% (EUS-FNA/EBUS). **Conclusion: EUS-FNA/EBUS plus mediastinoscopy resulted in fewer unnecessary thoracotomies and increased sensitivity for nodal metastases compared to mediastinoscopy or EBUS alone.**

MEDICALLY OPERABLE PATIENTS

■ **What is the surgery of choice? Is wedge resection sufficient?**

Ginsberg showed that wedge is inferior local therapy to lobectomy and that distant metastases are the driver of cancer-related death.

Ginsberg (*Ann Thorac Surg* 1995, PMID 7677489): PRT of 247 patients comparing limited resection (segmentectomy or wedge resection) vs. lobectomy in peripheral T1N0 NSCLC. RML tumors were excluded due to the small size of this lobe. At least 2 cm of normal lung tissue was required to be resected. Note: Patients were randomized intraoperatively. Forty percent of patients who were registered (but ultimately not enrolled) had benign disease. **Conclusion: Lobectomy is surgery of choice (see Table 27.3).**

Table 27.3: Results of Ginsberg Trial of Limited vs. Lobar Surgery for Early-Stage Lung Cancer				
	LRR	**Nonlocal Recurrence**	**Death With Cancer**	**Death From All Causes**
Limited Resection	17%	14%	25%	39%
Lobectomy	6%	12%	17%	30%
P value	.008	.672	.094	.088

■ **Can we improve surgical outcomes with sublobar resection + brachytherapy?**

Although the following ACOSOG trial was negative, it is useful to note that "modern" wedge resection is better than wedge resection in era of Ginsberg.

Fernando, ACOSOG Z4032 (*JCO*** 2014, PMID 24982457):** PRT of wedge resection ± I-125 mesh brachytherapy for medically high-risk patients. Results: The crude LF rate, defined by staple-line, lobar or hilar nodal failure, was 7.7%. There were no differences in time to LR or types of LR between arms. Moreover, in patients with a potentially compromised margin (margin <1 cm, margin-to-tumor ratio <1, positive staple-line cytology, or wedge resection nodule size >2.0 cm), brachytherapy did not reduce LF. 3-year OS was 71% in both arms. **Conclusion: Brachytherapy does not reduce local recurrence after sublobar resection, but the risk of recurrence is low in the modern era.**

■ **Which patients with early-stage lung cancer may benefit from adjuvant postoperative RT (PORT)?**

PORT is not indicated in completely resected stage I-II patients. Refer to PORT meta-analysis in Chapter 28, which showed a detriment to routine PORT for patients without N2 disease. The Trodella study discussed next is notable because it did show a benefit in stage I, but this is not routine practice, as it has not been reproduced.

Trodella, Italian Trial (*Radiother Oncol*** 2002, PMID 11830308):** PRT of adjuvant RT vs. observation in 104 patients with completely resected (R0) pathologic stage I NSCLC. RT was 50.4 Gy/28 fx. Target volume included the bronchial stump and ipsilateral hilum. Results: There were no treatment-related deaths. 5-year DFS favored the RT arm (71% vs. 60%, p = .039). 5-year OS favored RT arm as well (67% vs. 58%, p = .048). **Conclusion: Adjuvant RT may be safe and beneficial in terms of DFS and OS in select stage I patients.**

■ **Which patients benefit from adjuvant CHT?**

Adjuvant CHT should be considered for stage II patients based on the LACE meta-analysis. Stage IB is debatable; the CALGB study (see following) suggested a benefit for tumors ≥4 cm (included in LACE analysis).The Japanese study showed a benefit to uracil-tegafur, but is not used in the United States.[8]

Pignon, LACE Pooled Analysis (*JCO*** 2008, PMID 18506026):** Pooled individual data from 4,584 patients included on 5 PRTs of adjuvant CHT in NSCLC. MFU 5.2 years. Results: Overall HR of death was 0.89 (p = .005), corresponding to 5-yr absolute benefit of 5.4%. Benefit varied with stage: detrimental for stage IA (HR 1.4), nonsignificant for IB (HR 0.93), and beneficial for stage II (HR 0.83) and III (HR 0.8). Benefit was higher in patients with better performance status. Type of CHT, sex, age, histology, type of surgery, planned RT, and dose of cisplatin were not associated with outcome. **Conclusion: CHT confers a survival advantage in stage II/III NSCLC. IB controversial—there may be subset who benefit based on size of primary (CALGB 9633). IA not indicated (except in Japan[8]).**

One notable study that was included in the LACE analysis:

Strauss, CALGB 9633 (*JCO*** 2008, PMID 18809614):** PRT of adjuvant paclitaxel (200 mg/m[2]) and carboplatin (AUC 6) day 1 every 3 weeks × 4 cycles vs. observation in completely resected stage IB NSCLC. 384 patients randomized. Results: 3-year OS was 79% vs. 70% favoring CHT (p = .045). No difference in 5-year OS (60% vs. 57%, p = .32). **Subgroup analysis showed that for tumors ≥4 cm, there was improved DFS (median DFS 96 vs. 63 months) and OS (MS 99 vs. 77 months) with CHT. Conclusion: Although trial initially closed early after planned interim analysis, 5-year data showed no significant OS benefit. However, for patients with tumors ≥4cm, CHT may improve OS.**

MEDICALLY INOPERABLE

■ **What are the outcomes with conventional RT for early NSCLC?**

Historically, medically inoperable patients received conventionally-fractionated definitive RT to 50–60 Gy or supportive care only. Conventional RT provided LC in the range of 40% to 60%, with 30% to 40% of patients dying of lung cancer within 2 years.[12] There was some evidence for benefit of dose escalation to 70.2 Gy and hypofractionation (60 Gy/15 fx), but ultimately, as technology improved, SBRT has rendered previous forms of definitive RT obsolete in most cases.

Cheung, NCIC CTG BR.25 (*JNCI*** 2014, PMID 25074417):** Multi-institution phase II trial of 80 patients with T1-T3N0 NSCLC treated to 60 Gy/15 fx using 3D-CRT (no IMRT) without heterogeneity correction. GTV was tumor only; PTV was 1.5 cm margin (could be decreased to 1.0 cm in transverse plane if close to critical structures). Primary endpoint was 2-year tumor control. MFU 49 months. Results: 2-year primary tumor control rate was 87.4%, and 2-year OS was 68.7%; 2-year regional relapse rate was 8.8% and distant relapse rate was 21.6%. Most common grade 3+ toxicities were fatigue (6.3%), cough (7.5%), dyspnea (13.8%), and pneumonitis (10.0%). **Conclusion: Conformal RT to 60 Gy/15 fx using 3D-CRT results in favorable LC and OS without severe toxicities.**

Nyman, SPACE Trial (*Radiother Oncol* 2016, PMID 27600155): Randomized phase II trial of 102 medically inoperable patients with Stage I NSCLC comparing SBRT (66 Gy/3 fx over 1 week) and 3D-CRT (70 Gy/35 fx over 7 weeks). MFU 37 months. Results: No difference between 1-, 2-, and 3-year PFS with: SBRT: 76%, 53%, 42% and 3D-CRT: 87%, 54%, 42%. By end of study, 70% of SBRT patients had not progressed compared to 59% of 3D-CRT (*p* = .26). Toxicity was lower in SBRT patients (pneumonitis: 19% [SBRT] and 34% [3DCRT, *p* = .26]; esophagitis: 8% [SBRT] and 30% [3DCRT, *p* = .006]). **Conclusion: No difference in PFS or OS, but trend toward improved control rate in SBRT group with better quality of life and lower toxicity, so SBRT should be standard.**

Ball, TROG 09.02 CHISEL (*Lancet Oncol* 2019, PMID 30770291): International multicenter PRT of 101 medically inoperable patients with PET-diagnosed, bx-confirmed, peripheral T1–T2aN0 NSCLC randomized 2:1 to SBRT (54 Gy/3 fx or 48 Gy/4 fx if <2 cm from chest wall) or conventional fractionation (66 Gy/33 fx or 50 Gy/20 fx per institutional preference). Primary endpoint: time to local treatment failure. MFU 2.6 years SBRT, 2.1 years conventional. Results: 14% of SBRT patients progressed locally vs. 31% of conventional patients; 39% in SBRT group died vs. 62% of conventional patients. Freedom from local failure (HR 0.32, *p* = .0077) improved in SBRT group. Median freedom from local failure and median lung cancer-specific survival were not calculable in either group. No significant differences in patient-reported symptoms or functioning. See additional results in Table 27.4. **Conclusion: In inoperable patients with peripheral Stage I NSCLC, SBRT yields better LC compared to conventional fractionation with mildly increased toxicities at ~2 years of follow-up and improves OS.**

Table 27.4: Results of TROG 09.02 CHISEL Randomized Trial			
	SBRT	**Conventional fractionation**	**Measure of significance**
Median OS (years)	5.0	3.0	HR 0.53, *p* = .027
2-yr LC	89%	65%	Not provided
2-yr local failure	10%	26%	Not provided
2-yr OS	77%	59%	Not provided
Number of grade 3+ AEs (*n*)	8	2	Not provided

■ What trials defined the role of SBRT?

SBRT, formally defined as high dose per fraction delivered in ≤5 fractions, was first developed in Sweden. Dr. Timmerman at Indiana University led a dose-escalation trial in 2003, which then led to a phase II trial discovering high rate of central toxicity for 60 Gy/3 fx. In 2002, RTOG 0236 opened, which defined the role of SBRT for early peripheral lesions. Since there is debate regarding the value of surgery, RTOG 0618 investigated SBRT for operable patients, reserving surgery for salvage if needed. Since central tumors are considered high risk using 60 Gy/3 fx (but not with 50 Gy/5 fx), RTOG 0813 studied safety and dose escalation for central tumors starting at 50 Gy/5 fx and going to 60 Gy/5 fx. RTOG 0915 investigated single-fraction SBRT for peripheral lesions.

Timmerman, Indiana (*Chest* 2003, PMID 14605072): Phase I dose-escalation trial of extracranial stereotactic radioablation (ESR) in 37 patients with T1-2N0 biopsy-confirmed NSCLC. Initial dose was 24 Gy/3 fx and increased to tolerated dose 60 Gy/3 fx. Abdominal compression was used to decrease respiratory motion. MFU 15.2 months. Results: 87% response rate (27% CR). Six patients experienced LF, all receiving doses <18 Gy/fx. One patient (treated at 14 Gy/fx) developed symptomatic pneumonitis. **Conclusion: ESR is feasible and results in good response rates.**

Timmerman, Central Toxicity (*JCO* 2006, PMID 17050868; Update *IJROBP* 2009, PMID 19251380): Phase II trial of 70 medically inoperable patients with cT1-2N0 NSCLC treated with SBRT 60-66 Gy/3 fx over 1 to 2 weeks. MFU 50.2 months. Results: 3-year LC 88%. Nodal and distant recurrence rates were 9% and 13%, respectively. MS 32.4 months. 3-year CSS 82%, 3-year OS 43%. MS for T1 vs. T2 tumors was 39 vs. 24.5 months, respectively ($p = .019$). Tumor size or location did not impact control outcomes. Grades 3+ toxicity occurred in 10% of patients with peripheral tumors and 27% of patients with central tumors. **Conclusion: High LC rates with this regimen, but high toxicity for central tumors.**

Onishi, Japan (*JTO* 2007, PMID 17603311): RR of 257 patients (either medically-inoperable or refusing surgery) from 14 institutions treated with SBRT. 164 T1N0, 93 T2N0, all tumors <6 cm, all tumor locations included. MFU 38 months. Median BED_{10} was 111 Gy; 5.4% of patients had grade 3+ pulmonary toxicity; 14% of patients had local progression. LR 8% vs. 43% for BED > 100 Gy vs. < 100 Gy ($p < .001$); 5-year OS for medically operable patients refusing surgery was 71% for BED ≥ 100 Gy and 30% for BED < 100 Gy ($p < .05$). **Conclusion: SBRT is safe and effective for stage I lung cancer. With BED ≥ 100 Gy, LC is excellent and 5-year OS for *medically operable* patients is similar to surgical series (compare with 70% OS in Ginsburg for lobectomy of only stage IA patients).**

■ **All of the preceding trials come from single institutions. Are there any cooperative group data?**

RTOG 0236 is the most notable cooperative SBRT trial.

Timmerman, RTOG 0236 (*JAMA* 2010, PMID 20233825; Update *JAMA Oncol* 2018, PMID 29852036): Phase II multi-institutional study of SBRT for medically inoperable stage I/II NSCLC (peripheral location, T1/T2 N0, tumors < 5 cm). EBUS not required. 55 evaluable patients, MFU 48 months. Prescription was 60Gy/3fx, though later analysis showed dose actually 54Gy/3fx (with significant variation depending on lung density and tumor size and location) after accounting for heterogeneity. Treatment duration was ≥8 and <14 days. Results: grade 3 and 4 adverse events 27% and 3.6%. No grade 5 adverse events at 5 years. See Table 27.5 for oncologic outcomes. **Conclusion: Patients with medically inoperable NSCLC treated with SBRT had a modest survival, high rates of local tumor control, and moderate treatment-related morbidity. Longer term follow-up has shown increased lobar and regional failures.**

Table 27.5: Outcomes from RTOG 0236	Initial Results (3-Yr)	Long-Term Results (5-Yr)
OS	56%	40%
DFS	48%	26%
MS	48 months	48 months
LC	98%	93%
Lobar control	91%	80%
LRC	87%	75%
Distant Failure	22%	24%

■ **Is SBRT an appropriate option for medically operable patients?**

SBRT is not standard. Multiple trials investigating this question have closed early due to poor accrual. Several analyses attempt to answer this question while we await additional randomized data.

Chang, Pooled Analysis of STARS and ROSEL (*Lancet Oncol* 2015, PMID 25981812): Pooled analysis of two independent phase III PRT of SBRT vs. lobectomy and mediastinal lymph node dissection, which closed early due to slow accrual. Total of 58 patients. Six surgery patients died compared to one SBRT patient. 3-year OS 95% in SBRT group vs. 79% in surgery group (HR 0.14, $p = .037$). RFS was similar: 86% SBRT vs. 80% surgery, $p = .54$. Grade 3+ events were 10% for SBRT compared to 44% for surgery, with one postoperative death. **Conclusion: SBRT appears viable in medically operable patients, but additional PRTs are warranted.**

Onishi, Japan (*IJROBP* 2011, PMID 20638194): Review of outcomes for *medically operable subset*. MFU 55 months. Cumulative LC rates for T1 and T2 tumors at 5 years after SBRT were 92% and 73%, respectively. Pulmonary complications above grade 2 arose in 1 patient (1.1%, grade 3). 5-year OS for stage IA and IB was 72% and 62%, respectively. One patient who developed local recurrence safely underwent salvage surgery. **Conclusion: SBRT is safe and promising for operable stage I NSCLC, with survival rate approximating that for surgery.**

Zheng, Meta-analysis (*IJROBP* 2014, PMID 25052562): Study-level meta-analysis of 7,071 patients treated with surgery or SBRT (BED ≥ 100). Median age for SBRT and surgery were 74 and 66. MFU 28 months for SBRT and 37 months for surgery. OS rates at 1, 3, and 5 years for SBRT vs. lobectomy were 83% vs. 92%, 56% vs. 77%, and 41% vs. 66%. After adjustment for proportion of operable patients and age, SBRT and surgery have comparable DFS and OS. **Conclusion: SBRT appears comparable to surgery for medically operable patients.**

Timmerman, RTOG 0618 (*JAMA* 2018, PMID 29852037): Single-arm phase II study of SBRT for patients with operable Stage I/II NSCLC (peripheral location, T1-3N0 < 5 cm). Treatment was 54 Gy/3 fx. Primary end point was tumor control. Early surgical salvage was planned per protocol in the event of a LR. Secondary end points: survival, adverse events, incidence and outcome of surgical salvage. Results: 33 patients with MFU of 48.1 months. 4-year LRC rate was 88%, and distant failure was 12%; 4-year DFS 57%, and OS 56%. Median DFS and OS were 55.2 months. **Conclusion: SBRT appears to be associated with high tumor control rates and infrequent need for surgical salvage.**

■ **Can SBRT be delivered safely in a single fraction?**

Yes. Mature Phase II data demonstrate durable safety and efficacy.

Videtic, RTOG 0915 (*IJROBP* 2015, PMID 26530743; Update *IJROBP* 2019, PMID 30513377): Randomized phase II study of 94 (84 evaluable) medically inoperable, biopsy-proven, peripheral, T1-2N0 by PET comparing 34 Gy/1 fx (arm 1) to 48 Gy/4 fx (arm 2). Primary outcome: rate of grade 3+ AEs. Secondary endpoints: LC, OS, and PFS. MFU 4 years (6 years for those still living); 3% of patients in arm 1 vs. 11% in arm 2 with grade 3+ AEs. See Table 27.6 for oncologic outcomes. **Conclusion: For medically inoperable peripheral T1-2N0 NSCLC, 34 Gy/1 fx and 48 Gy/4 fx offer comparable toxicities and primary tumor control rates. MS of ~4 years in each arm is comparable to RTOG 0236. OS was lower in arm 1, though study was not powered for OS. Both regimens may be appropriate in this population, though prospective validation needed.**

Table 27.6: Outcomes of RTOG 0915		
	Arm 1 (34 Gy in 1 fx)	**Arm 2 (48 Gy in 4 fx)**
Grade 3+ AE	3%	11%
Median survival (years)	4.1	4.6
5-yr local failure	11%	7%
5-yr OS	30%	41%
5-yr PFS	19%	33%
5-yr distant failure	38%	41%

Singh, Roswell Park 1509 (*IJROBP* 2019, PMID 31445956): A total of 98 medically inoperable peripheral cT1-T2N0 NSCLC by PET comparing 30 Gy/1 fx (arm 1) to 60 Gy/3 fx (arm 2). Primary endpoint: frequency of grade 3 or higher AEs. Secondary end points: LC, OS, PFS, QOL. Results: MFU 54 months. Incidence of AEs 17% in arm 1, 15% in arm 2. No higher grade AEs. No SS difference in: 2-year OS (73% vs. 62%), 2-year PFS (65% vs. 50%), or 2-year LC (95% vs. 97%), though T2a had poorer OS on MVA. Regarding QOL, no significant differences in overall global health or PFTs; arm 1 had better dyspnea and social functioning. **CONCLUSION: No differences between single vs. three fraction regimens in OS, LC, PFS, or lung function; some toxicities improved in single-fraction regimen.**

■ What data exist regarding the safety of SBRT for central lung tumors?

Central location was originally defined as within 2 cm of the proximal bronchial tree by Timmerman,[12] though other definitions of centrality and "ultracentrality" exist, as in the studies following, which found significant toxicity associated with the treatment of central or ultracentral tumors.

Bezjak, RTOG 0813 (*JCO* 2019, PMID 30943123): Phase I/II study of maximum tolerated dose (MTD) and efficacy of SBRT for cT1-2 (<5 cm) N0 NSCLC in medically inoperable patients. Centrality defined as tumors within 2 cm of the tracheal–bronchial tree or immediately adjacent to mediastinal or pericardial pleura (where PTV would touch the pleura). Dose started at 50 Gy/5 fx and was escalated by 0.5 Gy/fx increments to 60 Gy/5 fx every other day over 1.5 to 2 weeks. MTD defined as dose at which probability of DLT (any treatment-related grade 3+ AE within 1st year) is closest to 20% without exceeding it. Results: 120 patients with MFU 37.9 months. MTD was 12 Gy/fx, and DLT in this group was 7.2%. No patients receiving 11 Gy/fx or lower had DLTs; 12% of patients in both 11.5 and 12 Gy groups had DLTs; 2-year LC, PFS, and OS with 11.5 Gy/fx was 89%, 52%, and 68% vs. 88%, 55%, and 73% with 12 Gy/fx (all NS). **Conclusion: For SBRT, 60 Gy/5fx is associated with clinically significant incidence of DLT, but also with excellent local control at 2 years.** *Note: This trial used a broader definition of centrality than the original Timmerman definition.*

Lindberg, Nordic HILUS (*IASLC* 2017, Abstract Only): Prospective phase II trial of 74 patients treated with SBRT for central (≤1 cm from proximal bronchial tree, but not eroding wall of mainstem bronchi) tumors ≤5 cm, either NSCLC or metastasis from extrapulmonary primary. Subclassified by tumor location: near trachea or main bronchus (42 patients) or lobar bronchus (31 patients). Treatment was 56 Gy/8 fx. Primary outcome: Toxicity. Results: 88% of patients had any toxicity, and 28% had grade 3+ toxicity, including seven patients with grade 5 toxicities (six fatal hemoptysis, one fatal pneumonitis). Grade 4–5 toxicities more common in the main bronchus group (19%) than lobar bronchus group (3%). **Conclusion: Risk of serious or fatal toxicity with SBRT for central tumors, particularly those near the main bronchi, is significant.**

Tekatli, Netherlands (*JTO* 2016, PMID 27013408): A total of 47 patients, either medically inoperable or unfit for chemoRT, with "ultracentral" (defined as PTV overlapping trachea or main bronchi) NSCLC treated with 60 Gy/12 fx (BED_{10} = 90 Gy). MFU 29 months, MS 16 months, and 3-year OS 20%. No isolated local recurrences. 38% of patients had grade 3+ toxicity, including 21% with "possible" or "likely" death related to treatment. 15% of patients died of fatal pulmonary hemorrhage. **Conclusion: High rates of grade 3+ toxicity, including high number of grade 5 toxicities, for patients with ultracentral tumors receiving SBRT.**

REFERENCES

1. Siegel RL MK, Jemal A. Cancer statistics, 2020. *CA Cancer J Clin.* 2020;70(1):7–30. doi:10.3322/caac.21590
2. Lynch R, Pitson G, Ball D, Claude L, Sarrut D. Computed tomographic atlas for the new international lymph node map for lung cancer: a radiation oncologist perspective. *Pract Radiat Oncol.* 2013;3(1):54–66. doi:10.1016/j.prro.2012.01.007
3. Shaw AT, Ou SH, Bang YJ, et al. Crizotinib in ROS1-rearranged non-small-cell lung cancer. *N Engl J Med.* 2014;371(21):1963–1971. doi:10.1056/NEJMoa1406766
4. Lam S MR, Ruparel M, Atkar-Khattra S, et al. *Lung cancer screenee selection by USPSTF versus PLCOm2012 criteria - interim list findings.* IASLC 2019 World Conference on Lung Cancer; 2019. doi:10.1016/j.jtho.2019.08.055
5. Brunelli A, Kim AW, Berger KI, Addrizzo-Harris DJ. Physiologic evaluation of the patient with lung cancer being considered for resectional surgery: diagnosis and management of lung cancer, 3rd ed: American College of Chest Physicians evidence-based clinical practice guidelines. *Chest.* 2013;143(5 Suppl):e166S–e190S. doi:10.1378/chest.12-2395
6. Yokoi K, Kamiya N, Matsuguma H, et al. Detection of brain metastasis in potentially operable non-small cell lung cancer: a comparison of CT and MRI. *Chest.* 1999;115(3):714–719. doi:10.1378/chest.115.3.714
7. McGarry RC, Song G, des Rosiers P, Timmerman R. Observation-only management of early stage, medically inoperable lung cancer: poor outcome. *Chest.* 2002;121(4):1155–1158. doi:10.1378/chest.121.4.1155
8. Yan TD, Black D, Bannon PG, McCaughan BC. Systematic review and meta-analysis of randomized and nonrandomized trials on safety and efficacy of video-assisted thoracic surgery lobectomy for early-stage non-small-cell lung cancer. *J Clin Oncol.* 2009;27(15):2553–2562. doi:10.1200/JCO.2008.18.2733

9. Kato H, Ichinose Y, Ohta M, et al. A randomized trial of adjuvant chemotherapy with uracil-tegafur for adenocarcinoma of the lung. *N Engl J Med*. 2004;350(17):1713–1721. doi:10.1056/NEJMoa032792

10. Lagerwaard FJ, Verstegen NE, Haasbeek CJ, et al. Outcomes of stereotactic ablative radiotherapy in patients with potentially operable stage I non-small cell lung cancer. *Int J Radiat Oncol Biol Phys*. 2012;83(1):348–353. doi:10.1016/j.ijrobp.2011.06.2003

11. Videtic GMM, Woody N, Vassil AD. *Handbook of Treatment Planning in Radiation Oncology*. 3rd ed. Demos Medical; 2020. doi:10.1891/9780826168429

12. Timmerman R, McGarry R, Yiannoutsos C, et al. Excessive toxicity when treating central tumors in a phase II study of stereotactic body radiation therapy for medically inoperable early-stage lung cancer. *J Clin Oncol*. 2006;24(30):4833–4839. doi:10.1200/JCO.2006.07.5937

Aditya Juloori, Matthew C. Ward, and Gregory M. M. Videtic

QUICK HIT ■ Treatment of stage III NSCLC is heterogeneous due to a wide range of local and nodal presentations (see Table 28.1). Treatment is frequently impacted by patient performance and medical comorbidities. Treatment options involve appropriate selection of CHT, RT, immunotherapy, and surgery, alone or in combination.

Table 28.1: General Treatment Paradigm for Stage III Lung Cancer

Treatment Option	Ideal Candidate	Treatment Details
Neoadjuvant chemoRT followed by resection (trimodality)	Good performance, lobectomy-appropriate, nonbulky non-multistation mediastinal node	45 Gy/25 fx with concurrent CHT
Initial surgery	Good performance cT1–3N0–1	Adjuvant CHT for ≥stage II Consider chemoRT for occult N2; positive margins (54–60 Gy, CHT sequential or concurrent)
Definitive concurrent chemoRT	Good performance status, stage III, acceptable baseline pulmonary function	60 Gy/30 fx with concurrent cisplatin/etoposide or carboplatin AUC 2/paclitaxel 45 mg/m^2 followed by 1 year of durvalumab
Sequential chemoRT	Impaired performance status OR stage III (any T/N), impaired baseline pulmonary function	CHT +/– immunotherapy followed by 60 Gy/30 fx (or as determined by clinician)
RT alone	Marginal performance status	60 Gy/30 fx, 60 Gy/15 fx, 45 Gy/15 fx, 30 Gy/10 fx
Palliative care alone	Poor performance, poor risk IIIB NSCLC	

EPIDEMIOLOGY, RISK FACTORS, ANATOMY, PATHOLOGY, GENETICS, SCREENING: See Chapter 27.

CLINICAL PRESENTATION: Cough, dyspnea, wheeze, stridor, hemoptysis, anorexia, weight loss, decline in performance status, paraneoplastic syndromes such as hypercalcemia from PTHrP (SCC), or hypertrophic pulmonary osteoarthropathy. Hoarseness from recurrent laryngeal (left-sided more common), Horner's syndrome (ptosis, miosis, anhidrosis). Pancoast syndrome (Horner's, brachial plexopathy, shoulder pain). SVC syndrome.

WORKUP: H&P. PFT: ACCP guidelines define standard for PFT evaluation.[1] For any surgery, preoperative FEV_1 >2 L (or 80% predicted) and DLCO >80% predicted are generally safe. For stage III patients undergoing neoadjuvant therapy followed by surgery, if preoperative FEV_1 is <2 L, recommended preresection DLCO is ≥50% and predicted postresection FEV_1 is ≥0.8 L.[2] For pneumonectomy, current ACCP guidelines recommend predicted postoperative FEV_1 and DLCO to both be >60% predicted.[1] For definitive chemoRT, pretreatment FEV_1 ≥1–1.2 L has been used as criteria for clinical trials.[3,4] Note that these are different than criteria for early-stage lung undergoing lobectomy (see Chapter 27).

Labs: CBC, CMP.

Imaging: CT chest (with contrast if evaluating nodes, consider CT abdomen for metastatic workup but at least review liver and adrenals), PET/CT. "Pathologic" lymph nodes defined as short-axis diameter >1 cm and "bulky" lymphadenopathy as short-axis diameter >3 cm, multiple matted nodes, radiographic ECE, or ≥3 stations involved. MRI brain for stage II or higher.[5] CT brain with contrast sufficient if MRI is too difficult.[6] MRI of thoracic inlet for superior sulcus tumors and octreotide scan for carcinoid.

Procedures: Biopsy indicated (EBUS, CT-guided, or thoracentesis depending on location/presence of effusion; sputum pathology is unreliable but at least 3 needed to be negative), PET/CT scan (upstages ~20%, prevents unnecessary thoracotomies but no improvement in survival).[7] For T4 and/or superior sulcus tumors, obtain MRI to investigate degree of local invasion. EBUS/mediastinoscopy to confirm positive LN on CT or PET and for all T3 or central T1–2 tumors (EBUS/mediastinoscopy reaches stations 2, 4, 7; EBUS also reaches station 10). Chamberlain procedure (anterior mediastinotomy) or VATS is required to reach stations 5 and 6, EUS for stations 8 and 9.

PROGNOSTIC FACTORS: Stage, weight loss >5% in 3 months, KPS <90, age >70, LVSI, marital status.

STAGING: See Chapter 27 for AJCC 8th edition staging.

TREATMENT PARADIGM

Surgery: Surgery is the standard local therapy modality.[5] Sublobar resections are not recommended for stage III disease due to need for mediastinal lymphadenectomy. Surgical plan should be decided prior to initiation of treatment. Role of surgery in N2 disease is controversial (see the following). N3 disease, bulky N2 disease (>3 cm), and multiple N2 nodes are relative contraindications to surgery. Pneumonectomy carries increased risk of operative mortality.

Chemotherapy: CHT is indicated in essentially all stage III patients who are fit enough to tolerate treatment. CHT can be delivered in preoperative, postoperative, or sequenced along with RT either concurrently or sequentially. Common concurrent regimens with RT include cisplatin 50 mg/m² on days 1, 8, 29, and 36 and etoposide 50 mg/m² days 1 to 5 and 29 to 33 or carboplatin AUC 2 and paclitaxel 50 mg/m² weekly. The introduction of consolidation immunotherapy to stage III care has eliminated the role of consolidation CHT. No consensus on optimal regimen (see the following data). For definitive sequential chemoRT, give carboplatin AUC 6 and paclitaxel 200 mg/m² every 3 weeks for 2 cycles followed by RT. Cisplatin and pemetrexed (multitarget antimetabolite) is an option for nonsquamous histologies.

Immunotherapy: As the role for immunotherapy in metastatic NSCLC has become first line, its role in the definitive management of locally advanced NSCLC is evolving. The standard of care in patients undergoing definitive chemoRT is 1 year of durvalumab after completion of chemoRT, as per the PACIFIC trial.[8] Current studies are underway to determine the role of immunotherapy in the neoadjuvant and adjuvant setting before and after surgical resection, as well as concurrent with definitive chemoRT.

Targeted Therapy: The role of adjuvant anti-EGFR agents such as osimertinib is controversial. The ADAURA trial showed a significant DFS benefit, but OS results are immature.[9]

Radiation

Indications: RT is an option for definitive local therapy when surgery is not recommended or as adjunct delivered either before or after surgery; 45 Gy/25 fx is given for neoadjuvant chemoRT followed by resection. Postoperatively, for microscopic positive margins give 54 to 60 Gy and for gross residual give 60 Gy. For definitive chemoRT, concurrent RT provides survival benefit compared to sequential chemoRT. RT dose escalation for definitive chemoRT does not improve outcomes. For poor performance patients who are not candidates for combined chemoRT, options include 60 Gy/30 fx, 60 Gy/15 fx, 45 Gy/15 fx, or palliative treatment alone. RT was also commonly utilized in the adjuvant setting for resected N2 disease, though this was recently shown to not provide an OS benefit in the LungART randomized controlled trial.[10]

Toxicity: Acute: Fatigue, cough, shortness of breath, pneumonitis, esophagitis. Late: Pneumonitis, cardiac toxicity, brachial plexopathy.

Procedure: See *Treatment Planning Handbook*, Chapter 6.[11]

■ **EVIDENCE-BASED Q&A**

MEDICALLY OPERABLE STAGE IIIA WITH CLINICALLY NEGATIVE MEDIASTINAL NODES (cT3–4N1, cT4N0)

■ Which stage III patients are optimal candidates for initial surgery?

Medically operable patients with resectable T3–4N1 or T4N0 may be candidates for initial surgery, particularly if T category is due to multiple nodules in the same lobe or invasion of chest wall, mediastinum, or mainstem bronchus <2 cm from carina. Induction therapy may also be feasible for these patients to facilitate surgery. Patients felt not to be good candidates for surgery should be treated with definitive chemoRT as follows if tolerable.

■ Which patients should be offered PORT?

Historically, pN2 disease and positive margins were considered indications for PORT. ASTRO and ACR guidelines suggest consideration for pN2 patients following CHT but omission in pN0–1 patients.[12,13] The LungART randomized trial recently demonstrated in abstract form that there is no overall OS or DFS benefit to the use of adjuvant RT in pN2 patients, but does show improved LC as previously noted in other trials.

PORT Meta-analysis (*Lancet* 1998, PMID 9690404; Update Burdett *Lung Cancer* 2005, PMID 15603857): Meta-analysis of 9 PRTs between 1965 and 1995 consisting of 2,128 patients treated postoperatively to doses of 40 to 60 Gy. Results demonstrated detrimental effect overall (7% absolute reduction in 2-year OS). On subset analysis, this was limited to stage I–II patients but for those with stage III (N2) disease, no clear detriment was identified. Most recent update demonstrated benefit in LC for N2 patients. **Conclusion: PORT recommended in pN2 patients but not in others after negative-margin resection.** *Comment: RT was with older regimens and techniques.*

Douillard, ANITA 2nd Analysis (*IJROBP* 2008, PMID 18439766): ANITA (Adjuvant Navelbine International Trialist Association) was PRT of 799 patients with resected stage IB–IIIA NSCLC (39% stage IIIA) randomized to 4 cycles of vinorelbine and cisplatin vs. observation. PORT recommended but optional for pN+ disease. Twenty-four percent of CHT patients and 33% of observation patients received PORT. Overall, trial improved OS by 8.6% at 5 years, mostly in stage IIA–IIIA patients. This unplanned subset analysis investigated the role of PORT and found that pN1 patients who received CHT had deleterious effect, pN1 patients who did not receive CHT had beneficial effect, and those with pN2 disease had improved OS with PORT in both arms. **Conclusion: Consider PORT for pN2 disease.**

Robinson, NCDB pN2 Analysis (*JCO* 2015, PMID 25667283): RR of NCDB including 4,483 pN2 patients from 2006 to 2010 stratified by use of PORT (1,850 PORT, 2,633 no PORT). MFU 22 months. On MVA, PORT was associated with improved OS (MS 40.7 vs. 45.2 months).

■ Does CHT in addition to surgery improve survival?

Adjuvant CHT following surgery consistently provides 5% to 8% absolute benefit to 5-year OS. Many trials exist, but a few to be familiar with include IALT (cisplatin doublet vs. observation, 4% OS benefit at 5 years), ANITA (see the preceding text), and LACE meta-analysis (see Chapter 27).[14]

MEDICALLY OPERABLE WITH POSITIVE N2/MEDIASTINAL LYMPH NODE(S)

■ Does trimodality therapy improve survival compared to chemoRT for patients with N2 disease?

INT 0139 (Albain) did not show this overall, but trimodality may still be treatment of choice for select patients (controversial).

Albain, INT 0139 (*Lancet* 2009, PMID 19632716): PRT of 429 potentially resectable NSCLC patients with biopsy-proven N2 disease randomized to either induction chemoRT followed by surgery 3 to 5 weeks later or to definitive chemoRT. Induction therapy for both arms was cisplatin 50 mg/m^2 and etoposide 50 mg/m^2 for 2 cycles (weeks 1 and 5) concurrent with 45 Gy/25 fx; those on definitive arm continued RT to 61 Gy without interruption (CT and PFTs were performed midtreatment in both arms to assess for progression); 2 cycles of consolidation cisplatin/etoposide were given after local therapy. No significant difference in MS between groups (23.6 vs. 22.2 months); 5-year OS 27% for surgery and 20% for chemoRT. PFS improved in surgery arm (median 12.8 vs. 10.5 months). Treatment-related death rate was 8% for surgery and 2% for chemoRT. Exploratory analysis demonstrated that lobectomy patients showed improved OS compared to chemoRT but pneumonectomy patients did not. **Conclusion: No OS difference was demonstrated between approaches, so definitive chemoRT often favored, although for healthy lobectomy patients, trimodality may be considered.** *Comment: Pneumonectomy mortality rate was higher than expected at 26%.*

■ **For those who respond to CHT, is surgery superior to RT?**

Van Meerbeeck, EORTC 08941 (*JNCI 2007*, PMID 17374834): PRT of patients with N2 NSCLC treated with 3 cycles of platinum-doublet induction CHT and then randomized to surgery vs. 60 to 62.5 Gy. PORT (56 Gy) only delivered for positive margins; 61% responded and were randomized. In surgery arm, 42% showed nodal downstaging, 25% nodal clearance, and 5% pCR. Only 50% achieved R0 resection. MS was no different: 16.4 months surgery vs. 17.5 months for RT. **Conclusion: Sequential chemoRT is reasonable treatment option, but induction CHT alone may not provide optimal surgical outcomes (in comparison to induction chemoRT).**

■ **Is induction chemoRT superior to induction CHT followed by PORT?**

Likely not, provided adjuvant RT is delivered postoperatively. Caution is warranted for pneumonectomy patients.

Thomas, German Lung Cancer Cooperative Group (*Lancet Oncol* 2008, PMID 18583190): Phase III PRT randomizing 524 patients with stage IIIA–B NSCLC after invasive mediastinal staging to either cisplatin/etoposide for 3 cycles, then surgery, then RT (54 Gy) or cisplatin/etoposide (3 cycles), then concurrent RT (45 Gy/30 fx BID) with carboplatin/vindesine, and then surgery. Primary end point PFS. ChemoRT improved mediastinal downstaging (46% vs. 29%, $p = .02$) and pathologic response (60% vs. 20%, $p < .0001$) but no difference in PFS (9.5 vs. 10 months). Pneumonectomy required in 35% for both groups, but mortality after chemoRT was higher (14% vs. 6%). **Conclusion: Neoadjuvant chemoRT improved response rates but not OS.**

NONOPERATIVE MANAGEMENT

■ **Is RT alone an optimal strategy for stage III NSCLC?**

RT alone is an option for patients unable to tolerate multimodality therapy. Previous dose-escalation studies demonstrated inferior outcomes despite high-dose treatment. This study clarified 60 Gy/30 fx as standard regimen for NSCLC. In the modern era, RT alone is the option for poor performance patients, and 45 Gy/15 fx was alternative biologically equivalent regimen allowed on RTOG 0213 (see the following); 60 Gy/15 fx appears generally well tolerated for patients with ECOG 2 or worse in whom OAR constraints could be met, based on a phase 1 dose-escalation trial by Westover et al. (50 Gy/15, 55 Gy/15, 60 Gy/15 fx).[15]

Perez, RTOG 7301 (*IJROBP* 1980, PMID 6998937): Four-arm PRT of definitive RT dose escalation for stage III NSCLC: 40 Gy split course (20 Gy/5 fx, 2-week break, then another 20 Gy/5 fx) or 40 Gy, 50 Gy, or 60 Gy given 5 fx/week. OS at 2 years was 10% to 18% with split course giving worst rates. Response was better in 50 and 60 Gy arms. **Conclusion: 60 Gy is standard dose.**

Gore, RTOG 0213 (*Clin Lung Cancer* 2011, PMID 21550559): Phase I/II trial of celecoxib concurrent with 60 Gy/30 fx or 45 Gy/15 fx for stage IIB–IIIB lung cancer patients with "intermediate" prognosis (PS 2 or weight loss >5%). Closed early after 13 patients. MS 10 months. **Conclusion: Although underpowered, this gives one reference for management of "intermediate prognosis" patients.**

■ **Does CHT followed by RT improve survival?**

Multiple trials have demonstrated improved survival with sequential chemoRT; selected studies follow.

Dillman, CALGB 8433 (*NEJM* 1990, PMID 2169587; Update *JNCI* 1996, PMID 8780630): PRT of 155 patients with stage III NSCLC randomized to cisplatin with vinblastine followed by 60 Gy/30 fx vs.

immediate identical RT. Long-term results reported 5-year OS rate of 17% vs. 6% in favor of CHT arm and confirmed initial results. **Conclusion: Sequential chemoRT is superior to RT alone.**

Sause, RTOG 8808/ECOG 4588 (*JNCI* 1995, PMID 7707407): Three-arm PRT of 452 patients with stage II–IIIB unresectable NSCLC randomized to either 60 Gy/30 fx alone, induction cisplatin/vinblastine followed by 60 Gy/30 fx or hyperfractionated RT: 69.6 Gy/58 fx at 1.2 Gy/fx BID. MS in each arm was 11.4, 13.8, and 12.3 months, respectively, with statistically significant improvement in CHT arm. **Conclusion: Sequential chemoRT is superior to standard and hyperfractionated RT alone.**

■ Does CHT concurrent with RT improve survival?

Multiple trials have demonstrated improved survival with concurrent compared to sequential chemoRT at expense of increased acute toxicity. Selected studies follow.

Curran, RTOG 9410 (*JNCI* 2011, PMID 21903745): Three-arm PRT of 610 patients with unresectable stage III NSCLC. See Table 28.2. Statistical significance was demonstrated between sequential and concurrent daily arms. **Conclusion: Concurrent CHT is superior to sequential.**

Table 28.2: RTOG 9410 Stage III Lung Trial		
Arm	5-Yr OS	MS (mos)
Sequential cisplatin/vinblastine × 2C, then 63 Gy/34 fx	10%	14.6
Concurrent cisplatin/vinblastine × 2C with 63 Gy/34 fx	16%	17
Concurrent cisplatin/etoposide with 69.6 Gy at 1.2 Gy/fx BID	13%	15.6

Note: 63 Gy delivered 45 Gy/25 fx followed by 18 Gy/9 fx boost without heterogeneity corrections is comparable to 60 Gy/30 fx.

Aupérin, NSCLC Collaborative Group Meta-Analysis (*JCO* 2010, PMID 20351327): Individual patient data meta-analysis of 6 of 7 eligible trials, 1,205 patients. Concurrent chemoRT demonstrated 4.5% absolute survival benefit at 5 years compared to sequential chemoRT. Concurrent therapy decreased locoregional but not distant progression and increased esophageal but not pulmonary toxicity. **Conclusion: Concurrent chemoRT improves survival at cost of manageable but increased esophageal toxicity.**

■ What is the optimal CHT regimen when given concurrently with RT?

Many regimens have been used but cisplatin/etoposide and carboplatin/paclitaxel are the most common regimens used in the United States. Carboplatin/paclitaxel and cisplatin/pemetrexed (for nonsquamous cancers) may have similar efficacy with reduced toxicity. Retrospective data suggests that carboplatin/paclitaxel is associated with increased radiation pneumonitis, which was confirmed by Liang as follows.[16] However, others feel cisplatin/etoposide is more difficult to tolerate.

Liang, China (*Ann Oncol* 2017, PMID 28137739): PRT comparing cisplatin/etoposide to carboplatin/paclitaxel both with concurrent RT to 60 to 66 Gy. Primary end point OS, powered for 17% improvement in 3-year OS. 200 patients, MFU 73 months. 3-year OS improved in cisplatin/etoposide arm by 15% (*p* = .024), MS 23.3 vs. 20.7 months favoring cisplatin/etoposide. Grade ≥2 pneumonitis increased in carboplatin/paclitaxel arm (33.3% vs. 18.9%, *p* = .036), esophagitis increased in the cisplatin/etoposide arm (20.0% vs. 6.3%, *p* = .009). **Conclusion: Cisplatin/etoposide may be superior to carboplatin/paclitaxel.**

Senan, PROCLAIM (*JCO* 2016, PMID 26811519): PRT of 555 patients with unresectable stage IIIA/B nonsquamous NSCLC randomized to receive either (a) pemetrexed 500 mg/m² and cisplatin 75 mg/m² every 3 weeks for 3 cycles plus 60 to 66 Gy followed by consolidation pemetrexed every 3 weeks for 4 cycles or (b) cisplatin 50 mg/m² with etoposide 50 mg/m² every 4 weeks for 2 cycles plus same RT with consolidation platinum doublet. Trial stopped early due to futility. Pemetrexed was not superior but was associated with fewer grade 3 to 4 adverse events. **Conclusion: Pemetrexed is not superior but may be associated with fewer adverse events.**

Santana-Davila, VA Health Data (*JCO* 2015, PMID 25422491): RR of 1,842 patients from Veterans Health Administration data comparing cisplatin/etoposide with carboplatin/paclitaxel from 2001 to 2010. After adjustment methods, there was no survival advantage to cisplatin/etoposide but was associated with more hospitalizations.

■ Does RT dose escalation improve outcomes when given with concurrent CHT?

Dating back to the 1970s, RTOG 7301 demonstrated 60 Gy/30 fx to be standard regimen. RTOG 9311 was phase I/II dose-escalation trial that delivered escalated doses based on achieved V20 with doses ranging from 70.9 Gy to 90.3 Gy without concurrent CHT. This led to RTOG 0617.

Bradley, RTOG 0617 (*Lancet Oncol* 2015, PMID 25601342): 2×2 PRT of 544 patients randomized to either 60 Gy/30 fx or 74 Gy/37 fx with concurrent carboplatin AUC 2/paclitaxel 45 mg/m² weekly. Adjuvant CHT given 2 weeks after RT with carboplatin AUC 6/paclitaxel 200 mg/m² with second randomization to addition of cetuximab during adjuvant phase; 47% treated with IMRT. See Table 28.3. Overall, no difference in toxicity rates between 60 Gy and 74 Gy, but grade ≥3 esophagitis was increased in 74 Gy arm. Noncompliance was higher in 74 Gy arm. Cetuximab increased grade ≥3 toxicity but did not improve OS, PFS, or DM. **Conclusion: 60 Gy is standard of care. 74 Gy is harmful and not superior. No benefit to cetuximab.** *Comment: Hypotheses as to why 74 Gy survival was inferior: Treatment-related deaths were highest in 74 Gy + cetuximab arm, effect of RT on heart, PTV coverage was sacrificed in 74 Gy arm for safety thus leading to failures. Second analysis demonstrated dosimetric benefits to IMRT, reduced lung dosimetry, and correlation of heart V40 with survival.*[17]

Table 28.3: Results of RTOG 0617 for Stage III NSCLC						
Arms	MS (mos)	OS (1 yr)	PFS (Median, mos)	PFS (1 yr)	LF (1 yr)	DM (1 yr)
60 Gy/30 fx	28.7	80%	11.8	49.2%	16.3%	32.2%
74 Gy/37 fx	20.3	69.8%	9.8	41.2%	24.8%	35.1%
p value	.004	.004	.12	.12	.13	.48

Chun, RTOG 0617 IMRT 2nd Analysis (*JCO* 2016, PMID 28034064): Secondary analysis comparing IMRT with 3D-CRT planning. Results: The IMRT group had larger planning treatment volumes (median, 427 vs. 486 mL; *p* = .005); larger planning treatment volume/volume of lung ratio (median, 0.13 vs. 0.15; *p* = .013); and more stage IIIB disease (30.3% vs. 38.6%, *p* = .056); 2-year OS, PFS, LF, and DMFS were not different between IMRT and 3D-CRT. IMRT associated with less ≥grade 3 pneumonitis (7.9% vs. 3.5%, *p* = .039) and a reduced risk in adjusted analyses (OR: 0.41, 95% CI: 0.171–0.986, *p* = .046). IMRT also produced lower heart doses (*p* < .05), and the volume of heart receiving 40 Gy (V40) was significantly associated with OS on adjusted analysis (*p* < .05). Lung V5 was not associated with any ≥grade 3 toxicity, whereas lung V20 was associated with increased ≥grade 3 pneumonitis risk on MVA (*p* = .026). **Conclusion: Although with no OS benefit, IMRT was associated with lower rates of severe pneumonitis and cardiac doses, which supports consideration of IMRT for locally advanced NSCLC.**

■ What trial established the role of immunotherapy in the definitive management of locally advanced lung cancer?

The seminal PACIFIC trial has established a new standard of care for the nonoperative management of stage III NSCLC with its finding on the benefits of immunotherapy.

Antonia, PACIFIC (*NEJM* 2018, PMID 30280658; Update *JCO* 2020, PMID 31622733): PRT of stage IIIA/B NSCLC s/p definitive CRT randomized to consolidation durvalumab for up to 12 months vs. placebo. Coprimary end points were PFS and OS. Results: 712 patients, MFU 25.5 months. Durvalumab significantly prolonged OS (HR: 0.68; *p* = .0025). Median time to death or DM (28.3 vs. 16.2 months), ORR (30% vs. 17.8%; *p* < .001), and median duration of response (NR vs. 18.4 months) favored durvalumab (see Table 28.4). 15.4% vs. 9.8% discontinued drug due to AE in durvalumab and placebo, respectively. Though both subsets benefited, patients with higher PD-L1 seemed to derive the most benefit. **Conclusion: Adjuvant durvalumab is new standard of care following chemoRT for stage III NSCLC.**

Table 28.4: Results of PACIFIC Trial				
Arm	Median PFS	OS (2 yrs)	OS (3 yrs)	Grade 3/4 AE
Durvalumab	17.2 mos	66.3%	57.0%	30.5%
Placebo	5.6 mos	55.6%	43.5%	26.1%
p value	SS	0.005	SS	-

■ **Is there benefit to adding induction CHT prior to concurrent chemoRT or additional consolidation CHT after concurrent chemoRT?**

The use of consolidation CHT after definitive chemoRT was given in RTOG 0617 and is optional as per NCCN guidelines but is not standard and may increase toxicity without benefit. In addition, now that consolidation durvalumab has become standard of care, this has replaced the role of consolidation CHT. Induction provides no OS benefit but in selected cases may help in downsizing tumors to meet OAR constraints prior to definitive RT.

Belani, LAMP (*JCO* 2005, PMID 16087941): Phase II PRT of 276 patients with stage IIIA/B NSCLC randomized to induction carboplatin/paclitaxel followed by 63 Gy RT alone; induction carboplatin/paclitaxel followed by 63 Gy RT with concurrent carboplatin/paclitaxel or 63 Gy RT with concurrent carboplatin/paclitaxel followed by consolidation carboplatin/paclitaxel. MFU 39.6 months, MS 13.0, 12.7, and 16.3 months in favor of consolidation. Grade 3/4 esophageal toxicity was worse with concurrent arms. **Conclusion: RT with concurrent and adjuvant carboplatin/paclitaxel is associated with improved OS in this phase II study.**

Hanna, Hoosier Oncology Group (*JCO* 2008, PMID 19001323; Update Jalal, *Ann Oncol* 2012, PMID 22156624): Phase III PRT of 203 patients with stage IIIA/B NSCLC treated with cisplatin/etoposide concurrent with RT to 59.4 Gy, then randomized to adjuvant docetaxel vs. observation. Closed early due to futility. MS not significantly different (initial publication 21.7 vs. 21.2 months, no difference on update). Toxicity increased in docetaxel arm. **Conclusion: Consolidation docetaxel increases toxicity but not OS.**

Vokes, CALGB 39801 (*JCO* 2007, PMID 17404369): PRT comparing induction CHT followed by chemoRT vs. chemoRT alone. No statistically significant difference in OS. **Conclusion: No benefit to induction CHT prior to chemoRT.**

Ahn, Korean KCSG-LU05-04 (*JCO* 2015, PMID 26150444): PRT of 437 patients with stage III NSCLC treated to 66 Gy with cisplatin/docetaxel, then randomized to receive either 3 additional cycles of docetaxel/cisplatin or no further treatment; 62% in consolidation arm completed. PFS 8.1 months in observation vs. 9.1 months in consolidation arm (*p* = .36).

MS was also not different (20.6 vs. 21.8 months, *p* = .44). **Conclusion: Additional CHT did not improve outcomes after chemoRT.**

SUPERIOR SULCUS TUMORS

Superior sulcus tumors were classically associated with poor rates of complete resection. SWOG 9416 changed paradigm, and these tumors are recommended to undergo induction chemoRT to facilitate resection.

Rusch, SWOG 9416/INT 0160 (*J Thorac Cardiovasc Surg* 2001, PMID 11241082; Update *JCO* 2007, PMID 17235046): Single-arm phase II trial of 111 patients with mediastinoscopy-negative and supraclavicular node-negative T3–4N0–1 superior sulcus tumors treated with 2 cycles of cisplatin/etoposide with concurrent RT 45 Gy/25 fx. If disease was stable or responding on reassessment, thoracotomy was performed 3 to 5 weeks later. Thereafter, 2 more cycles of CHT was delivered. 111 enrolled, 95 eligible for surgery and 83 underwent thoracotomy, 72 had complete resection (92%). Sixty-five percent of thoracotomy specimens demonstrated CR. On update, 5-year OS 44% overall and 56% after complete resection. **Conclusion: Induction combined modality therapy became standard for superior sulcus tumors after this trial.**

REFERENCES

1. Brunelli A, Kim AW, Berger KI, Addrizzo-Harris DJ. Physiologic evaluation of the patient with lung cancer being considered for resectional surgery: diagnosis and management of lung cancer, 3rd ed: American College of Chest Physicians evidence-based clinical practice guidelines. *Chest*. 2013;143(5 Suppl):e166S–190S. doi:10.1378/chest.12-2395

2. Edelman MJ. NRG Oncology RTOG 0839 Randomized Phase II Study of Pre-operative Chemoradiotherapy +/- Panitumumab (IND #110152) Followed by Consolidation Chemotherapy in Potentially Operable Locally Advanced (Stage IIIA, N2+ Non-Small Cell Lung Cancer. 2014. https://www.nrgoncology.org/Clinical-Trials/Protocol/rtog-0839?filter=rtog-0839

3. Bradley JD, Bae K, Graham MV, et al. Primary analysis of the phase II component of a phase I/II dose intensification study using three-dimensional conformal radiation therapy and concurrent chemotherapy for patients with inoperable non-small-cell lung cancer: RTOG 0117. *J Clin Oncol*. 2010;28(14):2475–2480. doi:10.1200/JCO.2009.27.1205

4. Bradley JD, Paulus R, Komaki R, et al. Standard-dose versus high-dose conformal radiotherapy with concurrent and consolidation carboplatin plus paclitaxel with or without cetuximab for patients with stage IIIA or IIIB non-small-cell lung cancer (RTOG 0617): a randomised, two-by-two factorial phase 3 study. *Lancet Oncol*. 2015;16(2):187–199. doi:10.1016/S1470-2045(14)71207-0

5. NCCN Clinical Practice Guidelines in Oncology: Non-small Cell Lung Cancer. 2017(4.2017). https://www.nccn.org/guidelines/guidelines-detail?category=1&id=1450

6. Yokoi K, Kamiya N, Matsuguma H, et al. Detection of brain metastasis in potentially operable non-small cell lung cancer: a comparison of CT and MRI. *Chest*. 1999;115(3):714–719. doi:10.1378/chest.115.3.714

7. Fischer B, Lassen U, Mortensen J, et al. Preoperative staging of lung cancer with combined PET-CT. *N Engl J Med*. 2009;361(1):32–39. doi:10.1056/NEJMoa0900043

8. Antonia SJ, Villegas A, Daniel D, et al. Overall survival with durvalumab after chemoradiotherapy in stage III NSCLC. *N Engl J Med*. 2018;379(24):2342–2350. doi:10.1056/NEJMoa1809697

9. Wu YL, Tsuboi M, He J, et al. Osimertinib in resected EGFR-mutated non-small-cell lung cancer. *N Engl J Med*. 2020;383(18):1711–1723. doi:10.1056/NEJMoa2027071

10. Le Pechoux C, Pourel N, Barlesi F, et al. LBA3_PR An international randomized trial, comparing post-operative conformal radiotherapy (PORT) to no PORT, in patients with completely resected non-small cell lung cancer (NSCLC) and mediastinal N2 involvement: primary end-point analysis of LungART (IFCT-0503, UK NCRI, SAKK) NCT00410683. *Ann Oncol*. 2020;31:S1178. doi:10.1016/j.annonc.2020.08.2280

11. Videtic GMM, Woody N, Vassil AD. *Handbook of Treatment Planning in Radiation Oncology*. 3rd ed. Demos Medical; 2020. doi:10.1891/9780826168429

12. Rodrigues G, Choy H, Bradley J, et al. Adjuvant radiation therapy in locally advanced non-small cell lung cancer: executive summary of an American Society for Radiation Oncology (ASTRO) evidence-based clinical practice guideline. *Pract Radiat Oncol*. 2015;5(3):149–155. doi:10.1016/j.prro.2015.02.013

13. Willers H, Stinchcombe TE, Barriger RB, et al. ACR Appropriateness Criteria(®) induction and adjuvant therapy for N2 non-small-cell lung cancer. *Am J Clin Oncol*. 2015;38(2):197–205. doi:10.1097/COC.0000000000000154

14. Arriagada R, Bergman B, Dunant A, et al. Cisplatin-based adjuvant chemotherapy in patients with completely resected non-small-cell lung cancer. *N Engl J Med*. 2004;350(4):351–360. doi:10.1056/NEJMoa031644

15. Westover KD, Loo BW, Jr., Gerber DE, et al. Precision hypofractionated radiation therapy in poor performing patients with non-small cell lung cancer: phase 1 dose escalation trial. *Int J Radia Oncol Biol Phys*. 2015;93(1):72–81. doi:10.1016/j.ijrobp.2015.05.004

16. Palma DA, Senan S, Tsujino K, et al. Predicting radiation pneumonitis after chemoradiation therapy for lung cancer: an international individual patient data meta-analysis. *Int J Radia Oncol Biol Phys*. 2013;85(2):444–450. doi:10.1016/j.ijrobp.2012.04.043

17. Chun SG, Hu C, Choy H, et al. Impact of intensity-modulated radiation therapy technique for locally advanced non-small-cell lung cancer: a secondary analysis of the NRG oncology RTOG 0617 randomized clinical trial. *J Clin Oncol*. 2017;35(1):56–62. doi:10.1200/JCO.2016.69.1378

29 ■ SMALL-CELL LUNG CANCER

Camille A. Berriochoa and Gregory M. M. Videtic

QUICK HIT ■ SCLC is classically described as either limited (fits within one radiation portal; LS-SCLC) or extensive (metastatic; ES-SCLC). Treatment for LS-SCLC consists of concurrent chemoRT with 4 cycles of platinum-based regimens and early start RT, with PCI offered for those with response to therapy. Treatment for ES-SCLC consists of 4 cycles of CHT with concurrent IO followed by IO maintenance. In the IO era, the role and timing of post-CHT/IO thoracic RT and PCI are controversial. Outcomes are generally modest, with MS 20 to 30 months for LS-SCLC and 9 to 12 months for ES-SCLC.

Table 29.1: General Treatment Paradigm for Small-Cell Lung Carcinoma	
Disease Extent	**General Treatment Paradigm**
Limited stage (30% of SCLC)	• Concurrent chemoRT w/ EP CHT × 4C, with RT start w/ either C1 or C2 • CHT: cisplatin 60 mg/m^2 d1 and etoposide 120 mg/m^2 d1–3 q3w × 4C • RT standard: 45 Gy/30 fx in 3w at 1.5 Gy/fx BID • PCI: 25 Gy/10 fx for responders • T1–T2N0M0 disease (5% of cases): assessment by thoracic surgeon, primary resection with adjuvant CHT + consideration of PCI. Medically inoperable cases: consider SBRT as surgical surrogate

Extensive stage (70% SCLC)	• Cisplatin-based CHT (4C) with concurrent and then maintenance atezolizumab
	• Palliative RT to symptomatic sites
	• Areas of controversy:
	  1. In patients w/o brain metastases, PCI (25 Gy/10 fx) for those w/ *any* response to CHT
	  2. In selected patients, consolidative thoracic RT: post-CHT/IO (30 Gy/10 fx)

EPIDEMIOLOGY: SCLC represents ~15% of all lung cancer diagnoses with decreasing incidence.[1] Approximately 30,000 people are diagnosed in the United States each year.[2] More common in men although gender difference is narrowing.[1]

RISK FACTORS: Occurs almost exclusively in smokers (>98%)—typically heavy smokers.[3] Uranium mining is another risk factor (radon exposure from uranium decay).[4]

ANATOMY: See Chapter 27.

PATHOLOGY:[5,6] SCLC is of neuroendocrine origin and lies along spectrum of other lung neuroendocrine tumors including low-grade neuroendocrine carcinoma (typical carcinoid), intermediate grade (atypical carcinoid), and high grade (LCNEC and SCLC). Light microscopy classically reveals clusters or sheets of small round blue cells, twice the size of normal lymphocytes. "Crush artifact" classic descriptor on cytology and is considered diagnostic. Cytoplasm is sparse and nucleus manifests finely dispersed chromatin without distinct nucleoli. Mitotic rates are high and necrosis is common. Up to 30% of SCLC autopsy specimens have areas of differentiation into NSCLC, suggestive that carcinogenesis occurs in pluripotent stem cells capable of varied differentiation. Three groups of antigen clusters have been identified: neural, epithelial, and neuroendocrine. Epithelial markers include keratin, epithelial membrane antigen, and TTF1. Neuroendocrine and neural markers include DOPA decarboxylase, calcitonin, NSE, synaptophysin, chromogranin A, CD56 (NCAM), gastrin releasing peptide, and IGF-1. Though these are common in SCLC, they are not specific, with about 10% of NSCLCs being positive for these classic neuroendocrine markers[7]; 75% of SCLC will manifest at least one neural/neuroendocrine marker.

GENETICS: In contrast to NSCLC, driving alterations in EGFR, K-ras, ALK, and p16 are rarely seen.

CLINICAL PRESENTATION: SCLC arises submucosally in central airways, often obstructing bronchial lumen. Commonly appears on imaging as large hilar mass with bulky mediastinal adenopathy.[8] Two-thirds present with extensive stage disease, one-third with limited stage disease. Common symptoms include new or worsening cough, dyspnea, chest pain, hoarseness, hemoptysis, malaise, anorexia, and weight loss. If other thoracic structures are compromised by enlarging mass, dysphagia or SVC syndrome (facial edema/plethora, distension of superficial veins, laryngeal edema, altered mental status) may be present. Most common sites of distant spread are liver, adrenals, bone, and brain. Brain mets incidence: 10% to 20% at diagnosis, 50% to 80% at 2 years.[9,10] As detailed in Table 29.2, patients may present with paraneoplastic syndromes (SCLC is the most common solid tumor associated with paraneoplastic syndromes).[11] Fundamentally, treatment of underlying malignancy is necessary to manage these syndromes, but temporizing management steps are described as follows.

Table 29.2: Paraneoplastic Syndromes Commonly Diagnosed in SCLC	
SIADH	Overproduction of ADH with euvolemic hyponatremia. May present with altered mental status, seizures. Treat with water restriction, hypertonic saline, demeclocycline, vasopressin inhibitors, and/or lithium
Cushing's syndrome	Ectopic production of ACTH. Treat with ketoconazole
Lambert–Eaton	Auto-antibodies to presynaptic calcium channels. Proximal muscle weakness that improves later in day. Treat with pyridostigmine, prednisone, IVIG and by treating cancer
Others (rare)	Subacute cerebellar degeneration, subacute sensory neuropathy, limbic encephalopathy, encephalomyelitis (anti-Hu antibodies)

WORKUP:[6] H&P. Encourage smoking cessation.[12]

Labs: CBC, BMP, LFTs, LDH, alkaline phosphatase, PFTs.

Imaging: CT chest with contrast (including liver and adrenals) and PET/CT (nearly 100% sensitive for SCLC; note that PET upstages 19% of patients initially diagnosed with LS disease).[13] Forego bone scan if PET obtained. Contrast-enhanced brain MRI (preferred) or CT brain (CT brain positive in 10%; MRI brain positive in 20%).[10]

Biopsy: For tissue diagnosis: sputum, bronchoscopy with biopsy/FNA (though note that FNA may not always adequately differentiate SCLC from carcinoid tumors), CT-guided biopsy or thoracentesis for pleural effusion. Consider bone marrow biopsy if neutropenia/thrombocytopenia/nucleated RBCs on peripheral smear. About 5% of patients present with cT1–2N0 disease. In this setting, mediastinal staging is useful (see Chapter 27). If LNs are uninvolved, up-front resection (or SBRT in medically inoperable patients) can be considered.

PROGNOSTIC FACTORS: Favorable: limited stage, female gender, performance status (0–1), absence of weight loss, absence of paraneoplastic syndromes, normal labs (LDH, sodium, albumin), smoking cessation.[12,14,15] Hyponatremia (MS 9 months if Na <135, 13 months if Na ≥135, $p < .001$).[16] LDH has been shown to correspond with disease burden, can raise concern for bone marrow involvement, and may be risk factor for early death.[17] More than 5% weight loss is a poor prognostic factor.[18]

NATURAL HISTORY: Distant failure is common with brain metastases in up to 80%.[9,10] Although distant failure is predominant driver of mortality, local failure is also common. Untreated, MS for LS-SCLC is 12 weeks and for ES-SCLC is 6 weeks.[19]

STAGING: The VA system (Table 29.3) is relevant historically, but AJCC staging now standard; see Chapter 27.

TREATMENT PARADIGM

Surgery: Surgery is not standard for most LS-SCLC based on historic MRC trial published in 1973 randomizing patients to either surgery or RT, with improved survival observed in those who received RT (mean OS improved from ~7 to 10 months, $p = .04$).[20] However, ~4% to 5% of SCLC diagnoses

Table 29.3: VA Lung Cancer Study Group				
Limited stage	Tumor confined to one hemithorax (including both ipsilateral and contralateral mediastinum) and ipsilateral SCV nodes	MS: 20–30 mos	2-yr OS: 40%	5-yr OS: 20% to 30%
Extensive stage	Tumor beyond boundaries of limited disease, including distant metastases, malignant pericardial/pleural effusions, and contralateral SCV/hilar LN involvement	MS: 12 mos	2-yr OS: 5%	5-yr OS: <5%

Source: Adapted from Fox W, Scadding JG. Medical Research Council comparative trial of surgery and radiotherapy for primary treatment of small-celled or oat-celled carcinoma of bronchus: ten-year follow-up. *Lancet.* 1973;2(7820):63–65. doi:10.1016/S0140-6736(73)93260-1

present as SPN. For T1–2 SPN SCLC tumors, lobectomy with mediastinal LN dissection is recommended, followed by CHT and/or mediastinal radiation depending on pathologic nodal status. Note that adjuvant CHT is indicated even if pN0.[6] A 2017 NCDB analysis showed increasing use of definitive surgical management in clinical stage I disease from 15% in 2004 to almost 30% in 2013 (the use of SBRT also increased from 0.4% to 6% in this time frame).[21]

Chemotherapy: Compared with no therapy, CHT improves MS fivefold. Cisplatin and EP are standard and found to be equally effective and less toxic than older regimens.[22,23] Current standard is 4 cycles of EP with concurrent RT. Dose of cisplatin is 60 to 100 mg/m² on day 1, and EP 120 mg/m² on days 1 to 3, every 3 weeks. Japanese data showed improved survival with irinotecan + cisplatin vs. EP for ES-SCLC (2-year OS: 19.5% vs. 5.2%); however, this was not reproduced by randomized studies in the United States, Canada, or Australia, potentially due to biologic differences in Japanese study population.[24,25] Additional CHT strategies such as dose intensification, triplet therapy, high-dose consolidation, alternating/sequential regimens, and maintenance therapy all have not demonstrated improvements in OS. Some substitute cisplatin with carboplatin for more favorable side effect profile, with the 2012 COCIS meta-analysis of four randomized trials (including both LS and ES disease) showing no differences in either group in response rate (~70%), PFS (~5 months), or OS (~9 months) between two platinum-based regimens.[26]

Radiation

Indications: Radiation, when added to CHT, was found to reduce intrathoracic failures by 50% (from 75%–90% to 30%–60%). RT also improves survival by 5.4% at 2 to 3 years (see *Warde* and *Pignon in the following*). For regimens using EP, concurrent chemoRT appears superior to sequential. Advantages of concurrent chemoRT: early use of both treatment modalities, more accurate RT planning, high-intensity treatment in short time, and radiosensitization of tumor. Main disadvantage is higher tissue toxicity (esophagitis, pneumonitis, myelosuppression), potentially leading to treatment breaks or discontinuation. Most studies have demonstrated benefit to early RT with CHT cycles 1 and 2. LS-SCLC patients who have complete response or good partial response to primary therapy should be treated with PCI to 25 Gy/10 fx, as this reduces incidence of brain metastases and improves OS (see *Auperin* meta-analysis). Of note, SBRT may have a role similar to surgery in inoperable early-stage patients. A 2017 multi-institution RR demonstrated excellent 3-year LC (≥95%) for 74 T1–2N0 patients treated with SBRT.[27] This series also showed improved OS in those who also received subsequent CHT (31 vs. 14 months, $p = .02$). The role of PCI in those with ES-SCLC without brain mets at diagnosis who respond to initial CHT remains controversial, particularly in the new IO era.

Dose: Standard accelerated dose is 45 Gy/30 fx at 1.5 Gy/fx BID in 3 weeks with concurrent EP CHT based on results from the landmark Turrisi trial.[28] This schedule has been confirmed as standard by the CONVERT trial. Proposed radiobiologic advantages of BID fx in SCLC include high growth fraction, short cell cycle time, and small/absent shoulder on cell survival curve. Cycle 2 start RT dose can be utilized when delivering 40 Gy/15 fx at 2.67 Gy/fx.[29] Notwithstanding trial results, a 2003 patterns of care practice survey found that fewer than 10% of clinicians employ BID RT approach, with >80% of patients receiving daily RT to a median dose of 50.4 Gy.[30] NCCN states that if daily fractionation is used, 60 to 70 Gy should be given (not based on level 1 evidence), and hypofractionated regimens such as 40 Gy/15 fx at 2.67 Gy/fx as employed by Murray et al. are not included in most recent guidelines.[31]

Toxicity

Acute: Fatigue, esophagitis, pneumonitis, nausea. Chronic: Pneumonitis, cardiac injury, dysphagia.

■ **EVIDENCE-BASED Q&A**

LIMITED STAGE SMALL-CELL LUNG CANCER

■ **Is there a benefit to RT in addition to CHT?**

Multiple RCTs compared CHT alone to chemoRT, which formed the basis of the seminal Warde and Pignon meta-analyses, both of which showed 5% benefit in OS with addition of thoracic RT to CHT.[32,33]

Warde, Ontario Meta-Analysis (*JCO* 1992, PMID 1316951): Meta-analysis of 11 randomized trials of LS-SCLC patients treated with CHT alone vs. chemoRT. Demonstrated significant 25.3% improvement in LC (47% vs. 24%) and 5.4% improvement in 2-year OS (20% vs. 15%) with addition of RT, with patients under age 60 deriving greatest benefit. There was no significant difference in treatment-related death.

Pignon, French Meta-Analysis (*NEJM* 1992, PMID 1331787): Meta-analysis of 13 randomized trials of 2,140 patients with LS-SCLC treated with CHT alone vs. chemoRT. Addition of thoracic RT improved 3-year OS by 5.4% (14.3% vs. 8.9%) over CHT alone, with 14% relative reduction in mortality rate. Younger patients (age <55) had greater benefit from addition of radiation to CHT compared to patients over age 70.

■ **What is the ideal dose and fractionation for LS-SCLC?**

A schedule of 45 Gy with BID fractionation as initially defined by Turrisi's Intergroup trial is the current standard of care,[28] with the results of the CONVERT trial confirming this schedule.

Turrisi, RTOG 88-15/INT 0096 (*NEJM* 1999, PMID 9920950): Phase III PRT of 417 patients treated with concurrent CHT and either daily or BID RT. CHT was 60 mg/m^2 cisplatin on day 1 and 120 mg/m^2 EP on days 1 to 3 every 3 weeks for 4C. RT was started on day 1 of CHT and was based on University of Pennsylvania RT technique reported in 1988.[33] RT dose was 45 Gy/25 fx in 5 weeks at 1.8 Gy/fx daily vs. 45 Gy/30 fx in 3 weeks at 1.5 Gy/fx BID. Fields taken off spinal cord at 36 Gy. Patients with CR received PCI 25 Gy/10 fx. Note that there was 60% to 70% risk of esophagitis in the subgroup of patients aged >70, so altering dose for elderly patients may be important (see Table 29.4). **Conclusion: BID fractionation significantly improved OS, though with higher acute grade 3 esophageal toxicity but not late toxicity.** *Comment: Employing 45 Gy/25 fx as standard arm may represent suboptimal dose given that this represents low BED for patients with gross disease. Also, experimental arm tested two additional variables: (a) decreased time between doses; and (b) finishing treatment in shorter period of time—both of which may have independently improved outcomes.*

Table 29.4: Results of Turrisi RTOG 8815/INT 0096, Hyperfractionation for SCLC				
Turrisi	**MS (mos)**	**5-Yr OS**	**Local Failure (Thoracic Relapse)**	**Acute Grade 3 Esophagitis**
45 Gy QD	19	16%	52%	11%
45 Gy BID	23	26%	36%	27%
p value	.04	.04	.06	<.001

Faivre-Finn, CONVERT (*Lancet Oncol* 2017, PMID 28642008): Randomized 547 patients with LS-SCLC to CHT with either BID RT (45 Gy/30 fx delivered BID over 3 weeks) or daily chemoRT (66 Gy/33 fx over 6.5 weeks), both with RT starting on day 1 of C2 of EP CHT, followed by PCI if indicated. Primary end point: 2-year OS. MFU 45 months. Two-year OS and MS were 56% and 30 months for BID and 51% and 25 months for daily tx (*p* = .14). Toxicities were comparable except for grade 4 neutropenia (increased from 38% in daily RT group to 49% in BID group, $p = .05$). In each arm, grade 3 esophagitis was 19%. Grade 3 to 4 pneumonitis was rare (~2% in each arm). **Conclusion: The superiority design of the trial suggests the standard arm (BID) remains standard as equivalence was not demonstrated.**

■ What is the optimal timing of chemoRT?

In an appropriately fit patient, chemoRT should be given concurrently and SER (start of any treatment until end of RT) should be <30 days as per De Ruysscher's meta-analysis.[34] There has historically been some controversy as to whether early vs. delayed start is optimal. There are three trials (Murray, Jeremic, Takada) suggesting benefit to early RT, but three other trials (CALGB, Spiro, and Sun) suggesting no benefit. However, given findings of De Ruysscher's meta-analysis (with particular attention on SER <30 days) as well as theoretical radiobiologic advantages to early treatment in SCLC (rapid cell turnover makes this disease prone to repopulation, which can be more vulnerable to accelerated treatment), most clinicians prefer cycle 1 or 2 start.

Murray, NCIC (*JCO* 1993, PMID 8381164): PRT of 308 patients treated with concurrent CHT and randomized to early RT (cycle 2 at week 3) or delayed RT (cycle 6 at week 15). CHT was alternating CAV and EP for 6 cycles. RT dose was 40 Gy/15 fx at 2.67 Gy/fx. PCI in 25 Gy/10 fx was given to all patients w/o progressive disease after CHT. Results in Table 29.5. Toxicity was similar between arms. **Conclusion: Early thoracic RT with concurrent CHT is superior to delayed RT.** *Comment: Cycle 2 start was to avoid concurrent Adriamycin in CAV. Since then, a number of trials have compared CAV, CAV–EP, and EP alone, and found that response rate for EP alone is equivalent to CAV/EP and superior to CAV alone.[34] Thus, EP rather than combined EP–CAV is now standard in this setting and thus cycle 1 start, if feasible, may still be preferable to cycle 2.*

Table 29.5: Results of Murray NCIC Trial for Small-Cell Lung Cancer						
Murray	**CR**	**MS**	**2-Yr OS**	**3-Yr OS**	**5-Yr OS**	**Brain Mets**
Early RT	64%	21 mos	40%	30%	20%	18%
Delayed RT	56%	16 mos	34%	21.5%	11%	28%
p value	.14	.008			*p = .006*	.042

Jeremic, Yugoslavia (*JCO* 1997, PMID 9060525): PRT 107 patients treated with RT 54 Gy/36 fx at 1.5 Gy BID (36/24 AP/PA, then taken off spinal cord) with concurrent daily carboplatin/EP (30 mg/m² each) followed by 4 cycles of cisplatin (30 mg/m²)/EP (120 mg/m²). Group 1 started with concurrent carboplatin/EP + RT, then 4 cycles of EP. Group 2 started with 2 cycles of EP, then RT with carboplatin/EP, then additional 2 cycles of EP. All responders received PCI to 25 Gy/10 fx. MS 34 vs. 26 months, 5-year OS 30% vs. 15% both in favor of group 1 ($p = .052$ on univariate analysis, $p = .027$ on MVA). MS 53 vs. 15 months for KPS 90 to 100 vs. 50 to 80 ($p < .0001$). Ninety-six percent vs. 80% CR rates at 9 weeks. Grade 3 to 4 esophagitis 28% vs. 24% (NS). **Conclusion: Accelerated BID RT to total dose of 54 Gy/36 fx has similar toxicities to Turrisi trial, with encouraging survival data.**

Takada, JCOG 9104 (*JCO* 2002, PMID 12118018): Compared concurrent chemoRT to sequential CHT, then RT (specifically, cycle 1 chemoRT at 45 Gy BID vs. same RT followed by CHT). MS 27 months for cycle 1 start, 20 months for sequential, $p = .097$. **Conclusion: Per the authors, this study strong suggests that EP and concurrent RT more effective than EP and sequential RT.**

Perry, CALGB 8083 (*JCO* 1998, PMID 9667265): Compared cycle 1 chemoRT vs. cycle 4 chemoRT vs. CHT alone. CHT was cyclophosphamide, EP, and vincristine, with doxorubicin replacing EP later in trial. RT was 50 Gy in 5 weeks (40 Gy to tumor and mediastinum + 10 Gy boost). All patients received PCI to 30 Gy. MS was approximately 13 to 14 months for all three arms. However, via pairwise comparisons using log-rank test, authors showed that CHT alone was inferior to both RT-containing regimens (see Table 29.6). **Conclusion: With 10 years of follow-up, two arms that included thoracic RT remain superior to CHT alone. Addition of thoracic RT to combination CHT improved both CR rates and survival, with increased but acceptable toxicity.** *Comment: CHT regimen may have been inferior to EP.*

Table 29.6: Long-Term Results of CALGB 8083 for Small-Cell Lung Cancer

CALGB 8083, 10-Yr Update	MS (mos)	Time to clinical failure (mos)
Arm I (Cycle 1 start)	13	11
Arm II (Cycle 4 start)	14.5	11.2
Arm III (CHT alone)	13.6	8.7

Note: Both MS and time to clinical failure were worse in arm III than I + II (SS) but could not demonstrate whether arm I or II was superior.

Spiro, UK London Lung Cancer Group (*JCO* 2006, PMID 16921033): PRT of 325 patients treated using NCIC regimen and randomization earlier again with both CAV and EP CHT. More patients in early arm were treated with RT than late arm, 92% vs. 82% ($p = .01$). Fewer patients in early arm completed CHT than late arm, 69% vs. 80% ($p = .003$). MS same, 13.7 vs. 15.1 months ($p = .23$). **Conclusion: Failed to replicate survival advantage noted in NCIC trial.** *Comment: Lower rate of CHT completion in early arm could have obscured detection of survival advantage when utilizing early thoracic RT.*

Sun, South Korea (*Ann Oncol* 2013, PMID 23592701): Phase III trial comparing thoracic RT w/ first cycle vs. third cycle of EP CHT; 220 patients. Outcomes were essentially same between two arms (CR, PFS, and OS), but neutropenic fever was worse in early arm (22% vs. 10%, $p = .002$). **Conclusion: Later RT start may be favorable.**

■ **When combining the preceding trials, is there difference in early vs. late administration of thoracic RT?**

De Ruysscher, Netherlands Meta-Analysis (*Ann Oncol* 2006, PMID 16344277): Meta-analysis of seven trials to determine whether timing of chest RT may influence survival of patients with LS-SCLC. When including all seven trials, 2- and 5-year OS was not improved between early and late RT. Looking at only trials using concurrent platinum CHT w/ RT, 5-year OS was significantly improved with early RT, OR 0.64 ($p = .02$). In studies with short RT (<30 days treatment time), 2-year survival showed no difference, but 5-year OS better (OR 0.56, SS).

De Ruysscher, RTT-SCLC Collaborative Group (*Ann Oncol* 2016, PMID 27436850): Individual patient-level analysis of nine trials comprising 2,305 patients with MFU of 10 years. Authors rationalized this patient-level update based on Spiro's combined RCT/meta-analysis, which showed that early delivery of thoracic RT may contribute to improved survival if patients received CHT regimen as prescribed.[35] When all trials were analyzed together, "earlier or shorter" vs. "later or longer" thoracic RT did not affect OS. However, when limiting analysis to those who were compliant with planned CHT, benefit to those receiving "earlier or shorter" thoracic RT was observed compared to those who received "later or longer" RT regimens (HR for survival: 0.79, 95% CI: 0.69–0.91). Grade 3–5 toxicity was greater in "earlier or shorter" group: neutropenia increased from 59% to 69%, $p = .001$, and esophagitis increased from 8% to 14%, $p < .001$. Interestingly, the reverse was shown in those unable to complete their planned CHT regimen (better OS with later/longer: HR: 1.19, 95% CI: 1.05–1.34). **Conclusion: "Earlier or shorter" delivery of thoracic RT in those who complete planned CHT significantly improves 5-year OS at cost of increased toxicity.**

■ **Does "package time" for RT delivery matter?**

Yes, "start of any treatment until end of RT" (SER) <30 days is critical.

De Ruysscher (*JCO* 2006, PMID 16505424): Meta-analysis of four trials (Murray, Jeremic, Turrisi, Takada) to analyze influence of timing of chest RT on local tumor control, survival, and esophagitis. SER was most important predictor of outcome. 5-year OS improved in shorter (<30 days) vs. longer SER arms (RR: 0.62, $p = .0003$). Each week extension of SER beyond that of study arm w/ shortest SER resulted in absolute 5-year OS decrease of 1.83%. Shorter SER also associated with higher incidence of severe esophagitis (RR: 0.55, $p < .0001$). SER did not correlate with local control rates.

■ **What is the ideal field size? Should the pre- or post-CHT volume be targeted?**

Nearly four decades ago, SWOG 7924 suggested use of the post-CHT rather than pre-CHT for the RT target leads to equivalent LC and OS. Hu et al. have confirmed this in the modern era.

Kies, SWOG 7924 (JCO 1987, PMID 3031226): PRT of 473 LS-SCLC patients treated with induction CHT (VMV-VAC x 6C); 153 patients (33%) who had CR to induction CHT were randomized to chest RT 48 Gy split course w/ PCI 30 Gy followed by CHT vs. continuing CHT w/ no chest RT. OS for CR patients did not differ according to whether chest RT was used due to distant relapses. However, patterns of tumor relapse were affected by chest RT, as 38 of 42 relapsing patients who did not receive RT had intrathoracic recurrences, compared to 20 of 36 radiated patients. 191 patients with PR/SD to induction CHT were treated with RT, randomized to "large-field" pre-CHT volume vs. "small-field" post-CHT volume. No significant difference in relapse patterns or OS between large or small RT volumes. Myelosuppression was higher in patients treated with larger field, but no difference in radiation pneumonitis.

Hu, China, (Cancer 2020, PMID 31714592). PRT of 309 patients randomized after 2 cycles of EP and cisplatin, to receive RT to the post-CHT or pre-CHT tumor volume. RT was 45 Gy/1.5 Gy BID. PCI given to responding patients. Lymph node regions originally involved before induction CHT were included as a nodal CTV for both arms even if the lymph node disappeared after induction CHT. Study halted early because of slow accrual. Between 2002 and 2017, 159 and 150 patients were randomized to the study arm or the control arm, respectively; 21.4% and 19.1% of patients were staged using PET ($p = .31$). MFU was 19.6 months for all patients and 54.1 months for surviving patients. The 3-year local/regional progression-free probability was 58.2% and 65.5% in the study and control arms, respectively ($p = .44$). The 5-year OS was 22.8% and 28.1% for post- and pre-CHT arms, respectively ($p = .26$). **Conclusion: The use of post-CHT target volumes is valid for RT planning.**

■ **Should elective nodal volumes be included in the CTV?**

Designing SCLC targets without ENI had once been controversial[36] but is now considered accepted practice in most clinical centers, as long as PET imaging is used as a planning tool.

Baas, Netherlands (BJC 2006, PMID 16465191): Phase II study of 38 patients with LS-SCLC treated with carboplatin, EP, and paclitaxel × 4C with concurrent RT 45 Gy/25 fractions, starting cycle 2, treating only involved sites (primary and any involved nodes >1 cm) determined at simulation with IV contrast; PCI given to responders (30 Gy/10 fx). MS 19.5 months. 5-year OS 27%. Grade 3 esophagitis 27%. Grade 3 to 4 heme toxicity 57%. In-field LR 16%.

Van Loon, Netherlands (IJROBP 2010, PMID 19782478): Single arm prospective trial of 60 patients with LS-SCLC, RT dose 45 Gy/BID with EP. Only PET-avid primary and LN stations irradiated (SNI). PET altered nodal involvement in 30% of patients. Isolated nodal relapse occurred in only 3% (n = 2). Acute grade 3 esophagitis occurred in 12% (lower than on Turrisi trial). MS was 19 months. **Conclusion: PET appears to help in selection of nodal stations for irradiation, which may reduce toxicity and keep regional failures low.** *Note: Only prospective study to show value of PET for SNI in LS-SCLC.*

Colaco, UK (Lung Cancer 2012, PMID 22014897): Evaluated relapse patterns in patients whose CT-based treatment volumes included only primary tumor and involved nodes. All treatment was 3D-conformal and PET was not routinely used; 38 patients were recruited and of 31 evaluable following treatment, 14 relapsed but there were no isolated nodal relapses. Authors concluded that omitting ENI based on CT imaging was not associated with high risk of isolated nodal recurrence.

■ **Does the addition of IO to chemotherapy improve outcomes for LS-SCLC?**

There is no data currently supporting use of IO in LS-SCLC. This is being explored by NRG-LU005, which is an ongoing RCT randomizing patients with LS-SCLC to chemoRT with or without concurrent atezolizumab beginning cycle 2 followed by 1 year of maintenance atezolizumab.[37]

EXTENSIVE STAGE SMALL-CELL LUNG CANCER

■ **Should consolidative chest RT be delivered to ES-SCLC patients with response to CHT?**

With the addition of IO to standard of care CHT for ES-SCLC, the role, if any, and timing of chest RT is now highly controversial. Chest RT had been considered in favorable patients who had demonstrated response when only CHT was used. As per 2020 guidelines, if thoracic RT is given, it is advised to start after CHT is complete and to deliver it simultaneously with PCI (if given; more in the following).[31]

Jeremic, Yugoslavia (*JCO* 1999, PMID 10561263): PRT of 210 patients w/ ES-SCLC treated w/ EP × 3C. Patients w/ CR at distant level and either CR or PR at local level received either (Group 1) hyperfractionated RT to 54 Gy/36 fx over 18 days w/ concurrent carboplatin/EP followed by EP × 2C or (Group 2) EP × 4C. All patients w/ CR at distant level received PCI (25 Gy/10 fx). RT fields included gross disease and ipsilateral hilum w/ 2 cm margin, mediastinum w/ 1 cm margin, and bilateral SCV. Patients w/ PR at distant level were treated nonrandomly with CHT and/or later HFX chemoRT, and patients w/ progressive disease received supportive care or oral EP. Among all patients, MS was 9 months and 5-year OS 3.4%. MS and 5-year OS superior in Group 1: 17 vs. 11 months and 9.1% vs. 3.7% ($p = .041$). LC nonsignificantly better in Group 1 ($p = .062$). No difference in DM. Acute Gr 3/4 toxicity higher in Group 2 (See Table 29.7). **Conclusion: Addition of hyperfractionated RT for most favorable subset of patients leads to improved OS over CHT alone.**

Table 29.7: Results of Jeremic Trial for Consolidative Chest RT in ES-SCLC

210 ES-SCLC patients treated w/ 3 cycles of EP, 109 patients with CR or PR, all received PCI and randomized to CHT alone vs. chemoRT		5-Yr LRFS	5-Yr DMFS	MS (mos)	Nausea and Vomiting
	ChemoRT (RT + carboplatin/etoposide CHT; 54 Gy/36 fx BID) + EP x2C	20%	27%	17	4%
	CHT alone (EP x4C)	8.1%	14%	11	20%
		$p = .062$	$p = .35$	$p = .041$	$p = .0038$

Slotman, Netherlands (*Lancet* 2015, PMID 25230595): Phase III RCT of 498 patients with WHO performance status 0–2 and ES-SCLC who responded to CHT, all of whom received PCI and were then randomized to thoracic RT (30 Gy/10 fx) or observation. Primary end point was 1-year OS; PFS was secondary end point. MFU 24 months. OS at 1 year was not significantly different between groups: 33% for thoracic RT arm vs. 28% for control group (HR: 0.84, $p = .066$). However, in secondary analysis, 2-year OS was 13% vs. 3% ($p = .004$). At 6 months, PFS was 24% in thoracic RT group vs. 7% in control group ($p = .001$). No significant difference in toxicity between groups. **Conclusion: Thoracic RT + PCI should be considered for patients with ES-SCLC who respond to CHT.**

Gore, RTOG 0937 (*J Thorac Oncol* 2017, PMID 28648948): Randomized phase II of patients with ES-SCLC with one to four extracranial metastases randomized to either PCI alone vs. PCI with consolidative RT to the intrathoracic disease and extracranial metastases to 45 Gy/15 fx (acceptable alternative: 30–40 Gy in 10 fx). Ninety-seven patients, MFU 9 months. 1-year OS was 60.1% (PCI) vs. 50.8% (PCI + consolidation, $p = .21$); 12-month progression was 79.6% vs. 75%, favoring consolidation (HR: 0.53, $p = .01$). **Conclusion: OS analysis was underpowered due to high rate of survival. Consolidation may reduce progression but did not alter OS.**

■ **Does the addition of IO to chemotherapy improve outcomes for first-line treatment of ES-SCLC?**

The IMpower133 and CASPIAN RCTs demonstrated a 2- to 3-month improvement in OS with the incorporation of IO.

Horn, IMpower133 (*NEJM* 2018, PMID 30280641): Phase III, double-blind, placebo-controlled RCT of patients with ES-SCLC treated first line with carboplatin and EP with or without atezolizumab during both induction and maintenance phases. Coprimary end point OS and PFS; 403 patients at median f/u 14 months, median OS improved with atezolizumab vs. placebo, 12.3 vs. 10.3 months (HR: 0.70, $p = .007$), and median PFS 5.2 vs. 4.3 months (HR: 0.77, $p = .02$). Immune-related AEs 40% with atezolizumab vs. 25% with placebo (rash and hypothyroidism most common). **Conclusion: For first-line treatment of ES-SCLC, the addition of atezolizumab to carboplatin/EP improves OS and PFS.** *Comment: Only 22 patients in each arm received PCI. Thoracic RT was not permitted.*

Paz-Ares, CASPIAN (*Lancet* 2019, PMID 31590988): Phase III PRT of patients with ES-SCLC randomized 1:1:1 to durvalumab + EP, durvalumab + tremelimumab + EP, or EP alone. PCI was given at investigator's discretion in the EP group. Primary end point OS. Planned interim analysis of durvalumab + EP vs. EP alone is reported. OS improved with addition of durvalumab, 13.0 vs. 10.3

months with 34% vs. 25% of patients alive at 18 months. Grade 3/4 AEs were similar in the two groups (62%), AEs leading to death were 5% vs. 6%. **Conclusion: First-line durvalumab + platinum/ EP significantly improves OS compared with platinum/EP alone, with similar safety profile.**

PROPHYLACTIC CRANIAL IRRADIATION

■ Who should be treated with PCI?

Historically, patients with LS-SCLC with CR or good PR after chemoRT as per Auperin meta-analysis have received PCI. In ES-SCLC, some have relied on findings of Slotman's 2007 study to justify PCI for any responders to CHT in ES-SCLC patients, but this remains controversial as this study did not require prerandomization brain MRI to confirm absence of brain metastases prior to cranial irradiation. This is in contrast to the 2017 Takahashi study, which incorporated prerandomization brain MRI. The PCILESS prospective trial is a single-arm study of LS-SCLC after definitive treatment with at least a good response, utilizing watchful observation rather than PCI, with results awaited.[38] As per 2020 consensus guidelines, PCI is strongly recommended for stage II or III patients who respond to CRT, with a caveat that this should be a shared decision for those at higher risk of neurocognitive toxicities; PCI is "conditionally not recommended" for stage I patients; and for ES-SCLC, authors recommend consideration of PCI vs. MRI surveillance.[31]

Auperin, French Meta-analysis (*NEJM* 1999, PMID 10441603): Meta-analysis of 987 patients w/ SCLC from seven RCTs conducted between 1965 and 1995 comparing PCI to no PCI. Most patients on this meta-analysis were limited stage but ~15% were extensive stage. PCI was performed in varied doses and fractionations. An analysis of four dose groups was performed: 8 Gy/1 fx vs. 24–25 Gy/8– 12 fx vs. 30 Gy/10 fx vs. 36–40 Gy/18–20 fx. PCI improved 3-year OS and reduced incidence of brain mets (see Table 29.8). Effect of PCI on OS did not differ significantly according to total dose. However, there was a trend toward lower risk of brain mets as RT dose increased. There was also trend toward greater effect of PCI on incidence of brain mets in patients randomized sooner (<6 months) after CHT.

Table 29.8: Results of Auperin Meta-Analysis of PCI		
	Incidence of Brain Mets	3-Yr OS
PCI	33.3%	20.7%
No PCI	58.6%	15.3%
	$p < .001$	$p = .01$

Slotman, EORTC 08993-22993 (*NEJM* 2007, PMID 17699816): Phase III RCT of PCI in ES-SCLC, including patients aged 18 to 75, PS 0–2, any response to CHT, no previous RT, no clinical suggestion of brain mets (imaging not required), n = 286. Dose ranged from 20 to 30 Gy with fractionation that was variable but consistent within an institution. Median interval between diagnosis and randomization was 4.2 months. Primary end point was reduction in symptomatic brain metastases. There was no difference in extracranial disease progression between groups. There was no difference in cognitive and emotional function with PCI (See Table 29.9). **Conclusion: PCI reduces incidence of symptomatic brain metastases and prolongs DFS and OS.** *Comment: Brain imaging was not required prior to randomization.*

Table 29.9: Results of Slotman PCI for ES-SCLC				
	Symptomatic Brain Mets at 1 yr	Median DFS (weeks)	MS (mos)	1-Yr OS
No PCI	40.4%	12	5.4	13.3%
PCI	14.6%	14.7	6.7	27.1%
	$p < .001$	$p = .02$	$p = .03$	$p = .003$

Takahashi, Japan (*Lancet Oncol* 2017, PMID 28343976): Phase III RCT of PCI in ES-SCLC including patients aged ≥20, PS 0–2, any response to platinum-based doublet CHT, and no brain mets on MRI obtained within 4 weeks of PCI randomized to 25 Gy/10 fx vs. no PCI. Post-PCI brain MRI was obtained at 3-month intervals up to 12 months, then at 18 and 24 months. Primary end point was

OS. The trial was terminated early due to likely futility (See Table 29.10). **Conclusion: PCI does not improve OS in ES-SCLC in this prescreened population, though does reduce the incidence of MRI-detected brain mets at all time points.** *Comment: Close MRI surveillance was performed and should be considered necessary to replicate results if PCI is omitted.*

Table 29.10: Results of Takahashi PCI for ES-SCLC			
	MS (mos)	**Incidence of Brain Mets at 12 mos**	**Overall Grade 3–4 Toxicity**
PCI	11.6	32.9%	2.5%
No PCI	13.7	59.0%	4.0%
	p = .094	*p* < .0001	NS

■ What dose of PCI should be delivered?

25 Gy/10 fx is standard. This was investigated in the EORTC/RTOG 0212 prospective randomized trial[39] *composed of three treatment arms: 25 Gy/10 fx, 36 Gy/18 fx QD, and 36 Gy/24 fx BID. Incidence of brain mets at 2 years was approximately 25% in all arms with no statistical difference; rates of chronic neurotoxicity were greater in the 36 Gy cohort (p = .02).*[40,41]

■ Is there a role for hippocampal avoidance in PCI?

The PREMER RCT from Spain randomized patients receiving PCI for SCLC to PCI vs. HA-PCI and has been preliminarily reported in abstract form only, showing a decline in free delayed recall in PCI vs. HA-PCI (33% vs. 7% at 6 months, p = .008).[42] *NRG CC003 is an RCT investigating PCI vs. HA-PCI in LS-SCLC and ES-SCLC; outcomes include intracranial relapse rates and differences in delayed recall.43 Results are awaited.*

REFERENCES

1. Govindan R, Page N, Morgensztern D, et al. Changing epidemiology of small-cell lung cancer in the United States over the last 30 years: analysis of the surveillance, epidemiologic, and end results database. *J Clin Oncol.* 2006;24(28):4539–4544. doi:10.1200/JCO.2005.04.4859
2. Siegel RL, Miller KD, Jemal A. Cancer statistics, 2016. *CA Cancer J Clin.* 2016;66(1):7–30. doi:10.3322/caac.21387
3. Pesch B, Kendzia B, Gustavsson P, et al. Cigarette smoking and lung cancer: relative risk estimates for the major histological types from a pooled analysis of case-control studies. *Int J Cancer.* 2012;131(5):1210–1219. doi:10.1002/ijc.27339
4. Kreuzer M, Muller KM, Brachner A, et al. Histopathologic findings of lung carcinoma in German uranium miners. *Cancer.* 2000;89(12):2613–2621. doi:10.1002/1097-0142(20001215)89:12<2613::AID-CNCR14>3.0.CO;2-Y
5. Travis WD, Brambilla E, Noguchi M, et al. International association for the study of lung cancer/American Thoracic Society/European Respiratory Society international multidisciplinary classification of lung adenocarcinoma. *J Thorac Oncol.* 2011;6(2):244–285. doi:10.1097/JTO.0b013e318206a221
6. NCCN Clinical Practice Guidelines in Oncology: Small-Cell Lung Cancer. 2016. https://www.nccn.org/professionals/physician_gls/pdf/sclc.pdf
7. Travis WD. Advances in neuroendocrine lung tumors. *Ann oncol.* 2010;21(Suppl 7):vii65–vii71. doi:10.1093/annonc/mdq380
8. Rivera MP, Mehta AC, Wahidi MM. Establishing the diagnosis of lung cancer: diagnosis and management of lung cancer, 3rd ed: American College of Chest Physicians evidence-based clinical practice guidelines. *Chest.* 2013;143(5, Suppl):e142S–e165S. doi:10.1378/chest.12-2353
9. Nugent JL, Bunn PA Jr, Matthews MJ, et al. CNS metastases in small cell bronchogenic carcinoma: increasing frequency and changing pattern with lengthening survival. *Cancer.* 1979;44(5):1885–1893. doi:10.1002/1097-0142(197911)44:5<1885::AID-CNCR2820440550>3.0.CO;2-F
10. Seute T, Leffers P, ten Velde GP, Twijnstra A. Detection of brain metastases from small cell lung cancer: consequences of changing imaging techniques (CT versus MRI). *Cancer.* 2008;112(8):1827–1834. doi:10.1002/cncr.23361
11. Castillo JJ, Vincent M, Justice E. Diagnosis and management of hyponatremia in cancer patients. *Oncologist.* 2012;17(6):756–765. doi:10.1634/theoncologist.2011-0400
12. Videtic GMM, Stitt LW, Dar AR, et al. Continued cigarette smoking by patients receiving concurrent chemoradiotherapy for limited-stage small-cell lung cancer is associated with decreased survival. *J Clin Oncol.* 2003;21(8):1544–1549. doi:10.1200/JCO.2003.10.089
13. Kalemkerian GP. Staging and imaging of small cell lung cancer. *Cancer Imaging.* 2012;11: 253–258. doi:10.1102/1470-7330.2011.0036

14. Foster NR, Mandrekar SJ, Schild SE, et al. Prognostic factors differ by tumor stage for small cell lung cancer: a pooled analysis of North Central Cancer Treatment Group trials. *Cancer.* 2009;115(12):2721–2731. doi:10.1002/cncr.24314

15. Albain KS, Crowley JJ, LeBlanc M, Livingston RB. Determinants of improved outcome in small-cell lung cancer: an analysis of the 2,580-patient Southwest Oncology Group data base. *J Clin Oncol.* 1990;8(9):1563–1574. doi:10.1200/JCO.1990.8.9.1563

16. Hermes A, Waschki B, Reck M. Hyponatremia as prognostic factor in small cell lung cancer: a retrospective single institution analysis. *Respir Med.* 2012;106(6):900–904. doi:10.1016/j.rmed.2012.02.010

17. Lassen UN, Osterlind K, Hirsch FR, et al. Early death during chemotherapy in patients with small-cell lung cancer: derivation of a prognostic index for toxic death and progression. *Br J Cancer.* 1999;79(3-4):515–519. doi:10.1038/sj.bjc.6690080

18. Fearon K, Strasser F, Anker SD, et al. Definition and classification of cancer cachexia: an international consensus. *Lancet Oncol.* 2011;12(5):489–495. doi:10.1016/S1470-2045(10)70218-7

19. The Diagnosis and Treatment of Lung Cancer (Update). Cardiff (UK). National Collaborating Centre for Cancer. NICE Clinical Guidelines NC, Treatment of SCLC. www.ncbi.nlm.nih.gov/books/NBK99023

20. Fox W, Scadding JG. Medical Research Council comparative trial of surgery and radiotherapy for primary treatment of small-celled or oat-celled carcinoma of bronchus: ten-year follow-up. *Lancet.* 1973;2(7820):63–65. doi:10.1016/S0140-6736(73)93260-1

21. Stahl JM, Corso CD, Verma V, et al. Trends in stereotactic body radiation therapy for stage I small cell lung cancer. *Lung Cancer.* 2017;103:11–16. doi:10.1016/j.lungcan.2016.11.009

22. Roth BJ, Johnson DH, Einhorn LH, et al. Randomized study of cyclophosphamide, doxorubicin, and vincristine versus etoposide and cisplatin versus alternation of these two regimens in extensive small-cell lung cancer: a Phase III trial of the Southeastern Cancer Study Group. *J Clin Oncol.* 1992;10(2):282–291. doi:10.1200/JCO.1992.10.2.282

23. Sundstrom S, Bremnes RM, Kaasa S, et al. Cisplatin and etoposide regimen is superior to cyclophosphamide, epirubicin, and vincristine regimen in small-cell lung cancer: results from a randomized phase III trial with 5 years' follow-up. *J Clin Oncol.* 2002;20(24):4665–4672. doi:10.1200/JCO.2002.12.111

24. Noda K, Nishiwaki Y, Kawahara M, et al. Irinotecan plus cisplatin compared with etoposide plus cisplatin for extensive small-cell lung cancer. *N Engl J Med.* 2002;346(2):85–91. doi:10.1056/NEJMoa003034

25. Lara PN Jr, Natale R, Crowley J, et al. Phase III trial of irinotecan/cisplatin compared with etoposide/cisplatin in extensive-stage small-cell lung cancer: clinical and pharmacogenomic results from SWOG S0124. *J Clin Oncol.* 2009;27(15):2530–2535. doi:10.1200/JCO.2008.20.1061

26. Rossi A, Di Maio M, Chiodini P, et al. Carboplatin- or cisplatin-based chemotherapy in first-line treatment of small-cell lung cancer: the COCIS meta-analysis of individual patient data. *J Clin Oncol.* 2012;30(14):1692–1698. doi:10.1200/JCO.2011.40.4905

27. Verma V, Simone CB 2nd, Allen PK, et al. Multi-Institutional experience of stereotactic ablative radiation therapy for stage I small cell lung cancer. *Int J Radiat Oncol Biol Phys.* 2017;97(2):362–371. doi:10.1016/j.ijrobp.2016.10.041

28. Turrisi AT 3rd, Kim K, Blum R, et al. Twice-daily compared with once-daily thoracic radiotherapy in limited small-cell lung cancer treated concurrently with cisplatin and etoposide. *N Engl J Med.* 1999;340(4):265–271. doi:10.1056/NEJM199901283400403

29. Murray N, Coy P, Pater JL, et al. Importance of timing for thoracic irradiation in the combined modality treatment of limited-stage small-cell lung cancer. The National Cancer Institute of Canada Clinical Trials Group. *J Clin Oncol.* 1993;11(2):336–344. doi:10.1200/JCO.1993.11.2.336

30. Movsas B, Moughan J, Komaki R, et al. Radiotherapy patterns of care study in lung carcinoma. *J Clin Oncol.* 2003;21(24):4553–4559. doi:10.1200/JCO.2003.04.018

31. Simone C, Bogart J, Cabrera A. Radiation therapy for small cell lung cancer: an ASTRO clinical practice guideline. *Pract Radiat Oncol.* 2020;10(3):158–163. doi:10.1016/j.prro.2020.02.009

32. Perry MC, Eaton WL, Propert KJ, et al. Chemotherapy with or without radiation therapy in limited small-cell carcinoma of the lung. *N Engl J Med.* 1987;316(15):912–918. doi:10.1056/NEJM198704093161504

33. Bunn PA Jr, Lichter AS, Makuch RW, et al. Chemotherapy alone or chemotherapy with chest radiation therapy in limited stage small cell lung cancer: a prospective, randomized trial. *Ann Intern Med.* 1987;106(5):655–662. doi:10.7326/0003-4819-106-5-655

34. De Ruysscher D, Pijls-Johannesma M, Vansteenkiste J, et al. Systematic review and meta-analysis of randomised, controlled trials of the timing of chest radiotherapy in patients with limited-stage, small-cell lung cancer. *Ann Oncol.* 2006;17(4):543–552. doi:10.1093/annonc/mdj094

35. Spiro SG, James LE, Rudd RM, et al. Early compared with late radiotherapy in combined modality treatment for limited disease small-cell lung cancer: a London Lung Cancer Group multicenter randomized clinical trial and meta-analysis. *J Clin Oncol.* 2006;24(24):3823–3830. doi:10.1200/JCO.2005.05.3181

36. Videtic GMM, Belderbos JS, Spring Kong FM, et al. Report from the International Atomic Energy Agency (IAEA) consultants' meeting on elective nodal irradiation in lung cancer: small-cell lung cancer (SCLC). *Int J Radiat Oncol Biol Phys.* 2008;72(2):327–334. doi:10.1016/j.ijrobp.2008.03.075

37. Ross H, Hu C, Higgins K, et al. NRG Oncology/Alliance LU005: a phase II/III randomized clinical trial of chemoradiation versus chemoradiation plus atezolizumab in limited stage small cell lung cancer. *J Clin Oncol.* 2020;38(15 suppl):TPS9082. doi:10.1200/JCO.2020.38.15_suppl.TPS9082

38. U.S. National Library of Medicine. Watchful Observation of Patients With LD-SCLC Instead of the PCI (PCILESS). 2019. https://www.clinicaltrials.gov/ct2/show/NCT04168281

39. Le Pechoux C, Dunant A, Senan S, et al. Standard-dose versus higher-dose prophylactic cranial irradiation (PCI) in patients with limited-stage small-cell lung cancer in complete remission after chemotherapy and thoracic radiotherapy (PCI 99-01, EORTC 22003-08004, RTOG 0212, and IFCT 99-01): a randomised clinical trial. *Lancet Oncol.* 2009;10(5):467–474. doi:10.1016/S1470-2045(09)70101-9

40. Le Pechoux C, Laplanche A, Faivre-Finn C, et al. Clinical neurological outcome and quality of life among patients with limited small-cell cancer treated with two different doses of prophylactic cranial irradiation in the intergroup phase III trial (PCI99-01, EORTC 22003-08004, RTOG 0212 and IFCT 99-01). *Ann Oncol.* 2011;22(5):1154–1163. doi:10.1093/annonc/mdq576

41. Wolfson AH, Bae K, Komaki R, et al. Primary analysis of a phase II randomized trial radiation therapy oncology group (RTOG) 0212: impact of different total doses and schedules of prophylactic cranial irradiation on chronic neurotoxicity and quality of life for patients with limited-disease small-cell lung cancer. *Int J Radiat Oncol Biol Phys.* 2011;81(1):77–84. doi:10.1016/j.ijrobp.2010.05.013

42. De Dios N, Murcia M, Counago F, et al. Phase III trial of prophylactic cranial irradiation with or without hippocampal avoidance for SMALL-CELL LUNG cancer. *Int J Radiat Oncol Biol Phys.* 2019;105(1):S35–S36.

43. U.S. National Library of Medicine. *Whole-Brain Radiation Therapy With or Without Hippocampal Avoidance in Treating Patients With Limited Stage or Extensive Stage Small Cell Lung Cancer.* 2019. https://clinicaltrials.gov/ct2/show/NCT02635009

30 ■ MESOTHELIOMA

Sarah M. C. Sittenfeld, Bindu V. Manyam, and Gregory M. M. Videtic

QUICK HIT ■ Mesothelioma is a rare thoracic malignancy associated with progressive morbidity. Patients are rarely curable due to disease extent and comorbidity at diagnosis. EPP and P/D are surgical options for nonmetastatic, medically operable patients with epithelioid histology. CHT and RT are used mainly for palliation, though can be considered in the perioperative setting.

Table 30.1: General Treatment Paradigm for Mesothelioma[1]	
Patient	**Treatment Options**
Clinical stages I–III Epithelial or biphasic histology Medically operable Resectable disease	• Induction CHT (cisplatin/pemetrexed), reassessment, P/D followed by observation • Induction CHT (cisplatin/pemetrexed), reassessment, EPP followed by hemithoracic RT (54 Gy) • EPP, sequential adjuvant CHT, hemithoracic RT (54 Gy) • P/D, CHT +/− IMRT consolidation
Clinical stage IV Sarcomatoid histology Medically inoperable Unresectable	• CHT and palliative RT • Immunotherapy

EPIDEMIOLOGY: U.S. incidence of mesothelioma is 3,000 cases per year. Incidence peaked around 2000 and has been steadily declining secondary to OSHA limitations on acceptable asbestos exposure initiated in the 1970s.[2]

RISK FACTORS: Exposure to asbestos is the most significant risk factor, with 90% of cases related to asbestos. Exposure is most commonly occupational (used as a flame retardant in automobile brakes, shipbuilding, ceiling tiles, pool tiles), and more rarely environmental. Occult transmission of asbestos fibers may occur from workers to family members. Lifetime risk of an asbestos worker developing mesothelioma is as high as 10%. Dose–response relationship and latency period of 20 to 40 years exist between exposure and development of disease. Known synergistic effect of asbestos and smoking. Other risk factors include ionizing RT, carbon nanotubes, and potentially viral oncogenes and genetic susceptibility (BAP1 mutation).[2]

ANATOMY: Can arise from any mesothelial surface, including pleura (80%), and less commonly peritoneum, tunic vaginalis, or pericardium. Two areas of pleura particularly challenging to identify and adequately cover after EPP include ipsilateral diaphragmatic crura and lowest posterior point of diaphragm. Right crus extends to L3 and left crus extends to L2. Lowest point of pleural space can extend as low as L4. Distribution of pleural mesothelioma: 60% right-sided, 35% left-sided, 5% bilateral.[3]

PATHOLOGY: Three histologic variants: **epithelioid** (most common, 60% of cases), **sarcomatoid**, **biphasic** (combination of latter two), though several variations exist. Histology more prognostic than stage. Immunohistochemistry is crucial for diagnosis (mesothelin glycoprotein is 67% sensitive and 98% specific); osteopontin and gene expression assays may be helpful.[2]

CLINICAL PRESENTATION: Majority of patients affected are over age 60 and present 20 to 40 years after asbestos exposure. Symptoms include weight loss, fatigue, chest pain, dyspnea, cough, hoarseness, and dysphagia. Physical exam findings are usually indicative of pleural effusion with unilateral dullness to percussion or decreased air exchange. Features on CXR suggestive of mesothelioma include unilateral pleural density or thickening, persistent pleural effusion, mediastinal shift, lung volume loss, asbestosis demonstrated as bibasilar interstitial fibrosis, and warrant further workup.

WORKUP: H&P with risk-factor assessment.

Labs: Assess operability with PFTs with DLCO, perfusion scanning (if FEV1 <80%), cardiac stress test.[4]

Imaging: CT chest with contrast necessary. PET/CT. MRI chest is optional, but may be helpful in determining resectability.

Biopsy: Historically, thoracentesis used for histologic diagnosis, though only diagnostic in 26% of cases. In contrast, VATS biopsy diagnostic in 98% and provides evidence of stromal, fibroadipose, or lung parenchymal invasion needed to differentiate between reactive hyperplasia, fibrous pleurisy, and malignancy; 10% risk of seeding biopsy tract, and tract should be excised at surgery. For patients who are potentially resectable, mediastinal staging with mediastinoscopy or EBUS.

PROGNOSTIC FACTORS: Stage and histology are most significant prognostic factors. Sarcomatoid and biphasic histologies have worse prognosis compared to epithelioid histology. Poor performance status, age >75, elevated LDH, and hematologic abnormalities (thrombocytosis, leukocytosis, anemia) are associated with worse prognosis.[4]

NATURAL HISTORY: Prognosis is poor, with OS 9 to 17 months. Distant metastatic disease is less common, but can involve bone, liver, and CNS. Most patients succumb to local progression of disease with respiratory failure, arrhythmia, heart failure, or stroke.

STAGING

Table 30.2: AJCC 8th Edition (2017): Staging for Malignant Pleural Mesothelioma				
T/M	N	cN0	cN1	cN2
T1	• Ipsilateral parietal pleura with extension to visceral, mediastinal, or diaphragmatic pleura	IA		
T2	• Involving all ipsilateral pleural surfaces (parietal, mediastinal, diaphragmatic, and visceral) with at least one of the following: • Diaphragmatic muscle • Underlying pulmonary parenchyma	IB	II	
T3	• Involving all ipsilateral pleural surfaces with involvement of at least one of the following: • Endothoracic fascia • Mediastinal fat • Solitary, resectable focus of tumor extending into chest wall soft tissue • Nontransmural pericardium		IIIA	
T4	• Involving all ipsilateral pleural surfaces with involvement of at least one of the following: • Multifocal chest wall mass • Transdiaphragmatic extension to peritoneum • Direct extension to contralateral pleura • Direct extension to mediastinal organs • Direct extension into spine • Direct extension to inner surface of pericardium • Direct extension to myocardium	IIIB		
M1	• Distant metastasis	IV		

cN1, ipsilateral bronchopulmonary, hilar, mediastinal (including internal mammary, peridiaphragmatic, pericardial fat pad, or intercostal) LNs; cN2, contralateral mediastinal or any supraclavicular LNs.

TREATMENT PARADIGM

Surgery: Radical surgery should be limited to carefully selected patients, as it is associated with significant morbidity and mortality (early series demonstrate 31% mortality with EPP). Surgical candidates are those with resectable disease, limited to one hemithorax (clinical stages I–III), adequate cardiopulmonary function, and ECOG PS <2. Nearly all surgical series demonstrate OS benefit to surgery when limited to pure epithelioid subtype. Patients with biphasic or sarcomatoid subtypes often have OS similar to or shorter than expected with nonoperative management.

Definitive surgical procedures include EPP or P/D. P/D provides opportunity to preserve lung parenchyma. Decision is based on surgeon's judgment on obtaining R0 resection. RRs suggest P/D may have less mortality and morbidity compared to EPP, with comparable OS. See Flores data in the following regarding outcomes for EPP vs. P/D.

- EPP is an en bloc resection of parietal and visceral pleura, ipsilateral lung, pericardium, and diaphragm. If there is no involvement of pericardium or diaphragm, these structures can remain intact.
- Extended P/D is parietal and visceral pleurectomy, with removal of all gross tumor and resection of diaphragm and pericardium.
- P/D is parietal and visceral pleurectomy with removal of all gross tumor, without diaphragm and pericardial resection.

Pleurodesis is a surgical option used to palliate symptoms from pleural effusion, involves obliteration of pleural space through injection of sterile, asbestos-free talc to cause adhesion of visceral and parietal pleura. Complete drainage of pleural effusion by tube thoracostomy or video thoracoscopy usually precedes this procedure.

Systemic Therapy: Roles exist for CHT in neoadjuvant, adjuvant, and palliative settings. Cisplatin and pemetrexed demonstrate prolonged OS in patients with unresectable disease. A phase II multicenter study by Krug used neoadjuvant pemetrexed and cisplatin for four cycles, followed by EPP in those patients who did not have disease progression, followed by adjuvant RT (54 Gy) and demonstrated an MS of 16.8 months.[5] Those patients who were able to complete all therapy had MS of 29.1 months. Alternative CHT regimens include cisplatin + gemcitabine and carboplatin + pemetrexed. Immunotherapy is showing promise in stage IV mesothelioma compared to standard CHT, and further study is ongoing.[6]

Radiation

Indications: Adjuvant after EPP, consolidation therapy after P/D, and palliative.

Dose: For EPP, dose for negative margins is 50 to 54 Gy and for positive margins boost to 54 to 60 Gy. After P/D, total dose deliverable (to a maximum of 50.4 Gy) will be limited by mean lung dose to residual lungs of 20 Gy and mandates use of IMRT.

Toxicity: Fatigue, esophagitis, pneumonitis (caution with contralateral lung in postpneumonectomy patients).[7]

■ EVIDENCE-BASED Q&A

▒ What is the benefit of EPP?

Local control is the main goal of EPP. There is high rate of mortality with EPP; however, with careful selection of patients, there may be survival benefit.

Treasure, MARS Study (*Lancet Oncol* 2011, PMID 21723781): PRT of 50 patients from 12 UK hospitals who received neoadjuvant CHT, randomized to EPP or no EPP, followed by RT. Of 24 patients randomized to EPP, 16 underwent EPP; 30-day mortality rate was 12.5%. HR for OS with EPP was 1.90 ($p = .082$). After adjustment for sex, histologic subtype, stage, and age, HR for EPP was 2.75 ($p = .016$). **Conclusion: Despite study deficiencies, EPP had worse OS than no EPP suggesting importance of choosing EPP candidates carefully.**

▒ What are outcomes of EPP compared to P/D?

Data are conflicting, with some showing improved LC and OS with EPP, while others demonstrating improved outcomes with P/D. EPP shown to have higher perioperative morbidity and mortality.

Flores, MSKCC (*J Thorac Cardiovasc Surg* 2008, PMID 18329481): RR of 663 patients from three institutions treated between 1990 and 2006 with EPP or P/D. EPP had perioperative mortality rate of 7% vs. 4% with P/D. Stage ($p < .001$), epithelioid histology ($p < .001$), EPP ($p < .001$), and multimodality therapy ($p < .001$) were all significantly associated with improved survival. Multivariate analysis demonstrated HR of 1.4 for EPP ($p < .001$) controlling for stage, histology, gender, and multimodality therapy. **Conclusion: P/D is associated with improved OS, though subject to selection bias. EPP is associated with a higher risk of perioperative mortality.**

Lang-Lazdunski, UK (*J Thorac Oncol* 2012, PMID 22425923): Nonrandomized prospective study of 22 patients receiving neoadjuvant CHT, EPP, adjuvant RT and 54 patients receiving neoadjuvant CHT, P/D, and adjuvant CHT. 30-day mortality rate was 4.5% in EPP and 0% for P/D. Complications observed in 68% in EPP and 27.7% in P/D. Trimodality therapy completed by 68% in EPP and 100% in P/D. Survival was significantly better in P/D compared to EPP (2-year OS 49% vs. 18.2% and 5-year OS 30.1% vs. 9%; $p = .004$). Epithelioid histology, P/D, and R0 resection all associated with improved survival on MVA. **Conclusion: P/D with perioperative CHT has improved survival compared with multimodality therapy with EPP in this nonrandomized study.**

■ **Is trimodality therapy safe and effective? Which patients are best candidates?**

Trimodality therapy is generally safe and effective in very carefully selected patients. Epithelioid histology, R0 resection, and N0 patients have been shown to have 5-year OS as high as 50% with trimodality therapy.

Sugarbaker (*J Thorac Cardiovasc Surg* 1999, PMID 9869758): RR of 183 patients treated with EPP followed by adjuvant CHT and RT. MFU 13 months. Perioperative mortality rate 3.8% at 2 years with 50% morbidity. Survival was 37% at 1 year and 15% at 5 years. MS was 19 months. Three variables significantly associated with improved survival: (a) **epithelial** type (52% 2-year OS, 21% 5-year OS, 26-month MS); (b) **negative resection margins** (44% 2-year OS, 25% 5-year OS, 23-month); (c) **negative lymph nodes** (42% 2-year OS, 17% 5-year OS). Patients with all three variables had 62% 2-year OS, 46% 5-year OS, and MS 51 months. **Conclusion: Trimodality therapy is feasible and mediastinal lymph node evaluation is important in selecting optimal patients. Epithelioid type, R0 resection, and extrapleural node-negative patients have extended survival.**

Pagan (*J Thorac Cardiovasc Surg* 2006, PMID 17033611): Prospective nonrandomized trial of EPP followed by carboplatin/paclitaxel and RT (50 Gy). 30-day mortality rate was 4.5% and overall complication rate was 50%. No major complications observed. MS was 20 months and 5-year OS 19%. Patients with epithelioid histology, R0 resection, and N0–1 had 5-year OS 50%.

■ **What is the benefit of postoperative RT after EPP? Is there a role for IMRT?**

Local recurrence rates following EPP are reported as high as 80%. Addition of postoperative RT has been shown to decrease locoregional failure rates to 37%. Various studies have employed IMRT showing that it can be safely used when appropriate mean lung dose constraints are met for the remaining lung.

Rusch (*J Thorac Cardiovasc Surgery* 2001, PMID 11581615): Phase II trial of 88 patients who underwent EPP or P/D followed by postoperative hemithoracic RT (54 Gy/30 fx) in 55 patients. RT was AP/PA with photons and electron boost to areas requiring shielding. LRF in 12.7%, grade 4 pneumonitis in 9.1%. MS was 33.8 months for stage I and II, 10 months for stage III and IV tumors ($p = .04$).

Allen (*IJROBP* 2006, PMID 16751058): RR of 13 patients treated with hemithoracic IMRT (54 Gy/30 fx) after EPP and adjuvant CHT with cisplatin or cisplatin/pemetrexed. Fatal pneumonitis rate was 46%. Patients with fatal pneumonitis had V20 15.3% to 22.4%, V5 81% to 100%, and mean lung dose 13.3 Gy to 17 Gy.

Rice (*Ann Thorac Surg* 2007, PMID 17954086): RR of 63 patients who underwent EPP followed by IMRT (45 Gy), CHT not routinely administered. Nonepithelioid histology in 33%, stage III 72%, and ipsilateral nodal metastases in 54%. Perioperative mortality was 8%. MS was 14.2 months for patients who received IMRT and 10.2 months for 3D-CRT. Node-negative patients with epithelioid histology had median survival 28 months. Locoregional recurrence was 13% and only 5% had in-field recurrence. Rate of fatal lung events was 9.5% and V20 predicted for pulmonary-related death on MVA.

■ **Is there a role for postoperative RT after P/D?**

There are series evaluating its use, initially using 3D-CRT, which observed residual gross disease could not be eradicated. More recent studies employing IMRT have been done showing improvement in survival as compared to palliative approaches though at the cost of increased toxicity, and thus its use is generally limited to centers of expertise.

Chance (IJROPB 2015, PMID 25442335): Matched pair analysis of 24 patients who underwent P/D followed by adjuvant CHT and hemithoracic IMRT to 45 Gy. Outcomes were compared to 24 patients who received EPP followed by IMRT, matched for age, nodal status, performance status, and CHT. MFU 12.2 months. There was statistically significant decrease in FVC, FEV1, and DLCO both after P/D and then further after IMRT. MS was 28.4 vs. 14.2 months ($p = .04$) and median PFS was 16.4 vs. 8.2 months ($p = .01$) for PD/IMRT vs. EPP/IMRT, respectively. There was no significant difference in grade 4 to 5 toxicity between two groups (0% vs. 12.5%; $p = .23$).

Rimner, IMPRINT (JCO 2016, PMID 27325859): Phase II study of 27 patients who received neoadjuvant platinum CHT and pemetrexed, P/D, followed by adjuvant hemithoracic IMRT (median dose 46.8 Gy). MFU 21.6 months. Grade 2 pneumonitis was 22% and grade 3 pneumonitis was 7.4% and all resolved with steroids. Median PFS and OS were 12.4 and 23.7 months, respectively. Two-year OS was 59%. **Conclusion: Hemithoracic IMRT after P/D is safe and should be considered in the treatment paradigm in this patient population.**

Trovo (IJROBP 2020, PMID 33259933): Phase III study of 108 patients undergoing lung-sparing surgery with gross residual disease randomized to adjuvant hemithoracic IMRT (50 Gy/25 fx plus 60 Gy SIB to gross disease) vs. palliative RT (most commonly 30–35 Gy/10 fx). All patients received CHT. MFU 14.6 months. Hemithoracic IMRT improved LC with 2-year cumulative LRR incidence of 27% vs. 83% for palliative RT. Median OS was 35.6 months for hemithoracic RT vs. 12.4 months with palliative RT ($p ≤ .001$). No grade 3 toxicity with palliative RT, while 20% had ≥3 acute toxicity and 31% had grade 3 to 4 late toxicity, including 16% grade ≥2 pneumonitis including 1 possible fatal event. **Conclusion: Adjuvant hemithoracic IMRT with SIB to gross residual disease is feasible and improves LC and OS as compared to palliative RT with increased rates of both acute and late toxicities.**

■ **Which CHT regimens are most effective?**

Platinum-doublet CHT has shown good outcomes in both the neoadjuvant and palliative settings. The addition of bevacizumab to platinum doublet in the palliative setting showed a potential survival benefit.

Vogelzang, EMPHACIS (JCO 2003, PMID 12860938): Single-blind PRT of 456 patients not eligible for surgical resection, randomized to cisplatin vs. cisplatin and pemetrexed every 21 days. MS was 12.1 vs. 9.3 months ($p = .02$) for cisplatin/pemetrexed vs. cisplatin, respectively. Median time to progression was significantly longer in cisplatin/pemetrexed arm (5.7 vs. 3.9 months; $p = .001$) with significantly higher response rates (41.3% vs. 16.7%; $p < .0001$). Folic acid and vitamin B12 were added after 117 patients, resulting in significant reduction in toxicities.

Krug (JCO 2009, PMID 19364962): Phase II multicenter trial of 75 patients who received neoadjuvant cisplatin/pemetrexed, 50 received EPP, and 28 received adjuvant RT. Patients who had radiographic response to CHT had trend toward better OS (29.1 vs. 13.9 months, $p = .07$). MS was 16.6 months for whole cohort and median PFS was 13.1 months.

Zelman (Lancet 2016, PMID 26719230): PRT of 448 patients with unresectable disease randomized to cisplatin/pemetrexed +/– bevacizumab in 21-day cycles for up to six cycles. OS was significantly longer with the addition of bevacizumab (18.8 vs. 16.1 months; $p = .0167$). There was more grade 3 hypertension (23% vs. 0%) and thrombotic events (6% vs. 1%) with bevacizumab.

■ **If biopsy tract is not surgically excised, can RT reduce the risk of tract recurrence?**

Currently, the role of tract RT depends on the clinical setting and primary form of treatment.

Bydder (Br J Cancer 2004, PMID 15199394): PRT of 28 patients randomized to 10 Gy/1 fx with electrons following chest wall violation vs. observation. Tract metastasis was not significantly different

(10% vs. 7%; $p = .53$) for RT and observation, respectively. Crude rates of tract metastases were 22% for Abrams needles, 9% for thoracic drains, and 4% for FNA, and these were not significantly different ($p = .23$).

O'Rourke (*Radiother Oncol* 2007, PMID 17588698): PRT of 61 patients who underwent chest drain placement or pleural biopsy randomized to 21 Gy/3 fx after procedure vs. observation. There were four drain site metastases in RT arm and three in observation arm ($p = .75$). **Conclusion: No significant differences between rate of tract metastases with or without adjuvant RT.**

Clive, SMART Trial (*Lancet Oncol* 2016, PMID 27345639): PRT of 203 patients from 22 UK hospitals who underwent large-bore pleural intervention randomized to prophylactic RT (21 Gy/3 fx within 42 days of pleural intervention) vs. salvage RT (21 Gy/3 fx upon procedure tract metastasis). Primary outcome was incidence of procedure tract metastasis within 7 cm of site of pleural intervention within 12 months of randomization. **Conclusion: There was no significant difference in procedure tract metastasis between immediate and deferred RT (9% vs. 16%; $p = .14$).**

■ **Is there benefit to dose-escalated RT in mesothelioma?**

No evidence at this time to increase dose beyond 54 Gy in the adjuvant setting.

Allen (*IJROBP* 2007, PMID 17674974): RR of 39 patients treated with hemithoracic RT after EPP, with 24 treated to doses of 30 to 40 Gy and 15 treated with 54 Gy. Local failure was higher with lower doses of RT (50% vs. 27%), but was not statistically significant. There was no significant difference in OS.

■ **Is RT useful for treating pain in mesothelioma?**

Evidence supports palliative benefit of RT in MPM, with duration of symptom control possibly a function of dose.

McLeod (*J Thorac Oncol* 2015, PMID 25654216): Phase II, 40 patients, with assessments of pain and other symptoms at baseline, then received 20 Gy/5 fx to areas of pain. Primary end point was assessment of pain at the site of RT at 5 weeks. **Forty-seven percent of patients alive at week 5 had an improvement in their pain.**

de Graaf-Strukowska (*IJROBP* 1999, PMID 10078630): RR of 189 patients, higher local response rate for patients treated with 4 Gy per fx compared with less than 4 Gy per fx (50% vs. 39%). Duration of response was short, with pain recurring predominantly in the RT field after a median of 69 days (range 32–363).

■ **Are there alternative therapies available for unresectable mesothelioma?**

There is emerging evidence for the addition of TTF, but further study is warranted.

Ceresoli, STELLAR (*Lancet Oncol* 2019, PMID 31628016): Prospective single-arm trial of 80 patients with unresectable disease received platinum doublet plus Novo-TTF-100L. MS was 18.2 months, 21.2 months in epithelioid histology subset. No increase in serious toxicity. **Conclusion: Novo-TTF when added to standard CHT is safe with encouraging survival results, and future study is warranted.**

REFERENCES

1. NCCN Clinical Practice Guidelines in Oncology: Malignant Pleural Mesothelioma. 2019.
2. Ai J, Stevenson JP. Current issues in malignant pleural mesothelioma evaluation and management. *Oncologist.* 2014;19(9):975–984. doi:10.1634/theoncologist.2014-0122
3. Rosenzweig KE, Giraud P. Radiation therapy for malignant pleural mesothelioma. *Cancer Radiother.* 2017;21(1):73–76. doi:10.1016/j.canrad.2016.09.009
4. Patel SC, Dowell JE. Modern management of malignant pleural mesothelioma. *Lung Cancer (Auckl).* 2016;7:63–72. doi:10.2147/LCTT.S83338
5. Krug LM, Pass HI, Rusch VW, et al. Multicenter phase II trial of neoadjuvant pemetrexed plus cisplatin followed by extrapleural pneumonectomy and radiation for malignant pleural mesothelioma. *J Clin Oncol.* 2009;27(18):3007–3013. doi:10.1200/JCO.2008.20.3943
6. Reuss JE, Forde PM. Immunotherapy for mesothelioma: rationale and new approaches. *Clin Adv Hematol Oncol.* 2020;18(9):562–572.
7. Allen AM, Czerminska M, Jänne PA, et al. Fatal pneumonitis associated with intensity-modulated radiation therapy for mesothelioma. *Int J Radiat Oncol, Biol, Phys.* 2006;65(3):640–645. doi:10.1016/j.ijrobp.2006.03.012

31 ■ THYMOMA

Christopher W. Fleming, Jonathan M. Sharrett, and Gregory M. M. Videtic

QUICK HIT ■ Thymoma is a rare tumor of the anterior mediastinum associated with MG and managed primarily with surgery. PORT is indicated for Masaoka–Koga stage III disease or incomplete resection, and CHT is usually employed for potentially resectable tumors to facilitate surgery (see Table 31.1). Metastatic thymoma may have a very long natural history; systemic therapy has limited benefits, and "aggressive" local therapies (surgery, RT) may be appropriate as indicated by patient and tumor presentations. Thymic carcinoma is a more aggressive entity and generally warrants PORT for all stages.

Table 31.1: General Treatment Paradigm for Thymoma

Thymic neoplasm suspected and resection possible?	Yes: proceed to total thymectomy (biopsy may be omitted)	Stage I	No adjuvant therapy
		Stage II	No adjuvant therapy (PORT controversial)
		Stage III to IVA, + margin, or thymic carcinoma	PORT 45 to 50 Gy (negative/close margins), 54 Gy (microscopic margins), 60 Gy (gross residual). CHT controversial, may be considered for gross residual or thymic carcinomas
	No (locally advanced, solitary/ potentially resectable metastases)	Core needle biopsy followed by induction CHT	Individualized by disease burden and performance status, including CHT +/− local therapy (surgery/RT) as indicated

EPIDEMIOLOGY: 1.5 cases per million person-years in the United States.[1] Typically occurs in adults aged 40 to 60. Comprises around 20% of all mediastinal tumors but half of all anterior mediastinal tumors. Thymic carcinomas represent less than 1% of thymic tumors.

RISK FACTORS: No known etiologic factors.

ANATOMY: Thymus is an anterior mediastinal structure responsible for the maturation of T-cells. Lymphatic drainage is to the lower cervical, internal mammary, and hilar nodes. Structurally, thymus consists of capsule, cortex, and medulla. Histologically, it includes epithelial cells, epitheliore-ticular cells (form Hassall's corpuscles), myoid cells, early T lymphocytes ("thymocytes"), and B lymphocytes.

PATHOLOGY

Table 31.2: WHO Thymoma Grading

WHO Type[2,3]	Histology
A	Medullary thymoma
AB	Mixed thymoma
B1	Predominantly cortical thymoma
B2	Cortical thymoma
B3	Well-differentiated thymic carcinoma
C	Thymic carcinoma

CLINICAL PRESENTATION: Often incidental finding on imaging. Local symptoms due to mass effect may include chest pain, dyspnea, cough, phrenic nerve palsy, and SVC syndrome. Paraneoplastic syndromes may be present prior to or after diagnosis. Up to 50% of patients will present with MG; it is less common for MG patients to have associated thymoma. Other less common paraneoplastic syndromes include red cell aplasia, immunodeficiency, and multiorgan autoimmunity.

WORKUP: H&P. If thymoma suspected and considered resectable, biopsy may be omitted and resection performed. If unresectable/medically inoperable, obtain core needle biopsy to confirm diagnosis (open biopsy also possible; biopsy should not violate pleural space); multidisciplinary evaluation indicated.

Labs: As indicated by clinical and radiographic findings: Serum β-hCG and AFP (rule out germ cell tumor), CBC, CMP, serum level of anti-ACh antibodies to assess for MG.

Imaging: Chest CT with contrast, PET/CT (optional), PFTs.

PROGNOSTIC FACTORS: Masaoka stage, histology (see Table 31.2), degree of resection (R0, R1 vs. R2).[4] Thymoma is an indolent but locally aggressive disease, with a long natural history even in setting of metastases. Thymic carcinoma is a more aggressive disease, with poorer outcomes due to early metastatic spread.

STAGING: Historically, Masaoka Staging System and Koga Modification of Masaoka Staging System have been utilized (see Tables 31.3). TNM staging system was first implemented in 2017 with AJCC 8th edition (see Table 31.4).

Table 31.3: Masaoka–Koga Staging System for Thymoma[5]	
Stage	**Definition**
I	Grossly and microscopically completely encapsulated tumor
IIa	Microscopic transcapsular invasion
IIb	Macroscopic invasion into surrounding fatty tissue or grossly adherent to but not breaking through mediastinal pleura or pericardium
III	Macroscopic invasion into neighboring organ (e.g., pericardium, great vessels, or lung)
IVA	Pleural or pericardial dissemination
IVB	Distant metastasis

Table 31.4: AJCC 8th Edition (2017) Staging for Thymic Tumors				
T/M \ N		N0	N1	N2
T1	T1a: No mediastinal pleura involvement	I		
	T1b: Direct invasion of mediastinal pleura			
T2	• Direct invasion of the pericardium (either partial or full thickness)	II	IVA	IVB
T3	• Direct invasion into lung, brachiocephalic vein, superior vena cava, phrenic nerve, chest wall, or extrapericardial pulmonary artery or veins	IIIA		
T4	• Invasion into aorta, arch vessels, intrapericardial pulmonary artery, myocardium, trachea, esophagus	IIIB		
M1	M1a: Separate pleural or pericardial nodule(s)			
	M1b: Pulmonary intraparenchymal nodule or distant organ metastasis			
N1: Metastasis in anterior (perithymic) lymph nodes. N2: Metastasis in deep intrathoracic or cervical lymph nodes.				

TREATMENT PARADIGM

Surgery: Total thymectomy with negative margins is mainstay of therapy in resectable cases. This is typically performed with median sternotomy. Resection of both phrenic nerves should be avoided to prevent severe respiratory compromise. Signs and symptoms of MG should be controlled medically with anticholinesterase inhibitors prior to surgery.

Chemotherapy: Platinum-based CHT is indicated for thymic carcinoma, unresectable disease, medically inoperable with gross disease. CHT is often used for downstaging and postoperatively based on degree of resection. For diffuse metastases, consider CHT alone. No randomized trials have identified superior regimen. Common regimens include cyclophosphamide/adriamycin/cisplatin (CAP), cisplatin/etoposide (PE), or carboplatin/paclitaxel.

Radiation

Indications: PORT should be offered for positive surgical margins, stage III disease and considered for any thymic carcinoma.

Dose: RT dosing is based on degree of resection with 45 to 54 Gy, 55 to 60 Gy, and 60 to 70 Gy given for R0, R1, and R2, respectively. Definitive RT indicated for medically inoperable disease, with the addition of CHT and its sequencing empiric.

Toxicity: Acute: Fatigue, cough, skin erythema. Late: Cardiac morbidity, hypothyroidism, second malignancy.

■ EVIDENCE-BASED Q&A

■ What are outcomes for completely resected thymoma by stage and when should PORT be considered?

Surgery is the mainstay of therapy for operable patients with locoregional disease, with excellent LC and survival for R0 resections. PORT is always indicated for residual disease if repeat resection is not feasible. Conventionally, stage III/IVA disease has been managed by surgery followed by the addition of PORT, independent of margins. Some authors have recommended PORT for stage II/III disease with positive or close margin (<1 mm), gross fibrous adhesion to pleura, or WHO high grade (B3), but otherwise no PORT for R0 resected thymoma.[6] However, Rimner et al. found the use of PORT in completely resected stage II and III thymoma to be associated with improved OS. At present, PORT for stage III would be generally recommended.

Kondo, Japan (*Ann Thorac Surg* 2003, PMID 12963221): RR of 1,320 patients with thymic epithelial tumors from 115 special thoracic surgery institutes across Japan. Patients with stage I thymoma received surgery alone and patients with stage II and III thymoma and thymic carcinoid underwent surgery + PORT. Patients with stage IV thymoma and thymic carcinoma were treated with RT or CHT. In stage III and IV thymoma, 5-year survival rates of total resection, subtotal resection, and inoperable groups were 93%, 64%, and 36%, respectively. In thymic carcinoma, 5-year survival rates of total resection, subtotal resection, and inoperable groups were 67%, 30%, and 24%, respectively. PORT did not change LR rates in patients with totally resected stage II and III thymoma. Adjuvant therapy including RT or CHT did not improve prognosis in patients with totally resected III and IV thymoma and thymic carcinoma (see Table 31.5). **Conclusion: Total resection is the most important factor in treatment of thymic epithelial tumors. Adjuvant therapy may not improve outcomes for totally resected invasive thymoma and thymic carcinoma.**

Table 31.5: Results of Japanese Retrospective Study for Thymoma by Kondo et al.				
Masaoka Stage	I	II	III	IVA
Complete resection (%)	100	100	85	42
Recurrence (%)	1	4	28	34
5-yr OS (%)	100	98	89	71

Utsumi, Japan (*Cancer* 2009, PMID 19685527): RR of 324 patients from 1970 to 2005 who underwent complete resection of thymoma. PORT was performed for 134 patients; 10-year DSS with and without PORT was 92.8% and 94.4%, respectively ($p = .22$). Subset analyses after stratifying by Masaoka stage and WHO cell type: 10-year DSS for patients w/o PORT with Masaoka stage I and II, as well as WHO cell types A, AB, or B1, was 100%. For Masaoka stage III/IV and those with WHO cell types B2/B, PORT did not improve outcomes. **Conclusion: Surgical resection alone is sufficient for thymoma patients with Masaoka stage I and II, and those with WHO cell types A, AB, and B1. Optimal treatment strategy should be established for patients with Masaoka stage III/IV and WHO cell type B2/B3 thymoma.**

Omasa, Japan (*Cancer* 2015, PMID 25565590): Database study from JART including 1,265 patients with stage II or III thymoma or thymic carcinoma (12.3%). Majority (70.8%) were stage II. PORT delivered to 403 (31.9%) patients; those receiving PORT had significantly higher rates of incomplete surgery. For stage II and III thymoma, PORT was not associated with improved RFS or OS ($p = .350$). PORT for stage II and III thymic carcinoma was associated with increasing RFS ($p = .003$) but not OS ($p = .536$). **Conclusion: PORT did not increase RFS or OS for stage II or III thymoma but did increase RFS for stage II or III thymic carcinoma.** *Comment: Higher rates of incomplete resection without worse outcomes suggest potential benefit to PORT for stage II to III thymoma.*

Rimner, ITMIG group (*J Thorac Oncol* 2016, PMID 27346413): Database study from the ITMIG including 1,263 patients with completely resected stage II or III thymoma; 870 (69%) had stage II thymoma and 827 (70%) had grade of B1, B2, or B3. The 5- and 10-year OS rates for patients receiving PORT were 95% and 86%, respectively, compared with 90% and 79% for patients receiving resection alone ($p = .002$). OS benefit remained significant when stage II ($p = .02$) and III ($p = .0005$) patients were analyzed separately. On MVA, younger age, female gender, absence of paraneoplastic syndromes, stage II disease, and use of PORT were significantly associated with longer OS. **Conclusion: OS benefit was observed with the use of PORT in completely resected stage II and III thymoma.**

Jackson, NCDB (*J Thorac Oncol* 2017, PMID 28126540): NCDB study including 4,056 patients who underwent surgery for thymoma or thymic carcinoma. PORT delivered to 49%. MVA and propensity score–matched analyses found survival advantage associated with PORT. Subset analysis indicated longer OS in association with PORT for patients with positive margins or stage IIB to III thymoma ($p < .05$), but not for patients stage I to IIA ($p = .156$). **Conclusions: PORT associated with longer OS, with the greatest relative benefits observed for stage IIB to III disease and positive margins.**

■ **What are reported outcomes specifically for thymic carcinoma?**

Ahmad, ITMIG group (*J Thorac Cardiovasc Surg* 2015, PMID 25524678): ITMIG database study of 1,042 patients with thymic carcinoma; 370 patients (45%) were stage III and 274 (33%) stage IV. 166 patients (22%) underwent induction CHT, and 48 (6%) underwent preoperative RT. R0 resection in 447 (61%), R1 in 102 (14%), and R2 in 184 (25%). SCC was the predominant histologic subtype ($n = 560; 79\%$). RT utilized for the majority of patients (72%), with the exception of stage I patients (45% underwent RT). Likewise, CHT was utilized for most (65%), with the exception of stage I and II patients (42% and 34%, respectively). Median OS 6.6 years and the cumulative incidence of recurrence at 5 years was 35%. On MVA, R0 resection and use of RT were associated with prolonged OS. **Conclusion: R0 resection and RT are associated with improved OS for thymic carcinomas.**

■ **What are the management options for unresectable/inoperable thymic tumors?**

In the unresectable setting, downstaging with neoadjuvant therapy may be attempted with induction CHT +/– RT. With good response to CHT, RT is often deferred in favor of resection, allowing pathologic stage to dictate necessity for PORT. In those who are medically inoperable or remain unresectable, completion of definitive treatment using combined-modality therapy may be appropriate. Data for definitive RT is modest given this rare clinical scenario. Diffuse systemic metastatic disease is typically treated with CHT alone, with palliative RT considered for symptomatic progression.

Loehrer, SWOG/SECSG/ECOG (*JCO* 1997, PMID 9294472): Prospective single-arm study conducted from 1983 to 1995 involving 26 patients with limited-stage unresectable thymoma or thymic carcinoma. Patients received 2 to 4 cycles q3 weeks of cisplatin, doxorubicin, and cyclophosphamide (PAC) followed by RT with 54 Gy to primary tumor and regional lymph nodes for patients without progressive disease. 23 patients were evaluable. Toxicity was mild. There were 5 CR and 11 PR to CHT (overall response rate, 69.6%). Median time to treatment failure was 93.2 months, and MS was 93 months. 5-year OS 52.5%. **Conclusion: PAC combination CHT produces response rates in management of patients with unresectable thymoma. Combined-modality therapy is feasible and associated with prolonged PFS. Benefit of combined-modality therapy over RT alone is suggested for patients with unresectable thymoma.**

Shin, MD Anderson (*Ann Intern Med* 1998, PMID 9669967): Prospective cohort study from 1990 to 1996 of 13 patients with newly diagnosed, histologically proven, unresectable malignant thymoma. Patients treated with induction CHT (3 cycles of cyclophosphamide, doxorubicin, cisplatin, and prednisone), surgical resection, PORT, and consolidation CHT with 3 more cycles of same regimen. Twelve patients were evaluable. CR to CHT in 3 patients (25%), PR in 8 patients (67%), and 1 patient had minor response (8%). Eleven patients underwent surgical resection with one refusing surgery. R0 resection in 9 (82%) and incompletely in 2 (18%) of 11 patients who had been receiving RT and con-solidation CHT. All 12 patients alive at 7 years, with MFU of 43 months, while 10/12 are disease-free (7-year DFS 73%). **Conclusion: Aggressive multimodal treatment may be appropriate for locally advanced, unresectable malignant thymoma.**

When is concurrent chemoRT recommended?

There are very little data on concurrent chemotherapy for thymic neoplasms. The following phase 2 trial from China found 60 Gy with concurrent EP to be well tolerated and efficacious. There is no prospective data comparing definitive RT alone to concurrent or sequential CHT regimens.

Fan, China (*IJROBP* 2020, PMID 31987968): Phase 2 trial of 56 patients with unresectable thymic malignancies (22 thymoma, 34 thymic carcinoma) undergoing 60 Gy IMRT with concurrent and adjuvant etoposide and cisplatin. 75% were stage IVB. Objective response rate was 85.7%. 1-, 2-, and 5-year PFS rates were 66.1%, 48.0%, and 29.5%, and the 1-, 2-, and 5-year OS rates were 91.0%, 76.2%, and 56.2%, respectively. The most common grade 3 to 4 adverse event was leukopenia (42.9%). G3 esophagitis rate 5.4%, no radiation pneumonitis. G3 pulmonary fibrosis in 5.3%. **Conclusion: Concurrent RT and EP may be a suitable treatment option for patients with unresectable thymic neoplasms.**

REFERENCES

1. Engels EA. Epidemiology of thymoma and associated malignancies. *J Thorac Oncol.* 2010;5(10 Suppl 4):S260–S265. doi:10.1097/JTO.0b013e3181f1f62d
2. Falkson CB, Bezjak A, Darling G, et al. The management of thymoma: a systematic review and practice guideline. *J Thorac Oncol.* 2009;4(7):911–919. doi:10.1097/JTO.0b013e3181a4b8e0
3. Kondo K, Yoshizawa K, Tsuyuguchi M, et al. WHO histologic classification is a prognostic indicator in thymoma. *Ann Thorac Surg.* 2004;77(4):1183–1188. doi:10.1016/j.athoracsur.2003.07.042
4. Safieddine N, Liu G, Cuningham K, et al. Prognostic factors for cure, recurrence and long-term survival after surgical resection of thymoma. *J Thorac Oncol.* 2014;9(7):1018–1022. doi:10.1097/JTO.0000000000000215
5. Masaoka A, Monden Y, Nakahara K, Tanioka T. Follow-up study of thymomas with special reference to their clinical stages. *Cancer.* 1981;48(11):2485–2492. doi:10.1002/1097-0142(19811201)48:11<2485::AID-CNCR2820481123>3.0.CO;2-R
6. Wright CD. Management of thymomas. *Crit Rev Oncol Hematol.* 2008;65(2):109–120. doi:10.1016/j.critrevonc.2007.04.005

VI ■ GASTROINTESTINAL

32 ■ ESOPHAGEAL CANCER

Camille A. Berriochoa and Gregory M. M. Videtic

QUICK HIT ■ Most esophageal cancer patients present with either locally advanced or metastatic disease. Palliative RT is therefore commonly used to relieve pain or obstruction. In potentially curable patients, EBRT may be employed in the definitive, neoadjuvant, or adjuvant settings, as the individual roles and sequencing of surgery, CHT, and RT in contributing to cure remain controversial. Brachytherapy may be an option in selected curative cases as a boost treatment, or in advanced cases for palliation (Table 32.1).

Table 32.1: General Treatment Paradigm for Esophageal Cancer[1]	
Stage I	Tis/T1a (SCC or ACA): Endoscopic resection/ablation (preferred) vs. esophagectomy T1b (SCC): Endoscopic resection/ablation T1b (ACA): Esophagectomy
Stage II to IVA (T4a only)	1. Preoperative chemoRT (41.4–50.4 Gy with concurrent CHT) or 2. Definitive chemoRT (particularly for cervical esophagus), typically to a dose of 50.4 Gy but can consider 60 to 66 Gy for cervical location or 3. Postoperative chemoRT for pathologic stages IIA (T3N0)–IVA; any stage with R1/R2 resection Can consider esophagectomy for T2 low-risk lesions, <2 cm, well differentiated
Stage IVA (T4b)	Definitive chemoRT, 50.4 Gy; can consider CHT alone if invasion to trachea, great vessels, or heart
Stage IVB	Palliation with EBRT, brachytherapy, CHT, and/or best supportive care

EPIDEMIOLOGY: Approximately 18,000 new esophageal cancers diagnosed with nearly 16,000 deaths per year in the United States.[2] Incidence peaks in sixth and seventh decades. Globally, SCC accounts for 90% of cases with the majority of these cases arising in endemic regions of Eastern Europe and Asia. However, adenocarcinoma is more common in North America and Western European countries, comprising ~70% of cases.[3] Both histologic subtypes are more common in men but the relative increased incidence in males is more pronounced for adenocarcinoma.

RISK FACTORS: For squamous cell (mnemonic: ABCDEF):[3-5] achalasia, bad diet (nutritional deficiency, high fat, low fruit/vegetables, drinking beverages at high temperatures causing thermal injury to mucosa), caustic stricture (lye ingestion), cigarette smoking, dysplasia/diverticuli, esophageal webs (Plummer–Vinson syndrome includes iron-deficiency anemia, atrophic glossitis, webs), ethanol (alcohol), familial. For adenocarcinoma (mnemonic: BOG):[3-5] Barrett's esophagus (squamocolumnar metaplasia; risk approximately 0.5%/year for nondysplastic lesions; ranges from 1% to 5% for dysplastic lesions),[6,7] obesity, GERD (weekly symptoms increase risk by factor of 5, daily symptoms increase risk by factor of 7),[8] cigarette smoking (less so than squamous), also associated with hiatal hernia and EGFR polymorphisms. Rarely, hereditary predisposition syndromes may be implicated including tylosis, Bloom's syndrome, Fanconi anemia for squamous cell, and familial Barrett's syndrome for adenocarcinoma.[1]

ANATOMY: Esophagus anatomic key features include: no true serosa, nonkeratinized squamous epithelium superiorly that transitions to glandular epithelium inferiorly, and extensive submucosal lymphatic plexus that often results in skip metastases. Approximately 25 cm long, begins at cricopharyngeus muscle at about 15 cm from incisors to GEJ, about 40 cm from incisors (Table 32.2). Esophagus extends from vertebral levels C6 to T10. GEJ tumors defined as within 5 cm from true GEJ (epithelial change) are frequently classified according to modified Siewert system, with class I tumors originating from 1 to 5 cm superior to true GEJ, class II tumors originating from 1 cm above to 2 cm below, and class III tumors from 2 to 5 cm below GEJ.[9,10]

Table 32.2: Anatomic and Endoscopic Landmarks of the Esophagus		
Anatomic Site	**Description**	**Approximate Distance From Incisors**
Cervical	UES to thoracic inlet (sternal notch)	15–20 cm
Upper thoracic	Sternal notch to azygos vein	20–25 cm
Middle thoracic	Azygos vein to inferior pulmonary vein	25–30 cm
Lower thoracic	Inferior pulmonary vein to GEJ	30–40 cm
Lower abdominal	GEJ to 5 cm below GEJ (see Chapter 33)	40–45 cm
GEJ/Cardia	GEJ to 5 cm below GEJ	40–45 cm

PATHOLOGY: As noted earlier, SCC accounts for 90% of cases globally but ACA comprises 70% of cases in North America and Western Europe. "Mixed adenosquamous" and "carcinomas," NOS are categorized as SCC for purposes of staging. Rare histologies include small-cell carcinoma and sarcoma.

CLINICAL PRESENTATION:[3] Common symptoms include progressive dysphagia, weight loss, heartburn that does not respond to medical therapy, melena, and/or symptoms of asymptomatic blood loss. Less commonly, patients may present with symptoms of laryngeal nerve paralysis such as hoarseness, cough, and pneumonia. Note that asymptomatic cases may be detected due to Barrett's esophagus screening. Given association with other aerodigestive malignancies, it is important to evaluate for symptoms related to H&N SCC.

WORKUP:[1] H&P with careful neck and abdominal exam.

Labs: CBC, CMP. HER2-neu testing for unresectable, recurrent, or metastatic adenocarcinoma (~25% of esophageal cancers are HER2-neu positive).[11,12]

Imaging: Barium swallow, CT chest/abdomen/pelvis with oral and IV contrast; PET/CT for distant metastases (has poor sensitivity and specificity for nodal metastases: approximately 50% and 80%, respectively).[13] EUS more accurate than CT and PET-CT for local/nodal staging (Table 32.3).[14]

Procedures: Upper GI endoscopy with biopsy. EUS permits biopsy of suspicious nodes. Lesions at or above carina need bronchoscopy to rule out tracheoesophageal fistula.

PROGNOSTIC FACTORS: Age, KPS, stage, grade, weight loss, pretreatment, and postinduction dysphagia.[15] RPA of esophageal patients showed only weight loss, specifically loss of ≥10% in preceding 6 months, as prognostic.[16]

NATURAL HISTORY: 5-year OS is approximately 40% if confined to primary site, 20% if spread to regional LNs, and 4% if distant metastases present.

STAGING

Table 32.3: AJCC 8th Edition (2017) Staging for Esophageal Cancer							
Tumor		**Node**		**Distant Metastasis**		**Grade**	
T1	a. Invades lamina propria or muscularis mucosa	N0	• No regional LNs	M0	• No distant metastasis	G1	• Well differentiated
	b. Invades submucosa						

(continued)

Table 32.3: AJCC 8th Edition (2017) Staging for Esophageal Cancer (*continued*)

Tumor		Node		Distant Metastasis		Grade	
T2	• Invades muscularis propria	N1	• 1 to 2 regional LNs	M1	• Distant metastasis	G2	• Moderately differentiated
T3	• Invades adventitia	N2	• 3 to 6 regional LNs			G3	• Poorly differentiated
T4	a. Resectable[1]	N3	• ≥7 regional LNs				
	b. Unresectable[2]						

Notes: Resectable[1] = invades pleura, pericardium, diaphragm, azygos vein, or peritoneum. Unresectable[2] = invades aorta, vertebral body, airway. AJCC suggests ≥10 nodes removed for pT1 tumors, ≥20 for pT2, and ≥30 for pT3–4.

Stage Grouping (AJCC 8th Edition)
Note that the AJCC 8th Edition includes a pathologic TNM and postneoadjuvant pathologic TNM, which are not displayed here.

Squamous Cell Carcinoma		Adenocarcinoma	
Clinical Stage	Clinical TNM	Clinical Stage	Clinical TNM
0	Tis N0	0	Tis N0
I	T1 N0–1	I	T1 N0
II	T2 N0–1 T3 N0	IIA	T1 N1
		IIB	T2 N0
III	T3 N1 T1–3 N2	III	T2 N1 T3 N0–1 T4a N0–1
IVA	T4 N0–2 T any N3	IVA	T1–4a N2 T4b N0–2 T any N3
IVB	T any N any M1	IVB	T any N any M1

TREATMENT PARADIGM

Surgery: Surgery is a commonly utilized option for locoregionally confined disease and options are based on patient's medical condition, tumor location, and stage. Cervical tumors are typically treated nonoperatively because these lesions may also need laryngopharyngectomy with permanent stoma. For upper and middle thoracic tumors (>5 cm below cricopharyngeus), total esophagectomy with gastric pull-through is standard. Distal esophagogastrectomy is standard for lesions of GEJ and lower thoracic esophagus. Contraindications to surgery include distant metastases, T4b lesions (involvement of heart, great vessels, trachea, or other surrounding organs), bulky multistation adenopathy, and medical comorbidity.

Three techniques are commonly employed in North America for total esophagectomy: Ivor Lewis, McKeown (tri-incisional), and transhiatal. Both Ivor Lewis esophagogastrectomy and McKeown esophagogastrectomy require right thoracotomy incisions, with the latter permitting access to more superiorly located tumors. Transhiatal esophagogastrectomy can be used for cervical, thoracic, and GEJ lesions and requires abdominal and left cervical incisions; thoracotomy is not performed (often resulting in shorter operative times). There is some evidence of lower postoperative morbidity with transhiatal approach;[17] however, several disadvantages associated with this technique include difficulty in resecting large, midesophageal and/or paratracheal tumors as well as lower lymph node retrieval. Postoperative mortality at high-volume centers is typically less than 5%[18–20] but can be 10% or higher after neoadjuvant chemoRT.[21–23]

For most distal lesions, mediastinal and upper abdominal lymphadenectomy is performed. Minimum number of lymph nodes to optimize staging and survival is controversial, with recommendations varying widely from 6 to 23 LNs.[24–27] Retrospective evidence exists for improved survival with increased number of lymph nodes resected.[26]

Minimally invasive surgery is possible although data are evolving. Two randomized trials have reported reduction in POCs with use of minimally invasive surgery (thoracoscopy with upper abdominal laparoscopy) as compared to open technique with thoracotomy.[28,29]

Chemotherapy: CHT is commonly utilized for T2 to T4 or node-positive tumors in neoadjuvant, perioperative, adjuvant, or definitive settings.[30-35] In both preoperative and definitive settings, common regimens concurrent with RT include cisplatin + infusional 5-FU or carboplatin + paclitaxel. Infusional 5-FU is thought to be superior to bolus 5-FU based on data from gastric cancer.[1,36] Oral capecitabine can be substituted for infusional 5-FU.[1] Metastatic adenocarcinomas of GEJ should be tested for HER2-neu and trastuzumab can be considered if positive based on survival benefit demonstrated by TOGA trial.[37] If perioperative CHT alone is being considered in the management of GEJ tumors, FLOT (5-FU, leucovorin, oxaliplatin and docetaxel) should be regarded as the recommended regimen.[31] Irinotecan, etoposide, and oxaliplatin are all also under investigation. Addition of cetuximab to standard cytotoxic therapy has shown no benefit.[38,39] No benefit to the addition of trastuzumab to definitive chemoRT in HER2 + esophageal adenocarcinoma per RTOG 1010 (results in abstract form only).[40] Emerging evidence supports the addition of icotinib (oral EGFR inhibitor) to definitive RT in patients ≥70 with esophageal SCC who are not candidates for CHT (OS for RT alone: 16.3 months; RT + icotinib: 24 month, $p = .008$).41

Radiation

Indications: Typically delivered with concurrent CHT in preoperative or definitive setting for T2 to T4 or node-positive tumors.

Dose: With concurrent CHT, 50 to 50.4 Gy/25 to 28 fx is standard. Without CHT, 64 Gy/32 fx is standard (see Herskovic). Randomized trials show benefit to concurrent CHT and no benefit to dose escalation beyond 50.4 Gy.[34,42] In preoperative setting, 41.4 Gy is appropriate dose based on the CROSS trial. Brachytherapy boost can be selectively employed though does not improve survival and may be associated with morbidity.[43,44]

Palliation: EBRT and brachytherapy can be used. Other options include dilation, laser therapy, endoscopic injection therapies, EMR, PDT, stenting (preferable in those with malignant fistula). Safe to treat with palliative RT poststenting.

Toxicity: Acute: esophagitis, fatigue, weight loss, subacute pneumonitis. Late: strictures, pulmonary fibrosis, pericarditis, coronary artery disease.

Procedure: See *Treatment Planning Handbook*, Chapter 6.[45]

Endoscopic Therapy: Endoscopic management of early esophageal cancer may be performed using EMR or ESD. Both techniques allow resection of mucosa (and possibly a portion of the submucosa) containing early tumor without interruption of deeper layers. EMR can remove lesions <2 cm in size en bloc. Larger lesions may require resection in piecemeal fashion limiting assessment of margins. ESD offers en bloc dissection of tumor regardless of size. ESD is performed with specialized needle knives, which allow incision followed by careful dissection of lesion within submucosal layer. ESD is labor-intensive and has increased risk of perforation. Esophageal stenosis remains a concern after extensive EMR or ESD.

Locally Ablative Modalities: Include thermal destruction by laser, MPEC, APC, or radiofrequency ablation; cryotherapy; and PDT. PDT may eradicate high-grade dysplasia and Barrett's.

■ **EVIDENCE-BASED Q&A**

UNRESECTABLE/INOPERABLE ESOPHAGEAL CANCER

■ **Is RT alone sufficient for esophageal cancer or should concurrent CHT be added?**

RT alone is insufficient since OS is improved with the addition of CHT to RT.

Herskovic, RTOG 8501 (*NEJM* 1992, PMID 1584260; **Update Al-Sarraf** *JCO* 1997, PMID 8996153; **Update Cooper** *JAMA* 1999, PMID 10235156): Phase III PRT of 129 patients with ACA (12%) or SCC (88%) cT1–3N0–1 randomized to RT alone (64 Gy/32 fx) vs. chemoRT (concurrent cisplatin/5-FU +

50 Gy/25 fx). CHT was cisplatin 75 mg/m² and 5-FU 1,000 mg/m² on weeks 1, 5, 8, and 11. Initial RT field extended from SCV fossa to GEJ (except SCV was optional for distal-third tumors). For chemoRT arm, extended field was taken to 30 Gy followed by 20 Gy boost to tumor + 5 cm. For RT alone arm, extended field was taken to 50 Gy followed by 14 Gy boost to tumor + 5 cm. Trial stopped early due to survival difference. 5-year OS was 26% vs. 0% favoring chemoRT. Persistent disease was the most common mode of failure: 26% in chemoRT arm and 37% in RT alone arm. Severe/life-threatening acute toxicity were 44%/20% with chemoRT, and 25%/3% with RT alone. No differences in late toxicity. **Conclusion: When treating nonoperatively, concurrent chemoRT is superior to RT alone for T1–3N0–1 esophageal cancer.**

■ Does RT dose escalation improve survival in setting of CHT?

There is no evidence that dose escalation improves outcomes. Whether modern techniques may permit safer delivery of dose-escalated treatment was evaluated in a 2016 NCDB analysis.[46] This analysis reviewed patients with stage I to III esophageal cancer who received RT between 2004 and 2012 to doses ≥50 Gy and found no benefit to dose escalation, consistent with the results of the Minsky trial. The ARTDECO study from the Netherlands was a phase III PRT comparing dose escalation in the definitive chemoRT setting utilizing SIB to the primary tumor (61.6 Gy compared to 50.4 Gy in the standard arm, both with concurrent weekly carbo/ taxol). Results are in abstract form only but again confirmed no benefit to dose escalation.[47]

Minsky, RTOG 94-05/INT 0123 (*JCO* 2002, PMID 11870157): Phase III PRT of 218 patients with T1–4N0–1 ACA (15%) or SCC (85%) treated with low-dose (50.4 Gy) vs. high-dose (64.8 Gy) RT with both arms receiving concurrent CHT (cisplatin + 5-FU). For the high-dose arm, RT was 50.4 Gy/28 fx to tumor + 5 cm sup–inf (and 2 cm laterally), with 14.4 Gy boost to tumor + 2 cm. CHT was cisplatin 75 mg/m² and 5-FU 1,000 mg/m² on weeks 1, 5, 9, and 13 in low-dose arm, and weeks 1, 5, 11, and 15 in high-dose arm. Closed early because no benefit seen in high-dose arm. See Table 32.4. **Conclusion: No benefit to high-dose RT with concurrent CHT, with higher incidence of treatment-related death in this trial.** *Note: Some authors have commented that higher mortality observed in high-dose arm may not be related to RT dose given 7 of 11 deaths occurred at ≤50.4 Gy.*

Table 32.4: RTOG 9405 Minsky: RT Dose Escalation for Esophageal Cancer				
	MS (mos)	2-Yr OS	2-Yr LR	Treatment-Related Deaths
High-dose chemoRT (64.8 Gy)	13.0	31%	56%	10% (7/11 deaths at ≤50.4 Gy)
Low-dose chemoRT (50.4 Gy)	18.1	40%	52%	2%
p value	NS	NS	.71	

■ Should elective nodal stations be targeted when treating patients definitively?

There is no strong evidence to suggest that elective nodal stations should not be included and current NCCN guidelines suggest that the CTV should include elective nodes respective to the primary tumor location.[1] Of note is the randomized study from China suggesting nonelective treatment is safe.

Lyu (*Cancer Med* 2020, PMID 32841543): PRT of 228 stage II to III thoracic SCC esophageal patients randomized to IFI or ENI. RT was delivered once a day in 1.8 to 2 Gy fractions to a total dose of 60 to 66 Gy to the GTV and 50 to 54 Gy to the CTV. Initial results in 2018 revealed significant decreases in treatment-related esophagitis and pneumonitis in IFI arm. In this current report, for ENI and IFI groups, respectively, the results showed: median PFS (20.3 vs. 21.4 months), OS (32.5 vs. 34.9 months). **Conclusion: IFI was associated with similar survival as ENI and is an acceptable treatment method for patients with thoracic esophageal SCC.**

RESECTABLE/OPERABLE ESOPHAGEAL CANCER

■ Is there benefit to trimodality therapy as compared to definitive chemoRT?

To date, there is no phase III evidence to suggest that surgery improves overall survival, although PFS appears improved by reducing locoregional failure. Note that the Stahl trial limited inclusion criteria to SCC only and that 90% of patients in the Bedenne trial had SCC.

Stahl, "Stahl I" (*JCO* 2005, PMID 15800321): Phase III PRT of 172 patients with locally advanced SCC upper–midesophageal cancer, uT3–4N0–1M0, age ≤70, randomized to either (A) induction CHT, pre-op chemoRT (40 Gy/20 fx), then surgery, or (B) induction CHT, then definitive chemoRT (≥65 Gy) without surgery. Induction CHT was bolus 5-FU, LCV, etoposide, and cisplatin q3 weeks for 3 cycles. Concurrent CHT was EP. In arm B, T4 and obstructing T3 tumors received 50 Gy/25 fx, with EBRT boost to 65 Gy with 15 Gy/10 fx BID over last week. For nonobstructing T3 tumors, patients received 60 Gy/30 fx, with HDR brachytherapy boost of 4 Gy × 2 fx to 5 mm depth. MFU was 6 years. No difference in 2-year OS (40% vs. 35%) or MS (16.4 vs. 14.9 months). Surgery arm had better 2-year PFS (64% vs. 41%, p = .003) due to improved LC, but also higher treatment-related mortality (13% vs. 4%, p = .03). Of arm A, only 66% proceeded to surgery, but complete resection was possible in 82% of those who did. Seventy percent of surgery patients had at least one severe complication; 11% post-op hospital mortality; 35% had pCR. Response to induction CHT was associated with improved survival. **Conclusion: Adding surgery to chemoRT improves LC but does not improve OS. Patients who respond to induction treatment may be treated definitively with chemoRT, while poor responders may benefit from surgery.**

Bedenne, French FFCD 9102 (*JCO* 2007, PMID 17401004): Phase III PRT of operable patients with T3N0–1M0 thoracic esophageal cancer comparing (A) neoadjuvant chemoRT followed by surgery vs. (B) higher dose definitive chemoRT in those with response to up-front chemoRT. Patients received 2 cycles of 5-FU and cisplatin (days 1–5 and 22–26) and either conventional (46 Gy in 4.5 weeks) or split-course (15 Gy, days 1–5 and 22–26) concomitant RT (investigator choice). Patients with response and no contraindication to either treatment were randomly assigned to surgery (arm A) or continuation of chemoRT (arm B; 3 additional cycles of 5-FU/cisplatin and either conventional [20 Gy] or split-course [15 Gy] RT). chemoRT was considered equivalent to surgery if difference in 2-year survival rate was <10%. Histologic composition: 90% SCC, 10% ACA. Surgery arm: MS: 17.7 vs. 19.3 months in no surgery arm (p = .44); 2-year LC: 66.4% in surgery arm compared with 57.0% in definitive chemoRT arm (p = .03). Fewer stents were required in surgery arm (5% vs. 32% in chemoRT arm; p < .001). **Conclusion: LC is improved with surgery but no difference in OS.**

■ **Does CHT with surgery improve OS compared to surgery alone?**

Yes, multiple trials studied neoadjuvant and perioperative regimens with most demonstrating OS benefit.[33,48] However, local response was often inadequate (pCR rates typically <5%) and chemoRT may be superior. The MAGIC trial, investigating perioperative ECF for gastric and GEJ cancers, showed improved OS for ECF + surgery compared to surgery alone. FLOT-4, which compared perioperative FLOT to ECF, has established FLOT as the perioperative CHT standard since it is superior to ECF.[31]

■ **Does preoperative chemoRT improve OS compared to surgery alone?**

Yes. The CROSS PRT showed doubled OS with use of trimodality therapy compared to surgery alone.

Van Hagen, CROSS (*NEJM* 2012, PMID 22646630; Update Shapiro *Lancet Oncol* 2015, PMID 26254683): Phase III PRT of neoadjuvant chemoRT + surgery vs. surgery alone. 366 potentially resectable patients randomized to carboplatin (AUC 2 mg/mm/min)/paclitaxel (50 mg/m^2) and concurrent RT (41.4 Gy/23 fx) followed by surgery (transthoracic or transhiatal approach) vs. surgery alone. Surgery was performed within 4 to 6 weeks of completion of chemoRT; 75% ACA, 23% SCC, and 2% had large-cell undifferentiated carcinoma. Initial publication showed that MS improved from 24 to 49.4 months with the addition of pre-op chemoRT (p = .003). Updated publication: MFU 84 months. Complete resection (R0) rate was higher with chemoRT, 92% vs. 69% (p < .001). pCR was achieved in 29% overall (49% in SCC subgroup) of those treated with chemoRT. MS improved in chemoRT + surgery group vs. surgery alone (see Table 32.5); 5-year OS increased from 33% to 47% (p = .003). Estimated number needed to treat to prevent one additional death at 5 years was 7.1. **Conclusion: Preoperative chemoRT improved MS among patients with potentially curable esophageal or GEJ cancer.**

Table 32.5: CROSS Trial of Neoadjuvant chemoRT for Esophageal Cancer			
	Neoadjuvant chemoRT + Surgery	Surgery Alone	p Value
MS, all	48.6 mos	24 mos	.003
MS, SCC	81.6 mos	21.1 mos	.008
MS, ACA	43.2 mos	27.1 mos	.038

■ **Does neoadjuvant chemoRT improve OS as compared to neoadjuvant CHT?**

Yes, the Stahl trial supports benefit to chemoRT as compared to CHT alone though was underpowered. The recent Neo-AEGIS trial is specifically powered to compare outcomes in adenocarcinoma, with arms as follows: perioperative CHT (modified MAGIC regimen) vs. neoadjuvant chemoRT per CROSS.[49] Results are awaited. Multiple meta-analyses also support this concept.

Stahl, "Stahl II" (*JCO* 2009, PMID 19139439): Phase III PRT of neoadjuvant CHT vs. neoadjuvant chemoRT in patients with locally advanced ACA of the GEJ; 126 patients (goal 394, closed due to poor accrual), resectable T3–4N×M0 (staged by EUS, CT, and laparoscopy), randomized to (A) PLF × 2.5 cycles (cisplatin/leucovorin/fluorouracil) vs. (B) PLF × 2 cycles, then 3 weeks of combined chemoRT, 30 Gy/15 fx with cisplatin/etoposide. Both arms followed by tumor resection 3 to 4 weeks after induction. R0 resection in 70% vs. 72%, pCR 2% vs. 15.6% ($p = .03$), 3-year OS 28% vs. 47% ($p = .07$). **Conclusion: Preoperative chemoRT has trend to improved OS compared with preoperative CHT alone.** *Comment: Trial closed early and is underpowered.*

Gebski, Australasian Group Meta-analysis (*Lancet Oncol* 2007, PMID 17329193): Study-level meta-analysis included 10 PRTs comparing neoadjuvant chemoRT vs. surgery alone and 8 PRTs comparing neoadjuvant CHT vs. surgery alone. HR for all-cause mortality with neoadjuvant chemoRT vs. surgery alone was 0.81 (95% CI: 0.70–0.93; $p = .002$), corresponding to 13% absolute difference in survival at 2 years, HR for neoadjuvant CHT was 0.90 (0.81–1.00; $p = .05$), which indicates 2-year absolute survival benefit of 7%. **Conclusion: chemoRT demonstrates larger effect size than neoadjuvant CHT alone.**

Pasquali, Network Meta-analysis (*Ann Surg* 2016, PMID 27429017): Study-level network (compares ≥3 treatment approaches) meta-analysis, which included 33 RCTs in which 6,072 patients were randomized to receive either surgery alone or neoadjuvant CHT, RT, or chemoRT followed by surgery OR surgery followed by adjuvant CHT, RT, and chemoRT. Neoadjuvant chemoRT demonstrated strongest effect on OS of all treatments. HR for OS of neoadjuvant chemoRT vs. surgery alone was 0.77 ($p < .001$) whereas HR for OS of neoadjuvant CHT vs. surgery alone was 0.89 ($p = .051$). **Conclusion: Neoadjuvant chemoRT appears the most effective strategy for resectable esophageal cancers.**

■ **If a patient gets surgery up front, what is the role of adjuvant therapy?**

The McDonald trial (INT 0116) evaluated the role of adjuvant chemoRT in patients with GEJ or gastric cancer and demonstrated improvement in 3-year OS (from 41% to 50%, p = .005) in those who received adjuvant chemoRT (bolus 5-FU and leucovorin with concurrent RT, 45 Gy/25 fx).[50] A recent meta-analysis of over 6,000 patients from 33 RCTs with resectable esophageal carcinoma found no significant advantage in OS in patients who received surgery + adjuvant therapy (HR: 0.87, 95% CI: 0.67–1.14) whereas neoadjuvant therapies followed by surgery were associated with survival advantage (HR: 0.83, 95% CI: 0.76–0.90).[30]

■ **Is there benefit to IMRT for esophageal cancer?**

3D-conformal RT via 3 or 4 fields is standard technique for esophageal cancer, with NCCN suggesting IMRT in cases when OAR constraints cannot be met.[1] Retrospective data suggest IMRT benefit with respect to cardiac toxicity, but selection and follow-up bias remains the issue and further study is necessary. Guidelines for IMRT planning are available.[51]

Lin, MDACC (*IJROBP* 2012, PMID 22867894): RR of 676 patients treated at MDACC (413 3D-CRT, 263 IMRT) with stage IB–IVA esophageal cancer treated with chemoRT (46% also received surgery) from 1998 to 2008. Inverse probability weighted adjusted Cox model used to compare OS. OS was independently associated with stage, performance status, PET staging, induction CHT, and treatment modality (IMRT vs. 3D-CRT, HR: 0.72, $p < .001$). Compared with IMRT, 3D-CRT patients had significantly greater risk of dying (72.6% vs. 52.9%, $p < .0001$) and of LRR ($p = .0038$). No difference seen in cancer-specific mortality (Gray's test, $p = .86$) or DM ($p = .99$). Increased cumulative incidence of cardiac death in 3D-CRT group ($p = .049$), as well as undocumented deaths (5-year estimate: 11.7% in 3D-CRT vs. 5.4% in IMRT, $p = .0029$). **Conclusion: IMRT can be considered in treatment of esophageal cancer.**

PROTON THERAPY

Proton therapy in the setting of thoracic tumors, including esophageal cancer, remains investigational. However, the study by Lin et al. is the first published randomized study of proton vs. photon irradiation and bears knowing, even for its unusual end point.

Lin (*JCO* 2020, PMID 32160096): Phase IIB randomized trial of PBT or IMRT (50.4 Gy): unresectable and potentially resectable cases included, stages II to III, and eligible to receive concurrent CHT; 145 patients randomly assigned (72 IMRT, 73 PBT), and 107 patients (61 IMRT, 46 PBT) evaluable. Primary end points were TTB and PFS. TTB end point, as per the authors, synthesizes the cumulative severity of multiple AEs that patients with EC may experience after chemoradiotherapy with or without surgery. The posterior mean TTB was 2.3 times higher for IMRT (39.9; 95% highest posterior density interval, 26.2–54.9) than PBT (17.4; 10.5–25.0). The mean POC score was 7.6 times higher for IMRT (19.1; 7.3–32.3) vs. PBT (2.5; 0.3–5.2). The posterior probability that mean TTB was lower for PBT compared with IMRT was 0.9989, which exceeded the trial's stopping boundary of 0.9942 at the 67% interim analysis; 3-year PFS (51%) and OS (44.5%) were essentially identical in both arms. **Conclusion: PBT for neoadjuvant or definitive treatment of locally advanced EC produced a lower toxicity profile, but similar PFS, compared to IMRT.**

ESOPHAGEAL BRACHYTHERAPY

■ **What is the role for esophageal brachytherapy in the modern era?**

Classically, brachytherapy was developed as a boost to EBRT and for palliation of dysphagia related to esophageal cancer. ABS consensus guidelines have been established for brachytherapy.[42] *Brachytherapy is less utilized in the modern era, likely due to availability of other advanced RT techniques, limited indications, and potential complications.*

■ **Does brachytherapy boost improve outcomes when added to definitive chemoRT?**

This was investigated in RTOG 9207, a phase I/II study of definitive chemoRT to 50 Gy/25 fx with cis/5-FU followed by brachytherapy boost (if HDR: initially 15 Gy/3 fx, then reduced to 10 Gy/2 fx prescribed to 1 cm depth; if LDR: 20 Gy in 1 fx).[43] *Results showed a 12% fistula rate that was lethal in 50% of patients and outcomes that were no better than prior trials looking at chemoRT alone. Of note, CHT was given concurrently with brachytherapy in this trial, and may have contributed to high toxicity rates.*

■ **Which is the most effective method of palliation: metal stent or brachytherapy?**

Homs, Dutch SIREC (*Lancet* 2004, PMID 15500894): Phase III PRT, 209 patients with either metastatic disease or with medically inoperable esophageal or GEJ cancer. Randomized either to stent or to 12 Gy in 1 fx via brachytherapy (10 mm diameter applicator, prescribed to 1 cm from source axis, sucralfate ×4 weeks, lifelong omeprazole). Excluded tumors >12 cm, fistula, tumor within 3 cm of upper esophageal sphincter, previous RT or stent. Primary end point was physician-reported dysphagia; patient-reported outcomes recorded as well. Stenting demonstrated more rapid relief, brachytherapy demonstrated more long-term relief. Late hemorrhage occurred more with stenting (33% vs. 22%, *p* = .02); QOL scores favored brachytherapy, medical costs were similar; fistula formation occurred in 3 patients in each group. **Conclusion: Brachytherapy has more durable dysphagia relief and fewer complications than stenting.**

REFERENCES

1. NCCN Clinical Practice Guidelines in Oncology: Esophageal Cancer. 2020. https://www.nccn.org/professionals/physician_gls/pdf/esophageal.pdf
2. American Cancer Society, Cancer Statistics. 2020. https://acsjournals.onlinelibrary.wiley.com/doi/full/10.3322/caac.21590
3. Rustgi A, El-Serag HB. Esophageal carcinoma. *N Engl J Med.* 2015;372(15):1472–1473. doi:10.1056/NEJMc1500692
4. Lundell LR. Etiology and risk factors for esophageal carcinoma. *Dig Dis.* 2010;28(4–5):641–644. doi:10.1159/000320452
5. Esophageal cancer risk factors. American Cancer Society. https://www.cancer.org/cancer/esophagus-cancer/causes-risks-prevention/risk-factors.html. Published June 6, 2020.

6. Hvid-Jensen F, Pedersen L, Drewes AM, et al. Incidence of adenocarcinoma among patients with Barrett's Esophagus. *N Engl J Med*. 2011;365(15):1375–1383. doi:10.1056/NEJMoa1103042

7. de Jonge PJ, van Blankenstein M, Looman CW, et al. Risk of malignant progression in patients with Barrett's oesophagus: a Dutch nationwide cohort study. *Gut*. 2010;59(8):1030–1036. doi:10.1136/gut.2009.176701

8. Rubenstein JH, Taylor JB. Meta-analysis: the association of oesophageal adenocarcinoma with symptoms of gastro-oesophageal reflux. *Aliment Pharmacol Ther*. 2010;32(10):1222–1227. doi:10.1111/j.1365-2036.2010.04471.x

9. Siewert JR, Stein HJ. Classification of adenocarcinoma of the Oesophagogastric junction. *Br J Surg*. 1998;85(11):1457–1459. doi:10.1046/j.1365-2168.1998.00940.x

10. Rudiger Siewert J, Feith M, Werner M, Stein HJ. Adenocarcinoma of the esophagogastric junction: results of surgical therapy based on anatomical/topographic classification in 1,002 consecutive patients. *Ann Surg*. 2000;232(3):353–361. doi:10.1097/00000658-200009000-00007

11. Gowryshankar A, Nagaraja V, Eslick GD. HER2 status in barrett's esophagus & esophageal cancer: a meta analysis. *J Gastrointest Oncol*. 2014;5(1):25–35.

12. Bartley AN, Washington MK, Ismaila N, Ajani JA. HER2 testing and clinical decision making in gastroesophageal adenocarcinoma: guideline summary from the College of American Pathologists, American Society for Clinical Pathology, and American Society of Clinical Oncology. *J Oncol Pract*. 2017;13(1):53–57. doi:10.1200/JOP.2016.018929

13. van Westreenen HL, Westerterp M, Bossuyt PM, et al. Systematic review of the staging performance of 18F-fluorodeoxyglucose positron emission tomography in esophageal cancer. *J Clin Oncol*. 2004;22(18):3805–3812. doi:10.1200/JCO.2004.01.083

14. Lightdale CJ, Kulkarni KG. Role of endoscopic ultrasonography in the staging and follow-up of esophageal cancer. *J Clin Oncol*. 2005;23(20):4483–4489. doi:10.1200/JCO.2005.20.644

15. McNamara MJ, Adelstein DJ, Allende DS, et al. Persistent dysphagia after induction chemotherapy in patients with esophageal adenocarcinoma predicts poor post-operative outcomes. *J Gastrointest Cancer*. 2016;48(2):181–189. doi:10.1007/s12029-016-9881-x

16. Thomas CR Jr, Berkey BA, Minsky BD, et al. Recursive partitioning analysis of pretreatment variables of 416 patients with locoregional esophageal cancer treated with definitive concomitant chemoradiotherapy on Intergroup and Radiation Therapy Oncology Group trials. *Int J Radiat Oncol Biol Phys*. 2004;58(5):1405–1410. doi:10.1016/j.ijrobp.2003.09.022

17. Hulscher JB, van Sandick JW, de Boer AG, et al. Extended transthoracic resection compared with limited transhiatal resection for adenocarcinoma of the esophagus. *N Engl J Med*. 2002;347(21):1662–1669. doi:10.1056/NEJMoa022343

18. Karl RC, Schreiber R, Boulware D, et al. Factors affecting morbidity, mortality, and survival in patients undergoing ivor lewis esophagogastrectomy. *Ann Surg*. 2000;231(5):635–643. doi:10.1097/00000658-200005000-00003

19. Orringer MB, Marshall B, Chang AC, et al. Two thousand transhiatal esophagectomies: changing trends, lessons learned. *Ann Surg*. 2007;246(3):363–372; discussion 372–364. doi:10.1097/SLA.0b013e31814697f2

20. Orringer MB, Marshall B, Iannettoni MD. Transhiatal esophagectomy: clinical experience and refinements. *Ann Surg*. 1999;230(3):392–400; discussion 400–393. doi:10.1097/00000658-199909000-00012

21. Bosset JF, Gignoux M, Triboulet JP, et al. Chemoradiotherapy followed by surgery compared with surgery alone in squamous-cell cancer of the esophagus. *N Engl J Med*. 1997;337(3):161–167. doi:10.1056/NEJM199707173370304

22. Stahl M, Stuschke M, Lehmann N, et al. Chemoradiation with and without surgery in patients with locally advanced squamous cell carcinoma of the esophagus. *J Clin Oncol*. 2005;23(10):2310–2317. doi:10.1200/JCO.2005.00.034

23. Bedenne L, Michel P, Bouche O, et al. Chemoradiation followed by surgery compared with chemoradiation alone in squamous cancer of the esophagus: FFCD 9102. *J Clin Oncol*. 2007;25(10):1160–1168. doi:10.1200/JCO.2005.04.7118

24. Bogoevski D, Onken F, Koenig A, et al. Is it time for a new TNM classification in esophageal carcinoma? *Ann Surg*. 2008;247(4):633–641. doi:10.1097/SLA.0b013e3181656d07

25. Hu Y, Hu C, Zhang H, et al. How does the number of resected lymph nodes influence TNM staging and prognosis for esophageal carcinoma? *Ann Surg Oncol*. 2010;17(3):784–790. doi:10.1245/s10434-009-0818-5

26. Greenstein AJ, Litle VR, Swanson SJ, et al. Effect of the number of lymph nodes sampled on postoperative survival of lymph node-negative esophageal cancer. *Cancer*. 2008;112(6):1239–1246. doi:10.1002/cncr.23309

27. Peyre CG, Hagen JA, DeMeester SR, et al. The number of lymph nodes removed predicts survival in esophageal cancer: an international study on the impact of extent of surgical resection. *Ann Surg*. 2008;248(4):549–556. doi:10.1097/SLA.0b013e318188c474

28. Biere SS, van Berge Henegouwen MI, Maas KW, et al. Minimally invasive versus open oesophagectomy for patients with oesophageal cancer: a multicentre, open-label, randomised controlled trial. *Lancet*. 2012;379(9829):1887–1892. doi:10.1016/S0140-6736(12)60516-9

29. Mariette C, Meunier B, Pezet D, et al. Hybrid minimally invasive versus open oesophagectomy for patients with oesophageal cancer: a multicenter, open-label, randomized phase III controlled trial, the MIRO trial. *J Clin Oncol*. 2015;33(Suppl 3):5. doi:10.1200/jco.2015.33.3_suppl.5

30. Pasquali S, Yim G, Vohra RS, et al. Survival after neoadjuvant and adjuvant treatments compared to surgery alone for resectable esophageal carcinoma: a network meta-analysis. *Ann Surg*. 2016; 265(3):481–491. doi:10.1097/SLA.0000000000001905

31. Al-Batran SE, Homann N, Pauligk C, et al. Perioperative chemotherapy with fluorouracil plus leucovorin, oxaliplatin, and docetaxel versus fluorouracil or capecitabine plus cisplatin and epirubicin for locally advanced, resectable gastric or gastro-oesophageal junction adenocarcinoma (FLOT4): a randomised, phase 2/3 trial. *Lancet*. 2019;393(10184):1948–1957.

32. Allum WH, Stenning SP, Bancewicz J, et al. Long-term results of a randomized trial of surgery with or without pre-operative chemotherapy in esophageal cancer. *J Clin Oncol*. 2009;27(30):5062–5067. doi:10.1200/JCO.2009.22.2083

33. Boige V PJ, Saint-Aubert B. Final results of a randomized trial comparing preoperative fluorouracil/cisplatin to surgery alone in adenocarcinoma of the stomach and lower esophagus: FNLCC ACCORD 07–FFCD 9703 trial. *J Clin Oncol*. 2007;25(18S):4510. doi:10.1200/jco.2007.25.18_suppl.4510

34. Herskovic A, Martz K, al-Sarraf M, et al. Combined chemotherapy and radiotherapy compared with radio-therapy alone in patients with cancer of the esophagus. *N Engl J Med*. 1992;326(24):1593–1598. doi:10.1056/NEJM199206113262403

35. Stahl M, Walz MK, Stuschke M, et al. Phase III comparison of preoperative chemotherapy compared with chemo-radiotherapy in patients with locally advanced adenocarcinoma of the esophagogastric junction. *J Clin Oncol*. 2009;27(6):851–856. doi:10.1200/JCO.2008.17.0506

36. Wagner AD, Grothe W, Haerting J, et al. Chemotherapy in advanced gastric cancer: a systematic review and meta-analysis based on aggregate data. *J Clin Oncol*. 2006;24(18):2903–2909. doi:10.1200/JCO.2005.05.0245

37. Bang YJ, Van Cutsem E, Feyereislova A, et al. Trastuzumab in combination with chemotherapy versus chemother-apy alone for treatment of HER2-positive advanced gastric or gastro-oesophageal junction cancer (ToGA): a phase 3, open-label, randomised controlled trial. *Lancet*. 2010;376(9742):687–697. doi:10.1016/S0140-6736(10)61121-X

38. Crosby T, Hurt CN, Falk S, et al. Chemoradiotherapy with or without cetuximab in patients with oesophageal cancer (SCOPE1): a multicentre, phase 2/3 randomised trial. *Lancet Oncol*. 2013;14(7):627–637. doi:10.1016/S1470-2045(13)70136-0

39. Suntharalingam M, Winter, K, Ilson D et al. Effect of the addition of cetuximab to paclitaxel, cisplatin, and radiation therapy for patients with esophageal cancer, NRG/RTOC 0436. *JAMA Oncol*. 2017;3(11):1520–1528. doi:10.1001/jamaoncol.2017.1598

40. Safran H, Winter K, Wigle D, et al. Trastuzumab with trimodality treatment for esophageal adenocarcinoma with HER2 overexpression: NRG Oncology/RTOG 1010. *JCO*. 2020;38(15):4500. doi:10.1200/JCO.2020.38.15_suppl.4500

41. Luo H, Jiang W, Ma L, et al. Icotinib with concurrent radiotherapy vs radiotherapy alone in older adults with unresectable esophageal squamous cell carcinoma: a phase ii randomized clinical trial. *JAMA Netw Open*. 2020;3(10):e2019440 doi:10.1001/jamanetworkopen.2020.19440

42. Minsky BD, Pajak TF, Ginsberg RJ, et al. INT 0123 (radiation therapy oncology group 94–05) phase III trial of com-bined-modality therapy for esophageal cancer: high-dose versus standard-dose radiation therapy. *J Clin Oncol*. 2002;20(5):1167–1174. doi:10.1200/JCO.2002.20.5.1167

43. Gaspar LE, Winter K, Kocha WI, et al. A phase I/II study of external beam radiation, brachytherapy, and concurrent chemotherapy for patients with localized carcinoma of the esophagus (radiation therapy oncology group study 9207): final report. *Cancer*. 2000;88(5):988–995. doi:10.1002/(SICI)1097-0142(20000301)88:5<988::AID-CNCR7>3.0.CO;2-U

44. Gaspar LE, Nag S, Herskovic A, et al. American brachytherapy society (ABS) consensus guidelines for brachyther-apy of esophageal cancer: clinical research committee, American brachytherapy society, Philadelphia, PA. *Int J Radiat Oncol Biol Phys*. 1997;38(1):127–132. doi:10.1016/S0360-3016(97)00231-9

45. Videtic GMM, Woody N, Vassil AD. *Handbook of Treatment Planning in Radiation Oncology*, 3rd ed. Demos Medical; 2020. doi:10.1891/9780826168429

46. Brower JV, Chen S, Bassetti MF, et al. Radiation dose escalation in esophageal cancer revisited: a contemporary analysis of the national cancer data base, 2004 to 2012. *Int J Radiat Oncol Biol Phys*. 2016;96(5):985–993. doi:10.1016/j.ijrobp.2016.08.016

47. Hulshof M, Geijsen D, Rozema T, et al. A randomized controlled phase III multicenter study on dose escala-tion in definitive chemoradiation for patients with locally advanced esophageal cancer: ARTDECO study. *JCO*. 2020;38(4):281. doi:10.1200/JCO.2020.38.4_suppl.281

48. Medical Research Council Oesophageal Cancer Working Group. Surgical resection with or without preoperative chemotherapy in oesophageal cancer: a randomised controlled trial. *Lancet*. 2002;359(9319):1727–1733. doi:10.1016/S0140-6736(02)08651-8

49. Reynolds J, Preston S, O'Neill B, et al. ICORG 10-14: NEOadjuvant trial in adenocarcinoma of the oesopha-gus and oesophagogastric junction international study (Neo-AEGIS). *BMC Cancer*. 2017;17:401. doi:10.1186/s12885-017-3386-2

50. Macdonald JS, Smalley SR, Benedetti J, et al. Chemoradiotherapy after surgery compared with surgery alone for adenocarcinoma of the stomach or gastroesophageal junction. *N Engl J Med*. 2001;345(10):725–730. doi:10.1056/NEJMoa010187

51. Wu AJ, Bosch WR, Chang DT, et al. Expert consensus contouring guidelines for intensity modulated radiation therapy in esophageal and gastroesophageal junction cancer. *Int J Radiat Oncol Biol Phys*. 2015;92(4):911–920. doi:10.1016/j.ijrobp.2015.03.030

33 ■ GASTRIC CANCER

Bindu V. Manyam, Kevin L. Stephans, and Gregory M. M. Videtic

QUICK HIT ■ Most gastric patients present with locoregionally advanced or metastatic disease. For cT2-4 or N+ locoregionally confined disease, management involves surgery followed by perioperative CHT or postoperative chemoRT. Surgery can be either partial or total gastrectomy depending on disease location and extent, with regional LND (D2 dissection recommended including ≥15 LNs).

Table 33.1: General Treatment Paradigm for Gastric Cancer	
Tis/T1a (≤3 cm, nonulcerated, well differentiated)	• Endoscopic mucosal resection or endoscopic submucosal dissection
T1a-bN0	• Gastrectomy and regional LND • No adjuvant therapy indicated
T2-4N0-3 or T1N+	• Gastrectomy and regional LND • Adjuvant CHT and RT indicated for T2–T4 or lymph node-positive disease • Per INT 0116: 45 Gy/25 fx starting on day 29 of CHT (five cycles of bolus 5-FU/LCV)
T4N0-3	• Perioperative FLOT • Gastrectomy and regional lymph node dissection • Adjuvant CHT and RT • Bulk of disease may prompt consideration of neoadjuvant CHT alone (FLOT) or neoadjuvant CHT (5-FU and LCV) with RT (45 Gy/25 fx) for downstaging, followed by gastrectomy and regional LND
M1	• Palliative CHT and/or RT

EPIDEMIOLOGY: Gastric cancer has estimated incidence of 27,600 cases and estimated 11,010 deaths in the United States in 2020. Gastric cancer is the 15th leading cause of cancer death in the United States and 4th leading cause of cancer death worldwide. It is most common in East Asia (China, Japan, Korea, and Taiwan), with lowest incidence in the United States and Canada. In the United States, most common location is within proximal stomach (GEJ and cardia).[1]

RISK FACTORS: Increased salt intake, salt-preserved foods (salted fish, cured meat, and salted vegetables), nitrates, smoked and processed meats, fried food, low consumption of fruits and vegetables, and low vitamin A and C.[2-4] Obesity (BMI ≥ 25, OR 1.22),[5] smoking,[6] and pathogens such as *Helicobacter pylori* and Epstein–Barr virus.[7,8] Hereditary syndromes due to HDGC, GAPPS, and FIGC represent about 1% to 3% of cases.[9]

ANATOMY

Stomach: Starts at GEJ (40–45 cm from incisions) and ends at pylorus. There are three main parts: fundus/cardia, body, and antrum/pylorus. There are five layers of stomach (starting from luminal surface): mucosa, submucosa, muscularis (outer longitudinal, middle circular, inner oblique), subserosa, and serosa. Gastric submucosal plexus is rich and carcinoma can spread superficially along stomach to esophagus, which also has rich submucosal plexus. Access to subserosal channels allows distal tumor spread to duodenum via subserosal lymphatic plexus.

Vascular: Vascular supply is derived from **celiac axis**, which is composed of three branches (Table 33.2).

Table 33.2: Vascular Supply of Stomach		
Celiac axis	Branches	Supply
Left gastric	-	Lesser curvature/right portion of stomach
Common hepatic	Right gastric	Lesser curvature/inferior right stomach
	Right gastroepiploic	Greater curvature
Splenic	Left gastroepiploic	Upper portion of greater curvature
	Short gastrics	Fundus/proximal stomach

Lymphatics: JRSGC proposed 16 regional lymph node stations for stomach in 1963. (See Table 33.3.) N1/2 lymph node stations are considered regional and N3/4 are considered distant.[10]

PATHOLOGY: Adenocarcinoma is the most common histology (90%–95%) and MALT lymphoma is the second most common. Rare histologies include leiomyosarcoma (2%), carcinoid (1%), adenoacanthoma (1%), and squamous cell carcinoma (1%).

Lauren Histological Classification: There are two distinct types of adenocarcinoma (intestinal and diffuse types). Intestinal type is more likely to be associated with environmental exposures (*H. pylori*, chronic gastritis, tobacco, diet), is more prevalent in high-incidence areas, and has better prognosis. Diffuse type (also known as "linitis plastic") tends to present as diffuse involvement of gastric mucosa, is characterized by organized clusters of signet ring (mucin-rich) cells, is more predominant in younger women, and is associated with poorer prognosis.[11]

Siewert Classification of GEJ Tumors (Based on Location): Class I: arises from metaplasia of distal esophagus and invades distally into stomach; Class II: arises from gastric cardia; Class III: arises from subcardia and invades proximally into esophagus.[12]

Bormann Classification: Class I: polypoid/fungating; Class II: ulcerative with raised borders; Class III: ulceration with invasion into gastric wall; Class IV: diffuse infiltration (linitis plastic).[13]

GENETICS: Her2-positivity was seen in 22% of patients screened for ToGA trial.[14]

SCREENING: Observational studies suggest screening in high-incidence areas may reduce gastric cancer mortality; however, there are no randomized data to support this finding.[15,16] Population-based screening has been implemented in Japan, Korea, Venezuela, and Chile, though screening intervals and modalities vary, and randomized data has not established optimal program.[15,17,18] In Japan, universal screening is recommended for all individuals >50 years of age with upper endoscopy every 2 to 3 years or double-contrast barium study every year. Alternatively, in Korea, upper endoscopy is recommended every 2 years for those 40 to 75 years of age.[19] In the United States, screening can be considered for patients with atrophic gastritis, pernicious anemia, gastric adenomas, Barrett's esophagus, and familial gastric cancer syndromes.

CLINICAL PRESENTATION: Symptoms include weight loss, epigastric pain, nausea, vomiting, anorexia, dysphagia, early satiety, melena, weakness. Characteristic physical exam findings include palpable stomach, succussion splash, palpable lymphadenopathy: Virchow's node (left supraclavicular), Irish's node (left axillary node), Sister Mary Joseph node (periumbilical node), Blumer's shelf (rectal shelf), Krukenberg tumor (metastatic deposit to ovary).

WORKUP: H&P.

Labs: CBC, CMP.

Imaging: Includes CT chest, abdomen, pelvis with IV and oral contrast. Consider PET/CT in absence of M1 disease on CT scans.

Pathology: EGD with biopsies (six to eight biopsies should be obtained), and endoscopic ultrasound to assess for tumor invasion and lymph node staging. Diagnostic laparoscopy to assess peritoneal cavity prior to surgery is indicated for clinical stage T1b and higher.[20] Obtain Her2-Neu status if metastatic.

PROGNOSTIC FACTORS: Poor KPS, advanced T and N stage, subtotal resection or gross residual disease (R2 > R1 > R0), diffuse-type histology are all poor prognostic features.[21] Retrospective multi-center study from Italy demonstrated that patients with 0, 1 to 3, 4 to 6, and >6 lymph nodes involved had 10-year OS after surgery of 92%, 82%, 73%, and 27%, respectively.[21] Metabolic response (≥35% decrease in PET SUV max) after neoadjuvant CHT is associated with improved MS.[22]

NATURAL HISTORY: Majority of patients (90%) present with locally advanced or metastatic disease, with 80% presenting with nodal metastases, 40% peritoneal metastases, and 30% liver metastases, for which prognosis is poor. Patients with early-stage gastric cancer (≤T1bN0) have excellent outcomes: 5-year OS of 100% with mucosal invasion and 80% to 90% with submucosal involvement.[23]

STAGING: Cancers with midpoint in lower thoracic esophagus, GEJ, or within proximal 5 cm of stomach *and* extending to GE junction or esophagus are staged as *esophageal neoplasms*. Cancers with midpoint in stomach >5 cm distal to GEJ or within 5 cm of GEJ, but *not* involving GEJ or esophagus are staged as gastric cancer. AJCC is based on number of nodes, whereas JRSGC is based on anatomic location. Positive peritoneal cytology is defined as pM1 (see Tables 33.3 and 33.4).

Table 33.3: AJCC 8th ed. (2017) Gastric Cancer Staging[24]							
T/M	N	cN0	cN1	cN2	cN3a	cN3b
T1	a. Lamina propria or muscularis mucosae	I	IIA				
	b. Submucosa						
T2	• Muscularis propria						
T3	• Subserosal connective tissue	IIB	III				
T4	a. Visceral peritoneum						
	b. Adjacent organs	IVA					
M1	• Distant metastasis	IVB					

cN1, 1–2 regional LNs; cN2, 3–6 regional LNs; cN3a, 7–15 regional LNs; cN3b, ≥16 regional LNs.

TREATMENT PARADIGM

Surgery: Surgery is mainstay of therapy, which includes endoscopic resection (small subset of patients), partial or total gastrectomy. Endoscopic resection includes endoscopic mucosal resection and endoscopic submucosal dissection, both shown in retrospective data to have high rate of local control in appropriately selected patients.[25] Optimal selection criteria for endoscopic resection are evolving, with routine features being high likelihood of en bloc resection, intestinal type histology, tumor limited to mucosa, no LVSI, and tumor size <2 cm without ulceration.[26–28]

Survival is similar between partial and total gastrectomy in setting of satisfactory margins, with partial gastrectomy associated with improved nutritional status and quality of life, except in proximal lesions, in which partial gastrectomy was associated with higher rates of reflux and anastomotic stenosis compared to total gastrectomy.[29,30] Therefore, total gastrectomy is typically utilized for lesions in upper third of stomach and partial gastrectomy is utilized for lesions in lower two-thirds.[30] Total gastrectomy involves esophagojejunostomy with Roux-en-Y anastomosis to prevent reflux of bile and pancreatic fluid. Billroth I is end-to-end gastrojejunal anastomosis using gastric resection margin. Billroth II is end-to-side gastrojejunal anastomosis, with closure of duodenal stump and lesser curvature (gastric resection margin not used for anastomosis). Complications include anastomotic failure, bleeding, ileus, B-12 deficiency, dumping syndrome, and reflux.

LND: Extent of LND is controversial, but it is recommended that at least 15 lymph nodes be removed for adequate staging. See Table 33.5 for data regarding extent of LND. Gastrectomy with D2 LND is standard of care in eastern Asia.[31]

Table 33.3: JRSGC Nodal stations		
N1	1	Right Cardia
	2	Left Cardia
	3	Lesser Curvature
	4	Greater Curvature
	5	Suprapyloric
	6	Infrapyloric
N2	7	Left gastric artery
	8	Common hepatic artery
	9	Celiac axis
	10	Splenic hila
	11	Splenic artery
N3	12	Hepatoduodenal lig.
	13	Post. Pancreatic head
	14	Mesenteric root
N4	15	Transverse mesocolon
	16	Paraaortic

Table 33.5: Definition of Extent of Lymph Node Dissection for Gastric Cancer	
D0	No LND
D1	JRSGC N1 nodes
D2	D1 dissection + JRSGC N2 nodes with distal pancreatectomy and splenectomy
D3	D2 dissection + JRSGC N3 nodes
D4	D3 dissection + JRSGC N4 nodes

Chemotherapy: GASTRIC meta-analysis demonstrated OS benefit of about 6% with use of 5-FU-based CHT in adjuvant setting compared to surgery alone.[32] Historical option in the United states was peri-operative epirubicin, cisplatin, and 5-FU (ECF) per MAGIC trial, which has now been replaced with peri-operative FLOT per FLOT4-AIO trial showing an OS benefit to FLOT over ECF. [33] Alternatively, adjuvant CHT with bolus 5-FU and LCV concurrent with RT per INT 0116 may be used.[34] ToGA trial demonstrated OS benefit to trastuzumab in addition to standard CHT (5-FU or capecitabine with cisplatin, 13.8 vs. 11.1 months; $p = .0046$) for locally advanced, recurrent, or metastatic and inoperable Her-2 Neu amplified cancers of GEJ and stomach.[14]

Radiation

Indications: Indications for adjuvant RT include T2–4, node-positive disease, or positive margins. Preoperative RT is option for borderline resectable or definitive RT for unresectable disease.

Dose: Dosing for adjuvant RT is 45 Gy/25 fx. Consider 5.4 to 5.9 Gy boost for positive margins or gross residual disease.[20] Tumor bed is covered and coverage of gastric remnant is dependent on risk and organs at risk. Lymph node coverage in adjuvant setting is dependent on anatomic site of primary (see the following). Can consider omission of nodal coverage in patients with T2-3N0 and >15 lymph nodes removed.[35–37]

Perigastric lymph nodes: Always covered, except for proximal T1-2aN0 patients with negative margins >5 cm and 10 to 15 LNs removed.

Celiac and suprapancreatic lymph nodes: Cover for T4, N+, or T3N0 with <15 LN resected.

Porta-hepatic LN: Cover all T4 or N+, except proximal lesions with only one to two involved LN and >15 LN resected.

Splenic LN: Cover for all T4 or N+, except distal lesions with only one to two involved LN and >15 LN resected.

Distal paraesophageal LN: Lesions with esophageal extension.

Toxicity: Acute: Fatigue, nausea, vomiting, diarrhea, gastritis, esophagitis. Late: Stricture, renal insufficiency, second malignancy.

Procedure: See *Treatment Planning Handbook,* Chapter 7.[38]

■ **EVIDENCE-BASED Q&A**

■ **What is the optimal extent of LND?**

It is recommended that at least 15 lymph nodes be dissected for satisfactory staging with NCCN recommending D2 dissection. However, extent of LND is controversial. There are four randomized clinical trials and meta-analysis demonstrating no survival advantage and higher postoperative morbidity and mortality with extensive LND.[39–42] On the other hand, several nonrandomized clinical trials have suggested improvement in survival with more radical LND.[29,43]

Bonenkamp, Dutch Gastric Cancer Group (*NEJM* 1999, PMID 10089184): PRT of 711 patients with gastric cancer undergoing curative resection randomized to D1 LND ($N = 380$) or D2 LND ($N = 331$). Patients who received D2 LND had significantly higher rates of postoperative complications compared to D1 LND (43% vs. 25%; $p < .001$) and postoperative deaths (10% vs. 4%; $p = .004$). 5-yr OS was similar between groups (45% vs. 47%), for D1 and D2 LND, respectively. **Conclusion: D2 LND resulted in significantly higher toxicity and no survival benefit compared to D1 LND.**

■ **Is there benefit to neoadjuvant CHT compared to surgery alone and what is the optimal CHT regimen?**

There are two PRTs (MAGIC/FFCD), which demonstrate significant survival benefit with use of neoadjuvant CHT compared to surgery alone, while EORTC 40954 demonstrated no survival benefit.[44] Neoadjuvant CHT may be particularly beneficial in patients at high risk of developing distant metastases (T3/T4 tumors, high clinical nodal burden, diffuse histology). The most recent FLOT4-AIO trial compared FLOT with ECF, with FLOT having improved OS and now is the recommended standard of care peri-operative CHT in gastric cancer.

Cunningham, MAGIC (*NEJM* 2006, PMID 16822992): PRT of 503 patients with stage II to IV (M0) potentially resectable adenocarcinoma of stomach (74%), GEJ (11%), or lower third of esophagus (14%) randomized to surgery alone or preoperative epirubicin 50 mg/m², cisplatin 60 mg/m², 5-FU 200 mg/m²/day for three cycles, surgery, and postoperative ECF for three cycles. Extent of LND was at discretion of surgeon. MFU was 4 years. See Table 33.6. There was no significant difference in postoperative complications (45% vs. 46%) for perioperative CHT and surgery alone, respectively.

Ychou, French FFCD/FNCLCC Trial (*JCO* 2011, PMID 21444866): PRT of 224 patients with resectable adenocarcinoma of stomach, GEJ, lower third of esophagus randomized to surgery alone or perioperative cisplatin 100 mg/m² on day 1 and 5-FU 800 mg/m², on days 1 to 5 for two to three cycles every 28 days, surgery, and same postoperative CHT for three or four cycles. See Table 33.6. On MVA, perioperative CHT ($p = .01$) and stomach tumor location ($p < .01$) were favorable prognostic factors. Perioperative CHT significantly improved R0 resection rate (84% vs. 73%; $p = .04$) and postoperative morbidity was similar between two groups.

Table 33.6: Neoadjuvant/Perioperative CHT Phase III Trials in Gastric Cancer						
Trial	N	CHT	R0 Resection	Local Recurrence	Distant Metastasis	OS
MAGIC Perioperative CHT Surgery	250 253	Epirubicin/ Cisplatin/5-FU	69% 66%	14% 21%	24% 37%	5-yr 36%* 23%*

(continued)

Table 33.6: Neoadjuvant/Perioperative CHT Phase III Trials in Gastric Cancer (*continued*)						
FFCD/FNCLCC Perioperative CHT Surgery	113 111	Cisplatin/5-FU	87%* 74%*	24% 26%	42% 56%	5-yr 38%* 24%*
Trial	*N*	**CHT**	**R0 Resection**	**Local Recurrence**	**Distant Metastasis**	**OS**
EORTC 40954 Neoadjuvant CHT Surgery	72 72	Cisplatin/5-FU/ LCV	82%* 67%*	-	-	2-yr 72.7% 69.9%

*Statistically significant.

Xiong, China (*Cancer Invest* 2014, PMID 24800782): Meta-analysis that included the preceding three trials and nine other PRT (*N* = 1,820) comparing variety of neoadjuvant CHT regimens vs. surgery alone for resectable gastric and GEJ cancer. **Conclusion: Neoadjuvant CHT was associated with significantly improved OS (OR 1.32, *p* = .01), 3-yr PFS (OR 1.85, *p* < .0001), and R0 resection (OR 1.38, *p* = .01), with no significant increase in operative complications, perioperative morality, or grade 3 or 4 adverse effects.**

Al-Batran, FLOT4-AIO (*Lancet Oncol* 2019, PMID 30982686): Phase 2/3 PRT of 716 patients with resectable gastric and GE junction tumors,cT2 or N+ or both, randomized to perioperative ECF/ECX vs. FLOT. Improved OS with FLOT (HR 0.77, 95% CI 0.63-0.94) with median OS 50 months vs. 35 months. Serious adverse events similar between groups. Pathologic CR better with FLOT (16% vs. 6%), with the highest benefit seen in intestinal type. **Conclusion: Peri-operative FLOT is CHT of choice in gastric cancer and improves OS as compared to ECF.**

Is there benefit to neoadjuvant CHT and RT?

The impact of RT, in addition to neoadjuvant CHT, is unclear but Stahl and RTOG 9904 suggest some benefit. TOPGEAR trial, which is currently accruing, will assess neoadjuvant ECF with RT + adjuvant ECF vs. neoadjuvant and adjuvant ECF alone.

Stahl, Germany (*JCO* 2009, PMID 19139439): PRT of 354 patients with locally advanced adenocarcinoma of lower third of esophagus or gastric cardia undergoing surgery randomized to induction CHT for 15 weeks (cisplatin, 5-FU, LCV) followed by surgery or induction CHT for 13 weeks followed by concurrent CHT (cisplatin and etoposide) and RT (30 Gy/15 fx) followed by surgery. Neoadjuvant chemoRT demonstrated higher rate of pCR (15.6% vs. 2%) and N0 status (64.6% vs. 37.7%), compared to neoadjuvant CHT alone. Three-year OS was (47.7% vs. 27.7%; *p* = .07) for neoadjuvant chemoRT and neoadjuvant CHT, respectively. **Conclusion: Neoadjuvant chemoRT had higher pCR and trend toward improved survival, though not statistically significant compared to neoadjuvant CHT alone.**

Ajani, RTOG 9904 (*JCO* 2006, PMID 16921048): Phase II trial of 49 patients with potentially resectable T2-3NxM0 gastric adenocarcinoma treated with induction CHT (cisplatin, 5-FU, LCV) for two cycles, followed by concurrent CHT (5-FU, paclitaxel) and RT (45 Gy/25 fx) and then surgery (D2 LND recommended). pCR was 26% and R0 resection was obtained in 77% of patients. One-year OS was 82% for patients who had pCR and 69% for patients who had less than pCR. **Conclusion: Neoadjuvant chemoRT had 26% pCR rate, which may be associated with higher OS.**

Is there benefit to adjuvant CHT compared to surgery alone?

The role of adjuvant CHT is unclear for Western patients, as trials performed in European populations have not shown survival benefit (GOIRC/GOIM). Only one trial (ACTS-GC) has demonstrated OS benefit in Japanese population, while CLASSIC trial demonstrated DFS benefit in patients from South Korea, China, and Taiwan. Summary of these trials is provided in Table 33.7.

Table 33.7: Summary of Adjuvant CHT Trials in Gastric Cancer					
Trial	*N*	**CHT**	**LRR**	**DM**	**OS**
ACTS-GC Adjuvant CHT Surgery	529 530	Tegafur/gimeracil/ oteracil	8% 13%	26% 32%	5-yr 72%* 61%*

(*continued*)

Table 33.7: Summary of Adjuvant CHT Trials in Gastric Cancer (*continued*)

GOIM Adjuvant CHT Surgery	112 113	Epirubicin/LCV/5-FU/etoposide	-	-	5-yr 41% 34%
GOIRC Adjuvant CHT Surgery	130 128	Epirubicin/LCV/5-FU/cisplatin	-	-	5-yr 48% 49%
CLASSIC Adjuvant CHT Surgery	520 515	Oxaliplatin/capecitabine	-	-	3-yr DFS 74%* 60%*

*Statistically significant.

Sakuramoto, ACTS-GC (*NEJM* 2007, PMID 17978289): PRT of 1,059 patients with stage II to III gastric cancer who underwent surgical resection with D2 LND randomized to observation vs. 1 year of oral S-1 (combination of tegafur, gimeracil, and oteracil). Median follow-up was 3 yrs. Ninety-five percent of patients had D2 LND and 5% had D3 LND. OS at 3 yrs was significantly higher with adjuvant CHT compared to observation (80.1% vs. 70.1%; $p = .002$). **Conclusion: Adjuvant CHT with oral S-1 had significant OS benefit in East Asian population of patients who underwent D2 LND.**

GASTRIC Group Meta-analysis (*JAMA* 2010, PMID 20442389): Meta-analysis of 17 PRTs comparing surgery alone vs. surgery and adjuvant CHT in patients with resectable gastric cancer. Adjuvant CHT was associated with significant PFS benefit (HR 0.82; $p < .001$) and 5-yr OS benefit (55.3% vs. 49.6%; $p < .001$). **Conclusion: Adjuvant CHT was shown to provide survival benefit compared to surgery alone.**

■ **Is there benefit to adjuvant chemoRT compared to surgery alone?**

In the United States, for patients undergoing surgery first, adjuvant chemoRT is preferred.

MacDonald, INT0116 (*NEJM* 2001, PMID 11547741; Update Smalley *JCO* 2012, PMID 22585691): PRT of 556 patients with stage IB-IV (M0) gastric cancer or GEJ adenocarcinoma with R0 resection randomized to surgery alone vs. surgery followed by adjuvant chemoRT. CHT was bolus 5-FU 425 mg/m² and LCV 20 mg/m²/day on days 1 to 5 for two cycles. RT was 45 Gy/25 fx and was started on day 1 of cycle 2 with 5-FU dose reduced to 400 mg/m² during RT and cycle 3 as 5-FU alone. After completion of RT, bolus 5-FU and LCV was given for two more cycles. Median follow-up was 5 years. See Table 33.8. D0 LND (54%), D1 LND (36%), and D2 LND (10%). Sixty-nine percent were T3–4 and 85% N+. With MFU >10 years, OS remained significantly improved with chemoRT (HR 1.32, $p = .0046$) and there was benefit in all subsets except diffuse histology.

Table 33.8: Results of INT0116 Adjuvant ChemoRT for Gastric Cancer

	3-yr RFS	Median DFS	DM	LRR	MS	3-yr OS
Surgery	31%	19 months	18%	29%	27 months	41%
Surgery + Adjuvant chemoRT	48%	30 months	33%	19%	36 months	50%
p value	<.001	<.001	NS		.006	.005

■ **Is there benefit to adjuvant chemoRT compared to adjuvant CHT alone?**

CRITICS trial did not demonstrate a benefit to adjuvant chemoRT compared to adjuvant CHT alone. ARTIST trial demonstrated trend to DFS benefit for adjuvant chemoRT in patients who had R0 resection with D2 LND. Subset analysis demonstrated DFS benefit in N+ or intestinal-type histology patients. ARTIST II trial is currently accruing to evaluate adjuvant CHT vs. adjuvant chemoRT.

Lee, ARTIST Trial (*JCO* 2015, PMID 25559811): PRT of 458 patients with R0 resection and D2 LND randomized to adjuvant capecitabine and cisplatin (XP) for six cycles or XP for two cycles followed by RT (45 Gy/25 fx) with capecitabine, followed by XP for two cycles. OS was similar between two groups. Subgroup analysis demonstrated that addition of RT to XP significantly improved 3-year DFS for patients with node-positive disease (76% vs. 72%, p = .04) and intestinal histology (94% vs. 83%, p = .01). **Conclusion: Adjuvant chemoRT did not significantly improve DFS and OS compared to adjuvant CHT alone.** *Comment: There may be subset of patients with N+ and intestinal type histology who have DFS benefit from adjuvant chemoRT.*

Verheji, CRITICS (*Lancet, 2018, PMID 29650363*): PRT of 788 patients from Netherlands, Denmark, and Sweden with stage IB–IV (M0) gastric cancer who received neoadjuvant CHT (epirubicin, capecitabine, and cisplatin or oxaliplatin: ECX or EOX) for three cycles and resection with D2 dissection, then randomized to three cycles of ECX/EOX or chemoRT (45 Gy/25 fx with weekly XP). (See Table 33.9.) Eighty-seven percent of patients had ≥D1 LND and removal of median 20 lymph nodes. Only 47% of patients completed adjuvant CHT and 55% completed adjuvant chemoRT. **Conclusion: Adjuvant chemoRT did not significantly improve OS compared to adjuvant CHT alone after preoperative CHT and surgery.**

Table 33.9: Results of CRITICS Gastric Cancer Trial		
	Median OS	**≥Grade 3 GI Toxicity**
CHT + Surgery + Adjuvant CHT	43 months	37%
CHT + Surgery + Adjuvant chemoRT	37 months	42%
p value	.90	.14

REFERENCES

1. Siegel RL, Miller KD, Jemal A. Cancer statistics, 2020. *CA Cancer J Clin.* 2020;70(1):7–30. doi:10.3322/caac.21590
2. Kono S, Hirohata T. Nutrition and stomach cancer. *Cancer Causes Control.* 1996;7(1):41–55. doi:10.1007/BF00115637
3. Gonzalez CA, Jakszyn P, Pera G, et al. Meat intake and risk of stomach and esophageal adenocarcinoma within the european prospective investigation into cancer and nutrition (EPIC). *J Natl Cancer Inst.* 2006;98(5):345–354. doi:10.1093/jnci/djj071
4. Zhu H, Yang X, Zhang C, et al. Red and processed meat intake is associated with higher gastric cancer risk: a meta-analysis of epidemiological observational studies. *PLoS One.* 2013;8(8):e70955. doi:10.1371/journal.pone.0070955
5. Yang P, Zhou Y, Chen B, et al. Overweight, obesity and gastric cancer risk: results from a meta-analysis of cohort studies. *Eur J Cancer.* 2009;45(16):2867–2873. doi:10.1016/j.ejca.2009.04.019
6. Ladeiras-Lopes R, Pereira AK, Nogueira A, et al. Smoking and gastric cancer: systematic review and meta-analysis of cohort studies. *Cancer Causes Control.* 2008;19(7):689–701. doi:10.1007/s10552-008-9132-y
7. Fox JG, Dangler CA, Taylor NS, et al. High-salt diet induces gastric epithelial hyperplasia and parietal cell loss, and enhances helicobacter pylori colonization in C57BL/6 mice. *Cancer Res.* 1999;59(19):4823–4828.
8. Boysen T, Mohammadi M, Melbye M, et al. EBV-associated gastric carcinoma in high- and low-incidence areas for nasopharyngeal carcinoma. *Br J Cancer.* 2009;101(3):530–533. doi:10.1038/sj.bjc.6605168
9. Oliveira C, Pinheiro H, Figueiredo J, et al. Familial gastric cancer: genetic susceptibility, pathology, and implications for management. *Lancet Oncol.* 2015;16(2):e60–e70. doi:10.1016/S1470-2045(14)71016-2
10. Moron FE, Szklaruk J. Learning the nodal stations in the abdomen. *Br J Radiol.* 2007;80(958):841–848. doi:10.1259/bjr/64292252
11. Correa P. Human gastric carcinogenesis: a multistep and multifactorial process—first american cancer society award lecture on cancer epidemiology and prevention. *Cancer Res.* 1992;52(24):6735–6740.
12. Siewert JR, Holscher AH, Becker K, Gossner W. [Cardia cancer: attempt at a therapeutically relevant classification]. *Der Chirurg; Zeitschrift fur alle Gebiete der operativen Medizen.* 1987;58(1):25–32.
13. Hu B, El Hajj N, Sittler S, et al. Gastric cancer: classification, histology and application of molecular pathology. *J Gastrointest Oncol.* 2012;3(3):251–261.
14. Bang YJ, Van Cutsem E, Feyereislova A, et al. Trastuzumab in combination with chemotherapy versus chemotherapy alone for treatment of HER2-positive advanced gastric or gastro-oesophageal junction cancer (ToGA): a phase 3, open-label, randomised controlled trial. *Lancet.* 2010;376(9742):687–697. doi:10.1016/S0140-6736(10)61121-X
15. Mizoue T, Yoshimura T, Tokui N, et al. Prospective study of screening for stomach cancer in Japan. *Int J Cancer.* 2003;106(1):103–107. doi:10.1002/ijc.11183
16. Kunisaki C, Ishino J, Nakajima S, et al. Outcomes of mass screening for gastric carcinoma. *Ann Surg Oncol.* 2006;13(2):221–228. doi:10.1245/ASO.2006.04.028
17. Llorens P. Gastric cancer mass survey in Chile. *Semin Surg Oncol.* 1991;7(6):339–343. doi:10.1002/ssu.2980070604

18. Pisani P, Oliver WE, Parkin DM, et al. Case-control study of gastric cancer screening in venezuela. *Br J Cancer*. 1994;69(6):1102–1105. doi:10.1038/bjc.1994.216

19. Choi IJ. Endoscopic gastric cancer screening and surveillance in high-risk groups. *Clin Endosc*. 2014;47(6):497–503. doi:10.5946/ce.2014.47.6.490

20. National Comprehensive Cancer Network. Gastric Cancer (Version 3.2017). https://www.nccn.org/professionals/physician_gls/pdf/gastric_blocks.pdf

21. Roviello F, Rossi S, Marrelli D, et al. Number of lymph node metastases and its prognostic significance in early gastric cancer: a Multicenter Italian Study. *J Surg Oncol*. 2006;94(4):275–280; discussion 274. doi:10.1002/jso.20566

22. Lordick F, Ott K, Krause BJ, et al. PET to assess early metabolic response and to guide treatment of adenocarcinoma of the oesophagogastric junction: the MUNICON Phase II trial. *Lancet Oncol*. 2007;8(9):797–805. doi:10.1016/S1470-2045(07)70244-9

23. Okada K, Fujisaki J, Yoshida T, et al. Long-term outcomes of endoscopic submucosal dissection for undifferentiated-type early gastric cancer. *Endoscopy*. 2012;44(2):122–127. doi:10.1055/s-0031-1291486

24. Amin MB, Edge S, Greene F, et al., eds. *AJCC Cancer Staging Manual*. 8th ed. Springer Publishing Company; 2017.

25. Takekoshi T, Baba Y, Ota H, et al. Endoscopic resection of early gastric carcinoma: results of a retrospective analysis of 308 cases. *Endoscopy*. 1994;26(4):352–358. doi:10.1055/s-2007-1008990

26. Soetikno R, Kaltenbach T, Yeh R, Gotoda T. Endoscopic mucosal resection for early cancers of the upper gastrointestinal tract. *J Clin Oncol*. 2005;23(20):4490–4498. doi:10.1200/JCO.2005.19.935

27. Min YW, Min BH, Lee JH, Kim JJ. Endoscopic treatment for early gastric cancer. *World J Gastroenterol*. 2014;20(16):4566–4573. doi:10.3748/wjg.v20.i16.4566

28. Gotoda T. Endoscopic resection of early gastric cancer: the Japanese perspective. *Curr Opin Gastroenterol*. 2006;22(5):561–569. doi:10.1097/01.mog.0000239873.06243.00

29. Bozzetti F, Marubini E, Bonfanti G, et al. Subtotal versus total gastrectomy for gastric cancer: five-year survival rates in a Multicenter Randomized Italian Trial. Italian Gastrointestinal Tumor Study Group. *Ann Surg*. 1999;230(2):170–178. doi:10.1097/00000658-199908000-00006

30. Pu YW, Gong W, Wu YY, et al. Proximal gastrectomy versus total gastrectomy for proximal gastric carcinoma. a meta-analysis on postoperative complications, 5-year survival, and recurrence rate. *Saudi Med J*. 2013;34(12):1223–1228.

31. Degiuli M, De Manzoni G, Di Leo A, et al. Gastric cancer: current status of lymph node dissection. *World J Gastroenterol*. 2016;22(10):2875–2893. doi:10.3748/wjg.v22.i10.2875

32. Group G, Paoletti X, Oba K, et al. Benefit of adjuvant chemotherapy for resectable gastric cancer: a meta-analysis. *JAMA*. 2010;303(17):1729–1737. doi:10.1001/jama.2010.534

33. Cunningham D, Allum WH, Stenning SP, et al. Perioperative chemotherapy versus surgery alone for resectable gastroesophageal cancer. *N Engl J Med*. 2006;355(1):11–20. doi:10.1056/NEJMoa055531

34. Macdonald JS, Smalley SR, Benedetti J, et al. Chemoradiotherapy after surgery compared with surgery alone for adenocarcinoma of the stomach or gastroesophageal junction. *N Engl J Med*. 2001;345(10):725–730. doi:10.1056/NEJMoa010187

35. Tepper JE, Gunderson LL. Radiation treatment parameters in the adjuvant postoperative therapy of gastric cancer. *Semin Radiat Oncol*. 2002;12(2):187–195. doi:10.1053/srao.2002.30827

36. Smalley SR, Gunderson L, Tepper J, et al. Gastric surgical adjuvant radiotherapy consensus report: rationale and treatment implementation. *Int J Radiat Oncol Biol Phys*. 2002;52(2):283–293. doi:10.1016/S0360-3016(01)02646-3

37. Wo JY, Yoon SS, Guimaraes AR, et al. Gastric lymph node contouring atlas: a tool to aid in clinical target volume definition in 3-dimensional treatment planning for gastric cancer. *Pract Radiat Oncol*. 2013;3(1):e11–e19. doi:10.1016/j.prro.2012.03.007

38. Videtic GMM, Woody N, Vassil AD. *Handbook of Treatment Planning in Radiation Oncology*. 3rd ed. Demos Medical; 2020. doi:10.1891/9780826168429

39. Bonenkamp JJ, Hermans J, Sasako M, et al. Extended lymph-node dissection for gastric cancer. *N Engl J Med*. 1999;340(12):908–914. doi:10.1056/NEJM199903253401202

40. Cuschieri A, Weeden S, Fielding J, et al. Patient survival after D1 and D2 resections for gastric cancer: long-term results of the MRC randomized surgical trial. surgical co-operative group. *Br J Cancer*. 1999;79(9–10):1522–1530. doi:10.1038/sj.bjc.6690243

41. Sasako M, Sano T, Yamamoto S, et al. D2 lymphadenectomy alone or with para-aortic nodal dissection for gastric cancer. *N Engl J Med*. 2008;359(5):453–462. doi:10.1056/NEJMoa0707035

42. Seevaratnam R, Bocicariu A, Cardoso R, et al. A meta-analysis of D1 versus D2 lymph node dissection. *Gastric Cancer*. 2012;15(Suppl 1):S60–S69. doi:10.1007/s10120-011-0110-9

43. Schwarz RE, Smith DD. Clinical impact of lymphadenectomy extent in resectable gastric cancer of advanced stage. *Ann Surg Oncol*. 2007;14(2):317–328. doi:10.1245/s10434-006-9218-2

44. Schuhmacher C, Gretschel S, Lordick F, et al. Neoadjuvant chemotherapy compared with surgery alone for locally advanced cancer of the stomach and cardia: European organisation for research and treatment of cancer randomized trial 40954. *J Clin Oncol*. 2010;28(35):5210–5218. doi:10.1200/JCO.2009.26.6114

Shauna R. Campbell, Neil M. Woody, and Kevin L. Stephans

QUICK HIT ■ HCC is associated with liver disease, particularly cirrhosis and hepatitis B and C. Screening of patients with chronic hepatitis infection and those with cirrhosis may result in early detection and improved outcomes. Diagnosis is commonly clinical based on AFP and imaging characteristics. Patients are staged according to BCLC staging system and early tumors are treated with surgical resection or liver transplantation if within Milan criteria. Patients with multiple tumors, larger tumors, or reduced functional status may be treated with focal therapies including RFA, TACE, radioembolization (Y^{90}), or RT (proton or SBRT). Patients with advanced disease may be candidates for sorafenib, lenvatinib, or atezolizumab/bevacizumab, which has been shown to improve OS in advanced disease.

EPIDEMIOLOGY: Second leading cause of cancer death worldwide in men and sixth leading cause of cancer death in women. In the United States, incidence of primary liver cancer (HCC and intrahepatic bile duct) is 8.3 cases per 100,000.[1] HCC is more common in areas with high rates of HBV and HCV infection. Incidence has been increasing in the United States due to the prevalence of HCV infection as well as NASH contributing to cirrhosis.

RISK FACTORS: Most strongly associated with cirrhosis, and primarily related to HBV and HCV infection, which are present in ~80% of cases. Treatment of viral infection has been shown to reduce future cancer risk in HBV by 50% to 60% and in HCV by 70%.[2] Other risk factors include male gender (RR 2–3), diabetes (RR 2), smoking, hereditary hemochromatosis, alcohol use, chemical exposure, obesity, and exposure to environmental toxins including aflatoxin and microcystin.

ANATOMY: The liver is the largest solid organ in body, surrounded by the peritoneal membrane (Glisson's capsule) and can be divided based on vasculature into eight segments. On the left numbering begins with caudate lobe (segment 1), followed by lateral (segments 2 and 3), and medial portion (segment 4). On the right numbering starts with anterior inferior segment (5) and moves in clockwise direction; posterior inferior, posterior superior, and anterior superior segments are numbered 6, 7, and 8 respectively. There are no anatomic borders between segments, and thus no barriers to intrahepatic spread of disease. The liver receives a dual blood supply; the portal vein (75%) supplies the normal hepatic parenchyma and the hepatic artery (25%) supplies normal hepatic parenchyma but also preferentially supplies malignant tumors.

PATHOLOGY: HCC can be diagnosed clinically based on AFP and radiographic criteria (see workup section) or less commonly with biopsy. HCC can be conventional type, which is graded from I to IV, based on the presence of trabecular organization and nuclear appearance. Molecular markers including HepPar1, albumin, fibrinogen, α1-antitrypsin, AFP and GPC-3 can help confirm the diagnosis.

SCREENING: AASLD has developed screening guidelines (updated 2018) for patients with chronic HBV infection and/or cirrhosis.[3] All patients with cirrhosis (except Child–Pugh C not on transplant list) and high-risk HBV should undergo surveillance with US every 6 months and AFP. Patients on the transplant waiting list should continue to be screened to ensure they do not develop HCC while awaiting transplant. Patients found to have a lesion <1 cm on US should have a repeat US in 3 mos and patients with lesions ≥1 cm or AFP ≥20 ng/mL should receive diagnostic imaging with a four-phase CT or MRI. A randomized trial of 18,816 patients in China using AFP and US showed low compliance rate of 58.2% but achieved 37% reduction in HCC mortality (no equivalent U.S.-based study).[4] NCCN guidelines recommend screening with AFP and US every 6 mos.[5]

CLINICAL PRESENTATION: Most commonly asymptomatic whereas symptoms related to the predisposing chronic liver disease are most evident. Patients may have mild to moderate abdominal pain, weight loss, early satiety, diarrhea, fever, and fatigue. Signs and symptoms of decompensated cirrhosis include ascites, encephalopathy, jaundice, and variceal bleeding. May present with paraneoplastic syndrome including erythrocytosis, hypercalcemia, hypoglycemia, and watery diarrhea. Paraneoplastic symptoms, except erythrocytosis, are associated with worse prognosis. HCC can be associated with cutaneous features including dermatomyositis, pemphigus foliaceus, sign of Leser–Trelat, pityriasis rotunda, and porphyria cutanea tarda although these are not specific to HCC.

WORKUP: Detailed H&P including evaluation of prior liver disease and treatment history.

Labs: HBV and HCV serology, AFP, CMP, CBC, and PT/INR.

Imaging: Diagnostic four-phase CT or MRI to evaluate lesions ≥1 cm on US with or without an elevated AFP. Imaging must include hepatic arterial phase, portal venous phase, delayed phase, and may include a pre-contrast phase as well. For cirrhotic (or other high-risk) patients, multiple criteria have been suggested by AASLD, OPTN, EASL, and LI-RADS for lesions ≥1 cm (lesions <1 cm are indeterminate).[6-9] Features include arterial hyperenhancement, pseudocapsule, venous washout, and growth. Criteria do not apply to patients without risk factors for HCC. Lesions with vascular invasion may have different features. Systemic staging includes CT of chest, abdomen, pelvis, and bone scan if symptoms are present. PET/CT is not recommended.

Biopsy: Can be done for lesions that are not diagnostic based on imaging criteria. Biopsy may be associated with small risk of tract seeding and in cases where an indeterminate lesion is resectable, it may be preferable to resect for simultaneous diagnosis and treatment.

PROGNOSTIC FACTORS: Tumor stage, functional status, Child–Pugh score (Table 34.1), and presence of metastatic disease are all prognostic of survival, which in some cases is more determined by cirrhosis than HCC.

Table 34.1: Child–Pugh Functional Status for Chronic Liver Disease			
Measure	1 point	2 points	3 points
Total bilirubin (mg/dL)	<2	2–3	>3
Serum albumin (g/dL)	>3.5	2.8–3.5	<2.8
Prothrombin time or INR	<4.0	4.0–6.0	>6.0
	<1.7	1.7–2.3	>2.3
Ascites	None	Moderate	Severe
Encephalopathy	None	Grade 1 to 2 or controlled with medication	Grade 3 to 4 or refractory
Sum of all points: 5 to 6 (Class A), 7 to 9 (Class B), 10 to 15 (Class C). 2-yr OS for Child–Pugh Class A, B, and C is 85%, 57%, and 35%, respectively.			

STAGING: Although AJCC TNM staging system exists for HCC, patients are typically staged according to BCLC (Tables 34.2 and 34.3), which includes liver and patient functional status as well as tumor characteristics and is accompanied by recommended treatment strategy.[10]

TREATMENT PARADIGM: As per BCLC staging system, treatment is based on tumor, patient, and liver function. Surgical resection or transplantation is preferred as curative option for early-stage patients while non-surgical options including RFA, Y[90], TACE, and RT may be used for definitive treatment, down staging, or as bridge to liver transplantation.[11-14] Systemic therapy is reserved for advanced disease.

Prevention: Vaccination of infants reduces rates of development of HBV infection and reduces incidence of HCC. Studies of universal vaccination in Taiwan beginning in 1984 revealed 50% decline in pediatric cases of HCC.[15] Similarly, treatment of HBV and HCV should be undertaken in affected patients and precautions should be taken to avoid transmission.[5]

Table 34.2: BCLC Staging System for HCC

	Stage Characteristics	Suggested Treatment
Very early stage (0)	ECOG PS 0, Child–Pugh A, single tumor <2 cm	Resection
Early stage (A)	ECOG PS 0, Child–Pugh A–B, 1–3 tumors, each <3 cm	Liver transplantation, radiofrequency ablation
Intermediate stage (B)	ECOG PS 0, Child–Pugh A–B, multiple tumors not meeting stage A	TACE
Advanced stage (C)	ECOG PS 02, Child–Pugh A–B, portal invasion, nodal or distant metastasis	Sorafenib or Lenvatinib
Terminal stage (D)	ECOG PS >2 or Child–Pugh C	Supportive care

Surgery: For early-stage patients surgical resection is mainstay of cure. For very small early lesions partial hepatectomy can provide high rate of cure.[16] However, many patients are not candidates for partial hepatectomy based on tumor features or liver function. In such cases, orthotopic liver transplantation may be an alternative surgical approach. For patients without cirrhosis, partial hepatectomy has equivalent cure rates to liver transplantation.[17] Since liver transplantation is also used for benign indications, patients are carefully selected for transplantation based on Milan criteria defined as single tumor ≤5 cm or ≤3 tumors each ≤3 cm, with no extrahepatic spread or macrovascular involvement. The Milan criteria resulted in 5-year OS of ~70%, and recurrence rates <15%.[18] UCSF validated expanded transplant criteria for HCC: single lesion ≤6.5 cm in diameter or two lesions ≤4.5 cm each with total tumor diameter ≤8 cm, which has also demonstrated low rates of recurrence.[19] Patients listed for transplantation are stratified based on risk of death using the MELD scoring system, which is the sum of an equation using creatinine, bilirubin, and INR and serves similar purpose to the older Child–Pugh score.[20] In addition, patients with HCC can be listed based on exception points, reflecting the risk that their tumor could progress and make them ineligible for transplantation. The number of points granted has changed over time to balance access to organs for cancer and non-cancer transplant candidates.

Chemotherapy: CHT is difficult to administer in patients with HCC who often have associated poor liver function. Multiple agents have been studied with small benefits at cost of significant toxicity, but newer agents are promising. First line agents for unresectable HCC in patients with Child–Pugh A cirrhosis include lenvatinib, atezolizumab/bevacizumab, nivolumab, and sorafenib can be considered for Child–Pugh A–B7 patients.[5] Atezolizumab/bevacizumab and nivolumab have resulted in improved OS compared with sorafenib in separate phase III RCTs, although the level of evidence for atezolizumab/bevacizumab is superior to single agent nivolumab.[21,22] Subsequent line therapy includes regorafenib, cabozantinib, ramucirumab, nivolumab/ipilimumab, and pembrolizumab.[5]

Table 34.3: AJCC 8th ed. Staging System for HCC

T/M		N	cN0	cN1
T1	a. Solitary tumor ≤2 cm		IA	
	b. Solitary tumor >2 cm without vascular invasion		IB	
T2	• Solitary tumor >2 cm with vascular invasion • Multiple tumors <5 cm		II	IVA
T3	• Multiple tumors, at least one >5 cm		IIIA	
T4	• Involvement of major branch of portal or hepatic vein • Direct invasion of adjacent organs (other than gall bladder) • Perforation of visceral peritoneum		IIIB	
M1	• Distant metastasis		IVB	

cN1, regional LNs.

Radiation

Indications: Historically, RT played a minor role in treatment due to intrinsic sensitivity of the liver. However, improved techniques including SBRT and proton therapy permit adequate liver sparing and RT is now a favorable LC modality, and in some patients may be preferable to other ablative techniques. Although comparative data are evolving, RT may be preferred to interventional techniques for those with vascular invasion, tumor thrombosis, inaccessible lesions or those with vascular shunting. Caution is necessary for Child–Pugh B and C patients as decompensation after RT can pose significant risk.

Dose: Dose varies by technique. Three and 5 fx regimens have been described up to 54 to 60 Gy/3 fx or 50 Gy/5 fx with dose reduction based on dose limits to normal liver. For patients requiring palliation, 8 Gy/1 fx to the involved liver can provide symptomatic improvement in ~50% of patients.[23]

Toxicity: RILD is the most feared complication, occurring 1 to 2 months after RT (range 0.5–8 months). Two types: classic (fatigue, pain, hepatomegaly, anicteric ascites, elevated alkaline phosphatase but not AST/ALT) and non-classic (jaundice, elevated ALT/AST). No effective treatment for RILD exists.[24]

Procedure: See *Treatment Planning Handbook*, Chapter 7.[25]

RFA: Percutaneous or laparoscopic technique, which involves thermal ablation of lesion. One or more probes may be used to achieve optimal ablation. Larger lesions and difficult locations such as hepatic dome, caudate lobe, central biliary tree, proximal to major blood vessels, subcapsular location, abutting gall bladder, small bowel, kidney, and stomach can be problematic. Advantages include single-day treatment and high control rates, particularly for small tumors.[26,27]

TACE: Combines arterial embolization of tumor vasculature with infusion of chemotherapeutic agents, increasing transit time of chemotherapeutic agent, and thus increasing apoptosis and necrosis. Generally considered for patients with lesions without vascular invasion or extrahepatic spread and preserved liver function. Limited data for safety and efficacy of TACE in setting of portal vein thrombus. A RCT of 112 patients comparing TACE to bland embolization and conservative treatment showed OS advantage to TACE (HR 0.47, $p = .025$) and 2-year OS was 63% with TACE and 50% with bland embolization.[28] There is controversy regarding survival benefit of TACE as other randomized studies of TACE have not shown survival benefit over conservative management.[28] TACE can be given using either CHT mixed with lipiodol or on DEB. Studies have not shown significant difference between conventional and DEB TACE. Chemotherapeutic agents employed included cisplatin, doxorubicin, and MMC. Post embolization syndrome seen in 80% of patients and includes RUQ pain, nausea, ileus, fatigue, fever, and transaminitis lasting typically 3 to 4 days, as such many patients are observed in the hospital for 24 hours following treatment. As many as 15% of patients may develop irreversible hepatotoxicity.

Radioembolization: Yttrium-90 microspheres: Y^{90} is pure β-emitter, with average energy ~1 MeV delivered via hepatic artery. Prior to radioembolization patients undergo pretreatment ^{99}mTc macro-aggregated albumin scan, which facilitates prediction of distribution of radioactive beads. If lung exposure ≥30 Gy is anticipated, lung shunt fraction exceeds 20%, or significant GI tract dose is observed then the distribution catheter needs to be repositioned. If the target cannot be isolated without significant shunting the procedure is contraindicated. Encephalopathy, Child–Pugh C status, and biliary obstruction are other contraindications. A longitudinal cohort study of Y^{90} in 291 patients receiving 526 treatments revealed overall time to progression of 7.9 mos. Child–Pugh A patients had median survival of 17.2 mos vs. 7.7 mos for Child–Pugh B patients, and Child–Pugh B patients with portal vein thrombus had median survival of 5.6 mos.[29] Y^{90} may be particularly useful in the setting of portal vein thrombus and a prospective study of 30 patients was completed revealing MS of 13 mos.[30] Alternatively, iodine 131-labeled lipiodol has also been employed for radioembolization.

■ **EVIDENCE-BASED Q&A**

▪ **What are key studies defining current role of SBRT for HCC?**

Prospective and retrospective studies demonstrate high rates of LC and favorable OS for patients treated with SBRT, often after prior liver directed therapy.

Bujold, PMH Phase I and II (*JCO* 2013, PMID 23547075): Combined analysis of prospective phase I and II studies of liver SBRT in Canada; 102 patients with HCC unsuitable for TACE, RFA, and surgery enrolled and treated to doses of 24 to 54 Gy in 6 fx; 52% of patients had prior liver directed therapy and 55% had tumor vascular thrombus. One-year LC 87% and MS 17 months; 30% of patients experienced grade 3 toxicity and seven patients experienced possible grade 5 toxicity. OS significantly worse in patients with tumor vascular thrombosis at 1 year (44% vs. 67%) and 2 years (27% vs. 42%).

Sanuki, Japan (*Acta Oncol* 2014, PMID 23962244): RR of 185 patients with 277 HCC tumors not candidates for surgery or percutaneous ablative therapy treated with SBRT 35 Gy (Child–Pugh B) or 40 Gy (Child–Pugh A) in 5 fx. MFU 24 mos; 3-yr LC and OS were 91% and 70%, respectively. Thirteen percent of patients had grade 3 toxicity and 10% experienced worsening of Child–Pugh score by ≥2 points.

Yoon, Korea (*PLoS One* 2013, PMID 24255719): Registry study of 93 patients treated with SBRT for HCC <6 cm not candidates for surgery or other percutaneous therapies, Child–Pugh A or B, >2 cm from OARs. Dose was 30 to 60 Gy in 3 to 4 fx. Patients with vascular invasion or extrahepatic metastases were excluded. MFU 25.6 months and 3-year LC and OS were 92% and 54%, respectively; 7% of patients experienced hepatic toxicity.

■ Is SBRT safe in Child–Pugh B and C patients?

Original reports of SBRT in Child–Pugh B-C patients demonstrated high rates of toxicity, but newer series demonstrate that in carefully selected Child–Pugh B–C patients SBRT can be feasible.

Culleton, PMH (*Radiother Oncol* 2014, PMID 24906626): RR of 29 patients with Child–Pugh B (*N* = 28) and C (*N* = 1) patients treated to 30 Gy/6 fx. MS 7.9 months and for 16 patients with posttreatment liver function testing available, 63% of patients experienced decline in Child–Pugh index of ≥2 points at 3 months.

Lee, UMass (*Adv Radiat Oncol* 2020, PMID 33083650): Prospective registry of 23 Child–Pugh B and C patients treated with SBRT, 20 were B8-C10. Seventy-eight percent previously treated with TACE. MFU 14.5 months with 1-year LC and OS of 92% and 57%, respectively. MS 14.5 months, 7.3 months for patients not transplanted. Pathologic CR rate was 64% for nine transplanted patients. No classic RILD but four patients experienced ≥2 points Child–Pugh score increase by 6 months. Of seven liver-related deaths only one was attributed to SBRT.

■ Can SBRT be used as a bridge to liver transplantation?

In small RRs SBRT as a bridge to transplantation appears to be associated with favorable outcomes.

Andolino, Indiana University (*IJROBP* 2011, PMID 21645977): RR of 60 patients treated with SBRT for HCC confined to liver, 40 to 44 Gy in 3 to 5 fx. MFU 27 mos; 2-year LC and OS 90% and 67% respectively; 23 patients (38.3%) proceeded to transplantation.

Facciuto, Mount Sinai (*J Surg Oncol* 2012, PMID 21960321): RR of 27 patients with 39 lesions listed for liver transplant treated with SBRT, 24 to 36 Gy in 2 to 5 fx with most patients receiving 28 Gy/4 fx; 17 patients (63%) proceeded to transplantation and 37% of tumors exhibited CR or PR.

■ What data ARE available to compare efficacy of ablative treatments for HCC?

Data comparing efficacy of liver directed therapies are limited, but in most studies SBRT demonstrates very favorable LC.

Wahl, Michigan (*JCO* 2016, PMID 26628466): RR of 224 patients treated with RFA (161 patients with 250 tumors) or SBRT (63 patients with 83 tumors). Patients treated with SBRT had lower Child–Pugh scores, higher pretreatment AFP, and more prior treatments; 1-year FFLP was increased with SBRT 97% vs. 84% for RFA. Increasing size was associated with reduced control for RFA but not SBRT. For tumors >2 cm, SBRT has significantly higher FFLP (HR 3.35, *p* = .025). No differences in 1- or 2-year OS. **Conclusion: For tumors >2 cm SBRT is superior to RFA.**

Bush, Loma Linda (*IJROBP* 2016, PMID 27084661): PRT of 69 patients with new diagnosis of HCC meeting either Milan or UCSF criteria for transplantation randomized to TACE vs. proton therapy 70.2 Gy/15 fx. Median tumor size 3.2 cm. At MFU 28 months, 2-year LC higher in proton group 88%

vs. 45% (p = .06) and 2-year OS not significantly different. Total hospitalization days within 30 days of treatment was significantly higher with TACE (166 vs. 24 days, p < .001) and proton therapy was associated with numerically higher CR rate among patients proceeding to transplantation (25% vs. 10%, p = .38). **Conclusion: Proton therapy may have better efficacy and lower toxicity than TACE as bridge to transplantation.**

Su, China (*Front Oncol* 2020, PMID 32266136): Multi-institutional propensity score matched analysis of 95 patient pairs with BCLC stage A HCC comparing SBRT vs. TACE. SBRT had better LC, intrahepatic control, and PFS than TACE with comparable OS; 1-year PFS 63% vs. 54% for SBRT vs. TACE (p = .049). On MVA SBRT associated with improved LC (HR 1.59, p = .04) and intrahepatic control (HR 1.61, p = .009). **Conclusion: SBRT is an effective alternative to TACE with improved LC.**

■ **Can SBRT be combined with TACE to improve outcomes?**

It appears safe and effective to give SBRT either combined with TACE or as salvage treatment.

Jacob, UAB (*HPB [Oxford]* 2015, PMID 25186290): RR of patients with HCC >3 cm treated with TACE (N = 124) vs. TACE + SBRT 45 Gy/3 fx over 7 days (N = 37). LR significantly lower in patients receiving TACE + SBRT, 11% vs. 26% (p = .04). When censored for liver transplantation TACE + SBRT exhibited higher OS than TACE alone.

Su, China (*BMC Cancer* 2016, PMID 27809890): RR of 127 patients with unresectable HCC who received SBRT followed by transarterial embolization or TACE (N = 77) compared with SBRT alone (N = 50). SBRT was 30 to 50 Gy in 3 to 5 fx. Eligibility criteria included tumor >5 cm (median 8.5 cm) and Child–Pugh A/B. The PFS and LRFS were not significantly different between the groups. In the entire cohort, BED10 ≥ 100 Gy and EQD2 ≥ 74 Gy were significant prognostic factors for OS, PFS, LRFS, and DMFS. **Conclusion: SBRT combined with transarterial embolization/TACE may be an effective complementary treatment approach for HCC > 5 cm and attempt for BED$_{10}$ ≥ 100 Gy should be made.**

■ **Can hypofractionated RT or SBRT improve outcomes in setting of portal vein tumor thrombus and can it be safely combined with other treatments?**

Patient series out of Asia demonstrate improved outcomes with SBRT, with or without other therapies, in patients with portal vein tumor thrombus. SBRT is also superior to conventionally fractionated RT and is the preferred RT modality.[31]

Kang, Beijing (*Mol Clin Oncol* 2014, PMID 24649306): PRT of 101 patients with HCC and portal vein tumor thrombus randomized to SBRT followed by TACE, TACE followed by SBRT, or SBRT alone. SBRT ranged from 21 to 60 Gy/6 fx with median dose of 40 Gy; 1-year LC trended toward improvement in SBRT followed by TACE (56%) vs. TACE followed by SBRT (49%) and SBRT alone (43%). CR of tumor thrombus to SBRT was achieved in 18% and PR in 53%. TACE followed by SBRT associated with slightly higher rate of increase in Child–Pugh score of 41% vs. 30% in other arms. **Conclusion: SBRT improves outcomes in HCC with portal vein thrombus and can be safely combined with TACE. It may be most advantageous to sequence SBRT followed by TACE to preserve liver function.**

Yoon, Korea (*JAMA Oncol* 2018, PMID 29543938): PRT comparing TACE + RT vs. sorafenib in 90 treatment-naïve Child–Pugh A HCC patients with macroscopic vascular invasion. TACE given every 6 weeks, RT was 45 Gy/15 to 18 fx, and sorafenib was 400 mg BID. At 12 weeks, PFS significantly higher with TACE + RT than sorafenib (86.7% vs. 34.3%, p < .001). OS significantly improved with TACE + RT vs. sorafenib (55 vs. 43 weeks, p = .04). 11.1% of TACE + RT patients underwent curative surgical resection due to down-staging. **Conclusion: TACE + RT significantly improved PFS and OS compared to sorafenib alone in HCC patients with vascular invasion.**

Shen, China (*Cancers* 2018, PMID 30558224): RR of HCC patients with macroscopic vascular invasion treated with TACE + SBRT (n = 26) or TACE + sorafenib (N = 51). After propensity score matching, patients with TACE + SBRT responded better than TACE + sorafenib group, with significant OS benefit (HR 0.36, p = .007), and PFS benefit (HR 0.35, p < .001). **Conclusion: For HCC patients with vascular invasion, TACE + SBRT may provide improved OS and PFS compared to TACE + sorafenib.**

■ Is RT safe and effective in the setting of IVC and/or right atrium involvement?

Data are limited, however, a recently published multicenter trial suggests RT is safe and effective.

Rim, KROG 17-10 (*IJROBP* 2020, PMID 31977276): From 2009 to 2016, 49 HCC patients with IVC and/or right atrium involvement received RT with median dose of 46.7 Gy (range 35.4–71.5). MFU 9.3 months with MS 10.1 months. LC 89% and 75% at 1- and 2-year, respectively. 1- and 2-year OS 43.5% and 30.1%, respectively. Factors affecting OS were AFP ≥ 300 ng/mL, tumor multiplicity, and patient volume of institutions (all $p < .05$). One case of possible RILD noted. **Conclusion: RT can yield favorable LC in HCC with extensive vascular involvement.**

■ Is there data to support RT pre- or post-operatively for resectable HCC with portal vein tumor thrombus?

Recently published RCTs from China showed improved recurrence and survival outcomes for RT combined with surgery, however this is primarily in HBV patients where surgery is more common. One study evaluated neo-adjuvant 3D-CRT (18 Gy/6 fx) prior to hepatectomy and demonstrated statistically significant improvements in OS, and on MVA RT reduced HCC-related mortality and recurrence rates.[32] Similarly, in a RCT post-op-erative IMRT (50 Gy/25 fx) demonstrated improved DFS and OS with the addition to RT after hepatectomy +/- thrombectomy.[33]

■ Is there an advantage to proton therapy for HCC?

Given the dosimetric characteristics of protons, there may be an advantage to spare normal liver and reduce the risk of RILD. However, prospective studies have been limited to single arm investigations.[34,35]

Fukumitsu, Japan (*IJROBP* 2009, PMID 19304408): Prospective study of 51 patients with HCC > 2 cm from porta hepatis treated to 66 GyE/10 fx. 3-year OS 49% and LC 95%. Only three patients developed grade 2 toxicity.

Bush, Loma Linda (*Cancer* 2011, PMID 21264826): Phase II study of proton therapy for 67 Child–Pugh A–C HCC patients with 63 GyE/15 fx. MS for Child–Pugh A, B, and C patients was 34, 13, and 12 months, respectively. In all patients, median PFS was 36 months and 19 patients underwent liver transplantation with 33% pCR. For transplanted patients 3-year OS was 70% with average time from RT to transplantation of 13.2 months. No significant change in liver function seen within 6 months post-treatment. **Conclusion: Proton beam therapy is a safe and effective treatment for inoperable HCC.**

Hong, Proton Phase II (*JCO* 2016, PMID 26668346): Prospective phase II study of unresectable HCC or cholangiocarcinoma. Tumors ≤2 cm from porta hepatis received 58 GyE while more peripheral tumors received 67.5 GyE all in 15 fx. 42 HCC patients included with 2-year OS of 63% and only two patients experienced LF.

REFERENCES

1. Siegel RL, Miller KD, Jemal A. Cancer statistics, 2020. *CA Cancer J Clin.* 2020;70(1):7–30. doi:10.3322/caac.21590
2. Ioannou GN, Green PK, Berry K. HCV eradication induced by direct-acting antiviral agents reduces the risk of hepatocellular carcinoma. *J Hepatol.* 2018;68(1):25–32. doi:10.1016/j.jhep.2017.08.030
3. Marrero JA, Kulik LM, Sirlin CB, et al. Diagnosis, staging, and management of hepatocellular carcinoma: 2018 practice guidance by the American association for the study of liver diseases. *Hepatology.* 2018;68(2):723–750. doi:10.1002/hep.29913
4. Zhang BH, Yang BH, Tang ZY. Randomized controlled trial of screening for hepatocellular carcinoma. *J Cancer Res Clin Oncol.* 2004;130(7):417–422. doi:10.1007/s00432-004-0552-0
5. National Comprehensive Cancer Network. Hepatobiliary Cancers (Version 5.2020). 2020. https://www.nccn.org/professionals/physician_gls/pdf/hepatobiliary.pdf
6. Pomfret EA, Washburn K, Wald C, et al. Report of a national conference on liver allocation in patients with hepatocellular carcinoma in the united states. *Liver Transpl.* 2010;16(3):262–278. doi:10.1002/lt.21999
7. Chernyak V, Fowler KJ, Kamaya A, et al. Liver imaging reporting and data system (LI-RADS) version 2018: imaging of hepatocellular carcinoma in at-risk patients. *Radiology.* 2018;289(3):816–830. doi:10.1148/radiol.2018181494
8. Bruix J, Sherman M. Management of hepatocellular carcinoma: an update. *Hepatology.* 2011;53(3):1020–1022. doi:10.1002/hep.24199

9. European Association for the Study of the Liver, European Organisation for Research and Treatment of Cancer. EASL-EORTC clinical practice guidelines: management of hepatocellular carcinoma. *J Hepatol.* 2012;56(4):908–943. doi:10.1016/j.jhep.2011.12.001

10. Forner A, Reig ME, Rodriguez de Lope C, Bruix J. Current strategy for staging and treatment: the BCLC update and future prospects. *Semin Liver Dis.* 2010;30(01):061–074. doi:10.1055/s-0030-1247133

11. O'Connor JK, Trotter J, Davis GL, et al. Long-term outcomes of stereotactic body radiation therapy in the treatment of hepatocellular cancer as a bridge to transplantation. *Liver Transpl.* 2012;18(8):949–954. doi:10.1002/lt.23439

12. Llovet JM, Fuster J, Bruix J. Intention-to-treat analysis of surgical treatment for early hepatocellular carcinoma: resection versus transplantation. *Hepatology.* 1999;30(6):1434–1440. doi:10.1002/hep.510300629

13. Kulik LM, Atassi B, Van Holsbeeck L, et al. Yttrium-90 microspheres (TheraSphere®) treatment of unresectable hepatocellular carcinoma: downstaging to resection, RFA and bridge to transplantation. *J Surg Oncol.* 2006;94(7):572–586. doi:10.1002/jso.20609

14. Graziadei IW, Sandmueller H, Waldenberger P, et al. Chemoembolization followed by liver transplantation for hepatocellular carcinoma impedes tumor progression while on the waiting list and leads to excellent outcome. *Liver Transpl.* 2003;9(6):557–563. doi:10.1053/jlts.2003.50106

15. Amin J, O'Connell D, Bartlett M, et al. Liver cancer and hepatitis B and C in new south wales, 1990–2002: a linkage study. *Aust N Z J Public Health.* 2007;31(5):475–482. doi:10.1111/j.1753-6405.2007.00121.x

16. Poon RT, Fan ST, Lo CM, et al. Long-term survival and pattern of recurrence after resection of small hepatocellular carcinoma in patients with preserved liver function: implications for a strategy of salvage transplantation. *Ann Surg.* 2002;235(3):373–382. doi:10.1097/00000658-200203000-00009

17. Iwatsuki S, Starzl TE, Sheahan DG, et al. Hepatic resection versus transplantation for hepatocellular carcinoma. *Ann Surg.* 1991;214(3):221–228; discussion 228–229. doi:10.1097/00000658-199109000-00005

18. Mazzaferro V, Regalia E, Doci R, et al. Liver transplantation for the treatment of small hepatocellular carcinomas in patients with cirrhosis. *N Engl J Med.* 1996;334(11):693–699. doi:10.1056/NEJM199603143341104

19. Yao FY, Xiao L, Bass NM, et al. Liver transplantation for hepatocellular carcinoma: validation of the UCSF-expanded criteria based on preoperative imaging. *Am J Transplant.* 2007;7(11):2587–2596. doi:10.1111/j.1600-6143.2007.01965.x

20. Wiesner R, Edwards E, Freeman R, et al. Model for end-stage liver disease (MELD) and allocation of donor livers. *Gastroenterology.* 2003;124(1):91–96. doi:10.1053/gast.2003.50016

21. Hack SP, Spahn J, Chen M, et al. IMbrave 050: a phase III trial of atezolizumab plus bevacizumab in high-risk hepatocellular carcinoma after curative resection or ablation. *Future Oncol.* 2020;16(15):975–989. doi:10.2217/fon-2020-0162

22. Yau T, Park JW, Finn RS, et al. CheckMate 459: A randomized, multi-center phase III study of nivolumab (NIVO) vs sorafenib (SOR) as first-line (1L) treatment in patients (pts) with advanced hepatocellular carcinoma (aHCC). *Ann Oncol.* 2019;30:v874–v875. doi:10.1093/annonc/mdz394.029

23. Soliman H, Ringash J, Jiang H, et al. Phase II trial of palliative radiotherapy for hepatocellular carcinoma and liver metastases. *J Clin Oncol.* 2013;31(31):3980–3986. doi:10.1200/JCO.2013.49.9202

24. Benson R, Madan R, Kilambi R, Chander S. Radiation induced liver disease: a clinical update. *J Egypt Natl Canc Inst.* 2016;28(1):7–11. doi:10.1016/j.jnci.2015.08.001

25. Videtic GMM, Vassil AD, Woody NM. *Handbook of Treatment Planning in Radiation Oncology, Third Edition.* Springer Publishing Company; 2020.

26. Tateishi R, Shiina S, Teratani T, et al. Percutaneous radiofrequency ablation for hepatocellular carcinoma. an analysis of 1000 cases. *Cancer.* 2005;103(6):1201–1209. doi:10.1002/cncr.20892

27. Tanabe KK, Curley SA, Dodd GD, et al. Radiofrequency ablation: the experts weigh in. *Cancer.* 2004;100(3):641–650. doi:10.1002/cncr.11919

28. Llovet JM, Real MI, Montaña X, et al. Arterial embolisation or chemoembolisation versus symptomatic treatment in patients with unresectable hepatocellular carcinoma: a randomised controlled trial. *Lancet.* 2002;359(9319):1734–1739. doi:10.1016/S0140-6736(02)08649-X

29. Salem R, Lewandowski RJ, Mulcahy MF, et al. Radioembolization for hepatocellular carcinoma using Yttrium-90 microspheres: a comprehensive report of long-term outcomes. *Gastroenterology.* 2010;138(1):52–64. doi:10.1053/j.gastro.2009.09.006

30. Kokabi N, Camacho JC, Xing M, et al. Open-label prospective study of the safety and efficacy of glass-based yttrium 90 radioembolization for infiltrative hepatocellular carcinoma with portal vein thrombosis. *Cancer.* 2015;121(13):2164–2174. doi:10.1002/cncr.29275

31. Yang JF, Lo CH, Lee MS, et al. Stereotactic ablative radiotherapy versus conventionally fractionated radiotherapy in the treatment of hepatocellular carcinoma with portal vein invasion: a retrospective analysis. *Radiat Oncol.* 2019;14(1):180. doi:10.1186/s13014-019-1382-1

32. Wei X, Jiang Y, Zhang X, et al. Neoadjuvant three-dimensional conformal radiotherapy for resectable hepatocellular carcinoma with portal vein tumor thrombus: a randomized, open-label, multicenter controlled study. *J Clin Oncol.* 2019;37(24):2141–2151. doi:10.1200/JCO.18.02184

33. Sun J, Yang L, Shi J, et al. Postoperative adjuvant IMRT for patients with HCC and portal vein tumor thrombus: an open-label randomized controlled trial. *Radiother Oncol.* 2019;140:20–25. doi:10.1016/j.radonc.2019.05.006

34. Cheng JY, Liu CM, Wang YM, et al. Proton versus photon radiotherapy for primary hepatocellular carcinoma: a propensity-matched analysis. *Radiat Oncol.* 2020;15(1):159. doi:10.1186/s13014-020-01605-4

35. Sanford NN, Pursley J, Noe B, et al. Protons versus photons for unresectable hepatocellular carcinoma: liver decompensation and overall survival. *Int J Radiat Oncol Biol Phys.* 2019;105(1):64–72. doi:10.1016/j.ijrobp.2019.01.076

35 ■ PANCREATIC ADENOCARCINOMA

James R. Broughman and Ehsan H. Balagamwala

QUICK HIT ■ Pancreatic adenocarcinoma is the 4th leading cause of cancer death in the United States. Though it is prone to wide dissemination, up to a third of patients die of complications from local progression. For the 15% of patients with resectable disease at presentation, immediate surgery +/- neoadjuvant CHT is standard and represents the only means of cure. Adjuvant treatment consists of CHT +/- RT. Twenty percent present with borderline resectable disease; however, only ~60% of these patients will undergo surgery to a clear margin. Patients with borderline disease may undergo downstaging with CHT +/- RT to increase the likelihood of an R0 resection (see Table 35.1). Combined-agent CHT regimens such as FOLFIRINOX are preferred over single-agent regimens in fit patients. Pancreatic cancer is intrinsically radioresistant, so there is growing interest in utilizing SBRT to improve local control though this is technically challenging due to the proximity of tumors to duodenum, jejunum, and stomach.

Table 35.1: General Treatment Paradigm for Pancreatic Cancer

Setting	Initial Option	Additional Treatment(s)	
Resectable disease	Neoadjuvant CHT	Surgery followed by adjuvant CHT +/- RT	
	Surgery	CHT alone[1] - 5-FU - Gemcitabine +/- capecitabine - 5-FU-based multiagent regimen (e.g., FOLFIRINOX)	
		CHT followed by chemoRT to 45–54 Gy with concurrent 5-FU or gemcitabine for positive margins and/or LN+	
Borderline resectable	Neoadjuvant CHT followed by chemoRT (45–54 Gy), reassessment, then surgery		
	Neoadjuvant CHT followed by surgery. Adjuvant chemoRT for positive margins and/or LN+		
Locally advanced/ unresectable	Initial CHT	SBRT (preferred) or in select cases chemoRT	
	SBRT (if symptomatic)		CHT
	CHT Alone		
Metastatic	Treated with single or multiagent systemic therapy +/- palliative surgery/biliary stent/ RT		

EPIDEMIOLOGY: Estimated 57,600 new cases in 2020 in the United States, with 47,050 deaths; 4th leading cause of cancer mortality.[2] Higher incidence in males vs. females (1.3:1); higher incidence in Blacks vs. Caucasians, and more common in developed nations.[3–6] Rare under 40 years of age with median age of 60 at diagnosis.[7] Peak incidence sixth to seventh decade, which makes aggressive treatment challenging.

RISK FACTORS: Chronic pancreatitis (RR 16–69), cigarette smoking (RR 1–3), high BMI (RR 1–2), chronic diabetes (RR 1–3), heavy alcohol consumption (RR 2–4), red meat (RR 1–1.5), and exposure to hydrocarbon compounds/pesticides/heavy metals.[8–10] There is emerging evidence for increased risk in those previously infected with *Helicobacter pylori*, HBV, and HCV.[8,11] Hereditary conditions include familial predisposition, hereditary pancreatitis (*PRSS1/SPINK1*, RR 50–67), Peutz–Jeghers (*STK11/ LKB1*, RR 132), FAMMM syndrome (*CDKN2A/TP16*, RR 48), mutations in *BRCA1/BRCA2* (RR 2–7), Lynch syndrome (*MLH1/MSH2/MSH6/PMS2*), or ataxia telangiectasia.[8,12–17] Five to 10% of cases have inherited component although if one first-degree relative, RR 1.5 to 13; if two relatives RR 18; if three relatives RR 57.[18–21] Other risk factors include non-O blood type (RR 1–2), partial gastrectomy/cholecystectomy/appendectomy, and coffee/tea.[8,22–24]

ANATOMY: Pancreas: retroperitoneal and located anterior to L1/L2. It is divided into head (including uncinate process), neck, body, and tail. Head lies in duodenal flexure, to right of SMV, with tail extending toward spleen. Peritoneal involvement is more common with body and tail tumors. Venous drainage is via portal system. Tumor invasion posteriorly can lead to lung/pleural metastasis via vena cava drainage. Pancreatic duct and accessory duct combine with common bile duct and enter duodenum via sphincter of Oddi at ampulla of Vater. Pancreas is directly adjacent to or in close proximity to stomach, duodenum, jejunum, kidneys, spleen, and several blood vessels (celiac axis, superior mesenteric artery, splenic artery, and associated veins as well as portal vein), and common bile duct. Celiac axis at T11/T12, SMA at L1.

Lymphatics/patterns of spread: Regional drainage is to peripancreatic, celiac, superior mesenteric, porta hepatic, and para-aortic lymph nodes. Frequently metastasizes to liver via portal venous network. Tumors of head and neck drain along common bile duct, common hepatic artery, portal vein, posterior/anterior pancreaticoduodenal arcades, SMV, and right lateral wall of SMA. Tumors of body and tail drain along common hepatic artery, celiac axis, splenic artery, and splenic hilum.

PATHOLOGY: Greater than 80% are ductal adenocarcinoma.[25] Approximately 60% arise from head, 15% in body or tail, and 20% diffusely involve pancreas.[25] Periampullary tumors can originate from head of pancreas, distal common bile duct, ampulla of Vater, or adjacent duodenum. Acinar cell tumors associated with fat necrosis, elevated lipase, rash, eosinophilia, polyarthralgia, and poor prognosis. Others include mucinous cystadenoma and adenosquamous carcinoma.[26] Other histologies include signet ring, medullary, adenosquamous, serous, and mixed acinar/ductal/neuroendocrine carcinoma. Approximately 5% of all pancreatic tumors are indolent endocrine tumors with long natural history and circulating polypeptides.[27]

GENETICS: Can be defined by *KRAS* and *P53* oncogene mutation in >90%.[25,28] Overexpression of MMP or EGFR in 60% to 70%. *TP53* mutation in 60%. *SMAD4* tumor suppressor mutated/deleted in ~30% and is a poor prognostic marker linked to higher predisposition for metastatic disease and shortened survival.[25,28]

SCREENING: CAPS consortium recommends screening with EUS and/or MRI/MRCP for high-risk individuals defined as patients with Peutz–Jeghers; hereditary pancreatitis; first-degree relative with pancreatic cancer and three or more first-/second-/third-degree relatives with pancreatic cancer; carriers of *BRCA1/2, P16,* and *HNPCC* mutations with one or more first-degree relative with pancreatic cancer.[29,30] No consensus exists on age to initiate or terminate screening/surveillance, how to manage detected lesions, and interval of screening required. Higher detection rate when screened with EUS over MRI or CT imaging.[31]

CLINICAL PRESENTATION: *Pain* (40%–60%) particularly in upper abdomen radiating to the back, which is intermittent and can be exacerbated by eating and/or alleviated by specific positions such as leaning forward, lying on left side or in fetal position; *weight loss* (80%–85%); fatigue (85%); nausea (~25%); diarrhea/steatorrhea; *jaundice* (~55%), often with acholic stools and/or dark urine; hepatomegaly.[32–34] Classically, painless jaundice in resectable patients as associated with a pancreatic head mass has a more favorable prognosis than those with symptomatic jaundice. Patients may develop diabetes in 2 to 3 years prior to presentation.

Eponyms: Enlarged nontender gallbladder (Courvoisier's sign), migratory thrombophlebitis (Trousseau's sign), left SCV lymph node (Virchow's node), left axillary node (Irish's node), periumbilical node (Sister Mary Joseph node), rectal shelf (Blumer's shelf), periumbilical ecchymosis (Cullen's sign), or flank ecchymosis (Grey Turner sign).

WORKUP: H&P.

Labs: CBC, CMP (including LFTs), CA 19-9 (may be undetectable in Lewis antigen-negative patients).

Imaging: Pancreatic protocol CT (early arterial, late arterial, and venous phases), or MRI (abdomen and pelvis). Systemic staging with CT (PET/CT controversial, detected unsuspected CT-occult DM in 33% of patients).[35]

Biopsy: Via EUS, ERCP, or CT-guidance. Biopsy is not necessarily required before surgery in patients with resectable disease, however, is necessary before administration of neoadjuvant therapy, in patients with unresectable or metastatic disease (biopsy of metastatic site may be preferable), or enrollment in clinical trial. EUS provides optimal T/N staging, and is favored method of biopsy because of better diagnostic yield, safety, and potentially lower risk of peritoneal seeding.[31,36,37] ERCP (with brushing/biopsy) may be useful for symptomatic obstructive jaundice requiring stent placement. MRCP useful when looking for occult primary (benefits are no contrast and no increased risk of post-ERCP pancreatitis).[38] Staging laparoscopy may be considered to assess for peritoneal disease; however, this varies by institution as by quality of pre-op imaging.[39–41]

PROGNOSTIC FACTORS: Age, stage (Table 35.2), grade, KPS, histology, location (head lesions are more favorable and present earlier), visceral artery involvement, extent of resection, response to neoadjuvant therapy, perineural invasion, lymph node status/ratio, and both pre- and postoperative serum CA 19-9 levels.[42–46]

STAGING

Table 35.2 :AJCC 8th ed. (2017) Staging for Exocrine Pancreatic Cancer		N	cN0	cN1	cN2
T/M					
T1	a. ≤0.5 cm		IA	IIB	III
	b. >0.5 and <1 cm				
	c. 1–2 cm				
T2	• 2.1–4 cm		IB		
T3	• >4 cm		IIA		
T4	• Involvement[1]				
M1	• Distant metastasis		IV		

Notes: Involvement[1] = celiac axis, SMA, and/or common hepatic artery.
cN1, 1–3 LNs; cN2, ≥ 4 LNs.

TREATMENT PARADIGM

Surgery: Surgery is currently the only potentially curative option for pancreatic cancer (Table 35.3). Twenty percent present with apparently resectable disease, however ~20% of patients thought to have resectable disease do *not* have resectable disease at time of surgery (e.g., peritoneal involvement, etc.). Approximately 50% of patients present with disseminated disease (commonly liver, peritoneum, and lungs). Remainder have borderline resectable disease (i.e., tumor is neither clearly resectable nor clearly unresectable) or locally advanced unresectable disease. Ultimately, ~15% of patients with newly diagnosed pancreatic cancer have up-front resectable disease. Whipple procedure (pancreaticoduodenectomy) is standard therapeutic operation, and involves en bloc resection of pancreatic head/body, distal stomach, duodenum, proximal jejunum, gallbladder, and distal common bile duct. Four PRTs have shown no difference in survival between variations on pancreaticoduodenectomy including pylorus-preserving, subtotal stomach-preserving, and minimally invasive techniques.[47–50] In addition, more extensive surgery, including extended lymphadenectomy and arterial en bloc resection, does not improve outcomes.[50,51] Operative mortality at high-volume centers is <5%.[52] After Whipple, remnant organs are attached to jejunum (pancreaticojejunostomy, gastrojejunostomy, and choledochojejunostomy) with vagotomy. Most common site of positive margin is retroperitoneal margin. Tail lesions can be considered for distal pancreatectomy depending on disease involvement. For highly selected patients with body/tail lesions with celiac artery involvement, Appleby procedure may be an option (includes splenectomy, distal pancreatectomy and celiac artery resection, relies on collateral circulation for hepatic perfusion). Postoperative complications include anastomotic leaks, which can lead to peritonitis, abscess, autodigestion, hemorrhage, and delayed gastric emptying.

Table 35.3: NCCN Criteria for Resectability[53]	
Clearly resectable	1. No tumor contact with celiac axis, SMA, and common hepatic artery 2. No radiographic evidence of SMV or portal vein contact or ≤180° contact without vein contour irregularity

Borderline resectable	1. Involvement of SMV/portal vein of >180° OR ≤180° with contour irregularity of vein
	2. SMV/Portal impingement (distortion/narrowing/occlusion/thrombosis), which can be resected/reconstructed
	3. Head/uncinate process tumor:
	  a. Involvement of common hepatic artery without celiac axis or hepatic bifurcation involved.
	  b. Abutment of SMA of ≤180°.
	  c. Contact with anatomic arterial variant (e.g., replaced or accessory artery).
	4. Body/Tail tumors: Involvement of ≤180° of celiac axis or >180° without aorta involvement and uninvolved gastroduodenal artery
	5. Limited involvement of IVC

Unresectable	1. Distant metastases, including lymph nodes beyond field of resection 2. Contact with first jejunal SMA branch for head/uncinate process lesions OR contact with celiac axis and aortic involvement for body/tail lesions. 3. Involvement with >180 degrees of celiac axis 4. Unreconstructable SMV/portal vein occlusion due to tumor involvement or occlusion (even bland thrombus) 5. Aortic invasion or encasement 6. Contact with proximal draining jejunal branch into SMV for head/uncinate process tumors.

Chemotherapy: Used in neoadjuvant and adjuvant settings as well as in context of locally advanced unresectable disease or metastatic disease. Single-agent 5-FU or gemcitabine was utilized historically, but multiagent CHT is now strongly favored in fit patients. FOLFIRINOX was shown to improve survival compared to single-agent gemcitabine in the adjuvant and metastatic setting at the expense of higher toxicity.[54] Gemcitabine-based combination therapies (e.g., gem/nab-paclitaxel) have also shown survival advantage.[55,56] In Japanese population, the oral fluoropyrimidine S-1 vs. gemcitabine after resection has shown higher survival with reduced toxicity; however, this has not been replicated in the United States.[57]

Radiation

Indications: RT can be delivered in neoadjuvant, postoperative, definitive, or palliative settings. Neoadjuvant RT has been utilized for borderline resectable patients in an attempt to optimize downstaging and provide local control in event resection does not occur, however, continues to be controversial in the setting of multiagent neoadjuvant CHT. Adjuvant RT should be considered in patients with positive margins and/or positive lymph nodes.[58] Definitive RT for unresectable/locally advanced cases improves local control and reduces pain, however, survival benefit has not been shown in modern trials (see the following). For locally advanced tumors, many prefer initial CHT followed by SBRT or chemoRT in setting of local progression or stable disease to avoid progression to second- or third-line CHT (see ASCO Guidelines).[59]

Dose: Conventional RT: 50.4 Gy/25 fx. SBRT: 25–50 Gy/5 fx given every other day.

Toxicity: Acute: Fatigue, dermatitis, N/V, diarrhea, appetite loss, weight loss, stomach ulcers. Late: Fatigue, skin discoloration, liver/renal dysfunction, bowel obstruction, stomach/bowel ulcers, dry/hyperpigmented skin.

Procedure: See *Treatment Planning Handbook,* Chapter 7[60] or RTOG Contouring Guidelines.[61]

Palliation: Palliative RT can improve pain control in up to 50% to 65% of patients.[62] SBRT has been shown to help achieve pain relief in >85% patients and is the preferred palliative option when appropriate.[63] Whipple procedure can offer palliation for duodenal obstruction and jaundice. Other surgeries include hepaticojejunostomy ± gastrojejunostomy. Endoscopic stent placement (frequently plastic for resectable disease and expandable metal stent for unresectable disease) is preferred method (compared to percutaneous stents). Celiac plexus and intrapleural nerve blocks and neurolysis can provide effective pain relief for select patients, however, relief can be transient in those who respond and others derive minimal relief after procedure.[64-66]

■ **EVIDENCE-BASED Q&A**

RESECTABLE PANCREATIC CANCER

■ **Is surgery necessary in the management of pancreatic cancer?**

Surgery, if possible, carries a significant survival benefit. Retroperitoneal lymphadenectomy is not necessary as it provides no OS advantage; and pylorus preservation carries higher risk of positive margins (21% vs. 5%).[51]

Doi, Japan (*Surg Today* 2008, PMID 18958561): Japanese multi-institution RCT of resectable pancreatic ACA (no involvement of SMA/common hepatic artery, no para-aortic LN+) randomized to surgery (pancreaticoduodenectomy or distal pancreatectomy + regional LN dissection) vs. chemoRT (continuous infusion 5-FU at 200 mg/m^2/day with 50.4 Gy/28 fx, four-field technique, tumor + 1–3 cm margin covering regional LN). Closed early due to survival benefit (42/150 enrolled) favoring surgical resection. MS 12.1 vs. 8.9 months, 3-year OS 20% vs. 0% ($p < .03$); 5-year OS 10% vs. 0% (NS). LC not reported. **Conclusion: Surgery significantly improves OS in resectable pancreatic cancer.**

■ **Is there benefit to adjuvant chemoRT compared to surgery alone?**

The benefit to adjuvant chemoRT compared to surgery alone is controversial given results of the following two trials. Latest ASCO guidelines suggest consideration of adjuvant chemoRT in patients with positive margins and/or positive LNs.[58]

Kalser, GITSG 91-73 (*Arch Surg* 1985, PMID 4015380; Confirmation Arm, *Cancer* 1987, PMID 3567862): PRT of 43 patients with negative margins following resection without peritoneal mets randomized to post-op chemoRT vs. observation. Treatment was split-course 40 Gy with 2-week break + 5-FU 500 mg/m^2 d1-3 with each 20 Gy course, then weekly 5-FU for 2 years or until recurrence. RT covered pancreas, pancreatic bed and regional LNs. Subtotal Whipple in 68%, total Whipple in 32%; 25% did not start adjuvant treatment for >10 weeks post-op. ChemoRT increased MS (20 vs. 11 mos) and 2-year OS (42% vs. 15%) (Table 35.4). **Conclusion: Combined use of chemoRT as adjuvant therapy after curative resection is effective and is preferred to no adjuvant therapy.** *Comment: Terminated early after 8 years due to poor accrual and early benefit to chemoRT presented in 1985. Additional 30 patients were accrued to receive adjuvant chemoRT after closure were presented in 1987 to demonstrate replication of results ("confirmation arm").*

Table 35.4: Results of GITSG 91-73 Adjuvant Pancreas Trial			
GITSG	MS (mos)	2-yr OS	5-yr OS
Surgery alone	11	15%	5%
Adjuvant chemoRT	20	42%	15%
Confirmation arm	18	46%	17%

Klinkenbijl, EORTC 40891 (*Ann Surg* 1999, PMID 10615932; Reanalysis Garofalo, *Ann Surg* 2006, PMID 16858208; Update Smeenk, *Ann Surg* 2007, PMID 17968163): PRT of 218 patients with T1-2N0-1a pancreatic head ACA (N = 114) or T1-3N0-1a periampullary ACA (N = 104) s/p resection. N1a was defined as LNs within resection specimen. Positive margins were included. Randomized to adjuvant concurrent chemoRT (40 Gy split course, with 5-FU 25 mg/kg on d1-5 and 29–34) vs. no adjuvant therapy. CHT was similar to GITSG 9173 with no maintenance CHT. Adjuvant treatment arm had more pancreatic head tumors than observation arm, and fewer periampullary tumors. Overall, no difference in OS, but study was underpowered (Table 35.5). Trend of benefit to adjuvant chemoRT for pancreatic head tumors (excluding periampullary). **Conclusion: Routine use of post-op chemoRT not recommended; 12-year update confirmed no benefit.** *Comment: Study limitations included: patients with positive margins, no maintenance CHT, split-course RT, low RT dose, no RT QA, and inclusion of periampullary and N1a patients. 20% of patients randomized to chemoRT did not receive it.*

Table 35.5: Results of EORTC 40891 Adjuvant ChemoRT for Pancreas Cancer							
EORTC 40891 (12-Year Update)	MS (yrs)	5-yr OS	10-yr OS	Median PFS (yrs)	5-yr PFS	10-yr PFS	MS Pancreatic Head (yrs)
Surgery alone	1.6	22%	18%	1.2	20%	17%	1
Adjuvant chemoRT	1.8	25%	17%	1.5	21%	16%	1.3
p value	NS	NS	NS	NS	NS	NS	NS

■ **Is there benefit to postoperative chemoRT compared to postoperative CHT?**

On basis of ESPAC-1, postoperative chemoRT is not beneficial and possibly detrimental compared to postoperative CHT.[67] However, both ESPAC-1 and EORTC 40891 had several flaws and thus results do not preclude chemoRT as an acceptable choice in adjuvant setting based on GITSG 91 to 73. Systemic therapy has greatly improved since these trials were conducted, and the ongoing Phase III trial RTOG 0848 is investigating the role of RT in the setting of modern systemic therapy. Current guidelines support consideration of adjuvant chemoRT in the setting of positive margins and/or positive lymph nodes.

Neoptolemos, ESPAC-1 (*Lancet* 2001, PMID 11716884; Update *NEJM* 2004, PMID 15028824): PRT of 541 patients with grossly resected pancreatic ductal carcinoma randomized to 2×2 factorial design to surgery followed by observation vs. CHT alone vs. chemoRT vs. chemoRT + consolidative CHT. Altered to boost accrual with randomization into one of main treatment comparisons (chemoRT vs. no chemoRT or CHT vs. no CHT). CHT was 5-FU 425 mg/m^2 d1-5 + LCV 20 mg/m^2 q28d × 6 cycles. ChemoRT regimen was 40 Gy split course (20 Gy/10 fx + bolus 5-FU 500 mg/m^2 followed by 2-week break followed by 20 Gy/10 fx + bolus 5-FU 500 mg/m^2); 285 patients randomized to 2×2 design: 68 to +/− chemoRT and 188 to +/− CHT. MFU 47 months. Eighty-one percent with R0 resection, 19% had positive margins. Median time from resection to treatment was 46 days in CHT arm and 61 days in chemoRT arm. Prognostic factors were higher grade, LN+, tumor >2 cm. QOL parameters were equivalent between groups. When adjusted for prognostic factors, there was no benefit for adjuvant chemoRT (MS 16.1 vs. 15.5 for chemoRT, *p* = .24). There was survival benefit for adjuvant CHT (MS 14 vs. 19.7 for CHT, HR 0.66, *p* = .0005) (Table 35.6). **Conclusion: CHT alone improved survival compared to observation. Adjuvant 5-FU-based chemoRT did not improve survival, and may have had deleterious effect.** *Comment: Study limitations included: no central QA, selection bias (physician allowed to select which randomization), background treatment allowed by clinician choice (CHT or chemoRT), nearly 1/3 of observation arm and 1/3 of CHT arm received RT, and RT dose was inconsistent— designed at 40 Gy, but choice of up to 60 Gy allowed.*

Table 35.6: Results of ESPAC 1 for Pancreas Cancer			
ESPAC 1: 2×2 Subset Only (2004)	MS (mos)	TTF (mos)	5-yr OS
ChemoRT	15.9	10.7	10%
No chemoRT	17.9	15.2	20%
p value (+/− chemoRT)	.05	.04	
CHT	20.1	15.3	21%
No CHT	15.5	10.5	8%
p value (+/− CHT)	.009	.02	

Stocken, Pancreatic Cancer Meta-Analysis Group (*Br J Cancer* 2005, PMID 15812554): Systematic review and meta-analysis of 5 RCT (GITSG, Norway, EORTC, Japan, ESPAC-1) of adjuvant CHT and chemoRT for 1,136 patients. CHT showed reduction in risk of death by 25% (HR 0.75, CI: 0.64– 0.90, *p* = .001) and improved MS of 19 months vs. 13.5 months without CHT. No significant difference in risk of death with chemoRT (HR 1.09, CI: 0.89–1.32, *p* = .43) (Table 35.7). Subgroup analysis showed chemoRT more effective with positive margins and CHT alone less effective. **Conclusion: CHT is effective adjuvant therapy while chemoRT is not unless patient has margin-positive disease.**

Table 35.7: Results of Stocken Meta-analysis			
Stocken Meta-analysis	MS (mos)	2-yr OS	5-yr OS
CHT alone	19.0	38%	19%
Observation (CHT)	13.5	28%	12%
ChemoRT	15.8	30%	12%
Observation (chemoRT)	15.2	34%	17%

Abrams, RTOG 0848 (*Am J Clin Oncol* 2020, PMID 31985516): Two-step phase III trial evaluating both erlotinib (part 1) and chemoRT (part 2) as adjuvant treatment for resected head of pancreas. Part 1: patients randomized to adjuvant CHT +/- erlotinib for six cycles. Part 2: patients without progression at the end of cycle 5 were randomized to concurrent chemoRT vs. no additional treatment. CHT initially consisted of gemcitabine alone, but was later modified to include mFOLFIRINOX or gemcitabmine–capecitabine. In outcomes from step 1, erlotinib did not improve OS (median 29.9 mos vs. 28.1 mos, $p = .62$) but did increase grade 3 diarrhea (2% vs. 10%; $p = .002$). **Conclusion: The addition of erlotinib to gemcitabine did not improve outcomes, but did increase toxicity. Part 2 investigating the role of adjuvant chemoRT is pending.**

▪ What is the optimal adjuvant CHT regimen?

ESPAC-1[68] and German CONKO-001[69,70] demonstrated a survival benefit to adjuvant CHT as compared to surgery alone and used 5-FU and gemcitabine monotherapy, respectively. In the modern era, mFOLFIRINOX and gemcitabine/capecitabine are preferred regimens based on results of PRODIGE-24[71] and ESPAC-4,[72] respectively, which both demonstrated an OS advantage to multiagent CHT as compared to gemcitabine alone. Gemcitabine/nab-paclitaxel as well as gemcitabine and 5-FU/LCV are acceptable alternatives.

▪ What is optimal adjuvant chemoRT regimen?

Regine, RTOG 97-04 (*JAMA* 2008, PMID 18319412; Update *Ann Surg Oncol* 2011, PMID 21499862): PRT of 451 patients s/p GTR of T1-4N0-1M0 pancreatic ACA (excluded ampullary cancers) with KPS >60 randomized to PVI 5-FU × 3 weeks → chemoRT → PVI 5-FU × 2 months or weekly gemcitabine × 3 → chemoRT → gemcitabine × 2 months. ChemoRT was 50.4 Gy/28 fx (cone-down after 45 Gy) with concurrent PVI 5-FU. Primary endpoint OS. MFU 1.5 years overall and 7 years for alive patients; 67% were N1, 75% were T3–4 (more in gemcitabine arm), 34% had positive margins (25% had unknown margin status), 86% pancreatic head tumors. Overall, no difference in OS or DFS. On MVA, no benefit of gemcitabine vs. 5-FU with MS of 20.5 vs. 17.1 months and 5-yr OS of 22% vs. 18% respectively (HR 0.84, $p = .12$) (Table 35.8). **Conclusion: No difference in OS of patients with gemcitabine or 5-FU given before/after chemoRT. Gemcitabine was associated with greater heme toxicity.** *Comment: Second analysis demonstrated effect between RT QA and protocol compliance on OS.[73] Furthermore, significantly worse OS reported in patients with postresection CA19-9 >90 U/mL (HR 3.1, $p < .0001$).[74]*

Table 35.8: Results of RTOG 97-04				
RTOG 97-04 (All Patients)	LR	MS	3-yr OS	Grade 4 Heme Toxicity
5-FU arm	28%	16.9 m	22%	1%
Gemcitabine arm	23%	20.5 m	31%	14%
p value	NS	.09		<.001

BORDERLINE RESECTABLE

▪ What is the rationale for neoadjuvant chemoRT?

Neoadjuvant chemoRT may help downstage patients, reduce nodal burden, reduce rate of positive margins, and improve resectability in borderline patients. CHT regimens include concurrent 5-FU or gemcitabine. Recently, attention is being paid to neoadjuvant regimens incorporating more aggressive CHT with or without RT, such as FOLFIRINOX, mFOLFIRINOX, gemcitabine/docetaxel/capecitabine, or gemcitabine/capecitabine and continues to be evaluated on trials.[75-77] Emerging data (ALLIANCE A021501) suggest that preoperative SBRT in an unselected patient population in the setting of neoadjuvant mFOLFIRINOX may not be helpful.

Versteijne, PREOPANC-1 (*JCO* 2020, PMID 32105518): Phase III RCT of 246 patients with resectable or borderline resectable pancreatic cancer randomized to immediate surgery (arm A) vs. preop chemoRT (arm B; 3 cycles gemcitabine with 36Gy/15fx during cycle 2). Both arms received adjuvant gemcitabine (6 cycles in arm A; 4 cycles in arm B). No difference in the primary endpoint OS overall (arm A: 14.3 mos vs. arm B: 16 mos; $p = .096$). However, on subset analysis of borderline resectable patients there was an OS benefit for preop chemoRT (13.2 vs. 17.6 mos; $p = .029$). Preop chemoRT also improved R0 resection rate (40% vs. 71%; $p < .001$). No difference in serious adverse events. **Conclusion: ChemoRT improves OS among borderline resectable pancreatic cancer patients.**

Laurence, Australian Meta-Analysis (*J Gastrointest Surg* 2011, PMID 21913045): Systematic review and meta-analysis of 19 studies to evaluate benefits and complications associated with neoadjuvant chemoRT for both resectable and initially unresectable pancreatic cancer. Patients with unresectable pancreatic cancer showed similar OS to patients with resectable disease. Only 40% ultimately resected after neoadjuvant therapy. Neoadjuvant chemoRT was associated with reduced margin+ rate. Increase risk of perioperative death, but no significant increase in pancreatic fistula formation or total complications. **Conclusion: Available data for OS of given studies was poor and unable to draw definitive conclusion. However, neoadjuvant therapy may reduce risk of positive margins while increasing risk of perioperative complications/death.**

Jang, Korea (*Ann Surg* 2018, PMID 29462005): PRT of 50 patients with borderline resectable pancreatic cancer randomized to pre-op chemoRT or post-op chemoRT. ChemoRT consisted of 54 Gy/30 fx with concurrent gemcitabine. Study was terminated early after interim analysis showed the pre-op chemoRT arm had significantly improved R0 resection rates (26% vs. 52%; $p = .004$) and OS (12 mos vs. 21 mos; $p = .03$). **Conclusion: Neoadjuvant chemoRT improves OS and R0 resection rate compared to adjuvant chemoRT.**

Gillen, Munich Meta-Analysis (*PLoS Med* 2010, PMID 20422030): Systematic review and meta-analysis of prospective and retrospective studies evaluating neoadjuvant chemoRT, RT, or CHT followed by restaging and surgical exploration/resection. Totally 111 studies (4,934 patients) were divided according to whether they were assessing initially resectable tumors or tumors considered unresectable/borderline. MS 23.3 months after resection for initially resectable disease and 20.5 months for unresectable patients. Initially resectable tumors had CR rate of 3.6% and PR rate of 30.6% while initially unresectable tumors showed CR rate of 4.8% and PR rate of 30.2%. **Conclusion: Neoadjuvant therapy with reassessment should be considered for patients thought to be unresectable as one-third of patients ultimately underwent surgery with OS similar to initially resectable group.**

LOCALLY ADVANCED/UNRESECTABLE PANCREATIC CANCER

■ **What is the optimal CHT to palliate symptoms from advanced pancreatic cancer?**

Burris (*JCO* 1997, PMID 9196156): Multi-institution PRT of 126 patients with symptomatic unresectable or metastatic disease randomized to gemcitabine or 5-FU. Evaluated "clinical benefit response," which was composite measurement of pain (analgesic consumption and pain intensity), KPS, and weight. Clinical benefit required sustained (defined as ≥4 weeks) improvement in ≥1 parameter without decrease in others. Median time to clinical benefit response was 7 weeks for gemcitabine and 3 weeks for 5-FU, mean duration was 18 weeks vs. 13 weeks, respectively. Gemcitabine demonstrated more treatment-related side effects. **Conclusion: Gemcitabine increased clinical benefit of response in advanced, symptomatic patient population while also improving OS. Treatment was well tolerated.**

■ **What is rationale for definitive chemoRT in locally advanced unresectable pancreatic cancer?**

As with resectable pancreatic cancer, use of chemoRT as part of standard management of locally advanced or unresectable disease is controversial because of conflicting results of randomized studies. In general, biliary stent (if jaundice) can be performed first followed by induction CHT with restaging followed by chemoRT or continued CHT alone (see ASCO guidelines).[58] The following trials (Table 35.9) support use of chemoRT, whereas later trials (Chauffert, Krishnan, and Hammel) do not support chemoRT.

Table 35.9: Trials Supporting Use of ChemoRT for Locally Advanced/Unresectable Pancreatic Cancer

Trial	Year	Arms	Results	Notes
Mayo Clinic[78]	1969	RT alone ChemoRT (35–40 Gy ± 5-FU)	MS 10.4 (chemoRT) vs. 6.3 mo (RT alone)	
GITSG 9273[79]	1981	RT alone (60 Gy) ChemoRT (40 Gy) ChemoRT (60 Gy)	1-yr OS 40% vs. 10%	RT given with 2-week break every 20 Gy, CHT 5-FU concurrent and maintenance
GITSG 9283[80]	1988	CHT alone ChemoRT	1-yr OS 41% vs. 19%	CHT alone: SMF (streptozocin, MMC, and 5-FU) ChemoRT was 54 Gy + 5-FU
ECOG E4201[81]	2008	CHT alone (gemcitabine) ChemoRT (gemcitabine + 50.4 Gy/28 fx)	MS 9.2 vs. 11.1 in favor of gem/RT (p = .017)	Closed early due to poor accrual

Chauffert, French FFCD-SFRO (*Ann Oncol* 2008, PMID 18467316): PRT of 119 patients with locally advanced pancreatic cancer and WHO PS-0 randomized to induction chemoRT (60 Gy/30 fx with PVI 5-FU, 300 mg/m^2, d1-5 ×6 weeks and cisplatin 20 mg/m^2, d1-5 during weeks 1 and 5) or induction gemcitabine alone (1,000 mg/m^2 weekly ×7 weeks). Maintenance gemcitabine (1000 mg/m^2 weekly, 3/4 weeks) given in both arms until disease progression or toxicity. Stopped early due to lower MS with chemoRT (8.6 vs. 13 months, p = .03), and higher toxicity (grade 3–4 toxicity 36% vs. 22% during induction and 32% vs. 18% during maintenance). **Conclusion: Induction chemoRT showed increased toxicity and decreased effectiveness than gemcitabine alone.** *Comment: ChemoRT regimen in this trial was nonstandard and toxic.*

Hammel, LAP07 (*JAMA* 2016, PMID 27139057): PRT of 442 patients. Two randomizations: first to either gemcitabine (1,000 mg/m^2 weekly ×3 weeks) or gemcitabine with erlotinib (100 mg/d for 4 months). Those with no progression after 4 months were randomized again to further CHT +/− RT (54 Gy and capecitabine 1600 mg/m^2/d). Patients receiving erlotinib received maintenance erlotinib after completion. MFU 36.7 mos. 269 patients had no progression after 4 months. MS was 16.5 with CHT and 15.2 months with CHT+RT (p = .83). MS was 13.6 mos in those undergoing gemcitabine and 11.9 mos for gemcitabine+erlotinib (p = .09). Reduced LR was noted with chemoRT (32% vs. 46%, p = .03) with no increased grade 3 to 4 toxicity except nausea. **Conclusion: No significant difference in OS with chemoRT vs. CHT or with addition of gemcitabine in conjunction with erlotinib used as maintenance CHT.** *Comment: After formal RT QA, only 32% of patients in chemoRT arm were treated per protocol, while 50% had minor deviations and 18% had major deviations.*

■ **What is the role of SBRT in locally advanced pancreatic cancer?**

Although there are no randomized trials comparing SBRT to chemoRT, there is growing interest in SBRT as a means to improve local control while minimizing interruption of systemic therapy. The ongoing PanCRS trial is investigating the role of SBRT among patients who do not progress on induction mFOLFIRINOX.

Chang, Stanford (*Cancer* 2009, PMID 19117351): RR of 77 patients with unresectable pancreatic cancer (58% locally advanced; 14% medically inoperable; 8% locally recurrent; 19% metastatic) treated with 25 Gy/1 fx with CyberKnife®. Twenty-one percent also received 45 to 54 Gy of fractionated EBRT. Various gemcitabine-based regimens in 96% of patients. Isolated local failure at 6 and 12 months was 5%. PFS at 6 and 12 months was 26% and 9%, respectively. OS at 6 and 12 months was 56% and 21%. Grade ≥2 acute toxicity was 5%. Grade ≥3 late toxicity was 9%. **Conclusion: 25 Gy/1 fx provides effective LC, though concerns about late toxicity, most commonly ulceration. A subsequent dose-volume analysis of duodenal toxicity (N = 73) showed the 12-month risk of duodenal toxicity was 29%.[82]**

Pollom, Stanford (*IJROBP* 2014, PMID 25585785): RR of 167 patients treated with SBRT with either single fx (45.5%) or 5 fx (54.5%) regimens. MFU 7.9 mo. No difference in recurrence by fractionation scheme with 6/12 month rates of LR 5.3%/9.5% for single fraction while 3.4%/11.7% for 5 fx, respectively. No difference in OS by fractionation scheme with 6/12 month rates of OS 67%/30.8% for single fraction while 75.7%/34.9% for 5 fx, respectively. Significantly less grade ≥2 toxicity with 5 fx regimen. In single fx group, 6/12 month rates of GI toxicity grade ≥3 were 8.1%/12.3%, respectively, while both were 5.6% in 5 fx group (NS). **Conclusion: Multifraction SBRT reduces GI toxicity without detriment in LC.**

Moningi, Johns Hopkins (*Ann Surg Oncol* 2015, PMID 25564157): RR of 88 patients with pancreatic ACA receiving SBRT (25–33 Gy/5 fx) from 2010 to 2014. 74 locally advanced and 14 borderline resectable. MFU 14.5 months for locally advanced and 10.3 months for borderline resectable. Most patients received pre-SBRT CHT. MS 18.4 months and median PFS 9.8 months. Only three patients had ≥grade 3 toxicity and five patients had late ≥grade 2 GI toxicity; 19 patients underwent resection, of whom 15 (79%) had locally advanced disease and 16 (84%) had R0 resection. **Conclusion: SBRT after CHT for either locally advanced or borderline resectable pancreatic cancer results in low acute and late toxicity. Majority of patients completed resection without significant radiographic response.**

REFERENCES

1. Twombly R. Adjuvant chemoradiation for pancreatic cancer: few good data, much debate. *J Natl Cancer Inst.* 2008;100(23):1670–1671. doi:10.1093/jnci/djn428
2. Siegel RL, Miller KD, Jemal A. Cancer statistics, 2017. *CA Cancer J Clin.* 2017;67(1):7–30. doi:10.3322/caac.21387
3. Boyle P, Hsieh CC, Maisonneuve P, et al. Epidemiology of pancreas cancer (1988). *Int J Pancreatol.* 1989;5(4):327–346. doi:10.1007/BF02924298
4. Hariharan D, Saied A, Kocher HM. Analysis of mortality rates for pancreatic cancer across the world. *HPB (Oxford).* 2008;10(1):58–62. doi:10.1080/13651820701883148
5. Yao JC, Eisner MP, Leary C, et al. Population-based study of islet cell carcinoma. *Ann Surg Oncol.* 2007;14(12):3492–3500. doi:10.1245/s10434-007-9566-6
6. Ma J, Siegel R, Jemal A. Pancreatic cancer death rates by race among US men and women, 1970–2009. *J Natl Cancer Inst.* 2013;105(22):1694–1700. doi:10.1093/jnci/djt292
7. Yao JC, Hassan M, Phan A, et al. One hundred years after "carcinoid": epidemiology of and prognostic factors for neuroendocrine tumors in 35,825 cases in the United States. *J Clin Oncol.* 2008;26(18):3063–3072. doi:10.1200/JCO.2007.15.4377
8. Barone E, Corrado A, Gemignani F, Landi S. Environmental risk factors for pancreatic cancer: an update. *Arch Toxicol.* 2016;90(11):2617–2642. doi:10.1007/s00204-016-1821-9
9. Fuchs CS, Colditz GA, Stampfer MJ, et al. A prospective study of cigarette smoking and the risk of pancreatic cancer. *Arch Intern Med.* 1996;156(19):2255–2260. doi:10.1001/archinte.1996.00440180119015
10. Michaud DS, Giovannucci E, Willett WC, et al. Physical activity, obesity, height, and the risk of pancreatic cancer. *JAMA.* 2001;286(8):921–929. doi:10.1001/jama.286.8.921
11. Hassan MM, Li D, El-Deeb AS, et al. Association between hepatitis B virus and pancreatic cancer. *J Clin Oncol.* 2008;26(28):4557–4562. doi:10.1200/JCO.2008.17.3526
12. Giardiello FM, Brensinger JD, Tersmette AC, et al. Very high risk of cancer in familial peutz-jeghers syndrome. *Gastroenterology.* 2000;119(6):1447–1453. doi:10.1053/gast.2000.20228
13. van Lier MG, Wagner A, Mathus-Vliegen EM, et al. High cancer risk in Peutz-Jeghers syndrome: a systematic review and surveillance recommendations. *Am J Gastroenterol.* 2010;105(6):1258–1264. doi:10.1038/ajg.2009.725
14. Lim W, Olschwang S, Keller JJ, et al. Relative frequency and morphology of cancers in STK11 mutation carriers. *Gastroenterology.* 2004;126(7):1788–1794. doi:10.1053/j.gastro.2004.03.014
15. de Snoo FA, Bishop DT, Bergman W, et al. Increased risk of cancer other than melanoma in CDKN2A founder mutation (p16-Leiden)-positive melanoma families. *Clin Cancer Res.* 2008;14(21):7151–7157. doi:10.1158/1078-0432.CCR-08-0403
16. Roberts NJ, Jiao Y, Yu J, et al. ATM mutations in patients with hereditary pancreatic cancer. *Cancer Discov.* 2012;2(1):41–46. doi:10.1158/2159-8290.CD-11-0194
17. Iqbal J, Ragone A, Lubinski J, et al. The incidence of pancreatic cancer in BRCA1 and BRCA2 mutation carriers. *Br J Cancer.* 2012;107(12):2005–2009. doi:10.1038/bjc.2012.483
18. Olson SH, Kurtz RC. Epidemiology of pancreatic cancer and the role of family history. *J Surg Oncol.* 2013;107(1):1–7. doi:10.1002/jso.23149
19. Klein AP. Genetic susceptibility to pancreatic cancer. *Mol Carcinog.* 2012;51(1):14–24. doi:10.1002/mc.20855
20. Klein AP, Hruban RH, Brune KA, et al. Familial pancreatic cancer. *Cancer J.* 2001;7(4):266–273.
21. Solomon S, Das S, Brand R, Whitcomb DC. Inherited pancreatic cancer syndromes. *Cancer J.* 2012;18(6):485–491. doi:10.1097/PPO.0b013e318278c4a6

22. Amundadottir L, Kraft P, Stolzenberg-Solomon RZ, et al. Genome-wide association study identifies variants in the ABO locus associated with susceptibility to pancreatic cancer. *Nat Genet.* 2009;41(9):986–990. doi:10.1038/ng.429

23. Wolpin BM, Chan AT, Hartge P, et al. ABO blood group and the risk of pancreatic cancer. *J Natl Cancer Inst.* 2009;101(6):424–431. doi:10.1093/jnci/djp020

24. Genkinger JM, Li R, Spiegelman D, et al. Coffee, tea, and sugar-sweetened carbonated soft drink intake and pancreatic cancer risk: a pooled analysis of 14 cohort studies. *Cancer Epidemiol Biomarkers Prev.* 2012;21(2):305–318. doi:10.1158/1055-9965.EPI-11-0945-T

25. Esposito I, Konukiewitz B, Schlitter AM, Kloppel G. Pathology of pancreatic ductal adenocarcinoma: facts, challenges and future developments. *World J Gastroenterol.* 2014;20(38):13833–13841. doi:10.3748/wjg.v20.i38.13833

26. La Rosa S, Sessa F, Capella C. Acinar Cell carcinoma of the pancreas: overview of clinicopathologic features and insights into the molecular pathology. *Front Med (Lausanne).* 2015;2:41. doi:10.3389/fmed.2015.00041

27. Klimstra DS. Nonductal neoplasms of the pancreas. *Mod Pathol.* 2007;20(Suppl 1):S94–S112. doi:10.1038/modpathol.3800686

28. Winter JM, Maitra A, Yeo CJ. Genetics and pathology of pancreatic cancer. *HPB (Oxford).* 2006;8(5):324–336. doi:10.1080/13651820600804203

29. Canto MI, Goggins M, Hruban RH, et al. Screening for early pancreatic neoplasia in high-risk individuals: a prospective controlled study. *Clin Gastroenterol Hepatol.* 2006;4(6):766–781; quiz 665. doi:10.1016/j.cgh.2006.04.003

30. Canto MI, Harinck F, Hruban RH, et al. International cancer of the pancreas screening (CAPS) consortium summit on the management of patients with increased risk for familial pancreatic cancer. *Gut.* 2013;62(3):339–347. doi:10.1136/gutjnl-2012-303108

31. Canto MI, Hruban RH, Fishman EK, et al. Frequent detection of pancreatic lesions in asymptomatic high-risk individuals. *Gastroenterology.* 2012;142(4):796–804; quiz e714–e795. doi:10.1053/j.gastro.2012.01.005

32. Porta M, Fabregat X, Malats N, et al. Exocrine pancreatic cancer: symptoms at presentation and their relation to tumour site and stage. *Clin Transl Oncol.* 2005;7(5):189–197. doi:10.1007/BF02712816

33. Kalser MH, Barkin J, MacIntyre JM. Pancreatic cancer: assessment of prognosis by clinical presentation. *Cancer.* 1985;56(2):397–402. doi:10.1002/1097-0142(19850715)56:2<397::AID-CNCR2820560232>3.0.CO;2-I

34. Bakkevold KE, Arnesjo B, Kambestad B. Carcinoma of the pancreas and papilla of vater: presenting symptoms, signs, and diagnosis related to stage and tumour site: a prospective multicentre trial in 472 patients. norwegian pancreatic cancer trial. *Scand J Gastroenterol.* 1992;27(4):317–325. doi:10.3109/00365529209000081

35. Chang JS, Choi SH, Lee Y, et al. Clinical usefulness of (1)(8)F-fluorodeoxyglucose-positron emission tomography in patients with locally advanced pancreatic cancer planned to undergo concurrent chemoradiation therapy. *Int J Radiat Oncol Biol Phys.* 2014;90(1):126–133. doi:10.1016/j.ijrobp.2014.05.030

36. Poley JW, Kluijt I, Gouma DJ, et al. The yield of first-time endoscopic ultrasonography in screening individuals at a high risk of developing pancreatic cancer. *Am J Gastroenterol.* 2009;104(9):2175–2181. doi:10.1038/ajg.2009.276

37. Langer P, Kann PH, Fendrich V, et al. Five years of prospective screening of high-risk individuals from families with familial pancreatic cancer. *Gut.* 2009;58(10):1410–1418. doi:10.1136/gut.2008.171611

38. Hennedige TP, Neo WT, Venkatesh SK. Imaging of malignancies of the biliary tract: an update. *Cancer Imaging.* 2014;14:14.

39. Ahmed SI, Bochkarev V, Oleynikov D, Sasson AR. Patients with pancreatic adenocarcinoma benefit from staging laparoscopy. *J Laparoendosc Adv Surg Tech A.* 2006;16(5):458–463. doi:10.1089/lap.2006.16.458

40. Allen VB, Gurusamy KS, Takwoingi Y, et al. Diagnostic accuracy of laparoscopy following computed tomography (CT) scanning for assessing the resectability with curative intent in pancreatic and periampullary cancer. *Cochrane Database Syst Rev.* 2013;(11):CD009323. doi:10.1002/14651858.CD009323.pub2

41. Warshaw AL, Gu ZY, Wittenberg J, Waltman AC. Preoperative staging and assessment of resectability of pancreatic cancer. *Arch Surg.* 1990;125(2):230–233. doi:10.1001/archsurg.1990.01410140108018

42. Gillen S, Schuster T, Meyer Zum Buschenfelde C, et al. Preoperative/neoadjuvant therapy in pancreatic cancer: a systematic review and meta-analysis of response and resection percentages. *PLoS Med.* 2010;7(4):e1000267. doi:10.1371/journal.pmed.1000267

43. Andren-Sandberg A. Prognostic factors in pancreatic cancer. *N Am J Med Sci.* 2012;4(1):9–12. doi:10.4103/1947-2714.92893

44. Bilici A. Prognostic factors related with survival in patients with pancreatic adenocarcinoma. *World J Gastroenterol.* 2014;20(31):10802–10812. doi:10.3748/wjg.v20.i31.10802

45. Tas F, Sen F, Keskin S, et al. Prognostic factors in metastatic pancreatic cancer: older patients are associated with reduced overall survival. *Mol Clin Oncol.* 2013;1(4):788–792. doi:10.3892/mco.2013.131

46. Eloubeidi MA, Desmond RA, Wilcox CM, et al. Prognostic factors for survival in pancreatic cancer: a population-based study. *Am J Surg.* 2006;192(3):322–329. doi:10.1016/j.amjsurg.2006.02.017

47. Tran KT, Smeenk HG, van Eijck CH, et al. Pylorus preserving pancreaticoduodenectomy versus standard Whipple procedure: a prospective, randomized, multicenter analysis of 170 patients with pancreatic and periampullary tumors. *Ann Surg.* 2004;240(5):738–745. doi:10.1097/01.sla.0000143248.71964.29

48. Lin PW, Shan YS, Lin YJ, Hung CJ. Pancreaticoduodenectomy for pancreatic head cancer: PPPD versus whipple procedure. *Hepatogastroenterology.* 2005;52(65):1601–1604.

49. Seiler CA, Wagner M, Bachmann T, et al. Randomized clinical trial of pylorus-preserving duodenopancreatectomy versus classical whipple resection-long term results. *Br J Surg.* 2005;92(5):547–556. doi:10.1002/bjs.4881

50. Yeo CJ, Cameron JL, Lillemoe KD, et al. Pancreaticoduodenectomy with or without distal gastrectomy and extended retroperitoneal lymphadenectomy for periampullary adenocarcinoma, part 2: randomized controlled trial evaluating survival, morbidity, and mortality. *Ann Surg.* 2002;236(3):355–366; discussion 366–358. doi:10.1097/00000658-200209000-00012

51. Riall TS, Cameron JL, Lillemoe KD, et al. Pancreaticoduodenectomy with or without distal gastrectomy and extended retroperitoneal lymphadenectomy for periampullary adenocarcinoma—Part 3: update on 5-year survival. *J Gastrointest Surg.* 2005;9(9):1191–1204; discussion 1204–1196. doi:10.1016/j.gassur.2005.08.034

52. Langer B. Role of volume outcome data in assuring quality in HPB surgery. *HPB (Oxford).* 2007;9(5):330–334. doi:10.1080/13651820701611234

53. NCCN Clinical Practice Guidelines in Oncology: Pancreatic Adenocarcinoma. 2020. https://www.nccn.org

54. Conroy T, Desseigne F, Ychou M, et al. FOLFIRINOX versus gemcitabine for metastatic pancreatic cancer. *N Engl J Med.* 2011;364(19):1817–1825. doi:10.1056/NEJMoa1011923

55. Goldstein D, El-Maraghi RH, Hammel P, et al. nab-Paclitaxel plus gemcitabine for metastatic pancreatic cancer: long-term survival from a phase III trial. *J Natl Cancer Inst.* 2015;107(2). doi:10.1093/jnci/dju413

56. Moore MJ, Goldstein D, Hamm J, et al. Erlotinib plus gemcitabine compared with gemcitabine alone in patients with advanced pancreatic cancer: a phase III trial of the national cancer institute of Canada clinical trials group. *J Clin Oncol.* 2007;25(15):1960–1966. doi:10.1200/JCO.2006.07.9525

57. Maeda A, Boku N, Fukutomi A, et al. Randomized phase III trial of adjuvant chemotherapy with gemcitabine versus S-1 in patients with resected pancreatic cancer: Japan adjuvant study group of pancreatic cancer (JASPAC-01). *Jpn J Clin Oncol.* 2008;38(3):227–229. doi:10.1093/jjco/hym178

58. Khorana AA, McKernin SE, Berlin J, et al. Potentially curable pancreatic adenocarcinoma: ASCO clinical practice guideline update. *J Clin Oncol.* 2019;37(23):2082–2088. doi:10.1200/JCO.19.00946

59. Balaban EP, Mangu PB, Khorana AA, et al. Locally advanced, unresectable pancreatic cancer: ASCO clinical practice guideline. *J Clin Oncol.* 2016;34(22):2654–2668. doi:10.1200/JCO.2016.67.5561

60. Videtic GMM, Woody N, Vassil AD. *Handbook of Treatment Planning in Radiation Oncology.* 3rd ed. Demos Medical; 2020. doi:10.1891/9780826168429

61. Goodman KA, Regine WF, Dawson LA, et al. Radiation therapy oncology group consensus panel guidelines for the delineation of the clinical target volume in the postoperative treatment of pancreatic head cancer. *Int J Radiat Oncol Biol Phys.* 2012;83(3):901–908. doi:10.1016/j.ijrobp.2012.01.022

62. Morganti AG, Trodella L, Valentini V, et al. Pain relief with short-term irradiation in locally advanced carcinoma of the pancreas. *J Palliat Care.* 2003;19(4):258–262. doi:10.1177/082585970301900407

63. Buwenge M, Macchia G, Arcelli A, et al. Stereotactic radiotherapy of pancreatic cancer: a systematic review on pain relief. *J Pain Res.* 2018:11:2169–2178. doi:10.2147/JPR.S167994

64. Arcidiacono PG, Calori G, Carrara S, et al. Celiac plexus block for pancreatic cancer pain in adults. *Cochrane Database Syst Rev.* 2011;(3):CD007519. doi:10.1002/14651858.CD007519.pub2

65. Wong GY, Schroeder DR, Carns PE, et al. Effect of neurolytic celiac plexus block on pain relief, quality of life, and survival in patients with unresectable pancreatic cancer: a randomized controlled trial. *JAMA.* 2004;291(9):1092–1099. doi:10.1001/jama.291.9.1092

66. Eisenberg E, Carr DB, Chalmers TC. Neurolytic celiac plexus block for treatment of cancer pain: a meta-analysis. *Anesth Analg.* 1995;80(2):290–295. doi:10.1097/00000539-199502000-00015

67. Neoptolemos JP, Dunn JA, Stocken DD, et al. Adjuvant chemoradiotherapy and chemotherapy in resectable pancreatic cancer: a randomised controlled trial. *Lancet.* 2001;358(9293):1576–1585. doi:10.1016/S0140-6736(01)06651-X

68. Neoptolemos JP, Stocken DD, Friess H, et al. A randomized trial of chemoradiotherapy and chemotherapy after resection of pancreatic cancer. *N Engl J Med.* 2004;350(12):1200–1210. doi:10.1056/NEJMoa032295

69. Oettle H, Neuhaus P, Hochhaus A, et al. Adjuvant chemotherapy with gemcitabine and long-term outcomes among patients with resected pancreatic cancer: the CONKO-001 randomized trial. *JAMA.* 2013;310(14):1473–1481. doi:10.1001/jama.2013.279201

70. Oettle H, Post S, Neuhaus P, et al. Adjuvant chemotherapy with gemcitabine vs observation in patients undergoing curative-intent resection of pancreatic cancer: a randomized controlled trial. *JAMA.* 2007;297(3):267–277. doi:10.1001/jama.297.3.267

71. Conroy T, Hammel P, Hebbar M, et al. FOLFIRINOX or gemcitabine as adjuvant therapy for pancreatic cancer. *N Engl J Med.* 2018;379(25):2395–2406. doi:10.1056/NEJMoa1809775

72. Neoptolemos JP, Palmer DH, Ghaneh P, et al. Comparison of adjuvant gemcitabine and capecitabine with gemcitabine monotherapy in patients with resected pancreatic cancer (ESPAC-4): a multicentre, open-label, randomised, phase 3 trial. *Lancet.* 2017;389(10073):1011–1024. doi:10.1016/S0140-6736(16)32409-6

73. Abrams RA, Winter KA, Regine WF, et al. Failure to adhere to protocol specified radiation therapy guidelines was associated with decreased survival in RTOG 9704: a Phase III trial of adjuvant chemotherapy and chemoradiotherapy for patients with resected adenocarcinoma of the pancreas. *Int J Radiat Oncol Biol Phys.* 2012;82(2):809–816. doi:10.1016/j.ijrobp.2010.11.039

74. Berger AC, Winter K, Hoffman JP, et al. Five year results of US intergroup/RTOG 9704 with postoperative CA 19-9 >90 U/mL and comparison to the CONKO-001 trial. *Int J Radiat Oncol Biol Phys.* 2012;84(3):e291–e297. doi:10.1016/j.ijrobp.2012.04.035

75. Paniccia A, Edil BH, Schulick RD, et al. Neoadjuvant FOLFIRINOX application in borderline resectable pancreatic adenocarcinoma: a retrospective cohort study. *Medicine (Baltimore)*. 2014;93(27):e198. doi:10.1097/MD.0000000000000198

76. Blazer M, Wu C, Goldberg RM, et al. Neoadjuvant modified (m) FOLFIRINOX for locally advanced unresectable (LAPC) and borderline resectable (BRPC) adenocarcinoma of the pancreas. *Ann Surg Oncol*. 2015;22(4):1153–1159. doi:10.1245/s10434-014-4225-1

77. Sherman WH, Chu K, Chabot J, et al. Neoadjuvant gemcitabine, docetaxel, and capecitabine followed by gemcitabine and capecitabine/radiation therapy and surgery in locally advanced, unresectable pancreatic adenocarcinoma. *Cancer*. 2015;121(5):673–680. doi:10.1002/cncr.29112

78. Moertel CG, Childs DS Jr, Reitemeier RJ, et al. Combined 5-fluorouracil and supervoltage radiation therapy of locally unresectable gastrointestinal cancer. *Lancet*. 1969;2(7626):865–867. doi:10.1016/S0140-6736(69)92326-5

79. Moertel CG, Frytak S, Hahn RG, et al. Therapy of locally unresectable pancreatic carcinoma: a randomized comparison of high dose (6000 rads) radiation alone, moderate dose radiation (4000 rads + 5-fluorouracil), and high dose radiation + 5-fluorouracil: the gastrointestinal tumor study group. *Cancer*. 1981;48(8):1705–1710. doi:10.1002/1097-0142(19811015)48:8<1705::AID-CNCR2820480803>3.0.CO;2-4

80. Gastrointestinal Tumor Study Group. Treatment of locally unresectable carcinoma of the pancreas: comparison of combined-modality therapy (chemotherapy plus radiotherapy) to chemotherapy alone. gastrointestinal tumor study group. *J Natl Cancer Inst*. 1988;80(10):751–755. doi:10.1093/jnci/80.10.751

81. Loehrer PJ Sr, Feng Y, Cardenes H, et al. Gemcitabine alone versus gemcitabine plus radiotherapy in patients with locally advanced pancreatic cancer: an eastern cooperative oncology group trial. *J Clin Oncol*. 2011;29(31):4105–4112. doi:10.1200/JCO.2011.34.8904

82. Murphy JD, Christman-Skieller C, Kim J, et al. A dosimetric model of duodenal toxicity after stereotactic body radiotherapy for pancreatic cancer. *Int J Radiat Oncol Biol Phys*. 2010;78(5):1420–1426. doi:10.1016/j.ijrobp.2009.09.075

Ian W. Winter, Ehsan H. Balagamwala, and Sudha R. Amarnath

QUICK HIT ■ CRC is the third most common cancer in the United States. Patients with FAP or HNPCC are at increased risk for developing CRC at younger age. Surgical resection is standard and involves TME accomplished by either LAR (sphincter sparing) or APR (not sphincter sparing). Neoadjuvant RT is standard for high-risk patients, typically defined as either node-positive or cT3–4 and reduces LRR. Typical RT dose is 50.4 Gy/28 fx with concurrent continuous infusion 5-FU or capecitabine followed by surgery ~7 to 8 weeks later, although short-course RT (25 Gy/5 fx) alone followed by surgery 7 to 10 days later is also an accepted standard. TNT with preoperative chemoRT/short-course RT and preoperative CHT followed by surgery is an emerging paradigm (Table 36.1).

Table 36.1: General Treatment Paradigm for Rectal Cancer

	Treatment Options
Stage I	cT1N0: consider transanal local excision alone followed by observation for low-risk lesions (Pt1 lesion <3 cm, <30% circumference, within 8 cm of anal verge, grades 1–2, margin >3 mm, no LVSI).[1] If pT1 with high-risk features (+margins, LVSI, poorly differentiated tumors) or pT2, proceed with APR/LAR with TME followed by adjuvant therapy as indicated. cT2N0: APR/LAR as indicated with TME. No adjuvant treatment if pT1-2N0. If pT3N0 or pT1-3N1-2, adjuvant CHT ± adjuvant chemoRT.
Stage II/III	Preoperative chemoRT/short-course RT, then LAR/APR with TME, then adjuvant CHT *or* Preoperative chemoRT/short-course RT before or after preoperative CHT, then LAR/APR with TME *Short-course RT with immediate surgery not recommended for T4 or multiple positive clinical LNs. Short-course RT with delayed surgery as a part of TNT may be appropriate in this setting. If obstructed may need diverting colostomy prior to induction therapy.*
Stage IVA (resectable metastasis)	Individualize therapy based on multidisciplinary discussion and presentation. General options include the following: Short-course RT followed by combination CHT, then staged or synchronous resection (primary and metastasis) and adjuvant CHT *or* Combination CHT followed by RT (short or long course), then staged or synchronous resection (primary with metastasis) and adjuvant CHT *or* ChemoRT followed by staged or synchronous resection (primary and metastasis) and adjuvant CHT
Isolated pelvic or anastomotic recurrence	Resectable: preoperative chemoRT → resection ± IORT Unresectable: CHT ± RT If prior pelvic RT, consider BID re-irradiation. May also consider SBRT in the unresectable setting.

EPIDEMIOLOGY: CRC is the third most common cancer and the third leading cause of cancer-related deaths in the United States in both males and females. In 2020, estimated incidence of CRC was 147,950, of which 43,340 were rectal cancers.[2] Incidence of CRC is higher in men and in Blacks compared to women and Caucasians. Incidence is declining in both genders but has risen sharply in young patients.[3] In the United States, average lifetime risk of developing CRC is 4% to 5%.[2]

RISK FACTORS: Age, male sex, IBD (especially UC[4]), high fat, low fiber, alcohol use, tobacco, family history, genetic syndromes (Table 36.2), diabetes, red meat, cholecystectomy. Protective factors: NSAIDs, fiber, vitamin B_6.

Table 36.2: Familial Colorectal Cancer Syndromes	
FAP	Autosomal dominant germline mutation in *APC* gene located on chromosome 5. CRC occurs at younger age than in the general population and usually does not arise from adenoma. Variants include Gardener's (sarcomas, osteomas, desmoid tumors) and Turcot's (GBM, medulloblastoma).
HNPCC (Lynch)	Due to microsatellite instability as result of mutations in mismatch repair genes, most commonly *hMLH1*, *hMSH2*, *hMSH6*, or *PMS2*. Synchronous and metachronous tumors are possible. Patients with HNPCC also have increased risk of endometrial, ovarian, stomach, small bowel, hepatobiliary system, brain, renal pelvis, and ureteral cancers.

ANATOMY: Rectal cancer defined as lesion straddling or inferior to peritoneal reflection (landmark is middle transverse fold at ~11 cm from anal verge) OR lesion within 12 cm of verge. If lesion is completely above this level, it is treated as colon cancer (note: trials have used anywhere up to 16 cm from verge). Layers of rectum: mucosa, muscularis mucosa, submucosa, muscularis propria, serosa, fat. Rectum is ~12 to 15 cm in length, beginning proximally at rectosigmoid junction (~S3) and extending to anorectal ring, just proximal to dentate line. Proximal third is peritonealized anteriorly and laterally, supplied by superior rectal artery (from IMA). Middle third is peritonealized anteriorly, and is supplied by middle rectal artery from internal iliac. Lower rectum is not peritonealized, and is supplied by inferior rectal artery from internal pudendal artery. Anorectal ring is composed of internal and external sphincters and levator ani muscles. Mesorectum is not true mesentery but rather loose connective tissue that is thicker posteriorly. It contains terminal branches of IMA and needs to be removed for adequate surgery (see TME in the following). Anorectal ring: (a) represents internal anal sphincter muscle and is necessary for anal continence, (b) represents inferior limit for functional sphincter preservation surgery, and (c) defines lymphatic watershed for rectal cancer spread. *Nodal drainage*: Superior half of rectum drains along superior rectal artery to pararectal, presacral, sigmoidal, and inferior mesenteric nodes. Inferior half of rectum drains along middle rectal artery to internal iliac nodes. Tumors extending to anal canal (below dentate line) may drain to superficial inguinal nodes. Tumors that invade anteriorly (into pelvic organs) can drain to external iliac nodes. *Pattern of metastasis*: Liver is the most common site of metastatic disease in both colon and rectal cancers. However, rectal cancer has increased propensity for lung as compared to colon cancer. Upper rectal tumors spread along the superior rectal vein to portal system and into liver. Middle and inferior rectal tumors spread along middle and inferior rectal veins, into internal iliac lymph nodes, into systemic circulation, and into lung.

PATHOLOGY: More than 90% of rectal cancers are adenocarcinomas. Approximately 15% to 20% of adenocarcinomas have colloid (extracellular mucin); however, there is no prognostic significance. Tumors with signet ring (intracellular mucin) compose 1% to 2% of adenocarcinomas and have worse prognosis. Other histologies: small cell, carcinoid, leiomyosarcoma, lymphoma.

SCREENING:[5,6] For average-risk patients, NCCN suggests colonoscopy at 50 years of age and every 10 years if negative. If polyps identified, repeat colonoscopy every 3 or 5 years depending on risk of polyp. Other options include stool-based testing, imaging with CT colonoscopy, or combination of flexible sigmoidoscopy with stool guaiac. Stool-based tests include stool guaiac, FIT, or fecal DNA; if positive, proceed to colonoscopy. In high-risk patients, start screening at 40 years of age or 10 years before first diagnosis in affected first-degree relative, then repeat colonoscopy every 5 years. If IBD, annual colonoscopy starting 8 to 10 years after symptom onset. If FAP, elective colectomy or proctocolectomy after onset of polyposis. If HNPCC, colonoscopy every 1 to 2 years starting at 20 to 25 years of age.

CLINICAL PRESENTATION: Hematochezia is the most common presenting symptom in rectal and lower sigmoid cancers. Abdominal pain is more common in colon cancer. Other symptoms are constipation, diarrhea, reduced stool caliber and in locally advanced disease, tenesmus, rectal urgency, inadequate emptying, urinary symptoms, buttock and perineal pain.

WORKUP: H&P, including DRE (size, location, mobility, sphincter function) and pelvic exam in women.

Labs: CBC, LFTs, CEA.

Procedures: Colonoscopy w/ biopsies.

Imaging: CT chest, abdomen, pelvis. MRI rectum with contrast is standard for clinical staging. Rectal ultrasound can be utilized if MRI not available. PET/CT is not routine, but is utilized in many practices.

PROGNOSTIC FACTORS: Stage (both T and N classifications) (Table 36.3), CRM, and LVSI are most important factors. Performance status, AJCC stage, grade (G3 worse), surgery, administration of CHT and hemoglobin levels before (<12 vs. ≥12 g/dL) and during RT all predicted for improved OS.[7] Preoperative CEA >5 ng/mL has been associated with inferior RFS and OS.

STAGING

Table 36.3: AJCC 8th ed. (2017): Staging for Rectal Cancer								
T/M \ N		cN0	cN1a	cN1b	cN1c	cN2a	cN2b
T1	Invades submucosa	I	IIIA				
T2	Invades muscularis propria						
T3	Invades into pericolorectal soft tissue	IIA	IIIB				
T4	a. Invades into visceral peritoneum[1]	IIB					
	b. Invades or adherent to adjacent organs/structures	IIC	IIIC				
M1a	Distant metastasis to 1 organ without peritoneal metastasis	IVA					
M1b	Distant metastasis to 2 organs without peritoneal metastasis	IVB					
M1c	Metastasis to peritoneal surface with or without other organ or site	IVC					

Notes: Peritoneum[1] = Includes gross perforation of bowel through tumor and continuous invasion of tumor through areas of inflammation to surface of visceral peritoneum.
cN1a, 1 regional LN; cN1b, 2–3 regional LNs; cN1c, no positive regional LNs, but subserosal, mesenteric, non-peritoneal peri-colic or peri-rectal tumor deposits; cN2a, 4–6 regional LNs; cN2b, ≥7 regional LNs.

TREATMENT PARADIGM

Surgery: Surgery is mainstay of treatment. T1 tumors can be initially managed with transanal excision. All other tumors should undergo transabdominal resection (LAR or APR) with sharp TME with at least 12 lymph nodes resected for staging.

Local Excision (Transanal Excision or Transanal Endoscopic Microsurgery): Possible for T1 tumors <3 cm in greatest diameter, <30% of rectal circumference, within 8 cm of dentate line or below middle rectal valve, low-grade histology and no LVSI.[1]

LAR: Sphincter-sparing surgery with coloanal anastomosis (or alternatively colonic J-pouch or coloplasty). With modern surgical techniques, distal margin of 2 cm or even less is now adequate and crucial margin is CRM.

APR: Historically for tumor <5 cm from anal verge where sphincter sparing was not thought possible. Rectosigmoid is oversewn via abdominal incision and pulled out with anal canal via perineal incision. Requires permanent colostomy. NSABP R-04 did not show worse QOL at 1 year between APR compared to sphincter-sparing surgery but profiles of QOL were different.[8]

Total Mesorectal Excision: Standard of care regardless of APR or LAR. Involves sharp *en bloc* removal of mesorectum including associated vascular and lymphatic structures, fatty tissue, and mesorectal fascia as "package" through sharp dissection, designed to spare autonomic nerves. TME improves LC and reduces autonomic nerve damage (impotence, retrograde ejaculation, and urinary incontinence) compared with standard blunt dissection of conventional surgery, but with higher rate of anastomotic leaks.

Chemotherapy: Utilization of CHT leads to improved LC and OS as well as decreased risk for developing DM.[9]

Indications: In pre/post-op setting for T3/T4, N1/N2 disease, positive margins or at high risk for local recurrence (high-grade positive or close margin).

Concurrent CHT:

1. PVI 5-FU: With concurrent RT improves LC, DFS, and OS (per Mayo Clinic/NCCTG study, in the following); PVI 5-FU with concurrent RT, when compared to bolus 5-FU, had lower rate of recurrence and DM, with improvement in 4-year OS from 60% to 70%.[10] PVI 5-FU dose is 225 mg/m^2 c throughout RT (7 days/week).
2. Capecitabine: Several trials suggest noninferiority relative to PVI 5-FU.[11] German phase III trial (included pre- and post-op chemoRT) showed significant reduction in DM and trend toward OS and DFS benefit.[12] Capecitabine is associated with more hand foot syndrome, fatigue, proctitis, and less leukopenia compared to 5-FU. Concurrent dose is 825 mg/m^2 BID 5 days per week. Without RT, dose is 1,000 to 1,250 mg/m^2 BID days 1 to 14, q3 weekly cycle.
3. Oxaliplatin: Not recommended as no benefit was observed on multiple trials despite increased toxicity.[11,13–15]
4. Irinotecan and bevacizumab: Multiple phase II trials showing good tolerability in combination with capecitabine as part of long-course chemoRT; however, use remains investigational.[16–18]

Adjuvant CHT: Role for adjuvant CHT is presently controversial but often performed given German rectal trial (see Sauer et al.). Common regimens included FOLFOX, CAPEOX, 5-FU, or 5-FU+LCV. ADORE trial showed improved 3-year DFS (72% vs. 63%) with adjuvant FOLFOX.[19] Similarly, CAO/ARO/AIO-04 trial comparing preoperative chemoRT with 5-FU ± oxaliplatin followed by surgery and adjuvant 5-FU+LCV ± oxaliplatin showed improved DFS with oxaliplatin.[20] In contrast, recent patient level meta-analysis shows no benefit to adjuvant CHT over no adjuvant CHT in patients who underwent concurrent pre-op chemoRT followed by surgery.[21,22] RAPIDO trial showed reduced risk for DM with preoperative CHT compared to adjuvant CHT supporting the emerging paradigm of TNT.[23]

Radiation: RT improves LC, reduces deaths from rectal cancer as well as possibly improves OS.[24]

Preoperative RT: Indications include cT3–4 or cN1–2. Options include short course (25 Gy/5 fx with surgery within 7 to 10 days and adjuvant CHT if node-positive) or long course (50.4 Gy/28 fx with concurrent CHT followed by surgery 7 to 8 weeks later). After short-course RT, postoperative complications increase after 5 days and substantially increase after 10 days (between surgery and RT). Although waiting 4 to 5 weeks after short course leads to improved downstaging (44% vs. 13%), there is no improvement in sphincter-sparing surgery.[25]

Postoperative RT: Indications include pT3–4, pN1–2 (stages II–III), positive margin, poor differentiation.[26] Consider boost to 55 to 60 Gy for gross residual disease. Consider colostomy prior to RT in select patients including patients with severe obstruction.

Procedure: See *Handbook of Treatment Planning in Radiation Oncology*, Chapter 7.[27]

Other Modalities: Other options for small T1 tumors include thermal electrocoagulation, endocavitary RT, or HDR brachytherapy.

■ EVIDENCE-BASED Q&A

LONG-COURSE RT

■ Why is addition of chemoRT to surgery standard for rectal cancer?

GITSG 7175 (*NEJM* 1985, PMID 2859523; Update Thomas, *Radiother Oncol* 1988, PMID 3064191): PRT of 227 patients with Dukes B2 and C rectal (T3–4 or N+) ACA, R0 resection, no mets, distal edge of tumor <12 cm from verge randomized to (a) surgery alone, (b) post-op CHT (bolus IV 5-FU/Me-CCNU), (c) post-op RT 40 or 48 Gy standard fraction, or (d) post-op chemoRT: 40 or 44 Gy standard fraction + 5-FU 500 mg/m² followed by adjuvant 5-FU/Me-CCNU. Trial ended early due to significant benefit to chemoRT. Overall, CHT reduced DM (20% vs. 30%) and RT decreased LR (16% vs. 25%) (Table 36.4). **Conclusion: Adjuvant chemoRT improves LR and OS in rectal cancer.**

Table 36.4: Results of GITSG 7175 Rectal Cancer	7-Yr LR	7-Yr OS
Surgery	24%	36%
Surgery + RT	27%	46%
Surgery + CHT	20%	46%
Surgery + chemoRT + adjuvant CHT	11%	56%

Fisher, NSABP R-01 (*JNCI* 1988, PMID 3276900): PRT of 555 patients with Dukes B (T3N0) and C (node-positive) rectal cancer after curative resection randomized to (a) surgery alone, (b) post-op CHT with Me-CCNU, vincristine, and 5-FU (MOF), or (c) post-op RT alone (46–47 Gy). CHT improved 5-year OS (53% vs. 43%, $p = .05$) and 5-year DFS (42% vs. 30%, $p = .006$) while RT improved 5-year LR (16% vs. 25%, $p = .06$) but did not improve OS. **Conclusion: Adjuvant CHT improves OS while RT reduces LR.**

Krook, NCCTG 794751 (*NEJM* 1991, PMID 1997835): PRT of 204 patients with T3–4 or N+, within 12 cm of anal verge randomized to (a) post-op RT 45 Gy/25 fx + 5.4 Gy boost to tumor bed and adjacent LN or (b) post-op chemoRT with 5-FU bolus + Me-CCNU ×1 month, then bolus 5-FU 500 mg/m² concurrent with RT, then 2 months consolidative 5-FU/Me-CCNU. ChemoRT improved OS, DFS, LR, and rate of DM compared to RT alone. **Conclusion: Adjuvant chemoRT is preferred to RT alone.**

■ What is the value of adding RT to CHT in adjuvant setting?

Wolmark, NSABP R-02 (*JNCI* 2000, PMID 106990969): PRT of 694 patients with resected Dukes B (T3N0) and C (node-positive) rectal cancer randomized to receive either (a) postoperative adjuvant CHT alone (N = 348) or (b) CHT with postoperative RT (N = 346). All female patients (N = 287) received 5-FU plus LCV; male patients received either MOF (N = 207) or 5-FU plus LCV (N = 200). RT significantly improved LC (Table 36.5). **Conclusion: Addition of RT to CHT improves LC but not OS.**

Table 36.5: Results of NSABP R-02 Rectal Trial			
NSABP R-02	5-Yr OS	5-Yr DFS	5-Yr LR
Post-op CHT	60%	54%	13%
Post-op chemoRT	62%	56%	8%
p value	.38	.90	.02

■ What is the benefit of preoperative chemoRT over postoperative chemoRT?

Sauer, German Rectal Study (*NEJM* 2004, PMID 15496622, Update *JCO* 2012, PMID 22529255): PRT of 823 patients ≤75 years of age with cT3–4 or cN+ rectal ACA with inferior margin ≤16 cm from anal verge, randomized to (a) pre-op chemoRT 50.4 Gy/28 fx and concurrent continuous infusion 5-FU followed by TME in 6 weeks, (b) post-op chemoRT 50.4 Gy/28 fx with 5.4 Gy boost to tumor bed 4 weeks following surgery. All patients had TME, and adjuvant CHT started 4 weeks after surgery or after completion of post-op chemoRT composed of four cycles of 5-FU 500 mg/m² intravenous bolus. Primary end point OS. Compliance higher in pre-op arm 90% vs. ~50% in post-op arm. Overall, sphincter-preserving surgery was not more common in pre-op group, although pre-op therapy improved likelihood of sphincter-sparing operation via downstaging (39% vs. 19% $p = .004$). Pre-op chemoRT improved acute and late toxicity as well as 10-year LR. pCR was 8%, nodal involvement decreased (40% vs. 25%). No improvement in DR, OS, or DFS (Table 36.6); 18% of patients in post-op arm were clinically overstaged. **Conclusion: Preoperative chemoRT improves LC and tumor down-staging, reduces late effects, and is preferred to postoperative chemoRT.**

Table 36.6: Long-term Results of German Rectal Study						
	10-Yr LR	10-Yr DM	10-Yr OS	10-Yr DFS	Acute Grades 3–4	Late Grades 3–4
Pre-op chemoRT	7%	29.8%	59.6%	68.1%	27%	14%
Post-op chemoRT	10%	29.6%	59.9%	67.8%	40%	24%
p value	.048	.9	.85	.65	.001	.01

Roh, NSABP R-03 (*JCO* 2009, PMID 19770376): PRT of 267 patients (900 planned) with cT3–4 or N+ rectal ACA, lesion <15 cm from verge, M0 randomized to (a) pre-op 5-FU 500 mg/m² and LCV 500 mg/m² ×6 weeks followed by chemoRT 50.4 Gy/28 fx with concurrent 5-FU+LCV or (b) post-op chemoRT (same as pre-op) with primary endpoints DFS and OS. Trial was underpowered with improved DFS with pre-op chemoRT 64.7% vs. 53.4% *p* = .01 but no difference in OS; 15% pCR rate. **Conclusion: Although underpowered, supports pre-op chemoRT as preferred approach.**

■ **Does concurrent CHT improve outcomes over long-course RT alone?**

Gérard, FFCD 9203/France (*JCO* 2006, PMID 17008704): PRT of T3–4NxM0 rectal ACA, accessible by DRE randomized to (a) pre-op RT 45 Gy/25 fx or (b) pre-op chemoRT with bolus 5-FU + LCV on weeks 1 and 5. Fifty percent of patients in both arms received adjuvant 5-FU and primary end point was OS. ChemoRT reduced LR and improved pCR at cost of increased grade 3 to 4 toxicity (Table 36.7). No change in sphincter preservation.

Table 36.7: Results of the FF9203 Study					
	5-Yr OS	5-Yr DFS	5-Yr LR	pCR Rate	Grades 3–4 Toxicity
Pre-op RT	67.9%	55.5%	16.5%	3.6%	3%
Pre-op CRT	67.4%	59.4%	8.1%	11.4%	15%
p value	NS	NS	.004	<0.0001	.05

Bosset, EORTC 22921 (*NEJM* 2006, PMID 16971718, **Update** *JCO* 2007, PMID 17906203): PRT of 1,011 patients (≤80 y/o) with T3 or resectable T4 rectal ACA within 15 cm of anal verge, randomized to (a) pre-op RT, (b) pre-op CHT, (c) pre-op RT and post-op CHT, or (d) pre-op chemoRT and post-op CHT. RT was 45 Gy/25 fx to posterior pelvis and 5-FU given 350 mg/m²/day. TME not routine. Primary endpoint OS; 5-year incidence of LR was 17.1%, 8.7%, 9.6%, and 7.6% per arms of study, respectively. There was no effect on OS. **Conclusion: Preoperative chemoRT is superior to long-course RT alone with respect to LC.**

■ **Does increased interval of time between pre-op chemoRT and surgery impact pCR rates?**

Lefevre, GRECCAR-6 (*JCO* 2016, PMID 27432930; **Update** *Ann Surg* 2019, PMID 31634178): PRT of 265 patients from 24 centers with cT3/4 or cN+ of mid or lower rectum. All received chemoRT to 45 to 50 Gy with 5-FU or capecitabine, then randomized to surgery at either 7 or 11 weeks. Primary end point pCR rate; 82% cT3. Surgery not performed in 3.4% of patients due to development of met-astatic disease or other reasons. Overall, 47 patients (18.6%) achieved pCR, which were not different between 7 and 11 weeks (15% vs. 17.4%, *p* = .598). However, morbidity was significantly increased in 11-week group (44.5% vs. 32%, *p* = .04) and quality of TME was also worse (complete mesorectum 78.7% vs. 90%, *p* = .02). At mean follow-up of 32 months, 3-year OS was 89%, with no difference between groups. No difference in DFS, distant, or local recurrences. **Conclusion: Waiting 11 weeks after chemoRT did not increase rate of pCR or OS at 3 years. Longer waiting period may be asso-ciated with higher morbidity and more difficult surgical resection.**

■ Since pCR is associated with improved outcomes, can additional CHT after pre-op long-course chemoRT increase pCR rates?

Garcia-Aguilar (Lancet Oncol 2015, PMID 26187751): Phase II, nonrandomized study with four consecutive groups: group 1 underwent chemoRT followed by surgery 6 to 8 weeks later; groups 2, 3, and 4 received 2, 4, or 6 cycles of mFOLFOX6, respectively, after long-course chemoRT followed by surgery. Primary end point pCR (intention to treat); 292 patients registered, 259 analyzable. pCR rates: 18% (group 1), 25% (group 2), 30% (group 3), 38% (group 4), *p* = .0036. Study group was independently associated with pCR (*p* = .011). Grades 3 and 4 toxicities were increased with TNT: group 2 (3%), group 3 (18%), group 4 (28%). **Conclusion: mFOLFOX6 prior to surgery is being evaluated for nonoperative management of rectal cancer.**

■ Does chemoRT with mFOLFOX6 provide a benefit over 5-FU?

Deng, FOWARC (JCO 2019, PMID 31557064): Phase III, multicenter PRT in China with 495 patients with stage II/III rectal cancer randomized to 5 cycles 5-FU + RT (46–50.4 Gy/23–28 fx) followed by surgery and 7 cycles of adjuvant 5-FU vs. the same treatment with neoadjuvant and adjuvant mFOLFOX6 vs. neoadjuvant mFOLFOX6 alone followed by surgery and adjuvant mFOLFOX6. Primary end point was 3-year DFS: 72.9%, 77.2% and 73.5% in the three arms (*p* = .709). No difference in 3-year OS: 91.3%, 89.1%, and 90.7% in the three arms (*p* = .971). There was a higher pCR rate in the mFOLFOX6 + RT arm (27.5%) vs. 5-FU + RT (14.0%) and mFOLFOX6 group (6.5%). **Conclusion: mFOLFOX6 with or without RT did not impact OS compared to neoadjuvant chemoRT with 5-FU in patients with stage II/III rectal cancer.**

■ In patients who achieve cCR after pre-op therapy, can surgery be omitted?

This is an active area of investigation on protocol but is not standard off protocol.

Habr-Gama, Brazil (Semin Radiat Oncol 2011, PMID 21645869): Review and RR of 173 patients from 1991 to 2009 treated with neoadjuvant chemoRT 50.4–54 Gy with concurrent 5-FU; 63% cT3/T4, 21% cTxN1-2. MFU 65 months. Sixty-seven patients (39%) developed cCR. Of these 67 patients, 13% underwent rectal biopsy and 87% were managed without surgical procedures. Recurrences in 15 patients (21%): eight patients developed local only recurrence and seven developed DM. Median time to recurrence was 38 months. Of eight patients who recurred locally, seven were successfully salvaged; 5-year OS 96% and 5-year DFS 72%. **Conclusion: Early retrospective data suggest it may be feasible to reserve surgery for salvage after cCR to chemoRT.**

Renehan, OnCoRe (Lancet Oncol 2016, PMID 26705854): Propensity-matched cohort study from UK evaluating "watch and wait" strategy in patients who achieve cCR after pre-op chemoRT. A total of 259 patients included, of which 228 underwent surgery and 31 (12%) had cCR and underwent watch and wait. Additional 98 patients with cCR were included via national registry for total of 129 patients managed by watch and wait. MFU 33 months. Of 129 patients, 44 (34%) had LR and 36 of 41 patients were salvaged. In matched analysis, there was no difference in non-regrowth DFS between watch and wait and immediate post-chemoRT surgery (88% and 78%, *p* = .04). No difference in 3-year OS (96% vs. 87%, *p* = .02). Improved 3-year colostomy-free survival in WW cohort (74% vs. 47%). **Conclusion: Watch and wait can be considered in many patients without detriment in 3-year OS.**

Smith, MSKCC (JAMA Oncol 2019, PMID 30629084): Retrospective case series with 113 patients with stage II/III rectal cancer who underwent neoadjuvant therapy (various regimens, most commonly RT 45–54 Gy/25–28 fx with concurrent 5-FU or capecitabine) who achieved cCR were followed by WW, compared with patients who underwent neoadjuvant therapy followed by TME found to have pCR. Twenty-two local regrowths occurred in the WW group, of which 20 (91%) were controlled with salvage surgery; 5-year OS was 73% in the WW group vs. 94% in the surgery group, DFS 75% vs. 92%. Rate of DM 36% in WW patients with local regrowth vs. 1% in WW patients without local failure (*p* < .001). **Conclusion: Excellent rectal preservation and pelvic tumor control with WW for patients achieving cCR after neoadjuvant therapy, but with worse OS and higher risk of DM in those with local regrowth.**

▪ Are there data assessing the utility and outcomes of total neoadjuvant therapy?

This new paradigm involves administering all CHT upfront, either prior to, or following, chemoRT/short-course RT, but prior to surgery, also known as total neoadjuvant therapy. This is being investigated with both long-course and short-course RT regimens with the goals of obtaining higher pCR rates and greater CHT compliance rates with lower toxicity. Several studies have demonstrated positive results in preliminary or abstract form, although mature published results are pending.[23,28–30]

Fernandez-Martos, GCR-3 (*Ann Oncol* **2015, PMID 25957330**): Phase II PRT of 108 patients with distal or middle third, T3–T4 and/or N+ rectal ACA by MRI randomized to arm A (*N* = 52): pre-op chemoRT followed by surgery and four cycles of adjuvant capecitabine and oxaliplatin (CAPOX) or arm B (*N* = 56): 4 cycles CAPOX followed by chemoRT and surgery. MFU 69.5 months. No differences in 5-year DFS (64% vs. 62%), or OS (78% vs. 75%); 5-year cumulative incidence of LR was 2% and 5% (*p* = .61) and 5-year cumulative incidence of DM was 21% and 23%; (*p* = .79) in arms A and B, respectively. **Conclusion: Both treatment approaches yield similar outcomes. Given the lower acute toxicity and improved compliance with induction CHT compared with adjuvant CHT, integrating effective systemic therapy before chemoRT and surgery is a promising strategy and should be examined in phase III trials.**

Bahadoer, RAPIDO (*Lancet Oncol* **2020, PMID 33301740**): Phase III PRT of 912 patients in Europe and the United States with primary locally advanced rectal cancer with high-risk features on MRI (cT4a/b, extramural vascular invasion, cN2, mesorectal fascia involvement, or enlarged lateral LNs) randomized to TNT vs. standard therapy. TNT arm was treated with short course RT (25 Gy/5 fx) followed by either six cycles of CAPOX or nine cycles of FOLFOX4, followed by TME. Standard arm was treated with chemoRT, 50 to 50.4 Gy/25 to 28 fx, with concurrent capecitabine, followed by TME and adjuvant CHT (if stipulated by hospital policy), either 8 cycles of CAPOX or 12 cycles of FOLFOX4. Primary end point was 3-year disease-related treatment failure. At MFU 4.6 years, 3-year cumulative probability of disease-related treatment failure was 23.7% vs. 30.4 %, favoring the TNT arm (HR 0.75, 95% CI 0.60–0.95). Rates of DM also favored the TNT arm (HR 0.69, 95% CI 0.54–0.90). pCR achieved in 28% of TNT arm vs. 14% for standard (OR 2.37, 95% CI 1.67–3.37). No difference in locoregional failure or OS. Serious adverse events were similar, 38% for TNT vs. 34% for standard arm, with four treatment-related deaths in each arm. **Conclusion: TNT with short course RT followed by CHT and delayed surgery is associated with decreased disease-related treatment failure vs. standard therapy.** *Comment: 52% of patients in the standard arm did not receive adjuvant CHT; however, on subset analysis there was no difference in DM or locoregional failure with and without CHT in the standard arm.*

▪ Can RT be omitted in patients with cT3N0 rectal cancer?

This cohort is considered "borderline" risk for local recurrence and may not benefit from RT in all cases. However, given concerns with accuracy of preoperative staging and nonequivalence of postoperative RT, most clinicians continue to recommend pre-op RT for cT3N0 patients.[31]

▪ Is tumor response after pre-op chemoRT predictive of outcomes?

Patel, Mercury Study (*JCO* **2011, PMID 21876084**): Prospective cohort study of 111 patients treated with pre-op long-course RT alone or long-course chemoRT who underwent pre-op MRI 4 to 6 weeks following pre-op treatment. All patients had to have at least 5 mm of initial tumor extension beyond muscularis propria. Tumor regression on MRI was significantly predictive of OS (HR 4.4) and DFS (HR 3.3). If CRM was involved based on posttreatment MRI, there was significantly increased risk of LR (28% vs. 12%, *p* < .05); 5-year OS for patients with involved pCRM was 30% vs. 63% (*p* = .001), DFS was 34% vs. 63% (*p* < .001), and LR was 26.4% vs. 6.5% (*p* < .001). **Conclusion: Tumor regression as documented by MRI predicts DFS and OS and MRI predicted CRM involvement is associated with increased risk of LR.**

Fokas, German Rectal Trial Posthoc Analysis (*JCO* **2014, PMID 24752056**): See trial details previously. Authors evaluated pathologic response based on viable tumor vs. fibrosis—Tumor Regression Grading (TRG): grade 0, no regression; grade 1, minor regression (dominant tumor mass with obvious fibrosis in ≤25% of tumor mass); grade 2, moderate regression (dominant tumor mass with obvious fibrosis in 26%–50% of tumor mass); grade 3, good regression (dominant fibrosis outgrowing tumor mass [i.e., >50% tumor regression]); and grade 4, total regression (no viable tumor cells; fibrotic mass only). MFU 132 months. MVA showed that ypN+ and TRG were only independent prognosticators for DM and DFS. ypN+ and LVSI were predictive of LR. Cienfuegos et al. also showed that in patients with PNI/LVSI, TRG had no impact on OS. However, in patients without PNI/LVSI, TRG was predictive for OS and DFS.[32] Finally, pathologic response correlated with DFS, LR, and DM (Table 36.8).

Table 36.8: German Rectal Trial Secondary Analysis on Tumor Regression Grade		
10-Yr results	DM	DFS
TRG 4	10.5%	89.5%
TRG 2/3	29.3%	73.6%
TRG 0/1	39.6%	63%
p value	.005	.008

SHORT-COURSE RT

■ **Is short course of preoperative RT effective compared to surgery alone?**

Folkesson, Swedish Rectal Cancer Trial (*NEJM* 1997, PMID 9091798; Update *JCO* 2005, PMID 16110023): PRT of 1,168 patients with resectable rectal carcinoma, age <80, planned abdominal surgery, and no mets randomized to (a) 25 Gy/5 fx followed by surgery within 1 week or (b) surgery alone. Primary endpoints were LR and postoperative mortality. See Table 36.9 for results. **Conclusion: Pre-op RT is associated with significantly improved LC and OS compared to surgery alone.** *Comment: Study criticized because it was unclear how many T1 patients were included, non-TME surgery was used, and there was an increase risk of late small bowel obstruction in RT group.*

Table 36.9: Results of Short-Course Swedish Rectal Trial			
	13-Yr LR	13-Yr OS	13-Yr CSS
Pre-op 25 Gy/5 fx	9%	38%	72%
Surgery alone	26%	30%	62%
p value	<.001	.004	<.001

■ **If TME is performed, is short-course RT still beneficial?**

Kapiteijn, Dutch CKVO 9504 (*NEJM* 2001, PMID 11547717; Updates *Ann Surg* 2007 PMID 17968156, *Lancet Oncol* 2011, PMID 21596621): PRT of 1,861 patients with clinically resectable ACA of rectum, no mets, inferior tumor margin <15 cm from anal verge randomized to (a) 25 Gy/5 fx followed by TME or (b) TME alone. Primary end point LR; 10-year LR was reduced from 11% to 5% (p < .0001) with no change in OS or DM. Of note, there was statistically significant OS benefit in stage III patients who had negative CRM (50% vs. 40%, p = .03). **Conclusion: Preoperative RT with 25 Gy/5 fx significantly improves LC, even with good surgery (TME), but does not improve OS.**

■ **Is pre-op short course better than post-op chemoRT?**

Sebag-Montefiore, MRC CR 07 (*Lancet* 2009, PMID 19269519): PRT of 1,350 patients with resectable rectal ACA, (distal tumor <15 cm from verge), no mets randomized to (a) 25 Gy/5 fx followed by surgery or (b) surgery followed by post-op chemoRT (45 Gy/25 fx with concurrent 5-FU) for those with positive CRM. Primary end point LR. Most node-positive patients received adjuvant CHT. Pre-op short course was associated with improved LR (4.4% vs. 10.6%, p < .0001) and DFS (77.5% vs. 71.5%, p = .013) but not OS (70.3% vs. 67.9%, p = .40). **Conclusion: Pre-op short course is superior to selected post-op chemoRT.**

■ **How does pre-op long-course chemoRT compare to short-course pre-op RT?**

Bujko, Polish Study (*Br J Surg* 2006, **PMID 16983741**): PRT of 312 patients with cT3–4 with no evidence of sphincter involvement randomized to (a) 25 Gy/5 fx followed by TME within 7 days or (b) 50.4 Gy/28 fx with concurrent bolus 5-FU+LCV followed by TME 4 to 6 weeks later. Primary endpoint was sphincter preservation. No difference in sphincter preservation, LR, OS, or DFS (Table 36.10). **Conclusion: Long-course chemoRT did not improve OS, LC, or late toxicity compared to short-course RT.** *Comment: Limitations to this study include clinical staging (no US or MRI), no standard post-op CHT, not all TME, and no RT QA.*

Table 36.10: Polish Rectal Cancer Short-Course Trial						
	4-Yr LR	4-Yr DFS	5-Yr OS	Grades 3–4 Early Toxicity	Grades 3–4 Late Toxicity	Positive CRM
Pre-op chemoRT	15.5%	55.6%	66%	18%	7%	4.4%
Pre-op short-course RT	10.6%	58.4%	67%	3%	10%	12.9%
p value	.2	NS	NS	<.001	.36	.017

Ngan, TROG Intergroup Trial (*JCO* 2012, **PMID 23008301**): PRT of 326 patients with cT3N0-2M0 rectal ACA, within 12 cm of verge (US or MRI staged) randomized to (a) 25 Gy/5 fx, surgery in 3 to 7 days, six cycles 5-FU with folinic acid, or (b) 50.4 Gy/28 fx + continuous infusion 5-FU (225 mg/m²), surgery in 4–6 weeks, four cycles of 5-FU with folinic acid. Primary end point LR. MFU 5.9 years. No differences in LR, DR, OS, or late grades 3–4 toxicity (Table 36.11). For distally located tumors, LR was 12.5% in arm 2 vs. 3% in arm 1 (NS). **Conclusion: Short-course pre-op RT is equivalent to pre-op chemoRT without increased late toxicity. Unclear if short course is equivalent to long course for distally located tumors.**

Table 36.11: Results of TROG Short vs. Long-Course Rectal Trial				
TROG 01.04	3-Yr LR	5-Yr DR	5-Yr OS	Late Grades 3–4 Toxicity
Long course	4.4%	30%	70%	8.2%
Short course	7.5%	27%	74%	5.8%
p value	.24	.92	.62	NS

Bujko, Polish II Trial (*Ann Oncol* 2016, **PMID 26884592; Update Cisel,** *Ann Oncol* 2019, **PMID 31192355**): Phase III PRT of 515 patients with either fixed cT3 or cT4 rectal cancer, randomized to 25 Gy/5 fx followed by three cycles of FOLFOX4 (group A, *n* = 261) or 50.4 Gy/28 fx combined with two 5-day cycles of bolus 5-FU 325 mg/m²/day and LCV 20 mg/m²/day during the 1st and 5th weeks of RT along with five infusions of oxaliplatin 50 mg/m² once weekly (group B, *N* = 254). Protocol amended in 2012 to allow oxaliplatin to be optional in both groups. At MFU 35 months, pre-op treatment acute toxicity was lower in group A than group B, *p* = .006; any toxicity being, respectively, 75% vs. 83%; grades 3–4 23% vs. 21% and toxic deaths 1% vs. 3%. R0 resection rates (primary end point) and pCR rates in groups A and B were, respectively, 77% vs. 71%, *p* = .07, and 16% vs. 12%, *p* = .17; 3-year OS and DFS in groups A and B were, respectively, 73% vs. 65% (*p* = .046) and 53% vs. 52% (*p* = .85), together with the cumulative incidence of LF and DM being 22% vs. 21% (*p* = .82), and 30% vs. 27% (*p* = .26). These differences disappeared with longer follow-up, with 8-year OS 49% in both groups, and no difference in DFS (43% vs. 41%), or cumulative incidence of LF or DM. There was no difference in post-op complications, 29% vs. 25% (*p* = .18) or grade ≥3 late complications, 11% vs. 9% (*p* = .66). **Conclusion: With long-term follow-up, 25 Gy/5 fx with consolidation CHT is not superior to long-course chemoRT.**

■ **How long after short-course RT should surgery be performed?**

Pach, Polish (*Langenbecks Arch Surg* **2012, PMID 22170083):** Polish study of 154 patients randomized to early surgery (7–10 days) vs. delayed (4–5 weeks) after short-course RT. Significantly higher rate of downstaging was achieved (44% vs. 13%), for those who underwent delayed surgery. No differences seen in sphincter sparing procedures, LC or OS. **Conclusion: In limited-size prospective trial, delayed surgery after short-course RT is feasible and associated with higher rate of downstaging.**

Erlandsson, Stockholm III Trial (*Lancet Oncol* **2017, PMID 28190762):** PRT (noninferiority) of 840 patients with resectable, M0 rectal ACA. Patients randomized to (1) short-course RT (25 Gy/5 fx) then surgery (within 1 week), (2) short-course RT then surgery (4–8 weeks after RT), or (3) long-course RT only (50 Gy/25 fx) then surgery (4–8 weeks after RT). LR was 2.2%, 2.8%, 5.5% per arms of study, respectively (*p* = NS). Post-op complications were similar between three arms of study. However, when evaluating only short-course patients, risk of post-op complications was lower in arm 2 compared to arm 1 (41% vs. 53%, *p* = .001). **Conclusion: Oncologic outcomes were similar between immediate surgery and delayed surgery after short-course RT, and long-course RT is similar to both short-course regimens. Postoperative complications were lower in patients who underwent delayed surgery after short-course RT.** *Comment: No CHT in long-course arm, protocol amendment allowed centers to enroll only on short-course arm; use of neoadjuvant CHT not reported; very few patients (<20%) received adjuvant CHT. Due to these deficiencies, it is difficult to interpret the results of this trial.*

■ **Is IMRT for rectal cancer safe and effective?**

Hong, RTOG 0822 (*IJROBP* **2015, PMID 26163334):** Phase II study of cT3–4, N0–2 low- to mid-rectal cancers treated with IMRT 45 Gy/25 fx followed by 3D-CRT boost of 5.4 Gy/3 fx with concurrent capecitabine and oxaliplatin. Primary end point was improvement in grade II GI toxicity seen on RTOG 0247. Seventy-nine patients enrolled, 68 analyzable, 51% of patients developed grade II or higher GI toxicity, which was not significantly improved relative to historical controls; 15% of patients developed pCR and 4-year LRF was 7.4%. **Conclusion: IMRT is feasible but did not demonstrate significant toxicity improvement relative to historical controls.**

Arbea, Spain (*IJROBP* **2012, PMID 22079731):** Phase II study of T3/T4 and/or N+ rectal cancer treated with pre-op IMRT 47.5 Gy/19 fx with concurrent capecitabine and oxaliplatin. One hundred patients enrolled. pCr in 13% and downstaging in 78%. **Conclusion: Preoperative IMRT with concurrent capecitabine and oxaliplatin is feasible.**

RECURRENT RECTAL CANCER

■ **Is re-irradiation of recurrent rectal cancer feasible?**

Valentini, STORM (*IJROBP* **2006, PMID 16414206):** Phase II nonrandomized trial of pelvic recurrences of rectal cancer in patients with previous RT <55 Gy and KPS ≥60. Pre-op RT: PTV2 (GTV + 4 cm) 30 Gy/25 fx at 1.2 Gy/fx BID followed by boost to PTV1 (GTV + 2 cm) to 10.8 Gy/9 fx at 1.2 Gy/fx BID with concurrent PVI 5-FU. Patients who were resectable underwent surgery 6 to 8 weeks later. Fifty-nine patients enrolled. Median time to reRT was 27 months (minimum 9 mos). Majority of patients (86.4%) completed therapy; 8.5% of patients developed pCR. Grade III GI toxicity was 5.1%. Overall response rate was 44.1%.

Guren, Norway (*Radiother Oncol* **2014, PMID 25613395):** Systematic review of reRT identified seven prospective and retrospective studies. Median initial dose was 50.4 Gy. Most studies used 1.2 Gy BID or 1.8 Gy daily fractionation with concurrent 5-FU. Median total dose was 30 to 40 Gy to GTV + 2 to 4 cm margin. Among patients who could be resected, MS was 39 to 60 months and 12 to 16 months for unresectable patients. Good symptomatic relief in 82% to 100%. Acute diarrhea reported in 9% to 20% of patients; however, late toxicity was insufficiently reported.

REFERENCES

1. NCCN. Clinical Practice Guidelines in Oncology: Rectal Cancer. 2020;6.2020.
2. Siegel RL, Miller KD, Jemal A. Cancer statistics, 2020. *CA Cancer J Clin.* 2020;70(1):7–30. doi:10.3322/caac.21387
3. Siegel RL, Fedewa SA, Anderson WF, et al. Colorectal cancer incidence patterns in the United States, 1974–2013. *J Natl Cancer Inst.* 2017;109(8). doi:10.1093/jnci/djw322
4. Ekbom A, Helmick C, Zack M, Adami HO. Ulcerative colitis and colorectal cancer: a population-based study. *N Engl J Med.* 1990;323:1228–1233. doi:10.1056/NEJM199011013231802
5. NCCN. Clinical Practice Guidelines in Oncology: Colorectal Cancer Screening. 2020;2.2020.
6. NCCN. Clinical Practice Guidelines in Oncology: Genetic/Familial High-Risk Assessment: Colorectal. 2020;1.2020.
7. Rades D, Kuhn H, Schultze J, et al. Prognostic factors affecting locally recurrent rectal cancer and clinical significance of hemoglobin. *Int J Radiat Oncol Biol Phys.* 2008;70:1087–1093. doi:10.1016/j.ijrobp.2007.07.2364
8. Russell MM, Ganz PA, Lopa S, et al. Comparative effectiveness of sphincter-sparing surgery versus abdominoperineal resection in rectal cancer: patient-reported outcomes in national surgical adjuvant breast and bowel project randomized trial R-04. *Ann Surg.* 2015;261:144–148. doi:10.1097/SLA.0000000000000594
9. Buyse M, Zeleniuch-Jacquotte A, Chalmers TC. Adjuvant therapy of colorectal cancer. why we still don't know. *JAMA.* 1988;259:3571–3578. doi:10.1001/jama.259.24.3571
10. O'Connell MJ, Martenson JA, Wieand HS, et al. Improving adjuvant therapy for rectal cancer by combining protracted-infusion fluorouracil with radiation therapy after curative surgery. *N Engl J Med.* 1994;331:502–507. doi:10.1056/NEJM199408253310803
11. Allegra CJ, Yothers G, O'Connell MJ, et al. Neoadjuvant 5-FU or capecitabine plus radiation with or without oxaliplatin in rectal cancer patients: a phase III randomized clinical trial. *J Natl Cancer Inst.* 2015;107:djv248.
12. Hofheinz R-D, Wenz F, Post S, et al. Chemoradiotherapy with capecitabine versus fluorouracil for locally advanced rectal cancer: a randomised, multicentre, non-inferiority, phase 3 trial. *Lancet Oncol.* 2012;13:579–588. doi:10.1016/S1470-2045(12)70116-X
13. Aschele C, Cionini L, Lonardi S, et al. Primary tumor response to preoperative chemoradiation with or without oxaliplatin in locally advanced rectal cancer: pathologic results of the STAR-01 randomized phase III trial. *J Clin Oncol.* 2011;29:2773–2780. doi:10.1200/JCO.2010.34.4911
14. Gérard J-P, Azria D, Gourgou-Bourgade S, et al. Comparison of two neoadjuvant chemoradiotherapy regimens for locally advanced rectal cancer: results of the phase III trial ACCORD 12/0405-prodige 2. *J Clin Oncol.* 2010;28:1638–1644. doi:10.1200/JCO.2009.25.8376
15. Hong TS, Moughan J, Garofalo MC, et al. NRG oncology radiation therapy oncology group 0822: a phase 2 study of preoperative chemoradiation therapy using intensity modulated radiation therapy in combination with capecitabine and oxaliplatin for patients with locally advanced rectal cancer. *Int J Radiat Oncol Biol Phys.* 2015;93:29–36. doi:10.1016/j.ijrobp.2015.05.005
16. Cai G, Zhu J, Palmer JD, et al. CAPIRI-IMRT: a phase II study of concurrent capecitabine and irinotecan with intensity-modulated radiation therapy for the treatment of recurrent rectal cancer. *Radiat Oncol (London, England).* 2015;10:57. doi:10.1186/s13014-015-0360-5
17. García M, Martinez-Villacampa M, Santos C, et al. Phase II study of preoperative bevacizumab, capecitabine and radiotherapy for resectable locally-advanced rectal cancer. *BMC Cancer.* 2015;15:59. doi:10.1186/s12885-015-1052-0
18. Salazar R, Capdevila J, Laquente B, et al. A randomized phase II study of capecitabine-based chemoradiation with or without bevacizumab in resectable locally advanced rectal cancer: clinical and biological features. *BMC Cancer.* 2015;15:60. doi:10.1186/s12885-015-1053-z
19. Hong YS, Nam B-H, Kim K-P, et al. Oxaliplatin, fluorouracil, and leucovorin versus fluorouracil and leucovorin as adjuvant chemotherapy for locally advanced rectal cancer after preoperative chemoradiotherapy (ADORE): an open-label, multicentre, phase 2, randomised controlled trial. *Lancet Oncol.* 2014;15:1245–1253. doi:10.1016/S1470-2045(14)70377-8
20. Rodel C, Liersch T, Fietkau R, et al. Preoperative chemoradiotherapy and postoperative chemotherapy with 5-fluorouracil and oxaliplatin versus 5-fluorouracil alone in locally advanced rectal cancer: results of the german CAO/ARO/AIO-04 randomized phase III trial. *J Clin Oncol.* 2014;32:5s. doi:10.1200/jco.2014.32.15_suppl.3500
21. Breugom AJ, Swets M, Bosset J-F, et al. Adjuvant chemotherapy after preoperative (chemo)radiotherapy and surgery for patients with rectal cancer: a systematic review and meta-analysis of individual patient data. *Lancet Oncol.* 2015;16:200–207. doi:10.1016/S1470-2045(14)71199-4
22. Colorectal Cancer Collaborative Group. Adjuvant radiotherapy for rectal cancer: a systematic overview of 8,507 patients from 22 randomised trials. *Lancet (London, England).* 2001;358:1291–1304. doi:10.1016/S0140-6736(01)06409-1
23. Bahadoer RR, Dijkstra EA, van Etten B, et al. Short-course radiotherapy followed by chemotherapy before total mesorectal excision (TME) versus preoperative chemoradiotherapy, TME, and optional adjuvant chemotherapy in locally advanced rectal cancer (RAPIDO): a randomised, open-label, phase 3 trial. *Lancet Oncol.* 2021;22(1):29–42. doi:10.1016/S1470-2045(20)30555-6
24. Cammà C, Giunta M, Fiorica F, et al. Preoperative radiotherapy for resectable rectal cancer: a meta-analysis. *JAMA.* 2000;284:1008–1015. doi:10.1001/jama.284.8.1008
25. Pach R, Kulig J, Richter P, et al. Randomized clinical trial on preoperative radiotherapy 25 Gy in rectal cancer--treatment results at 5-year follow-up. *Langenbecks Arch Surg.* 2012;397:801–807. doi:10.1007/s00423-011-0890-8

26. Song C, Song S, Kim J-S, et al. Impact of postoperative chemoradiotherapy versus chemotherapy alone on recurrence and survival in patients with stage II and III upper rectal cancer: a propensity score-matched analysis. *PLoS One*. 2015;10:e0123657. doi:10.1371/journal.pone.0123657

27. Videtic GMM, Woody N, Vassil AD. *Handbook of Treatment Planning in Radiation Oncology*. 3rd ed. Demos Medical; 2020. doi:10.1891/9780826168429

28. Garcia-Aguilar J, Patil S, Kim JK, et al. Preliminary results of the organ preservation of rectal adenocarcinoma (OPRA) trial. *J Clin Oncol*. 2020;38(15_suppl):4008–4008. doi:10.1200/JCO.2020.38.15_suppl.4008

29. Conroy T, Lamfichekh N, Etienne P-L, et al. Total neoadjuvant therapy with mFOLFIRINOX versus preoperative chemoradiation in patients with locally advanced rectal cancer: final results of PRODIGE 23 phase III trial, a UNICANCER GI trial. *J Clin Oncol*. 2020;38(15_suppl):4007–4007. doi:10.1200/JCO.2020.38.15_suppl.4007

30. Fokas E, Allgauer M, Polat B, et al. Randomized phase II trial of chemoradiotherapy plus induction or consolidation chemotherapy as total neoadjuvant therapy for locally advanced rectal cancer: CAO/ARO/AIO-12. *J Clin Oncol*. 2019;37(34):3212–3222. doi:10.1200/JCO.19.00308

31. Wo JY, Mamon HJ, Ryan DP, Hong TS. T3N0 rectal cancer: radiation for all? *Semin Radiat Oncol*. 2011;21(3):212–219. doi:10.1016/j.semradonc.2011.02.007

32. Cienfuegos JA, Rotellar F, Baixauli J, et al. Impact of perineural and lymphovascular invasion on oncological outcomes in rectal cancer treated with neoadjuvant chemoradiotherapy and surgery. *Ann Surg Oncol*. 2015;22(3):916–923. doi:10.1245/s10434-014-4051-5

37 ■ ANAL CANCER

Kristine Bauer-Nilsen, Aditya Juloori, and Sudha R. Amarnath

QUICK HIT ■ Squamous cell carcinoma of the anal canal is a relatively rare but often curable cancer (Table 37.1). Standard of care is concurrent chemoRT with 5-FU and MMC. Select T1N0 patients with well-differentiated anal margin cancers may be treated with WLE with 1 cm margins. Acute treatment-related toxicities are often severe, but treatment breaks should be avoided as prolonged treatment time has been associated with increased failure rates. IMRT has been shown to reduce hematologic, GI, and skin toxicities, but expertise is required with this approach.

Table 37.1: General Treatment Paradigm for Anal Cancer	
Stage	**Treatment Recommendations***
T1N0 (anal margin, well differentiated)	WLE ± chemoRT if inadequate margins
T1–T2N0 (anal canal)	50.4 Gy/28 fx to primary, 42 Gy/28 fx to LN Per NCCN, can consider excision alone if the tumor meets criteria for "superficial SCC," i.e., <3 mm invasion past basement membrane and <7 mm horizontal spread
T3/T4N0	54 Gy/30 fx to primary, 45 Gy/30 fx to LN
Node positive	54 Gy/30 fx to primary **Nodes**: ≤3 cm: 50.4 Gy/28 fx >3 cm: 54 Gy/30 fx

*IMRT doses per RTOG 0529[1]

EPIDEMIOLOGY: Approximately 8,600 new diagnoses with 1,400 anal cancer–related deaths in the United States in 2020.[2] Lifetime risk 1 in 500.[3] Comprises 2.6% of GI malignancies[2] (rectal cancer is 5× as common). Incidence in men and women has increased over past 30 years. Average age at diagnosis is in early 60s.[3] Incidence of anal cancer is more than twice as high in females as it is in males.[2] Incidence has not decreased in the era of HAART.[4]

RISK FACTORS: HPV (most commonly HPV-16, but also 18, 31, 33, and 45).[3] High-risk HPV DNA has been detected in up to 84% of specimens in large-scale anal cancer studies.[5] Other risk factors include HIV infection, history of cervical, vulvar, or vaginal cancer (HPV-related), immunosuppression after organ transplant, smoking, and history of receptive anal intercourse.

ANATOMY: The *anal canal* is 4 cm long and extends proximally from *anal verge* (palpable junction between non–hair-bearing and hair-bearing squamous epithelium) to *dentate line* (line between simple columnar epithelium proximally to stratified squamous epithelium distally). *Anal margin* is skin within 5 cm of anal verge. Canal is surrounded by internal and external anal sphincters.

Histology: Three zones: *Cutaneous zone* is anal margin. *Transition zone* is in canal and ends at dentate line, contains squamous epithelium without hair. *True mucosa* starts at dentate line and contains columns of Morgagni and holds transitional epithelium for about 2 cm before true mucosa of rectum begins.

Lymphatics: For tumors that arise below dentate line, drainage pattern is to inguinal and femoral nodes that arise from external iliacs. Above dentate line, nodal drainage pattern is similar to that of rectal cancer: perirectal and internal iliacs.

PATHOLOGY: About 75% to 80% are squamous cell carcinoma. Other, more rare anal cancers include adenocarcinoma (treated like rectal cancer), melanoma, neuroendocrine, carcinoid, Kaposi's, leiomyosarcoma, and lymphoma. Perianal skin tumors (SCC, BCC, melanoma, Bowen's, Paget's) should be treated as skin cancer.

CLINICAL PRESENTATION: About 45% of patients present with rectal bleeding; 30% will experience either pain or sensation of rectal mass.[6] Patients with more proximally located tumors can also present with alteration in bowel movements. At presentation, roughly 50% will present with localized disease, 30% with regional LN involvement, and 10% with distant metastases (most commonly liver and lung).[7] Risk of nodal involvement is higher in patients with sphincter involvement or poorly differentiated tumors.

WORKUP: H&P (with careful attention to inguinal node exam and digital rectal exam to determine extent of tumor and sphincter function). GYN exam/cervical screening for females (see Table 37.2).

Labs: CBC, BMP, LFTs, CEA, HIV if there are risk factors (and CD4 if HIV+). Anoscopy with biopsy of primary, excisional biopsy, or FNA of suspicious inguinal LNs and HPV status. Sigmoidoscopy/colonoscopy often performed as well.

Imaging: CT chest, abdomen, and pelvis, MRI of pelvis with contrast, PET/CT.

PROGNOSTIC FACTORS: Male sex, positive nodes, and tumor size >5 cm were independently prognostic for worse OS on analysis of RTOG 98-11.

STAGING

Table 37.2: AJCC 8th ed. (2017): Staging for Anal Cancer					
T/M		**cN0**	**cN1a**	**cN1b**	**cN1c**
T1	• ≤2 cm	I			
T2	• 2.1–5 cm	IIA		IIIA	
T3	• >5 cm	IIB			
T4	• Invasion into adjacent organs[1]	IIIB		IIIC	
M1	• Distant metastasis			IV	

Notes: Organs[1] = Invasion of vagina, urethra, bladder. Invasion of rectal wall, perirectal skin, subcutaneous tissue, or sphincter muscle are not always T4.

cN1a, metastasis in inguinal, mesorectal, or internal iliac nodes; cN1b, metastasis in external iliac nodes; cN1c, metastasis in external iliac node as well as any of inguinal, mesorectal, or internal iliac node involvement.

TREATMENT PARADIGM

Surgery: Before the 1970s, anal cancer was treated with APR and permanent colostomy with historical 5-year OS rates of 60% for T1/2 disease, 40% for T3 disease, and 20% for LN+ disease. In the 1970s, the Nigro regimen was established after high CR rates to neoadjuvant chemoRT were noted. Concurrent chemoRT is now standard but has never been prospectively compared with surgery. Local excision is a treatment option per NCCN for those with T1N0 well-differentiated tumors of anal margin.[8] Patients with adequate margins (>1 cm) can be observed. Those resected with positive margins require re-excision, adjuvant RT, or chemoRT.

Chemotherapy: Definitive chemoRT, as established by Nigro, is indicated for T2+ or any N+ disease. Standard of care is two cycles of 5-FU/MMC concurrent with RT; 5-FU dose is 1,000 mg/m² days 1 to 4 and 29 to 32 (start of week 5). MMC is often given concurrently with 5-FU, two cycles on d1 and 29, 10 mg/m² IV bolus. Some providers are currently using single-dose MMC (12 mg/m²) in week 1 with 5-FU given on weeks 1 and 5 per the ACT I trial or replacing 5-FU with daily Xeloda during radiation, which is similar to rectal cancer CHT administration, but with the addition of MMC. Major limiting toxicity of MMC is neutropenia.

Cisplatin is used at some institutions as the ACT II trial demonstrated the replacement of MMC for cisplatin yielded equivalent response rates. However, no trials to date have demonstrated an oncologic benefit to the use of cisplatin.

Radiation

Indications: RT is indicated in all cases except T1N0 tumors of anal margin treated with WLE, although RT alone may be appropriate for T1N0 (controversial). For others (cT2–4 or N+), organ-preservation therapy is standard with concurrent chemoRT.

Dose: No prospective data exist to guide RT dosing strategies. One common standard is as defined by RTOG 0529 (see Table 37.1 for dosing). IMRT is standard of care.

Toxicity: Acute: Skin desquamation, fatigue, nausea, vomiting, diarrhea, urethritis, cystitis, pain, neutropenia.

Late: Cystitis, proctitis, sexual dysfunction (females), infertility, sacral insufficiency fracture, second malignancy, bowel stricture, fistula, hyperpigmentation, bowel incontinence.

■ EVIDENCE-BASED Q&A

■ What is the basis for nonsurgical management of anal cancer?

Historically, primary treatment was APR. Use of preoperative chemoRT in Wayne State study demonstrated excellent rates of CR and thus established that chemoRT alone was adequate. There has not been direct phase III comparison with surgery, though definitive chemoRT compares favorably in retrospective reviews with the benefit of allowing for sphincter preservation. T1 patients were not included in original Nigro studies.

Leichman, Wayne State "Nigro Regimen" (*Am J Med* 1985, PMID 3918441): RR of 45 patients (T2 or greater) treated with continuous infusion 5-FU (1,000 mg/m²) for 96 hours × 2 cycles days 1 to 4 and 29 to 32, as well as 1 cycle bolus MMC (15 mg/m²) on day 1. RT was 30 Gy/15 fx over 3 weeks using AP/PA technique to pelvis and inguinal nodes. Post-treatment biopsy was taken 4 to 6 weeks.after completion of chemoRT. Originally APR was required for all patients but the first 5 out of 6 patients had pCR. Thus, in the remainder of study, APR was required only for those with positive post-treatment biopsy. Eighty-four percent of patients had negative biopsy after chemoRT, and there were no recurrences observed in this population with rate of 89% OS at 50 months. Overall, 5-year OS was 67% and 5-year CFS was 59%. **Conclusion: Definitive treatment with chemoRT alone is effective treatment for anal cancer.**

■ Is concurrent chemoRT superior to RT alone?

Two major randomized trials have been performed to answer this question. Both trials included more locally advanced patients and demonstrated that addition of CHT to RT improves pCR rates, LC, CFS, and DSS, though there was no noted improvement in OS. Addition of CHT did not significantly increase late toxicity. Update of ACT I shows that benefit provided by adjuvant chemoRT persists at 13 years.

UK ACT I (*Lancet* 1996, PMID 8874455; Update Northover, *Br J Cancer* 2010, PMID 20354531): PRT of 577 patients with stages II to IV anal SCC randomized to RT alone vs. chemoRT. RT regimen was either 45 Gy/20 fx or 45 Gy/25 fx depending on institutional preference. In chemoRT arm, regimen was two cycles of continuous infusion 5-FU (1,000 mg/m² days 1–4 or 750 mg/m² days 1–5) during first and last week of RT. One cycle of bolus MMC was given on day 1 (12 mg/m²). Clinical response was assessed at 6 weeks and those with response received additional 15Gy boost with EBRT or 25Gy boost with Ir-192 brachytherapy. Those without response had salvage surgery. Primary end point was LF. See Table 37.3. Addition of concurrent CHT to RT significantly improved LC and CSS. Acute toxicity was worse with CHT, but there was no observed increase in late toxicity; 13-year update demonstrated that for every 100 patients treated with chemoRT, there were 25 fewer locoregional relapses and 12.5 fewer anal cancer deaths with no difference in late toxicity. Though there was initial increase in non-anal cancer–related deaths in first 5 years in patients treated with chemoRT, this was not seen in long-term FU. **Conclusion: CHT in addition to RT improves LC and CSS without increasing late toxicity.**

Table 37.3: Initial Results of ACT I Concurrent ChemoRT for Anal Cancer					
	3-Yr LF	3-Yr OS	3-Yr CSS	Acute Morbidity	Late Morbidity
RT	61%	58%	61%	39%	38%
RT + 5-FU/MMC	39%	65%	72%	48%	42%
P value	<.0001	.25	.02	.03	.39

Bartelink, EORTC 22861 (*JCO* 1997, PMID 9164216): PRT of 103 patients with T3/T4 or N+ disease randomized to RT vs. chemoRT. RT was 45 Gy/25 fx, with assessment at 6 weeks followed by 20Gy boost for PR and 15Gy boost for CR. APR was used if there was no response. CHT was continuous infusion 5-FU 750 mg/m² on days 1 to 5 and days 29 to 33 and single dose of MMC 15 mg/m² on day 1. See Table 37.4. Addition of concurrent CHT improves LC, CFS, and CR rates, but not OS. No significant difference in severe toxicities. **Conclusion: ChemoRT improves oncologic outcomes over use of definitive RT alone.**

Table 37.4: Results of EORTC ChemoRT for Anal Cancer				
	5-Yr CR	**5-Yr LC**	**5-Yr CFS**	**5-Yr OS**
RT (N = 52)	54%	50%	40%	56%
RT + 5-FU/MMC (N = 51)	80%	68%	72%	56%
p value	.02	.02	.002	.17

■ Is concurrent 5-FU alone sufficient in comparison to 5-FU/MMC?

Multiple studies have shown that addition of MMC to 5-FU-based chemoRT improves outcomes of LC, CFS, and OS despite greater toxicity. Most notable is RTOG 87-04 as follows, but the Princess Margaret study also confirmed importance of adding MMC.[9]

Flam, ECOG 1289/RTOG 8704 (*JCO* 1996, PMID 8823332): PRT of 291 patients with anal cancer of any T/N-stage treated with definitive chemoRT and randomized to either concurrent 5-FU and MMC or 5-FU alone. Regimen was 5-FU 1,000 mg/m² continuous infusion days 1 to 4 and 28 to 33, MMC 10 mg/m² bolus days 1 and 28. RT was 45 Gy/25 fx to pelvis with 5.4 Gy boost if palpable disease present at end of initial RT course. Biopsy was performed 4 to 6 weeks after chemoRT. If biopsy positive, further 9 Gy was given with concurrent 5-FU and cisplatin. Patients with residual tumor underwent APR. With concurrent MMC, rates of colostomy were lower (9% vs. 22%, P = .002), CFS was higher (71% vs. 59%, P = .014), and DFS was higher (73% vs. 51%, p = .003) at 4 years. No significant differences in OS. Grades 4 and 5 toxicity was higher with MMC (23% vs. 7%, P ≤ .001). Of 24 patients who underwent salvage chemoRT after initial course of chemoRT, 50% were cured. **Conclusion: Though it is associated with greater toxicity, use of MMC improves DFS and CFS. Salvage chemoRT may be reasonable for patients with residual disease as opposed to salvage APR.**

■ Can MMC be replaced with cisplatin?

RTOG 98-11 showed that replacing MMC with cisplatin and addition of induction CHT significantly decreased hematologic toxicities but also increased colostomy rates and reduced DFS and OS. However, ACT II trial established that replacement of MMC with cisplatin does not affect rate of complete response. Because of ACT II showing that CHT regimens are equal in terms of response rate, some have suggested results of 98 to 11 show that induction CHT may be detrimental.

Ajani, RTOG 98-11 (*JAMA* 2008, PMID 18430910; Update Gunderson *JCO* 2012, PMID 23150707): PRT of 649 patients with T2–T4, N0–N3 disease randomized to (a) RT + concurrent 5-FU/MMC or (b) RT + induction/concurrent 5-FU/cisplatin. RT was 45 Gy/25 fx with boost to primary tumor and involved nodes to 55–59 Gy for those with T3–T4, N+ or T2 patients with residual disease after 45 Gy. Elective nodal sites were treated to 30.6 to 36 Gy/17-20 fx. CHT in arm A was 5-FU 1,000 mg/m² continuous infusion days 1 to 4 and 29 to 32 and MMC 10 mg/m² bolus days 1 and 29. In arm B, two cycles of induction 5-FU were given and RT started on day 57 with the 3rd cycle of 5-FU and was continued through the end of 4th cycle. Cisplatin was also given in four bolus administrations: 75 mg/m² days 1, 29, 57, and 85, with 2 cycles prior to start of RT. See Table 37.5. OS and DFS were superior in arm A. **Conclusion: Use of concurrent 5-FU/MMC without induction CHT should remain standard of care.**

James, UK ACT II (*Lancet Oncol* 2013, PMID 23578724): PRT of 940 T1–T4 patients randomized in 2 × 2 fashion to either concurrent 5-FU/cisplatin or concurrent 5-FU/MMC, followed by second randomization to 5-FU × 2 cycles after completion of chemoRT (maintenance) or observation. RT dose was 50.4 Gy/28 fx. MFU 5.1 years. CR was ~90% with either concurrent CHT regimen; 3-year PFS was 74% with maintenance CHT vs. 73% with observation (*P* = NS). **Conclusion: MMC/5-FU + RT remains stand-ard. There was no benefit to addition of maintenance CHT after completion of standard therapy.**

Table 37.5: Results of RTOG 98-11					
	5-Yr OS	5-Yr CFS	5-Yr DFS	Grades 3–4 Heme Toxicity	Grades 3–4 Non-heme Toxicity
RT + concurrent 5-FU/ MMC	78.3%	71.9%	67.8%	61%	74%
RT+ induction/concurrent 5-FU/cisplatin	70.7%	65%	57.8%	42%	74%
p value	.026	.05	.006	.0013	NS

Are there any advantages to dose escalation?

RTOG 9208[10] *demonstrated that there is no role for dose escalation, though study was limited because of treat-ment break. Patients were treated to 59.4 Gy with concurrent 5-FU/MMC with mandatory 2-week break (then amended to be continuous without break). Higher dose in this study was associated with increased colostomy rate and no significant difference in OS or LC compared to historical standards (RTOG 8704). These findings are supported by the ACCORD 03 trial, which also showed no improvement in oncologic outcomes with high dose boost (see the following).*

Should we add induction CHT or high dose boost?

The results of ACCORD 03 are in line with findings of RTOG 98-11—there is no benefit to induction CHT. One retrospective study has suggested there may be benefit in colostomy-free survival with use of induction CHT in T4 patients, though this has not been validated prospectively.[11] There is no role for high dose boost at this time.

Peiffert, ACCORD 03 (*JCO* 2012, PMID 22529257): PRT of 307 patients with anal SCC (either ≥ 4 cm or N+) randomized in 2 × 2 fashion: ±induction CHT and either standard or high dose boost in addition to concurrent chemoRT (45 Gy/25 fx with concurrent 5-FU/cisplatin). Standard boost was 15 Gy. High-dose boost was 20 Gy for CR or greater than 80% reduction and 25 Gy for PR (less than 80% reduction). See Table 37.6. At MFU 50 months, there was no statistically significant difference between four arms. CFS was main end point with no advantage of induction CHT (*P* = .37) or high dose (*P* = .067) RT boost. **Conclusion: No benefit to induction CHT or high dose boost. Authors concluded that there should be further evaluation of dose intensification, given that high dose boost trends to improved CFS.**

Table 37.6: Results of ACCORD 03 for Anal Cancer			
Arm	5-Yr CFS	5-Yr LC	5-Yr DSS
Induction + chemoRT + standard boost	69.6%	72.0%	76.6%
Induction + chemoRT + high dose boost	82.4%	87.9%	88.8%
chemoRT + standard boost	77.1%	83.7%	80.6%
chemoRT + high dose boost	72.7%	78.0%	75.9%

Is there benefit to IMRT?

RTOG 0529[1] *was a phase II trial evaluating use of IMRT for anal cancer and demonstrated significant reduc-tion in hematologic, GI, and skin toxicity, compared to historic 3D-CRT standards. NCCN consensus is that IMRT is preferred over 3D-CRT; however, IMRT requires expertise in its application as 81% of patients on study required replanning on central review. RTOG 0529 is appropriate guideline for use of IMRT in anal cancer.*

■ **What salvage options are available for recurrence after definitive chemoRT?**

APR is used for salvage in setting of failure after definitive chemoRT. Salvage surgery results vary widely in literature due to small patient populations and selection bias. One study performed in the Netherlands of 47 patients undergoing salvage APR demonstrated negative margin resections in 81% with a 5-year OS rate of 42%. However, 45% of the cohort ultimately recurred.[12]

■ **For incomplete post-treatment response, when should biopsy be performed?**

Initial guidelines recommended response assessment at 6 to 12 weeks after treatment; however, post-hoc analysis of ACT II showed that there can be a delayed clinical response up to 26 weeks without negative impact on survival.

Glynne-Jones (*Lancet* 2017, PMID 28209296): Post-hoc analysis of ACT II to determine optimal response assessment time point. cCR was evaluated at 3 time points measured from start of CRT: 11 weeks, 18 weeks, and 26 weeks. cCR was defined as no evidence of residual tumor or nodal disease by clinical exam. At 11, 18, and 26 weeks, cCR rates were 52%, 71%, and 78%, respectively. Five-year OS for cCR at each time point was 83%, 84%, and 87% vs. 72%, 59%, and 46% for those who did not have a cCR at each time point. **Conclusion: Many patients without cCR at 11 weeks will respond by 26 weeks, and any salvage interventions should be delayed until after this time point to avoid unnecessary surgeries.**

■ **What is the recommendation for T1N0 patients?**

This patient subset was not included in the original Nigro studies and were also excluded from RTOG 9811, ACT I, ACT II, and EORTC 22861. NCCN recommends local excision with adequate margins (defined as 1 cm) for anal margin cancers and chemoRT for anal canal lesions. Options for inadequate margins include re-excision (preferred) or local radiation with or without concurrent CHT. Retrospective series have suggested good outcomes with definitive RT in this patient subset.

■ **What are the outcomes with non-regional lymph node metastasis (PA lymph nodes) treated definitively?**

There may be a small subset of patients who have good outcomes with extended DFS when treated definitively with extended field RT and CHT.

Holliday (*IJROPB* 2018, PMID 29907489): RR of 30 patients with denovo SCC of the anal canal metastatic to PA lymph nodes, treated with extended field chemoRT (median dose 51 Gy) and cis/5-FU/ Xeloda, 5-FU/MMC, or daily Xeloda; 3-year OS and DFS was 67% and 42%; 3-year rate of distant metastasis was 50%. **Conclusion: In patients presenting with SCC of the anal canal with metastases limited to the PA lymph nodes, extended field chemoRT is a viable treatment option.**

REFERENCES

1. Kachnic LA, Winter K, Myerson RJ, et al. RTOG 0529: phase 2 evaluation of dose-painted intensity modulated radiation therapy in combination with 5-fluorouracil and mitomycin-C for reduction of acute morbidity in carcinoma of anal canal. *Int J Radiat Oncol Biol Phys.* 2013; 86(1):27–33. doi:10.1016/j.ijrobp.2012.09.023
2. Siegel RL, Miller KD, Jemal A, et al. Cancer statistics, 2020. *CA Cancer J Clin.* 2020;70(1):7–30. doi:10.3322/caac.21590
3. American Cancer Society-Anal Cancer. Key Statistics for Anal Cancer. 2020. https://www.cancer.org/cancer/anal-cancer/about/what-is-key-statistics.html
4. Crum-Cianflone NF, Hullsiek KH, Marconi VC, et al. Anal cancers among HIV-infected persons: HAART is not slowing rising incidence. *AIDS (London, England).* 2010; 24(4):535–543. doi:10.1097/QAD.0b013e328331f6e2
5. Frisch M, Glimelius B, van den Brule AJ, et al. Sexually transmitted infection as cause of anal cancer. *N Engl J Med.* 1997;337(19):1350–1358. doi:10.1056/NEJM199711063371904
6. Ryan DP, Compton CC, Mayer RJ. Carcinoma of anal canal. *N Engl J Med.* 2000;342(11):792–800. doi:10.1056/NEJM200003163421107
7. Altekruse SF, Kosary CL, Krapcho M, et al., eds. *SEER Cancer Statistics Review, 1975–2007, National Cancer Institute.* Bethesda, MD. (Based on November 2009 SEER data submission, posted to the SEER website, 2010). https://seer.cancer.gov/explorer/application.html?site=34&data_type=1&graph_type=4&compareBy=sex&chk_sex_3=3&chk_sex_2=2&race=1&age_range=1&advopt_precision=1

8. NCCN Clinical Practice Guidelines in Oncology: Anal Carcinoma. 2017. https://www.nccn.org
9. Cummings BJ, Keane TJ, O'Sullivan B, et al. Epidermoid anal cancer: treatment by radiation alone or by radiation and 5-fluorouracil with and without mitomycin C. *Int J Radiat Oncol Biol Phys*. 1991; 21(5):1115–1125. doi:10.1016/0360-3016(91)90265-6
10. Konski A, Garcia M Jr, John M, et al. Evaluation of planned treatment breaks during radiation therapy for anal cancer: update of RTOG 92-08. *Int J Radiat Oncol Biol Phys*. 2008;72(1):114–118. doi:10.1016/j.ijrobp.2007.12.027
11. Moureau-Zabotto L, Viret F, Giovaninni M, et al. Is neoadjuvant chemotherapy prior to radio-chemotherapy beneficial in T4 anal carcinoma? *J Surg Oncol*. 2011;104(1):66–71. doi:10.1002/jso.21866
12. Hagemans JAW, Blinde SE, Nuyttens JJ, et al. Salvage abdominoperineal resection for squamous cell anal cancer: a 30-year single-institution experience. *Ann Surg Oncol*. 2018;25(7):1970–1979. doi:10.1245/s10434-018-6483-9

38 ■ CHOLANGIOCARCINOMA

Christopher W. Fleming, Shauna R. Campbell, and Kevin L. Stephans

QUICK HIT ■ CC is a rare and highly lethal cancer, with a propensity for both local and distant recurrence. Surgery is required for cure, though the majority of patients present with advanced, unresectable disease. CC is categorized based on three sites of origin: intrahepatic, perihilar, and distal extrahepatic. The general treatment paradigm for resectable CC consists of surgery, followed by adjuvant CHT, with RT reserved for positive margins or positive lymph nodes. Unresectable patients receive CHT and can be considered for dose-escalated hypofractionated RT. Transplant protocols, consisting of neoadjuvant CRT, brachytherapy boost, and OLT, have shown excellent outcomes for patients with perihilar CC with unresectable disease or arising in the setting of PSC.

EPIDEMIOLOGY: Incidence in the United States is 2 per 100,000 people annually and appears to be increasing due to a rise in intrahepatic CC.[1] Worldwide, the highest incidence is found in Thailand and Southeast Asia, with nearly 20 times higher incidence than Western countries.[2] Patients are typically diagnosed between ages 50 and 70, though patients with PSC often present at a younger age.

RISK FACTORS: PSC is the strongest risk factor, with an estimated lifetime risk of 5% to 20%.[3] Other established risk factors include hepatobiliary lithiasis, congenital biliary duct cysts (seen in Caroli's disease), infection with the liver flukes Opisthorchis viverrini and Clonorchis sinensis (most commonly found in Southeast Asia and Thailand), and exposure to Thorotrast, a radiologic contrast agent banned in the 1960s. Other risk factors include genetic disorders such as Lynch syndrome and cystic fibrosis, smoking, diabetes, obesity, nitrosamine intake, inflammatory bowel disease, cirrhosis, and hepatitis B and C.[4]

ANATOMY: CC originates from the bile duct epithelium and is classified based on site of origin: intrahepatic, perihilar, and distal extrahepatic. Perihilar tumors have been further classified based on extent of ductal involvement using the Bismuth–Corlette system; those involving the common hepatic duct bifurcation are referred to as Klatskin tumors. One-third of patients will have regional lymph node metastases at diagnosis.[5-7]

PATHOLOGY: The vast majority are adenocarcinoma. Tumors often develop significant peritumoral desmoplasia, lowering the diagnostic yield of biopsy and cytology. Perihilar tumors are particularly challenging, as only half of the patients will have a diagnostic biopsy. The need for tissue diagnosis has been questioned, as patients diagnosed using clinical criteria alone (see Workup section) have similar likelihood of malignancy found on explanted livers.[8] CC is often multifocal and has a strong propensity for perineural invasion.[9] CK7 is generally positive by IHC, though not specific to biliary cancers. FISH testing for chromosomal abnormalities may aid in diagnosis when cytology is inconclusive for malignancy, increasing the diagnostic yield. Combined hepatocellular-cholangiocarcinoma, also referred to as hepatocholangiocarcinoma or primary liver carcinoma with biphenotypic differentiation, is considered a subtype of intrahepatic CC.

SCREENING: PSC patients are generally recommended at least annual surveillance with CA 19-9 and US, CT, or MRI.

CLINICAL PRESENTATION: Perihilar and distal extrahepatic CC often present due to obstructive symptoms of jaundice, pruritus, malabsorption, and dark urine. Intrahepatic CC is less likely to cause obstruction unless very advanced, and generally presents with RUQ pain, weight loss, and fever.

WORKUP: H&P, with attention to symptoms as previously noted. EUS with FNA (for distal lesions) and/or ERCP with brush cytology for pathologic confirmation. ERCP and PTHC (percutaneous transhepatic cholangiography) allow for visualization of the biliary tree and therapeutic drainage.

Staging laparoscopy should be performed prior to surgery to assess for resectability and peritoneal metastases.

Labs: CBC, CMP, CA 19-9, CEA, AFP (elevated in HCC and mixed hepatocholangiocarcinoma). Patients presenting with cholangitis should have tumor markers redrawn after infection and obstruction have resolved, as these can spuriously elevate marker levels.

Imaging: Patients often have undergone CT and US of the liver during workup but should undergo MRI or MRCP for assessment of local tumor extent and resectability. If stent placement is required for obstruction, MRI is ideally performed prior to avoid artifact. CT chest or PET/CT to evaluate for distant metastases, most commonly to liver, peritoneum, bone, and lungs.

Criteria for diagnosis of perihilar CC: Presence of a malignant-appearing stricture on percutaneous or endoscopic cholangiography *and* one of the following: malignant cytology or histology on transluminal brushings or biopsy, polysomy on FISH, CA 19-9 > 100 U/mL, or mass on cross-sectional imaging at the site of the malignant-appearing stricture.[8]

PROGNOSTIC FACTORS: Age, stage, grade, margin status, tumor markers.[10] Overall, 5-year OS is estimated between 2% and 30%.[11]

STAGING: AJCC's 8th edition has separate TNM and group staging for each site of origin (Table 38.1).

Table 38.1: AJCC's 8th Edition: Staging for Cholangiocarcinoma			
	Intrahepatic	Perihilar	Distal
T1	a: ≤5 cm, no vascular invasion b: >5 cm, no vascular invasion	Confined to bile duct, extension up to muscle layer or fibrous tissue	Invades bile duct wall, depth <5 mm
T2	Single tumor with vascular invasion, or multiple tumors	a. Invasion into surrounding fat b. Invasion into adjacent liver	Invades bile duct wall, depth 5–12 mm
T3	Perforates visceral peritoneum	Invades unilateral branches of portal vein or hepatic artery	Invades bile duct wall, depth >12 mm
T4	Invasion[1]	Invasion[2]	Invasion[3]
N0	No regional lymph node metastases		
N1	Involves regional nodes	1–3 regional nodes	
N2	N/A	4 + regional nodes	
M0	No distant metastases		
M1	Distant metastases present		

Note: Invasion[1] = invasion into local extrahepatic structures. Invasion[2] = invasion into main portal vein or its bilateral branches, common hepatic artery, or unilateral second-order biliary radicals with contralateral portal vein or hepatic artery involvement. Invasion[3] = invasion of celiac axis, SMA, or common hepatic artery.
Group staging also varies for each location; see AJCC staging manual.[12]

TREATMENT PARADIGM

Surgery: Surgery is performed for all resectable patients. Patients considered for resection are those without distance metastases, in whom margin negative resection would maintain adequate hepatic function post-operatively; this unfortunately represents the minority of patients. Variable degrees of vascular, biliary tree, and diaphragmatic involvement are considered resectable based on center experience. PVE may be used to induce hypertrophy of the future liver remnant to allow for more extensive resections. Intrahepatic tumors are resected via partial hepatectomy. At least 1 cm margins are preferred, as smaller margins are associated with higher risk of recurrence.[13] Distal extrahepatic tumors are resected via pancreaticoduodenectomy (Whipple procedure) and are more likely to be resectable at diagnosis.[14] Perihilar tumors are often unresectable due to degree of bile duct involvement. Some may be amenable to bile duct excision and partial hepatectomy, though recurrence rates after local excision are high,[15] as is peri-operative mortality.[16] These factors have led to increasing adoption of OLT for early stage perihilar CC, as well as for CC arising in the setting of PSC (see Transplant Protocol).

Chemotherapy

Adjuvant: CC is prone to both locoregional and distant recurrence, highlighting the need for adjuvant therapies. Adjuvant CHT is indicated for all patients with positive margins or regional lymph nodes. Management of node-negative patients after R0 resection is controversial; while 2020 NCCN Guidelines allow for observation, 2019 ASCO Clinical Practice Guidelines recommend all patients with resected biliary tract cancers undergo 6 months of adjuvant capecitabine based on results of the phase III BILCAP trial.[11] Gemcitabine, cisplatin, and 5-FU/leucovorin have also been utilized. The ACTICCA-1 trial is an ongoing phase III trial comparing combination gemcitabine/cisplatin to capecitabine in the adjuvant setting.[17]

Unresectable or metastatic: Combination gemcitabine/cisplatin is preferred due to OS benefit compared to cisplatin alone in ABC-02 trial.[18] Patients received cisplatin 25 mg/m^2 followed by gemcitabine 1,000 mg/m^2 each administered on days 1 and 8, every 3 weeks for 8 cycles. Gemcitabine/capecitabine is another option per SWOG 0809 trial (see adjuvant RT section).

Radiotherapy

Adjuvant: Traditional indications include positive margins and consideration for positive lymph nodes. Dose, volume, and elective nodal irradiation are not standardized. For extrahepatic biliary cancers with R1 resection, ASCO guidelines recommend consideration of adjuvant CRT with capecitabine based on results of the SWOG 0809 trial.[11] Patients received 4 cycles of gemcitabine (1,000 mg/m^2 on days 1 and 8) and capecitabine (1,500 mg/m^2 per day on days 1–14) every 21 days, followed by concurrent capecitabine (1,330 mg/m^2 per day) and RT, consisting of 45 Gy to the regional lymphatics with a boost to 54 to 59.4 Gy to the resection bed. Intrahepatic tumors were not included in this recommendation due to the challenge of identifying the area of positive margin. Concurrent 5-FU (225 mg/m^2 daily) or capecitabine (825 mg/m^2 BID) alone are reasonable alternatives.

Unresectable: Unresectable patients will often start treatment with CHT alone, with locoregional therapy considered for those who do not progress distantly. Dose-escalated hypofractionated RT, with or without concurrent CHT, has shown promising results in single-institution studies for unresectable intrahepatic CC.[19,20] NRG GI-001 is investigating the benefit of RT following three cycles of gemcitabine/cisplatin, with doses up to 67.5 Gy/15 fx, with dose reductions based on mean liver dose and proximity to porta hepatis.[19] SBRT has also been used in this setting; common prescriptions include 40 to 60 Gy/5 fx and 30 to 45 Gy/3 fx.[21] A small proportion of patients will convert to resectable disease after RT.

Mayo Clinic Transplant Protocol for Perihilar CC: Mayo Clinic has pioneered the use of OLT for perihilar tumors and CC arising in a setting of PSC. This protocol consists of neoadjuvant CRT, brachytherapy boost, maintenance CHT, followed by OLT. Staging laparoscopy is required prior to transplant.[22]

Inclusion criteria:

- Diagnosis of CC either pathologically or with clinical criteria as noted previously
- Perihilar CC arising in the setting of PSC or anatomically unresectable
- Radial tumor diameter ≤ 3 cm
- Absence of intra- and extrahepatic metastases, including regional lymph nodes
- Candidate for OLT

Chemoradiation: 45 Gy/30 fx BID with concurrent 5-FU or capecitabine.

Brachytherapy: 15 Gy/3 fx HDR or 20 to 30 Gy/3 fx LDR. For patients not candidates for brachytherapy (e.g., unable to place biliary catheters), SBRT has been utilized as replacement for brachytherapy[23] and the external RT component as well.[24]

Maintenance CHT: 5-FU or capecitabine until transplant.

■ **EVIDENCE-BASED Q&A**

▦ **What is the benefit of adjuvant CHT?**

Adjuvant CHT is indicated for all patients with positive margins or positive regional lymph nodes. There is controversy regarding its use in N0 patients after R0 resection (see Chemotherapy section).

Primrose, BILCAP (*Lancet Oncol* 2017, PMID 30922733): Multicenter phase III trial randomizing 447 patients with CC or gallbladder carcinoma after macroscopically complete resection to adjuvant capecitabine vs. observation; 62% had R0 resection, 53% were pN0. By intention to treat, median OS 51 vs. 36 months in favor of adjuvant capecitabine, *P* = .097. Per-protocol analysis showed OS 53 vs. 36 months, *p* = .028. **Conclusion: Adjuvant capecitabine can improve OS in resected biliary tract cancer.**

▦ **What are the indications for adjuvant RT?**

General indications for consideration of adjuvant RT include positive margins and lymph nodes. Controversy exists regarding the use of adjuvant RT for intrahepatic CC (see Radiotherapy section). SWOG 0809 enrolled extrahepatic CC and showed favorable outcomes compared to historical reports, providing an evidence-based adjuvant regimen for clinicians.

Ben-Josef, SWOG 0809 (*JCO* 2015, PMID 25964250): Prospective single-arm phase II trial including 79 patients with extrahepatic CC or gallbladder carcinoma, surgically resected with pT2–T4, positive nodes, or positive margins. Patients received four cycles adjuvant gemcitabine/capecitabine, followed by RT (45 Gy to regional lymphatics; 54–59.4 Gy to tumor bed) with concurrent capecitabine. Eighty-six percent completed treatment per protocol; 2-year OS 65% and 2-year LR 11%, neither of which was different between R0/R1 patients, suggesting potential efficacy of the treatment regimen. **Conclusion: This combination was well tolerated, has promising efficacy, and provides a well-supported adjuvant regimen for clinical use.**

▦ **How should RT be delivered for unresectable CC?**

For patients who remain free of metastatic disease after initial CHT, RT can be added to prolong LC and potentially OS. The best evidence exists for dose-escalated hypofractionated RT, which is being investigated on NRG GI-001, randomizing patients with intrahepatic CC to observation vs. hypofractionated RT after initial gemcitabine/cisplatin. Outcomes after SBRT have been reported as well.[21]

Tao, MD Anderson (*JCO* 2016, PMID 26503201): RR of 79 patients with inoperable intrahepatic CC treated with definitive RT between 2002 and 2014. Doses ranged from 35 to 100 Gy in 3 to 30 fractions, with a median BED of 80.5 Gy. Eighty-nine percent received CHT prior to RT. Median OS 30 months, 3-year OS 44%. For patients receiving BED > 80.5 Gy, 3-year OS 73% vs. 38%, *p* = .017, and 3-year LC 78% vs. 45%, *p* = .04. No significant RT-related toxicities. **Conclusion: Higher BED is associated with improved LC and OS.**

Hong, Multi-institutional (*JCO* 2016, PMID: 26668346). Phase II study of 92 patients with unresectable HCC or intrahepatic CC (*n* = 41), undergoing high dose hypofractionated proton beam therapy. Median RT dose 58 GyE (range 15.1–67.5) in 15 fx; 2-year LC 94% for both HCC and CC; 2-year OS 63.2% for HCC and 46.5% CC. Five percent rate of grade 3 adverse effects. **Conclusion: High-dose hypofractionated proton therapy demonstrated high LC with low rates of toxicity.**

▦ **What studies have led to the adoption of OLT for unresectable hilar CC?**

Early experiences with transplantation alone were disappointing, with 5-year OS <30%.[25] The University of Nebraska then pioneered a neoadjuvant regimen with CRT, followed by OLT, showing 45% long-term survival.[26] This approach was later adopted by the Mayo Clinic, which published excellent initial outcomes, with 5-year OS of 82% for those completing the protocol.[27] Several other institutions adopted this protocol, with reproducible results. Due to the success of this paradigm, some have suggested implementation of OLT for resectable hilar and intrahepatic CC.[28–30]

Rosen, Mayo Clinic (*HPB* 2008, PMID 18773052): Review of 148 patients enrolled on prospective institutional protocol, 61% underwent OLT; 5-year OS for all patients 55%, 71% for those who proceeded to transplant. **Conclusion: Transplant protocol achieves significantly lower recurrence and higher long-term survival rates than resection, OLT alone, or medical treatment in hilar CC.**

Darwish Murad, Multi-Institutional (*Gastroenterology* 2012, PMID 22504095): RR of 287 patients from 12 U.S. transplant centers (67% from Mayo Clinic) enrolled on OLT protocols. Seventy-five percent underwent OLT with 5-year RFS of 65% in those patients; 5-year OS 53% in all patients. No difference in outcomes between centers. **Conclusion: Transplant protocol proved to be reproducible across multiple transplant centers.**

Ethun, Multi-Institutional (*Ann Surg* 2018, PMID 29064885): RR of 304 patients with hilar CC treated at 10 U.S. institutions; 234 underwent attempted resection, and 70 enrolled on transplant protocols. Patients who underwent transplant had improved OS, compared with resection (3-yr 72% vs. 33%; 5-yr 64% vs. 18%; $p < .001$). Among patients who underwent resection for tumors <3cm with lymph node-negative disease, and excluding PSC patients, transplant was still associated with improved OS (3-yr 54% vs. 44%; 5-yr 54% vs. 29%; $P = .03$). Transplant remained associated with improved OS on intention-to-treat analysis, even after accounting for tumor size, lymph node status, and PSC ($p = .049$). **Conclusion: Resection for hilar CC meeting criteria for transplantation (<3cm, lymph node negative) is associated with substantially decreased OS compared to transplant for unresectable disease.**

REFERENCES

1. Patel N, Benipal B. Incidence of Cholangiocarcinoma in the USA from 2001–2015: a US Cancer Statistics Analysis of 50 States. *Cureus*. 2019;11(1):e3962. doi:10.7759/cureus.3962
2. Sripa B, Pairojkul C. Cholangiocarcinoma: lessons from Thailand. *Curr Opin Gastroenterol*. 2008;24(3):349–356. doi:10.1097/MOG.0b013e3282fbf9b3
3. Fung BM, Lindor KD, Tabibian JH. Cancer risk in primary sclerosing cholangitis: epidemiology, prevention, and surveillance strategies. *World J Gastroenterol*. 2019;25(6):659–671. doi:10.3748/wjg.v25.i6.659
4. Tyson GL, El-Serag HB. Risk factors for cholangiocarcinoma. *Hepatology*. 2011;54(1):173–184. doi:10.1002/hep.24351
5. Kiriyama M, Ebata T, Aoba T, et al. Prognostic impact of lymph node metastasis in distal cholangiocarcinoma. *Br J Surg*. 2015;102(4):399–406. doi:10.1002/bjs.9752
6. Bagante F, Tran T, Spolverato G, et al. Perihilar cholangiocarcinoma: number of nodes examined and optimal lymph node prognostic scheme. *J Am Coll Surg*. 2016;222(5):750–759 e752. doi:10.1016/j.jamcollsurg.2016.02.012
7. Jutric Z, Johnston WC, Hoen HM, et al. Impact of lymph node status in patients with intrahepatic cholangiocarcinoma treated by major hepatectomy: a review of the National Cancer Database. *HPB (Oxford)*. 2016;18(1):79–87. doi:10.1016/j.hpb.2015.07.006
8. Rosen CB, Darwish Murad S, Heimbach JK, et al. Neoadjuvant therapy and liver transplantation for hilar cholangiocarcinoma: is pretreatment pathological confirmation of diagnosis necessary? *J Am Coll Surg*. 2012;215(1):31–38; discussion 38–40. doi:10.1016/j.jamcollsurg.2012.03.014
9. Li CG, Zhou ZP, Tan XL, Zhao ZM. Perineural invasion of hilar cholangiocarcinoma in Chinese population: one center's experience. *World J Gastrointest Oncol*. 2020;12(4):457–466. doi:10.4251/wjgo.v12.i4.457
10. Mavros MN, Economopoulos KP, Alexiou VG, Pawlik TM. Treatment and prognosis for patients with intrahepatic cholangiocarcinoma: systematic review and meta-analysis. *JAMA Surg*. 2014;149(6):565–574. doi:10.1001/jamasurg.2013.5137
11. Shroff RT, Kennedy EB, Bachini M, et al. Adjuvant therapy for resected biliary tract cancer: ASCO Clinical Practice Guideline. *J Clin Oncol*. 2019;37(12):1015–1027. doi:10.1200/JCO.18.02178
12. Amin MB, American Joint Committee on Cancer, American Cancer Society. *AJCC cancer staging manual*. 2017.
13. Spolverato G, Yakoob MY, Kim Y, et al. The impact of surgical margin status on long-term outcome after resection for intrahepatic cholangiocarcinoma. *Ann Surg Oncol*. 2015;22(12):4020–4028. doi:10.1245/s10434-015-4472-9
14. Nakeeb A, Pitt HA, Sohn TA, et al. Cholangiocarcinoma: a spectrum of intrahepatic, perihilar, and distal tumors. *Ann Surg*. 1996;224(4):463–473; discussion 473–465. doi:10.1097/00000658-199610000-00005
15. Groot Koerkamp B, Wiggers JK, Allen PJ, et al. Recurrence rate and pattern of perihilar cholangiocarcinoma after curative intent resection. *J Am Coll Surg*. 2015;221(6):1041–1049. doi:10.1016/j.jamcollsurg.2015.09.005
16. Loehrer AP, House MG, Nakeeb A, et al. Cholangiocarcinoma: are North American surgical outcomes optimal? *J Am Coll Surg*. 2013;216(2):192–200. doi:10.1016/j.jamcollsurg.2012.11.002
17. Stein A, Arnold D, Bridgewater J, et al. Adjuvant chemotherapy with gemcitabine and cisplatin compared to observation after curative intent resection of cholangiocarcinoma and muscle invasive gallbladder carcinoma (ACTICCA-1 trial): a randomized, multidisciplinary, multinational phase III trial. *BMC Cancer*. 2015;15:564. doi:10.1186/s12885-015-1498-0
18. Valle J, Wasan H, Palmer DH, et al. Cisplatin plus gemcitabine versus gemcitabine for biliary tract cancer. *N Engl J Med*. 2010;362(14):1273–1281. doi:10.1056/NEJMoa0908721

19. Hong TS, Wo JY, Yeap BY, et al. Multi-institutional phase ii study of high-dose hypofractionated proton beam therapy in patients with localized, unresectable hepatocellular carcinoma and intrahepatic cholangiocarcinoma. *J Clin Oncol.* 2016;34(5):460–468. doi:10.1200/JCO.2015.64.2710

20. Tao R, Krishnan S, Bhosale PR, et al. Ablative radiotherapy doses lead to a substantial prolongation of survival in patients with inoperable intrahepatic cholangiocarcinoma: a retrospective dose response analysis. *J Clin Oncol.* 2016;34(3):219–226. doi:10.1200/JCO.2015.61.3778

21. Lee J, Yoon WS, Koom WS, Rim CH. Efficacy of stereotactic body radiotherapy for unresectable or recurrent cholangiocarcinoma: a meta-analysis and systematic review. *Strahlenther Onkol.* 2019;195(2):93–102. doi:10.1007/s00066-018-1367-2

22. Rosen CB, Heimbach JK, Gores GJ. Liver transplantation for cholangiocarcinoma. *Transpl Int.* 2010;23(7):692–697. doi:10.1111/j.1432-2277.2010.01108.x

23. Broughman R, Sittenfeld S, Bauer-Nilsen K, Stephans K. Substituting stereotactic body radiation therapy boost for brachytherapy in Mayo protocol for peri-hilar cholangiocarcinoma. *Appl Rad Oncol.* 2019;8(3):43–45.

24. Welling TH, Feng M, Wan S, et al. Neoadjuvant stereotactic body radiation therapy, capecitabine, and liver transplantation for unresectable hilar cholangiocarcinoma. *Liver Transpl.* 2014;20(1):81–88. doi:10.1002/lt.23757

25. Iwatsuki S, Todo S, Marsh JW, et al. Treatment of hilar cholangiocarcinoma (Klatskin tumors) with hepatic resection or transplantation. *J Am Coll Surg.* 1998;187(4):358–364. doi:10.1016/S1072-7515(98)00207-5

26. Sudan D, DeRoover A, Chinnakotla S, et al. Radiochemotherapy and transplantation allow long-term survival for nonresectable hilar cholangiocarcinoma. *Am J Transplant.* 2002;2(8):774–779. doi:10.1034/j.1600-6143.2002.20812.x

27. Rea DJ, Heimbach JK, Rosen CB, et al. Liver transplantation with neoadjuvant chemoradiation is more effective than resection for hilar cholangiocarcinoma. *Ann Surg.* 2005;242(3):451–458; discussion 458–461. doi:10.1097/01.sla.0000179678.13285.fa

28. Ethun CG, Lopez-Aguiar AG, Anderson DJ, et al. Transplantation versus resection for hilar cholangiocarcinoma: an argument for shifting treatment paradigms for resectable disease. *Ann Surg.* 2018;267(5):797–805. doi:10.1097/SLA.0000000000002574

29. Goldaracena N, Gorgen A, Sapisochin G. Current status of liver transplantation for cholangiocarcinoma. *Liver Transpl.* 2018;24(2):294–303. doi:10.1002/lt.24955

30. Lunsford KE, Javle M, Heyne K, et al. Liver transplantation for locally advanced intrahepatic cholangiocarcinoma treated with neoadjuvant therapy: a prospective case-series. *Lancet Gastroenterol Hepatol.* 2018;3(5):337–348. doi:10.1016/S2468-1253(18)30045-1

VII ■ GENITOURINARY

Timothy D. Smile and Rahul D. Tendulkar

QUICK HIT ■ Low-risk prostate cancer includes organ-confined disease typically detected by a screening PSA or on DRE (T1-T2a), with a PSA < 10 ng/mL and GS ≤ 6. Standard treatment options include active surveillance, prostatectomy, EBRT, or brachytherapy (see Table 39.1). Prostate cancer–specific survival is >95% for each. Therefore, treatment selection is guided by side effect profiles and patient preference. Most guidelines recommend treatment only if life expectancy is >10 years. Dose-escalated RT improves biochemical control, compared to "conventional" doses. Concurrent ADT is not indicated in low-risk prostate cancer. The PROST-QA and ProtecT trials included patient-reported outcomes and are helpful to inform patient decisions.

Table 39.1: General Overview of Treatment Options for Low-Risk Prostate Cancer				
Treatment Option	**General Overview/ Example**	**Pros**	**Cons**	**Patient Selection**
Watchful waiting	No further testing; treatment only when symptoms develop	Avoids overtreatment, reduces cost	Progression may occur without notice	Patients with severe comorbidity and/or limited life span
Active surveillance	Regimented follow-up with PSA testing and repeat biopsies; consider genomic testing and MRI-guided biopsy	Avoids immediate side effects and cost of treatment	Patient anxiety; risk of disease progression; costs increase over time	Compliant patients with low-risk or favorable intermediate-risk disease motivated toward deferring treatment
Radical prostatectomy	Robotic or open, usually with pelvic lymph node dissection	Removes all tumor/ prostate; relieves obstructive symptoms; obtains pathologic staging; avoids radiation exposure	Operative risk; higher risk of ED and incontinence than nonoperative options	Younger, healthier patients motivated toward avoiding RT or with significant obstructive symptoms or concern regarding urinary or bowel effects of RT

(continued)

Table 39.1: General Overview of Treatment Options for Low-Risk Prostate Cancer (continued)

Treatment Option	General Overview/ Example	Pros	Cons	Patient Selection
IMRT (standard fractionation)	74–80 Gy over 7–9 weeks	"Historic gold standard" RT regimen with long-term follow-up	Protracted course is inconvenient; potential late effects include cystitis, proctitis, ED, second malignancy	Patients motivated toward nonoperative intervention or specific concerns of erectile dysfunction or incontinence from RP
IMRT (moderate hypofractionation)	60–70 Gy over 4–5.5 weeks	Reduces treatment time, large randomized trials supporting treatment; reduced cost over conventional IMRT	Treatment time still moderately protracted; potential late effects include cystitis, proctitis, ED, second malignancy	
SBRT (extreme hypofractionation)	35–40 Gy/5 fx QOD	Significantly reduces overall treatment time; late effects appear favorable	Long-term follow-up data not available; potential late effects include cystitis, proctitis, ED, second malignancy	
Brachytherapy	LDR with I-125/P-103 or HDR with Ir-192	Single-day procedure (LDR); minimally invasive; long-term follow-up available	Pronounced acute LUTS; potential late effects include urinary retention, cystitis, ED, second malignancy	

EPIDEMIOLOGY: Estimated 248,530 new cases and 34,130 deaths predicted for 2021.[1] Prostate cancer is the most common non-cutaneous malignancy in U.S. men (lifetime risk 1 in 7) and second-most common cause of cancer death in men (after lung cancer). Due to screening, the median age of diagnosis is 60 years of age. The incidence is highest in Scandinavia and lowest in Asia.

RISK FACTORS: Age and family history are the strongest known factors.[2] Black men have worse outcomes than White men, though the contribution of biological vs. nonbiological factors is under investigation.[2-6] Mutations in genes responsible for DNA repair (e.g., germline BRCA2 mutation) may be associated with higher GS and worse prognosis.[7,8] Other general syndromes associated with increased risk of prostate cancer are Lynch syndrome, BRCA2, Fanconi's anemia, and HOXB13.[9-11]

ANATOMY: The prostate is composed of two thirds glandular elements and one third fibromuscular stroma. The glandular part is divided into three zones: peripheral zone (comprises 70% of prostate volume, with the majority of prostate cancer arising from this zone), central zone (comprises 25% of prostate volume, with 5% of prostate cancer arising from this zone), and transition zone (comprises

5% of the prostate volume and is the site of benign prostatic hyperplasia). The neurovascular bundles are located posterolaterally. The fibromuscular stroma (or anterior zone) extends superiorly from the smooth muscle of the bladder neck and inferiorly to the urethra, prostate apex, and external sphincter. The SVs are coaxial with the gland and adjacent to the posterolateral aspect of the prostate, joining the vas deferens to the ejaculatory duct and entering the prostatic urethra at the verumontanum. The position of the prostate and SVs varies w/ filling of the rectum and bladder. Typical prostate variability is as follows (standard deviation): A-P—2.4 mm, Inf-Sup—2.1 mm, and Med-Lat—0.4 mm; SV displacement: A-P—3.5 mm, Inf-Sup—2.1 mm, and Med-Lat—0.8 mm.[12] Lymphatic drainage of the prostate includes internal iliac, external iliac, obturator, and presacral lymph nodes, with occasional drainage directly to the common iliac nodes. The lymphatics of the SVs typically drain to the external iliac nodes.

PATHOLOGY: Ninety-five percent of prostate cancers are adenocarcinomas. Other histologies such as small cell (neuroendocrine) carcinoma, ductal adenocarcinoma, transitional cell carcinoma, sarcomatoid carcinoma, and sarcoma are associated with a worse prognosis.[13–16] The GS is based on the architectural structure of the malignant cells. Current recommendation for core needle biopsies is that the most prevalent and highest grade are summed together for the GS since any amount of high-grade tumor may indicate a more significant amount within the prostate. Tertiary grades are given only in RP specimens if there is a component (< 5%) of higher grade tumor than the two predominant patterns (see Table 39.2).[17] ECE is seen in ~45% of patients with clinically localized disease and is within 2.5 mm in 96% of cases.[18] SV involvement increases with risk group: low risk ~1%, intermediate risk ~15%, and high risk ~30%, with a median 1 cm length of involvement and ~1% risk of SV involvement beyond 2 cm.[19] A grade grouping system was developed by the International Society of Urological Pathology based on GS, which demonstrated an increased risk of biochemical recurrence with increasing grade group (see Table 39.2).[20]

Table 39.2: ISUP Consensus Grouping[20]		
Grade Group	Gleason Score(s)	HR of Biochemical Recurrence
1	≤6	Reference
2	3 + 4 = 7	1.9
3	4 + 3 = 7	5.4
4	8	8.0
5	9 or 10	11.7

GENETICS: Several tissue-based tests have been developed to determine prognosis, including Oncotype DX Genomic Prostate Score (Genomic Health, Redwood City, California), which is a 17-gene expression panel used in patients with very low, low, and "modified intermediate" risk cancer, which predicts risk of recurrence, prostate cancer death, and aggressive features on pathology (Gleason ≥ 4 + 3 or pT3) after RP.[21] This test, as well as others, can be used in patients with at least 10-year life expectancy, who might be candidates for active surveillance (AS) or definitive therapy.[22] Another novel genomic classifier test was observed to predict 10-year DM rates in conjunction with NCCN risk groups.[23]

SCREENING: The AUA recommends PSA screening every 1 to 2 years for men aged 55 to 69 years of age with life expectancy >10 years. Screening decisions should be individualized for men 40 to 54 years of age with other risk factors.[24] Free PSA (ratio of free PSA/total PSA, with lower free PSA predicting higher risk of cancer) and PSA velocity (> 0.75 ng/mL/year) can increase the positive predictive value of screening.[25] PSA velocity of >2 ng/mL in the year previous to diagnosis has been associated with increased risk of death due to prostate cancer.[26] The half-life of PSA is ~2.2 days. PSA levels can be increased by prostatitis, urinary retention, DRE, ejaculation, TRUS biopsy, TURP, and BPH. Medical treatment for BPH with 5α-reductase inhibitors such as finasteride decreases PSA by ~50% within 6 months of use, and thus correct PSA by multiplying by 2 in the first 2 years and by 2.3× for longer-term use.[27,28] National screening guidelines do not recommend DRE alone for screening (poor PPV of 4%–11%).[29] Combined DRE and PSA screening is left to the discretion of physicians, and DRE is recommended in any patient with suspicious PSA.[24] DRE palpates only the posterior and lateral aspects of the prostate gland, which inherently limits its screening utility, but 85% of prostate cancers arise from these locations. DRE has a sensitivity of 53% and specificity of 86% in one study.[30] A multicenter screening study demonstrated that PSA detected significantly more prostate cancer than DRE (82% vs. 55%; $p = .001$).[31] PCA3 is an RNA biomarker overexpressed by malignant cells and can be found in urine after an "attentive" DRE, with a "minimum of 6 pressed strokes on the prostate from lateral to medial"; this test may be a useful surrogate to repeat biopsies in the detection of cancer with a high negative predictive value (88%), but its use is not routine.[32] The 4K score is a blood test that measures prostate-specific kallikrein used to determine patient-specific probability of finding GS $\geq$7 on biopsy.[33] Serum levels are combined with an algorithm including patient age, presence of palpable nodule on DRE, and prior negative biopsy to give a percent risk score (1%–95%) of having aggressive cancer on biopsy.

CLINICAL PRESENTATION: Prostate cancer is usually asymptomatic, with the majority diagnosed by PSA value or as an incidental finding on TURP. Suspicious DRE findings include areas of nodularity, asymmetry, or induration. Some patients with locally advanced disease may present with obstructive urinary symptoms (weak or interrupted stream), polyuria, and less frequently, dysuria and hematuria. Unexplained bony pain may suggest metastatic disease, but this is rare in patients with otherwise low-risk prostate cancer.

WORKUP: H&P, including DRE and assessment of baseline urinary, bowel, and sexual function. The AUA score (a.k.a. International Prostate Symptom Score or IPSS) can be used to assess urinary function (range 0–5 points for 7 questions; total score 35, with higher score implying worse symptoms) based on incomplete emptying, frequency, intermittency, urgency, weak stream, straining, and nocturia. The SHIM score is commonly used to assess baseline erectile function (range 0/1–5 points for 5 questions; total score 25, with higher score signifying better erections).

Labs: PSA, preoperative workup if surgery indicated.

Biopsy: TRUS-guided random biopsy involving removal of 8 to 12 cores of tissue is the most common approach for diagnosis. A systematic review suggested that MRI-targeted biopsy may detect clinically significant cancers with less core samples compared to conventional prostate biopsy techniques.[34]

Imaging: No role for routine staging scans in low-risk prostate cancer. Multi-parametric MRI may be used in patients considering AS as it may detect lesions concerning for GS $\geq$7 cancer or ECE.

PROGNOSTIC FACTORS: Risk stratification of prostate cancer is based primarily upon clinical staging by DRE, pre-treatment PSA, GS/grade group on biopsy, and the number of biopsy cores involved with cancer. Several risk classifications exist, including the NCCN, D'Amico, and AJCC risk categories (Tables 39.3 and 39.4). Further discussion of favorable- and unfavorable-intermediate risk classification can be found in Chapter 40. Other prognostic factors also exist, including cancer volume (>4 cm³ demonstrated shorter time to PSA failure),[35] PNI on biopsy (associated with higher rate of positive margin, but has not been shown to be an independent predictor of PSA recurrence),[36] and the presence of disseminated cancer cells (>5 disseminated cancer cells per 7.5 mL associated with shorter OS in three randomized trials).[37] The UCSF–CAPRA nomogram includes age ($\geq$50 years vs. <50 years), PSA, GS, clinical stage (T1/T2 vs. T3a), percentage of biopsy core involved (<34% vs. $\geq$34%) to predict likelihood of disease recurrence or progression.[38]

NATURAL HISTORY: The risk of death from early-stage, low-risk disease is ~1% at 10 years (per active monitoring arm of the ProtecT trial). Many tumors follow an indolent course for the first 10 to 15 years after diagnosis, but beyond 15 years, the PCSM rate triples (15/1,000 person-years to 44/1,000 person-years).[39] Per the Pound study of patients with biochemical failure after prostatectomy, metastases developed at a median of 8 years after biochemical failure and death occurred at a median of 5 years from the development of DM.[40]

STAGING

Table 39.3: AJCC 8th ed. (2017): Prostate Cancer Staging							
cT		**pT**		**N**		**M**	
T1	a. Incidental finding in ≤5% of tissue resected			**N0**	• No regional LNs	**M1a**	• Nonregional LNs
	b. Incidental finding in >5% of tissue resected						
	c. Identified by needle biopsy (e.g., PSA), but not palpable						
T2	a. Palpable ≤½ of one lobe or less	**T2**	• Organ-confined disease	**N1**	• Metastasis in regional LNs	**M1b**	• Metastasis to bone
	b. Palpable >½ of one lobe, but not both lobes						
	c. Palpable both lobes						
T3	a. EPE	**T3**	a. EPE or microscopic bladder neck invasion			**M1c**	• Metastasis to other sites with or without bone disease
	b. SV invasion		b. SV invasion				
T4	Invasion[1]	**T4**	• Invasion[1]				

AJCC 8th edition (2017): Prognostic Stage Groups	
I	cT1a-c, cT2a or pT2 + PSA < 10 ng/mL + grade group 1
IIA	cT1a-c or cT2a + PSA ≥ 10 and < 20 ng/mL + grade group 1 cT2b-c + PSA < 20 ng/mL + grade group 1
IIB	T1-T2, PSA < 20 ng/mL, grade group 2
IIC	T1-T2, PSA< 20 ng/mL, grade group 3 T1-T2, PSA< 20 ng/mL, grade group 4
IIIA	T1-T2, PSA ≥ 20, grade groups 1–4
IIIB	T3-T4, Any PSA, grade groups 1–4
IIIC	Any T, Any PSA, grade group 5
IVA	Any T, N1, Any PSA, any grade group
IVB	Any T, M1, Any PSA, any grade group

Notes: Invasion[1] = Invasion into bladder, external sphincter, rectum, levator muscles, pelvic wall.

Table 39.4: Risk Stratifications for Prostate Cancer (Other Than AJCC Staging)		
NCCN Risk Classification[41]		**D'Amico Risk Categories**[42]
Very low risk	T1 GS ≤ 6 PSA < 10 ng/mL <3 positive biopsy cores <50% cancer in any core PSA density <0.15 ng/mL/g	**Low risk** T1–2a, and GS ≤ 6, and PSA < 10 ng/mL
Low risk	T1–T2a, and GS ≤ 6/grade group 1, and PSA < 10 ng/mL	
Favorable intermediate risk	T2b–T2c, or GS 3 + 4 = 7/grade group 2, or PSA 10–20 ng/mL, and Percent of positive biopsy cores < 50%	**Intermediate risk** T2b, or GS 7, or PSA 10–20 ng/mL
Unfavorable intermediate risk	2 or 3 intermediate risk factors (above), and/or Grade group 3, and/or ≥50% cores positive	
High risk	T3a, or GS 8/grade group 4, or GS 9–10/grade group 5, or PSA > 20 ng/mL	**High risk** ≤T2c, or GS 8–10, or PSA > 20 ng/mL
Very high risk	T3b–T4, or Primary Gleason pattern 5/grade group 5, or > 4 cores with GS 8–10/grade group 4 or 5	

TREATMENT PARADIGM

AS and WW: AS involves regular monitoring of patients with PSA, DRE, and biopsy, and evidence of progression will prompt conversion to potentially curative treatment. This is different from WW, in which monitoring continues but treatment is typically initiated only when symptoms develop. Recommendations for AS criteria vary but can include most patients who have low-risk disease (GS ≤ 6) with a "reasonable" life expectancy,[43] while NCCN recommends it for very low-risk disease and life expectancy ≤20 years.[41] Genomic profiling may help identify patients appropriate for AS. WW recommendations also vary and can be considered for patients with low-risk cancer and limited life expectancy (<10 years).[41,43]

Prevention: The role of 5-α-reductase inhibitors to prevent cancer progression in the setting of AS is debatable among consensus guidelines, but the REDEEM trial revealed lower 3-year rates of prostate cancer progression with dutasteride, compared to placebo (38% vs. 48%, $p = .009$).[44] Finasteride is currently not approved by the FDA for prevention of prostate cancer.

Surgery: RP approaches include retropubic or laparoscopic/robotic approach. Robotic surgery has been compared to open surgery in one single-institution RCT, which reported early outcomes at 6 and 12 weeks and demonstrated similar rates of positive surgical margins, postoperative complications, intraoperative adverse events, and similar patient-reported urinary and sexual function scores for both techniques.[45] A perineal approach omits lymphadenectomy and SV removal, and has been shown to be associated with higher rates of biochemical failure, +margins, capsular incisions, and rectal injury.[46] The positive margin rates for open, laparoscopic, and robotic techniques are estimated to be 23%, 15%, and 14%, respectively.[47] Perioperative complications are rare and include mortality (<1%), rectal injury (<1%), thromboembolism (1%–3%), myocardial infarction (1%–8%), wound infection (<1%), <1 L blood loss, and pelvic pain.[48,49] Impotence and incontinence are the most common postoperative adverse effects. Bilateral nerve-sparing procedure is associated with an estimated ~50% rate of impotence and unilateral nerve-sparing procedure is associated with impotence rate of ~75%. In one study, an estimated 32% of patients reported total urinary control, 40% occasional leakage,

7% frequent leakage, and 1%–2% no urinary control.[50] A standard lymph node dissection involves sampling of the obturator and external iliac lymph nodes. It is uncertain whether an extended lymph node dissection improves outcomes.

Radiation

Indications: Definitive RT is an option for low-risk prostate cancer, without contraindications such as prior pelvic RT or inflammatory bowel disease.

Dose: Dose escalation with conventional EBRT has been shown to improve biochemical outcomes in several randomized trials, but without an improvement in OS. Dose and fractionation vary widely in practice. Common conventionally fractionation regimens: 78 Gy/39 fx or 79.2 Gy/44 fx. Moderately hypofractionated options such as 70 Gy/28 fx or 60 Gy/20 fx have been tested in large prospective trials. For SBRT, 36.25 to 40 Gy in 5 fx delivered QOD is a commonly utilized regimen, although SBRT has not been tested against IMRT in a randomized trial. Brachytherapy is frequently used for low-risk prostate cancer with comparable outcomes to surgery and EBRT, but no randomized trial has compared these modalities head to head for assessment of clinical outcomes. Dose for LDR brachytherapy is 144 to 145 Gy for I-125 or 125 Gy for Pd-103. For low-risk and favorable intermediate-risk prostate cancer, there is no role for combining EBRT with brachytherapy boost or with ADT; monotherapy is sufficient. Recent evidence suggests HDR brachytherapy monotherapy delivered in two fractions is well tolerated with favorable 5-year outcomes, and is superior to single-fraction HDR brachytherapy.[51] After RT, PSA surveillance should occur ~q6 months. Per RTOG-ASTRO Phoenix Consensus, the definition of biochemical failure is a rise of 2 ng/mL above the post-treatment nadir PSA.[52] A PSA "bounce" phenomenon may occur in some patients, particularly after brachytherapy, and is not associated with worse outcomes.

Toxicity: Acute: Fatigue, dysuria, urgency, frequency, retention, rectal urgency, diarrhea. Late: Stricture, cystitis, proctitis, sexual dysfunction, second malignancy. QOL outcomes have been compared between these therapies and each modality is associated with distinct patterns of change in terms of urinary, bowel, and sexual function (see the ProtecT and PROST-QA trials).

Procedure: See *Handbook of Treatment Planning in Radiation Oncology*, Chapter 8.[53,54]

Other: Other treatments such as HIFU and cryotherapy are emerging techniques but are not recommended as first-line options per NCCN guidelines.

■ **EVIDENCE-BASED Q&A**

SCREENING AND PREVENTION

▪ **What is the value of PSA screening? Why did the U.S. Preventive Services Task Force (USPSTF) previously recommend against PSA screening?**

Despite stage migration toward early localized disease and a decrease in metastatic rates in the PSA era, the USPSTF recommended against routine PSA screening in 2018 for men over 70 years old, but recommended that the screening decision for men aged 55 to 69 years be "an individual one."[55] There are three major screening trials, and the methodology suggests that the magnitude of screening may be likely larger than represented. The ERSPC and Swedish Trial shows a PCSM benefit for PSA screening, while PLCO did not. Notably, it is difficult to keep people in the "observation" arm from being screened, which is one of the criticisms of the PLCO trial.

Schröder, ERSPC (*NEJM* 2009, PMID 19297566; Update *Lancet* 2014, PMID 25108889): A total of 162,388 men (55–69 years of age) randomized to PSA q4 years (on average) vs. no screening. PSA ≥ 3 ng/mL was indication for biopsy in most centers; 1° endpoint PCM. Incidence of prostate cancer was 9.55/1,000 person-years for screening vs. 6.23/1,000 person-years for control group; 355 men in screening group and 545 men in control died from prostate cancer, yielding a PCM rate ratio of 0.79 at 13 years (*p* = .001), corresponding to an NNS of **781** and an NNT of **27** to prevent one death. No difference in ACM. **Conclusion: Reduction in PCM was observed in the cohort randomized to PSA screening.** *Comment: Did not report treatment type, assumed arms were balanced, and overall rate of screening in control group was not reported; there was variance among European centers for recruiting, use of DRE, TRUS, and screening intervals. There is increased survival and decreased progression but at a cost of overdetection and overtreatment.*

Hugosson, Swedish Trial (*Lancet Oncol* 2010, PMID 20598634): A total of 20,000 men 50 to 64 years of age living in Göteborg, Sweden, randomly selected by computer to be screened by PSA every other year or not (no informed consent). PSA > 3 ng/mL was indication for DRE and biopsies; 1° endpoint was PCM; 78% reached maximum follow-up of 14 years, 76% compliance with screening. Incidence and metastatic burden decreased by screening. Prostate cancer incidence of 12.7% in screening group vs. 8.2% in control group (HR 1.64; 95% CI 1.50%–1.80; $P < .0001$). Rate ratio for PCM was 0.56 (95% CI 0.39%–0.82; $P = .002$) for screening vs. control group; 46 screened men vs. 87 controls were dx with metastatic disease ($P = .003$). NNS = 293, NNT = 12 to prevent one prostate cancer death. Risk of prostate cancer was only 2.6% if the first PSA was < 1. **Conclusion: PSA screening is worth it and reduces risk of death by almost half.** *Comment: This is the most "pure" trial because of the randomization and lack of informed consent with good follow-up, and also had the lowest NNS.*

Andriole, PLCO Cancer Screening Trial (*NEJM* 2009, PMID 19297565; Update *J Natl Cancer Inst* 2012, PMID 22228146; Update Shoag, *NEJM* 2016, PMID 27144870): 76,693 men 55 to 74 years of age randomized to annual screening with PSA + DRE vs. usual care. PSA > 4 ng/mL or abnormal DRE was indication for biopsy. Ninety-two percent of participants followed for 10 years. Incidence of prostate cancer was 108 vs. 97 per 10,000 person-years for screening arm vs. control arm, which is a 12% relative increase in incidence rates (RR 1.12), but there was no statistical difference in PCM in screening vs. control arm, 3.7 vs. 3.4 deaths per 10,000 person-years. **Conclusion: No evidence of PCM benefit from annual screening.** *Comment: 45% men had PSA in the 3 years preceding randomization, eliminating prostate cancer prior to randomization; 52% (85% at the update) of men in control arm underwent PSA testing. Because of the crossover contamination and prescreening PSA, many feel these data are insufficient to conclude PSA screening is not useful.*

■ **Can prostate cancer be prevented with 5-α-reductase inhibitors?**

Yes, although 5-a-reductase inhibitors reduce primarily the risk of low-grade cancer.

Thompson, PCPT Trial (*NEJM* 2003, PMID 12824459; Update *NEJM* 2013, PMID 23944298): 18,880 men randomized to finasteride (5 mg/day) vs. placebo. Cutoff level PSA ≤ 3 ng/mL; 10.5% in the finasteride arm vs. 14.9% in the placebo arm were diagnosed with prostate cancer (RR 0.7, 95% CI 0.65–0.76; $P < .001$). Finasteride group compared to placebo had a significant relative risk reduction of low-grade cancers (GS 2-6) (RR 0.57; 95% CI 0.52–0.63; $p < .001$). The finasteride group compared to placebo had more high-grade cancers (GS 7-10; 3.5% vs. 3.0%, RR 1.17, $P = .05$), with no difference in survival between groups for this subset of patients; 15-year OS rates did not differ for finasteride vs. placebo (78% vs. 78.2%). **Conclusion: Finasteride decreases the risk of prostate cancer by about one-third and is "due entirely to a relative reduction of 43% in the risk of low-grade cancer."**

Andriole, REDUCE Trial (*NEJM* 2010, PMID 20357281): 6,729 men randomized to dutasteride 0.5 mg daily vs. placebo. Included men with PSA of 2.5 to 10 ng/mL (ages 50–60) or 3 to 10 ng/mL (> 60 y/o). During study period of 4 years, 19.9% in dutasteride vs. 25.1% in placebo group had a diagnosis of prostate cancer, with relative risk reduction for prostate cancer of 22.8% and absolute risk reduction of 5.1% with dutasteride. The dutasteride group had less GS 5 to 6 cancers compared to placebo (13.2% vs. 18.1%, $P < .001$) and accounted for 70% of cancers. GS 7 to 10 tumors did not differ between groups. During years 3 and 4, there were more GS 8 to 10 tumors in dutasteride group vs. placebo ($P = .003$). No difference in OS between groups. **Conclusion: Dutasteride reduced the risk of prostate cancer mainly due to reduction in GS 5 to 6 cancers.** *Comment: Increase in high GS tumors may be due to gland shrinkage and increased biopsy yield.*

ACTIVE SURVEILLANCE

■ **What are the long-term outcomes of men on active surveillance?**

Klotz (*JCO* 2010, PMID 19917860; Update *JCO* 2015, PMID 25512465): Single-arm cohort of 993 patients followed under AS. Between 1995 and 1999, included all GS ≤ 6 and PSA ≤ 10 ng/mL. If > 70 years of age, PSA ≤ 15 ng/mL or GS ≤ 3+4. From 2000, restricted to GS ≤ 6 and PSA ≤ 10 ng/mL or patients with favorable intermediate-risk disease (PSA 10–20 ng/mL and/or GS 3 + 4) with significant comorbidities and life expectancy < 10 years. Excellent 10- and 15-year actuarial prostate cancer survival rates of 98.1% and 94.3%, respectively. Only 15 of 933 (1.5%) died of prostate cancer and 2.8%

developed metastatic disease. The 10- and 15-year OS rates were 80% and 62%, respectively. At 5, 10, and 15 years, 75.7%, 63.5%, and 55.0% of patients remained untreated and on AS. Patients were 9.2 times more likely to die of causes other than prostate cancer. **Conclusion: AS for low-risk and select favorable intermediate-risk patients seems safe.**

■ Can a 5-α-reductase inhibitor aid patients undergoing active surveillance?

Fleshner, REDEEM Trial (*Lancet* 2012, PMID 22277570): 302 men with Gleason 5 to 6, PSA ≤ 11 placed on AS randomized to dutasteride 0.5 mg daily vs. placebo. Patients followed q3 months for 1 year, then q6 months with a PSA and DRE at each visit q18 months. All patients had repeat biopsy at 18 months and 3 years or if concerning PSA/DRE. Progression defined as ≥ 4 cores involved, ≥ 50% of one core or Gleason pattern 4. At 3 years, prostate cancer progression decreased from 48% to 38% with dutasteride (HR 0.62, 95% CI 0.43–0.89; p = .009). **Conclusion: Dutasteride may be beneficial for reducing progression in AS patients.**

■ Is early treatment better than active surveillance or watchful waiting?

Bill-Axelson, SPCG-4 (*NEJM* 2011, PMID 21542742; QOL *Lancet Onc* 2011, PMID 21821474; *NEJM* 2018, PMID 30575473): PRT of 695 patients with early prostate cancer randomized to RP vs. WW. Progression for WW group defined as palpable ECE or symptoms of obstruction w/ voiding requiring intervention. T2 were 76%, T1c were 12% (not the current population in post-PSA era). Eligibility: age <75 years of age, T1–2, PSA < 50 ng/mL, and life expectancy > 10 years; 6.6% were LN+ at RP. RP had higher rates of at least once-daily urinary leakage (41% vs. 11%) and reported ED (84% vs. 80%) but lower rates of urinary obstruction (29% vs. 40%). Rates of bowel dysfunction, anxiety, depression, well-being, and subjective QOL were similar. NNT to prevent one death at 18-year FU was 8. Update at 23-year FU revealed a mean of 2.9 extra life-years gained with RP, and that ECE and Gleason 7 were associated with higher risk of death from prostate cancer compared to no ECE and Gleason 6, respectively (see Table 39.5). **Conclusion: RP is associated with a statistically significant reduction in all end points.** *Comment: Due to stage migration, these results may not be readily applicable to a modern low-risk population.*

Table 39.5: Results of SPCG-4 Prostatectomy Trial			
	18-Yr DSM	**18-Yr DM**	**18-Yr OM**
WW	28.7%	38.3%	68.9%
RP	17.7%	26.1%	56.1%
p value	.001	<.001	<.001

Wilt, PIVOT Trial (*NEJM* 2012, PMID 22808955; Update *NEJM* 2017, PMID 28700844): PRT of 731 men randomized to AS vs. RP. Included T1–2, any grade, PSA <50, <75 years of age, life expectancy >10 years; 40% low-risk, 34% intermediate, 21% high-risk. AS group: definitive treatment offered for patients with a PSA doubling of <3 yrs, GS progression to ≥ 4 + 3 or clinical progression. MFU 12.7 years (update). In RP arm, 7.4% died from prostate cancer or treatments vs. 4% in observation arm (p = .06). No difference in ACM for RP vs. AS (61.3% vs. 66.8%, p = .06) but RP reduced ACM in intermediate but not low-risk. **Conclusion: RP did not significantly reduce ACM or PCM as compared with AS.** *Comment: Effect size is reasonable (5.5% absolute risk reduction in ACM), and more power may have led to a significant p value.*

Hamdy, UK ProtecT (*NEJM* 2016, PMID 27626136; QOL Donovan *NEJM* 2016, PMID 27626365; Update *Eur Urol* 2020, PMID 31771797): 1,643 patients 50 to 69 years of age with localized prostate cancer randomized to "active monitoring" (AM, PSA monitoring only), surgery (RP), or RT with ADT. Median age 62 years of age, median PSA 4.6 ng/mL (range 3–19.9), 77% had GS 6, 76% had T1c. AM group had PSA q3 months 1st year, q6–12 months thereafter; increase in 50% PSA in previous 12 months triggered a review to continue monitoring or pursue treatment. RT arm had ADT for 3 to 6 months before and concurrent with 3D-CRT to 74 Gy/37 fx. RP arm had post-op PSA q3 months for 1st year, then q6 to 12 months. 1° outcome: PCSS. MFU 10 years. PCSM rates for AM, RP and RT groups were 1.85%, 0.67% and 0.73%, respectively, without any significant difference among groups (P = .08). More DM and disease progression in AM groups than RP or RT group. In AM arm (N = 545): 54.8% received a radical treatment at 10 years. RP arm (N = 391): 2% had PSA > 0.2 ng/mL post-op, 5 had salvage RT, 9 had adjuvant RT within a year after surgery due to pT3 (29%) or +margins (24%). RP NNT = 27 and RT NNT = 33 to avoid one patient having metastatic disease. NNT = 9 with either RP or RT to avoid one patient having clinical progression (see Table 39.6). **Conclusion: Irrespective of treatment arm, PCM remained low at ~1%. Rates of disease progression and metastatic disease were significantly lower for RP or RT compared to AM. ACM and PCSM were much lower in the ProtecT trial than SPCG-4 or PIVOT trials.**

Table 39.6: Results of ProtecT Randomized Trial					
	5-Yr PCSS	10-Yr PCSS	10-Yr Clinical Progression	10-Yr Metastatic Disease	All-Cause Deaths
Active monitoring	99.4%	98.8%	20.4%	5.6%	10.9
Surgery	100%	99%	5.9%	2.4%	10.1
Radiation	100%	99.6%	6.6%	2.7%	10.3
P value	.48	.48	< 0.001	.004	.87

EXTERNAL BEAM RADIATION THERAPY

■ With conventional EBRT, does dose escalation improve outcomes?

There have been at least five major randomized trials investigating "dose escalation" with each one showing a biochemical control benefit (but no difference in OS) for higher doses compared to "conventional" lower doses (~70 Gy at 1.8–2.0 Gy/fx), but also higher rates of rectal bleeding. The current standard dose is 78 to 80 Gy with conventional fractionation (see Table 39.7).

Table 39.7: Summary of Phase III Dose-Escalation Trials for Prostate Cancer					
	Pasalic, MDACC[56]	Zietman, MGH[57]	Heemsbergen, Dutch[58]	Dearnaley, MRC[59]	Michalski, RTOG 0126[60]
Doses	70 vs. 78 Gy	70.2 vs. 79.2 Gy	68 vs. 78 Gy	64 vs. 74 Gy	70.2 vs. 79.2 Gy
N	301	393	669	843	1,499
Technique	4-field box and 3D-CRT	4-field box and proton boost	3D	3D	3D or IMRT
MFU (yrs)	14.3	8.9	9.1	10	7
Biochemical Control	81% vs. 88%, P = .042	67.6% vs. 83.3%, P < .0001	49% vs. 43%, P = .046	43% vs. 55%, P = .0003	55% vs. 70%, P < .0001

■ Is moderate hypofractionation safe and effective?

There have been several randomized trials examining moderate hypofractionation (2.4–4 Gy/fx to 60–70 Gy) compared to conventional fractionation (see Table 39.8). The potential advantages include improved convenience for patients, lower cost, and potentially improved outcomes (due to hypothesized low α/β ratio). Follow-up is moderate, with MFU ranging from 5 to 10 years. This is a reasonable option but longer follow-up will be helpful to establish noninferiority for clinical effectiveness and toxicity profiles.

Table 39.8: Summary of Moderate Hypofractionation Trials in Prostate Cancer

Author, Institution	MFU	Eligibility	Hypofx Arm	Conventional Arm	Outcome
Hoffman, MDACC[61]	8.4 yrs	LR-IR	72 Gy at 2.4 Gy/fx	75.6 at 1.8 Gy/fx	8-yr bRFS 89.3% vs. 84.6%, 10-yr 89.3% vs. 76.3%, P = .036 favoring hypofx arm. No diff in OS or late GI or GU toxicity (but hypofx arm had nonsignificantly more rectal bleeding after treatment). Better control emerged after 5 yrs
Avkshtol, Fox Chase[62]	10.2 yrs	IR-HR	70.2 Gy at 2.7 Gy/fx	76 Gy at 2 Gy/fx	10-yr biochemical/clinical disease failure: 30.6% vs. 25.9% (P = NS). No diff in late toxicity (except those with poor urinary function IPSS > 12 had higher toxicity in hypofx arm). No diff in bF, PCSM, or OS, but trend toward higher DM in hypofx arm
Lee, RTOG 0415[63]	5.8 yrs	LR	70 Gy at 2.5 Gy/fx	73.8 at 1.8 Gy/fx	No SS difference in DFS (HR 0.85; CI 0.64–1.14) or bF (HR 0.77; CI 0.51–1.17). Hypofx arm noninferior to conventional arm. Hypofx arm more late grade 2 GI (18.3% vs. 11.4%, P = .002) and GU toxicity (26.2% vs. 20.5%, P = .06), but this was not clinically significant in patient-reported outcomes (ASTRO 2016)
Dearnaley, CHHiP[64]	5.2 yrs	All (most IR)	60 or 57 Gy at 3 Gy/fx	74 at 2 Gy/fx	5-yr bRFS: 88.3% (74 Gy) vs. 90.6% (60 Gy) vs. 85.9% (57 Gy). 60 Gy not inferior to 74 Gy but noninferiority could NOT be claimed for 57 Gy vs. 74 Gy. No diff in GI/GU toxicity between arms
Incrocci, HYPRO/ Dutch[65]	5 yrs	IR-HR	64.6 Gy at 3.4 Gy/fx	78 Gy at 2 Gy/fx	Treatment failure: 20% hypofx vs. 22% conventional. 5-yr RFS: 80.5% hypofx arm vs. 77.1% conventional arm (P =.36). Grade ≥ 3 late GU toxicity significantly greater for hypofx vs. conventional (19.0% vs. 12.9%; P = .021)
Arcangeli, Italian[66,67]	9 yrs	HR	62 Gy at 3.1 Gy/fx	80 at 2 Gy/fx	10-yr FFBF 72% hypofx vs. 65% conventional (P = .148). No difference in late effects.
Catton, PROFIT[68]	6 yrs	IR	60 Gy at 3 Gy/fx	78 at 2 Gy/fx	5-yr bF in both arms was 15% (HR = 0.96; 90% CI 0.77–1.2). Hypofx arm not inferior to conventional arm. No SS difference in late grade 3 + GI and GU toxicity.

HR, high risk; IR, intermediate risk; LR, low risk.

■ **Is extreme hypofractionation (> 4–10 Gy/fx) delivered with SBRT safe and effective?**

Biochemical control and toxicity outcomes with SBRT are comparable to historical outcomes of dose-escalated 3D/IMRT but longer follow-up is needed (see Table 39.9). Patients should be aware of the shorter follow-up and lack of randomized data with SBRT.

Widmark, HYPO-RT-PC (*Lancet* 2019, PMID 31227373): PRT of 1,180 men undergoing RT for intermediate- (89%) or high-risk (11%) prostate cancer, randomized to conventional fractionation (78 Gy/39 fx) vs. ultra-hypofractionation (42.7 Gy/7 fx QOD). No ADT allowed, and primary endpoint was time to biochemical or clinical failure. MFU 5 years, the estimated failure-free survival was 84% in both arms with adjusted HR of 1.002 (p = .99). There was a trend toward higher incidence of > G2 acute urinary toxicity in ultra-hypofractionation arm (28% vs. 23%, P = .057), and urinary toxicity was higher in ultra-hypofractionation arm at 1 year (6% vs. 2%, P = .0037). **Conclusion: Ultra-hypofractionation is noninferior to conventionally fractionated RT, with regard to failure-free survival, although acute toxicity is slightly more pronounced.**

Jackson, Meta-Analysis (*IJROBP* 2020, PMID 30959121): Meta-analysis of 6,116 men receiving prostate SBRT in 38 prospective trials of which 92% included low-risk, 78% included intermediate-risk, and 38% included high-risk patients. MFU 39 mo. Overall, 5- and 7-year bRFS rates were 95.3% and 93.7%, respectively. Late grade > 3 GU and GI toxicity was 2.0% and 1.1%, respectively. Increased SBRT dose was associated with improved biochemical control (p = .018) but worse late grade > 3 GU toxicity (p = .014). **Conclusion: Prostate SBRT achieves favorable biochemical control and toxicity outcomes.**

Table 39.9: Summary of Select SBRT Series for Prostate Cancer						
Study	N	Dose (Gy/Fx)	Fx	Total Dose	MFU (Years)	Biochemical Control
Meier et al.[69]	309	7.25–8	5	36.25 Gy to PTV and 40 Gy (SIB) to prostate	5.1	97.1%
Parsai et al.[70]	35	7.25–10	5	36.25 Gy to PTV and 50 Gy (SIB) to prostate (sparing urethra, bladder, rectum)	3.8	3 yrs: 88.0%
Katz et al.[71]	515	7–7.25	5	35–36.25 Gy	7	8 yrs: Low risk: 93.6%, Intermediate risk: 84.3% High risk: 65%
Chen et al.[72]	100	7–7.25	5	35–36.25 Gy	2.3	99%
King et al.[73]	67	7.25	5	36.25 Gy	2.7	94%
Boike et al.[74]	45	9–10	5	45–50 Gy	2.5	100%
Freeman et al.[75]	41	7.25	5	35–36.25 Gy	5	93%
Madsen et al.[76]	40	6.7	5	33.5 Gy	3.4	90%

■ **What data exist regarding adverse effects of SBRT?**

Many studies have published low rates of late GI/GU toxicity in short follow-up, but longer follow-up is necessary to observe late effects (see Table 39.10)[77] found that 90% of toxicity events occurred within 3 years of treatment. The early experience from Stanford found that QOD treatment resulted in less toxicity than once daily SBRT (nonrandomized), and so most have adopted a QOD schedule.[73] The preliminary toxicity report from the phase III prospective PACE B Trial, which randomized men with early stage prostate cancer to EBRT (78 Gy/39 fx or 62 Gy/20 fx) vs. SBRT (36.25 Gy/5 fx over 1–2 weeks), revealed similar rates of grade ≥ 2 acute GI (10% vs. 12%) and GU (23% vs. 27%) toxicity between SBRT and EBRT cohorts, respectively, neither of which was statistically significant.[78]

Table 39.10: Summary of Toxicity Outcomes in Select Prostate SBRT Series

Study	Dose	MFU (Years)	Late GI Toxicity	Late GU Toxicity
Zelefsky et al.[79]	Four dose-escalation Rx: 32.5, 35, 37.5, and 40 Gy/5 fx	3.5–5.9	0% > G2	Dose 1: 23% (G2) Dose 2: 26% Dose 3: 28% Dose 4: 31%
Meier et al.[69]	36.25 Gy (SIB to 40 Gy)/5 fx	5.1	2% G2	12% G2
Parsai et al.[70]	36.25 Gy (SIB to 50 Gy)/5 fx	3.8	5.7% ≥ G3	2.9% ≥ G3
Katz et al.[77]	35–36.25 Gy/5 fx	6	4% G2	9% G2 2% G3
King et al.[73]	36.25 Gy/5 fx	2.7	16% G1-2	23% G1 5% G2 3% G3
Freeman et al.[75]	36.25 Gy/5 fx	5	15.5% G1-2	32% G1-2 2.5% G3

■ **Does the fractionation schedule of SBRT affect toxicity outcomes?**

The prospective PATRIOT trial reported decreased patient-reported acute bowel QOL decrement with once-weekly compared to QOD fractionation in men receiving 40 Gy/5 fx.[80] Long-term follow-up, however, revealed similarly low rates of late GI and GU toxicity with either fractionation regimen.[81]

■ **How does the side effect profile compare between RP, EBRT, and brachytherapy?**

Generally, RP has worse incontinence and impotence, EBRT has worse bowel/rectal irritation (without rectal spacer use), and brachytherapy has worse urinary irritation/obstruction. Placement of a rectal spacer can significantly reduce rectal dose and side effects from RT.[70]

Sanda, PROST-QA (*NEJM* 2008, PMID 18354103): First major prospective study (nonrandomized) to document patient- and partner-reported QOL outcomes. Prospective questionnaire of 1,201 patients and 625 spouses given pre- and post- (up to 24 months) definitive RP, brachytherapy, and EBRT for localized T1–T2 cancer. Patients who received EBRT had greatest number of baseline comorbidities, followed by brachytherapy and RP. RP associated with worse sexual and urinary incontinence scores despite higher baseline function. Nerve-sparing surgical procedures had better recovery of sexual QOL. EBRT associated with more irritative and obstructive side effects, as well as bowel toxicity. Large prostates had greater urinary irritation with brachytherapy and greater relief w/ RP. The use of ADT decreased vitality scores. On MVA, the most important factors associated with overall patient satisfaction were sexual function, vitality, and urinary function, in descending order. Patient-related factors that diminished health-related QOL included obesity, large prostate size, elevated initial PSA, older age, and African American race.

Donovan, ProtecT Trial QOL (*NEJM* 2016, PMID 27626365): Same trial as noted previously (Hamdy et al). Patient-reported outcomes through questionnaires given before diagnosis, 6 and 12 months, then annually and reported through 6 years. RP had greatest negative effect on sexual function (erections firm enough for intercourse at 6 months: 52% AM, 22% RT, 12% surgery) and urinary incontinence. RT had peak negative effect on sexual function at 6 months but recovered and stabilized (note: all patients received short-term ADT). RT had little effect on urinary continence but urinary voiding and nocturia problems peaked at 6 months, then recovered by 12 months to be similar to other groups. RT had worse bowel function at 6 months compared to other arms but then recovered (except for frequency of bloody stools, which remained ~5%), while other groups had stable bowel function. Sexual function gradually declined in AM group (erections firm enough for intercourse: 41% yr 3 and 30% at yr 6) as well as urinary function. No differences among groups for anxiety, depression, general health-related or cancer-related QOL.

■ **Is daily image guidance necessary?**

There have been many data reporting inter- and intra-fraction prostate motion signifying the importance of image guidance during treatment.

De Crevoisier (*IJROBP* 2018, PMID 30071296): PRT of daily vs. weekly (days 1, 2, and 3 then weekly) IGRT in N0 localized prostate cancer, treating prostate only with IMRT (mean dose 78 Gy); 470 men enrolled, primary end point 5-year RFS, secondary outcomes OS and toxicity. No difference in RFS. OS worse in the daily IGRT group compared to weekly group ($p = .042$), with more secondary cancer events (11 vs. 24). Acute rectal bleeding and late rectal toxicity lower in daily IGRT group (6% vs. 11%, $p = .014$). Biochemical progression-free interval and clinical progression-free interval both improved with daily IGRT, risk of biochemical and clinical recurrence reduced by a factor of 2 with daily IGRT. **Conclusion: Daily IGRT improves biochemical control and reduces toxicity compared to weekly IGRT, with potential increase in second malignancies, though too few events to conclude.**

REFERENCES

1. Siegel RL, Miller KD, Fuchs HE, Jemal A. Cancer Statistics, 2021. *CA: a cancer journal for clinicians*. 2021;71(1):7-33.
2. Hoffman RM, Gilliland FD, Eley JW, et al. Racial and ethnic differences in advanced-stage prostate cancer: the Prostate Cancer Outcomes Study. *J Natl Cancer Inst*. 2001;93(5):388–395. doi:10.1093/jnci/93.5.388
3. Deka R, Courtney PT, Parsons JK, et al. Association between African American race and clinical outcomes in men treated for low-risk prostate cancer with active surveillance. *JAMA*. 2020;324(17):1747–1754. doi:10.1001/jama.2020.17020
4. Butler S, Muralidhar V, Chavez J, et al. Active surveillance for low-risk prostate cancer in black patients. *N Engl J Med*. 2019;380(21):2070–2072. doi:10.1056/NEJMc1900333
5. Dess RT, Hartman HE, Mahal BA, et al. Association of black race with prostate cancer-specific and other-cause mortality. *JAMA Oncol*. 2019;5(7):975–983. doi:10.1001/jamaoncol.2019.0826
6. Hamilton RJ, Aronson WJ, Presti JC Jr, et al. Race, biochemical disease recurrence, and prostate-specific antigen doubling time after radical prostatectomy: results from the SEARCH database. *Cancer*. 2007;110(10):2202–2209. doi:10.1002/cncr.23012
7. Agalliu I, Gern R, Leanza S, Burk RD. Associations of high-grade prostate cancer with BRCA1 and BRCA2 founder mutations. *Clin Cancer Res*. 2009;15(3):1112–1120. doi:10.1158/1078-0432.CCR-08-1822
8. Castro E, Goh C, Olmos D, et al. Germline BRCA mutations are associated with higher risk of nodal involvement, distant metastasis, and poor survival outcomes in prostate cancer. *J Clin Oncol*. 2013;31(14):1748–1757. doi:10.1200/JCO.2012.43.1882
9. Raymond VM, Mukherjee B, Wang F, et al. Elevated risk of prostate cancer among men with Lynch syndrome. *J Clin Oncol*. 2013;31(14):1713–1718. doi:10.1200/JCO.2012.44.1238
10. Tischkowitz M, Easton DF, Ball J, Hodgson SV, Mathew CG. Cancer incidence in relatives of British Fanconi Anaemia patients. *BMC Cancer*. 2008;8:257. doi:10.1186/1471-2407-8-257
11. Ewing CM, Ray AM, Lange EM, et al. Germline mutations in HOXB13 and prostate-cancer risk. *N Engl J Med*. 2012;366(2):141–149. doi:10.1056/NEJMoa1110000
12. Deurloo KE, Steenbakkers RJ, Zijp LJ, et al. Quantification of shape variation of prostate and seminal vesicles during external beam radiotherapy. *Int J Radiat Oncol Biol Phys*. 2005;61(1):228–238. doi:10.1016/j.ijrobp.2004.09.023
13. Epstein JI, Egevad L, Amin MB, et al. The 2014 International Society of Urological Pathology (ISUP) consensus conference on gleason grading of prostatic carcinoma: definition of grading patterns and proposal for a new grading system. *Am J Surg Pathol*. 2016;40(2):244–252. doi:10.1097/PAS.0000000000000530
14. Tetu B, Ro JY, Ayala AG, et al. Small cell carcinoma of the prostate. Part I. A clinicopathologic study of 20 cases. *Cancer*. 1987;59(10):1803–1809. doi:10.1002/1097-0142(19870515)59:10<1803::AID-CNCR2820591019>3.0.CO;2-X
15. Robinson B, Magi-Galluzzi C, Zhou M. Intraductal carcinoma of the prostate. *Arch Pathol Lab Med*. 2012;136(4):418–425. doi:10.5858/arpa.2011-0519-RA
16. Palou J, Wood D, Bochner BH, et al. ICUD-EAU International Consultation on Bladder Cancer 2012: Urothelial carcinoma of the prostate. *Eur Urol*. 2013;63(1):81–87. doi:10.1016/j.eururo.2012.08.011
17. Markowski MC, Eisenberger MA, Zahurak M, et al. Sarcomatoid carcinoma of the prostate: retrospective review of a case series from the Johns Hopkins Hospital. *Urology*. 2015;86(3):539–543. doi:10.1016/j.urology.2015.06.011
18. Gordetsky J, Epstein J. Grading of prostatic adenocarcinoma: current state and prognostic implications. *Diagn Pathol*. 2016;11:25. doi:10.1186/s13000-016-0478-2
19. Davis BJ, Pisansky TM, Wilson TM, et al. The radial distance of extraprostatic extension of prostate carcinoma: implications for prostate brachytherapy. *Cancer*. 1999;85(12):2630–2637. doi:10.1002/(SICI)1097-0142(19990615)85:12<2630::AID-CNCR20>3.0.CO;2-L

20. Kestin L, Goldstein N, Vicini F, et al. Treatment of prostate cancer with radiotherapy: should the entire seminal vesicles be included in the clinical target volume? *Int J Radiat Oncol Biol Phys*. 2002;54(3):686–697. doi:10.1016/S0360-3016(02)03011-0

21. Cullen J, Rosner IL, Brand TC, et al. A biopsy-based 17-gene genomic prostate score predicts recurrence after radical prostatectomy and adverse surgical pathology in a racially diverse population of men with clinically low- and intermediate-risk prostate cancer. *Eur Urol*. 2015;68(1):123–131. doi:10.1016/j.eururo.2014.11.030

22. Ross JR, Saunders Y, Edmonds PM, et al. Systematic review of role of bisphosphonates on skeletal morbidity in metastatic cancer. *BMJ (Clinical research ed)*. 2003;327:469. doi:10.1136/bmj.327.7413.469

23. Spratt DE, Zhang J, Santiago-Jiménez M, et al. Development and validation of a novel integrated clinical-genomic risk group classification for localized prostate cancer. *J Clin Oncol*. 2018;36(6):581–590. doi:10.1200/JCO.2017.74.2940

24. Gershman B, Van Houten HK, Herrin J, et al. Impact of Prostate-specific Antigen (PSA) screening trials and revised PSA screening guidelines on rates of prostate biopsy and postbiopsy complications. *Eur Urol*. 2017;71(1):55–65. doi:10.1016/j.eururo.2016.03.015

25. Catalona WJ, Partin AW, Slawin KM, et al. Use of the percentage of free prostate-specific antigen to enhance differentiation of prostate cancer from benign prostatic disease: a prospective multicenter clinical trial. *JAMA*. 1998;279(19):1542–1547. doi:10.1001/jama.279.19.1542

26. D'Amico AV, Chen MH, Roehl KA, Catalona WJ. Preoperative PSA velocity and the risk of death from prostate cancer after radical prostatectomy. *N Engl J Med*. 2004;351(2):125–135. doi:10.1056/NEJMoa032975

27. Guess HA, Heyse JF, Gormley GJ. The effect of finasteride on prostate-specific antigen in men with benign prostatic hyperplasia. *Prostate*. 1993;22(1):31–37. doi:10.1002/pros.2990220105

28. Thompson IM, Goodman PJ, Tangen CM, et al. The influence of finasteride on the development of prostate cancer. *N Engl J Med*. 2003;349(3):215–224. doi:10.1056/NEJMoa030660

29. Schroder FH, van der Maas P, Beemsterboer P, et al. Evaluation of the digital rectal examination as a screening test for prostate cancer. Rotterdam section of the European Randomized Study of Screening for Prostate Cancer. *J Natl Cancer Inst*. 1998;90(23):1817–1823. doi:10.1093/jnci/90.23.1817

30. Mistry K, Cable G. Meta-analysis of prostate-specific antigen and digital rectal examination as screening tests for prostate carcinoma. *J Am Board Fam Pract*. 2003;16(2):95–101. doi:10.3122/jabfm.16.2.95

31. Catalona WJ, Richie JP, Ahmann FR, et al. Comparison of digital rectal examination and serum prostate specific antigen in the early detection of prostate cancer: results of a multicenter clinical trial of 6,630 men. *J Urol*. 1994;151(5):1283–1290. doi:10.1016/S0022-5347(17)35233-3

32. Wei JT, Feng Z, Partin AW, et al. Can urinary PCA3 supplement PSA in the early detection of prostate cancer? *J Clin Oncol*. 2014;32(36):4066–4072. doi:10.1200/JCO.2013.52.8505

33. Parekh DJ, Punnen S, Sjoberg DD, et al. A multi-institutional prospective trial in the USA confirms that the 4Kscore accurately identifies men with high-grade prostate cancer. *Eur Urol*. 2015;68(3):464–470. doi:10.1016/j.eururo.2014.10.021

34. Moore CM, Robertson NL, Arsanious N, et al. Image-guided prostate biopsy using magnetic resonance imaging-derived targets: a systematic review. *Eur Urol*. 2013;63(1):125–140. doi:10.1016/j.eururo.2012.06.004

35. D'Amico AV, Whittington R, Malkowicz SB, et al. Calculated prostate cancer volume greater than 4.0 cm^3 identifies patients with localized prostate cancer who have a poor prognosis following radical prostatectomy or external-beam radiation therapy. *J Clin Oncol*. 1998;16(9):3094–3100. doi:10.1200/JCO.1998.16.9.3094

36. D'Amico AV, Wu Y, Chen MH, Nash M, Renshaw AA, Richie JP. Perineural invasion as a predictor of biochemical outcome following radical prostatectomy for select men with clinically localized prostate cancer. *J Urol*. 2001;165(1):126–129. doi:10.1097/00005392-200101000-00031

37. Goldkorn A, Ely B, Quinn DI, et al. Circulating tumor cell counts are prognostic of overall survival in SWOG S0421: a phase III trial of docetaxel with or without atrasentan for metastatic castration-resistant prostate cancer. *J Clin Oncol*. 2014;32(11):1136–1142. doi:10.1200/JCO.2013.51.7417

38. Punnen S, Freedland SJ, Presti JC Jr, et al. Multi-institutional validation of the CAPRA-S score to predict disease recurrence and mortality after radical prostatectomy. *Eur Urol*. 2014;65(6):1171–1177. doi:10.1016/j.eururo.2013.03.058

39. Johansson JE, Andren O, Andersson SO, et al. Natural history of early, localized prostate cancer. *JAMA*. 2004;291(22):2713–2719. doi:10.1001/jama.291.22.2713

40. Pound CR, Partin AW, Eisenberger MA, et al. Natural history of progression after PSA elevation following radical prostatectomy. *JAMA*. 1999;281(17):1591–1597. doi:10.1001/jama.281.17.1591

41. National Comprehensive Cancer Network. Prostate Cancer (Version 2.2017). 2017. https://www.nccn.org/professionals/physician_gls/pdf/prostate.pdf

42. D'Amico AV, Whittington R, Malkowicz SB, et al. Biochemical outcome after radical prostatectomy, external beam radiation therapy, or interstitial radiation therapy for clinically localized prostate cancer. *JAMA*. 1998;280(11):969–974. doi:10.1001/jama.280.11.969

43. Chen RC, Rumble RB, Loblaw DA, et al. Active surveillance for the management of localized prostate cancer (Cancer Care Ontario Guideline): American Society of Clinical Oncology Clinical Practice Guideline Endorsement. *J Clin Oncol*. 2016;34(18):2182–2190. doi:10.1200/JCO.2015.65.7759

44. Fleshner NE, Lucia MS, Egerdie B, et al. Dutasteride in localised prostate cancer management: the REDEEM randomised, double-blind, placebo-controlled trial. *Lancet*. 2012;379(9821):1103–1111. doi:10.1016/S0140-6736(11)61619-X

45. Yaxley JW, Coughlin GD, Chambers SK, et al. Robot-assisted laparoscopic prostatectomy versus open radical retropubic prostatectomy: early outcomes from a randomised controlled phase 3 study. *Lancet*. 2016;388(10049):1057–1066. doi:10.1016/S0140-6736(16)30592-X

46. Boccon-Gibod L, Ravery V, Vordos D, et al. Radical prostatectomy for prostate cancer: the perineal approach increases the risk of surgically induced positive margins and capsular incisions. *J Urol*. 1998;160(4):1383–1385. doi:10.1097/00005392-199810000-00045

47. Sooriakumaran P, Srivastava A, Shariat SF, et al. A multinational, multi-institutional study comparing positive surgical margin rates among 22393 open, laparoscopic, and robot-assisted radical prostatectomy patients. *Eur Urol*. 2014;66(3):450–456. doi:10.1016/j.eururo.2013.11.018

48. Alibhai SM, Leach M, Tomlinson G, et al. 30-day mortality and major complications after radical prostatectomy: influence of age and comorbidity. *J Natl Cancer Inst*. 2005;97(20):1525–1532. doi:10.1093/jnci/dji313

49. Van Hemelrijck M, Garmo H, Holmberg L, et al. Thromboembolic events following surgery for prostate cancer. *Eur Urol*. 2013;63(2):354–363. doi:10.1016/j.eururo.2012.09.041

50. Stanford JL, Feng Z, Hamilton AS, et al. Urinary and sexual function after radical prostatectomy for clinically localized prostate cancer: the Prostate Cancer Outcomes Study. *JAMA*. 2000;283(3):354–360. doi:10.1001/jama.283.3.354

51. Morton G, McGuffin M, Chung HT, et al. Prostate high dose-rate brachytherapy as monotherapy for low and intermediate risk prostate cancer: efficacy results from a randomized phase II clinical trial of one fraction of 19 Gy or two fractions of 13.5 Gy. *Radiother Oncol*. 2020;146:90–96. doi:10.1016/j.radonc.2020.02.009

52. Roach M 3rd, Hanks G, Thames H Jr, et al. Defining biochemical failure following radiotherapy with or without hormonal therapy in men with clinically localized prostate cancer: recommendations of the RTOG-ASTRO Phoenix Consensus Conference. *Int J Radiat Oncol Biol Phys*. 2006;65(4):965–974. doi:10.1016/j.ijrobp.2006.04.029

53. Videtic GMM, Woody N, Vassil AD. *Handbook of Treatment Planning in Radiation Oncology*. 2nd ed. Demos Medical; 2015. doi:10.1891/9781617051975

54. Videtic GMM, Woody N, Vassil AD. *Handbook of Treatment Planning in Radiation Oncology*. 3rd ed. Demos Medical; 2020. doi:10.1891/9780826168429

55. Fenton JJ, Weyrich MS, Durbin S, et al. Prostate-specific antigen-based screening for prostate cancer: evidence report and systematic review for the US Preventive Services Task Force. *JAMA*. 2018;319(18):1914–1931. doi:10.1001/jama.2018.3712

56. Pasalic D, Kuban DA, Allen PK, et al. Dose escalation for prostate adenocarcinoma: a long-term update on the outcomes of a Phase 3, Single Institution Randomized Clinical Trial. *Int J Radiat Oncol Biol Phys*. 2019;104(4):790–797. doi:10.1016/j.ijrobp.2019.02.045

57. Zietman AL, Bae K, Slater JD, et al. Randomized trial comparing conventional-dose with high-dose conformal radiation therapy in early-stage adenocarcinoma of the prostate: long-term results from proton radiation oncology group/american college of radiology 95–09. *J Clin Oncol*. 2010;28(7):1106–1111. doi:10.1200/JCO.2009.25.8475

58. Heemsbergen WD, Al-Mamgani A, Slot A, et al. Long-term results of the Dutch randomized prostate cancer trial: impact of dose-escalation on local, biochemical, clinical failure, and survival. *Radiother Oncol*. 2014;110(1):104–109. doi:10.1016/j.radonc.2013.09.026

59. Dearnaley DP, Jovic G, Syndikus I, et al. Escalated-dose versus control-dose conformal radiotherapy for prostate cancer: long-term results from the MRC RT01 randomised controlled trial. *Lancet Oncol*. 2014;15(4):464–473. doi:10.1016/S1470-2045(14)70040-3

60. Michalski JM, Moughan J, Purdy J, et al. Effect of standard vs dose-escalated radiation therapy for patients with intermediate-risk prostate cancer: the NRG Oncology RTOG 0126 Randomized Clinical Trial. *JAMA Oncol*. 2018;4(6):e180039. doi:10.1001/jamaoncol.2018.0039

61. Hoffman KE, Voong KR, Levy LB, et al. Randomized trial of hypofractionated, dose-escalated, Intensity-Modulated Radiation Therapy (IMRT) versus conventionally fractionated IMRT for localized prostate cancer. *J Clin Oncol*. 2018;36(6):2943–2949. doi:10.1200/JCO.2018.77.9868

62. Avkshtol V, Ruth KJ, Ross EA, et al. Ten-year update of a randomized, prospective trial of conventional fractionated versus moderate hypofractionated radiation therapy for localized prostate cancer. *J Clin Oncol*. 2020;38(15):1676–1684. doi:10.1200/JCO.19.01485

63. Lee WR, Dignam JJ, Amin MB, et al. Randomized phase III noninferiority study comparing two radiotherapy fractionation schedules in patients with low-risk prostate cancer. *J Clin Oncol*. 2016;34(20):2325–2332. doi:10.1200/JCO.2016.67.0448

64. Dearnaley D, Syndikus I, Mossop H, et al. Conventional versus hypofractionated high-dose intensity-modulated radiotherapy for prostate cancer: 5-year outcomes of the randomised, non-inferiority, phase 3 CHHiP trial. *Lancet Oncol*. 2016;17(8):1047–1060. doi:10.1016/S1470-2045(16)30102-4

65. Incrocci L, Wortel RC, Alemayehu WG, et al. Hypofractionated versus conventionally fractionated radiotherapy for patients with localised prostate cancer (HYPRO): final efficacy results from a randomised, multicentre, open-label, phase 3 trial. *Lancet Oncol*. 2016;17(8):1061–1069. doi:10.1016/S1470-2045(16)30070-5

66. Arcangeli S, Strigari L, Gomellini S, et al. Updated results and patterns of failure in a randomized hypofractionation trial for high-risk prostate cancer. *Int J Radiat Oncol Biol Phys*. 2012;84(5):1172–1178. doi:10.1016/j.ijrobp.2012.02.049

67. Arcangeli G, Saracino B, Arcangeli S, et al. Moderate hypofractionation in high-risk, organ-confined prostate cancer: final results of a phase III randomized trial. *J Clin Oncol*. 2017;35(17):1891–1897. doi:10.1200/JCO.2016.70.4189

68. Catton CN, Lukka H, Gu CS, et al. Randomized trial of a hypofractionated radiation regimen for the treatment of localized prostate cancer. *J Clin Oncol*. 2017;35(17):1884–1890.

69. Meier RM, Bloch DA, Cotrutz C, et al. Multicenter trial of stereotactic body radiation therapy for low- and inter-mediate-risk prostate cancer: survival and toxicity endpoints. *Int J Radiat Oncol Biol Phys.* 2018;102(2):296–303. doi:10.1016/j.ijrobp.2018.05.040

70. Parsai S, Juloori A, Sedor G, et al. Heterogenous dose-escalated prostate stereotactic body radiation therapy for all risk prostate cancer: quality of life and clinical outcomes of an institutional pilot study. *Am J Clin Oncol.* 2020;43(7):469–476. doi:10.1097/COC.0000000000000693

71. Katz A, Formenti SC, Kang J. Predicting biochemical disease-free survival after prostate stereotactic body radio-therapy: risk-stratification and patterns of failure. *Front Oncol.* 2016;6:168. doi:10.3389/fonc.2016.00168

72. Chen LN, Suy S, Uhm S, et al. Stereotactic body radiation therapy (SBRT) for clinically localized prostate cancer: the Georgetown University experience. *Radiat Oncol.* 2013;8:58. doi:10.1186/1748-717X-8-58

73. King CR, Brooks JD, Gill H, Presti JC Jr. Long-term outcomes from a prospective trial of stereotactic body radio-therapy for low-risk prostate cancer. *Int J Radiat Oncol Biol Phys.* 2012;82(2):877–882. doi:10.1016/j.ijrobp.2010.11.054

74. Boike TP, Lotan Y, Cho LC, et al. Phase I dose-escalation study of stereotactic body radiation therapy for low- and intermediate-risk prostate cancer. *J Clin Oncol.* 2011;29(15):2020–2026. doi:10.1200/JCO.2010.31.4377

75. Freeman DE, King CR. Stereotactic body radiotherapy for low-risk prostate cancer: five-year outcomes. *Radiat Oncol.* 2011;6:3. doi:10.1186/1748-717X-6-3

76. Madsen BL, Hsi RA, Pham HT, et al. Stereotactic hypofractionated accurate radiotherapy of the prostate (SHARP), 33.5 Gy in five fractions for localized disease: first clinical trial results. *Int J Radiat Oncol Biol Phys.* 2007;67(4):1099–1105. doi:10.1016/j.ijrobp.2006.10.050

77. Katz AJ, Kang J. Quality of life and toxicity after SBRT for organ-confined prostate cancer, a 7-year study. *Front Oncol.* 2014;4:301. doi:10.3389/fonc.2014.00301

78. Brand DH, Tree AC, Ostler P, et al. Intensity-modulated fractionated radiotherapy versus stereotactic body radio-therapy for prostate cancer (PACE-B): acute toxicity findings from an international, randomised, open-label, phase 3, non-inferiority trial. *Lancet Oncol.* 2019;20(11):1531–1543. doi:10.1016/S1470-2045(19)30569-8

79. Zelefsky MJ, Kollmeier M, McBride S, et al. Five-year outcomes of a phase 1 dose-escalation study using stereotac-tic body radiosurgery for patients with low-risk and intermediate-risk prostate cancer. *Int J Radiat Oncol Biol Phys.* 2019;104(1):42–49. doi:10.1016/j.ijrobp.2018.12.045

80. Quon HC, Ong A, Cheung P, et al. Once-weekly versus every-other-day stereotactic body radiotherapy in patients with prostate cancer (PATRIOT): a phase 2 randomized trial. *Radiother Oncol.* 2018;127(2):206–212. doi:10.1016/j.radonc.2018.02.029

81. Alayed Y, Quon H, Ong A, et al. Accelerating prostate stereotactic ablative body radiotherapy: efficacy and toxicity of a randomized phase II study of 11 versus 29 days overall treatment time (PATRIOT). *Radiother Oncol.* 2020;149:8–13. doi:10.1016/j.radonc.2020.04.039

40 ■ INTERMEDIATE- AND HIGH-RISK PROSTATE CANCER

Rahul D. Tendulkar, Bindu V. Manyam, and Omar Y. Mian

QUICK HIT ■ Prostate cancer demonstrates heterogeneous clinical behavior. Most patients with intermediate-risk and nearly all with high-risk disease are treated with local therapy (as opposed to active surveillance). Multimodality therapy is often required, consisting of either prostatectomy ± postoperative RT (depending on pathology findings and PSA kinetics) or definitive RT combined with ADT (4–6 months for intermediate-risk and 18–36 months for high risk) and/or brachytherapy boost (Table 40.1).

Table 40.1: General Treatment Paradigm for Intermediate- and High-Risk Prostate Cancer[1]	
Definitions (NCCN)	**Treatment Options**
IR One or more IRFs but no high-risk features: T2b–T2c or Grade group 2 or 3 or PSA 10–20 ng/mL **FIR** 1 IRF AND Grade group 1 or 2 AND <50% + biopsy cores **UIR** 2 or 3 IRFs and/or Grade group 3 and/or ≥ 50% biopsy cores positive	• Active surveillance (if life expectancy < 10 yrs) • EBRT ± short-term ADT (4–6 months) • Brachytherapy alone (FIR) • EBRT + brachytherapy (UIR) • RP: Consider early salvage RT for adverse features (+ margins, seminal vesicle invasion, extracapsular extension) and detectable postoperative PSA
HR cT3a or GS 8–10 or PSA > 20 ng/mL **VHR** T3b–4 or Primary GS 5 or >4 cores with GS 8–10	• EBRT + long-term ADT (18–36 months) • EBRT + brachytherapy boost + ADT (12–36 months) • RP: Consider early salvage RT for adverse features (+margins, seminal vesicle invasion, extracapsular extension) and detectable postoperative PSA. If lymph node positive, consider ADT + pelvic EBRT • ADT alone reserved for select patients who are not otherwise candidates for local therapy (e.g., if limited life expectancy)
Clinically node positive	• RT + long-term ADT (24–36 months) • ADT ± antiandrogen (if limited life expectancy)

Source: Adapted from Mohler JL, Antonarakis ES, Armstrong AJ, et al. Prostate Cancer, Version 2.2019, NCCN Clinical Practice Guidelines in Oncology. *J Natl Compr Canc Netw: JNCCN.* 2019;17(5):479–505. doi:10.6004/jnccn.2019.0023

EPIDEMIOLOGY: See Chapter 39. About 15% of new prostate cancer diagnoses are comprised of HR disease.[2]

RISK FACTORS: See Chapter 39. Family history, specifically having a father who survived <24 months from prostate cancer, has been associated with higher risk disease.[3] Germline mutations in DNA repair genes occur in about 5% of localized cases, and in particular, germline *BRCA2* mutations are associated with a higher GS and a worse prognosis.[4-6] NCCN guidelines recommend germline genetic testing for patients with a family history of prostate cancer, intraductal/cribriform histology, high-risk localized, lymph node-positive, or metastatic prostate cancer to assess for mutations including *BRCA1, BRCA2, ATM, PALB2, MLH1, MSH2, MSH6,* and *PMS2,*[5] as well as other germline alterations associated with familial prostate cancer.[7] Syndromes associated with increased risk of prostate cancer are Lynch syndrome, Fanconi's anemia, and HOXB13.[8–10]

ANATOMY, PATHOLOGY, SCREENING, CLINICAL PRESENTATION: See Chapter 39. The risk of pelvic nodal involvement has been estimated by both Partin tables and the Roach formula (2/3*PSA+[Gleason-6]*10, which tends to over-stimate risk in the modern era).[11,12]

WORKUP: H&P including DRE and assessment of baseline urinary, bowel, and sexual function.

Labs: PSA, preoperative workup as indicated. Molecular biomarkers such as Decipher, Oncotype, or Prolaris provide prognostic value beyond traditional factors, and NCCN guidelines recommend that such molecular assays be considered for men with UIR and HR prostate cancer and life expectancy >10 years.[13,14]

Imaging: Bone scan indicated for patients at high risk for metastases (indications per NCCN guidelines include any of the following: UIR [if T2 and PSA >10], HR, or VHR). Per NCCN, CT or MRI pelvis is indicated for patients with IR or HR and nomogram-indicated probability of lymph node involvement > 10%.[1] PET-CT with prostate-specific radionuclide tracers (e.g., fluciclovine or PSMA-based) has higher sensitivity and specificity in the detection of metastatic disease, although this is not presently approved in the up-front setting.[15]

NATURAL HISTORY: The Connecticut Tumor Registry demonstrated the probability of dying from untreated prostate cancer within 15 years in a patient with GS 8 to 10 disease was 60% to 87%.[16] Most men treated for HR prostate cancer live >10 years, and remain at risk of death from other causes.[17]

PROGNOSTIC FACTORS, STAGING: See Chapter 39 for prognostic factors, AJCC 8th Edition staging and risk classifications.

TREATMENT PARADIGM

Active surveillance: Not a standard management option for men with UIR and HR prostate cancer but may has a role in select patients with low-volume, FIR prostate cancer, and/or those with a limited life expectancy and multiple medical comorbidities.[18]

Surgery: Radical prostatectomy is an option for IR and HR prostate cancer although some patients will require postoperative RT. There have been no prospective randomized trials comparing RP with EBRT for HR prostate cancer, and retrospective comparisons are difficult to interpret due to significant selection biases. Thus, either operative or non-operative approaches may be considered. See Chapter 39 for details regarding surgical options.

ADT: The decision to use ADT, timing, and sequencing are dependent on disease characteristics and patient factors (Table 40.2). In combination with EBRT, generally 18 to 36 months of ADT are recommended for HR, while 4 to 6 months of ADT should be considered for IR prostate cancer.[1] Most commonly used are GnRH agonists (e.g., leuprolide) alone or with oral antiandrogens (combined androgen blockade). Testosterone recovery after treatment with GnRH agonists can be delayed by several months to years.[19,20] Relugolix is an oral GnRH antagonist as effective as leuprolide for long-term castration, with fewer cardiovascular events and the advantage of rapid reversibility.[21] Systemic therapy alone is used for treatment of metastatic prostate cancer or for select patients who are not otherwise candidates for definitive local therapy. Side effects include impotence, decreased libido, fatigue, weight gain, hot flashes, cognitive changes, depression, osteoporosis, sarcopenia, and potentially cardiovascular disease.

Radiation

Indications: Unless contraindicated (e.g., prior pelvic RT or inflammatory bowel disease), EBRT is an appropriate option for all patients with IR and HR prostate cancer, and is typically delivered by IMRT or SBRT. EBRT plus brachytherapy boost can be considered in select UIR and HR patients. Pelvic ENI should be considered for HR patients.[24,25] When nodal RT is performed, the updated NRG Oncology guidelines recommend including the common iliac (up to L4-L5), external iliac, internal iliac, presacral (S1-S3), and obturator lymph nodes.[26] Concurrent/adjuvant ADT with EBRT should be given.

Table 40.2: Androgen Deprivation Therapy Medications		
Method	**Mechanism**	**Examples**
Surgical castration	Removes 90%–95% of circulating testosterone and results in prompt decline in testosterone	Bilateral orchiectomy
GnRH agonists (a.k.a. LHRHa)	Induce stimulation of LH and an initial testosterone surge, followed by gradual decline to castrate levels over 3–4 weeks. A testosterone surge can exacerbate pain in patients with metastatic disease. An antiandrogen is commonly used concurrently with initiation of LHRHa to avoid this flare reaction	Leuprolide (7.5 mg/month), goserelin acetate (3.6 mg/month), buserelin, triptorelin
GnRH antagonists	Suppresses testosterone while avoiding flare reaction	Degarelix, relugolix
Steroidal antiandrogens	Inhibition of testosterone and DHT from binding to the androgen receptor in prostatic nuclei	Megestrol acetate, cyproterone acetate
Nonsteroidal antiandrogens	Competitive inhibitors of androgen binding to androgen receptors. Next-generation antiandrogens prevent nuclear translocation of androgen receptors and binding of androgen receptors to DNA response elements. Associated with gynecomastia	Bicalutamide (50 mg), flutamide (*hepatotoxicity*), enzalutamide, apalutamide, darolutamide
Adrenal suppression	Suppresses synthesis of multiple adrenal steroids	Ketoconazole (*most rapid drug for reducing testosterone*)
5-α-reductase inhibitors	Suppresses the enzyme that catalyzes the conversion of testosterone to DHT	Finasteride, dutasteride
CYP17A1 inhibitors	Inhibits the formation of DHEA and androstenedione, precursors of testosterone. Approved for use in castrate-resistant metastatic prostate cancer and castrate sensitive prostate cancer[22,23]	Abiraterone (must be given with prednisone)

Dose: With standard fractionation, dose escalation to 74 to 81 Gy improves biochemical PFS but has not improved OS (see Chapter 39 for details).[27–30] Moderate hypofractionation options include 70 Gy/28 fx, 70.2 Gy/26 fx, or 60 Gy/20 fx. The 2020 NCCN guidelines endorsed SBRT as an appropriate option for all risk groups including HR and VHR, to a dose of 36.25 to 40 Gy/5 fx. If combined EBRT and brachytherapy boost is planned, EBRT dose is 45 to 50 Gy, followed by LDR (110–115 Gy for I-125 or 90-100 Gy for Pd-103) or HDR (15 Gy x 1 fx or 10.75 Gy x 2 fx).[31]

Due to an elevated risk of SVI, the proximal 1 to 2 cm of the seminal vesicles are typically included within the CTV for IR and HR patients.[32] In an analysis of prostatectomy specimens, extracapsular extension extended to 4 mm in 90% of cases, which has implications for CTV margins (typically ≥ 5 mm).[33]

Toxicity: Common acute effects of EBRT include fatigue, dysuria, urinary frequency, urinary, and rectal urgency. If treating pelvic nodes, diarrhea and cramping are more common. Late effects are less common and include radiation cystitis, urethral stricture, radiation proctitis, bowel obstruction, fistula, and secondary malignancies.

Procedure: See *Handbook of Treatment Planning in Radiation Oncology*, Chapter 8.[34]

■ **EVIDENCE-BASED Q&A**

■ **For patients with IR prostate cancer, is there a benefit to ADT with EBRT over EBRT alone? Does the benefit to ADT persist in the setting of EBRT dose escalation?**

RTOG 9408, which consisted of a majority of IR patients, demonstrated an improvement in all outcomes with the addition of 4 months ADT to 66.6 Gy EBRT. A Canadian trial demonstrated that 6 months ADT with 70 or

76 Gy resulted in superior biochemical control and PCSM than 76 Gy alone. RTOG 0815 investigated the role of ADT in the setting of modern, dose-escalated RT, with results pending. Alternatively, dose escalation with a brachytherapy boost is an option for UIR patients although it is controversial whether ADT may be omitted in this setting or not.[35]

Jones, RTOG 9408 (*NEJM* 2011, PMID 21751904): PRT of 1,979 patients with prostate cancer T1b-T2b and PSA ≤ 20 ng/mL randomized to EBRT (46.8 Gy to whole pelvis with 19.8 Gy boost to prostate, for total 66.6 Gy) alone or with neoadjuvant and concurrent ADT (goserelin or leuprolide × 4 months, starting 2 months before RT); 35% LR, 54% IR, 11% HR. **Conclusion: The use of short-term neoadjuvant and concurrent ADT with EBRT significantly decreased BF, DM, and PCSM and improved OS (Table 40.3). Post hoc risk analysis demonstrated that benefit was limited to IR patients, but not LR patients. Comment: 66.6 Gy is low by modern standards.**

Table 40.3: RTOG 9408 Results				
10-Yr Data	BF	DM	PCSM	OS
EBRT	41%	8%	8%	57%
EBRT + ADT (4 months)	26%	6%	4%	62%

All results are statistically significant.

Nabid, Canadian PCS III (*Eur J Cancer* 2021, PMID 33279855): PRT of 600 patients with IR prostate cancer (23% FIR, 77% UIR) randomized to short-term ADT (bicalutamide and goserelin for 6 months, with 4 months given neoadjuvantly) with conventional dose EBRT (70 Gy, arm 1) or short-term ADT with dose-escalated EBRT (76 Gy, arm 2) or dose-escalated EBRT alone (76 Gy, arm 3) with 3D-CRT. The primary end point of bF was higher in arm 3 (30% at 10 yrs) than in arm 1 (16%) or arm 2 (13%), $p < .001$. Rates of prostate cancer progression (4.5% vs. 3.3% vs. 12%, for arms 1 vs. 2 vs. 3, respectively; $p = .001$) and PCSM (3.0% vs. 1.5% vs. 6.0%, $P = .03$) were also worse with dose-escalated RT alone than either arm with ADT. No significant difference in OS between the three arms. Grade ≥ 2 GI toxicity was higher with 76 Gy than 70 Gy (16% vs. 5%, $p < .001$). **Conclusion: Combination of short-term ADT and EBRT, even with lower RT doses, leads to superior biochemical control and PCSM compared to dose-escalated EBRT alone in IR prostate cancer (77% of whom were UIR).**

Bolla, EORTC 22991 (*JCO* 2016, PMID 26976418): PRT of 819 patients with IR (75%) or HR (25%) prostate cancer (T1b-c and PSA > 10 ng/mL or GS ≥ 7 or cT2aN0 and PSA ≤ 50 ng/mL) randomized to concurrent and adjuvant ADT (GnRH agonist × 6 months) and EBRT (70, 74, or 78 Gy, per institution preference) or EBRT alone. RT was 3D-CRT (83%) or IMRT (17%); 25% received 70 Gy, 50% 74 Gy, and 25% 78 Gy (IMRT used in > 50% of 78 Gy patients). The addition of ADT improved 5-year bDFS (HR 0.52, $P < .001$) and 5-year cDFS (HR 0.63, $P = .001$), with a similar effect across all three dose groups (Table 40.4). **Conclusion: 6 months' ADT improves bDFS and cDFS, even for dose-escalated RT.**

Table 40.4: EORTC 22991 Results				
5-Yr Data	bDFS	cDFS	DM	OS
EBRT	70%	81%	8%	88%
EBRT + ADT	83%	89%	4%	91%
p value	<.001	.001	.05	NA

■ **For IR prostate cancer, does longer term ADT improve outcomes?**

For patients with IR prostate cancer receiving ADT, short-term ADT (4 months) has been shown to be similar to longer term regimens (9 months on RTOG 9910, 28 months on DART).

Pisansky, RTOG 9910 (*JCO* 2015, PMID 25534388): PRT of 1,579 patients with IR prostate cancer randomized to neoadjuvant ADT for 8 weeks vs. 28 weeks prior to EBRT (70.2 Gy/39 fx) followed by 8 weeks of concurrent ADT (total 4 months vs. 9 months). Both arms yielded similar rates of bF, CSS, and OS (Table 40.5). **Conclusion: Longer duration of ADT does not improve outcomes in patients with IR prostate cancer.**

Table 40.5: RTOG 9910 Results			
10-Yr Data	bF	CSS	OS
4-month ADT + EBRT	27%	95%	66%
9-month ADT + EBRT	27%	96%	67%
p value	.77	.45	.62

■ **What is the optimal sequencing of short-term ADT and RT?**

Historically, ADT has often been given neoadjuvantly for ~2 months prior to starting RT. Recent evidence suggests that when short-term ADT is utilized, it should be given concurrently/adjuvantly with the start of RT.[36,37] There are no such comparative data in the setting of long-term ADT.

Malone, Canadian (*JCO* 2019, PMID 31829912): PRT of 432 patients with primarily IR prostate cancer (GS 6–7, T1b-T3a, and PSA < 30) randomized to 6 months of neoadjuvant/concurrent ADT, starting 4 months before RT, or RT with concurrent/adjuvant ADT (6 months total). Primary end point was bRFS but also measured OS and late grade 3 + toxicity. No SS difference in 10-year bRFS, OS, or grade 3 + toxicity. **Conclusion: Timing of short-term ADT in relation to RT does not impact biochemical control, OS, or toxicity. Neoadjuvant ADT is not necessary: RT and ADT can be started concurrently.**

■ **Is LDR brachytherapy alone sufficient treatment for FIR prostate cancer?**

Prestige, RTOG 0232 (*ASTRO* 2016, abstract 7): PRT of 579 patients with primarily FIR prostate cancer (T1c–T2b; GS 2–6 with PSA 10–19 ng/mL or GS 7 with PSA < 10 ng/mL) randomized to EBRT (45 Gy/25 fx to prostate and SVs; lymph nodes optional), followed by LDR brachytherapy boost with Pd-103 (100 Gy) or I-125 (110 Gy) vs. brachytherapy alone with Pd-103 (125 Gy) or I-125 (145 Gy). Freedom from progression was not improved at 5 years with the addition of EBRT. Grade ≥ 2 and grade ≥ 3 acute toxicities were similar, but grade ≥ 2 (53% vs. 37%; *p* = .0001) and grade ≥3 (12% vs. 7%; *p* = .039) late toxicities were higher in the EBRT + brachytherapy arm. **Conclusion: The addition of EBRT to brachytherapy did not significantly improve 5-year freedom from progression but did increase late toxicity in patients with FIR prostate cancer; brachytherapy alone is appropriate.**

■ **For HR or locally advanced prostate cancer, what is the benefit of combining ADT with EBRT over EBRT alone?**

Multiple trials have demonstrated a survival benefit from the addition of ADT to EBRT. These trials largely did not utilize dose-escalated EBRT, and all historically included pelvic ENI (Table 40.6). These trials used heterogeneous inclusion criteria and sequencing and duration of ADT.

Table 40.6: Summary of Major RT ±ADT Trials				
Trial	*N*	Inclusion	Arms	Findings
EORTC 22863 Bolla	415	T1–2 Grade 3 or T3–4	70 Gy ± LHRHa 36 months	ADT improved all endpoints including OS
RTOG 8531 Pilepich	977	T3N0-1	65–70 Gy ± orchiectomy or lifelong LHRHa	ADT improved all endpoints including OS
RTOG 8610 Pilepich	456	T2-4N0-1	65-70 Gy ±4 months LHRHa + flutamide	ADT improved all endpoints except OS (4 months may be insufficient)

Bolla, EORTC 22863 (*Lancet Oncol* 2010, PMID 20933466): PRT of 415 patients with T1-2N0 and grade 3 (17%) or T3-T4N0-1 (93%) randomized to EBRT (50 Gy/25 fx to whole pelvis with 20 Gy/10 fx cone down to prostate and SVs) + ADT (goserelin × 3 yrs on day 1 of EBRT + concurrent cyproterone acetate × 1 month) or EBRT alone. **Conclusion: Immediate androgen suppression with GnRH agonist for 3 years with EBRT improves bPFS, DFS, and OS in patients with HR or locally advanced prostate cancer (Table 40.7).**

Table 40.7: EORTC 22863 Results			
10-Yr Data	bPFS	DFS	OS
EBRT	18%	23%	40%
EBRT + ADT (3 yrs)	38%	48%	58%

All results are statistically significant.

Pilepich, RTOG 8531 (*IJROBP* 2005, PMID 15817329): PRT of 945 patients with T3 or N1 prostate cancer randomized to EBRT (44–46 Gy to whole pelvis with boost to prostate of 20 to 25 Gy) + ADT (goserelin during last day of RT, then monthly indefinitely) or EBRT alone. MFU 7.6 years; 10-year bF was not significantly different for GS ≤ 6 (57% vs. 51%; $P = .26$), but was significantly higher with EBRT alone for GS ≥ 7 (52% vs. 42%; $P = .026$). Cardiovascular mortality was not significantly different between the groups (8% ADT vs. 11% no ADT). **Conclusion: The addition of ADT to EBRT improved outcomes, particularly in patients with GS ≥7 (Table 40.8).**

Table 40.8: RTOG 8531 Results				
10-Yr Data	LF	DM	bNED	OS
EBRT	38%	39%	9%	39%
EBRT + ADT (lifelong)	23%	24%	31%	49%

All results are statistically significant.

Roach, RTOG 8610 (*JCO* 2008, PMID 18172188): PRT of 456 patients with T2-T4N0-1 prostate cancer randomized to EBRT (44–46 Gy whole pelvis with boost to prostate of 20–25 Gy, for total 65–70 Gy) + neoadjuvant and concurrent ADT (goserelin × 4 months starting 2 months before EBRT + flutamide × 4 months). **Conclusion: The addition of 4 months of neoadjuvant and concurrent ADT improved DFS and PCSM but had no OS benefit, with no increase in cardiovascular mortality (Table 40.9).** *Comment: Subset of GS 2 to 6 patients had improved OS, but those with GS 7 to 10 did not, suggesting that 4 months ADT may be insufficient in HR patients.*

Table 40.9: RTOG 8610 Results					
10-Yr Data	LF	DM	PCSM	OS	Cardiovascular Mortality
EBRT	42%	47%	3%	34%	9%
EBRT + ADT (4 months)	30%	35%	11%	43%	12.5%
All results are statistically significant except OS.					$p = .32$

D'Amico, Dana Farber 95-096 (*JAMA* 2004, PMID 15315996; Update D'Amico *JAMA* 2008, PMID 18212313; Update D'Amico *JAMA* 2015, PMID 26393854): PRT of 206 patients with IR and HR prostate cancer randomized to 70 Gy (without nodal RT), with or without 6 months of ADT. The first two reports suggested improved OS and CSS with ADT. Final results suggested no long-term difference overall, but men with no-to-minimal comorbidity benefited from ADT; whereas in men with moderate to severe comorbidity, OM was worse with ADT. **Conclusion: ADT benefits men with minimal comorbidity; use caution in those with comorbidity.**

Denham, TROG 9601 (*Lancet Oncol* 2011, PMID 21440505): PRT of 802 patients with cT2b-4N0 randomized to neoadjuvant and concurrent ADT (goserelin and flutamide × 3 months) + EBRT (66 Gy to prostate and SVs) or neoadjuvant and concurrent ADT (6 months) + EBRT or EBRT alone. 85% HR. Compared to EBRT alone, 3 months of ADT decreased PSA progression (HR 0.72, p = .003) and improved EFS (HR 0.63, p < .0001); 6 months of ADT further reduced PSA progression (HR 0.57, p < .0001) and led to a greater improvement in EFS (HR 0.51, p < .0001), compared with EBRT alone. While 3-month ADT had no effect on distant progression, PCSM, or ACM, 6-month ADT significantly decreased distant progression (HR 0.49, p = .001), PCSM (HR 0.49, p = .0008), and ACM (HR 0.63, p = .0008), compared to EBRT alone. **Conclusion: 6-month ADT had superior overall outcomes compared to no ADT for patients with HR prostate cancer, while 3-month ADT had no significant effect.**

■ **What is the optimal duration of hormone therapy for HR prostate cancer?**

For patients with HR prostate cancer, an OS benefit has been demonstrated with long-term ADT (28–36 months) compared to short-term regimens (4–6 months), even in the dose-escalated era (DART trial). One trial (PCS IV) found similar oncologic outcomes between 18 months and 36 months of ADT, although it was not powered to demonstrate non-inferiority. The RADAR trial found that 18 months of ADT was superior to 6 months of ADT for HR prostate cancer.

Hanks, RTOG 9202 (*JCO* 2003, PMID 14581419; Update Horwitz *JCO* 2008, PMID 18413638): PRT of 1,554 patients with cT2c-4 prostate cancer and PSA < 150 ng/mL randomized to neoadjuvant and concurrent short-term ADT (goserelin and flutamide × 4 months) and EBRT (45 Gy to whole pelvis and boost to 65–70 Gy to prostate) or long-term ADT × 28 months and EBRT. **Conclusion: Long-term ADT provided DFS benefit for all patients, but not OS benefit (Table 40.10). Long-term ADT had significant OS benefit for the subset with GS 8 to 10 disease.**

Table 40.10: RTOG 9202 Results							
10-Yr Data	**DFS**	**BF**	**LF**	**DM**	**DSS**	**OS (all GS)**	**OS (GS 8–10)**
4-month ADT + EBRT	13%	68%	22%	26%	84%	52%	32%
28-month ADT + EBRT	22%	52%	12%	18%	89%	54%	45%
p value	.0001	<.0001	.0002	.0002	.0001	.25	.006

Bolla, EORTC 22961 (*NEJM* 2009, PMID 19516032): PRT of 970 patients with cT2c-4 or N1 and PSA <150 ng/mL prostate cancer randomized to short-term ADT (triptorelin × 6 months) and EBRT (50 Gy to whole pelvis with boost to prostate and SVs to 70 Gy) or long-term ADT (36 months) and EBRT (Table 40.11). **Conclusion: Long-term ADT (3 yrs) demonstrated significant OS benefit compared to short-term ADT (6 months), with comparable quality of life and no difference in fatal cardiac events (4% vs. 3%).**

Table 40.11: EORTC 22961 Results					
5-Yr Data	**bPFS**	**CSS**	**OS**	**Gynecomastia**	**Incontinence**
6-month ADT + EBRT	59%	95%	81%	7%	10%
36-month ADT + EBRT	78%	97%	85%	18%	18%

All results are statistically significant.

Zapatero, DART 01/05 GICOR (*Lancet Oncol* 2015, PMID 25702876; Update IJROBP 2016, PMID 27598804): PRT of 355 patients with IR (47%) and HR (53%) prostate cancer (cT1c-T3aN0M0 and PSA < 100 ng/mL) randomized to neoadjuvant and concurrent short-term ADT (goserelin × 4 months) and dose-escalated EBRT (76–82 Gy) or long-term ADT (goserelin × 28 months) and EBRT. Pelvic ENI was optional, and used in 15% (mostly HR). On MVA, long-term ADT (HR 2.09, 95% CI 1.17–3.72, p = .012) and history of MI (HR 2.08, 95% CI 1.13–3.81, P = .018) were the only factors associated with elevated risk of CV event. No difference in rectal or urinary toxicity rates. **Conclusion: Long-term ADT significantly improved outcomes, including OS, compared to short-term ADT, even with dose-escalated EBRT (Table 40.12). The OS benefit was evident in patients with HR prostate cancer (p = .01) but not in the subset with IR disease.**

Table 40.12: DART 01/05 GICOR Results			
5-Yr Data	bDFS	MFS	OS
4-month ADT + EBRT	81%	83%	86%
28-month ADT + EBRT	89%	94%	95%
p value	.019	.009	.009

Nabid, PCS IV (*Eur Urol* 2018, PMID 29980331): PRT of 630 patients with HR prostate cancer (cT3-T4, Gl 8–10, PSA > 20) who received pelvic (44 Gy) and prostate RT (70 Gy/35 fx) and randomized to ADT for either 36 or 18 months (bicalutamide 50 mg for 1 month, goserelin 10.8 mg every 3 months); 10-year OS with 36 months of ADT was 62.4% vs. 62% with 18 months of ADT (HR 1.02, P = .8). QOL significantly favored 18 months of ADT (p < .001) for hot flashes and enjoyable sex. Only 53% of 36-month arm patients received full duration compared with 88% of 18-month arm. Median time to testosterone recovery from randomization was 3.6 years for 18-month ADT and 6.6 years for 36-month ADT (P < .001). **Conclusion: In HR prostate cancer treated with RT, 36 months ADT is not superior to 18 months (study was not designed to evaluate if 18 months was non-inferior).**

Denham, TROG 03.04 RADAR (*Lancet Oncol* 2019, PMID 30579763): PRT comparing short-term ADT (6 months) + RT vs. intermediate term ADT (18 months) + RT, with or without zolendronic acid in men with locally advanced prostate cancer. All patients received RT to the prostate and SVs, starting from the end of the 5th month of ADT. Dosing options: 66, 70, and 74 Gy in 2 Gy/fx, or 46 Gy in 2 Gy/fx, followed by a HDR brachytherapy boost dose of 19.5 Gy in 6.5 Gy/fx. Primary endpoint PCSM. The addition of zolendronic acid did not affect PCSM. Regarding ADT, PCSM was 13.3% vs. 9.7%, favoring 18 months of ADT. **Conclusion: 18 months of ADT + RT is a more effective treatment option for locally advanced prostate cancer than 6 months of ADT + RT. The addition of zoledronic acid is not beneficial.**

■ **Is there significant cardiovascular toxicity associated with ADT?**

Multiple pooled analyses have been performed, with mixed results. Some demonstrated no significant difference in cardiovascular mortality with the use of ADT, while others demonstrated increased cardiovascular death and shorter time to fatal myocardial infarction, particularly in men over 65 years of age. Studies have consistently demonstrated that the duration of ADT does not seem to significantly influence cardiovascular risk.[38–40]

Nguyen, Meta-Analysis (*JAMA* 2011, PMID 22147380): Systematic review of 4,141 patients from eight randomized trials. Demonstrated that cardiovascular death was not significantly different between patients who received ADT and those who did not, but PCSM and OM were improved with ADT. There was no excess risk of cardiovascular death in long-term ADT (> 3 years) vs. short-term ADT (≤6 months). **Conclusion: In patients with IR and HR prostate cancer, use of ADT was not associated with an increased risk of cardiovascular death; however, ADT did reduce PCSM and OM.**

■ **Is there a role for ADT prior to prostatectomy?**

A meta-analysis demonstrated improved surgical margin status but no difference in PFS or OS with the addition of neoadjuvant ADT before prostatectomy.[41] *Additional studies are ongoing to assess whether newer agents or CHT improve outcomes over prostatectomy alone.*

■ **Is there a benefit to elective pelvic nodal RT and which patients should be considered?**

The data are conflicting regarding the benefit of pelvic ENI. RTOG 9413 has been a difficult trial to interpret but demonstrates a small PFS benefit to ENI in patients with ≥15% risk of lymph node metastasis. Because most of the seminal high-risk trials used whole pelvic fields, virtually all HR patients can be considered candidates for ENI. Preliminary results of the POP-RT trial suggest favorable outcomes with hypofraction-ated IMRT with simultaneous treatment of pelvic nodes.[25] The question of ENI is being further investigated on RTOG 0924.

Roach, RTOG 9413 (*JCO* 2003, PMID 12743142; Update Roach *IJROBP* 2006, PMID 17011443; Update Lawton *IJROBP* 2007, PMID 17531401; Update Roach *Lancet Oncol* 2018, PMID 30507486): PRT of 1,275 patients with clinically localized prostate cancer with PSA ≤ 100 ng/mL and an estimated ≥ 15% risk of LN-positive disease according to Roach formula. Primary endpoint PFS. Randomization was 2 × 2 design, testing NHT vs. AHT and PORT vs. WPRT. ADT was goserelin or leuprolide with flutamide for 2 months before EBRT and 2 months during EBRT in the NHT arm. AHT was also 4 months but started at end of EBRT. EBRT dose was 50.4 Gy to the whole pelvis with 4-field box and boost of 19.8 Gy to the prostate in the WPRT arm, and 70.2 Gy in the PORT arm. Initial publication demonstrated PFS improvement with WPRT (both arms) compared to PORT (both arms). In the 2018 update, the NHT plus WPRT arm had improved 10-year PFS (28%) compared to NHT plus PORT (24%) and compared to AHT plus WPRT (19%), but not compared to AHT plus PORT (30%), p = .0002. There were no differences between arms in OS (p = .07) or DM (P = .32). Late grade 3 toxicity was also higher in the NHT plus WPRT arm. **Conclusion: In patients with ≥15% risk of lymph node metastasis, NHT and WPRT appears to improve PFS compared to NHT plus PORT and AHT plus WPRT arms, but not compared to AHT plus PORT.** Comment: This trial is controversial due to the 2 × 2 design, short duration of ADT, and low dose to the primary tumor, which may limit the ability to detect a potential effect of ENI.

Murthy, POP-RT, Tata Memorial (*JCO* 2021, PMID 33497252): PRT of 224 high risk patients ran-domized to PORT vs. WPRT. Treatment was 68 Gy/25 fx to the prostate +/- 50 Gy to pelvic LNs (including common iliacs) via SIB, with minimum 2 years ADT. 80% were cT3-T4 (only 1% T1). 80% underwent staging PSMA PET-CT to exclude cN1 or M1. **Conclusion: WPRT had higher late grade 2 GU toxicity, but improved BFFS, DFS, and MFS (but not OS) over PORT alone.** Comment: This small, single institutional trial may not be representative of a U.S. population (not screen detected, yet 80% PET staged).

■ **Is hypofractionation safe and effective for IR and HR prostate cancer?**

The published hypofractionation trials enrolled a variety of risk groups, and generally found similar outcomes as standard fractionation (with the exception of higher toxicity with 64.6 Gy/19 fx on HYPRO). Patients with IR and HR were included on the PROFIT trial (all IR), the CHHiP trial (73% IR, 12% HR), the HYPRO trial (26% IR, 74% HR), and the Arcangeli trial (all HR).[42-45] NCCN guidelines endorse hypofractionation for all risk groups. See <u>Chapter 39</u> for additional details.

■ **For HR or locally advanced prostate cancer, is there a benefit to combined EBRT and ADT over ADT alone?**

Two trials demonstrated an OS benefit to combined EBRT plus ADT over ADT alone. One older MRC trial did not demonstrate an advantage to the addition of EBRT to ADT, but this trial was underpowered.[46]

Widmark, SPCG-7/SFU0-3 (*Lancet* 2009, PMID 19091394): PRT of 875 patients from 47 centers with T1b-T2 and G2-G3 disease or T3, PSA < 70 ng/mL, N0, M0 randomized to ADT (3 months total androgen blockage followed by continuous flutamide 250 mg) or ADT + EBRT (70 Gy) to prostate/ SVs. **Conclusion: The addition of EBRT to flutamide improved bPFS, CSS, and OS for patients with HR prostate cancer (Table 40.13).**

Table 40.13: SPCG-7 Trial Results							
10-Yr Data	**bPFS**	**CSS**	**OS**	**Erectile Dysfunction**	**Urethral Stricture**	**Urgency**	**Incontinence**
ADT	25%	76%	61%	81%	0%	8%	3%
ADT + EBRT	74%	88%	70%	89%	2%	14%	7%

All results are statistically significant.

Warde, NCIC CTG PR.3/MRC UK PR 07 (*Lancet* 2011, PMID 22056152; **Update Mason** *JCO* 2015, PMID 25691677): PRT of 1,205 patients with T3-4N0, or T1-2 and PSA > 40 ng/mL, or PSA > 20 ng/mL and GS > 8 randomized to lifelong ADT (bilateral orchiectomy or GnRH agonist) or ADT + EBRT (64–69 Gy to prostate, SVs, and 45 Gy to pelvic nodes). The addition of EBRT to ADT improved OS at 7 years (74% vs. 66%; *p* = .033). Deaths from prostate cancer were significantly reduced by the addition of RT to ADT (HR 0.46, *p* < .001). **Conclusion: The addition of EBRT to lifelong ADT improves OS in patients with HR prostate cancer.**

■ **Can brachytherapy boost improve outcomes when added to EBRT?**

Brachytherapy boost is associated with improved biochemical control but increased toxicity. There may be a benefit to combined EBRT and brachytherapy in higher grade patients.[47]

Morris, ASCENDE-RT (*IJROBP* 2016, PMID 28262473; **Rodda** *IJROBP* 2016, PMID 28433432): PRT of 398 patients with IR (31%) and HR (69%) prostate cancer treated with neoadjuvant and concurrent ADT for 8 months and EBRT (46 Gy/23 fx to the whole pelvis) and then randomized to conformal EBRT boost to prostate (32 Gy/16 fx) or I-125 LDR brachytherapy boost (prescribed to minimum peripheral dose of 115 Gy). The 9-year RFS (defined as nadir + 2 ng/mL) was significantly higher for the brachytherapy boost arm compared to EBRT boost arm (83% vs. 62%; *p* < .001), but also had higher risk of GU toxicity (grade 3 rate at 5 years was 18% with brachytherapy boost and 5% with EBRT boost). **Conclusion: LDR brachytherapy boost significantly increased biochemical control compared to EBRT boost in patients with IR and HR prostate cancer, but also had higher risk of GU toxicity.**

Kishan, Multi-Institutional (*JAMA* 2018, PMID 29509865): Retrospective cohort study in 1,809 men with GS 9-10 prostate cancer. 3 cohorts: prostatectomy (*N* = 639; 35%), EBRT (*N* = 734; 41%), EBRT + BT (*N* = 436; 24%). Patients treated with RP were significantly younger, had lower PSA, were less likely to have GS 10, and more likely to have cT1-2 (all *p* < .001). ADT used in ~90% of patients receiving EBRT and EBRT+BT, although for shorter duration with EBRT+BT (12 months vs. 21.9 months; *p* < .001). Systemic salvage was given in 24% of RP, 12% of EBRT, and 6% of EBRT+BT patients. Within the first 7.5 years, EBRT+BT was associated with significantly lower ACM (cause-specific HR 0.66 [95% CI 0.46–0.96] compared to RP and 0.61 [95% CI 0.45–0.84] compared to EBRT). No significant differences in PCSM, DM, or ACM were found between men treated with EBRT or RP. **Conclusion: Gleason 9 to 10 treated with EBRT + BT is associated with lower PCSM and DM compared with RP or EBRT, despite having more adverse factors at baseline (Table 40.14). RP and EBRT appeared similar. Prospective study is warranted.**

Table 40.14: Multi-institutional Gleason 9 to 10 Results			
	5-Yr PCSM	5-Yr DM	7.5-Yr ACM
RP	12%	24%	17%
EBRT	13%	24%	18%
EBRT + BT	3%	8%	10%

■ **Is there a role for the use of CHT in HR prostate cancer?**

The OS benefit of the addition of CHT to long-term ADT and dose-escalated EBRT in the modern era for patients with HR prostate cancer is unclear. PRTs currently have limited follow-up but demonstrate significantly improved biochemical control, and NCCN guidelines currently suggest consideration of CHT for VHR prostate cancer. The decision to use CHT should be individualized, based on patient and disease characteristics.[48]

Rosenthal, RTOG 9902 (*IJROBP* 2015, PMID 26209502): PRT of 397 patients with HR prostate cancer randomized to EBRT + long-term ADT (GnRH agonist × 24 months) with adjuvant paclitaxel, estramustine, oral etoposide CHT vs. EBRT + ADT alone. **Conclusion: The addition of CHT to standard-of-care EBRT + long-term ADT did not improve outcomes in patients with HR prostate cancer (Table 40.15).**

Table 40.15: RTOG 9902 Results

10-Yr Results	BF	LF	DM	DFS	OS
EBRT + ADT + CHT	54%	7%	14%	26%	63%
EBRT + ADT	58%	11%	16%	22%	65%
p value	.82	.09	.42	.61	.81

Rosenthal, RTOG 0521 (*JCO* 2019, PMID 30860948): PRT of 612 patients with HR prostate cancer randomized to EBRT (75.6 Gy) + long-term ADT (24 months), followed by CHT (docetaxel × 6 cycles) or EBRT + long-term ADT alone. EBRT + ADT + CHT had significantly higher 4-year OS (93% vs. 89%; one-sided $p = .04$) and 6-year DFS (65% vs. 55%; two-sided $P = .04$), compared to EBRT + ADT alone. **Conclusion: Adjuvant docetaxel, in addition to EBRT and long-term ADT, may provide a benefit in patients with HR prostate cancer.**

Fizazi, GETUG 12 (*Lancet Oncol* 2015, PMID 26028518): PRT of 207 patients with HR or N1 prostate cancer randomized to long-term ADT (GnRH agonist × 3 yrs) with CHT (docetaxel and estramustine × 4 cycles) or ADT alone. Local therapy with RP or EBRT was performed 3 months after systemic treatment; 8-year RFS was significantly higher with the addition of CHT (62% vs. 50%; $P = .017$). **Conclusion: Docetaxel and estramustine CHT, in combination with long-term ADT and local therapy (RP or EBRT), significantly improved RFS in patients with HR prostate cancer.**

LYMPH NODE-POSITIVE PROSTATE CANCER

▇ What is the management of patients with clinically lymph node–positive disease?

Current NCCN guidelines endorse combined modality therapy for lymph node-positive prostate cancer. RTOG 8531 found that combined ADT + RT had better outcomes than RT alone in a small subset of node-positive patients.[49] The STAMPEDE trial demonstrated that adding RT to ADT was associated with improved FFS for N + M0 disease (HR 0.48, 95% CI 0.29–0.79).[50]

LOCALLY RECURRENT PROSTATE CANCER AFTER RADIATION

▇ What are treatment options for local recurrence of prostate cancer after previous RT?

Several salvage options exist after prior EBRT, including RP, cryotherapy, brachytherapy, or SBRT. The MASTER meta-analysis demonstrated that estimated rates of 5-year bRFS on meta-regression were similar between various local salvage therapies, ranging from 50% to 60% after RP, cryotherapy, SBRT, or brachytherapy, with no significant differences between any modality and RP. Severe GU toxicity was lower after all three forms of RT salvage than with RP (21% for RP, 15% for cryotherapy, 5.6% for SBRT, 9.6% for HDR brachytherapy, and 9.1% for LDR brachytherapy; $P < 0.001$). GI toxicity was lower with salvage HDR brachytherapy than with RP but was < 2% across all modalities.[51]

Crook, RTOG 0526 (*IJROBP* 2019, PMID 30312717): Phase II trial of 92 patients with initially LR or IR prostate cancer treated with EBRT, with biopsy-proven local-only recurrence > 30 months after EBRT and PSA < 10, treated with salvage LDR brachytherapy. Median EBRT dose was 74 Gy, with median interval of 85 months. Brachytherapy was I-125 140 Gy or Pd-103 120 Gy. The primary end point of grade 3 GI/GU toxicity was observed in 14%, with no grade 4 or 5 toxicities.

REFERENCES

1. Mohler JL, Antonarakis ES, Armstrong AJ, et al. Prostate Cancer, Version 2.2019, NCCN Clinical Practice Guidelines in Oncology. *J Natl Compr Canc Netw.* 2019;17(5):479–505. doi:10.6004/jnccn.2019.0023
2. Cooperberg MR, Broering JM, Carroll PR. Time trends and local variation in primary treatment of localized prostate cancer. *J Clin Oncol.* 2010;28(7):1117–1123. doi:10.1200/JCO.2009.26.0133
3. Hemminki K, Ji J, Forsti A, Sundquist J, Lenner P. Concordance of survival in family members with prostate cancer. *J Clin Oncol.* 2008;26(10):1705–1709. doi:10.1200/JCO.2007.13.3355

4. Agalliu I, Gern R, Leanza S, Burk RD. Associations of high-grade prostate cancer with BRCA1 and BRCA2 founder mutations. *Clin Cancer Res.* 2009;15(3):1112–1120. doi:10.1158/1078-0432.CCR-08-1822

5. Castro E, Goh C, Olmos D, et al. Germline BRCA mutations are associated with higher risk of nodal involvement, distant metastasis, and poor survival outcomes in prostate cancer. *J Clin Oncol.* 2013;31(14):1748–1757. doi:10.1200/JCO.2012.43.1882

6. Pritchard CC, Mateo J, Walsh MF, et al. Inherited DNA-repair gene mutations in men with metastatic prostate cancer. *N Engl J Med.* 2016;375(5):443–453. doi:10.1056/NEJMoa1603144

7. Schumacher FR, Al Olama AA, Berndt SI, et al. Association analyses of more than 140,000 men identify 63 new prostate cancer susceptibility loci. *Nat Genet.* 2018;50(7):928–936. doi:10.1038/s41588-018-0142-8

8. Raymond VM, Mukherjee B, Wang F, et al. Elevated risk of prostate cancer among men with Lynch syndrome. *J Clin Oncol.* 2013;31(14):1713–1718. doi:10.1200/JCO.2012.44.1238

9. Tischkowitz M, Easton DF, Ball J, et al. Cancer incidence in relatives of British Fanconi Anaemia patients. *BMC Cancer.* 2008;8:257. doi:10.1186/1471-2407-8-257

10. Ewing CM, Ray AM, Lange EM, et al. Germline mutations in HOXB13 and prostate-cancer risk. *N Engl J Med.* 2012;366(2):141–149. doi:10.1056/NEJMoa1110000

11. Eifler JB, Feng Z, Lin BM, et al. An updated prostate cancer staging nomogram (Partin tables) based on cases from 2006 to 2011. *BJU Int.* 2013;111(1):22–29. doi:10.1111/j.1464-410X.2012.11324.x

12. Nguyen PL, Chen MH, Hoffman KE, et al. Predicting the risk of pelvic node involvement among men with prostate cancer in the contemporary era. *Int J Radiat Oncol Biol Phys.* 2009;74(1):104–109. doi:10.1016/j.ijrobp.2008.07.053

13. Berlin A, Murgic J, Hosni A, et al. Genomic classifier for guiding treatment of intermediate-risk prostate cancers to dose-escalated image guided radiation therapy without hormone therapy. *Int J Radiat Oncol Biol Phys.* 2019;103(1):84–91. doi:10.1016/j.ijrobp.2018.08.030

14. Spratt DE, Zhang J, Santiago-Jimenez M, et al. Development and validation of a novel integrated clinical-genomic risk group classification for localized prostate cancer. *J Clin Oncol.* 2018;36(6):581–590. doi:10.1200/JCO.2017.74.2940

15. Hofman MS, Lawrentschuk N, Francis RJ, et al. Prostate-specific membrane antigen PET-CT in patients with high-risk prostate cancer before curative-intent surgery or radiotherapy (proPSMA): a prospective, randomised, multi-centre study. *Lancet.* 2020;395(10231):1208–1216. doi:10.1016/S0140-6736(20)30314-7

16. Albertsen PC, Hanley JA, Fine J. 20-year outcomes following conservative management of clinically localized prostate cancer. *JAMA.* 2005;293(17):2095–2101. doi:10.1001/jama.293.17.2095

17. Tendulkar RD, Hunter GK, Reddy CA, et al. Causes of mortality after dose-escalated radiation therapy and androgen deprivation for high-risk prostate cancer. *Int J Radiat Oncol Biol Phys.* 2013;87(1):94–99. doi:10.1016/j.ijrobp.2013.05.044

18. Chen RC, Rumble RB, Loblaw DA, et al. Active surveillance for the management of localized prostate cancer (Cancer Care Ontario Guideline): American Society of Clinical Oncology Clinical Practice Guideline Endorsement. *J Clin Oncol.* 2016;34(18):2182–2190. doi:10.1200/JCO.2015.65.7759

19. Nabid A, Carrier N, Martin AG, et al. Duration of androgen deprivation therapy in high-risk prostate cancer: a randomized phase III trial. *Eur Urol.* 2018;74(4):432–441. doi:10.1016/j.eururo.2018.06.018

20. Nabid A, Carrier N, Vigneault E, et al. Androgen deprivation therapy and radiotherapy in intermediate-risk prostate cancer: a randomised phase III trial. *Eur J Cancer* (Oxford, 1990). 2021;143:64–74. doi:10.1016/j.ejca.2020.10.023

21. Shore ND, Saad F, Cookson MS, et al. Oral relugolix for androgen-deprivation therapy in advanced prostate cancer. *N Engl J Med.* 2020;382(23):2187–2196. doi:10.1056/NEJMoa2004325

22. James ND, de Bono JS, Spears MR, et al. Abiraterone for prostate cancer not previously treated with hormone therapy. *N Engl J Med.* 2017;377(4):338–351. doi:10.1056/NEJMoa1702900

23. Fizazi K, Tran N, Fein L, et al. Abiraterone plus prednisone in metastatic, castration-sensitive prostate cancer. *N Engl J Med.* 2017;377(4):352–360. doi:10.1056/NEJMoa1704174

24. Zapatero A, Guerrero A, Maldonado X, et al. High-dose radiotherapy with short-term or long-term androgen deprivation in localised prostate cancer (DART01/05 GICOR): a randomised, controlled, phase 3 trial. *Lancet Oncol.* 2015;16(3):320–327. doi:10.1016/S1470-2045(15)70045-8

25. Murthy V, Maitre P, Kannan S, et al. Prostate-only versus whole-pelvic radiation therapy in high-risk and very high-risk prostate cancer (POP-RT): outcomes from phase III randomized controlled trial. *J Clin Oncol.* 2021;39(11):1234–1242. doi: 10.1200/JCO.20.03282

26. Hall WA, Paulson E, Davis BJ, et al. NRG oncology updated international consensus atlas on pelvic lymph node volumes for intact and postoperative prostate cancer. *Int J Radiat Oncol Biol Phys.* 2021;109(1):174–185. doi:10.1016/j.ijrobp.2020.08.034

27. Pasalic D, Kuban DA, Allen PK, et al. Dose escalation for prostate adenocarcinoma: a long-term update on the outcomes of a phase 3, single institution randomized clinical trial. *Int J Radiat Oncol Biol Phys.* 2019;104(4):790–797. doi:10.1016/j.ijrobp.2019.02.045

28. Zietman AL, Bae K, Slater JD, et al. Randomized trial comparing conventional-dose with high-dose conformal radiation therapy in early-stage adenocarcinoma of the prostate: long-term results from proton radiation oncology group/American College of Radiology 95–09. *J Clin Oncol.* 2010;28(7):1106–1111. doi:10.1200/JCO.2009.25.8475

29. Dearnaley DP, Jovic G, Syndikus I, et al. Escalated-dose versus control-dose conformal radiotherapy for prostate cancer: long-term results from the MRC RT01 randomised controlled trial. *Lancet Oncol.* 2014;15(4):464–473. doi:10.1016/S1470-2045(14)70040-3

30. Heemsbergen WD, Al-Mamgani A, Slot A, et al. Long-term results of the Dutch randomized prostate cancer trial: impact of dose-escalation on local, biochemical, clinical failure, and survival. *Radiother Oncol.* 2014;110(1):104–109. doi:10.1016/j.radonc.2013.09.026

31. Orio PF, 3rd, Nguyen PL, Buzurovic I, et al. The decreased use of brachytherapy boost for intermediate and high-risk prostate cancer despite evidence supporting its effectiveness. *Brachytherapy.* 2016;15(6):701–706. doi:10.1016/j.brachy.2016.05.001

32. Kestin L, Goldstein N, Vicini F, et al. Treatment of prostate cancer with radiotherapy: should the entire seminal vesicles be included in the clinical target volume? *Int J Radiat Oncol Biol Phys.* 2002;54(3):686–697. doi:10.1016/S0360-3016(02)03011-0

33. Sohayda C, Kupelian PA, Levin HS, Klein EA. Extent of extracapsular extension in localized prostate cancer. *Urology.* 2000;55(3):382–386. doi:10.1016/S0090-4295(99)00458-6

34. Videtic GMM, Woody N, Vassil AD. *Handbook of Treatment Planning in Radiation Oncology.* 3rd ed. *Demos Medical;* 2020. doi:10.1891/9780826168429

35. Jackson WC, Hartman HE, Dess RT, et al. Addition of androgen-deprivation therapy or brachytherapy boost to external beam radiotherapy for localized prostate cancer: a network meta-analysis of randomized trials. *J Clin Oncol.* 2020;38(26):3024–3031. doi:10.1200/JCO.19.03217

36. Malone S, Roy S, Eapen L, et al. Sequencing of androgen-deprivation therapy with external-beam radiotherapy in localized prostate cancer: a phase III randomized controlled trial. *J Clin Oncol.* 2020;38(6):593–601. doi:10.1200/JCO.19.01904

37. Spratt DE, Malone S, Roy S, et al. Prostate radiotherapy with adjuvant Androgen Deprivation Therapy (ADT) improves metastasis-free survival compared to neoadjuvant ADT: an individual patient meta-analysis. *J Clin Oncol.* 2021;39(2):136–144. doi:10.1200/JCO.20.02438

38. Nguyen PL, Je Y, Schutz FA, et al. Association of androgen deprivation therapy with cardiovascular death in patients with prostate cancer: a meta-analysis of randomized trials. *JAMA.* 2011;306(21):2359–2366. doi:10.1001/jama.2011.1745

39. D'Amico AV, Denham JW, Crook J, et al. Influence of androgen suppression therapy for prostate cancer on the frequency and timing of fatal myocardial infarctions. *J Clin Oncol.* 2007;25(17):2420–2425. doi:10.1200/JCO.2006.09.3369

40. Tsai HK, D'Amico AV, Sadetsky N, et al. Androgen deprivation therapy for localized prostate cancer and the risk of cardiovascular mortality. *J Natl Cancer Inst.* 2007;99(20):1516–1524. doi:10.1093/jnci/djm168

41. Shelley MD, Kumar S, Wilt T, et al. A systematic review and meta-analysis of randomised trials of neo-adjuvant hormone therapy for localised and locally advanced prostate carcinoma. *Cancer Treat Rev.* 2009;35(1):9–17. doi:10.1016/j.ctrv.2008.08.002

42. Catton CN, Lukka H, Gu CS, et al. Randomized Trial of a Hypofractionated Radiation Regimen for the Treatment of Localized Prostate Cancer. *J Clin Oncol.* 2017;35(17):1884–1890. doi:10.1200/JCO.2016.71.7397

43. Dearnaley D, Syndikus I, Mossop H, et al. Conventional versus hypofractionated high-dose intensity-modulated radiotherapy for prostate cancer: 5-year outcomes of the randomised, non-inferiority, phase 3 CHHiP trial. *Lancet Oncol.* 2016;17(8):1047–1060. doi:10.1016/S1470-2045(16)30102-4

44. Incrocci L, Wortel RC, Alemayehu WG, et al. Hypofractionated versus conventionally fractionated radiotherapy for patients with localised prostate cancer (HYPRO): final efficacy results from a randomised, multicentre, open-label, phase 3 trial. Lancet Oncol. 2016;17(8):1061–1069. doi:10.1016/S1470-2045(16)30070-5

45. Arcangeli G, Saracino B, Arcangeli S, et al. Moderate Hypofractionation in High-Risk, Organ-Confined Prostate Cancer: Final Results of a Phase III Randomized Trial. *J Clin Oncol.* 2017;35(17):1891–1897. doi:10.1200/JCO.2016.70.4189

46. Fellows GJ, Clark PB, Beynon LL, et al. Treatment of advanced localised prostatic cancer by orchiectomy, radiotherapy, or combined treatment. A Medical Research Council Study. Urological Cancer Working Party--Subgroup on Prostatic Cancer. *British journal of urology.* 1992;70(3):304–309. doi:10.1111/j.1464-410X.1992.tb15736.x

47. Hoskin PJ, Rojas AM, Bownes PJ, et al. Randomised trial of external beam radiotherapy alone or combined with high-dose-rate brachytherapy boost for localised prostate cancer. *Radiother Oncol.* 2012;103(2):217–222. doi:10.1016/j.radonc.2012.01.007

48. Vale CL, Burdett S, Rydzewska LHM, et al. Addition of docetaxel or bisphosphonates to standard of care in men with localised or metastatic, hormone-sensitive prostate cancer: a systematic review and meta-analyses of aggregate data. *Lancet Oncol.* 2016;17(2):243–256. doi:10.1016/S1470-2045(15)00489-1

49. Lawton CA, Winter K, Grignon D, Pilepich MV. Androgen suppression plus radiation versus radiation alone for patients with stage D1/pathologic node-positive adenocarcinoma of the prostate: updated results based on national prospective randomized trial Radiation Therapy Oncology Group 85–31. *J Clin Oncol.* 2005;23(4):800–807. doi:10.1200/JCO.2005.08.141

50. James ND, Spears MR, Clarke NW, et al. Failure-free survival and radiotherapy in patients with newly diagnosed nonmetastatic prostate cancer: data from patients in the control arm of the STAMPEDE trial. *JAMA Oncol.* 2016;2(3):348–357. doi:10.1001/jamaoncol.2015.4350

51. Valle LF, Lehrer EJ, Markovic D, et al. A systematic review and meta-analysis of local salvage therapies after radiotherapy for prostate cancer (MASTER). *Eur Urol.* 2020. doi:10.1016/j.eururo.2020.11.010

James R. Broughman, Camille A. Berriochoa, and Rahul D. Tendulkar

QUICK HIT ■ After RP, approximately 25% to 30% will have PSA progression postoperatively (over 50% among men with pT3 disease or positive margins). Three historical randomized trials (SWOG 8794, German ARO 9602, and EORTC 22911) showed that immediate RT improves bRFS by ~20% to 25% over observation among patients with positive margins, ECE (pT3a), or SVI (pT3b). Of these, only the SWOG study detected an improvement in DMFS and OS. The ARTISTIC meta-analysis combined the results of three more recent trials (RAVES, RADICALS-RT, and GETUG-AFU 17) and suggests that early salvage RT may reduce toxicity and avoid unnecessary treatment without compromising EFS compared to adjuvant RT. The addition of ADT to RT improved outcomes in RTOG 9601 and GETUG-AFU 16 though patient selection for treatment intensification remains controversial (see Table 41.1). Salvage RT typically consists of 64 to 72 Gy in 1.8 to 2 Gy fractions delivered to the prostate bed. RTOG 0534 supports nodal RT in men with higher PSA. Emerging genomic classifiers and PET imaging may help guide decisions for post-prostatectomy RT.

TABLE 41.1: General Treatment Paradigm for Postoperative Prostate Cancer

Initial Treatment	Pathologic Findings	Subsequent Treatment Options
Radical prostatectomy	No adverse features or LN mets	Close monitoring and early salvage RT*
	Adverse features (positive margin, SVI, ECE)	Adjuvant RT if multiple risk factors (e.g., SVI, high grade, genomic classifier score, LN+)
		Close monitoring and early salvage RT*
	Positive for LN mets	ADT ± RT
		Close monitoring and early salvage RT*
	Detectable postoperative PSA and no evidence of distant metastases	Salvage RT ± ADT
		Close monitoring* (if low grade with slow PSA doubling time and/or limited life expectancy)

*Close monitoring: PSA q6–12 mos + annual DRE. Early salvage RT indicated if PSA rises to 0.2 ng/mL, or >2 consecutive rises above 0.1 ng/mL.

EPIDEMIOLOGY: Approximately 230,000 diagnoses of prostate cancer and 30,000 deaths in the United States annually.[1] Over 90% have localized disease and over half undergo RP as initial treatment. Following RP, PSA is highly sensitive and biochemical failure is not uncommon: for men with intermediate-risk prostate cancer, 5-year bRFS ~80%, 10-year bRFS ~65%. For high/very high risk disease, 5-year bRFS ~70%, 10-year bRFS ~55%.[2] Laparoscopic/robotic surgery has become more common, with 85% undergoing this approach rather than open technique.[3] Overall, after RP, 25% to 30% have post-op PSA progression (>50% if pT3 or positive margins).

RISK FACTORS, ANATOMY, PATHOLOGY, SCREENING, CLINICAL PRESENTATION: See Chapter 39 for further details.

GENETICS: Role of multigene assays to improve selection for adjuvant RT is evolving.

WORKUP: H&P to rule out distant metastatic disease. Palpation of nodule on DRE is suggestive of anastomotic recurrence.

Labs: PSA should be undetectable following RP. A detectable/rising PSA postoperatively warrants investigation for locoregional or distant metastatic disease. The AUA definition of biochemical failure is PSA ≥0.2 ng/mL, followed by second confirmatory PSA ≥0.2 ng/mL.[4]

Imaging

Bone scan (Tc-99m): Consider for high PSA, short PSADT, symptomatic, or after prior ADT. Has poor sensitivity at PSA levels <10 ng/mL.[5] If negative but there is still strong suspicion for bone mets, next-generation nuclear imaging may be indicated.

CT abdomen/Pelvis: Consider preoperatively for T3-T4 disease or T1-T2 disease with a >10% risk of nodal metastases per nomogram. Postoperatively, consider if PSA does not fall to undetectable levels.

Nuclear imaging: There are four FDA-approved PET tracers for men with prostate cancer: F18 fluciclovine (Axumin), F18 sodium fluoride, C11 choline, and Ga68 PSMA-11 (prostate-specific membrane antigen). These are typically utilized when conventional imaging is equivocal. Although F18 sodium fluoride is more sensitive for detecting bone metastases compared to bone scan, it is not more specific and suffers from false positives from benign processes like arthritis.[6] Prospective data show improved detection rates with Ga68 PSMA compared to Axumin (OR 4.8; SS) with PSA ≤2.0 ng/mL.[6]

MRI: May help with visualization of postsurgical recurrence[7,8] and also with treatment planning.[9] Note that for a prostate MRI, a 3T magnet is preferred for sufficient resolution.

Procedures: Generally no role for biopsy unless a suspicious finding is discovered on exam or imaging. Pathology from prostatectomy sample should be analyzed.

PROGNOSTIC FACTORS: Per Stephenson and Tendulkar nomograms: surgical margins (positive margins are favorable for response to salvage RT), Gleason score, PSA level, PSADT, PSA response (ratio of rate of climb to rate of fall before and after ADT, ratio <1 has >3× OS), interval from surgery to bF, lack of SV involvement.[10,11] Tertiary pattern of 4 or 5 in prostatectomy specimens should be considered as having high-risk disease.

NATURAL HISTORY: Most common sites of local recurrence following RP: (a) vesicourethral anastomosis (approximately 2/3 of LR), (b) bladder neck, and (c) retrotrigone.[12] Survival following bF is highly variable ranging from 4 to 15+ years in various series.[13] Historically, median time to radiographic mets after post-prostatectomy bF is 8 years without treatment, and median time to death after developing macrometastatic disease is another 5 years.[14]

STAGING: See Chapter 39 for AJCC 8th edition's staging and risk classifications.[15]

TREATMENT PARADIGM

Surgery: See Chapter 39.

Chemotherapy: No current role for adjuvant cytotoxic CHT in the early salvage setting. The STAMPEDE trial found an OS benefit to the use of docetaxel administered at the time of first-line ADT in metastatic hormone-sensitive prostate cancer patients, although it is unclear if this applies in the nonmetastatic recurrent setting.[16]

Androgen Deprivation: Two trials demonstrated benefit to adding ADT to salvage RT for PSA >0.2 ng/mL.[17,18] However, a secondary analysis of RTOG 9601 showed benefit only for PSA >0.6 ng/mL.[19] See Chapter 40 for details on ADT dosing and administration.

Radiation

Indications

Adjuvant therapy: Treatment given to high-risk patients in absence of detectable disease, generally within 3 to 4 months after surgery so that incontinence or other post-op complications are allowed time for recovery. Rationale: to prevent recurrence in those at high risk when disease burden is minimal. Classic indications: positive margins, ECE (pT3a), SVI (pT3b).

Salvage therapy: Treatment in presence of detectable disease (elevated PSA or palpable nodule). Rationale: RT may eradicate locally recurrent/residual prostate cancer. Clinical indications: palpable local recurrence, persistently elevated post-op PSA, or rising PSA.

Pelvic nodal RT: Indicated in the pN+ setting (see the following for discussion). For pN0 patients, a biochemical control benefit of nodal RT was observed for men with PSA ≥0.34 ng/nL per preliminary results of RTOG 0534.[20]

Dose: Typically ranges from 64 to 72 at 1.8 to 2 Gy/fx. Doses of at least 66 Gy appear to be associated with improved outcomes, in retrospective series.[21]

Procedure: See *Handbook of Treatment Planning in Radiation Oncology*, Chapter 9.[22]

■ EVIDENCE-BASED Q&A

▓ Does immediate post-prostatectomy RT improve outcomes for patients with high-risk features?

Rates of bF after prostatectomy are >50% in those with pT3 disease, positive margins, and high Gleason score.[23,24] Therefore, three major trials evaluated the role of immediate ("adjuvant") RT to the prostate bed vs. observation. In all three, immediate RT improved bRFS by about 20% to 30%, but only the SWOG study detected an improvement in DMFS and OS. Two meta-analyses (Ontario and Cochrane) were also performed, with conflicting results.[25,26] However, none of these trials specified the timing or type of salvage treatment provided to patients who failed observation. This was instead left to the treating physician and ultimately a wide range of treatments were given, including no salvage therapy for some patients.[18]

Swanson, SWOG 8794 (*JCO* 2007, PMID 17105795; Update *J Urology* 2009, PMID 19167731): PRT of 425 patients w/ pT3N0 and/or positive margins randomized to immediate RT (60–64 Gy) vs. observation. No concurrent ADT. PSA q3 months for 1 year, q6 months for 2 years, then annually. Primary end point: metastasis-free survival. Secondary end point: bRFS (bF defined as PSA ≥0.4 ng/mL). MFU 12.7 years; 33% of observation patients eventually received RT, 50% of observation patients eventually required ADT. All end points improved with adjuvant RT: bF (decreased from 64% to 34%, $p < .005$), MFS (median 14.7 vs. 12.9 years, HR: 0.71, $p = .016$, NNT = 12 to prevent 1 death at 12.6 years), and OS (median 15.2 vs. 13.3 years, HR: 0.72, $p = .023$, NNT = 9.1 to prevent one death at 12.6 years). QOL was worse w/ RT at 6 months and 2 years but equivalent by 5 years. Benefit to RT seen in all three risk groups. **Conclusion: Immediate RT improved OS, DM, and bF for patients with pT3 or margin-positive prostate cancer.** *Comment: Approximately 30% had a detectable PSA >0.2 ng/mL prior to "adjuvant" RT, so not truly an adjuvant RT trial.*

Bolla, EORTC 22911 (*Lancet* 2005, PMID 16099293; Update *Lancet* 2012, PMID 23084481): PRT of 1,005 patients treated with immediate RT to 60 Gy vs. W&S after RP, pT3N0, and/or positive margins. RT started within 16 weeks after RP. RT was four-field to a dose of 50 Gy/25 fx + 10 Gy boost to the prostate bed. bF defined as increase of 0.2 ng/mL over nadir on 3 separate occasions 2 weeks apart. MFU 10.6 years. In the W&S group, 56% received salvage RT and 23% received ADT. Results shown in Table 41.2. **Conclusion: Immediate RT improved bF for patients for patients with pT3 or margin-positive prostate cancer.** *Comment: Like the SWOG study, ~30% of patients had a detectable PSA >0.2 ng/mL prior to "adjuvant" RT.*

TABLE 41.2: Results of EORTC 22911 Adjuvant RT for Prostate Cancer							
	10-Yr bRFS (1° End Point)	5-Yr Clinical PFS	10-Yr LRF	Grade 3 Acute Toxicity	10-Yr Toxicity	10-Yr OS	10-Yr DM
Adjuvant RT	62%	70%	7%	5.3%	70.8%	77%	10.1%
Wait and see	39%	65%	16%	2.5%	59.7%	80%	11%
p value	<.0001	.054	<.0001	.052	.001	NS	NS

Wiegel, German ARO 96-02 (*JCO* 2009, PMID 19433689; Update *Eur Urol* 2014, PMID 24680359): PRT of 385 patients w/ pT3N0 prostate cancer (any margin status) and PSA <0.1 ng/mL randomized to adjuvant RT vs. W&S. Primary end point: bRFS. RT (60 Gy/30 fx) with 3D-CRT to prostatic bed + SVs, 1 cm PTV margins, starting 8 to 12 weeks after surgery; 70 of 78 patients who did not reach "undetectable PSA" received 66.6 Gy RT and were excluded from randomization. bF defined as undetectable to detectable and another increase at 3 months. Nineteen percent of patients randomized to RT did not receive it. Neither DMFS nor OS was significantly improved by adjuvant RT. Only 1 grade 3 bladder toxicity, and 5 total grade 2 urinary and/or rectal toxicities reported. Results shown below (Table 41.3). **Conclusion: Adjuvant RT reduced the risk of biochemical progression with a hazard**

TABLE 41.3: Results of German ARO 9602 Adjuvant RT for Prostate Cancer

	5-Yr bRFS (PSA Undetectable)	≥Gr 1 Toxicity	10-Yr bRFS
Adjuvant RT	72%	22%	56%
Observation	54%	4%	35%
p value	.0015	<.001	<.0001

ratio of 0.51 in pT3 PCa and is safe. *Comment: ARO used the most modern RT technique and most sensitive PSA assay, required an undetectable PSA prior to randomization, and included only pT3 patients.*

Is early salvage RT superior to adjuvant RT?

The ARTISTIC meta-analysis combined the results of RAVES, RADICALS-RT, and GETUG-AFU 17 (Table 41.4) and suggests that early salvage RT may reduce toxicity and avoid unnecessary treatment without compromising EFS compared to adjuvant RT.[17,27–29] UCLA data shows that with every 0.1 ng/mL increase, the likelihood of cure decreases by ~3%, suggesting that earlier intervention may lead to better outcomes.[18]

Vale, ARTISTIC Meta-Analysis (*Lancet* 2020, PMID 33002431): The ARTISTIC collaboration is a planned series of reviews and meta-analyses for RAVES,[28] RADICALS-RT,[29] and GETUG-AFU 17.[17] This first series analyzed EFS defined as (a) PSA ≥0.4 after RT, (b) any PSA ≥2.0, (c) clinical or radiographic progression, (d) nontrial treatment, or (e) death from prostate cancer. Over 70% of patients had at least one of positive margins, ECE, or SVI. At the time of analysis, 39% of men assigned to early salvage therapy had received RT. Adjuvant RT did not improve EFS (89% vs. 88%) compared to salvage RT. Outcomes were consistent across all three included trials and across patient subgroups. Only 8% to 17% had GS 8-10 and 19% to 21% had SVI, suggesting that most enrolled patients had relatively favorable pathology findings. **Conclusion: Adjuvant RT does not improve EFS in men with localized or locally advanced prostate cancer compared to early salvage RT.**

TABLE 41.4: Randomized Trials of Adjuvant vs. Early Salvage RT

Trial	Post-Op PSA (ng/mL)	Salvage RT Threshold	RT Dose	5-Yr bPFS (Adjuvant vs. Salvage)
RAVES[28]	<0.1	0.2 ng/mL	64 Gy/32 fx	86% vs. 87%
RADICALS-RT[29]	<0.2	0.1 ng/mL or 3 successive increases	66 Gy/33 fx or 52.5 Gy/20 fx	85% vs. 88%
GETUG-AFU 17[17]	<0.1	0.2 ng/mL	66 Gy/33 fx	92% vs. 90%

Is there a nomogram that can be used to delineate which patients may be good candidates for salvage RT?

The Stephenson nomogram has been utilized to predict outcomes after salvage RT and was updated by Tendulkar to help elucidate the efficacy of salvage therapy in the ultrasensitive PSA era.

Tendulkar, Multi-Institution Nomogram (*JCO* 2016, PMID 27528718): Multi-institution RR of 2,460 LN-negative patients s/p RP with a detectable post-RP PSA treated with salvage RT w/ or w/o ADT including patients whose post-op PSA was <0.2 ng/mL. Both bRFS and DM rates improved when salvage RT delivered at lower PSA levels, even before meeting AUA criteria for bF of ≥0.2 ng/mL (see Table 41.5). On MVA, pre-RT PSA, GS, EPE, SVI, surgical margins, ADT use, and RT dose were associated with FFBF.

TABLE 41.5 Tendulkar Nomogram Results

PSA at Salvage RT	0.01–0.20 ng/mL	0.21–0.5 ng/mL	0.51–1.0 ng/mL	1.01–2 ng/mL	>2.0 ng/mL	p Value
5-yr bRFS	71%	63%	54%	43%	37%	<.001
10-yr DM	9%	15%	19%	20%	37%	<.001

■ How can advanced imaging impact postoperative radiation?

Jani, EMPIRE-1 (Lancet 2021, PMID 33971152): Phase 2-3 trial of 165 patients with detectable PSA after prostatectomy and negative conventional imaging randomized to F18 fluciclovine PET-CT for radiation decision making. Fluciclovine PET-CT improved 3-yr EFS compared to conventional imaging alone (76% vs. 63%, *p* = .0028).

■ Can genomic classifiers help risk-stratify patients?

There is growing evidence that genomic classifiers such as Decipher may improve selection for post-operative RT and/or ADT following prostatectomy.

Feng (*JAMA Oncol* 2021, PMID 33570548): Subset of 760 patients from RTOG 9601. Decipher GC score was independently associated with DM, PCSM, and OS. The addition of bicalutamide to early salvage RT (at PSA <0.7 ng/ml) was associated with better outcomes in patients with higher GC scores but not lower GC scores.

Dalela (*JCO* 2017, PMID 28350520): Cohort of 512 patients s/p RP with ≥pT3a, pN1, or positive margins. Twenty-two percent received adjuvant RT. Genomic classifier (Decipher) score >0.6 was an independent predictor of clinical recurrence. Adjuvant RT associated with decreased 10-year clinical recurrence (10% vs. 42%; SS) in those with ≥2 risk factors (pT3b/T4, Gleason 8–10, N+, or Decipher >0.6). **Conclusion: Decipher score may aid in patient selection for adjuvant RT.**

■ What is the benefit of adding ADT to salvage RT?

Two randomized trials comparing salvage RT ± ADT have both shown a bRFS benefit to the addition of ADT, and RTOG 9601 found an OS benefit of 5% at 12 years. RTOG 9601 utilized 2 years of bicalutamide whereas the GETUG trial used 6 months of goserelin. Some clinicians have used the GETUG trial to justify limiting ADT to 6 months, although the optimal duration and method of ADT in the postoperative setting is unknown. The RADICALS-RT study has a companion hormonal therapy study testing no ADT vs. 6 months ADT vs. 2 years ADT, which may help elucidate the optimal duration of ADT. GU006 is assessing the role of apalutamide in this setting.

Shipley, RTOG 9601 (*NEJM* 2017, PMID 28146658): PRT of 761 patients with biochemical failure (post-op PSA 0.2–4.0 ng/mL) and either pT2 w/ positive margins or pT3, N0, who received salvage RT (64.8 Gy/36 fx), then randomized to 24 months of 150 mg daily bicalutamide vs. placebo. Median PSA at entry 0.6 ng/mL. MFU 12.6 years. **Conclusion: The addition of ADT to salvage RT improved bF, DM, PCM, and OS with tolerable side effects.** *Comment: Relatively high PSA at entry, low RT dose by modern standards.*

TABLE 41.6: RTOG 9601 Clinical Outcomes							
	12-Yr bF	12-Yr DM	12-Yr PCM	12-Yr OS	Late Grade 3/4 Bladder Toxicity	Late Grade 3/4 Bowel Toxicity	Gynecomastia
RT + placebo	68%	23%	13%	71%	6.7%	1.6%	11%
RT + bicalutamide	44%	14%	6%	76%	7%	2.7%	70%
p value	<.001	<.001	<.001	.04	NS	NS	<.001

Spratt, Secondary Analysis of RTOG 9601 (*JAMA Oncol* 2020, PMID 32215583): See trial details in Table 41.6. This analysis demonstrated a significant OS benefit for bicalutamide in men with PSA >1.5 ng/mL (HR 0.45; 0.25–0.81), but not for PSA 0.2 to 1.5 ng/mL (HR 0.87; 0.66–1.16). In a subset analysis of men with PSA of 0.61 to 1.5 ng/mL, bicalutamide was associated with improved OS (HR 0.61; 0.39–0.94). Men receiving bicalutamide with PSA ≤0.6 ng/mL had increased other-cause mortality (HR 1.94; 1.17–3.20) and grades 3 to 5 cardiac events (OR 3.57; 1.09–15.97). **Conclusion: Long-term ADT did not improve OS in patients receiving early salvage RT (PSA ≤0.6 ng/mL), and may be associated with increased risk of other-cause mortality.**

Carrie, GETUG-AFU 16 (*Lancet* 2019, PMID 31629656): PRT of 743 men s/p RP with initially unde-tectable and subsequently rising post-op PSA between 0.2 and 2.0 ng/mL, randomized to RT alone vs. RT + 6 months of goserelin. RT was 66 Gy/33 fx via 3D-CRT or IMRT. MFU, 112 months. RT + ADT improved 5-year bRFS (49% vs. 64%; SS) and 10-year DMFS (69% vs. 75%; SS). **Conclusion: Salvage RT plus short-term ADT improves DMFS.** *Comment: Men with PSA >0.5 ng/ml had a greater bRFS benefit compared with those with <0.5 ng/ml.*

▪ Is there a hypofractionated regimen that can be considered when delivering salvage RT?

A University of Wisconsin study (Kruser et al.) evaluated 108 patients treated with salvage RT to 65 Gy/26 fx of 2.5 Gy/fx. The 4-year bRFS was 67%, and authors concluded that "hypofractionation may provide a con-venient, resource-efficient, and well-tolerated salvage approach."[30] Additionally, the German PRIAMOS trial utilized 54 Gy/18 fx to the prostate bed; toxicity outcomes were favorable at 10 weeks post-RT.[31] Gladwish et al. (Toronto) published their phase I/II toxicity results using 51 Gy/17 fx.[32] These two trials each included 40 or fewer patients, and oncologic outcomes are pending. NRG GU003 is a recently closed trial that randomized patients to 66.6 Gy/37 fx (1.8/fx) vs. 62.5 Gy/25 fx (2.5/fx).

▪ How should we treat patients with lymph node–positive disease following prostatectomy?

The Messing trial established ADT as standard of care for pN1 disease.[33] The role of RT is controversial, though retrospective data suggest benefit particularly for patients with (a) ≤2 +LNs, GS 7 to 10, pT3b/pT4 disease, or positive margins or (b) 3 to 4 +LNs.[25,34]

Messing (*NEJM* 1999, PMID 10588962; Update *Lancet Oncol* 2006, PMID 16750497): Multi-institution PRT of 98 men with pT1b–T2 prostate cancer s/p RP found to have LN+ disease randomized to imme-diate (monthly goserelin or bilateral orchiectomy) vs. delayed ADT (initiated at disease progression). MFU 11.9 years. Immediate ADT improved OS (HR: 1.84, $p = .04$), PCSS (HR: 4.09, $p = .0004$), and PFS (HR: 3.42, $p < .0001$). Seventy-nine percent of those in the delayed ADT arm entered an active treat-ment by 5 years. **Conclusion: Immediate postoperative ADT improves OS for LN+ prostate cancer.** *Comment: Study conducted in the pre-PSA era and PSA was not used to guide decision-making (i.e., only clinically palpable nodules were considered local failures); average pretreatment PSA in the delayed ADT arm was 14 ng/mL at time of initiating ADT; Gleason score information was not available from 14 of 36 institutions; an imbalance may exist that accounts for differences in survival.*

Briganti (*Eur Urol* 2011, PMID 21354694): Retrospective matched pair analysis for pT2–4, LN+ pros-tate cancer comparing ADT + RT vs. ADT alone; 703 patients matched for age, T stage, GS, margin status, number of nodes, follow-up time. MFU 100 months; 10-year OS 55% vs. 74% ($p < .001$) and 10-year CSS 70% vs. 86% ($p = .004$) in favor of ADT + RT. **Conclusion: Adding RT to ADT may improve CSS and OS for LN+ disease.** *Comment: retrospective; lack of standardized RT dose and length of ADT; PSA data at time of RT not available.*

Abdollah (*JCO* 2014, PMID 25245445): RR of 1,100 patients with pN1 prostate cancer treated with RP and PLND between 1988 and 2010 treated with ADT with or without RT. Investigators found four variables that could be used to stratify patients according to PCM risk: the number of involved LNs, pathologic GS, tumor stage, and margin status. Men with either (a) ≤2 +LNs, GS 7 to 10, pT3b/ pT4 disease, or positive margins (HR: 0.30, $p = .002$) or (b) 3 to 4 +LNs (HR: 0.21, $p = .02$) appeared to benefit from combined ADT + RT. These results were confirmed when OS was examined as an end point. **Conclusion: Postoperative RT appears to provide benefit in carefully selected men with pathologically node-positive prostate cancer.**

REFERENCES

1. Siegel RL, Miller KD, Jemal A. Cancer statistics, 2020. *CA Cancer J Clin.* 2020;70(1):7–30. doi:10.3322/caac.21387
2. Boorjian SA, Karnes RJ, Rangel LJ, et al. Mayo Clinic validation of the D'amico risk group classification for pre-dicting survival following radical prostatectomy. *J Urol.* 2008;179(4):1354–1360; discussion 1360–1351. doi:10.1016/j.juro.2007.11.061
3. Barry MJ, Gallagher PM, Skinner JS, Fowler FJ Jr. Adverse effects of robotic-assisted laparoscopic versus open retro-pubic radical prostatectomy among a nationwide random sample of medicare-age men. *J Clin Oncol.* 2012;30(5):513–518. doi:10.1200/JCO.2011.36.8621

4. Cookson MS, Aus G, Burnett AL, et al. Variation in the definition of biochemical recurrence in patients treated for localized prostate cancer: the American Urological Association Prostate Guidelines for Localized Prostate Cancer Update Panel report and recommendations for a standard in the reporting of surgical outcomes. *J Urol.* 2007;177(2):540–545. doi:10.1016/j.juro.2006.10.097

5. Dotan ZA, Bianco FJ, Jr., Rabbani F, et al. Pattern of prostate-specific antigen (PSA) failure dictates the probability of a positive bone scan in patients with an increasing PSA after radical prostatectomy. *J Clin Oncol.* 2005;23(9):1962–1968. doi:10.1200/JCO.2005.06.058

6. Tateishi U, Morita S, Taguri M, et al. A meta-analysis of (18)F-Fluoride positron emission tomography for assessment of metastatic bone tumor. *Ann Nucl Med.* 2010;24(7):523–531. doi:10.1007/s12149-010-0393-7

7. Sella T, Schwartz LH, Swindle PW, et al. Suspected local recurrence after radical prostatectomy: endorectal coil MR imaging. *Radiology.* 2004;231(2):379–385. doi:10.1148/radiol.2312030011

8. Silverman JM, Krebs TL. MR imaging evaluation with a transrectal surface coil of local recurrence of prostatic cancer in men who have undergone radical prostatectomy. *AJR Am J Roentgenol.* 1997;168(2):379–385. doi:10.2214/ajr.168.2.9016212

9. Miralbell R, Vees H, Lozano J, et al. Endorectal MRI assessment of local relapse after surgery for prostate cancer: a model to define treatment field guidelines for adjuvant radiotherapy in patients at high risk for local failure. *Int J Radiat Oncol Biol Phys.* 2007;67(2):356–361. doi:10.1016/j.ijrobp.2006.08.079

10. Tendulkar RD, Stephans K. Contemporary external beam radiotherapy. In: Klein EA, Jones JS. *Management of Prostate Cancer.* 3rd ed. Humana Press; 2012;243–261. doi:10.1007/978-1-60761-259-9_15

11. Stephenson AJ, Scardino PT, Kattan MW, et al. Predicting the outcome of salvage radiation therapy for recurrent prostate cancer after radical prostatectomy. *J Clin Oncol.* 2007;25(15):2035–2041. doi:10.1200/JCO.2006.08.9607

12. Connolly JA, Shinohara K, Presti JC Jr, Carroll PR. Local recurrence after radical prostatectomy: characteristics in size, location, and relationship to prostate-specific antigen and surgical margins. *Urology.* 1996;47(2):225–231. doi:10.1016/S0090-4295(99)80421-X

13. Freedland SJ, Humphreys EB, Mangold LA, et al. Risk of prostate cancer-specific mortality following biochemical recurrence after radical prostatectomy. *JAMA.* 2005;294(4):433–439. doi:10.1001/jama.294.4.433

14. Pound CR, Partin AW, Eisenberger MA, et al. Natural history of progression after PSA elevation following radical prostatectomy. *JAMA.* 1999;281(17):1591–1597. doi:10.1001/jama.281.17.1591

15. *AJCC Cancer Staging Manual, Eighth Edition.* 8th ed. Springer Publishing Company; 2017. doi:10.1093/annonc/mdz396

16. Clarke NW, Ali A, Ingleby FC, et al. Addition of docetaxel to hormonal therapy in low- and high-burden metastatic hormone sensitive prostate cancer: long-term survival results from the STAMPEDE trial. *Ann Oncol.* 2019;30(12):1992–2003. doi:10.1093/annonc/mdz396

17. Sargos P, Chabaud S, Latorzeff I, et al. Adjuvant radiotherapy versus early salvage radiotherapy plus short-term androgen deprivation therapy in men with localised prostate cancer after radical prostatectomy (GETUG-AFU 17): a randomised, phase 3 trial. *Lancet Oncol.* 2020;21(10):1341–1352. doi:10.1016/S1470-2045(20)30454-X

18. King CR. The timing of salvage radiotherapy after radical prostatectomy: a systematic review. *Int J Radiat Oncol Biol Phys.* 2012;84(1):104–111. doi:10.1016/j.ijrobp.2011.10.069

19. Dess RT, Sun Y, Jackson WC, et al. Association of presalvage radiotherapy psa levels after prostatectomy with outcomes of long-term antiandrogen therapy in men with prostate cancer. *JAMA Oncol.* 2020;6(5):735–743. doi:10.1001/jamaoncol.2020.0109

20. Pollack A, Karrison TG, Balogh AG, et al. Short term androgen deprivation therapy without or with pelvic lymph node treatment added to prostate bed only salvage radiotherapy: the NRG Oncology/RTOG 0534 SPPORT Trial. *Int J Radiat Oncol Biol Phys.* 2018;102:1605. doi:10.1016/j.ijrobp.2018.08.052

21. Pisansky TM, Agrawal S, Hamstra DA, et al. Salvage radiation therapy dose response for biochemical failure of prostate cancer after prostatectomy-a multi-institutional observational study. *Int J Radiat Oncol Biol Phys.* 2016;96(5):1046–1053. doi:10.1016/j.ijrobp.2016.08.043

22. Videtic GMM, Woody N, Vassil AD. *Handbook of Treatment Planning in Radiation Oncology.* 3rd ed. Demos Medical; 2020. doi:10.1891/9780826168429

23. Han M, Partin AW, Zahurak M, et al. Biochemical (prostate specific antigen) recurrence probability following radical prostatectomy for clinically localized prostate cancer. *J Urol.* 2003;169(2):517–523. doi:10.1016/S0022-5347(05)63946-8

24. Nguyen CT, Reuther AM, Stephenson AJ. The specific definition of high risk prostate cancer has minimal impact on biochemical relapse-free survival. *J Urol.* 2009;181(1):75–80. doi:10.1016/j.juro.2008.09.027

25. Briganti A, Karnes RJ, Da Pozzo LF, et al. Combination of adjuvant hormonal and radiation therapy significantly prolongs survival of patients with pT2-4 pN+ prostate cancer: results of a matched analysis. *Eur Urol.* 2011;59(5):832–840. doi:10.1016/j.eururo.2011.02.024

26. Daly T, Hickey BE, Lehman M, Francis DP, See AM. Adjuvant radiotherapy following radical prostatectomy for prostate cancer. *The Cochrane database of systematic reviews.* 2011(12):Cd007234.

27. Vale CL, Fisher D, Kneebone A, et al. Adjuvant or early salvage radiotherapy for the treatment of localised and locally advanced prostate cancer: a prospectively planned systematic review and meta-analysis of aggregate data. *Lancet Oncol.* 2020;396:1422–1431. doi:10.1016/S0140-6736(20)31952-8

28. Kneebone A, Fraser-Browne C, Duchesne GM, et al. Adjuvant radiotherapy versus early salvage radiotherapy following radical prostatectomy (TROG 08.03/ANZUP RAVES): a randomised, controlled, phase 3, non-inferiority trial. *Lancet Oncol.* 2020;21(10):1331–1340. doi:10.1016/S1470-2045(20)30456-3

29. Parker CC, Clarke NW, Cook AD, et al. Timing of radiotherapy after radical prostatectomy (RADICALS-RT): a randomised, controlled phase 3 trial. *Lancet.* 2020;396:1413–1421. doi:10.1016/S0140-6736(20)31553-1

30. Kruser TJ, Jarrard DF, Graf, AK, et al. Early hypofractionated salvage radiotherapy for postprostatectomy biochemical recurrence. *Cancer.* 2011;117(12):2629–2636. doi:10.1002/cncr.25824

31. Katayama S, Striecker T, Kessel K, et al. Hypofractionated IMRT of the prostate bed after radical prostatectomy: acute toxicity in the PRIAMOS-1 trial. *Int J Radiat Oncol Biol Phys.* 2014;90(4):926–933. doi:10.1016/j.ijrobp.2014.07.015

32. Gladwish A, Loblaw A, Cheung P, et al. Accelerated hypofractioned postoperative radiotherapy for prostate cancer: a prospective phase I/II study. *Clin Oncol.* 2015;27(3):145–152. doi:10.1016/j.clon.2014.12.003

33. Messing EM, Manola J, Yao J, et al. Immediate versus deferred androgen deprivation treatment in patients with node-positive prostate cancer after radical prostatectomy and pelvic lymphadenectomy. *Lancet Oncol.* 2006;7(6):472–479. doi:10.1016/S1470-2045(06)70700-8

34. Abdollah F, Karnes RJ, Suardi N, et al. Impact of adjuvant radiotherapy on survival of patients with node-positive prostate cancer. *J Clin Oncol.* 2014;32(35):3939–3947. doi:10.1200/JCO.2013.54.7893

42 ■ BLADDER CANCER

Winston Vuong, Omar Y. Mian, and Rahul D. Tendulkar

QUICK HIT ■ Bladder cancer is the second most common GU malignancy, and >90% are urothelial carcinomas. About 70% have superficial disease and are managed with TURBT ± intravesical therapy (Table 42.1). Patients with MIBC are most often managed with radical cystectomy and perioperative CHT. SBP may be utilized in certain patients. Up to 80% achieve a CR to induction chemoRT, and 70% to 80% will remain free of local recurrence and retain their native bladder.

Table 42.1: General Treatment Paradigm for Bladder Cancer	
	Treatment Options
Superficial tumors (Ta, Tis, T1)	TURBT followed by surveillance OR intravesical therapy (BCG vs. mitomycin) OR cystectomy (for high risk)
T2–T4a (cystectomy candidates)	Radical cystectomy ± neoadjuvant cisplatin-based CHT OR SBP: maximal TURBT, then chemoRT 40–45 Gy, then cystoscopy, then if CR* boost to 64 Gy, then surveillance; hypofractionation to 55 Gy/20 fractions is an acceptable alternative
T2–T4 (inoperable)	ChemoRT (preferred, if CHT candidate) OR RT alone (if not CHT candidate)
Metastatic	CHT (e.g., cisplatin/gemcitabine) + palliative RT as needed; immunotherapy with PD-1 inhibitor (atezolizumab or pembrolizumab) is first line if cisplatin-ineligible

*CR = T0/Tis/Ta; if ≥T1 on cystoscopy after induction chemoRT, salvage cystectomy.
Optimal candidates for selective bladder preservation: unifocal tumor <5 cm after complete TURBT, cT2–T3 (and selected T4a), cN0, adequate bladder function, compliant with surveillance protocol, no hydronephrosis, no associated CIS, no IBD, no prior RT.

EPIDEMIOLOGY: In 2020, ~81,400 new cases (76% male), ~18,000 deaths.[1] Median age 70 years.[2] Highest rates in North America/Western Europe.[3]

RISK FACTORS: Majority of cases are related to environmental exposures. Smoking is most important with RR of 2 to 5 compared with nonsmokers and is associated with about 50% of cases. Others include chemical exposures (industrial aromatic amines, polycyclic aromatic hyrdrocarbons, hair dyes, chlorinated water, arsenic), drugs (phenacetin-containing analgesics, cyclophosphamide), schistosomiasis (associated with squamous cell carcinoma), chronic inflammation (chronic UTIs, cystitis, stones), radiation exposure.[3]

ANATOMY: The bladder can be divided into the body (above the ureteral orifices), the trigone (area between the ureteral and urethral orifices), and bladder neck. Layers from internal to external: urothelium (epithelial lining made up of transitional cells bounded by a thin basement membrane), lamina propria (thick layer of fibroelastic connective tissue), and detrusor muscle (smooth muscle arranged in inner longitudinal, middle circular, and outer longitudinal layers). The bladder is anchored to anterior abdominal wall by the urachus. It is bounded superiorly by peritoneum, and anteriorly/inferiorly/laterally by perivesical fat. Primary lymph node drainage includes external iliac, internal iliac, obturator, perivesical, and presacral nodes. The common iliacs are a secondary drainage site.[4]

PATHOLOGY: Urothelial carcinoma (>90% of cases in the United States), squamous cell carcinoma (~3%), adenocarcinoma (~2%), small-cell carcinoma (~1%), all others <1% (sarcomas, lymphomas, melanoma, mets). More aggressive urothelial variants include micropapillary, plasmacytoid, nested, and sarcomatoid histologies, which may warrant more aggressive management. In *Schistosoma haematobium* endemic areas, squamous cell carcinomas comprise the majority of cases. Urachal tumors are commonly adenocarcinomas, and have better outcomes than nonurachal adenocarcinoma.

CLINICAL PRESENTATION: Gross or microscopic hematuria most common presenting symptoms. If gross hematuria, risk of a bladder tumor is 10% to 20%. Less commonly, patients may note obstructive/irritative bladder symptoms or pain.

WORKUP: H&P.

Labs: Urine cytology. Cytology has poor sensitivity (34%) but high specificity (>98%).[5] CBC, CMP, alkaline phosphatase.

Procedures: Cystoscopy. If a suspicious lesion is noted in the bladder, proceed to TURBT. TURBT is diagnostic and often therapeutic for T1 disease. Random or targeted biopsies of sites adjacent to tumor are performed to assess for field defect/CIS, as well as biopsy of the prostate. Biopsy specimen should include muscle to assess for invasion.

Imaging: If cystoscopic appearance of the tumor is solid, high grade, or MIBC, consider CT or MRI of abdomen and pelvis prior to TURBT. The entire urinary tract should be imaged (e.g., CT urogram with and without contrast including delayed images or MRI urogram). Obtain chest imaging if muscle invasive. Bone scan if alkaline phosphatase elevated or bone pain. No role for PET/CT. Neuroimaging only for symptomatic or high-risk patients, such as those with small-cell histology.

PROGNOSTIC FACTORS: Stage (Table 42.2), grade, multicentricity, size, recurrence, presence of CIS, LVI, growth pattern, histology.

STAGING

TABLE 42.2: AJCC 8th Edition (2017): Staging for Urinary Bladder Cancer						
T/M		N	cN0	cN1	cN2	cN3
T1	• Invades lamina propria (subepithelial connective tissue)		I	IIIA	IIIB	
T2	a Invades muscularis propria (inner half)		II			
	b Invades muscularis propria (outer half)					
T3	a Invades perivesical tissue (microscopic)					
	b Invades perivesical tissue (macroscopic)					
T4	a Invades prostatic stroma, seminal vesicles, uterus, vagina					
	b Invades pelvic wall or abdominal wall		IVA			
M1a	Nonregional LNs					
M1b	Distant metastasis		IVB			

cN1, single pelvic node (true pelvis, perivesicular, obturator, internal iliac, external iliac, or sacral); cN2, multiple LNs in the true pelvis; cN3, common iliac LNs.

TREATMENT PARADIGM

Surgery

TURBT: First step in diagnosis, and is therapeutic for Ta/Tis/T1 non–muscle-invasive disease. Observation can be considered after TURBT in select patients with Ta or low-grade T1 disease without risk factors. Adjuvant intravesical therapy recommended for Tis, high-grade Ta or T1, positive cytology, recurrent disease, or multifocality. TURBT for maximal debulking is recommended as the initial step in patients considering SBP for MIBC.

Cystectomy: Radical cystectomy with urinary diversion is a standard of care for multiple recurrent superficial tumors, high-grade T1 tumors with CIS, and MIBC, as well as variant histologies. The technique includes en bloc resection of bladder, peritoneal covering, urachus, perivesical fat, lower ureters, bilateral pelvic LNs, proximal urethra (men), entire urethra (all women, and men with CIS/multicentric tumors/involvement of bladder neck or prostatic urethra), prostate, seminal vesicles, pelvic vas deferens (men), uterus, fallopian tubes, ovaries, cervix, vaginal cuff (women). Per NCCN, bilateral pelvic lymphadenectomy should be performed and include at a minimum the obturator, external iliac, internal iliac, and common iliac lymph nodes.[6] SWOG 8710 demonstrated improved survival when at least 10 LNs were removed.[7] A 2016 ASCO guideline stated that the standard treatment for cT2–T4a bladder cancer is neoadjuvant cisplatin-based combination CHT followed by radical cystectomy, reserving chemoRT as an alternative in appropriately selected patients and in patients for whom cystectomy is not an option.[8]

Urinary Diversions: Diversion may be either noncontinent or continent. Historically, noncontinent diversions were standard (e.g., ileal conduit). Advances in technique resulted in continent diversion for most patients in the modern era. Broadly, these techniques are categorized as continent cutaneous diversions (e.g., Kock, Indiana, Miami pouches) that require self-catheterization or (more commonly) orthotopic neobladders that connect directly to the native urethra using the external sphincter for continence.

Intravesical Therapy: Allows for high concentrations of agents to be delivered locally in an effort to eradicate viable tumor and prevent recurrences. BCG is a live attenuated *mycobacterium bovis* that functions via an antitumor immunostimulatory mechanism, and is considered the adjuvant treatment of choice for high-grade Ta, Tis, or T1 tumors after TURBT. BCG is initiated 3 to 4 weeks after resection, and given weekly for 6 weeks. Meta-analyses have shown BCG to be superior to mitomycin C in Tis as well as Ta and T1 disease.[9,10] Common toxicities of BCG include urinary frequency (71%), cystitis (67%), fever (25%), and hematuria (23%).[10] Note that the frequency and dysuria associated with BCG treatment can be severe and that many patients do not complete the full 6-week course due to acute toxicity.

Chemotherapy: Can be used perioperatively before or after cystectomy, concurrent with RT as part of bladder preservation therapy, or in the metastatic setting. Evidence is stronger for neoadjuvant CHT rather than for adjuvant—a meta-analysis demonstrated a 5% survival benefit with neoadjuvant platinum-based CHT compared to surgery alone.[11] Current and future trials are assessing the addition of immunotherapy in the nonmetastatic setting.

Perioperative: Cisplatin-based regimens including dose-dense methotrexate, vinblastine, doxorubicin, and cisplatin (DD-MVAC), gemcitabine/cisplatin, and methotrexate, cisplatin, and vinblastine (MCV). The different regimens have not been directly compared in randomized trials.

Concurrent With RT: NCCN endorsed regimens for concurrent CHT include: cisplatin 15 mg/m^2 days 1 to 3, 8 to 10, 15 to 17 and paclitaxel 50 mg/m^2 on days 1, 8, and 15; cisplatin 15 mg/m^2 on days 1 to 3, 8 to 10, 15 to 17, and 5-FU 400 mg/m^2 on days 1 to 3, 8 to 10, and 15 to 17; or 5-FU 500 mg/m^2 on days 1 to 5 and 16 to 20 and mitomycin C 12 mg/m^2 on day 1.

Metastatic: Gemcitabine/cisplatin or DD-MVAC followed by avelumab maintenance therapy. Immunotherapy is second line in cisplatin-eligible patients. In cisplatin-ineligible patients, options include gemcitabine/carboplatin followed by avelumab maintenance, and atezolizumab or pembrolizumab for patients with PDL-1 expressing tumors or those not eligible for platinum-based therapy regardless of PDL-1 expression.

Radiation

Indications: RT may be given for organ preservation as an alternative to cystectomy (SBP), as definitive management in nonsurgical candidates or those who refuse cystectomy, or palliatively. The role for adjuvant RT after cystectomy is evolving but may be considered for select cases of pT3–4, positive margins, or ECE (54–60 Gy to positive margin with tumor bed and pelvic nodes to 45 to 50.4 Gy; see adjuvant guidelines).[12]

Selective Bladder Preservation: Ideal candidates include those with a unifocal tumor <5 cm after complete TURBT, cT2–T3 (and selected T4a), cN0, adequate bladder function, compliant with surveillance protocol, no hydronephrosis, no associated CIS, no IBD, and no prior pelvic RT. SBP can be considered in patients with unilateral hydronephrosis, typically following ureteral stenting.

Schema: Maximal TURBT → chemoRT 40 to 45 Gy → cystoscopy → if CR (T0/Tis/Ta) boost to ~64 Gy → surveillance. If ≥T1 on cystoscopy after induction chemoRT, proceed to salvage cystectomy. Interim cystoscopy may be avoided in patients who are not surgical candidates.

Dose: Multiple regimens have been used, typically treating the pelvis to 40–45 Gy followed by a boost to ~64 Gy at 1.8 to 2.0 Gy/fraction. An alternative fractionation is 55 Gy/20 fx as per BC2001.[13] ENI was typically utilized in RTOG trials, but not in BC2001. ENI is appropriate in high-risk patients, for example, T3/T4 tumors, micropapillary, plasmacytoid, or small-cell histology or clinically N1 patients. For clinical node-positive disease, consider boosting the involved node up to 64 Gy if safely achievable.

Toxicity: Acute: fatigue, nausea, diarrhea, urinary urgency, frequency. Late: cystitis, fibrosis, proctitis, enteritis.

Procedure: See *Handbook of Treatment Planning in Radiation Oncology*, Chapter 8.[14]

■ EVIDENCE-BASED Q&A

▨ What is the rationale for SBP?

Strategies to preserve the native bladder and avoid the potential complications of radical cystectomy and urinary diversion are appealing, particularly for those who are older adults or with significant comorbidities. A series of phase II trials were conducted by the RTOG in the 1980s and 1990s.[15-21] Pooled analysis of these trials demonstrated low rates of toxicity with survival outcomes similar to historical cystectomy series for clinically staged patients.[22,23] There have been no randomized trials directly comparing SBP with radical cystectomy. Of note, clinical understaging is common and SBP patients are generally older with more comorbidities; therefore, caution must be taken when comparing retrospective series of SBP vs. cystectomy.

Mak, RTOG pooled analysis (*JCO* 2014, PMID 25366678): Pooled analysis of 5 RTOG prospective phase II trials; 468 patients, clinical T2 (61%), T3 (35%), T4 (4%). Following chemoRT, CR was observed in 69% of patients; 5-year OS associated with T stage: 62% for T2 vs. 49% for T3–4 (p = .002); see Table 42.3 for overall results. **Conclusion: Long-term DSS is comparable to cystectomy series and can be considered as an alternative to surgery.**

TABLE 42.3: RTOG Pooled Analysis of Selective Bladder Trials					
	OS	DSS	Muscle-Invasive LF	Non–Muscle-Invasive LF	DM
5 years	57%	71%	13%	31%	31%
10 years	36%	65%	14%	36%	35%

▨ Are the rates of toxicity after SBP prohibitive?

Although survival rates are comparable to cystectomy, there is concern regarding late effects. RTOG pooled analysis suggests high-grade toxicity is uncommon.[24] Furthermore, patient-reported QOL outcomes from the BC2001 trial discussed in the following reported similar reductions in QOL between arms immediately following treatment, which improved to pretreatment baseline after 6 months, with no evidence that the addition of CHT impairs QOL long term.[25]

Efstathiou, RTOG pooled analysis (*JCO* 2009, PMID 19636019): A total of 285 patients from 4 RTOG trials. MFU 5.4 years. The late grade ≥3 toxicity rates were 5.7% GU and 1.9% GI. There were no late grade 4 events, and no patients required a cystectomy due to treatment-related toxicity. **Conclusion: Late effects do not appear prohibitive after SBP.**

▨ Is there a benefit to neoadjuvant/induction CHT prior to SBP?

Neoadjuvant CHT improves survival when delivered prior to radical cystectomy.[11] RTOG 8903 tested this concept in the SBP setting, but both this trial and other retrospective series showed no benefit to neoadjuvant CHT prior to definitive chemoRT.[26]

Shipley, RTOG 8903 (*JCO* 1998, PMID 9817278): PRT to assess the addition of neoadjuvant CHT to SBP. 123 patients with cT2–4a MIBC received TURBT and then randomized to ± 2 cycles of neoadjuvant MCV (methotrexate, cisplatin, vinblastine). All patients were treated to a dose of 39.6 Gy at 1.8 Gy/fx to pelvic field with cisplatin, then underwent cystoscopy at 4 weeks. If <CR, patients proceeded to cystectomy. If CR, patients received a 25.2 Gy tumor boost with cisplatin. No difference

in CR rate (61% vs. 55%), 5-year OS (48% vs. 49%), DM (33% vs. 39%), or survival with intact bladder (36% vs. 40%). **Conclusion: Neoadjuvant CHT prior to SBP increased toxicity without improving outcomes.**

■ **Does the addition of CHT to RT improve outcomes with definitive (nonoperative) management?**

LR rates with RT alone are high, and early data suggested a benefit to concurrent CHT.[27] This led to the UK Bladder Cancer 2001 (BC2001) trial.[13]

James, BC2001 (*NEJM* 2012, PMID 22512481): PRT of 360 patients with T2–T4a bladder cancer (adenocarcinoma, TCC, and SCC included). Allowed but did not require neoadjuvant CHT. Randomized to RT alone vs. RT and concurrent CHT with 5-FU 500 mg/m² days 1 to 5 and 16 to 20 and mitomycin C 12 mg/m² on day 1. RT either 55 Gy/20 fx or 64 Gy/32 fx, and the pelvic nodes were not electively targeted. Of note, midtreatment cystoscopy was not performed on this protocol; as a result, all patients were treated definitively. Primary end point was LRFS. **Conclusion: The addition of 5-FU/MMC to RT improves LRFS over RT alone (Table 42.4), without significant difference in OS (but not powered for OS).**

BC2001	2-Yr LRFS	Invasive LR	Noninvasive LR	2-Yr Cystectomy	5-Yr OS
RT	54%	19%	17%	17%	35%
ChemoRT	67%	11%	14%	11%	48%
p value	.03	.01		.03	.16

Table 42.4: UK BC2001 Trial of Definitive RT for Bladder Cancer

---

■ **What are some of the CHT regimens utilized for SBP in the modern era?**

Cisplatin-based CHT regimens predominate in North America because these are the regimens that have been evaluated by the RTOG. For patients who may not be candidates for platinum-based CHT due to hearing impairment, renal dysfunction, or poor performance status, there have been recent efforts to establish platinum-free chemoRT regimens. Per BC2001, 5-FU/MMC is an option. Most recently, the RTOG 0712 trial utilized 5-FU/cisplatin plus BID RT vs. low-dose gemcitabine plus daily RT.[28] RTOG 0233 examined cisplatin-based induction with either paclitaxel or 5-FU with concurrent BID RT followed by response-driven consolidation, then adjuvant cis/gem/paclitaxel, and found similar treatment completion and toxicity rates.[29]

Coen, NRG/RTOG 0712 (*JCO* 2019, PMID 30433852): Phase II PRT in MIBC randomizing 66 patients to FCT (5-FU/cisplatin) concurrent with RT delivered BID vs. GD (gemcitabine) concurrent with RT delivered once daily. Patients underwent TURBT and induction chemoRT to 40 Gy. Those achieving CR received consolidation chemoRT to 64 Gy. Non-CR had cystectomy performed. Patients on both arms were to receive adjuvant gemcitabine + cisplatin (GC). Primary end point: rate of freedom from distant metastasis at 3 years (DMF3). DMF3 was 78% and 84% for FCT and GD, respectively. Postinduction CR rates were 88% and 78%, respectively. In the FCT arm, 64% experienced treatment-related grade 3/4 acute toxicities, majority hematologic. In the GD arm, grade 3/4 acute toxicity was 55%, majority hematologic. **Conclusion: Both regimens exceeded the primary end point demonstrating a DMF3 greater than 75%. The trial was not powered to compare regimens. Fewer toxicities seen in the GD arm. Either arm would be acceptable to use as a base in future trials.**

■ **Do target volumes need to include the entire bladder? Is there a benefit to ENI?**

Given the difficulties with tumor localization as well as the propensity for multifocality of bladder cancer, standard RT techniques included the entire bladder in the target volume, even in localized disease. However, sparing the uninvolved bladder could potentially reduce toxicity, leading to interest in partial bladder-sparing techniques, which was assessed by the BC2001 trial. Most RTOG trials incorporate ENI using a "mini-pelvis" field, with the superior border at S2 to S3 to allow sparing of bowel in the potential future event of a urinary diversion. BC2001 did not intentionally target elective nodes, but did include the low pelvis/obturator nodes given the field design of whole bladder + 1.5 cm margin. Only 10 of 76 locoregional recurrences were in the pelvic nodes.

Huddart, BC2001 (IJROBP 2013, PMID 23958147): A total of 219 patients (subset of BC2001) randomized to standard whole bladder RT (PTV included outer bladder wall plus extravesical extent of tumor + 1.5 cm) vs. reduced high-dose volume RT (2 PTVs defined: PTV1 was the same as the control group and was treated to 80% of the prescribed dose, and PTV2 was defined as GTV + 1.5 cm). Patients were simulated with bladder empty. No difference in 2-year LRFS (61% vs. 64%), grades 3 to 4 acute toxicity (23% vs. 23%), 2-year grades 3 to 4 late toxicity (2.4% vs. 5.4%), or reduction in bladder capacity (76 mL difference in reduction favoring the reduced RT volume group was not statistically significant). **Conclusion: No differences in 2-year LRFS or late toxicity with reduced high-dose volume RT.**

Is there a benefit to hypofractionation?

The two most common fractionation schemes, 64 Gy/32 fx and 55 Gy/20 fx, have not been directly compared head-to-head in an RCT; however, a meta-analysis of the BC2001 and BCON trials support the use of the hypofractionated schedule.[30]

Choudury, BC2001/BCON Meta-Analysis (Lancet Oncol 2021, PMID 33539743): An individual patient data meta-analysis of 782 patients from the BC2001 trial (456 patients) and the BCON trial (326 patients) who had undergone SBP with either 64 Gy/32 fx or 55 Gy/20 fx (48% and 52% of the total cohort, respectively). With a median follow-up of 10 years, 55 Gy/20 fx was non-inferior to 64 Gy/32 fx with respect to invasive locoregional recurrence and bowel or bladder toxicity (adjusted RD -3.37%, 95% CI -11.85-5.10); and notably, a significantly lower risk of locoregional recurrence [adjusted HR 0.71, 95% CI 0.52-0.96]. **Conclusion: SBP with hypofractionation, 55 Gy/20 fx, has superior invasive locoregional control and is iso-toxic with 64 Gy/32 fx.**

Is there a benefit to hyperfractionation?

Evidence for hyperfractionation is mixed, as two older PRTs showed improved outcomes with hyperfractionation over standard fractionation, while a more recent PRT demonstrated no benefit and increased toxicity.[25] None of these trials included concurrent CHT, and thus the role of hyperfractionation is unclear in this setting. However, hyperfractionated chemoRT was one of the arms in the completed RTOG 0712 phase II randomized trial and may be considered in select patients.

Is there a benefit to adjuvant RT after cystectomy?

Adjuvant RT after cystectomy is rarely utilized. However, certain patient populations are known to have high rates of local failure (~30% for T3-4, ~70% for positive margins).[7] A randomized trial published in 1992 demonstrated an LC and DFS benefit in patients with T3-T4 disease; however, 80% of the patients on this study had squamous cell carcinoma.[31] A patterns-of-failure analysis showed that in patients with negative margins and >PT3 disease, 76% of all LF sites would have been covered within a small CTV covering only the iliac/obturator nodes, which would limit dose to bowel and neobladder. In patients with positive margins, failure in the cystectomy bed and presacral nodes increases substantially, necessitating larger CTV and the subsequent increase in potential toxicity, leading to consensus contouring guidelines.[12,32] An NCDB analysis found that PORT was associated with improved OS although this must be confirmed in prospective trials.[33]

Baumann, NCDB (Cancer Med 2019, PMID 31119885): NCDB analysis of ≥pT3pN0-3M0 LABC patients diagnosed from 2004 to 2014 who underwent RC ± PORT. Of 15,124 patients, PORT was given in 512 (3%). Overall, MS was 20.0 months for PORT vs. 20.8 months for no PORT (NS). After propensity matching, MS was 19.8 months for PORT vs. 16.9 months for no PORT (p = .03). For the subset of documented urothelial carcinoma patients (n = 1,460), PORT was associated with improved OS for pT4, pN+, and positive margins (p < .01 for all). **Conclusion: In this observational cohort, PORT was associated with improved OS in LABC after propensity matching.**

Is there a role for RT in select cases of T1 non–muscle-invasive disease?

TURBT followed by intravesical therapy is the standard of care for most patients with high-grade superficial cancers. However, many will still recur locally after this approach. For recurrent disease, standard therapy is cystectomy. RT may offer a bladder-sparing option for some patients with high-grade T1 or recurrent T1 cancers after BCG. The evidence supporting this approach is mixed, and RTOG 0926 is addressing this question.

■ Is there a role for palliative radiation?

Duchesne, MRC BA09 (*IJROBP* 2000, PMID 10802363): PRT of 500 patients (272 evaluable) with symptomatic MIBC considered unsuitable for curative treatment due to staging (T4b, N1, or M1) or comorbidity. Randomized to 21 Gy/3 fx QOD vs. 35 Gy/10 fx QD. Primary end point was symptomatic improvement at 3 months. Results: At 3 months, there was no statistically significant difference in symptomatic improvement between the two arms (71% for 35 Gy vs. 64% for 21 Gy). **Conclusion: 21 Gy/3 fx delivered QOD is a reasonable option for palliation of MIBC.**

REFERENCES

1. Siegel RL, Miller KD, Jemal A. Cancer statistics, 2020. *CA Cancer J Clin.* 2020;70(1):7–30. doi:10.3322/caac.21590
2. Scosyrev E, Noyes K, Feng C, Messing E. Sex and racial differences in bladder cancer presentation and mortality in the US. *Cancer.* 2009;115(1):68–74. doi:10.1002/cncr.23986
3. Pelucchi C, Bosetti C, Negri E, et al. Mechanisms of disease: the epidemiology of bladder cancer. *Nat Clin Pract Urol.* 2006;3(6):327–340. doi:10.1038/ncpuro0510
4. Amin M, Edge S, Greene F, et al. American Joint Committee on Cancer. *AJCC Cancer Staging Manual.* 8th ed. Springer International Publishing; 2017.
5. Lotan Y, Roehrborn CG. Sensitivity and specificity of commonly available bladder tumor markers versus cytology: results of a comprehensive literature review and meta-analyses. *Urology.* 2003;61(1):109–118; discussion 118. doi:10.1016/S0090-4295(02)02136-2
6. NCCN Clinical Practice Guidelines in Oncology: Bladder Cancer v6.2020. *J Natl Compr Canc Netw.* 2020.
7. Herr HW, Faulkner JR, Grossman HB, et al. Surgical factors influence bladder cancer outcomes: a cooperative group report. *J Clin Oncol.* 2004;22(14):2781–2789. doi:10.1200/JCO.2004.11.024
8. Milowsky MI, Rumble RB, Booth CM, et al. Guideline on muscle-invasive and metastatic bladder cancer (European Association of Urology Guideline): American Society of Clinical Oncology Clinical Practice Guideline Endorsement. *J Clin Oncol.* 2016;34(16):1945–1952. doi:10.1200/JCO.2015.65.9797
9. Sylvester RJ, van der Meijden AP, Witjes JA, Kurth K. Bacillus calmette-guerin versus chemotherapy for the intravesical treatment of patients with carcinoma in situ of the bladder: a meta-analysis of the published results of randomized clinical trials. *J Urol.* 2005;174(1):86–91; discussion 91-82. doi:10.1097/01.ju.0000162059.64886.1c
10. Shelley MD, Court JB, Kynaston H, et al. Intravesical Bacillus Calmette-Guerin in Ta and T1 Bladder Cancer. *Cochrane Database Syst Rev.* 2000;2000(4):Cd001986. doi:10.1002/14651858.CD001986
11. Vale C. Neoadjuvant chemotherapy in invasive bladder cancer: a systematic review and meta-analysis. *Lancet.* 2003;361(9373):1927–1934. doi:10.1016/S0140-6736(03)13580-5
12. Baumann BC, Bosch WR, Bahl A, et al. Development and validation of consensus contouring guidelines for adjuvant radiation therapy for bladder cancer after radical cystectomy. *Int J Radiat Oncol Biol Phys.* 2016;96(1):78–86. doi:10.1016/j.ijrobp.2016.04.032
13. James ND, Hussain SA, Hall E, et al. Radiotherapy with or without chemotherapy in muscle-invasive bladder cancer. *N Engl J Med.* 2012;366(16):1477–1488. doi:10.1056/NEJMoa1106106
14. Videtic GMM, Vassil AD, Woody NM. *Handbook of Treatment Planning in Radiation Oncology.* 3rd ed. Demos Medical; 2020.
15. Shipley WU, Prout GR Jr, Einstein AB, et al. Treatment of invasive bladder cancer by cisplatin and radiation in patients unsuited for surgery. *JAMA.* 1987;258(7):931–935. doi:10.1001/jama.258.7.931
16. Kaufman DS, Shipley WU, Griffin PP, et al. Selective bladder preservation by combination treatment of invasive bladder cancer. *N Engl J Med.* 1993;329(19):1377–1382. doi:10.1056/NEJM199311043291903
17. Tester W, Porter A, Asbell S, et al. Combined modality program with possible organ preservation for invasive bladder carcinoma: results of RTOG protocol 85-12. *Int J Radiat Oncol Biol Phys.* 1993;25(5):783–790. doi:10.1016/0360-3016(93)90306-G
18. Tester W, Caplan R, Heaney J, et al. Neoadjuvant combined modality program with selective organ preservation for invasive bladder cancer: results of Radiation Therapy Oncology Group phase II trial 8802. *J Clin Oncol.* 1996;14(1):119–126. doi:10.1200/JCO.1996.14.1.119
19. Kaufman DS, Winter KA, Shipley WU, et al. The initial results in muscle-invading bladder cancer of RTOG 95-06: phase I/II trial of transurethral surgery plus radiation therapy with concurrent cisplatin and 5-fluorouracil followed by selective bladder preservation or cystectomy depending on the initial response. *Oncologist.* 2000;5(6):471–476. doi:10.1634/theoncologist.5-6-471
20. Hagan MP, Winter KA, Kaufman DS, et al. RTOG 97-06: initial report of a phase I-II trial of selective bladder conservation using TURBT, twice-daily accelerated irradiation sensitized with cisplatin, and adjuvant MCV combination chemotherapy. *Int J Radiat Oncol Biol Phys.* 2003;57(3):665–672. doi:10.1016/S0360-3016(03)00718-1

21. Kaufman DS, Winter KA, Shipley WU, et al. Phase I-II RTOG study (99-06) of patients with muscle-invasive bladder cancer undergoing transurethral surgery, paclitaxel, cisplatin, and twice-daily radiotherapy followed by selective bladder preservation or radical cystectomy and adjuvant chemotherapy. *Urology*. 2009;73(4):833–837. doi:10.1016/j.urology.2008.09.036

22. Stein JP, Lieskovsky G, Cote R, et al. Radical cystectomy in the treatment of invasive bladder cancer: long-term results in 1,054 patients. *J Clin Oncol*. 2001;19(3):666–675. doi:10.1200/JCO.2001.19.3.666

23. Mak RH, Hunt D, Shipley WU, et al. Long-term outcomes in patients with muscle-invasive bladder cancer after selective bladder-preserving combined-modality therapy: a pooled analysis of Radiation Therapy Oncology Group protocols 8802, 8903, 9506, 9706, 9906, and 0233. *J Clin Oncol*. 2014;32(34):3801–3809. doi:10.1200/JCO.2014.57.5548

24. Efstathiou JA, Bae K, Shipley WU, et al. Late pelvic toxicity after bladder-sparing therapy in patients with invasive bladder cancer: RTOG 89-03, 95-06, 97-06, 99-06. *J Clin Oncol*. 2009;27(25):4055–4061. doi:10.1200/JCO.2008.19.5776

25. Huddart RA, Hall E, Lewis R, et al. Patient-reported quality of life outcomes in patients treated for muscle-invasive bladder cancer with radiotherapy ± chemotherapy in the BC2001 phase III randomised controlled trial. *Eur Urol*. 2020;77(2):260–268. doi:10.1016/j.eururo.2019.11.001

26. Shipley WU, Winter KA, Kaufman DS, et al. Phase III trial of neoadjuvant chemotherapy in patients with invasive bladder cancer treated with selective bladder preservation by combined radiation therapy and chemotherapy: initial results of Radiation Therapy Oncology Group 89-03. *J Clin Oncol*. 1998;16(11):3576–3583. doi:10.1200/JCO.1998.16.11.3576

27. Coppin CM, Gospodarowicz MK, James K, et al. Improved local control of invasive bladder cancer by concurrent cisplatin and preoperative or definitive radiation. The National Cancer Institute of Canada Clinical Trials Group. *J Clin Oncol*. 1996;14(11):2901–2907. doi:10.1200/JCO.1996.14.11.2901

28. Coen JJ, Zhang P, Saylor PJ, et al. Bladder preservation with twice-a-day radiation plus fluorouracil/cisplatin or once daily radiation plus gemcitabine for muscle-invasive bladder cancer: NRG/RTOG 0712-A Randomized Phase II Trial. *J Clin Oncol*. 2019;37(1):44–51. doi:10.1200/JCO.18.00537

29. Mitin T, Hunt D, Shipley WU, et al. Transurethral surgery and twice-daily radiation plus paclitaxel-cisplatin or fluorouracil-cisplatin with selective bladder preservation and adjuvant chemotherapy for patients with muscle invasive bladder cancer (RTOG 0233): a randomised multicentre phase 2 trial. *Lancet Oncol*. 2013;14(9):863–872. doi:10.1016/S1470-2045(13)70255-9

30. Choudhury A, Porta N, Hall E, et al. Hypofractionated radiotherapy in locally advanced bladder cancer: an individual patient data meta-analysis of the BC2001 and BCON trials. *Lancet Oncol*. 2021;22(2):246–255. doi:10.1016/S1470-2045(20)30607-0

31. Zaghloul MS, Awwad HK, Akoush HH, et al. Postoperative radiotherapy of carcinoma in bilharzial bladder: improved disease free survival through improving local control. *Int J Radiat Oncol Biol Phys*. 1992;23(3):511–517. doi:10.1016/0360-3016(92)90005-3

32. Baumann BC, Guzzo TJ, He J, et al. Bladder cancer patterns of pelvic failure: implications for adjuvant radiation therapy. *Int J Radiat Oncol Biol Phys*. 2013;85(2):363–369. doi:10.1016/j.ijrobp.2012.03.061

33. Fischer-Valuck BW, Michalski JM, Mitra N, et al. Effectiveness of postoperative radiotherapy after radical cystectomy for locally advanced bladder cancer. *Cancer Med*. 2019;8(8):3698–3709. doi:10.1002/cam4.2102

43 ■ TESTICULAR CANCER

Zachary Mayo, Ehsan H. Balagamwala, and Rahul D. Tendulkar

QUICK HIT ■ Testicular cancer is a relatively uncommon genitourinary malignancy with excellent prognosis. The majority of testicular malignancies are GCT (95%), of which approximately 50% to 60% are seminomatous and 40% to 50% are nonseminomatous GCT. Eighty-five percent of seminomas present as clinical stage I disease. Initial management is inguinal orchiectomy with high ligation of the spermatic cord (not transscrotal biopsy). Treatment paradigm for seminomatous testicular cancer is summarized in Table 43.1. Depending on stage, adjuvant therapy for NSGCT after inguinal orchiectomy is surveillance, nsRPLND, or CHT.

Table 43.1: General Treatment Paradigm for Testicular Seminoma

Seminoma	Initial Treatment	Adjuvant Treatment Options
Stage I	Radical inguinal orchiectomy with high ligation of spermatic cord	Active surveillance: 15%–20% relapse Carboplatin (AUC 7 x1–2C): <5% relapse (TE19 trial) RT (para-aortic strip, 20 Gy/10 fx): <5% relapse (TE10/TE18 trials)
Stage II		Stage IIA: Modified dogleg RT, 20 Gy/10 fx with boost to 30 Gy Stage IIB: CHT preferred (NCCN): EP x 4C or BEP x 3C RT for select nonbulky disease (nodes ≤3 cm).[1] Modified dogleg RT, 20 Gy/10 fx with boost to 36 Gy Stage IIC: EP × 4C or BEP × 3C RT/surgery for salvage
Stage III		EP × 4C or BEP × 3C RT/surgery for salvage

EPIDEMIOLOGY: Approximately 9,600 cases diagnosed annually with ~440 deaths.[2] Accounts for 1% of male cancers overall, but is the most common solid tumor in men 15 to 34 years of age. NSGCTs typically present between 20 and 30 years of age while seminomas present between 30 and 40 years of age. Up to 5% are bilateral (synchronous or metachronous). Excellent prognosis with 10-year survival >95%. Worldwide incidence has more than doubled in the past four decades. Lymphoma is the most common testicular tumor in men over 60.[2,3]

RISK FACTORS: Abdominal cryptorchid testes have 1/20 (5%) risk of cancer and must be resected. Inguinal cryptorchid testes have 1/80 (1.3%) risk of cancer and should undergo orchiopexy before puberty. Risk of cancer increases with age at which cryptorchidism is detected/reversed. Twenty percent of GCTs in patients with a history of cryptorchidism occur in the contralateral, normally descended testicle. Untreated carcinoma in situ of the testis has a 50% risk of progression to invasive malignancy within 5 years.[4] Other risk factors include hypospadias, androgen insensitivity syndrome, gonadal dysgenesis, previous contralateral testicular cancer,[5] extragonadal GCT, family history, White race, HIV, marijuana use, and Peutz–Jeghers syndrome.

ANATOMY: Layers (from external to internal): Skin, dartos fascia, external spermatic fascia, cremasteric fascia, internal spermatic fascia, parietal layer of tunica vaginalis, visceral layer of tunica vaginalis, and tunica albuginea. Seminiferous tubules merge to form the rete testis. Testicular arteries arise directly from abdominal aorta. Right testicular vein joins IVC inferior to right renal vein; left testicular vein joins left renal vein. Lymphatic drainage is from rete testes via spermatic cord along testicular veins to retroperitoneal/para-aortic LNs at vertebral levels T11–L4, then via cisterna chyli and thoracic duct to posterior mediastinum, left SCV, and axilla. Inguinal nodes are not involved in testicular cancer unless the scrotum is surgically disrupted (usually by trans-scrotal biopsy, hernia repair, vasectomy, etc.).

PATHOLOGY:[6] Majority (95%) of testicular cancers are GCTs (Table 43.2): seminomas (50%–60%) and NSGCTs (40%–50%). Minority (5%) are non-GCTs including Leydig cell, Sertoli cell, rhabdomyosarcoma, or lymphoma. Seminomas include classic (85%), anaplastic (10%), or spermatocytic (5%), which are all treated the same. Anaplastic has high mitotic activity but does not have worse outcomes. Spermatocytic type occurs in older men (age >50) and has a favorable prognosis. Pure seminomas with syncytiotrophoblastic cells (still considered pure) may have elevated β-hCG in 10% to 15%. NSGCTs include embryonal, teratoma, choriocarcinoma, yolk sac (endodermal sinus tumors), and mixed tumors. CIS precedes invasive GCTs by 3 to 5 years and is found adjacent to invasive tumor in nearly 100% (except spermatocytic seminoma and infant tumors). AFP is never elevated in pure seminoma. AFP can also be elevated in hepatocellular carcinoma and liver disease. β-hCG is very high with choriocarcinoma and can also be elevated with high luteinizing hormone, GI, GU, lung, and breast cancers. LDH is nonspecific and can be elevated in about half of germ cell tumors.

Table 43.2: Characteristics of Testicular Histologies				
GCT Histology	Age	Characteristics	% With AFP Elevation	% With β-hCG Elevation
Seminoma (50%–60%)	30–40	Radiosensitive; 80% local at presentation; lymphatic spread; relapse occurs later	0%	9%
NSGCTs (40%–50%)	20–30	Radioresistant; 70% distant at presentation; often hematogenous spread; relapse occurs earlier	50%	60%
• Embryonal	25–35	Most common pure NSGCT; more aggressive, >60% DM (lung, liver) at presentation	70%	60%
• Teratoma	25–35	Second most common NSGCT; multiple germ layers; mature vs. immature; >75% NSGCTs have teratoma component	38%	25%
• Choriocarcinoma	20–30	Rare; very high β-hCG (gynecomastia), AFP always normal; most aggressive; spreads hematogenously; may hemorrhage	0%	100%
• Yolk sac	<10	Most common pediatric GCT, 80% <2 y/o; in adults, presents in mediastinum and is chemoresistant; Schiller–Duval bodies	75%	25%

CLINICAL PRESENTATION: Classically presents as a painless testicular mass or painless testicular swelling. Other presentations include a dull ache, heavy sensation in lower abdomen or perianal area, or fullness of the scrotum. A minority (10%) will present with acute pain. Symptoms associated with distant metastasis seen in 10%. Infertility seen in 50%. Gynecomastia (5%) secondary to estrogenic effect of β-hCG. Tumor size and epididymal invasion are associated with higher risk of metastatic disease at time of presentation.[7]

DIFFERENTIAL DIAGNOSIS: Testicular cancer, testicular torsion, epididymitis, hydrocele, varicocele, hernia, hematoma, or spermatocele.

WORKUP: H&P with bimanual exam of scrotal contents. A firm or fixed mass is cancer until proven otherwise. Palpate abdomen for nodal disease or visceral involvement. Examine chest for gynecomastia and palpate for SCV nodes.

Labs: CBC, CMP, serum tumor markers (AFP, β-hCG, LDH).

Imaging: Bilateral scrotal color Doppler ultrasound demonstrates a hypoechoic mass. Seminomas are well defined without cystic areas while NSGCTs are inhomogeneous with calcifications, cystic areas, and indistinct margins. Surgery required for staging as ultrasound is insufficient (accuracy 44% of seminomas and 8% in NSGCTs).[8] CXR, CT abdomen/pelvis (add CT chest if suspicious). PET is of limited utility for workup; may be more useful for seminoma than NSGCTs and alters staging in 10%.[9] Brain imaging if symptomatic, significant lung metastases, or with high β-hCG.

Other: Trans-scrotal biopsy or orchiectomy is absolutely contraindicated because of risk of tumor seeding into the scrotal sac, lymphatic disruption, or metastatic spread of tumor into the inguinal lymph nodes. RPLND for select patients with NSGCT. Repeat serum tumor markers (AFP, β-hCG, and LDH) since S stage in the AJCC system is based on postorchiectomy values. The half-life of β-hCG is 24 to 36 hours and of AFP is 5 to 7 days.[10] Offer semen analysis/sperm banking prior to treatment.

PROGNOSTIC FACTORS

Seminoma: stage, NPVM.

NSGCT: LVI, NPVM, S3, mediastinal primary, embryonal predominant.[11]

NATURAL HISTORY: Risk for relapse after orchiectomy approximately 12% for stage I seminoma with size <3 cm and 20% with size ≥3 cm. However, for patients who did not suffer a relapse in the first 2 years, their risk for relapse in the next 5 years was 3.9% and 5.6%, respectively[12]; 90% of nodal relapses on surveillance occur in the para-aortic lymph nodes ("landing zone") and 10% also have positive pelvic LN.[13] Nodal crossover may occur from right to left (~15%), but rarely from left to right. Late distant relapses are possible.

STAGING

TABLE 43.3: AJCC 8th Edition (2017): Staging for Testicular Cancer [14]

Pt		cN		pN		M	
Tis	• Germ cell neoplasia in situ	N1	• Regional LNs ≤2 cm (single or multiple)	N1	• Regional LN ≤2 cm • ≤5 LNs positive	M1a	• Non retroperitoneal LNs • Pulmonary metastasis
T1	a. Limited to testis (including rete testis invasion), no LVSI, <3 cm	N2	• Regional LN >2 cm and ≤5 cm	N2	• Regional LN >2 cm and ≤5 cm • >5 regional LNs, ≤5 cm and no ECE	M1b	• Non pulmonary visceral metastasis
	b. Limited to testis (including rete testis invasion), no LVSI, ≥3 cm						
T2	• Limited to testis with LVSI or involves hilar soft tissue or involves epididymis or penetrating visceral mesothelial layer covering the external surface of tunica albuginea	N3	• Regional LNs >5 cm	N3	• Regional LN >5 cm		
T3	• Invasion of spermatic cord*			**S Staging (Serum Tumor Markers)**			
T4	• Invasion of scrotum				**AFP (ng/mL)**	**LDH**	**β-hCG (mIU/mL)**
				S0	WNL	WNL	WNL
				S1	<1,000 and	<5,000 and	<1.5× normal
				S2	1,000–10,000 or	5,000–50,000 or	1.5–10× normal
				S3	>10,000 or	>50,000 or	>10× normal

Stage Grouping				
IA	T1	N0	M0	S0
IB	T2–4	N0	M0	S0
IS	Any T	N0	M0	S1–3
IIA	Any T	N1	M0	S0–1
IIB	Any T	N2	M0	S0–1
IIC	Any T	N3	M0	S0–1
IIIA	Any T	Any N	M1a	S0–1
IIIB	Any T	N1–3	M0	S2
	Any T	Any N	M1a	S2
IIIC	Any T	N1–3	M0	S3
	Any T	Any N	M1a	S3
	Any T	Any N	M1b	Any S

*Discontinuous involvement of the spermatic cord is considered M1.

SEMINOMA TREATMENT PARADIGM: Mixed seminomas/NSGCT are treated based on the NSGCT component. In NSGCT, RT is reserved for salvage/palliation. Seminomas may have an indication for RT, and therefore this discussion will focus on the treatment of seminoma.

Surgery: The standard surgery is a radical inguinal orchiectomy with high ligation of the spermatic cord. RPLND is indicated for select NSGCT but not in seminoma.

Active Surveillance: Recommended option for stage I patients after orchiectomy. Must be compliant with follow-up. NCCN recommends H&P every 3 to 6 months for year 1, every 6 months for year 2, every 6 to 12 months for year 3, and then annually. Serum tumor markers optional and ultrasound recommended for equivocal exam. CT abdomen/pelvis is recommended at 3, 6, and 12 months in the first year, every 6 months in year 2, every 6 to 12 months in year 3, then every 12 to 24 months in years 4 to 5. CXR as clinically indicated in years 1 to 5. Consider CT chest if symptomatic.[1]

Chemotherapy: Adjuvant CHT is based on stage. Single-agent carboplatin (AUC 7) × 1–2 cycles is an option for stage I patients. BEP (bleomycin, etoposide, cisplatin) × 3 cycles or EP (etoposide, cisplatin) × 4 cycles are options for stages II–III patients. CHT preferred for stages IIB, IIC, and III.

Radiation Therapy: For stage I patients, a PAS may be treated to 20 Gy/10 fx. For stage IIA patients, a modified DL field to include the para-aortic and ipsilateral internal iliac lymph nodes can be delivered to 20 Gy/10 fx with a boost to 30 Gy for gross disease. For stage IIB patients, a modified DL field to 20 Gy/10 fx is followed by boost to 36 Gy to the gross disease.[6] Most recommend coverage of the left renal hilum (see TE10 in the following). Contraindications to RT include horseshoe kidney, inflammatory bowel disease, prior radiation, and genetic syndromes with an increased risk of further malignancies. Side effects include nausea, vomiting, diarrhea, fatigue, and second malignancy.

Procedure: See *Handbook of Treatment Planning in Radiation Oncology*, Chapter 8 for details.

■ **EVIDENCE-BASED Q&A**

STAGE I SEMINOMA

■ **What data support active surveillance as an option for patients with stage I seminoma?**

The risk of relapse and death from a stage I seminoma is small. Although no prospective trials support this approach directly, a systematic literature review (14 studies with 2,060 men) showed that relapse occurred in 17% (9% relapsed >2 years) and mortality from seminoma was 0.3% due to effective salvage therapies.[15] Another study demonstrated that the risk of relapse can be as low as 6% if tumor size <4 cm and no rete testis invasion.[16] *A Danish retrospective cohort study of 1,954 men showed that the median time to relapse was 13.7 months with 73.4% of patients developing relapse during the first 2 years, 22.2% between years 3 and 5, and 4.3% after year 5. The 15-year DSS and OS were 99.3% and 91.6%, respectively.[17] Despite the push toward increasing surveillance in these patients, approximately 40% of patients continue to receive adjuvant therapy.[18,19]*

■ **Is a full DL field necessary for stage I patients treated with adjuvant RT, or will a PAs suffice?**

For stage I patients, pelvic relapse is rare. MRC TE10 showed that PAS is the standard RT field and DL fields should be reserved for patients with prior inguinal or scrotal surgery due to aberrant lymphatic drainage.

Fossa, MRC TE10 (*JCO*** 1999, PMID 10561173):** Equivalence study of 478 patients with stage I (T1–T3) seminoma randomized to DL (PAS plus ipsilateral iliac lymph node) vs. PAS (T11–L5) fields. All treated to 30 Gy/15 fx. MFU 4.5 years. No difference in 3-year RFS or OS. Each group had nine relapses, although the PAS group had four pelvic relapses compared to none in the DL group. PAS had less acute toxicity (N/V, diarrhea, leukopenia) and higher sperm counts than DL fields. One patient in the para-aortic arm died of seminoma. **Conclusion: PAS irradiation is considered standard treatment for stage I (T1–T3), with DL fields reserved for patients with prior inguinal or scrotal surgery.**

TABLE 43.4: Results of MRC TE10				
MRC TE10	3-Yr RFS	3-Yr OS	Number of Pelvic Relapses	Azoospermia
PAS	96.0%	99.3%	4 (2%)	11%
DL	96.6%	100%	0 (0%)	35%
p value	NS	NS	–	<.001

■ **What is the optimal RT dose for patients with stage I seminoma?**

Based on MRC TE18, the standard dose for stage I seminoma is 20 Gy in 10 fx.

Jones, MRC TE18 (*JCO*** 2005, PMID 15718317):** Noninferiority trial of 625 patients with stage I seminoma (pT1–3N0) randomized to 20 Gy/10 fx vs. 30 Gy/15 fx, all to PAS (T11–L5). Designed to assess noninferiority and powered to exclude a 4% difference in 2-year relapse rates. MFU 61 months. No difference in OS or RFS; 30 Gy arm had 10 relapses, compared to 11 relapses in the 20 Gy arm (*p* = NS); 20 Gy arm had less acute side effects (moderate–severe fatigue and inability to conduct normal work) at 4 weeks, but differences returned to baseline by 12 weeks. Six new primary cancers diagnosed, all in the 30 Gy arm. **Conclusion: 20 Gy/10 fx is as effective as 30 Gy/15 fx, with less acute SE.**

TABLE 43.5: Results of MRC TE18			
MRC TE18	2-Yr RFS	Moderate–Severe Lethargy	Inability to Work at 4 Weeks
20 Gy	97.0%	5%	28%
30 Gy	97.7%	20%	46%
p value	NS	<.001	<.001

■ **What is the role for CHT in patients with stage I seminoma?**

Based on MRC TE19, carboplatin is noninferior to RT, and has reduced side effects. Single-agent carboplatin is given for 1 to 2 cycles.[20]

Oliver, MRC TE19 (*Lancet*** 2005, PMID 16039331; Oliver *JCO* 2011, PMID 21282539):** PRT of 1,477 patients with stage I seminoma randomized to adjuvant carboplatin (1 cycle, AUC 7) vs. adjuvant RT (20 Gy/10 fx [36%] or 30 Gy/15 fx [54%] or an intermediate dose [10%]; DL [13%] or PAS [87%]) after orchiectomy. Powered to exclude absolute differences in 2-year relapse rates of >3%. MFU 6.5 years. Carboplatin had more para-aortic node-only relapses, but fewer pelvic, mediastinal, or SCV relapses compared to RT. Carboplatin arm had fewer second GCTs (carboplatin: $n = 2$, RT: $n = 15$, HR: 0.22, $p = .03$) and significantly less acute dyspepsia (8% vs. 17%), moderate–severe lethargy (7% vs. 24%), and inability to do normal work (19% vs. 38%), but more thrombocytopenia (12% vs. 2%). Only one seminoma death, which was in the RT arm. Those getting more of the prescribed CHT (>99% AUC 7) had improved RFS (96.1% vs. 92.6%) than those who received less CHT. **Conclusion: Adjuvant carboplatin is not inferior to RT for stage I seminoma, and has fewer acute SE.**

Table 43.6: Results of MRC TE19				
MRC TE19	2-Yr RFS	3-Yr RFS	5-Yr RFS (Not SS)	New GCT
RT	96.7%	95.9%	96%	15 (1.7%)
Carboplatin	97.7%	94.8%	94.7%	2 (0.3%)

■ **What are the outcomes in patients with stage I seminoma who experience a relapse?**

Choo, Toronto (*IJROBP* 2005, PMID 15708251): Prospective, single-arm observational study in 88 patients with stage I seminoma. MFU 12.1 years; 15-year RFS rate was 80%. Seventeen patients relapsed, 88% of which were below the diaphragm. Salvage therapy: 14 treated with RT (25–35 Gy), 3 treated with CHT (3–4 cycles of BEP). All 17 ultimately were salvaged successfully. **Conclusion: Surveillance with the reservation of RT or CHT for salvage is a safe alternative to up-front adjuvant therapy for stage I testicular seminoma.**

Mead, UK TE Pooled Analysis (*JNCI* 2011, PMID 21212385): Pooled analysis of the TE10, TE18, TE19 trials. A total of 3,049 patients included in these three noninferiority studies. MFU 6.4 to 12 years in the three trials; 99.8% CSS overall; 98 relapses, but only 4 (0.2%) relapsed after 3 years. Four died of metastatic failure. Among patients treated with DL who relapsed, 11/16 (65%) failed in the mediastinum or neck. Of those treated with a PAS who relapsed, 20/54 (37%) failed in the pelvis and 14/54 (26%) failed in the mediastinum or neck. In patients treated with carboplatin who relapsed, 18/27 (67%) failed in the retroperitoneum. **Conclusion: Patterns of relapse depend on adjuvant treatment received.**

STAGE II SEMINOMA

■ **What are the potential advantages of RT over CHT in patients with stage IIA/B seminoma?**

Per the 2020 NCCN guidelines, adjuvant RT to the para-aortic and ipsilateral pelvic LN or chemotherapy is recommended for stage II seminoma. RT is given to 30 Gy for stage IIA and 36 Gy for stage IIB. Chemotherapy is BEP × 3C or EP × 4C. Per NCCN, chemo is preferred for stage IIB or higher (category 1 recommendation for stage IIC or III). Notably, radiation is not considered a preferred option for bulky nodal disease due to higher failure rates.

Krege, German Testicular Cancer Study Group (*Ann Oncol* 2006, PMID 16254023): Phase II trial of single-agent carboplatin (AUC 7) q4 weeks × 3C in stage IIA ($n = 51$) or × 4C in stage IIB ($n = 57$). CR was achieved in 81% of patients, 16% with PR, and 2% had no change; 13% who initially achieved a CR relapsed and required salvage therapy. Overall failure rate was 18%. OS 99% and DSS 100%. **Conclusion: Single-agent carboplatin was not effective in eradicating RP metastasis in stage IIA/B seminoma.**

TOXICITY AND SECONDARY MALIGNANCY RISK

■ **What is the risk for developing secondary malignancy after adjuvant therapy for testicular cancer?**

After adjuvant therapy (CHT or RT), patients with testicular cancer are at a higher risk for developing secondary malignancy. Given the increased risk of mortality from secondary malignancies, it is important to appropriately select patients for adjuvant therapy.

Travis, NIH (*JNCI* 2005, PMID 16174857): Population-based registries of >40,000 testicular cancer survivors used to calculate relative and absolute risks of second solid cancers. Among 10-year survivors diagnosed at age 35, the relative risk of a second solid tumor was 1.9, and remained statistically significantly elevated for 35 years. Cancers of the lung (RR = 1.5), colon (RR = 2), bladder (RR = 2.7), pancreas (RR = 3.6), and stomach (RR = 4) accounted for ~60% of the excess malignancies. There was also an increased risk of pleural (malignant mesothelioma, RR = 3.4) and esophageal (RR = 1.7) cancers. Overall, RR of second solid malignancy for patients treated with RT alone was 2, CHT alone 1.9, and both 2.9. For patients diagnosed with seminoma or NSGCT at 35 years of age, cumulative risk of solid cancer in the next 40 years was 36% or 31%, respectively (corresponding risk of solid cancer in the general population was 23%). Note that the authors estimate ~16% of the evaluated patients received chest RT. **Conclusion: Testicular cancer survivors treated with RT and/or CHT are at increased risk of solid tumors for at least 35 years.**

Kier, Danish Nationwide Cohort (*JAMA Oncology* **2016, PMID 27711914):** Danish nationwide cohort of 5,190 patients (2,804 seminoma, 2,386 nonseminoma) treated with adjuvant therapy. Patients underwent surveillance, retroperitoneal RT, BEP, CHT, or MTOL (more than one line) of CHT. MFU 14.4 years. The 20-year cumulative incidence of second malignancy (death used as a competing risk) was 7.8% for surveillance, 7.6% for BEP (HR 1.7), 13.5% for RT (HR 1.8), 9.2% for MTOL (HR 3.7), and 7.0% for controls. Excess mortality due to second malignancy was found with BEP (HR 1.6), RT (HR 2.1), and MTOL (HR 5.8). **Conclusion: Excess mortality due to second malignancy from adjuvant therapy suggests that approaches to define the best candidates for adjuvant therapy are needed.**

REFERENCES

1. NCCN Clinical Practice Guidelines in Oncology: Testicular Cancer. 2020. https://www.nccn.org/professionals/physician_gls/pdf/testicular.pdf
2. Siegel RL, Miller KD, Jemal A. Cancer statistics, 2020. *CA Cancer J Clin.* 2020;70(1):7–30. doi:10.3322/caac.21590
3. Yacoub JH, Oto A, Allen BC, et al. ACR appropriateness criteria staging of testicular malignancy. *J Am Coll Radiol.* 2016;13:1203–1209. doi:10.1016/j.jacr.2016.06.026
4. von der Maase H, Rørth M, Walbom-Jørgensen S, et al. Carcinoma in situ of contralateral testis in patients with testicular germ cell cancer: study of 27 cases in 500 patients. *BMJ.* 1986;293:1398–1401. doi:10.1136/bmj.293.6559.1398
5. Fosså SD, Chen J, Schonfeld SJ, et al. Risk of contralateral testicular cancer: a population-based study of 29,515 U.S. men. *J Natl Cancer Inst.* 2005;97:1056–1066. doi:10.1093/jnci/dji185
6. Wilder RB, Buyyounouski MK, Efstathiou JA, Beard CJ. Radiotherapy treatment planning for testicular seminoma. *Int J Radiat Oncol Biol Phys.* 2012;83:e445–e452. doi:10.1016/j.ijrobp.2012.01.044
7. Scandura G, Wagner T, Beltran L, et al. Pathological risk factors for metastatic disease at presentation in testicular seminomas with focus on the recent pT changes in AJCC TNM eighth edition. *Hum Pathol.* 2019;94:16–22. doi:10.1016/j.humpath.2019.10.004
8. Marth D, Scheidegger J, Studer UE. Ultrasonography of testicular tumors. *Urol Int.* 1990;45:237–240. doi:10.1159/000281715
9. Ng SP, Duchesne G, Tai KH, et al. Can Positron Emission Tomography (PET) complement conventional staging of early-stage testicular seminoma? *Int J Radiat Oncol Biol Phys.* 2016;96:E253. doi:10.1016/j.ijrobp.2016.06.1258
10. *AJCC cancer staging manual.* Springer Science+Business Media; 2016.
11. International Germ Cell Consensus Classification: a prognostic factor-based staging system for metastatic germ cell cancers. International Germ Cell Cancer Collaborative Group. *J Clin Oncol.* 1997;15:594–603. doi:10.1200/JCO.1997.15.2.594
12. Nayan M, Jewett MAS, Hosni A, et al. Conditional risk of relapse in surveillance for clinical stage I testicular cancer. *Eur Urol.* 2017;71(1):120–127.
13. von der Maase H, Specht L, Jacobsen GK, et al. Surveillance following orchidectomy for stage I seminoma of the testis. *Eur J Cancer.* 1993;29A:1931–1934. doi:10.1016/0959-8049(93)90446-M
14. *AJCC Cancer Staging Manual, Eighth Edition.* 8th ed: Springer Publishing; 2017.
15. Groll RJ, Warde P, Jewett MAS. A comprehensive systematic review of testicular germ cell tumor surveillance. *Crit Rev Oncol Hematol.* 2007;64:182–197. doi:10.1016/j.critrevonc.2007.04.014
16. Albers P, Albrecht W, Algaba F, et al. Guidelines on testicular cancer: 2015 update. *Eur Urol.* 2015;68:1054–1068. doi:10.1016/j.eururo.2015.07.044
17. Mortensen MS, Lauritsen J, Gundgaard MG, et al. A nationwide cohort study of stage I seminoma patients followed on a surveillance program. *Eur Urol.* 2014;66:1172–1178. doi:/10.1016/j.eururo.2014.07.001
18. Matulewicz RS, Oberlin DT, Sheinfeld J, Meeks JJ. The evolving management of patients with clinical stage I seminoma. *Urology.* 2016;98:113–119. doi:10.1016/j.urology.2016.07.037
19. Wymer KM, Pearce SM, Harris KT, et al. Adherence to National Comprehensive Cancer Network Guidelines for Testicular Cancer. *J Urol.* 2017;197(3 Pt 1):684–689. doi:10.1016/j.juro.2016.09.073
20. Dieckmann KP, Dralle-Filiz I, Matthies C, et al. Testicular seminoma clinical stage 1: treatment outcome on a routine care level. *J Cancer Res Clin Oncol.* 2016;142(7):1599–1607. doi:10.1007/s00432-016-2162-z

44 ■ PENILE CANCER

Rahul D. Tendulkar, Rupesh Kotecha, and Omar Y. Mian

QUICK HIT ■ Penile cancer is rare. The primary nodal drainage is to inguinal LNs—about 50% of clinically enlarged LNs are pathologically involved (the rest are reactive). Surgical management can include a partial or total penectomy, with inguinal and/or pelvic LND depending on clinical risk factors and staging outcomes (Table 44.1). Organ preservation can be performed for select early-stage patients with either EBRT or brachytherapy (ideally for T1–T2 tumors <4 cm and <1 cm of corpora invasion). Locally advanced patients should be evaluated for neoadjuvant CHT (TIP × 4 cycles) followed by surgery or definitive chemoRT.

TABLE 44.1: General Treatment Paradigms for Penile Cancer	
Stage	**Treatment Options**
Tis or Ta	Topical therapy, WLE, laser therapy, glansectomy, Mohs surgery
T1	Grades 1–2: WLE, glansectomy, Mohs, laser therapy, RT Grade 3: WLE, partial penectomy, total penectomy, RT, chemoRT
T2–T4	Partial penectomy, total penectomy, RT, chemoRT, neoadjuvant CHT (TIP), and surgery

EPIDEMIOLOGY: Rare cancer in the United States, accounting for ~0.1% of all solid tumors with ~2,200 new cases and 440 deaths annually.[1] More common in the less developed world. Mean age 60. A significant proportion of men have delayed treatment due to incorrect diagnosis or perceptions of social stigma.

RISK FACTORS: Epidemiologic factors: single, never married, lack of circumcision. Medical factors: HPV exposure, genital warts, UTI, penile injury, urethral stricture, phimosis (circumferential fibrosis of the prepuce causing inability to retract the foreskin over the glans), HIV, tobacco exposure, psoralen, and UVA photochemotherapy; 30% to 50% are HPV+ (most commonly 16 and 18) with some suggestion of a more favorable prognosis.

ANATOMY: Generally divided into the root, shaft, and glans. Penis is anchored to the pubic ramus. Two corporal bodies share a perforated midline septum terminating at the glans. The urethra is surrounded by the corpus spongiosum. Two layers of fascia cover the corpora: the superficial fascia is continuous with the dartos fascia of the scrotum and the deep fascia (Buck's) surrounds the erectile bodies (acts as barrier to corporal invasion). Blood supply is from the common penile artery from the internal pudendal artery, which is a branch of the internal iliac. LN drainage occurs bilaterally and sequentially, from the superficial inguinal to the deep femoral LNs, then into the pelvis. Regional LNs include superficial inguinal, deep inguinal, and iliac LNs. The sentinel LNs (Cloquet) are located anteromedial to the superficial epigastric and saphenous vessels.

PATHOLOGY: Ninety-five percent are squamous cell carcinoma. Other rarer subtypes include melanoma, TCC, BCC, Kaposi sarcoma, lymphoma, extramammary Paget's disease, or metastasis from other sites. Penile squamous cell carcinomas can be subclassified by microscopic histologic features: usual type SCC (most common), papillary, warty, basaloid, verrucous, and sarcomatoid subgroups. Low-grade (1–2) carcinomas comprise 80% of cases. Poorly differentiated (grade 3), basaloid and sarcomatoid subgroups have poorer prognosis. Verrucous and low-grade tumors are more commonly local diseases and rarely metastasize.

CLINICAL PRESENTATION: Often presents with a penile mass or skin abnormality, occurring typically on the glans, in the coronal sulcus, or prepuce (involvement of the shaft is rare, <10%). Presenting symptoms include rash, ulceration, bleeding, or secondary infection. May be mistaken for premalignant lesions such as bowenoid papulosis (papules on the penile shaft), Bowen's disease (plaque on follicle-bearing epithelium of penile shaft), erythroplasia of Queyrat (red lesion on mucocutaneous epithelium of the glans or prepuce), lichen sclerosis, condylomas, Buschke–Lowenstein (giant condyloma), and Kaposi sarcoma. Bowenoid papulosis, Bowen's disease, and erythroplasia of Queyrat are associated with HPV+ and are considered in situ lesions. Locoregionally advanced cases typically progress in an orderly fashion to inguinal LNs, followed by spread to pelvic or RP LNs. Only 50% of clinically apparent inguinal lymphadenopathy is due to metastatic nodal disease (other 50% are reactive adenopathy, often from infection); <10% have DM at presentation.

WORKUP: H&P with careful examination of penile lesion and inguinal LNs. If infection is suspected, consider a 4- to 6-week course of antibiotics.

Labs: CBC, CMP, alkaline phosphatase.

Imaging: CT abdomen/pelvis and CXR are standard. MRI and ultrasound may clarify depth of invasion. MRI should be performed if corporal involvement is suspected. Bone scan if advanced disease is suspected. PET/CT should be considered in high-risk patients, particularly those with LN+ by FNA or LND.

Procedures: Punch or incisional biopsy of the penile lesion can usually be performed, reserving excisional biopsy if the initial biopsy is not diagnostic. Assessment of HPV status is recommended. Cystourethroscopy should be performed to examine lower urinary tract.

PROGNOSTIC FACTORS: LN+ (correlates with T stage and grade, p53+, LVSI, PNI, tumor emboli in venous/lymphatic channel), ENE. There is some evidence that HPV may have better prognosis (but not reproducible across series).

STAGING

T/M		N	cN0	cN1	cN2	cN3
TABLE 44.2: AJCC 8th Edition (2017): Staging for Penile Cancer[2]						
T1[1]	a No LVSI, PNI, or Grade 3/sarcomatoid		I	IIIA	IIIB	IV
	b LVSI, PNI or Grade 3/sarcomatoid		IIA			
T2	• Invades corpus spongiosum with or without urethral invasion					
T3	• Invades corpus cavernosum with or without urethral invasion		IIB			
T4	• Invades adjacent structures (scrotum, prostate, pubic bone)		IV			
M1	• Distant metastasis					

Notes: T1[1] = Glans: invades lamina propria; foreskin: invades dermis, lamina propria or dartos fascia; shaft: invades connective tissue between epidermis and corpora.
cN1, palpable, mobile unilateral inguinal LN; cN2, palpable, mobile, ≥ 2 unilateral inguinal or bilateral inguinal LN; cN3, palpable, fixed inguinal nodal mass or pelvic lymphadenopathy.

TREATMENT PARADIGM: The European Association of Urology published guidelines, which are summarized as follows.[3]

Surgery: In general, men with low-risk operable tumors (Tia, Ta, T1a) should undergo organ-preserving treatment (Table 44.3). High-risk patients with T1 G3 or T2–T4 tumors should undergo penile amputation with either a total penectomy or partial penectomy (removal of the glans ± underlying corpora cavernosa), depending on extent of disease and location of tumor. For T1 G3 without involvement of the glans or underlying corporal tissues, can consider excision of the penile shaft skin alone. Distal T2–3 tumors can be treated with limited excision if a negative margin can be attained (need to leave >2 cm for standing void). In a large review, most patients are able to undergo partial penectomy (total penectomy accounted for 23%).[4] LR is <10% in most series. The most common side effect is meatal stenosis (4%–9%). Psychological trauma is also common and some patients have attempted or committed suicide after penectomy. Men should be counseled about penile reconstruction options. For patients who refuse surgery, interstitial brachytherapy can be considered. Those with unresectable primary tumors or bulky lymphadenopathy should receive neoadjuvant CHT ± RT prior to consideration of surgery.

TABLE 44.3: Management Options for Early-Stage Penile Cancer

Candidates	Treatment	Notes
Tis, Ta, or T1a	Limited excision	Goal is to preserve penile length and sexual function
Tis	Topical therapy	5-FU cream and imiquimod cream for 4–6 weeks
Tis	Laser ablation	CO_2, argon, Nd:YAG, and potassium titanyl phosphate laser ablation; high rate of preserving sexual activity and satisfaction
Tis	Total glans resurfacing	Removal of epithelial and subepithelial layers of glans down to corpus spongiosum, followed by skin graft
Tis or T1	Mohs surgery	Layer-by-layer excision to maximize organ preservation
Tis or T1	RT	Brachytherapy or EBRT

LN assessment: In addition to assessment of the primary tumor, evaluation of LNs should be performed, noting high rates of false positives and negatives on clinical exam (**Tables 44.4 and 44.5**).[5] Factors such as T stage, grade, and LVSI predict for LN involvement and risk categories have been identified to guide management of the inguinal LNs. If no palpable or radiographic adenopathy, consider dynamic SLNB (high sensitivity, but requires expertise in technique).[6] A superficial inguinal LND or modified inguinal LND may be performed by clinicians without experience in dynamic SLNB, but have higher complication rates than SLNB. For patients with palpable inguinal adenopathy or enlarged LNs on imaging, perform FNA first. If FNA is positive, then perform a complete (superficial and deep) ipsilateral inguinal node dissection. All patients with pLN+ should also undergo a contralateral superficial inguinal LND and cross-sectional imaging for staging. After inguinal LND, if only a single LN is positive without ENE, no pelvic LND is needed. If multiple LN+ or ENE is present, then pelvic LND is indicated. For N2 disease, consider neoadjuvant CHT (TIP × 4 cycles) ± RT followed by surgery. For patients who are ineligible for neoadjuvant CHT, LND or RT or chemoRT is recommended.

TABLE 44.4: Inguinal Node Evaluation in Clinically LN– patients

Risk Category	Primary Tumor Factors (all cN0)	Management of cN0 Inguinal LNs
Low risk	pTis, Ta, or T1 G1, and no LVSI	Surveillance (consider SLNB, or superficial or modified inguinal LND for noncompliant patients)
Intermediate risk	pT1a G2 and no LVSI	SLNB (alternatively, superficial or modified inguinal LND; surveillance in well-informed and compliant patients) • If LN– → surveillance • If 1 LN+, no ENE → complete inguinal LND • If 2 LN+ or ENE → complete inguinal and pelvic LND
High risk	pT1b or higher (G3 or LVSI)	SLNB or superficial or modified inguinal LND • If LN– → surveillance • If 1 LN+, no ENE → complete inguinal LND • If 2 LN + or ENE → complete inguinal and pelvic LND

Table 44.5 Inguinal Node Evaluation in Clinically LN+ Patients After Initial FNA of Suspicious LN(s)

Clinical scenario (all cN+)	Management of cN+ inguinal LNs
Single enlarged LN <4 cm, low-risk primary tumor (pTis, pTa, pT1 G1)	If FNA– → excisional biopsy of enlarged LN If FNA+ → complete inguinal LND • If 1 LN+, no ENE → surveillance • If 2 LN+ or ENE → pelvic LND
Single enlarged LN <4 cm, high-risk primary tumor (pT1 or higher with G3 or LVSI)	If FNA– → superficial or modified inguinal LND If FNA+ → complete inguinal LND • If 1 LN+, no ENE → surveillance • If 2 LN+ or ENE → pelvic LND
Multiple or bilateral enlarged LNs	If FNA– → superficial inguinal LND with intra-op frozen evaluation If FNA+ → complete inguinal (and pelvic LND if 2 LN+ or ENE) OR neoadjuvant CHT (TIP×4C) followed by surgery

Chemotherapy: CHT options are summarized in Table 44.6. TIP resulted in a response in 39/60 men in a phase II study of men with advanced penile cancer with 10 patients ypN0.[7] The 5-year OS for those who responded to neoadjuvant CHT was 50% vs. 8% for those who progressed during CHT. TPF has relatively poor response rates and tolerance. Adjuvant CHT recommendations are largely extrapolated from the neoadjuvant and metastatic setting, but may be applied to men with high-risk features.

TABLE 44.6: CHT Options for Penile Cancer		
Type	**Indications**	**CHT Options**
Neoadjuvant	Unresectable primary tumor Bulky inguinal LN+ Bilateral inguinal LN+	• TIP (paclitaxel [175 mg/m² d1], ifosfamide [1,200 mg/m² d1–3], cisplatin [25 mg/m² d1–3]) q3–4 weeks × 4C • TPF (docetaxel, cisplatin and 5-FU)
Adjuvant	Pelvic LN+ ENE Bilateral inguinal LN+ >3 LN+	• TIP
Metastatic	KPS ≥80	• TIP • Cisplatin (100 mg/m² d1) + 5-FU (1000 mg/m²/day d1–5) q3–4 weeks • Cisplatin (80 mg/m² on day 1) + irinotecan (60 mg/m² d1/8/15) on a 28-day cycle • Consider panitumumab, cetuximab alone, or in combo with CHT

Radiation: Used in the definitive setting for organ preservation (either RT alone or concurrent chemoRT, extrapolating from cervical and anal cancer), neoadjuvant setting if locally advanced unresectable disease, or for symptom palliation in those with metastatic disease (Table 44.7). First step in management is circumcision, which allows for full exposure and can prevent radiation balanitis and phimosis. Definitive RT for organ preservation of early-stage lesions can consist of either EBRT (LC 44%–65%, penile preservation 58%–86%) or brachytherapy (LC 70%–86%, penile preservation 74%–88%). Brachytherapy alone can be considered for lower risk (T1–T2) lesions <4 cm with corpora invasion <1 cm. For more advanced lesions, either EBRT alone or combined EBRT and CHT or brachytherapy boost may be considered.

Table 44.7 General Principles of RT for Penile Cancer	
Group	**RT Treatment Options**
Early stage (T1–T2, N0) <4 cm	Definitive brachytherapy alone or EBRT or chemoRT to primary site ± LNs
Early stage (T1–T2, N0) >4 cm	Definitive chemoRT (primary site + LNs)
Locally advanced (T3–4 or N+)	Definitive chemoRT (primary site + LNs)
Resected with positive margins	Adjuvant EBRT to primary site and surgical scar ± LNs if inadequate LND
Resected LN+	Adjuvant chemoRT to primary site and regional LNs, including pelvic LNs (extrapolating from vulvar cancer trials)

EBRT: For details, see *Handbook of Treatment Planning in Radiation Oncology,* Chapter 8.[8] Setup may be prone or supine with immobilizing bolus to position the penis (wax mold, Perspex block, plastic cylinder, water bath, etc.). Setup frog-leg if planning on inguinal node treatment via AP/PA technique (wide AP fields with electron supplementation). The entire length of the penis should be covered, with LNs included if clinically involved or at risk.

Dose: Historically, doses of 50 to –55 Gy were used,[9,10] but in the modern era 45 to 50 Gy is given to the entire penile shaft followed by a boost to 65 to 70 Gy to treat gross disease. A hypofractionated schedule of 52.5 Gy/16 fx may be considered.[11] When electively treating LNs, uninvolved nodes should receive 45 to 50 Gy and gross/unresected groin nodes should be boosted to 65 to 70 Gy.

Brachytherapy: ABS-GEC-ESTRO guidelines have been summarized by Crook et al.[12] Brachytherapy is ideally restricted to lesions <4 cm with <1 cm invasion of the corpora cavernosa (typically T1–T2 lesions and select T3 cases). Larger size associated with higher LR and increased risk of late effects. Superficial molds may be created to contain sources or interstitial implant. Patient placed under general anesthesia or penile block with systemic sedation. Foley catheter is placed to aid in urethral identification. Templates placed on either side of the penis for stabilization. Up to six needles inserted perpendicular to penis, 1 cm apart and in planes. Target volume includes tumor plus 1.5 to 2 cm margin for small lesions; include glans and shaft for larger lesions. Needles are loaded after edema has subsided. LDR dose is 60 to 65 Gy, limiting urethra to 50 Gy over 6 to 7 days. Dose rates with PDR technique are typically ~50 to 60 cGy/hr. If using HDR brachtherapy, no consensus standard dosing exists. A common HDR dose is 54 Gy in BID fx of 3 Gy each delivered over 9 days and 38.4 Gy in BID fx of 3.2 Gy/fx over 6 days is well tolerated. Interfraction interval should be ≥6 hours. To reduce risk of penile necrosis, limit V125 <40% and V150 <20%. To decrease risk of urethral strictures, limit urethra V115 <10% and V90 <95%. Minimize confluent areas of 125%.

Toxicity: Dermatitis, dysuria, skin telangiectasia, urethral stricture (10%–40%), urethral fistula, impotence, penile fibrosis, penile necrosis (3%–15%, higher with interstitial technique), bowel obstruction.

■ EVIDENCE-BASED Q&A

■ What are the general outcomes of penile cancer? Does surgery or RT provide better outcomes?

Surgery and RT are both appropriate modalities. Some retrospective series suggest better LC with surgical resection; however, psychosexual morbidity with penectomy is high.

Sarin (*IJROBP* 1997, PMID: 9240637): RR of 101 patients with stages I–IV disease treated with EBRT (59), brachytherapy (13), or penectomy (29). In 36 failures, 23 received partial penectomy, 3 had penectomy, 2 had RT, and 6 received CHT. 5-yr and 10-yr OS were 57% and 39%; 5-yr and 10-yr CSS were 66% and 57%; 5-yr and 10-yr LC were 60% and 55%. No difference between surgery and RT in LC after salvage. Among EBRT patients, five had moderate stricture, two had severe stricture, and two had penectomy (one for necrosis and one for urethral damage). In surgical patients, there were two suicide attempts after penectomy.

Ozsahin (*IJROBP* 2006, PMID: 16949770): RR of 60 men with SCC s/p either surgery (*n* = 27) or RT (*n* = 29); 70% cN0. Twenty-two patients received post-op RT for either + margins or LNs. Twenty-nine patients received RT for organ preservation and four patients refused RT. Median EBRT dose 52 Gy (26–74.5 Gy) with brachytherapy boost given in 7 (15–25 Gy). One patient treated with brachytherapy alone. Nineteen of 29 patients received nodal RT (36–66 Gy). LF was 13% in surgery group and 56% in organ sparing. Clinically positive LNs controlled in 9/11 patients with lymphadenectomy and 5/7 patients with RT alone; 73% of LF salvaged with surgery; 5-yr OS 43%, 10-yr OS 25%.

■ What are the expected outcomes with limited excision?

Limited excision has been used more recently for patients with early-stage disease with a low risk for LR (Tis, Ta, or T1a). Recent long-term data show low rates of LR. Importantly, the historical standard was for a 2-cm margin, but in the current era, negative margin excision with a goal of 5 mm is appropriate.

Philippou (*J Urol* 2012, PMID: 22818137): UK study of 179 patients with invasive penile cancer treated from 2002 to 2010 with organ-preserving surgery: circumcision (involving skin shaft), WLE with primary closure, removal of the glans, or removal of the glans and distal corpora. Median distance to resection margin was 5 mm. After excision, LR in 9%, regional recurrence in 11%, and DM in 5%. 5-yr DSS 55%. For patients with isolated LR, 5-yr DSS 92% vs. 38% for those with a regional recurrence; 5-yr LRFS 86%. On MVA, tumor grade, stage, and LVSI were independent predictors of LR. Distance to margin was not a significant predictor of recurrence. **Conclusion: Penile-conserving surgery is safe and excision with 5-mm margin is still associated with low risk of LR. LR has no impact on OS.**

■ Is RT alone an adequate modality for early-stage lesions?

RT alone is an option for organ preservation. Nodal disease has poor prognosis. Close follow-up is required as relapses are frequent.

McLean (*IJROBP* 1993, PMID: 8454480): RR of 26 patients with invasive SCC stage I–II and 11 patients with CIS from 1970 to 1985. RT dose ranged from 35 to 60 Gy. Nodal dose ranged from 38 to 51 Gy. 5-yr OS 62% and was 79% for LN– vs. 12% for LN+. Twenty-one of 26 patients had initial CR but 11/21 responders recurred (3 in penis alone, 2 in penis + LNs, 4 in LNs alone, 2 DM). Seven patients developed meatal stenosis/phimosis, seven patients had other late effects (severe telangiectasia, fibrosis, urethral stenosis, ulceration), and eight patients later underwent penectomy (six for recurrence, two for RT complications).

■ **What is the efficacy of brachytherapy for early-stage penile cancer?**

Brachytherapy is effective with high rates of LC for early-stage tumors.

Crook (*World J Urol* 2009, PMID: 18636264): RR of 67 patients; 5-yr OS 59%, 10-yr CSS 84%; 5-yr and 10-yr penile preservation rates were 88% and 67%. Soft tissue necrosis in 12% and urethral stenosis in 9%. Six of 11 patients with regional recurrence salvaged by LND ± EBRT.

de Crevoisier (*IJROBP* 2009, PMID: 19395183): RR of 144 patients with SCC of glans treated with brachytherapy to median dose of 65 Gy; 10-yr penile recurrence 20%, inguinal node recurrence 11%, inguinal node met 6%. 10-yr CSS 92%; 10-yr probability of avoiding penile surgery was 72%. Stenosis in 23% and pain/necrosis in 22%,

---

■ **Are there data to support adjuvant RT in patients with LN+ penile cancer?**

Given the rarity of penile cancer, data on the benefit of adjuvant RT in patients with LN+ disease are often extrapolated from vulvar cancer trials, which showed a benefit in LC and OS to pelvic RT. One series from the Netherlands provides support when compared to older series and also highlights shortcomings of RT in patients with ENE and pelvic LN+ disease.

Graafland (*J Urol* 2010, PMID: 20723934): RR of 156 patients with LN+ penile cancer s/p therapeutic regional LND. Post-op RT (50 Gy/25 fx) was given to inguinal ± pelvic nodes if >1 pLN+ per institution paradigm and was performed in 45% of patients; 5-yr CSS was 61%. Men with ENE had decreased 5-yr CSS (42% vs. 80%). On MVA, ENE and pelvic LN+ disease were associated with decreased CSS. **Conclusion: Despite RT, ENE and pelvic LN+ disease are associated with inferior survival.**

Robinson (*Eur Urol* 2018, PMID: 29703686): Systematic review of seven retrospective studies including 1,605 patients with positive inguinal LNs. Due to wide variability in data, there was insufficient evidence to assess whether adjuvant inguinal nodal RT improved outcomes. Regional recurrence rates were high, and toxicity assessments were limited.

REFERENCES

1. Siegel RL, Miller KD, Jemal A. Cancer statistics, 2020. *CA Cancer J Clin.* 2020;70(1):7–30. doi:10.3322/caac.21590
2. *AJCC Cancer Staging Manual, Eighth Edition.* 8th ed. Springer Publishing; 2017.
3. Hakenberg OW, Comperat EM, Minhas S, et al. EAU guidelines on penile cancer: 2014 update. *Eur Urol.* 2015;67(1):142–150. doi:10.1016/j.eururo.2014.10.017
4. Solsona E, Bahl A, Brandes SB, et al. New developments in the treatment of localized penile cancer. *Urology.* 2010;76(2 Suppl 1):S36–S42. doi:10.1016/j.urology.2010.04.009
5. Heyns CF, Fleshner N, Sangar V, et al. Management of the lymph nodes in penile cancer. *Urology.* 2010;76(2 Suppl 1):S43–S57. doi:10.1016/j.urology.2010.03.001
6. Graafland NM, Lam W, Leijte JA, et al. Prognostic factors for occult inguinal lymph node involvement in penile carcinoma and assessment of the high-risk EAU subgroup: a two-institution analysis of 342 clinically node-negative patients. *Eur Urol.* 2010;58(5):742–747. doi:10.1016/j.eururo.2010.08.015
7. Dickstein RJ, Munsell MF, Pagliaro LC, Pettaway CA. Prognostic factors influencing survival from regionally advanced squamous cell carcinoma of the penis after preoperative chemotherapy. *BJU Int.* 2016;117(1):118–125. doi:10.1111/bju.12946
8. Videtic GMM, Woody N, Vassil AD. *Handbook of Treatment Planning in Radiation Oncology.* 3rd ed. Demos Medical; 2020. doi:10.1891/9780826168429
9. Neave F, Neal AJ, Hoskin PJ, Hope-Stone HF. Carcinoma of the penis: a retrospective review of treatment with iridium mould and external beam irradiation. *Clin Oncol (R Coll Radiol).* 1993;5(4):207–210. doi:10.1016/S0936-6555(05)80230-4

10. Munro NP, Thomas PJ, Deutsch GP, Hodson NJ. Penile cancer: a case for guidelines. *Ann R Coll Surg Engl.* 2001;83(3):180–185.

11. Azrif M, Logue JP, Swindell R, et al. External-beam radiotherapy in T1-2 N0 penile carcinoma. *Clin Oncol (R Coll Radiol).* 2006;18(4):320–325. doi:10.1016/j.clon.2006.01.004

12. Crook JM, Haie-Meder C, Demanes DJ, et al. American Brachytherapy Society–Groupe Europeen de Curietherapie–European Society of Therapeutic Radiation Oncology (ABS-GEC-ESTRO) consensus statement for penile brachytherapy. *Brachytherapy.* 2013;12(3):191–198. doi:10.1016/j.brachy.2013.01.167

45 ■ URETHRAL CANCER

Rahul D. Tendulkar, Rupesh Kotecha, and Omar Y. Mian

QUICK HIT ■ Rare tumor that often presents with locally advanced disease, particularly proximal tumors, which have a worse prognosis. Urothelial carcinomas are most common followed by squamous cell carcinomas. Management involves surgery for early-stage disease (with organ preservation if possible) and combined modality therapy for advanced stage. Unfortunately, no prospective randomized trials guide management.

EPIDEMIOLOGY: Very rare tumor (<1% of GU malignancies). In a SEER registry from 1973 to 2002, there were 1,075 urethral carcinomas in men and 540 in women.[1] Annual incidence is ~500 cases. Up to 50% die of their disease.[2]

RISK FACTORS: Chronic inflammation: prior history of STD, urethritis, urethral strictures (potentially secondary to trauma), urethral diverticuli, urinary stasis, recurrent infection. HPV, prior urothelial cancer, or prior radiation therapy.[3]

ANATOMY

Men: Male urethra extends from bladder neck proximally to urethral meatus distally (~20–21 cm in length), and is divided into the prostatic urethra (10% of cancer cases; composed of transitional epithelium), bulbomembranous (60%; transitional epithelium), and penile (30%; pseudostratified columnar epithelium) portions, with squamous epithelium at the meatus.

Women: Female urethra is shorter than males (3–4 cm) and is divided into the posterior segment (proximal one-third, transitional cells) and anterior segment (distal two-thirds, squamous epithelium).

PATHOLOGY: In general, the majority of urethral cancers are urothelial carcinomas, followed by squamous cell carcinomas. Adenocarcinomas are rare and typically arise from periurethral glandular tissue (Skene's glands). Mixed tumors can also be seen.

CLINICAL PRESENTATION: May present with symptoms of a urethral stricture (urinary retention, difficulty voiding, dysuria), hematuria, urethral discharge, pain, swelling, priapism, irritative urinary symptoms, or dyspareunia. Often presents late because symptoms can be attributed to benign causes (e.g., UTI or strictures). Cancers can extend locally into the penis, spread to pelvic LNs (primary drainage for the proximal one third urethra) or to inguinal LNs (primary drainage for the distal two thirds urethra), which can present with palpable nodal metastasis. Clinically suspicious LNs are usually involved by urethral cancer metastases (in contrast to penile cancer where only ~50% of cN+ are pN+). DM present in only 10% at diagnosis (lung, liver, bone).

WORKUP: H&P with full GU exam (also GYN exam for women). EUA (palpation of the genitalia, urethra, rectum, perineum) and cystourethroscopy to evaluate extent of disease. Consider retrograde urethrogram.

Labs: CBC, CMP, urine cytology (more sensitive for urothelial carcinomas in pendulous urethra).[4]

Imaging: CT or MRI of the primary site and pelvis. Chest CT ± bone scan. PET/CT is not standard.

Biopsy: Transurethral biopsy.

PROGNOSTIC FACTORS: Poor prognosis associated with advanced age, tumor location (proximal worse than distal), tumor size (>2 cm vs. <2 cm), higher clinical nodal stage, higher histologic grade, presence of metastatic disease.[5–8]

STAGING

TABLE 45.1 (A): AJCC 8th Edition (2017): Staging for Male Penile Urethra and Female Urethra				
T/M	N	cN0	cN1	cN2
T1	• Invades subepithelial connective tissue	I	III	IV
T2	• Invades corpus spongiosum or periurethral muscle	II		
T3	• Invades corpus cavernosum or anterior vagina			
T4	• Invades adjacent organs			
M1	• Distant metastasis			

Notes: Regional LNs include inguinal (superficial or deep), perivesical, obturator, internal, and external iliac cN1, single regional LN; cN2, multiple regional LNs.

TABLE 45.1 (B): AJCC 8th Edition (2017): Staging for Prostatic Urethra	
Tis	Carcinoma in situ involving prostatic urethra or periurethral or prostatic ducts without stromal invasion
T1	Invades subepithelial connective tissue
T2	Invades prostatic stroma surrounding ducts by direct extension from urothelial surface or prostatic ducts
T3	Invades periprostatic fat
T4	Invades other adjacent organs (e.g., bladder wall, rectal wall)

TREATMENT PARADIGM: Without prospective trials to guide management, only retrospective series are available. Treatment based on gender, location, extent of disease, and histology (Table 45.2).

General Principles

Localized disease: Surgical management, with transurethral resection for small lesions or segmental resection for larger lesions (partial or total urethrectomy). Consider RT for organ preservation.

Locally advanced disease: Neoadjuvant CHT ± RT followed by surgery.

Metastatic disease: CHT ± immunotherapy ± palliative local therapy.

Surgery: In both men and women, inguinal LND is generally recommended in patients with clinically or radiographically positive LNs. No definitive data on SLNB, although performed at some centers.

Men: For small Tis-T1 tumors, endoscopic resection is appropriate. Distal tumors can undergo distal urethrectomy. For larger tumors or if unable to obtain a negative margin resection endoscopically, perform a segmental resection with anastomosis. Subtotal urethrectomy and perineal urethrostomy for T2 cancers (spongiosum but not cavernosa involvement). T3–T4 tumors often require total penectomy, cystoprostatectomy, and anterior exenteration with perineal reconstruction.

TABLE 45.2: General Treatment Paradigm for Urethral Cancer	
Men (Ta, Tis, T1 low grade)	Transurethral (endoscopic) resection or fulguration; distal urethrectomy for distal lesions
Men (T1 high grade)	Segmental resection with primary anastomosis
Men (T2)	Subtotal urethrectomy and perineal urethrostomy
Women (Ta, T1, and T2)	Local excision vs. definitive RT
T3/T4 or LN+	Neoadjuvant CHT ± RT followed by surgery (likely exenteration), or definitive chemoRT (reserving surgery for salvage). Inguinal LN dissection for patients with LN+ disease

Women: T1 tumors can be treated with endoscopic resection (must maintain urethral sphincter to preserve continence). More advanced tumors are treated by total urethrectomy with bladder neck closure and urinary diversion. Extensive locoregional disease may require pelvic exenteration and vaginectomy.

Chemotherapy: Neoadjuvant CHT indicated for locally advanced disease ± RT prior to surgery based on histology. Squamous cell carcinomas often treated with 5-FU + cisplatin or 5-FU + MMC. Urothelial carcinomas typically receive cisplatin-based regimens such as gemcitabine + cisplatin or ddMVAC (dose-dense methotrexate, vinblastine, doxorubicin, and cisplatin).

Radiation: Prior to RT, perform circumcision in men to prevent balanitis and phimosis.

Adjuvant: Consider post-op RT for patients with locally-advanced (pT3–4) primary disease depending on surgery extent or positive margins.

Neoadjuvant: Consider pre-op RT or chemoRT to reduce tumor burden and/or extent of surgery required.

Definitive: Consider organ preservation for distal tumors in men and proximal tumors in women. T1–T2 tumors can potentially be treated with RT alone, but for more advanced disease consider sequential or concurrent chemoRT.

Palliative: Indicated for symptomatic locally advanced disease not amenable to curative therapy.

Dose: EBRT dose is 45 to 50.4 Gy to primary site and inguinal, external and internal iliac LNs. Brachytherapy may be considered for lesions <2 to 3 cm with negative LNs or prior to EBRT for patients with larger tumors or LN + disease. Brachytherapy dose is generally ~20 to 25 Gy after EBRT.

Toxicities: Acute: Radiation dermatitis, local pain, fibrosis, radiation cystitis, urethritis. Late: Chronic penile edema, fistula, and urethral stricture (consider biopsy to rule out recurrent disease).

Procedure: See *Handbook of Treatment Planning in Radiation Oncology*, Chapter 8.[9]

■ **EVIDENCE-BASED Q&A**

■ **Can an organ-preservation approach be used for patients with early-stage urethral cancer?**

Select series show promising outcomes with definitive RT (brachytherapy ± EBRT) as an alternative to surgery.

Sharma, All India Institute (*J Contemp Brachytherapy* 2016, PMID 26985196): RR of 10 female patients with periurethral cancer (5 recurrent and 5 primary cancers) treated with HDR brachytherapy (2–3 plane free-hand implant with plastic catheters to tumor + 5 mm margin) ± EBRT (primary site, inguinal LNs, external iliac LNs, internal iliac LNs). Brachytherapy alone 42 Gy/14 fx over 7 days BID for patients with lesions <3 cm in size, and brachytherapy boost 18 to 21 Gy/6 to 7 fx BID after EBRT (50.4 Gy up-front or 36 Gy for recurrent cases after prior RT) for patients with lesions >3 cm. Brachytherapy performed prior to EBRT since tumors are well-delineated and easier to implant; no desquamation from EBRT to delay treatment and higher dose able to be delivered over a short period. Six patients were disease-free and four patients recurred. All five patients treated with brachytherapy developed moist desquamation. Grade II toxicity 30%. **Conclusion: Small sample size but brachytherapy provides good LRC with expected toxicity. Regional nodal RT recommended for patients with tumors >2 cm given the higher than expected nodal failure rate.**

■ **Can an organ-preservation approach be used for patients with locally advanced urethral cancer?**

Select series show promising outcomes with definitive chemoRT for patients who refuse surgery or are not surgical candidates (as an alternative to surgery). However, those who do not respond to therapy have dismal outcomes (despite salvage surgery).

Kent, Lahey Clinic (*J Urol* 2015, PMID 25088950): RR of 26 male patients treated with 2 cycles of 5-FU 1,000 mg/m² + MMC 10 mg/m² with concurrent EBRT 45 to 55 Gy/25 fx to genitals, perineum, and inguinal and external iliac LN. All but one patient had squamous histology; 88% had at least T3 or LN + disease; 79% had CR, and 21% had no response to treatment (all of these patients died of their disease, regardless of salvage surgery). Of the CR patients, 42% ultimately had disease recurrence at median 12.5 mos. 5-yr DSS 68%, DFS 43%, and OS 52%. **Conclusion: ChemoRT may allow for organ preservation in select patients.**

■ **Are there any data supporting the use of neoadjuvant CHT or chemoRT in patients with locally advanced urethral cancer?**

For significant locally advanced disease, neoadjuvant therapy can decrease the burden of disease and reduce the extent of surgery needed.

Gakis, Multi-Institutional (*Ann Oncol* 2015, PMID 25969370): Multicenter RR of 124 patients (86 men, 38 women) with urethral cancer treated at 10 centers from 1993 to 2012. Thirty-one percent received neoadjuvant CHT, 15% neoadjuvant chemoRT + adjuvant CHT, and 54% received adjuvant CHT. Neoadjuvant therapy was more likely to be used in patients with LN + disease and reduced extent of surgery (avoiding cystectomy). RR to neoadjuvant CHT was 25% and to neoadjuvant chemoRT was 33%; 3-yr OS 100% for those who received neoadjuvant CHT or neoadjuvant chemoRT, but only 50% after surgery and 20% after surgery + adjuvant CHT. Neoadjuvant treatment was associated with improved 3-yr RFS and OS. **Conclusion: Neoadjuvant CHT or chemoRT for patients with T3 or LN+ disease was associated with improved outcomes compared to up-front surgery or surgery + CHT.**

■ **What is the role of adjuvant RT in patients with locally advanced urethral cancer?**

Son, Multi-Institutional (*IJROBP* 2018, PMID 29908944): RR of 2614 patients, with 5-yr OS 54%. Among 501 patients with locally advanced urethral cancer, surgery + RT was associated with improved OS compared to surgery alone (especially for adenocarcinomas HR 0.20 and transitional cell carcinomas HR 0.45). For 1,705 patients with early stage disease, no OS difference was noted with the addition of post-operative RT.

REFERENCES

1. Swartz MA, Porter MP, Lin DW, Weiss NS. Incidence of primary urethral carcinoma in the United States. *Urology.* 2006;68(6):1164–1168. doi:10.1016/j.urology.2006.08.1057
2. Visser O, Adolfsson J, Rossi S, et al. Incidence and survival of rare urogenital cancers in Europe. *Eur J Cancer.* 2012;48(4):456–464. doi:10.1016/j.ejca.2011.10.031
3. Gakis G, Bruins HM, Cathomas R, et al. European association of urology guidelines on primary urethral carcinoma-2020 update. *Eur Urol Oncol.* 2020;3(4):424–432. doi:10.1016/j.euo.2020.06.003
4. Touijer AK, Dalbagni G. Role of voided urine cytology in diagnosing primary urethral carcinoma. *Urology.* 2004;63(1):33–35. doi:10.1016/j.urology.2003.08.007
5. Gakis G, Morgan TM, Efstathiou JA, et al. Prognostic factors and outcomes in primary urethral cancer: results from the international collaboration on primary urethral carcinoma. *World J Urol.* 2016;34(1):97–103. doi:10.1007/s00345-015-1583-7
6. Rabbani F. Prognostic factors in male urethral cancer. *Cancer.* 2011;117(11):2426–2434. doi:10.1002/cncr.25787
7. Champ CE, Hegarty SE, Shen X, et al. Prognostic factors and outcomes after definitive treatment of female urethral cancer: a population-based analysis. *Urology.* 2012;80(2):374–381. doi:10.1016/j.urology.2012.02.058
8. Dalbagni G, Zhang ZF, Lacombe L, Herr HW. Female urethral carcinoma: an analysis of treatment outcome and a plea for a standardized management strategy. *Br J Urol.* 1998;82(6):835–841. doi:10.1046/j.1464-410X.1998.00878.x
9. Videtic GMM, Woody N, Vassil AD. *Handbook of Treatment Planning in Radiation Oncology.* 3rd ed. Demos Medical; 2020. doi:10.1046/j.1464-410X.1998.00878.x

46 ■ RENAL CELL CARCINOMA

Sarah M.C. Sittenfeld and Rahul D. Tendulkar

> **QUICK HIT** ■ Renal cell carcinoma is a relatively common primary tumor of the kidney. Surgical resection alone is recommended for localized disease. Radiotherapy has historically had minimal role in the adjuvant setting due to the rarity of locoregional failure and the frequency of distant failure. Historically, radical nephrectomy was performed even in the setting of metastatic disease based on randomized data showing a survival benefit in the pre-VEGF era. With the advent of VEGF-directed therapy, survival has been dramatically extended, and surgical resection in the setting of metastatic disease may not be necessary. For medically inoperable patients, RFA or cryotherapy are commonly used for small tumors, with increasing evidence to suggest a role for definitive SBRT.

EPIDEMIOLOGY: Expected incidence of 73,750 cases and 14,830 deaths in 2020.[1] Incidence of 16.6 per 100,000 continues to increase, predominately for early localized disease likely related to incidental findings on imaging.[2] Median age at diagnosis is 65 years with a slight male preponderance.

RISK FACTORS: Cigarette smoking (50% increased risk in males, 20% in females as compared to non-smokers), obesity, phenacetin-containing analgesics (cancer usually follows prolonged and heavy use, with resultant renal papillary necrosis), and low fruit/vegetable diet.[3–5]

ANATOMY: The kidneys and renal pelvis are encapsulated retroperitoneal structures that are enveloped in perinephric fat and Gerota's fascia. They are centered at L1 or L2, and lie between T12 and L3 with the right kidney slightly more inferior due to the liver. Centrally, minor and major calyces drain urine into the renal pelvis which then convey urine into the ureters. The lymphatics of the right kidney are to renal hilar, paracaval, and interaortocaval nodes. The lymphatics of the left kidney are to renal hilar and paraaortic nodes.

PATHOLOGY: RCC arises within the renal cortex and represents 80% to 85% of primary renal neoplasms. Several RCC subtypes exist, including clear cell (75%–85%), papillary (10–15%), chromophobe (5%–10%), oncocytic (3%–5%), and collecting duct (Bellini duct, <1%). The distinct sarcomatoid subtype, representing <10% of renal tumors, is associated with worse OS than other subtypes, and 50% to 70% of patients with sarcomatoid tumors present with bone metastases. While tumors <3 cm have historically been characterized as renal adenomas, data have shown small tumors can still represent malignancy and often definitive management is warranted.[6,7]

GENETICS: Hereditary diseases: (a) von Hippel-Lindau: mutation/deletion in the *VHL* gene located on the short arm of chromosome 3 (3p25) that predisposes the development of characteristic red birthmarks, renal cancer, CNS hemangioblastoma, retinal angioma, pheochromocytoma, epididymal cystadenoma, and pancreatic tumors; 30% to 45% of patients develop clear cell RCC. The VHL protein is responsible for ubiquitinating HIF-1α under normoxic conditions marking it for proteasomal degradation. The absence of functional VHL simulates hypoxia, causing upregulation of hypoxia-responsive genes such as *VEGF, PDGF, EGFR, GLUT-1, TGF-β*, and *EPO*. (b) HCRC: rare, AD disease associated with mutation in *VHL* gene. (c) HPRC: rare, AD disease associated with germline abnormality in MET proto-oncogene.[8]

CLINICAL PRESENTATION: Common symptoms are painless gross or microscopic hematuria. Uncommon symptoms are pain, flank mass, and paraneoplastic syndromes. The classic triad of *gross hematuria, flank mass, and pain* occurs in only 10% of patients and usually indicates advanced disease. Up to 25% to 40% are asymptomatic and discovered incidentally. Paraneoplastic syndromes may cause anemia, polycythemia (EPO), pyrexia, amyloidosis, liver dysfunction, hypertension, or hypercalcemia (PTH-rp). The sudden onset of a left-sided varicocele should raise the possibility of a renal tumor obstructing the testicular vein at its entry point into the left renal vein (occurs in 2% of male patients).

WORKUP: H&P.

Labs: CBC, CMP.

Imaging: Ultrasound or abdominal CT based on presenting symptoms. MRI is useful when US or CT are inconclusive or patient is unable to receive IV contrast. CT chest for staging. Bone scan indicated only in patients with symptoms or elevated alkaline phosphatase.

Biopsy: CT-guided biopsy may be performed for indeterminate tumor on radiographic workup. A nephrectomy is usually done without obtaining tissue biopsy because diagnosis is frequently obvious from radiographic workup. Selective renal arteriogram should be done if considering a partial nephrectomy.

PROGNOSTIC FACTORS: Stage is the most important factor. KPS <80, time from diagnosis to initiation of targeted therapy <1 year, low hemoglobin, high calcium, high neutrophil count, and high platelet count are all associated with worse survival.

STAGING: AJCC 8th edition (Table 46.1).

Table 46.1: AJCC 8th Edition: Staging for RCC				
T/M		**N**	**cN0**	**cN1**
T1	**a** ≤4 cm, limited to the kidney		I	III
	b >4 and ≤7 cm, limited to kidney			
T2	**a** 7–10 cm, limited to kidney		II	
	b >10 cm, limited to kidney			
T3	**a** Tumor extends into the renal vein or its segmental branches, or invades the pelvicalyceal system, or invades perirenal and/or renal sinus fat but not beyond Gerota's fascia		III	
	b Tumor extends into the vena cava below the diaphragm			
	c Tumor grossly extends into the vena cava above the diaphragm or invades the wall of the vena cava			
T4	Tumor invades beyond Gerota's fascia (including contiguous extension to the ipsilateral adrenal gland)		IV	
M1	Distant metastasis			

TREATMENT PARADIGM

Surgery: Mainstay of treatment of non-metastatic disease. Surgical choice depends on tumor and patient factors.

Radical nephrectomy (RN): En bloc removal of the kidney along with Gerota's fascia and its contents (including adrenal gland, kidney, and perinephric fat, and often hilar lymph nodes). RN has not been compared to a simple nephrectomy in a randomized trial, but it allows a more reliable margin around tumor. The surgical approach depends on the patient's body habitus and position of tumor. Tumor within the IVC does NOT preclude a curative resection.

Partial nephrectomy (PN): Indicated for early-stage (IA/IB) disease and poor renal reserve, absence of normally functioning contralateral kidney, and bilateral renal cancer with PN performed on the lesser involved kidney. PN may be considered electively for small tumors (<4 cm), as well as for patients with von Hippel–Lindau disease, renal artery stenosis, hydronephrosis, ureteral reflux, and nephrosclerosis. PN is a more complicated procedure than RN with a greater risk of bleeding complications. PN patients are candidates for surgical salvage in the event of a local failure (<10% of cases).

Palliative nephrectomy: Indicated for intractable bleeding and pain. Debulking nephrectomy prior to systemic therapy in patients with metastatic disease has been shown to improve survival when compared to IFN-α alone in two randomized trials[9,10]; however, with more effective systemic therapy options, there appears to be a more limited role for this approach in the modern era.[11] Debulking surgery induces spontaneous regression of metastases in <1% of cases. Lymph node dissection remains controversial as it does provide useful staging information but has been shown to have no impact on survival.

Cryoablation/RFA: Minimally invasive option for localized disease especially those with a single kidney or comorbidities. Contraindications include tumor >5 cm, distant metastases, and hilar or central tumors.

Systemic therapy: Multiple trials have investigated the role of adjuvant therapy in non-metastatic disease with low response rates and no clear benefit seen. Sunitinib has been approved for adjuvant treatment in high-risk disease after resection based on an improvement in DFS (59.3% vs. 51.3%) over placebo, though no OS has been seen and therapy is associated with toxicity.[12] Various immunotherapies are currently under investigation for their role in the adjuvant setting. Significant advances have been made with immunotherapy in the metastatic setting and several options are available for the first-line treatment of metastatic disease including: nivolumab plus ipilimumab, pembrolizumab plus axitinib, or avelumab plus axitinib.[13-15]

Radiation

Adjuvant RT: After radical nephrectomy, the risk of LR is less than 5%; therefore, adjuvant therapy is not generally recommended. Two early randomized trials of postoperative RT (50–55 Gy) vs. observation showed no benefit in LC or OS with the addition of RT, with a significant increase in toxicity and complications.[16,17] Although these studies were done in the 2D era, there have not been data to support adjuvant RT in more modern series. Some retrospective series suggest a potential LC benefit for adjuvant RT in patients with T3–T4 disease, positive margins, or positive LNs; however, given low rates of LR without RT, adjuvant treatment is generally not employed.

Definitive SBRT: Several institutional series of SBRT have reported excellent rates of local control with favorable toxicity profiles in patients who are inoperable or have unresectable RCC. Various dose and fractionation schemes have been employed and further study is needed to refine dose and fractionation recommendations.

■ EVIDENCE-BASED Q&A

▨ What data are available to support the use of SBRT for the treatment of inoperable RCC?

Multiple single institutional retrospective and small prospective single-arm series have reported efficacy and toxicity of SBRT for RCC in patients who are inoperable, with overall favorable results to date. More recent pooled data confirm the early favorable reports, even in larger tumor sizes. Larger phase II studies are under way to provide more evidence to support the use of SBRT in the medically inoperable patient population.

Siva, IROCK (*Cancer* **2017, PMID: 29266183):** Pooled analysis from 9 institutions of 223 patients with inoperable RCC. Average age 72 years, and tumor size 4.36 cm. A total of 118 received single-fraction SBRT (14–26 Gy, median 25 Gy) and 105 received multifraction (24–70 Gy in 2–10 fx; median 40 Gy in 5 fx). Median follow up 2.6 years; 2 year LC, PFS, and OS was 98%, 77%, and 82%, respectively. Tumor size and multi-fraction SBRT significantly predicted for worse outcomes. Multifraction SBRT was associated with greater likelihood of distant failure. Grade 3 toxicity rate of 3.8%. **Conclusion: SBRT for inoperable RCC has excellent LC and is well tolerated. Further prospective study is needed.**

Siva, IROCK (*IJROBP* **2020, PMID 32562838):** Pooled analysis from 9 institutions of 95 inoperable patients with tumors >4 cm treated with SBRT. CSS, OS, and PFS were 96%, 84%, and 81% at 2 years and 91%, 69%, and 65% at 4 years, respectively. No grades 3 to 5 toxicities were reported. On MVA, increasing tumor size was associated with inferior CSS (HR per 1 cm increase 1.3; $p < .001$). **Conclusion: SBRT for inoperable RCC >4 cm appears to be safe and effective, with larger tumors associated with inferior survival.**

REFERENCES

1. Siegel RL, Miller KD, Jemal A. Cancer statistics, 2020. *CA Cancer J Clin*. 2020;70(1):7–30. doi:10.3322/caac.21590
2. King SC, Pollack LA, Li J, et al. Continued increase in incidence of renal cell carcinoma, especially in young patients and high grade disease: United States 2001 to 2010. *J Urol*. 2014;191(6):1665–1670. doi:10.1016/j.juro.2013.12.046
3. Chow WH, Dong LM, Devesa SS. Epidemiology and risk factors for kidney cancer. *Nat Rev Urol*. 2010;7(5):245–257. doi:10.1038/nrurol.2010.46
4. Zeegers MP, Tan FE, Dorant E, et al. The impact of characteristics of cigarette smoking on urinary tract cancer risk: a meta-analysis of epidemiologic studies. *Cancer*. 2000;89(3):630–639. doi:10.1002/1097-0142(20000801)89:3<630::AID-CNCR19>3.0.CO;2-Q
5. Oh SW, Yoon YS, Shin SA. Effects of excess weight on cancer incidences depending on cancer sites and histologic findings among men: Korea National Health Insurance Corporation Study. *J Clin Oncol*. 2005;23(21):4742–4754. doi:10.1200/JCO.2005.11.726
6. Bosniak MA, Birnbaum BA, Krinsky GA, Waisman J. Small renal parenchymal neoplasms: further observations on growth. *Radiology*. 1995;197(3):589–597. doi:10.1148/radiology.197.3.7480724
7. Schlomer B, Figenshau RS, Yan Y, et al. Pathological features of renal neoplasms classified by size and symptomatology. *J Urol*. 2006;176(4 Pt 1):1317–1320; discussion 1320. doi:10.1016/j.juro.2006.06.005
8. Haas NB, Nathanson KL. Hereditary kidney cancer syndromes. *Adv Chronic Kidney Dis*. 2014;21(1):81–90. doi:10.1053/j.ackd.2013.10.001
9. Flanigan RC, Salmon SE, Blumenstein BA, et al. Nephrectomy followed by interferon alfa-2b compared with interferon alfa-2b alone for metastatic renal-cell cancer. *N Engl J Med*. 2001;345(23):1655–1659. doi:10.1056/NEJMoa003013
10. Mickisch GH, Garin A, van Poppel H, et al. Radical nephrectomy plus interferon-alfa-based immunotherapy compared with interferon alfa alone in metastatic renal-cell carcinoma: a randomised trial. *Lancet*. 2001;358(9286):966–970. doi:10.1016/S0140-6736(01)06103-7
11. Méjean A, Ravaud A, Thezenas S, et al. Sunitinib alone or after nephrectomy in metastatic renal-cell carcinoma. *N Engl J Med*. 2018;379(5):417–427. doi:10.1056/NEJMoa1803675
12. Ravaud A, Motzer RJ, Pandha HS, et al. Adjuvant sunitinib in high-risk renal-cell carcinoma after nephrectomy. *N Engl J Med*. 2016;375(23):2246–2254. doi:10.1056/NEJMoa1611406
13. Motzer RJ, Tannir NM, McDermott DF, et al. Nivolumab plus ipilimumab versus sunitinib in advanced renal-cell carcinoma. *N Engl J Med*. 2018;378(14):1277–1290. doi:10.1056/NEJMoa1712126
14. Rini BI, Plimack ER, Stus V, et al. Pembrolizumab plus axitinib versus sunitinib for advanced renal-cell carcinoma. *N Engl J Med*. 2019;380(12):1116–1127. doi:10.1056/NEJMoa1816714
15. Motzer RJ, Penkov K, Haanen J, et al. Avelumab plus axitinib versus sunitinib for advanced renal-cell carcinoma. *N Engl J Med*. 2019;380(12):1103–1115. doi:10.1056/NEJMoa1816047
16. Finney R. The value of radiotherapy in the treatment of hypernephroma: a clinical trial. *Br J Urol*. 1973;45(3):258–269. doi:10.1111/j.1464-410X.1973.tb12152.x
17. Micheletti E, Favardi U, Cozzoli A. Role of postoperative adjuvant radiotherapy in the treatment of class T2-3 N0 M0 adenocarcinoma of the kidney. *Radiol Med*. 1991;81(6):887–892.

47 ■ CERVICAL CANCER

Sudha R. Amarnath, Monica E. Shukla, and Sheen Cherian

QUICK HIT ■ The vast majority of cervical cancer cases are HPV mediated. Incidence and mortality significantly declined with introduction of screening with Pap smears. Three FDA-approved vaccines are available that prevent the development of cervical cancer. Treatment at early stages is often surgical, while RT ± CHT is employed in later stages. When treating definitively, EBRT is followed by an intracavitary or interstitial brachytherapy boost. Postoperative RT ± CHT is occasionally indicated for adverse pathologic features.

Table 47.1 Cervical Cancer General Treatment Paradigm[1,2]	
Early Stage	
IA1 (Non-fertility sparing)	Extrafascial hysterectomy or modified radical hysterectomy + PLND OR brachytherapy alone ± EBRT
IA1 (Fertility sparing)	*w/o LVSI:* CKC w/ 3 mm negative margins *w/LVSI:* CKC w/ 3 mm negative margins + PLND (± PALNS) OR Radical trachelectomy + PLND (± PALNS)
IA2 (Non-fertility sparing)	Modified radical hysterectomy + PLND (± PALNS) OR Pelvic EBRT + brachytherapy ± concurrent CHT (for high-risk features)
IA2 (Fertility sparing)	CKC w/ 3 mm negative margins + PLND (± PALNS) OR Radical trachelectomy + PLND (± PALNS)
IB1 or IB2 or IIA1 (Non-fertility sparing)	Radical hysterectomy + PLND (± PALNS) OR Definitive EBRT + brachytherapy ± concurrent CHT
IB1 and select IB2 (Fertility sparing)	Radical trachelectomy + PLND (± PALNS)
Locally Advanced	
IB3, IIA2 - IVA	Definitive EBRT + brachytherapy + concurrent CHT

EPIDEMIOLOGY: In the United States, there were an estimated 13,800 new cases of and 4,290 deaths due to invasive cervical cancer in 2020.[3] Disease burden in less developed countries is much higher (~85% of new cases). With screening, precancerous lesions are diagnosed far more often than invasive lesions. Incidence and death rate have decreased steadily over decades due to screening, which detects earlier lesions. Median age at diagnosis is 49.

RISK FACTORS: HPV infection is associated with >90% of cervical cancer cases. HPV 16/18 confer highest risk of carcinogenesis and account for 65% to 70% of cases (other cancer-causing strains are 31, 33, 45, 52, 58).[4] Other risk factors include smoking, immunocompromised status (transplant, AIDS), history of STDs, young age at first intercourse, multiple sexual partners, multiparity, low SES, DES exposure in utero (associated with clear cell adenocarcinoma of cervix/vagina).

ANATOMY: Cervix: Lower part of uterus that is cylindrical in shape. Endocervical canal, lined by columnar epithelium, runs through it and connects uterine cavity to vagina. Distal part of cervix projects into vagina (called ectocervix) and is lined by squamous epithelium. Squamo-columnar junction is located at external os and is most common site for carcinogenesis. Broad and cardinal ligaments attach uterus and cervix, respectively, to pelvic sidewall. Uterosacral ligament attaches low uterus to sacrum. Lymphatic drainage of cervix is through these ligaments to following lymphatic beds: presacral, obturator, internal iliac, external iliac, common iliac, and para-aortic LNs. Most common sites of distant spread are lungs, supraclavicular LNs (via thoracic duct), bones, and liver.

PATHOLOGY: Squamous cell carcinoma (70%–75%); adenocarcinoma (20%–25%); adenosquamous (5%). Higher incidence of adenocarcinoma histologies in younger patients. Adenocarcinoma often presents with larger tumors ("barrel cervix") with higher risk of local failure. Incidence is increasing and Pap screening is less sensitive for this histology. HPV testing may increase sensitivity. Less common histologies: clear-cell adenocarcinoma, small cell, neuroendocrine, sarcoma (rhabdomyosarcoma in adolescents), melanoma, adenoid cystic carcinoma.

SCREENING: Screening guidelines vary between ACS, USPSTF, and ACOG. Current ACOG recommendations (2017):[5] **Ages 21 to 29**—Pap test alone q3 years, HPV testing is not recommended. **Ages 30 to 65:** Pap test with HPV test (cotesting) q5 years (preferred) or Pap test alone q3 years; **≥65 years:** No further screening if no history of moderate/severe dysplasia and three negative Paps in row or two negative cotests in row within 10 years, most recent within 5 years. Having HPV vaccination does not alter screening recommendations.

CLINICAL PRESENTATION: Asymptomatic and detected on screening, abnormal vaginal discharge, post-coital bleeding, dyspareunia, pelvic pain.

WORKUP: H&P with focus on GYN history and careful abdomen/pelvic exam with attention to inferior extension into vagina, lateral extension into parametria, posterior extension into uterosacral ligament or rectum, examine supraclavicular and inguinal LNs. Smoking cessation counseling.

Labs: CBC/CMP, pregnancy test, consider HIV testing.

Procedures: Colposcopy with cervical biopsy, CKC if cervical biopsy is inadequate to determine DOI or if part of lesion is not well visualized on colposcopy or as definitive procedure in select early cases desiring fertility preservation. EUA with cystoscopy/rectosigmoidoscopy (for advanced disease or if bladder or rectal extension is suspected), ureteral stent placement if necessary.

Imaging: PET/CT (nodal staging),[6] pelvic MRI (to delineate local disease extent and guide decisions on fertility vs. non-fertility sparing approaches).

PROGNOSTIC FACTORS: Stage, age, tumor size (≥4 cm worse), lymph node involvement, LVSI, persistent uptake on posttreatment PET/CT,[7] prolonged treatment time (>56 days), low hemoglobin (<10 g/dL).

STAGING:

Table 47.2 AJCC 9th Edition (2021) and FIGO 2018: Staging for Cervical Cancer		
AJCC		**FIGO**
T1	Confined to cervix, microscopic lesion **1a1** ≤3 mm DOI **1a2** 3–5 mm DOI	I
	Confined to cervix, >5 mm DOI **1b1** <2 cm **1b2** ≥2 and <4 cm **1b3** ≥4 cm	

AJCC		FIGO
Table 47.2 AJCC 9th Edition (2021) and FIGO 2018: Staging for Cervical Cancer (*continued*)		
T2	**Extension beyond uterus, but not to side wall or lower one-third vagina** **2a1** ≤4 cm, no parametrial invasion **2a2** >4 cm, no parametrial invasion **2b** Parametrial invasion	II
T3	**3a** Involves lower one-third vagina, no extension to pelvic side wall **3b** Extends to pelvic side wall and/or causes hydronephrosis or non-functioning kidney	III
T4	Invasion of bladder, rectum, and/or extends beyond true pelvis	IVA
N0	No regional LNs	
N0 (i +)	Isolated tumor cells ≤0.2 mm	
N1a	Pelvic LN metastases only	IIIC1
N2	Para aortic LN metastases with or without positive pelvic LNs	IIIC2
M0	No distant metastasis	
M1	Distant metastasis	IVB

Notes: When in doubt, the lower staging should be assigned.
FIGO 2018 staging update: IA no longer includes horizontal spread; IB doesn't need to be visible; prior staging had only IB1 (<4 cm) and IB2 (>4cm); now there is IB1–IB3, IIIC added; advanced imaging can now be used with extra annotation ("r" for imaging and "p" for pathology). AJCC 9th edition was updated in 2021 to mirror FIGO 2018 staging changes.

TREATMENT PARADIGM

Observation: Refer to current ACOG guidelines on management for ASCUS, LSIL, HSIL, ASC-H, AGC.

Prevention: ACS, CDC, and ACOG recommend routine vaccination of 11- to 12-year-old boys and girls with 9-valent HPV vaccine (covers: 6, 11, 16, 18, 31, 33, 45, 52, 58), with "catch-up" vaccination through age 26. Adults ages 27 to 45 may be vaccinated, as clinically indicated. HPV 6 and 11 cause ~90% cases of anogenital warts.

Surgery: Reserved mainly for IA1–IB2 and IIA. BSO is optional, but spared when fertility preservation is desired. Goal of up-front surgery is to select patients at low risk of needing adjuvant RT since bimodality therapy increases morbidity.

CKC: Removal of cone-shaped piece of tissue containing ectocervix and endocervical canal en bloc with scalpel to avoid electrosurgical artifact. This facilitates accurate margin status assessment.

Radical Trachelectomy: Fertility-sparing surgery that removes cervix, upper vagina, and parametria, while leaving uterine body in place. Cerclage or "purse-string stitch" is made at distal end of uterine body.

Class I a.k.a. "Simple" or "Extrafascial" hysterectomy: Removal of uterus and cervix, parametria left intact.

Class II a.k.a. "Modified-Radical" Hysterectomy: Removes uterus, cervix, 1–2 cm vagina, and WLE of parametria.

Class III a.k.a. "Radical" Hysterectomy: Removal of uterus, cervix, one-fourth to one-third of vagina, parametria divided at pelvic sidewall or sacral origin.

Adjuvant hysterectomy: Not generally performed, no additional benefit seen in DFS and OS.[8] Caveat: Persistent metabolic activity following up-front RT or chemoRT, and otherwise non-metastatic, surgery is often performed as salvage in the hope of improving outcomes.

Chemotherapy

Definitive: Concurrent CHT with RT for locally advanced disease improves DFS and OS over RT alone (see the following). Weekly cisplatin 40 mg/m² has become standard of care. Common alternative is cisplatin/5-FU. Other concurrent regimens: weekly cisplatin + gemcitabine (increased pCR rate, PFS, and OS compared to cisplatin alone at the cost of very high acute toxicity)[9] and weekly cisplatin + bevacizumab (evaluated in RTOG 0417, proved to be tolerable with encouraging results, OS of 81%).[10]

Adjuvant: Concurrent CHT with postoperative RT improves OS in patients with positive margins, parametrial involvement, and positive lymph nodes (see the following). Adjuvant CHT following definitive chemoRT is active area of study (OUTBACK Trial—GOG 274/RTOG 1174/ANZGOG0902, which is phase III trial of definitive cisplatin with RT randomized to ± adjuvant carboplatin/paclitaxel × 4C) with initial results showing no OS benefit to additional adjuvant CHT.

Metastatic: Doublet CHT shows better outcomes than single-agent therapy.[11] GOG 240 showed significant improvement in PFS (2 months) and OS (3.7 months) with addition of bevacizumab to cisplatin/paclitaxel or topotecan/paclitaxel.[12]

Radiation

Definitive EBRT

Indications: EBRT is indicated in all cases stage ≥IA2 (and IA1 with LVSI) when treated non-operatively. Ensure coverage of uterus, cervix, parametria, uterosacral ligament, lymph nodes at risk determined by imaging and/or surgical nodal staging. Give sufficient vaginal margin (2–3 cm below inferior most extent of gross disease). For LN negative cases, cover external and internal iliac, obturator, and presacral LNs (superior border L4-5, some routinely cover common iliac LNs). For pelvic LN+, add common iliac coverage. For high-pelvic LN+, extended field RT to renal vessels or higher is indicated. Add inguinal coverage for distal one third vaginal extension.

Dose: 45 Gy/25 fx. Consider conformal boost to 50 to 54 Gy for parametrial involvement or grossly involved LNs. For bulky lymph nodes theoretically requiring ≥65 to 66 Gy to control, consider excision followed by microscopic dose RT. Central primary tumor is boosted to 80 Gy (small volume) or 85 to 90 Gy (large volume) with brachytherapy (see the following). Use of IMRT for intact cervix is evolving and conditionally recommended by ASTRO,[2] but is more standardly used in the setting of extended field RT and nodal boosts. If considering IMRT in the definitive setting, it is important to have a thorough imaging workup to understand full extent of disease, contouring must be complete and accurate, and one must account for daily pelvic organ motion due to bowel/bladder filling and use daily image guidance.[13]

Postoperative EBRT

Indications: Recommended following hysterectomy for those at higher risk for recurrence. Post-op RT alone recommended for any two of three Sedlis risk factors (simplified): LVSI, middle or deep one third stromal invasion and tumor size ≥4 cm. Rotman update showed RT improved outcomes in adenocarcinoma or adenosquamous histology as well (see the following). Add concurrent CHT for 3 Ps: positive LNs, positive surgical margins, and parametrial involvement (see Peters later). Consider vaginal brachytherapy boost for close or positive vaginal margin or deep one third stromal invasion.

Dose: 45 to 50.4 Gy/25 to 28 fx. IMRT reduces small bowel and iliac crest (bone marrow) dose, especially when treating extended field to cover PA LNs and/or when boosting grossly involved nodes.[14] IMRT is now recommended in the postoperative setting as it may decrease acute and late toxicities.[2,15] See RTOG 0418 and accompanying atlas for details.

Brachytherapy: Can be used as monotherapy for select early-stage cases (IA1), but more commonly following pelvic EBRT to boost gross residual primary to curative intent dose. Vaginal cuff brachytherapy considered postoperatively following EBRT as vaginal apex boost in cases of close or positive vaginal margin. EBRT + brachytherapy improves OS over EBRT alone even in setting of concurrent CHT.[16] Proper applicator placement and dosing are critical to achieving optimal outcomes.[17] Repeat clinical exam and imaging prior to first insertion allows selection of applicator. Generally, intracavitary therapy is employed, but interstitial technique may be necessary in certain circumstances (e.g., narrow anatomy not accommodating intracavity applicator, wide lateral extent of disease, distal vaginal involvement, inaccessible cervical os). Hybrid devices exist that combine intracavitary and interstitial components. Anesthesia is often needed for patient comfort and to achieve high-quality insertion. ABS 2012 guidelines recommend 3D imaging for volume delineation and planning.[18] MRI-based planning is preferred; better coverage of tumor, while potentially limiting dose to bladder, sigmoid, and rectum as compared to conventional planning.[19] GEC-ESTRO guidelines[20] define high-risk CTV (HR-CTV) and intermediate-risk CTV (IR-CTV) for 3D planning.

Dose: Intended dose should cover ≥90% of HR-CTV (D_{90}). ABS recommends EQD2 of ≥80 Gy (~5.5 Gy × 5 fx) for <4 cm of residual disease and EQD2 of 85 to 90 Gy (~6 Gy × 5 fx) for nonresponders or ≥4 cm residual disease.[21] IR-CTV should receive ≥60 Gy. It is still required to report dose to point A.

Toxicity: Acute: Fatigue, diarrhea, rectal urgency, bloating/cramping, bladder/urethral irritation, skin erythema, and possible desquamation if inguinal LNs or distal vagina/vulva covered in fields. Late: Rectal bleeding, bowel obstruction, hematuria, fistula (GI or urinary), vaginal ulceration/necrosis (5%–10% within 1 year, generally heals within 6 months with local care), vaginal stenosis (use dilators) and sexual dysfunction, infertility (~2 Gy), ovarian failure (5–10 Gy), osteopenia leading to hip and sacral insufficiency fractures.

Procedure: See *Handbook of Treatment Planning in Radiation Oncology*, Chapter 9.[22]

■ **EVIDENCE-BASED Q&A**

SURGICAL MANAGEMENT

▦ **What factors portend higher risk of pelvic LN involvement or unfavorable outcome?**

Delgado, GOG 49 (*Gynecol Oncol* 1989, PMID 2599466; *Gynecol Oncol* 1990, PMID 2227547): Prospective registry of stage I patients with ≥3 mm invasion treated with radical hysterectomy with pelvic and para-aortic nodal dissection. A total of 645 SCC patients with negative para-aortic LNs were included. Factors associated with positive lymph nodes included: DOI, parametrial invasion, tumor grade and gross vs. occult tumors. Three-year DFI for positive nodes was 74% and for negative nodes was 86%. Factors associated with worse 3-year DFI were DOI (deep 1/3 < middle 1/3 < superficial 1/3 invasion), tumor size (occult vs. <3 cm vs. ≥3 cm), parametrial invasion, and LVSI. Led to development of GOG 92 (see the following).

▦ **What are indications for adjuvant RT after hysterectomy?**

The Sedlis trial defined these risk factors. Although inclusion criteria are challenging to remember, "any two of three risk factors" is good way of simplifying it and will often be correct. Risk factors: LVSI, middle or deep one-third stromal invasion, and tumor size ≥4 cm.

Sedlis, GOG 92 (*Gynecol Oncol* 1999, PMID 10329031; Update Rotman *IJROBP* 2006, PMID 16427212): Phase III PRT of 277 patients with FIGO IB cervical cancer randomized to radical hysterectomy + pelvic LND ± adjuvant RT. Postoperatively, patients had negative nodes and (a) +LVSI and deep 1/3 stromal invasion; (b) +LVSI, middle 1/3 stromal invasion, and tumor ≥2 cm; (c) +LVSI, superficial one third, and tumor ≥5 cm; *OR* (d) no LVSI, deep or middle 1/3, and tumor ≥4 cm. Whole-pelvis RT given 4–6 weeks postoperatively to 46 to 50.4 Gy/23 to 28 fx. RT decreased LR (28% to 15%, $p = .019$) and improved RFS (79% to 88%, $p = .008$). At longer term follow-up, LR benefit persisted and post-op RT also decreased risk of recurrence for adenocarcinoma/adenosquamous histologies (44–9%).

▦ **What factors postoperatively are indications for adjuvant chemoRT rather than RT alone?**

The Peters criteria include any one of three factors ("three Ps"): positive margins, parametrial involvement, and positive nodes and serve as indications for adjuvant chemoRT.

Peters, GOG 109 (*JCO* 2000, PMID 10764420; Monk *Gynecol Oncol* 2005, PMID 15721417): Phase III PRT of 243 patients with FIGO IA2-IIA cervical cancer with positive margins, positive pelvic nodes, or microscopic parametrial involvement randomized to adjuvant RT 49.3 Gy/29 fx with or without concurrent cisplatin 70 mg/m² and 5-FU 1,000 mg/m²/day over 96 hours. Four cycles of CHT were given, first two concurrent with RT. 95% were FIGO IB. **Conclusions: CHT improved OS (71%–81%, $p = .007$) and PFS (63%–80%, $p = .003$). Subsequent retrospective analysis by Monk questioned CHT benefit for smaller (≤2 cm) tumors and for patients with only one LN+.**

▦ **Should FIGO IB-IIA patients be managed with surgery or RT?**

Stage IA patients can easily be managed with extrafascial hysterectomy and stage IIB-IVA are typically better candidates for chemoRT given extent of disease. However, management of stage IB-IIA tumors is challenging and patient specific. Main advantages of surgery over RT are preserved sexual and ovarian function and elimination of secondary malignancy risk.

Landoni, Italian Trial (*Lancet* 1997, PMID 9284774): Phase III PRT of 343 patients with FIGO stage IB or IIA cervical cancer randomized to radical hysterectomy or definitive RT. 69% of IBs were ≤4 cm. EBRT was 40 to 53 Gy followed by Cs-137 LDR implant to 70-90 Gy to point A. When lymphangiography showed common iliac or PA LNs+, 45 Gy was given to these beds; involved LNs boosted another 5 to 10 Gy. In surgical arm, adjuvant RT recommended for >pT2a disease, <3 mm of "safe" cervical stroma, tumor cut-through, or positive nodes. Adjuvant RT was 50.4 Gy to WP (± 45 Gy to PA LNs based on pathologic involvement). MFU 87 months. Identical 5-year OS and DFS in both groups, 83% and 74%, respectively. Recurrence rates 25% in surgery group and 26% in RT group. Severe toxicity seen in 28% of surgery group and 12% of RT group ($p = .0004$). Adenocarcinoma had inferior outcomes with RT as compared to surgery (DFS 66% vs. 47%, $p = .05$; OS 70% vs. 59%, $p = .02$). **Conclusion: Both surgery and RT are options for stage IB-IIA cervical cancer. Although RT may be better tolerated, surgery may improve outcomes for adenocarcinoma. Toxicity with combined treatment is worse than RT alone.** *Note: In the surgical arm, adjuvant RT was required in 64% (84% for those with tumors >4 cm).*

■ **Does adjuvant hysterectomy following RT improve overall survival?**

Keys, GOG 71 (*Gynecol Oncol* 2003, PMID 12798694): Phase III PRT of 256 patients with FIGO IB "suboptimal or bulky" (current IB2) cervical cancer randomized to RT ± adjuvant simple extrafascial hysterectomy. Whole-pelvis RT was 40 Gy for RT arm and 45 Gy for hysterectomy arm; both were followed by intracavitary boost to 40 Gy (RT only arm) or 30 Gy (hysterectomy arm) to point A. Extrafascial hysterectomy was performed 2–6 weeks later. No difference in OS (58% vs. 56%) or PFS (62% vs. 53%, $p = .09$); 10% grades 3 to 4 toxicity in both arms. Interaction was demonstrated with tumor sizes of 4, 5, and 6 cm possibly benefitting from surgery. **Conclusion: Adjuvant hysterectomy did not improve survival.**

DEFINITIVE MANAGEMENT

■ **Is there benefit to concurrent CHT in addition to RT compared to RT (EFRT) alone?**

Yes. Based on mounting evidence, NCI issued clinical alert in 1999 recommending concurrent cisplatin be administered with RT for invasive cervical cancer. In addition to the following classic trials, there have been several randomized trials and meta-analyses demonstrating DFS and OS benefit for concurrent chemoRT over RT alone in invasive cervical cancer.[23,24]

Morris, RTOG 9001 (*NEJM* 1999, PMID 10202164; Update Eifel *JCO* 2004, PMID 14990643): Phase III PRT of 389 cervical cancer patients, stage IIB-IV or stage IB/IIA with tumor size ≥5 cm or biopsy-proven pelvic nodal metastasis randomized to EFRT or whole-pelvis RT with concurrent cisplatin 75 mg/m^2 and 5-FU 4,000 mg/m^2 over 96 hours for three cycles given every 3 weeks. Patients in CHT arm treated from L4/5 interspace down to midpubis or 4 cm below distal edge of tumor. Patients in EFRT arm received RT to L1/2 interspace. Both arms received 45 Gy/25 fx. Updated results with MFU of 6.6 years showed 8-year OS improved from 41% to 67% with CHT. Late toxicity was similar; 5-year LR and DM were also improved. **Conclusions: Concurrent cisplatin/5-FU improved OS without significant increase in late effects.**

Keys, GOG 123 (*NEJM* 1999, PMID 10202166): Phase III PRT of 369 women with bulky IB cervical cancer (current IB3) w/o radiographic lymphadenopathy treated with RT (45 Gy + LDR boost) ±– concurrent CHT (weekly cisplatin 40 mg/m^2 for up to 6 cycles) followed by extrafascial hysterectomy. PFS and OS were improved in CHT group (PFS HR 0.51, OS HR 0.54, both $p < .01$). **Conclusion: Concurrent cisplatin improves OS.**

Shrivastava, Tata Memorial (*JAMA Onc* 2018, PMID 29423520): Phase III PRT of 850 women with FIGO IIIB cervical cancer randomized to RT ± weekly cisplatin. Primary endpoint of 5-year DFS was significantly improved with RT + cisplatin vs. RT alone (52.3% vs. 43.8%, respectively, HR 0.81, $p = .03$), as well as 5-year OS (54% vs. 46%, HR 0.82, $p = .04$). **Conclusion: For women with stage IIIB cervical cancer, the addition of cisplatin to RT improves DFS and OS.**

■ **To whom should concurrent CHT be added?**

NCCN recommends addition of concurrent platinum-based CHT for "bulky" tumors (stage IB3, IIA2, and higher). For stage IB1–2 and IIA1, CHT is optional. For IA1 with LVSI or IA2 tumors, surgery is good option, but if treated nonoperatively, CHT can be omitted.[1]

■ **What is standard concurrent CHT regimen?**

Multiple single- and multi-agent regimens have been studied but currently single-agent cisplatin, given weekly, is most common. Cisplatin/5-FU is common alternative.

Rose, GOG 120 (*NEJM* 1999, PMID 10202165; Update *JCO* 2007, PMID 17502627): Three-arm PRT of 526 women with stage IIB-IVA cervical carcinoma without para-aortic involvement randomized to either concurrent cisplatin (40 mg/m² weekly for 6 weeks), concurrent hydroxyurea or combination cisplatin, 5-FU, and hydroxyurea. EBRT delivered to dose of 40.8 Gy/24 fx (or 51 Gy/30 fx for stages IIB, IIIB-IVA) followed by brachytherapy boost. Superior border of pelvic field was L4/5 interspace. MFU 35 months. Hydroxyurea alone arm demonstrated worse PFS and OS, but cisplatin and multi-agent arms were similar. Acute toxicity was worse in three-drug arm. **Conclusion: Cisplatin-based chemoRT improves PFS and OS. No increased late toxicity seen at long-term follow-up.**

■ **What is impact of overall treatment time (OTT) on outcomes of patients treated definitively?**

OTT for EBRT + brachytherapy should be ≤56 days.[25] Other OTT limits have been identified: ≤49 days;[26] ≤63 days.[27] Brachytherapy should begin no more than 7 days post-EBRT if downsizing of bulky disease is required. Alternatively, for favorable anatomy or small primary tumor, practitioners can interdigitate brachytherapy during last couple weeks of EBRT. It is generally recommended to avoid CHT and EBRT administration on brachytherapy days.

■ **Is there benefit to IMRT in postoperative setting?**

Early reports of phase III data confirm benefit, safety, and efficacy of IMRT for gynecologic malignancies after hysterectomy[28,29] and is recommended by ASTRO guidelines.[2] See Chapter 48 for details.

■ **What are the differences between high-dose rate (HDR) and low-dose rate (LDR) brachytherapy?**

LDR is generally administered over 1 to 2 fx, each over 1 to 3 days during which patient stays on strict bed rest with applicator and sources held in place. Despite best efforts, it is difficult to keep patients comfortable and immobilized for prolonged period of time. Change in applicator position can lead to changes in dose distribution. RT exposure to health care personnel is also major issue. Main theoretical advantage to LDR over HDR is much lower dose rate, which allows for enhanced sublethal damage repair. Concerns over years about HDR leading to increased toxicity have not consistently been borne out in studies.[30] HDR, used by 85% of surveyed U.S. institutions,[31] requires more frequent insertions, but treatment time is short (~10 min). Remote afterloading by and large eliminates exposure risk to health care personnel. Several different dwell positions and times allow for shaping of dose to treat target and avoid OARs. PDR used in some institutions combines advantages of LDR and HDR. LDR: Dose rate 0.6 to 0.8 Gy/hr, generally with Cs-137 source, T½ = 30 years, β-decay, energy 662 keV. HDR: Dose rate >12 Gy/hr with Ir-192 source, T½ = 74 days, γ-decay with ~380 keV.

■ **What is the difference between brachytherapy dose prescriptions to HR-CTV vs. point A?**

Before CT/MRI were readily available, applicator placement was confirmed via AP and lateral films. Dose prescription was to 2D point A (2 cm superior and 2 cm lateral to os, in plane of tandem), roughly corresponding to medial aspect of broad ligament (where uterine artery and ureter cross). Dose was estimated to point B (5 cm lateral to midline at level of point A), which represented pelvic sidewall/obturator LNs. Based on ICRU 38 report, maximum doses to bladder and rectum were recorded at following points: Bladder: posterior surface of Foley balloon on lateral film; Rectum: 0.5 cm posterior to vaginal wall at intersection of tandem and ovoids/ring. CT/MRI studies have shown that adequate dose to point A does not always indicate good coverage of HR-CTV[32] and ICRU bladder and rectal points do not always accurately estimate max doses to these OARs.[33,34] In volumetric planning era, targets (HR-CTV, IR-CTV) and OARs (bladder, rectum, sigmoid, small bowel) can be accurately contoured in 3D and dose to these structures evaluated spatially and quantitatively using DVHs.

Dose distribution during planning can be modified to adequately cover target while avoiding OARs. This is now the preferred method of planning/reporting.

REFERENCES

1. National Comprehensive Cancer Network. Cervical cancer (Version I.2021). https://www.nccn.org
2. Chino J, Annunziata C, Beriwal S, et al. Radiation therapy for cervical cancer: an ASTRO clinical practice guideline. *Pract Radiat Oncol.* 2020;10(4):220–234. doi:10.1016/j.prro.2020.04.002
3. National Cancer Institute: Surveillance, Epidemiology and End Results Program. Cancer Stat Facts: Cervix Uteri Cancer. https://seer.cancer.gov/statfacts/html/cervix.html. 2020.
4. Cancer NCI-C. Causes and Prevention–HPV and Cancer. https://www.cancer.gov/about-cancer/causes-prevention/risk/infectious-agents/hpv-fact-sheet
5. The American College of Obstetricians and Gynecologists. Cervical Cancer Screening. http://www.acog.org/Patients/FAQs/Cervical-Cancer-Screening. 2017.
6. Tsai CS, Lai CH, Chang TC, et al. Prospective randomized trial to study impact of pretreatment FDG-PET for cervical cancer patients with MRI-detected positive pelvic but negative para-aortic lymphadenopathy. *Int J Radiat Oncol Biol Phys.* 2010;76(2):477–484. doi:10.1016/j.ijrobp.2009.02.020
7. Schwarz JK, Siegel BA, Dehdashti F, Grigsby PW. Metabolic response on post-therapy FDG-PET predicts patterns of failure after RTy for cervical cancer. *Int J Radiat Oncol Biol Phys.* 2012;83(1):185–190. doi:10.1016/j.ijrobp.2011.05.053
8. Keys HM, Bundy BN, Stehman FB, et al. Radiation therapy with and without extrafascial hysterectomy for bulky stage IB cervical carcinoma: randomized trial of Gynecologic Oncology Group. *Gynecol Oncol.* 2003;89(3):343–353. doi:10.1016/S0090-8258(03)00173-2
9. Duenas-Gonzalez A, Cetina-Perez L, Lopez-Graniel C, et al. Pathologic response and toxicity assessment of chemoRTy with cisplatin versus cisplatin plus gemcitabine in cervical cancer: randomized phase II study. *Int J Radiat Oncol Biol Phys.* 2005;61(3):817–823. doi:10.1016/j.ijrobp.2004.07.676
10. Schefter T, Winter K, Kwon JS, et al. RTOG 0417: efficacy of bevacizumab in combination with definitive radiation therapy and cisplatin CHT in untreated patients with locally advanced cervical carcinoma. *Int J Radiat Oncol Biol Phys.* 2014;88(1):101–105. doi:10.1016/j.ijrobp.2013.10.022
11. Long HJ 3rd, Bundy BN, Grendys EC Jr, et al. Randomized phase III trial of cisplatin with or without topotecan in carcinoma of uterine cervix: gynecologic oncology group study. *J Clin Oncol.* 2005;23(21):4626–4633. doi:10.1200/JCO.2005.10.021
12. Tewari KS, Sill MW, Long HJ 3rd, et al. Improved survival with bevacizumab in advanced cervical cancer. *N Engl J Med.* 2014;370(8):734–743. doi:10.1056/NEJMoa1309748
13. Lim K, Small W, Jr., Portelance L, et al. Consensus guidelines for delineation of clinical target volume for intensity-modulated pelvic RTy for definitive treatment of cervix cancer. *Int J Radiat Oncol Biol Phys.* 2011;79(2):348–355. doi:10.1016/j.ijrobp.2009.10.075
14. Vargo JA, Kim H, Choi S, et al. Extended field intensity modulated radiation therapy with concomitant boost for lymph node-positive cervical cancer: analysis of regional control and recurrence patterns in positron emission tomography/computed tomography era. *Int J Radiat Oncol Biol Phys.* 2014;90(5):1091–1098. doi:10.1016/j.ijrobp.2014.08.013
15. Klopp AH, Moughan J, Portelance L, et al. Hematologic toxicity in RTOG 0418: phase 2 study of postoperative IMRT for gynecologic cancer. *Int J Radiat Oncol Biol Phys.* 2013;86(1):83–90. doi:10.1016/j.ijrobp.2013.01.017
16. Gill BS, Lin JF, Krivak TC, et al. National cancer data base analysis of radiation therapy consolidation modality for cervical cancer: impact of new technological advancements. *Int J Radiat Oncol Biol Phys.* 2014;90(5):1083–1090. doi:10.1016/j.ijrobp.2014.07.017
17. Viswanathan AN, Moughan J, Small W Jr, et al. Quality of cervical cancer brachytherapy implantation and impact on local recurrence and disease-free survival in radiation therapy oncology group prospective trials 0116 and 0128. *Int J Gynecol Cancer.* 2012;22(1):123–131. doi:10.1097/IGC.0b013e31823ae3c9
18. Viswanathan AN, Thomadsen B, American Brachytherapy Society Cervical Cancer Recommendations Committee; American Brachytherapy Society. American brachytherapy society consensus guidelines for locally advanced carcinoma of cervix. Part I: general principles. *Brachytherapy.* 2012;11(1):33–46. doi:10.1016/j.brachy.2011.07.003
19. Zwahlen D, Jezioranski J, Chan P, et al. Magnetic resonance imaging-guided intracavitary brachytherapy for cancer of cervix. *Int J Radiat Oncol Biol Phys.* 2009;74(4):1157–1164. doi:10.1016/j.ijrobp.2008.09.010
20. Potter R, Haie-Meder C, Van Limbergen E, et al. Recommendations from gynaecological (GYN) GEC ESTRO working group (II): concepts and terms in 3D image-based treatment planning in cervix cancer brachytherapy-3D dose volume parameters and aspects of 3D image-based anatomy, radiation physics, radiobiology. *Radiother Oncol.* 2006;78(1):67–77. doi:10.1016/j.radonc.2005.11.014
21. Viswanathan AN, Beriwal S, De Los Santos JF, et al. American brachytherapy society consensus guidelines for locally advanced carcinoma of cervix. Part II: high-dose–rate brachytherapy. *Brachytherapy.* 2012;11(1):47–52. doi:10.1016/j.brachy.2011.07.002

22. Videtic GMM, Woody N, Vassil AD. *Handbook of Treatment Planning in Radiation Oncology.* 3rd ed. Demos Medical; 2020. doi:10.1891/9780826168429

23. Green JA, Kirwan JM, Tierney JF, et al. Survival and recurrence after concomitant CHT and RTy for cancer of uterine cervix: systematic review and meta-analysis. *Lancet.* 2001;358(9284):781–786. doi:10.1016/S0140-6736(01)05965-7

24. Chemoradiotherapy for Cervical Cancer Meta-Analysis Collaboration. Reducing uncertainties about effects of chemoRTy for cervical cancer: systematic review and meta-analysis of individual patient data from 18 randomized trials. *J Clin Oncol.* 2008;26(35):5802–5812. doi:10.1200/JCO.2008.16.4368

25. Song S, Rudra S, Hasselle MD, et al. Effect of treatment time in locally advanced cervical cancer in era of concurrent chemoRTy. *Cancer.* 2013;119(2):325–331. doi:10.1002/cncr.27652

26. Perez CA, Grigsby PW, Castro-Vita H, Lockett MA. Carcinoma of uterine cervix: I. impact of prolongation of overall treatment time and timing of brachytherapy on outcome of radiation therapy. *Int J Radiat Oncol Biol Phys.* 1995;32(5):1275–1288. doi:10.1016/0360-3016(95)00220-S

27. Chen SW, Liang JA, Yang SN, et al. adverse effect of treatment prolongation in cervical cancer by high-dose-rate intracavitary brachytherapy. *Radiother Oncol.* 2003;67(1):69–76. doi:10.1016/S0167-8140(02)00439-5

28. 28. Klopp AH, Yeung AR, Deshmukh S, et al. Patient-reported toxicity during pelvic intensity-modulated radiation therapy: NRG oncology-RTOG 1203. *J Clin Oncol.* 2018;36(24): 2538 –2544. doi:10.1200/JCO.2017.77.4273

29. Shih KK, Hajj X, Kollmeier M, et al. Impact of post-operative intensity-modulated radiation therapy (IMRT) on the rate of bowel obstruction in gynecologic malignancy. *Gynecol Oncol.* 2016;143:18 –21. doi:10.1016/j.ygyno.2016.07.116

30. Liu R, Wang X, Tian JH, et al. High dose rate versus low dose rate intracavity brachytherapy for locally advanced uterine cervix cancer. *Cochrane Database Syst Rev.* 2014(10):CD007563. doi:10.1002/14651858.CD007563.pub3

31. Viswanathan AN, Erickson BA. Three-dimensional imaging in gynecologic brachytherapy: survey of American brachytherapy society. *Int J Radiat Oncol Biol Phys.* 2010;76(1):104–109. doi:10.1016/j.ijrobp.2009.01.043

32. Potter R, Kirisits C, Fidarova EF, et al. Present status and future of high-precision image-guided adaptive brachytherapy for cervix carcinoma. *Acta Oncologica.* 2008;47(7):1325–1336. doi:10.1080/02841860802282794

33. Pelloski CE, Palmer M, Chronowski GM, et al. Comparison between CT-based volumetric calculations and ICRU reference-point estimates of radiation doses delivered to bladder and rectum during intracavitary RTy for cervical cancer. *Int J Radiat Oncol Biol Phys.* 2005;62(1):131–137. doi:10.1016/j.ijrobp.2004.09.059

34. Hashim N, Jamalludin Z, Ung NM, et al. CT based 3-dimensional treatment planning of intracavitary brachytherapy for cancer of cervix: comparison between dose-volume histograms and ICRU point doses to rectum and bladder. *Asian Pac J Cancer Prev.* 2014;15(13):5259–5264. doi:10.7314/APJCP.2014.15.13.5259

48 ■ UTERINE CANCER: ENDOMETRIAL CANCER AND UTERINE SARCOMA

Shireen Parsai, Sarah M. C. Sittenfeld, Michael Weller, and Sudha R. Amarnath

QUICK HIT ■ Endometrial cancer is the most common gynecologic malignancy in the United States. Medically operable patients should undergo TAH/BSO (or radical hysterectomy if cervical stromal involvement) with peritoneal cytology. Need for pelvic and PA lymphadenectomy for staging is controversial and could be considered for risk factors such as large, deeply invasive, or high-grade tumors. Postoperative management is dictated by pathologic features. Early-stage patients are grouped into low-, intermediate-, or high-risk groups, which were defined by GOG 33, GOG 99, and PORTEC studies. Management paradigm for locally advanced endometrial cancer is evolving but generally consists of surgery followed by CHT or combination chemoRT.

Table 48.1: General Treatment Paradigm for Endometrial Cancer (See ASCO/ASTRO Guidelines for Details)[1,2]

Stage	Adjuvant Treatment Options (After TAH/BSO)
Stage IA, grades I–II	Observation*
Stage IA, grade III or stage IB, grade I–II	Favor vaginal cuff brachytherapy†
Stage IB, grade III	Favor pelvic RT
Stage II	Pelvic RT + VBT boost ± CHT
Stages III–IV	ChemoRT vs. CHT ± tumor-directed RT
Medically inoperable	Tumor-directed EBRT to uterus, cervix, upper vagina, pelvic LN, other involved areas (45–50.4 Gy) + intracavitary boost ± CHT

*Can consider vaginal cuff brachytherapy if higher risk features (age >60, LVSI).
†Can consider pelvic RT if other high-risk factors are present (age >60, LVSI) and surgical staging was inadequate.

EPIDEMIOLOGY: Malignancy of the uterine corpus is the most common gynecologic malignancy in the United States with >65,000 new cases and >12,000 deaths projected in 2020 (second most common cause of gynecologic cancer deaths after ovarian cancer).[3] Uterine cancer accounts for 3.6% of all new cancer cases in the United States.[4] Median age at diagnosis is 63 years of age with ~6% of cases occurring in patients <45 years of age.[4]

RISK FACTORS: Main risk factor is excess endogenous/exogenous estrogen without opposing progestin: (a) *physiologic*: obesity, nulliparity, early menarche, and late menopause;[5-7] (b) *pathologic*: diabetes mellitus, polycystic ovarian syndrome;[5,7] (c) *exposure*: unopposed estrogen therapy, tamoxifen;[8] (d) *protective*: combined OCPs, progestin, exercise;[5,9] (e) *family history/genetics*: Lynch II, subset of HNPCC has been associated with increased risk of endometrial cancer. HNPCC is autosomal dominant mutation in DNA *MMR* genes and increases lifetime risk of endometrial cancer to 27% to 71% as compared to 3% lifetime risk in general population.[10,11] In patients diagnosed with endometrial cancer <50 years of age, consider screening for HNPCC.[12] Prophylactic TAH/BSO can be considered for HNPCC carriers.[13]

ANATOMY: Uterine corpus is defined as the upper two thirds of uterus above internal cervical os (composed of fundus and body). Cervix and lower uterine segment comprise the lower one third of uterus. Oviducts (aka fallopian tubes) and round ligaments enter uterus at upper outer corners (cornu). Fundus and body of uterus are separated by line connecting tubouterine orifices. Uterine wall is composed of endometrium, myometrium, and serosa from innermost to outermost layers. Cancer arising from the epithelial lining of the uterine cavity is referred to as endometrial cancer. The first site of local extension for endometrial cancer is into the myometrium. Cancers arising from the stromal and muscle tissues of the myometrium are referred to as uterine sarcomas.[14] There are three major ligaments that support the uterus: the broad ligament, uterosacral ligament, and transverse (a.k.a. Mackenrodt's or cardinal) ligament.

Lymphatics: Regional lymphatics include bilateral parametrial, obturator, internal iliac (aka hypogastric), external iliac, common iliac, PA, presacral, and sacral.[15] Fundal lesions can drain directly to PA lymph nodes, but are uncommon, whereas cervical lesions drain laterally to parametrium, obturator, and pelvic nodes.[14]

PATHOLOGY: Two distinct pathologic types have been described:

- **Type I** (~80%): Favorable course, presents at early stage. Grades 1 to 2. Endometrioid histology. Estrogen responsive (and therefore main risk factors are related to excess of estrogen without opposing progestin as described previously). Diploid. Type I malignancies are thought to have multistep process leading to carcinogenesis: simple endometrial hyperplasia progresses to complex atypical hyperplasia, which becomes precursor lesion, and subsequently develops into endometrial intraepithelial neoplasia, which ultimately becomes endometrial carcinoma.[16]
- **Type II** (10%–20%): Aggressive course. Grade 3. Nonendometrioid histologies including serous, clear cell. Independent of estrogen or endometrial hyperplasia and develops from atrophic endometrium. Aneuploid. *TP53* is mutated early (81% of cases) and may account for different rates of progression in these two subtypes.[5,14,17]

In addition to appropriate staging, grade of tumor must also be reported. Grading system reports degree of glandular differentiation (which is described as percentage of nonsquamous or nonmorular solid growth pattern) and corresponds to aggressiveness of tumor. **Grades 1, 2, and 3 tumors have ≤5%, 6% to 50%, and >50% nonsquamous or nonmorular solid growth patterns, respectively.** In addition, papillary serous and clear cell histologies are considered grade 3. Note: nuclear atypia out of proportion to architectural grade raises grade by 1 for grade 1 and 2 tumors.[14] "MELF" pattern (microcystic, elongated, and fragmented) has been described as correlating with more advanced pathologic features and may necessitate nodal staging, although its impact on survival outcomes is unclear.[18,19]

GENETICS: Many genetic mutations have been identified, most commonly in PIK3CA pathway and more specifically *PTEN* mutations, which are thought to be early events in carcinogenesis. *TP53* mutations are only seen in grade 3 endometrioid carcinomas (may represent late step in carcinogenesis though pathway not completely elucidated as of yet); 30% to 40% of cases have loss of DNA mismatch repair mechanisms resulting from loss of MLH1 promoter hypermethylation both among sporadic cases and hereditary Lynch syndrome (HNPCC).[5,14,20,21]

SCREENING: Cancer Genetics Consortium recommends screening for patients with HNPCC with annual endometrial sampling and TVUS beginning at 30 to 35 years of age.[22]

CLINICAL PRESENTATION: The most common presenting symptom is postmenopausal vaginal bleeding (~90%). Other symptoms including abdominal/pelvic pain, abdominal distension, urinary/rectal bleeding, and constipation may be symptoms of advanced disease.[5,12,15]

WORKUP

H&P: Careful inspection of external genitalia, vagina, and cervix, rectal exam, and bimanual pelvic exam. Attention for enlargement of uterus, or tumor extension to cervix, vagina, or parametrium.

Labs: CBC; optional: LFTs and CA-125 for high-risk subtypes.[12]

Imaging: Goal is to guide surgical approach based on risk of recurrence as estimated per myometrial/cervical invasion and LN metastases. Endometrial stripe should be assessed with TVUS. If endometrial stripe is abnormally thickened, it should be further evaluated with a biopsy. Chest imaging with CXR. MRI is preferred imaging modality for assessing preoperative local extent of disease. However, it is *not* particularly helpful in detecting LN or peritoneal involvement and is performed only for suspicion of locally advanced disease or in medically inoperable setting. PET/CT remains best imaging modality for detecting LN metastases but is not routinely performed. May consider CT chest/abdomen/pelvis for high-grade tumors.[5,12]

Procedures: Gold standard is biopsy under hysteroscopy. Endometrial biopsy for histologic information as preoperative evaluation. If endometrial biopsy nondiagnostic and concern for malignancy persists, fractional D&C should be performed.[5,12]

PROGNOSTIC FACTORS: Poor prognostic factors include age, grade, tumor size, LVSI, depth of invasion, clear cell/papillary serous histology, lymph node involvement, and tumor involvement of lower uterine segment.[23,24] Since the mid-1970s, survival has improved for all of the most common cancers except uterine corpus and cervix cancers, likely due to the lack of major treatment advances at the time of disease recurrence or development of metastatic disease.[3]

NATURAL HISTORY: May arise from background of hyperplasia. Simple hyperplasia is associated with ~1% risk of malignancy, complex hyperplasia ~3%, simple atypia ~10%, and complex atypia ~30% to 40%. In general, complexity refers to glandular structure whereas atypia refers to cellular morphology. At diagnosis, disease is localized/organ confined in 67%, spread to regional LN and organs in 21%, and metastatic in 8%.[5] Most common metastatic sites are vagina, ovaries, and lung.[14] Clear cell tumors have been associated with metastases to abdominal or pelvic peritoneal surfaces or omentum.[3] The most common site of locoregional recurrence is the vagina.[25]

STAGING: AJCC staging system is both clinical and pathologic whereas FIGO staging system uses surgical and pathologic data (Table 48.2). The clinical staging system is assigned before CHT or RT if those are initial modalities of therapy.[3]

Table 48.2: AJCC 8th Edition (2017): Staging for Corpus Uteri Carcinoma and Carcinosarcoma		
AJCC		**FIGO**
T1	**T1a** Tumor limited to endometrium or invades <50% of myometrium	**IA**
	T1b Tumor invades ≥50% of myometrial invasion	**IB**
T2	• Invades cervical stroma, but does not extend beyond uterus	**II**
T3	**T3a** Invades serosa and/or adnexa via direct extension or metastasis*	**IIIA**
	T3b Invades vagina via direct extension or metastasis or parametrial involvement*	**IIIB**
N0 (I+)	• Isolated tumor cells ≤0.2 mm	
N1mi	• Positive pelvic LNs (0.2–2.0 mm)	**IIIC1**
N1a	• Positive pelvic LNs (>2.0 mm)	
N2mi	• Positive PA LNs (with or without pelvic LNs) (0.2–2.0 mm)	**IIIC2**
N2a	• Positive PA LNs (with or without pelvic LNs) (>2.0 mm)	
T4	• Invasion of bladder and/or bowel mucosa (bullous edema not sufficient)	**IVA**
M1	• Distant metastasis	**IVB**

*Positive cytology should be reported, but it does not change stage.

TREATMENT PARADIGM

Surgery: TAH/BSO (a.k.a. simple or type I hysterectomy) is standard of care for early disease. Laparoscopic approaches are becoming increasingly utilized. Radical hysterectomy is done for cases of gross cervical invasion. Surgical staging requires evaluation of peritoneal surfaces. Omental and peritoneal biopsies are performed for high-risk disease.[5] Pelvic and PA lymphadenectomy is controversial (see the following ASTEC trial) and if performed, most appropriate technique remains unknown ranging from sentinel lymph node mapping to complete pelvic and PA lymphadenectomy. To avoid overtreatment, surgeon should consider patients at low risk for LN metastases including (a) <50% myometrial invasion; (b) tumor size <2 cm; (c) well-differentiated or moderately differentiated histology.[26,27] Per FIGO, any suspicious LNs should be removed and complete pelvic lymphadenectomy with resection of enlarged PA nodes should be performed for high-risk patients.[14]

Complications: Lymphedema (8%–50% risk depending on number of LNs removed, adjuvant CHT/RT, preoperative NSAID use).[28]

Chemotherapy: Adjuvant CHT is standard in patients with stage III/IV disease, but generally not indicated in patients with low- or intermediate-risk disease. High-risk patients should be encouraged to participate in ongoing clinical trials. Carboplatin/paclitaxel is most common adjuvant regimen. Cisplatin is most common therapy given concurrently with RT (see the following trials).

Radiation

Indications: RT is used as adjuvant therapy after TAH/BSO or as primary therapy for patients who are not surgical candidates. Indications for VCB include HIR disease, generally defined as grade 1 to 2 tumors with ≥50% myometrial invasion or grade 3 tumors with <50% invasion (see the following trials and ABS guidelines)[1,29] or as boost following pelvic EBRT (not generally warranted except when risk factors such as cervical stromal invasion or positive margin). Pelvic EBRT is given to early-stage patients at high risk (grade 3 tumors with ≥50% invasion).

Dose: To treat the whole pelvis adjuvantly, 45 to 50 Gy is given via EBRT with IMRT.[12] For VCB, PORTEC 2 (see the following) used 21 Gy/3 fx prescribed to 0.5 cm depth given weekly, but other regimens are also common (see ABS guidelines). For a vaginal brachytherapy boost following EBRT, 18 Gy/3 fx prescribed to the vaginal mucosa is acceptable among other regimens. For medically inoperable patients, see ABS consensus statement for guidelines.[30]

Toxicity: Acute: Fatigue, diarrhea, nausea, myelosuppression, dysuria, urinary frequency. Late: Vaginal stenosis, vaginal dryness, rarely RT cystitis, proctitis, sacral insufficiency fractures, bowel obstruction, fistula.

Procedure: See *Handbook of Treatment Planning in Radiation Oncology,* Chapter 9.[31]

■ **EVIDENCE-BASED Q&A**

EARLY-STAGE ENDOMETRIAL CANCER

■ **How are women with endometrial cancer categorized?**

Endometrial cancers are historically classified into low-, intermediate-, and high-risk groups. Aalders trial (see the following) was one of the first to demonstrate differences by risk group. GOG 33 (see the following) was a surgical study that demonstrated noninvasive (old stage IA) tumors were "low" risk, invasive cancers (old stage IB, IC, and occult stage IIA–B) were "intermediate" risk, and any stage III or IV or invasive clear cell/papillary were "high" risk. GOG 33 further subdivided "intermediate" risk into low- and high-intermediate risk (see GOG 99). The HIR group benefited from adjuvant therapy as demonstrated in GOG 99 and PORTEC 1/2.

■ **What pathologic findings correlate with risk of nodal involvement?**

Early studies from GOG suggest that depth of invasion and grade highly correlate with nodal involvement.

Creasman, GOG 33 Staging (*Cancer* 1987, PMID 3652025): Prospective observational study of 681 women treated with TAH/BSO, pelvic, and PA dissection with peritoneal cytology from 1977 to 1983. On MVA, grade, depth of invasion, and intraperitoneal disease were predictive of LN metastasis. See Table 48.3.

Table 48.3: Results of GOG 33 for Endometrial Cancer						
Depth of Invasion	**% PA and Pelvic LN Involvement**					
	Grade 1		**Grade 2**		**Grade 3**	
	PA	Pelvic	PA	Pelvic	PA	Pelvic
Endometrium Only	0%	0%	3%	3%	0%	0%
Superficial Myometrial Invasion	1%	3%	4%	5%	4%	9%
Middle Myometrial Invasion	5%	0%	0%	9%	0%	4%
Deep Myometrial Invasion	6%	11%	14%	19%	23%	34%

Note: Risk of PA LN involvement is two-thirds the risk of pelvic LN involvement; 30% to 55% of +pelvic LNs have +PA LNs.

Morrow, GOG 33 (*Gynecol Oncol* 1991, PMID 1989916): Same study as the preceding but correlated surgical pathology findings and recurrence patterns prospectively; 895 patients with FIGO stage I and II (occult), endometrioid type. (a) Isolated positive PA LNs in setting of negative pelvic LNs is uncommon (2.2%). (b) Only 5.4% ($n = 48$) had positive PA LNs. Of these, 47 had >1 of grossly positive pelvic LNs, grossly positive adnexal mets, or deep myometrial penetration (accounted for 98% of cases with positive PA LNs and could be used to select patients for nodal staging). (c) **Conclusion: Among patients without metastases, LVSI, depth of invasion, and grade correlate with recurrence-free interval.** (d) LRF rate (32.4% vs. 48.4%) appears to favor adjuvant RT for patients with >one-third myometrial invasion and Gr 2–3 tumor.

Katsoulakis, SEER (*Int J Gynaecol Obstet* 2014, PMID 25194213): SEER analysis from 1998 to 2003 ("contemporary era") including 4,052 patients. Pelvic nodal metastases identified as per Table 48.4.

Table 48.4: SEER Patterns of Nodal Spread						
	Grade 1		Grade 2		Grade 3	
	Pelvic	Para-Aortic	Pelvic	Para-Aortic	Pelvic	Para-Aortic
IA	1%	0%	2%	0%	1%	1%
IB	2%	0%	3%	1%	3%	2%
IC	3%	3%	8%	5%	12%	8%
IIA	7%	3%	10%	4%	10%	5%
IIB	8%	4%	13%	8%	19%	12%

■ **Is pelvic nodal dissection necessary in early-stage disease?**

Without suspicious intraoperative lymph nodes, elective pelvic and PA nodal dissection likely does not change oncologic outcomes but may help guide treatment in few who are upgraded pathologically. Two trials did not show differences in DFS or OS.

Kitchener, ASTEC Trial (*Lancet* 2009, PMID 19070889). PRT of 1,408 women who underwent TAH/BSO, then randomized to ± lymphadenectomy; 80% stage I/IIA; 40% had EBRT in both arms. MFU 37 months. OS similar in both arms (HR: 1.04, $p = .83$). RFS was slightly better in "no lymphadenectomy" arm (HR: 1.25, $p = .14$). **Conclusion: No significant OS or RFS benefit for lymphadenectomy in early-stage endometrial cancer.**

Bendetti, Italian Trial (*JNCI* 2008, PMID 19033573): PRT of 514 women with clinical stage I randomized to TAH/BSO ± lymphadenectomy. Excluded if grade I <50% invasion; ~80% stage I/IIA. MFU 49 months; 13% vs. 3% of patients were found to have nodal involvement ($p < .001$). No improvement with LND in 5-year DFS (82% vs. 81%) or 5-year OS (90% vs. 86%). **Conclusion: LND improves staging but did not change DFS or OS.**

■ **Which patients benefit from adjuvant RT after TAH/BSO?**

Early-stage patients with adverse path features are at risk for extrauterine disease and recurrence. High-risk features vary but overall include deep myometrial invasion, tumor grade, cervical involvement, older age, LVSI, and tumor size (from GOG 33).

Keys, GOG 99 (*Gynecol Oncol* 2004, PMID 14984936): PRT of 392 patients with "intermediate-risk" endometrial cancer evaluating TAH/BSO with pelvic and PA nodal sampling, and cytology randomized to no adjuvant therapy or WPRT. Eligibility: old FIGO IB-occult stage II (2009 FIGO stages IA, IB, and occult II) disease. Inclusion criteria were revised during trial to include only HIR subgroup (based on GOG 33): (a) age >70 years with one risk factor (grade 2 or 3, LVSI, outer one-third myometrial invasion); (b) age >50 years with two risk factors; and (c) any age with three risk factors. All others were LIR. RT 50.4 Gy/28 fx. Primary end point was cumulative incidence of recurrence (CIR) and study not powered for OS. MFU 69 months. Fifty-nine percent of patients had stage IA disease and 82% had grade 1 or 2 disease. Greatest benefit in LR was in HIR patients from 26% vs. 6% vs. LIR patients from 6% vs. 2%. Of three pelvic and vaginal recurrences in RT arm, two actually refused RT. RT had worse hematologic, GI, GU, and cutaneous toxicities. **Conclusion: Adjuvant RT**

in early-stage intermediate-risk endometrial cancer decreases risk of recurrence in HIR patients. *Comment: Grade 2 was grouped with grade 3 even though grade 2 tends to behave more similarly to grade 1.*

Table 48.5: Results of GOG 99			
GOG 99	2-Yr Any Recurrence (All Patients)	2-Yr Any Recurrence for HIR Patients	4-Yr OS
Surgery	12%	26%	86%
Surgery + RT	3%	6%	92%
p value	.007	.007	.557

Scholten, PORTEC 1 (*IJROBP*** 2005, PMID 15927414; Update Creutzberg ***IJROBP*** 2011, PMID 21640520):** PRT of 714 patients with stage I disease evaluating TAH/BSO + cytology ± pelvic RT (no PLND). Eligibility: <½ MI and G2–3 OR ≥½ MI and G1–2 (stage IB/IC at time); 99 patients w/ stage IC, G3 disease not randomized, but received post-op RT. RT 46 Gy/23 fx in 2 to 4 fields within 8 weeks post-op. MFU 97 months. On MVA, RT and age <60 were favorable prognostic factors for LRR. Patients w/ ≥2 of 3 risk factors (age ≥60 y/o, >50% MI, and Gr 3) had highest benefit from RT. In patients w/ isolated vaginal relapse, CR was obtained in 31/35 patients (89%), and 24 patients (77%) still had CR after further f/u; 3-year OS after vaginal relapse was 73%. On MVA of 15-year data (MFU 13.3 years), *grade 3, age >60, and invasion were prognostic for both LRR and endometrial cancer death.* **Conclusion: Post-op RT in stage IB, G1–2 or stage IA, G2–3 endometrial cancer reduces LRR with no impact on OS.** *Note: ~75% of LRs were in vaginal vault. On central pathology review, there was significant shift from G2 to G1.* Post-op RT is *not* indicated in patients w/ stage IA, G2 disease, or for patients <60 years of age w/ stage IB, G1–2 or stage IA, G2–3 disease. OS after relapse is significantly better in patient group w/o prior RT. Treatment for vaginal relapse is effective. Patients w/ stage IB, G3 disease have high risk of early DM and endometrial cancer–related death. Adjuvant WPRT should be avoided for patients at low or intermediate risk of recurrence.

Table 48.6: Results of PORTEC 1						
15-Yr Data	LRR	OS	DM	(–) Physical Function	Urinary/ Bowel Symptoms	Second Malignancy
NAT	16%	60%	7%	61.60%	23.6%/14.1%	13%
WPRT	6%	52%	9%	50.50%	28.1%/19.5%	19%
p Value	<.0001	.14	.26	.004	<.001	.12

■ **Is there benefit to adding pelvic RT to vaginal brachytherapy?**

Aalders, Norway (*Obstet Gynecol*** 1980, PMID 6999399):** PRT of 540 patients with stage I disease evaluating TAH/BSO (without LND/sampling or peritoneal cytology) followed by VBT, then randomized to no further treatment or pelvic EBRT (4,000 rads [sic] to pelvic LNs with midline block at 2,000 rads [sic]). Overall, pelvic RT arm had decreased 9-year LR (6.9% vs. 1.9%) but more DM (5.4% vs. 9.9%). There was no difference overall in 5-year OS. On subset analysis, pelvic RT improved 9-year OS for patients with G3 and >50% MI or LVSI (72% vs. 82%). **Conclusion: Only patients with Gr 3 tumors and >50% MI or LVSI may benefit from pelvic RT. All other stage I patients should receive VBT alone.**

Table 48.7: Results of Aalders (Norway) Trial of Pelvic RT for Endometrial Cancer					
	5-Yr OS	9-Yr OS	LRR	DM	Deaths From DM
No Pelvic RT	91%	90%	6.9%	5.4%	4.6%
Pelvic RT	89%	87%	1.9%	9.9%	9.5%
p Value	NS	NS	<.01	NS	.10 > *p* > .05

Blake, MRC ASTEC-NCIC EN.5 Pooled Results (*Lancet* 2009, PMID 19070891): PRT of 905 patients with *high-risk* endometrial cancer treated with TAH/BSO ± adjuvant EBRT. Lymphadenectomy was optional (29% of patients underwent lymphadenectomy, of which 4% were found to have positive LN) and intracavitary was optional but had to be stated up front whether institution would deliver it and it had to be offered to both arms if given (used in 51% vs. 52%). High-risk disease: Grade 3, stage IB, endocervical glandular involvement, serous papillary, or clear cell type; +PA nodes excluded. RT was 40 to 46 Gy/20 to 25 fx. Median age 65. EBRT had higher acute (60% vs. 26%) and late (7% vs. 3%) toxicity; 5-year OS 84%, DSS 89%, RFS 78%. No difference between arms. Isolated vaginal/pelvic relapse (3.2% vs. 6.1% favoring EBRT, p = .038). **Conclusion: EBRT should not be routinely recommended for intermediate- or high-risk patients and although EBRT reduces local recurrence, it is not without toxicity.**

Kong (*J Natl Cancer Inst* 2012, PMID 22962693): Meta-analysis of seven RCTs comparing EBRT vs. no EBRT (includes VBT) and one trial comparing VBT to no additional treatment. EBRT significantly reduced LRR (HR: 0.36, p < .001) but did not improve OS (HR: 0.99, p = .95), CSS, or DM. EBRT associated with increased severe acute and late toxicity. **Conclusion: EBRT reduces LRR but has no impact on survival and is associated with significant morbidity and reduction in QOL.**

Sorbe, Swedish Intermediate Risk (*IJROBP* 2012, PMID 21676554): PRT of 527 patients randomized to TAH/BSO + VBT ± WPRT. *Eligibility:* Stage I endometrioid histology with one risk factor (G3, IB, or DNA aneuploidy), 46 Gy + VBT or VBT alone (3 Gy × 6, 5.9 Gy × 3, or 20 Gy × 1 to 5 mm); 15 pelvic recurrences in VBT-alone arm, one in WPRT + VBT (LR 5% vs. 1.5% at 5 years); 5-year OS was 89% and 90% (p = .548). Deep MI was prognostic but not grade or DNA ploidy. WPRT had low toxicity (<2%) but difference favored VBT alone. **Conclusion: Even with LR benefit for WPRT + VBT, combined RT should be reserved for high-risk cases with two or more high-risk factors given toxicity and no OS benefit. VBT alone should be adjuvant treatment option for purely medium-risk cases.**

■ **Does VCB reduce recurrence in low-risk women?**

Sorbe, Swedish Low Risk (*Int J Gyn Cancer* 2009, PMID 19574776). PRT of 645 patients randomized to TAH/BSO ± VBT (HDR or LDR). *Eligibility:* FIGO 1988 stage IA/B and G1–2. RT with Perspex applicators or ovoids Rx to 3 to 8 Gy with 3 to 6 fx 5 mm from surface. Vaginal recurrence 1.2% with VBT and 3.1% without (p = .114). Few side effects with G1–2 toxicity of 2.8% with VBT and 0.6% without. **Conclusion: VBT is associated with nonsignificant reduction in recurrence. Observation is appropriate for this subgroup.** *Comment: Possible that certain other subgroups of low- or medium-risk patients (only stage IB, G-2, or tumors w/ LVSI, or patients w/ higher age) may benefit from VBT.*

■ **How should one select between adjuvant VCB and adjuvant EBRT?**

Appropriate patient selection is key. Most recurrences in GOG 99 and PORTEC were in vaginal vault, though 28% were noncentral (sidewall). Also, GOG 99 patients were surgically staged. In PORTEC-2, however, after central pathology review, many of the patients on study were found to be lower risk.

Nout, PORTEC-2 (*Lancet* 2010, PMID 20206777): PRT of 427 HIR patients s/p TAH/BSO (no PLND) w/ EBRT (46 Gy /23) vs. VBT (21 Gy/3 fx HDR or 30 Gy LDR). *Eligibility:* Age ≥60 and IB G1–2 or IA G3; or endocervical glandular involvement grades 1–3, any age, but >50% *myometrial invasion w/ G3 excluded.* MFU 45 months. QOL better in VBT (social function, diarrhea, fecal incontinence, and limit of ADLs). Central path review: G2 tumors showed poor reproducibility and on re-review, many patients considered grade 1 (see Table 48.8). On MVA, high-risk profile and LVSI were only risk factors for OS and RFS. **Conclusion: No difference in vaginal recurrence, OS, and DFS for VBT vs. EBRT. In view of QOL benefit, VBT should be treatment for HIR endometrial cancer. Late Gr 3 GI toxicity was 2% vs. none.**

Table 48.8: Results of PORTEC-2 for Endometrial Cancer										
5-Yr Results	VR	LRR	Pelvic-Only Recurrence	DFS	OS	Gr 1–2 GI Toxicity	Path Distribution	G-1	G-2	G-3
EBRT	1.6%	2.1%	1.5%	82.7%	84.8%	53.8%	Original	48%	45%	7%
VBT	1.8%	5.1%	0.5%	78.1%	79.6%	12.6%	Review	79%	9%	12%
p Value	.74	.17	.30	.74	.57	NS after 24 mos				

Randall, GOG 249 (*JCO* 2019, PMID 30995174): Phase III PRT of 601 patients with FIGO stage I endometrioid meeting HIR criteria as per GOG 99, all stage II, or stage I/II serous/clear cell carcinoma randomized after surgery to whole-pelvis EBRT (45–50.4 Gy/25–28 fx) vs. VCB followed by carboplatin/paclitaxel for 3 cycles given q3 weeks (VCB/C). Optional cuff boost allowed on EBRT arm for stage II patients or papillary serous/clear cell histology; 74% of patients stage I, 71% endometrioid, and 20% serous/clear cell. Eighty-nine percent underwent lymphadenectomy. MFU 53 months; 60-month RFS 76% for both arms. Five-year OS was not statistically different between EBRT and VCB/C (87% and 85%, respectively). No differences were seen for vaginal or distant failures. However, pelvic or PA nodal recurrence was significantly more common in the VCB/C (9% vs. 4%, $p = .472$). Acute grade ≥3 toxicity significantly increased in the VCB/C group. Grade ≥3 late toxicity similar in both groups. No clear subset benefited from either regimen. **Conclusion: VCB/C is not superior to pelvic RT in terms of RFS or OS, and is associated with more acute toxicity (but similar late toxicity). VCB/C has higher rate of pelvic and PA nodal recurrences compared to EBRT, while both modalities have similar rates of vaginal and distant recurrence. Pelvic RT remains an effective adjuvant treatment modality for patients with high-risk, early-stage endometrial cancer of all histologies.**

- **How strong of a risk factor is LVSI?**

LVSI has consistently been shown to be a strong risk factor for local and distant recurrence.

Bosse, Pooled PORTEC 1 & 2 (*Eur J Cancer* 2015, PMID 26049688): Pooled analysis from PORTEC-1 and PORTEC-2 showed that substantial LVSI (diffuse or multifocal LVSI as opposed to focal or no LVSI) was the strongest independent prognostic factor for pelvic regional recurrence (HR 6.2), DM (HR 3.6), and OS (HR 2.0); 5-year risk of pelvic failure was 1.7%, 2.5%, and 15.3% for no, focal, and substantial LVSI, respectively. In patients with substantial LVSI, 5-year pelvic recurrence was 4.3% after EBRT vs. 27.1% with VBT alone and 30.7% after no additional treatment.

- **Does postoperative IMRT reduce treatment-related toxicity while maintaining control rates?**

IMRT may decrease risk of bowel, bladder, rectal toxicity as compared to conventional 4-field RT.

Klopp, RTOG 1203/TIME-C (*JCO* 2018, PMID 2998957): Phase III PRT of patient-reported toxicity and QOL during post-op RT in 278 patients with cervical or endometrial cancer randomized to IMRT vs. conventional four-field RT. Between baseline and end of RT, mean EPIC bowel score declined 23.6 points with standard RT vs. 18.6 points with IMRT ($p = .048$), mean EPIC urinary score declined 10.4 points with standard RT vs. 5.6 points with IMRT ($p = .03$). At end of RT, 51.9% in standard RT vs. 33.7% in IMRT arm reported frequent or almost constant diarrhea ($p = .01$). **Conclusion: IMRT improves acute effects and QOL.**

Klopp, RTOG 0418 (*IJROBP* 2013, PMID 23582248): Phase II trial of 83 patients who underwent postoperative pelvic IMRT vs. conventional four-field RT (included patients with cervical and endometrial cancer). Patients with endometrial cancer received IMRT alone, patients with cervical cancer received IMRT + weekly cisplatin. RT: IMRT to 50.4 Gy/28 fx to pelvic lymphatics and vagina. **Conclusion: In patients who received weekly cisplatin, V40 of bone marrow >37% was associated with grade 2 or higher hematologic toxicity compared to V40 of bone marrow <37% (75% vs. 40%, respectively).**

Viswanathan, RTOG 0921 (*Cancer* 2015, PMID 25847373): Phase II study of post-op IMRT w/ concurrent CDDP/bevacizumab followed by carboplatin/paclitaxel in 34 high-risk endometrial carcinoma patients. Eligible patients include Gr 3/papillary serous/clear cell carcinoma w/ stage IC or IIA; Gr 2/3 w/ stage IIB; or stages III–IVA, any grade. Objectives were AEs, OS, pelvic failure, regional failure, distant failure, and DFS; 30 evaluable patients; 23.3% grade >3 treatment-related nonhematologic toxicity within 90 days, with additional 20% within year from treatment; 2-year OS 96.7% and DFS 79.1%. No in-field failures and no FIGO stage I to IIIA had recurrence after MFU of 26 months. **Conclusion: IMRT and bevacizumab is safe and effective.**

ADVANCED ENDOMETRIAL CANCER

■ **What is definition of advanced endometrial cancer?**

The clearest definition of advanced endometrial cancer is any stage III–IVA although multiple trials also included high-risk early-stage patients typically defined by GOG 99 and PORTEC 1 as stage IB, grade 3, stage II, or those with aggressive histologies (papillary serous or clear cell).

■ **Is adjuvant CHT alone superior to adjuvant RT alone for locally advanced disease?**

Randall, GOG 122 (*JCO* 2006, PMID 16330675): PRT of 422 patients (396 assessable) with stages III to IV endometrial carcinoma receiving WART vs. doxorubicin–cisplatin (AP). *Eligibility*: Tumor invading beyond uterus s/p TAH/BSO, surgical staging w/ <2 cm residual tumor (PA LNs allowed). RT 30 Gy/20 fx AP/PA +15 Gy boost to pelvic ± PA LNs. AP was given every 3 weeks × 7 cycles followed by 1 additional cycle of cisplatin. Median age 63. MFU 74 months. 50% had endometrioid histology. Most (>75%) were IIIC to IVA/B; 84% completed RT, only 63% completed CHT. AP had more Gr 3–4 hematologic (88% vs. 14%), gastrointestinal, cardiac, and neurologic toxicity. However, AP improved 5-year PFS (50% vs. 38%; $p < .01$) and OS (55% vs. 42%; $p < .01$), and reduced crude percentage of initial extra-abdominal failures (10% vs. 19%) compared to WART. Pelvic failures in 13% of patients on WART arm and 18% on AP arm, and abdominal recurrences occurred in 16% and 14%, respectively. **Conclusion: Surgical stage III or IV treated w/ AP had improved OS and PFS, but also more toxicity.** *Comment: Results were questioned because, although this was randomized trial, post hoc stage adjustment without reporting PRT end point (unadjusted) weakens results. Additionally, for patients with unresected lesions up to 2 cm who received RT, dose delivered would be considered inadequate, which limits findings.*

Maggi, Italy (*Br J Ca* 2006, PMID 16868539): PRT of 345 patients w/ high-risk endometrial carcinoma comparing adjuvant CHT vs. RT. All patients underwent TAH/BSO and selective pelvic and PA LN sampling. *Eligibility*: FIGO stage IC G3, II G3 w/ >50% myometrial invasion, and III (224 patients) limited to pelvis. EBRT to 45 to 50 Gy to pelvis; LN+ disease also received lumboaortic RT to 45 Gy. CHT was cyclophosphamide 600 mg/m², doxorubicin 45 mg/m², and cisplatin 50 mg/m² q28d × 5 cycles. MFU 95.5 months. For RT and CHT, 7-year OS was 62% for both arms, and 7-year PFS was 56% vs. 60% (NS), respectively. While nonsignificant, cumulative incidence curves of local and distant relapse favor RT for LRC and CHT for DM. **Conclusion: No difference of improvement in PFS and OS between two protocols with acceptable toxicity for both. Randomized trials of pelvic RT combined with adjuvant cytotoxic therapy compared with RT alone are eagerly awaited.**

Susumu, JGOG 2033 (*Gynecol Oncol* 2008, PMID 17996926): Phase III PRT of adjuvant pelvic RT vs. cisplatin-based CHT in patients with intermediate- and high-risk endometrioid adenocarcinoma w/ >50% MI; 385 eligible patients were randomized to adjuvant pelvic RT (*n* = 193) of at least 40 Gy vs. cyclophosphamide–doxorubicin–cisplatin (CAP; *n* = 192). *Eligibility*: >50% MI, including patients with stages IC tp IIIC (only 11.9% IIIC) disease s/p TAH/BSO and surgical staging. RT 45 to 50 Gy AP/PA. CHT was given for >3 cycles. 5-year PFS in pelvic RT and CAP groups was 83.5% and 81.8% (NS), while 5-year OS was 85.3% and 86.7% (NS). Unplanned subset analysis of high-risk subgroup consisting of (a) stage IC in >70 years of age or G3 endometrioid adenocarcinoma or (b) stage II or IIIA (positive cytology), showed higher PFS rate (83.8% vs. 66.2%, $p = .024$) and OS rate (89.7% vs. 73.6%, $p = .006$) for CAP. **Conclusion: Adjuvant CHT may be useful as alternative to RT for HIR endometrial cancer.** *Comment: Study was not stratified for subset analysis; nor was it planned, limiting utility of this observation. Only 11.9% stage IIIC. Randomization was not stratified by stage of disease.*

Johnson (*Gynecol Oncol* 2010, PMID 21975736): Meta-analysis of 5 PRTs with over 2,000 women comparing adjuvant CHT with any other adjuvant treatment or no other treatment. Four of these trials compared platinum-based CHT vs. RT. Addition of Pt-based CHT is associated with 5% ARR for first recurrence outside pelvis and 4% ARR for relative risk of death regardless of addition of RT. **Conclusion: Postoperative platinum CHT associated with small benefit of PFS and OS irrespective of RT.** *Comment: Analysis of pelvic rate recurrences is underpowered, with no direct comparison against RT,* *so cannot determine if more effective based on this. Could be alternative to RT for select patients and has added value when used with RT.*

Galaal (*Cochrane Database Syst Rev* 2014, PMID 24832785): Pooled planned meta-analysis of four RCTs involving 1,269 women treated with adjuvant CHT compared with RT or chemoRT in those with FIGO stage III and IV endometrial carcinoma. *Eligibility:* JGOG 2033, Italian trial by Maggi et al. and GOG 122 were included. Only two of these trials (Maggi et al., GOG 122) provided survival data; thus only these two trials were combined, leaving 620 evaluable patients. Of note, the fourth trial was GOG 184, which was comparing cisplatin/doxorubicin/paclitaxel vs. cisplatin/doxorubicin following adjuvant RT. OS and PFS favored adjuvant CHT over RT (OS: HR 0.75, 95% CI: 0.57–0.99, and PFS: HR 0.74, 95% CI: 0.59–0.92). Sensitivity analysis for adjusted/unadjusted OS data and subgroup analysis showed results did not differ within stage III or between stages III and IV. Adverse effects were higher with CHT than RT, and no difference in treatment-related deaths. **Conclusion: Report increased survival time around 25% with adjuvant CHT vs. RT in stage III/IV endometrial carcinoma. CHT vs. chemoRT should be further explored with one large trial ongoing (see the following).**

■ **Is it safe and effective to give RT along with CHT?**

Multiple studies have demonstrated safety of various forms of CHT along with RT and compared to previous results, these regimens may be more effective.

Greven, RTOG 9708 (2 Years: *IJROBP* 2004, PMID 15093913; 4 Years: *Gynecol Oncol* 2006, PMID 16545437): Phase II study of 44 eligible patients w/ high-risk endometrial carcinoma evaluating safety and toxicity of CHT when combined w/ pelvic RT. All patients underwent TAH/BSO. *Eligibility*: Stage IB G2–3, II, or III disease. Pelvis RT consisted of 45 Gy/25 fx. CHT with cisplatin dose of 50 mg/m^2 was given on d 1 and 28. After pelvic RT, intracavitary RT was delivered with single-dose LDR 20 Gy or 3 HDR applications totaling 18 Gy to vaginal surface. After RT, four additional courses of cisplatin 50 mg/m^2 and paclitaxel 175 mg/m^2 at 28-day intervals. Protocol completion rate was 98%. At median of 4.3-year follow-up, maximum tolerated late toxicity was grade 1 in 16%, grade 2 in 41%, grade 3 in 16%, and grade 4 in 5%; 4-year pelvic, regional, and distant recurrence rates were 2%, 2%, and 19%, respectively; 4-year OS and DFS were 85% and 81%, respectively; 4-year OS and DFS for stage III patients were 77% and 72%, respectively. No recurrences for remaining stages. **Conclusion: LRC is excellent following combined-modality treatment in all patients, suggesting additive effects of CHT and RT.**

Homesley, GOG 184 (*Gynecol Oncol* 2009, PMID 19108877): PRT of 552 patients with stage III/IV (changed to exclude abdominal disease other than PAs) s/p hysterectomy/BSO. LN sampling was not required and pelvic/EFRT (50.4 Gy to pelvis, 43.5 Gy to PAs when +PA or inadequate LND) randomized to cisplatin + doxorubicin (CD) ± paclitaxel (P). RFS at 3 years: 62% for CD vs. 64% for CDP. In subgroup analysis, CDP associated with 50% reduction in risk of recurrence or death among patients with gross residual disease (95% CI: 0.26–0.92). **Conclusion: Addition of paclitaxel to cisplatin and doxorubicin following surgery and RT was not associated with significant improvement in RFS but was associated with increased toxicity.** *Comment: Difficult to compare to GOG 122, as stage IV patients became ineligible early in GOG 184.*

■ **Is combined chemoRT superior to either modality alone?**

The preceding trials seemed to support that RT reduces locoregional failure whereas CHT reduces distant metastases. Therefore, combined chemoRT may be superior regimen, although this has not been demonstrated clearly and details on sequencing are in flux.

De Boer, PORTEC-3 (*Lancet Oncol* 2018, PMID 29449189; Update: *Lancet Oncol* 2019, PMID 31345626): Phase 3 trial of 660 women with high-risk endometrial cancer (FIGO stage I grade 3 endometrioid with deep MI and/or LVSI, stage II/III endometrioid, or stage I-III serous or clear cell histology) randomized to RT (48.6 Gy/27fx) vs. CTRT (RT/cisplatin → carbo/tax x4 cycles). MFU 72.6 months. Coprimary end points were OS and FFS. 5-year OS significantly higher for CTRT vs. RT (81.4% vs. 76.1%, p = .034). Similarly, 5-year FFS was 75% for CTRT vs. 68% for RT (p = .01). Stage III patients had lower 5-year FFS and OS compared to stage I–II (FFS 64% vs. 79%, OS 74% vs. 83%, p < .0001). Stage III had greatest benefit to CTRT: 5-year FFS 69.3% for CTRT vs. 58% for RT (p = .031), and 5-year OS 78.7% vs. 69.8% (p = .11, Cox-adjusted p = .074). Serous histology had similar improvements with CTRT with 5-year FFS and OS of 59.7% and 71.4% vs. 52.8% and 47.9% with RT alone ($p =$ .037 and .008). Interestingly, patients ≥70 years old had significantly better OS and FFS with CTRT. **Conclusion: CHT given during and after pelvic RT significantly improved 5-year OS and FFS compared to that of RT alone in high-risk endometrial cancer patients. Subgroup analysis showed the most benefit in stage III patients and serous histology. Subgroup analysis showed stages I–II patients did not benefit, though this may be attributed to low numbers. Further follow-up is needed to evaluate outcomes.**

De Boer, PORTEC-3 QOL (*Lancet Oncol* 2016, PMID 27397040): Phase III PRT as in the aforementioned trial. Secondary end points of health-related QOL as assessed by EORTC QLC-C30 and symptom scales from CX 24 and OV28. During treatment, grade ≥2 and grade ≥3 toxicity occurred in 94% and 61% of patients in chemoRT arm vs. 44% and 13% in RT alone arm, respectively (SS). At 12 and 24 months, there was no statistically significant differences in grade ≥3 toxicity; only grade ≥2 neuropathy persisted in 10% of chemoRT group vs. RT alone group (SS). **Conclusion: At completion of RT and at 6 months, QOL was worse for chemoRT group. But at 12 and 24 months, QOL was similar and only physical functioning scores remained slightly lower in chemoRT arm.**

Matei, GOG 258 (*NEJM* 2019, PMID 31189035): Phase 3 trial of stage III and IVA w/ <2 cm residual OR those with positive cytology and serous/clear cell histology randomized to CHT alone (carbo/tax x 6C) vs. chemoRT (EBRT + Cis, then carbo/tax × 4C); 707 patients, MFU 47 months with 75% completing chemoRT and 85% completing CHT; 5-year RFS 59% in chemoRT vs. 58% in CHT (NS). ChemoRT significantly reduced 5-year vaginal recurrence (2% vs. 7% in CHT arm), and reduced pelvic/PA nodal recurrence at 5 years to 11% vs. 20% in CHT arm. Distant recurrences more common with chemoRT (27%) vs. CHT (21%; HR 1.36, [1.00–1.86]); 5-year OS 70% in chemoRT arm vs. 73% in CHT arm. **Conclusions: Although chemoRT reduced the rate of vaginal and nodal recurrence compared to CHT, the combined-modality regimen did not increase RFS in optimally debulked, stage III/IVA endometrial cancer patients.**

Kuoppala (*Gynecol Oncol* 2008, PMID 18534669): PRT of 156 patients s/p TAH/BSO (PLND in 80%) and randomized to split-course pelvic RT (28 Gy/14 fx with 3-week break) vs. interdigitated chemoRT (28 Gy → CHT → 28 Gy → CHT, where CHT was cisplatin/epirubicin/cyclophosphamide). *Eligibility*: Patients with (a) FIGO stages IA to B grade 3 or stages IC to IIIA grades 1 to 3. There was no difference in 5-year DFS, LR, DM, or OS. **Conclusion: Adjuvant CHT failed to improve OS or lower LR rate in patients operated on and radiated for high-risk endometrial carcinoma. CHT was associated with low rate of acute toxicity but appeared to increase risk of bowel complications.**

Hogberg, Pooled Results of MaNGO ILIADE-III and EORTC 55991 (*Eur J Cancer* 2010, PMID 20619634): Data from two PRTs of sequential adjuvant CHT and RT. Arm 1—adjuvant RT and arm 2—adjuvant CHT and RT. Patients with serous, clear cell, or anaplastic carcinomas were eligible regardless of risk factors; however, serous/clear cell carcinoma was excluded in ILIADE-III. RT was 45 Gy/25 fx. VBT was allowed if cervical stromal involvement. CHT was doxorubicin 60 mg/m^2 and cisplatin 50 mg/m^2 q3 weeks × 3 cycles; 5-year PFS was 69% vs. 78% and 5-year OS was 75% vs. 82% ($p = .07$) for arms 1 and 2, respectively. CSS was SS for chemoRT. Subset analysis showed no benefit to CHT for serous/clear cell carcinoma. **Conclusion: Addition of adjuvant CHT improves PFS with trend to OS improvement.** *Comment: Subset analysis was not planned and not powered to address question of endometrioid vs. serous/clear cell histology.*

■ What is ideal sequencing of CHT with RT?

Optimal sequencing of CHT is unclear, but Geller and Secord demonstrated benefit of "sandwich" regimen (CHT → RT → CHT); however, these were small and retrospective evaluations, with imbalances in histologic subtypes between treatment groups requiring complex modeling.

Geller (*Gynecol Oncol* 2011, PMID 21239048): Phase II trial of carboplatin and docetaxel followed by RT and then consolidation CHT given in "sandwich" method for stages III, IV, and recurrent endometrial cancer; 42 patients with surgically staged III to IV (excluding IIIA from cytology alone) or biopsy-proven recurrent disease were eligible; 3 cycles of docetaxel and carboplatin followed by IFRT (45 Gy) ± brachytherapy and 3 additional cycles of docetaxel and carboplatin; 7 patients expired with MFU of 28 months. KM estimates of OS at 1, 3, and 5 years were 95%, 90%, and 71%, respectively. KM estimates of PFS at 1, 3, and 5 years were 87%, 71%, and 64%, respectively. **Conclusion: "Sandwiching" RT between CHT for advanced or recurrent endometrial cancer should be further investigated in PRTs.**

Secord (*Gynecol Oncol* **2007, PMID 17688923**): RR of 356 patients from 1975 to 2006 at Duke/UNC with surgical stage III/IV with TAH/BSO ± pelvic/PA LND followed with CHT +/− RT. Subset of 51 patients treated with "sandwich regimen" CHT → RT → CHT had highest 3-year OS (91%) and PFS (69%) compared to 9 patients treated with CHT → RT (47% and 19%) or 15 patients treated with RT → CHT (65% and 60%), respectively. **Conclusion: Promising results warrant further investigation on sequencing of therapy.** *Comment: Retrospective study, small number of patients, histology imbalance, and complex modeling of study are significant limitations.*

Secord (*Gynecol Oncol* **2009, PMID 19560193**): Multicenter RR of 109 patients with surgical stages III and IV endometrial cancer treated from 1993 to 2007 who received postoperative adjuvant therapies. Subset of 44 patients (41%) received "sandwich" therapy; 17% received RT followed by CHT, and 42% CHT followed by RT. **Conclusion: SS better 3-year PFS (69% vs. 52% vs. 47%, p = .025) and 3-year OS (88% vs. 57% vs. 54%) for sandwich approach (CHT → RT → CHT) vs. CHT → RT or RT → CHT, respectively.**

■ **Can genetic or molecular features guide CHT treatment planning?**

Leon-Castillo, PORTEC-3 Molecular Classification (*JCO* **2020, PMID 32749941**): Molecular analysis of 410 evaluable tissue samples from PORTEC-3 analyzed for association of RFS after adjuvant chemoRT vs. adjuvant RT alone with molecular features as defined by TCGA prognostic molecular classification. Tumors were classified as p53 abnormal (p53abn, 23%), POLE-ultramutated (POLEmut, 12%), MMR-deficient (MMRd, 33%), or no specific molecular profile (NSMP, 32%). Primary end point: RFS. For p53abn patients, 5-year RFS 59% for chemoRT vs. 36% RT alone (p = .019). No significant difference in RFS after chemoRT vs. RT for the other molecular classes. Furthermore, regardless of treatment modality, molecular class was prognostic for RFS: at 5 years, RFS 48% for p53abn, 98% for POLEmut, 72% for MMRd, 74% for NSMP. **Conclusion: In high-risk endometrial cancer, molecular classification is strongly prognostic for RFS. In patients with p53abn disease, adjuvant chemoRT improves RFS over adjuvant RT alone.**

CARCINOSARCOMA

■ **What is carcinosarcoma and how does its management differ from that of other endometrial carcinomas?**

Carcinosarcoma is a high-grade carcinoma mixed with mesenchymal elements. Historically named "malignant mixed Müllerian tumor," it was considered one of the uterine sarcomas (see uterine sarcoma studies) but now is often treated similar to a high-grade carcinoma and staged as an endometrial cancer. General management is similar to that of other high-grade endometrial cancers: thorough workup followed by surgery, including omentectomy, peritoneal washings, pelvic and PA nodal dissection.

These are rare tumors, and often present at advanced stages, so evidence for adjuvant treatment is primarily retrospective. Carcinosarcomas were included in the EORTC 55874 study, which demonstrated an LC benefit to adjuvant pelvic RT (47% vs. 24%) compared to observation. Similarly, the French SARCGYN also included carcinosarcoma and demonstrated a DFS improvement to chemoRT over pelvic RT alone. Others prefer multiagent CHT alone based on GOG 150 in the following. However, multiple retrospective series including NCDB, SEER, and other large experiences have demonstrated a benefit to either pelvic RT or VBT in addition to CHT, so the optimal adjuvant treatment remains unclear.[32-38]

Wolfson, GOG 150 (*Gynecol Oncol* **2007, PMID 17822748**): PRT of stages I to IV uterine carcinosarcoma, <1 cm residual disease randomized to either WART or cisplatin/ifosfamide/mesna (CIM) × 3 cycles. WART delivered AP/PA, 30 Gy/30 fx BID, then due to slow accrual, changed to 30 Gy/20 fx QD. After WART, whole-pelvis boost to 20 Gy/20 fx BID but then changed to 19.8 Gy/11 fx QD boost (total 49.8 Gy); 232 patients, 44% stage I/II, 57% stage III/IV. MFU 5 years. After adjustment for age and stage, recurrence rate was 21% lower for CIM than WART and the death rate was 29% lower for CIM than for WART (relative hazard 0.712, p = .085). **Conclusion: Results favor multiagent CHT for carcinosarcoma.** *Comment: Trial used older obsolete RT techniques and does not answer the question in the modern era about combined CHT and pelvic RT.*

UTERINE SARCOMA

Uterine sarcomas are rare tumors, comprising ~3% of all uterine malignancies. They are stromal neoplasms arising from the myometrium and connective tissue elements (in contrast to endometrial carcinomas, which are epithelial), and generally behave more aggressively. They are broadly divided into nonepithelial tumors, including endometrial stromal sarcomas (ESS, low grade), leiomyosarcomas (LMS, high grade), and undifferentiated endometrial sarcoma(UES), and mixed epithelial–nonepithelial tumors, which include adenosarcomas. A separate staging system is used (Table 48.9). In general, patients with resectable disease should undergo total hysterectomy and BSO followed by adjuvant therapy depending on risk factors (Table 48.10).

Table 48.9: AJCC 8th Edition (2017) and FIGO Staging for Uterine Sarcoma[39]			
AJCC	Leiomyosarcoma and Endometrial Stromal Sarcoma	Adenosarcoma	FIGO
T1	a ≤5 cm in greatest dimension	Limited to endometrium/endocervix	IA
	b >5 cm in greatest dimension	Limited to <1/2 myometrium	IB
	c Not applicable	Limited to >1/2 myometrium	IC
T2	a Involves adnexa	Involves adnexa	IIA
	b Involves other pelvic tissue	Involves other pelvic tissue	IIB
T3	a Tumor infiltrates abdominal tissues (1 site)	Tumor infiltrates abdominal tissues (1 site)	IIIA
	b Tumor infiltrates abdominal tissues (>1 site)	Tumor infiltrates abdominal tissues (>1 site)	IIIB
N1	• Regional LNs	• Regional LNs	IIIC
T4	• Invades bladder or rectum	• Invades bladder or rectum	IVA
M1	• Distant metastasis	• Distant metastasis	IVB

Table 48.10: General Adjuvant Treatment Guidelines for Uterine Sarcoma Following Hysterectomy		
	LMS/UES	ESS/Adenosarcoma
Stage I	Observation (CHT under investigation)	Observation vs. endocrine therapy
Stage II	Observation (CHT under investigation)	Endocrine therapy ±– RT
Stages III–IVA	CHT ± RT	Endocrine therapy ± RT
Stage IVB	CHT ± palliative RT	Endocrine therapy ± palliative RT

■ **Should RT be offered as adjuvant treatment for patients with uterine sarcoma?**

Evidence supporting the use of RT in uterine sarcomas is sparse and generally limited to retrospective reviews. These generally show small benefits in LC and no difference in survival, though much of the benefit derived from patients with carcinosarcoma who were included on these trials.

Sampath, UC Davis (*IJROBP* 2010, PMID 19700247): RR of 3,650 patients with uterine sarcoma identified from the NODB (proprietary data set). Patients with sarcoma, myomatous neoplasm, and complex/mixed neoplasm identified. Of those included, 51% were carcinosarcomas, 25% LMS, 15% ESS, 4% AS, 5% other. 30% were stage I, 37% unknown stage; 7%, 12%, and 13% were stages II to IV, respectively. Adjuvant RT improved LC in the entire cohort as well as in all subgroups. No difference in OS (5-year OS 37%). On MVA, age, stage, grade, histology, and nodal status significantly influenced OS. **Conclusion: RT may improve LRFFS for patients with uterine sarcoma.**

Table 48.11: Results of Sampath Study: RT for Uterine Sarcoma

Group	5-Yr LRFFS (%)		Log-Rank *p* Value
	No RT	RT	
Carcinosarcoma	80	90	<.001
LMS	84	98	<.01
ESS	93	97	<.05
Overall	85	93	<.01

Reed, EORTC 55874 (*Eur J Cancer* 2008, PMID 18378136): Phase III PRT of 224 patients w/ stages I to II uterine sarcoma (99 LMS, 92 CS, 30 ESS, 3 other) s/p TAH BSO randomized to adjuvant pelvic RT (50.4 Gy/28 fx) vs. observation. Required 13 years to accrue. In all patients, the addition of RT decreased the rate of local recurrence (40% vs. 24%) with no impact on DFS or OS. On subgroup analysis, the improvement in local failure was driven by CS (47% vs. 24%) and there was no benefit in local recurrence in patients with LMS (24% vs. 20%). **Conclusion: The addition of adjuvant RT improves LC in patients with stages I to II carcinosarcoma, but not LMS. RT does not impact survival.**

■ Is chemoradiation more effective than RT alone?

Pautier, SARCGYN French Study (*Ann Oncol* 2013, PMID 23139262): Phase III PRT of 81 patients. Stages I to III CS (19), LMS (53), UDES (9) randomized to adjuvant CHT (4 cycles of doxorubicin 50 mg/m² day 1, ifosfamide 3 g/m²/day days 1 to 2, cisplatin 75 mg/m² day 3) followed by pelvic RT (45 Gy/25 fx) vs. RT alone. Primary end point DFS. 50 patients also received brachytherapy. Stopped early due to poor accrual (planned 256 patients). The addition of CHT improved 3-year DFS (55% vs. 41%, *p* = .048). OS improved but not statistically (81% vs. 69%, *p* = .41). Two toxic deaths, 76% grades 3 to 4 thrombocytopenia in CHT arm. **Conclusion: Adjuvant chemoRT improves DFS for uterine sarcoma.** *Comment: Approximately one fourth were carcinosarcoma.*

REFERENCES

1. Klopp A, Smith BD, Alektiar K, et al. The role of postoperative radiation therapy for endometrial cancer: executive summary of an American society for radiation oncology evidence-based guideline. *Pract Radiat Oncol.* 2014;4(3):137–144. doi:10.1016/j.prro.2014.01.003
2. Meyer LA, Bohlke K, Powell MA, et al. Postoperative radiation therapy for endometrial cancer: American society of clinical oncology clinical practice guideline endorsement of the American society for radiation oncology evidence-based guideline. *J Clin Oncol.* 2015;33(26):2908–2913. doi:10.1200/JCO.2015.62.5459
3. Siegel RL, Miller KD, Jemal A. Cancer statistics, 2020. *CA Cancer J Clin.* 2020;70(1):7–30. doi:10.3322/caac.21387
4. Cancer Stat Facts: Endometrial Cancer. https://seer.cancer.gov/statfacts/html/corp.html
5. Morice P, Leary A, Creutzberg C, et al. Endometrial cancer. *Lancet.* 2016;387(10023):1094–1108. doi:10.1016/S0140-6736(15)00130-0
6. Renehan AG, Tyson M, Egger M, et al. Body-mass index and incidence of cancer: a systematic review and meta-analysis of prospective observational studies. *Lancet.* 2008;371(9612):569–578. doi:10.1016/S0140-6736(08)60269-X
7. Hernandez AV, Pasupuleti V, Benites-Zapata VA, et al. Insulin resistance and endometrial cancer risk: a systematic review and meta-analysis. *Eur J Cancer.* 2015;51(18):2747–2758. doi:10.1016/j.ejca.2015.08.031
8. Shapiro S, Kelly JP, Rosenberg L, et al. Risk of localized and widespread endometrial cancer in relation to recent and discontinued use of conjugated estrogens. *N Engl J Med.* 1985;313(16):969–972. doi:10.1056/NEJM198510173131601
9. Beavis AL, Smith AJ, Fader AN. Lifestyle changes and the risk of developing endometrial and ovarian cancers: opportunities for prevention and management. *Int J Womens Health.* 2016;8:151–167. doi:10.2147/IJWH.S88367
10. Barrow E, Robinson L, Alduaij W, et al. Cumulative lifetime incidence of extracolonic cancers in lynch syndrome: a report of 121 families with proven mutations. *Clin Genet.* 2009;75(2):141–149. doi:10.1111/j.1399-0004.2008.01125.x
11. Koornstra JJ, Mourits MJ, Sijmons RH, et al. Management of extracolonic tumours in patients with lynch syndrome. *Lancet Oncol.* 2009;10(4):400–408. doi:10.1016/S1470-2045(09)70041-5
12. NCCN Clinical Practice Guidelines in Oncology: Uterine Neoplasms. 2019. https://www.nccn.org
13. Schmeler KM, Lynch HT, Chen LM, et al. Prophylactic surgery to reduce the risk of gynecologic cancers in the Lynch syndrome. *N Engl J Med.* 2006;354(3):261–269. doi:10.1056/NEJMoa052627
14. Amant F, Mirza MR, Koskas M, Creutzberg CL. Cancer of the corpus uteri. *Int J Gynaecol Obstet.* 2018;143(Suppl 2):37–50. doi:10.1002/ijgo.12612

15. Halperin EC, Wazer DE, Perez CA, Brady LW. *Perez and Brady's Principles and Practice of Radiation Oncology*. 6th ed. Lipincott Williams; 2013.

16. Owings RA, Quick CM. Endometrial intraepithelial neoplasia. *Arch Pathol Lab Med*. 2014;138(4):484–491. doi:10.5858/arpa.2012-0709-RA

17. Kuhn E, Wu RC, Guan B, et al. Identification of molecular pathway aberrations in uterine serous carcinoma by genome-wide analyses. *J Natl Cancer Inst*. 2012;104(19):1503–1513. doi:10.1093/jnci/djs345

18. Kihara A, Yoshida H, Watanabe R, et al. Clinicopathologic association and prognostic value of microcystic, elongated, and fragmented (MELF) pattern in endometrial endometrioid carcinoma. *Am J Surg Pathol*. 2017. doi:10.1097/PAS.0000000000000856

19. Sanci M, Gungorduk K, Gulseren V, et al. MELF pattern for predicting lymph node involvement and survival in grade I-II endometrioid-type endometrium cancer. *Int J Gynecol Pathol*. 2018; 37(1):17–21. doi:10.1097/PGP.0000000000000370

20. Mutter GL, Lin MC, Fitzgerald JT, et al. Altered PTEN expression as a diagnostic marker for the earliest endometrial precancers. *J Natl Cancer Inst*. 2000;92(11):924–930. doi:10.1093/jnci/92.11.924

21. Kandoth C, Schultz N, Cherniack AD, et al. Integrated genomic characterization of endometrial carcinoma. *Nature*. 2013;497(7447):67–73. doi:10.1038/nature12113

22. Lindor NM, Petersen GM, Hadley DW, et al. Recommendations for the care of individuals with an inherited predisposition to Lynch syndrome: a systematic review. *JAMA*. 2006;296(12):1507–1517. doi:10.1001/jama.296.12.1507

23. Benedetti Panici P, Basile S, Salerno MG, et al. Secondary analyses from a randomized clinical trial: age as the key prognostic factor in endometrial carcinoma. *Am J Obstet Gynecol*. 2014;210(4):363.e361–e363.e310.

24. Doll KM, Tseng J, Denslow SA, et al. High-grade endometrial cancer: revisiting the impact of tumor size and location on outcomes. *Gynecol Oncol*. 2014;132(1):44–49. doi:10.1016/j.ygyno.2013.10.023

25. Creutzberg CL, van Putten WL, Koper PC, et al. Surgery and postoperative radiotherapy versus surgery alone for patients with stage-1 endometrial carcinoma: multicentre randomised trial. PORTEC study group. post operative radiation therapy in endometrial carcinoma. *Lancet*. 2000;355(9213):1404–1411. doi:10.1016/S0140-6736(00)02139-5

26. Milam MR, Java J, Walker JL, et al. Nodal metastasis risk in endometrioid endometrial cancer. *Obstet Gynecol*. 2012;119(2 Pt 1):286–292. doi:10.1097/AOG.0b013e318240de51

27. Neubauer NL, Lurain JR. The role of lymphadenectomy in surgical staging of endometrial cancer. *Int J Surg Oncol*. 2011;2011:814649. doi:10.1155/2011/814649

28. Beesley VL, Rowlands IJ, Hayes SC, et al. Incidence, risk factors and estimates of a woman's risk of developing secondary lower limb lymphedema and lymphedema-specific supportive care needs in women treated for endometrial cancer. *Gynecol Oncol*. 2015;136(1):87–93. doi:10.1016/j.ygyno.2014.11.006

29. Small W, Jr., Beriwal S, Demanes DJ, et al. American brachytherapy society consensus guidelines for adjuvant vaginal cuff brachytherapy after hysterectomy. *Brachytherapy*. 2012;11(1):58–67. doi:10.1016/j.brachy.2011.08.005

30. Schwarz JK, Beriwal S, Esthappan J, et al. Consensus statement for brachytherapy for the treatment of medically inoperable endometrial cancer. *Brachytherapy*. 2015;14(5):587–599. doi:10.1016/j.brachy.2015.06.002

31. Videtic GMM WN, Vassil AD. *Handbook of Treatment Planning in Radiation Oncology*. 3rd ed. Demos Medical; 2020. doi:10.1891/9780826168429

32. Seagle BL, Kanis M, Kocherginsky M, et al. Stage I uterine carcinosarcoma: matched cohort analyses for lymphadenectomy, chemotherapy, and brachytherapy. *Gynecol Oncol*. 2017;145(1):71–77. doi:10.1016/j.ygyno.2017.01.010

33. Odei B, Boothe D, Suneja G, et al. Chemoradiation versus chemotherapy in uterine carcinosarcoma: patterns of care and impact on overall survival. *Am J Clin Oncol*. 2018;41(8):784–791. doi:10.1097/COC.0000000000000360

34. Cha J, Kim YS, Park W, et al. Clinical significance of radiotherapy in patients with primary uterine carcinosarcoma: a multicenter retrospective study (KROG 13-08). *J Gynecol Oncol*. 2016;27(6):e58. doi:10.3802/jgo.2016.27.e58

35. Zwahlen DR, Schick U, Bolukbasi Y, et al. Outcome and predictive factors in uterine carcinosarcoma using postoperative radiotherapy: a rare cancer network study. *Rare Tumors*. 2016;8(2):6052. doi:10.4081/rt.2016.6052

36. Manzerova J, Sison CP, Gupta D, et al. Adjuvant radiation therapy in uterine carcinosarcoma: a population-based analysis of patient demographic and clinical characteristics, patterns of care and outcomes. *Gynecol Oncol*. 2016;141(2):225–230. doi:10.1016/j.ygyno.2016.02.013

37. Sozen H, Çiftçi R, Vatansever D, et al. Combination of adjuvant chemotherapy and radiotherapy is associated with improved survival at early stage type II endometrial cancer and carcinosarcoma. *Aust N Z J Obstet Gynaecol*. 2016;56(2):199–206. doi:10.1111/ajo.12449

38. Guttmann DM, Li H, Sevak P, et al. The impact of adjuvant therapy on survival and recurrence patterns in women with early-stage uterine carcinosarcoma: a multi-institutional study. *Int J Gynecol Cancer*. 2016;26(1):141–148. doi:10.1097/IGC.0000000000000561

39. *AJCC Cancer Staging Manual*. 8th ed. Springer International Publishing; 2017.

Ahmed Halima and Sudha R. Amarnath

QUICK HIT ■ Vulvar cancers are rare, most commonly squamous cancer, and occur in older women with a history of either HPV or lichen sclerosis. Primary therapy is surgical with risk-adapted adjuvant RT as indicated. IMRT use postoperatively is becoming more routine but is technically challenging. Prospective data guiding the use of concurrent CHT are lacking except in the neoadjuvant setting.

Table 49.1 General Treatment Paradigm for Vulvar Cancer[1]

Stage	Initial Treatment	Subsequent Therapy
VIN	Local excision, skinning vulvectomy, imiquimod, topical 5-FU, laser ablation	N/A
Stage IA	Wide local excision	Excision alone is appropriate if final pathology demonstrates ≤1 mm of invasion, negative margins, and no additional risk factors
Stage IB–II	Radical local resection or modified radical vulvectomy with inguinal SLNB (can be unilateral SLNB for well-lateralized primary >2 cm from midline)	*RT to vulva*: margins <8 mm (also consider for LVSI, depth of invasion >5 mm, tumor size, diffuse or spray histology) *RT to inguinal and pelvic nodes*: ≥2 positive nodes, ECE. Consider treatment for 1 positive node, particularly if <12 nodes were dissected without SLNB. Consider concurrent CHT based on risk factors (no clear indications described)
Stage III/IVA	Surgical resection is preferred if feasible	Risk-adapted RT to primary and/or lymph nodes as in the preceding case
	If unresectable disease, neoadjuvant chemoRT with concurrent weekly cisplatin	Biopsy for pathologic confirmation of complete response, consider groin dissection as well for confirmation. If partial response, organ-sparing surgery if possible

EPIDEMIOLOGY: Rare cancer, estimated 6,120 cases and 1,350 deaths in 2020.[2,3] White women at slightly higher risk than Black or Hispanic women.[4] Peak incidence in the seventh decade of life.

RISK FACTORS: The two major etiologies are HPV infection and vulvar dystrophy.[4] Risk factors relating to HPV: younger age at first intercourse, number of sexual partners, genital warts. VIN is related to HPV. Most common high-risk HPV subtypes are HPV 16, 18, and 33. Vaginal dystrophies, such as lichen sclerosis, are chronic inflammatory lesions and associated with vulvar cancer in older patients. Risk of malignant transformation of lichen sclerosis is approximately 5%.[4] Risk of malignant transformation of VIN III is 80%.[5]

ANATOMY: Vulva consists of mons pubis, clitoris, labia majora, and labia minora. Fourchette is merging of labia minora posteriorly. Vulva is bounded posteriorly by perineal body. Innervation is provided by pudendal nerve (S2–S4). Bartholin glands are in posterior labia majora; Skene glands are periurethral. Lymphatic drainage is to superficial inguinal nodes but can travel directly to deep inguinal nodes. In addition to inguinal nodes, clitoral lesions can drain directly to pelvic nodes (obturator, internal, or external).[4] Cloquet's/Rosenmüller's node is superiormost deep inguinal node classically associated with additional pelvic metastases.[6] Per AJCC, pelvic nodes are distant (FIGO stage IVB), a finding supported by poor outcome on GOG 37 (Homesley in the following) but questioned in the modern era.[7]

PATHOLOGY: Approximately 90% are squamous cell carcinoma, 5% to 10% melanoma, and remaining are rare types such as adenocarcinomas arising from Bartholin gland. Basaloid carcinoma is associated with HPV; keratinizing associated with vulvar dystrophy. Verrucous carcinoma is squamous variant that is warty in appearance and rarely metastasizes. Of squamous carcinomas, two patterns of growth have been identified by NCCN as a risk factor after surgery: spray and diffuse. Spray pattern is associated with "fingers" of tumor extending deeper than main tumor and into dermis. Diffuse pattern is connected tumor of >1 mm in dimension and is often deeply invasive with stromal desmoplasia.[4] Extramammary Paget's disease of vulva may be associated with invasive carcinoma in approximately 80%.[8] Risk of groin lymph nodes is related to tumor thickness (as measured in GOG 36, similar to but not identical to depth of stromal invasion) with risk being 2.6% if ≤1 mm; 8.9%, 18.6%, 30.9%, 33.3% for 2 to 5 mm, respectively; and 47.9% if >5 mm (this is tumor thickness).[9] For unilateral lesions, risk of contralateral groin involvement was 8% on GOG 36. Inguinal nodal ratio of >20% is associated with 53% risk of contralateral nodal metastases.[10]

CLINICAL PRESENTATION: Erythematous, ulcerated lesion, may be associated with bleeding, pruritus, or pain. Groin nodes may be palpable and/or ulcerated. Dark discoloration should raise concern for melanoma. Synchronous cervical cancer may be present in ~20%. Lung is the most common site of distant metastases. Differential includes epidermal inclusion cyst, lentigo, benign Bartholin gland disorders, acrochordons, seborrheic keratoses, hidradenomas, lichen scleroses, condyloma acuminata.

WORKUP: H&P with pelvic and rectal exam.

Labs: CBC, LFTs. Pregnancy test as indicated.

Pathology: Biopsy with HPV testing. Consider EUA with proctoscopy or sigmoidoscopy if concerning.

Imaging: CXR is sufficient unless symptoms of metastatic disease. MRI pelvis with and without contrast, if helpful for surgical or RT planning. Accuracy values of contrasted MRI for tumor stage and lymph node metastases are both approximately 85%.[11] Consider PET/CT for clinically advanced or to evaluate for node-positive lesions.[1]

PROGNOSTIC FACTORS: Most important factor for nonmetastatic patients is lymph node involvement. Margin status, depth of invasion, extracapsular extension, tumor grade, LVSI, tumor size, perineural invasion, and p16 status.[12]

STAGING

Table 49.2 AJCC 8th Edition (2017) and FIGO 2009[13] Staging for Vulvar Cancer		
AJCC		FIGO
T1	a. Confined to vulva/perineum, ≤2 cm in size, stromal invasion ≤1 mm	IA
	b. Confined to vulva/perineum, >2 cm in size, stromal invasion >1 mm	IB
T2	• Adjacent spread to distal one-third of urethra and/or distal one-third vagina or anus	II
T3	• Extension to proximal two-thirds urethra and/or proximal two-thirds vagina, bladder/rectal mucosa or fixation to pelvic bones	IVA
N0 (I+)	• Isolated tumor cells <0.2 mm	
N1	a 1–2 LNs, <5 mm	IIIA
	b 1 LN, >5 mm	
N2	a >3 LNs, all <5 mm	IIIB
	b >2 LNs, >5 mm	
	c Any LN with ECE	IIIC
N3	• Fixed or ulcerated LNs	IVA
M1	• Distant metastasis	IVB

Note: Vulvar melanoma is staged separately.

TREATMENT PARADIGM

Surgery: Surgical excision prior to RT is standard and is determined by size and location of the lesion. For small T1 lesions, wide local excision is appropriate. For T2 or higher lesions, modified radical vulvectomy (also called "radical local excision"; spares uninvolved parts of vulva whereas radical vulvectomy removes entire vulva). For select well-localized lesions, hemivulvectomy is appropriate. For large T3 lesions in which degree of resection necessary would not be tolerated, definitive nonoperative management is appropriate. For primary, gross tumor should be excised to deep fascia and periosteum with at least 1 cm clinical margin and 8 mm pathologic margin (see Heaps).[14] For close or positive margins, re-excision should be considered. For clinically node-negative patients with depth of invasion ≤1 mm (FIGO stage IA), nodal dissection is likely unnecessary. For clinically node-negative stage IB–II patients, SLNB is usually appropriate. If both Tc-99m and blue dye are used, sensitivity is 91% with negative predictive value of 96%.[15] Unilateral nodal staging with sentinel biopsy can be performed for well-lateralized lesions (>2 cm from midline). If sentinel node is positive, NCCN recommends RT, chemoRT, or completion dissection followed by risk-adapted RT (see the following for indications). For clinically node-positive patients, at least SLNB is recommended as even MRI is inaccurate in approximately 15% (in pre-MRI era, false-negative rate of clinical exam was 23.9% on GOG 36).[9,11] If biopsy is positive and nodes are not fixed or ulcerated, inguinal node dissection is recommended (classically includes both superficial and deep inguinal nodes). If there are fixed nodal metastases, definitive RT is recommended and surgical management is variable based on surgeon preference. Historically, radical vulvectomy with bilateral groin dissection was common but associated with high wound complication rates (50%). Today, for those requiring full groin dissection, primary tumor is often managed independently from groin dissection with two to three separate incisions, thus improving recovery. Tumor recurrence between primary and groin incision is possible but rare.

Chemotherapy: No prospective data exist to confirm benefit of concurrent CHT with RT for vulvar cancer. NCDB data suggest survival benefit for node-positive patients in the adjuvant setting.[16] Although patterns of practice vary, most common regimen is concurrent weekly cisplatin (typically 40 mg/m²).[17] For locally advanced patients, neoadjuvant chemoRT is an option and has been prospectively evaluated with various regimens including cisplatin/5-FU or 5-FU/MMC.[17] NCCN allows for adjuvant chemoRT for stage T1b–2 patients with microscopic positive nodes and recommends neoadjuvant chemoRT for tumors >4 cm or patients requiring visceral organs to be resected.[1]

Radiation

Indications: Data most clearly support adjuvant RT for ≥2 positive nodes (GOG 37 in the following) or close (<8 mm) or positive margins.[18] Data are less clear for those with a single positive node, but RT may be beneficial when ≤12 nodes were removed on groin dissection (may not apply in sentinel era).[19] NCCN risk factors for primary tumor treatment include LVSI, margins <8 mm, tumor size, depth of invasion (cutoff unclear, some use >5 mm), diffuse or spray histology. Treatment to groin nodes indicated for ≥2 positive nodes, ECE, or clinically node-positive groin.

Dose (per NCCN and Gaffney consensus guidelines):[1,20] For postoperative treatment with negative margins, recommended vulvar dose is 45 to 50.4 Gy but higher doses may be necessary for LVSI or positive margins. Optimal positive margin dose may be 54 to 59.9 Gy as per NCDB.[21] For gross disease, 60 to >70 Gy is recommended (consider site, size, response, CHT, and toxicity when deciding dose). To uninvolved lymph nodes, 45 to 50 Gy is recommended. For gross unresectable nodal disease, 60 to 70 Gy is recommended based on size and safety.[1] For neoadjuvant RT with concurrent CHT, dose is classically 45 Gy to regional nodes with cone-down boost to total of 57.6 Gy/32 fx (as per GOG 205 in the following), although open trial GOG 279 boosts to 64 Gy/34 fx to gross tumor (60 Gy to high-risk groin and 45 Gy to low-risk nodes). For ECE, consider 54 to 64 Gy. Acute side effects include wound breakdown, skin moist desquamation, cystitis, proctitis. Late effects include pelvic insufficiency fracture, vaginal and skin fibrosis, lymphedema, RT proctitis, cystitis, bowel obstruction.

Procedure: See *Handbook of Treatment Planning in Radiation Oncology,* Chapter 9.[22]

Other modalities: Laser ablation, topical 5-FU, and imiquimod (immune response modulator) are options for VIN.

■ **EVIDENCE-BASED Q&A**

ADJUVANT THERAPY

■ **Which resected patients benefit from adjuvant RT to the vulva?**

Classically, strongest data are for patients with close (<8 mm) or positive margin.[23] *LVSI, tumor size, depth of invasion, and diffuse or spray histology are also factors to consider per NCCN.*[1] *Note that node-negative patients with risk factors are often treated to vulva alone rather than comprehensively.*

Heaps, UCLA (*Gynecol Oncol* 1990, PMID 2227541): Retrospective review of 135 patients with SCC of vulva treated surgically between 1957 and 1985. Ninety-one had margin ≥8 mm and 0 had local recurrence. Forty-four had margin <8 mm and 21 recurred locally. Other factors associated with higher local recurrence included LVSI, depth of invasion (>9.1 mm), and spray histologic pattern. **Conclusion: Final margin of <8 mm is associated with 50% chance of recurrence.**

Faul, Pittsburgh (*IJROBP* 1997, PMID 9226327): Retrospective review of 62 patients with vulvar carcinoma and margin <8 mm; 31 treated with RT, 31 observed. Local recurrence 58% vs. 16% in favor of RT. RT improved local recurrence for both close and positive margin cases (*p* < .01 for both). **Conclusion: Adjuvant RT is indicated for this high-risk cohort.**

Bedell, Minnesota (*Gynecol Oncol*, 2019, PMID 31171409): Retrospective review of 150 patients with FIGO stage I vulvar SCC treated with resection between 1995 and 2017. Forty-seven (31.3%) patients had close (<8mm) or positive margins. Of these, 21 (44.6%) underwent re-excision or vulvar RT. Two-year recurrence rates were similar between the no further therapy group vs. re-excision/RT groups (11.5% vs. 4.8%, *p* = .62), with no difference in RFS or OS. **Conclusion: Stage I resected vulvar cancer with close/positive margins have numerically higher rates of local recurrences without further re-excision or adjuvant RT, though not statistically significant different outcomes.**

■ **For patients with positive inguinal nodes, should pelvic nodes be managed surgically or with RT?**

Homesley, GOG 37 (*Obstet Gynecol* 1986, PMID 3785783; Kunos *Obstet Gyencol* 2009, PMID 19701032): Phase III PRT from 1977 to 1984 of SCC of vulva and one or more pathologically positive inguinal nodes (51% clinically node-positive) demonstrated on radical vulvectomy and bilateral groin dissection. (GOG 36 was overarching study looking at inguinal metastases.[9] If positive, patient was eligible for GOG 37.) Patients randomized intraoperatively to either pelvic node dissection or RT to 45–50 Gy to groins and pelvis in 5 to 6.5 weeks. Groin dose prescribed to 2 to 3 cm depth. Fields were from L5/S1 to top of obturator foramen. Primary vulvar site was omitted. Trial closed early at 114 patients due to significant survival difference. Twenty-eight percent of patients in surgery arm had positive pelvic nodes (14% for N0–1 patients and 45% for N2–3 patients). Initial report demonstrated improvement in 2-year OS from 54% to 68% (*p* = .03) with RT. Benefit to RT was particularly significant for those with ≥2 positive nodes. In 6-year update, OS difference not evident for all patients but difference remained for fixed or ulcerated groin nodes or ≥2 inguinal nodes. Isolated vulvar recurrence in 9% in RT arm (vulva not targeted) vs. 7% in surgery arm. Two-year OS for those with positive pelvic node was 23%, and hence pelvic nodes are staged as FIGO IVB (this has been questioned in the modern era[7]). Late effects were similar. **Conclusion: RT improves OS for patients with ≥2 positive groin nodes. Pelvic nodal dissection is not routinely indicated.**

Table 49.3 Results of GOG 37 for Vulvar Cancer				
	2-Yr OS	6-Yr OS	MS (N2/3)	2-Yr Groin Relapse
RT	68%	51%	40 mos	5%
Pelvic LND	54%	41%	12 mos	24%
p value	.03	.18	.01	.02

■ Which resected patients benefit from adjuvant RT to groin and pelvic nodes?

Homesley/GOG 37 provides strongest data and supports comprehensive nodal RT to groin and pelvic nodes for those with ≥2 positive nodes. NCCN recommends RT for any positive node, including sentinel lymph node, especially if node is >2 mm[1] as supported by SEER data.

Parthasarathy, SEER Analysis (*Gynecol Oncol* 2006, PMID 16889821): SEER data from 1988 to 2001 identified 208 patients with vulvar SCC with one positive node. Ninety-two percent treated with radical vulvectomy with either unilateral or bilateral inguinal dissection. Median of 13 nodes removed; 102 underwent adjuvant RT, 106 did not; 5-year DSS was 77% vs. 61% (*p* = .02) in favor of RT. RT particularly beneficial in those with ≤12 nodes removed (DSS 77% vs. 55%, *p* = .035) but in those with ≥12 nodes removed, difference did not reach significance (77% RT vs. 67% no RT, *p* = .23). **Conclusion: Adjuvant RT may improve DSS for patients with single positive node, particularly when ≤12 nodes resected.**

■ Is RT alone sufficient to treat groins or is groin dissection necessary?

Stehman, GOG 88 (*IJROBP* 1992, PMID 1526880): Phase III PRT of 52 patients with SCC and clinically negative/nonsuspicious nodes treated with radical vulvectomy and randomized to either groin dissection or RT. T1–3 tumors were included, but T1 tumors required LVSI or >5 mm of invasion to be eligible. RT was 50 Gy to depth of 3 cm with photons allowed but electrons recommended. Only inguinal nodes were treated; pelvic nodes and primary site were omitted. Patients in surgery arm with positive nodes received postoperative RT to groin and hemipelvis (based on GOG 37 in the preceding). Trial stopped early due to excessive recurrences in RT arm. Seventy-one percent of tumors were 2.1 to 4.0 cm. Five of 25 patients on groin dissection arm had positive nodes. PFS and OS were both inferior in RT arm. Lymphedema (28% vs. 0%) and acute grades 3 to 4 toxicity (22% vs. 10%) were both worse in groin dissection arm. **Conclusion: Radiation, as delivered in this study, is inferior to groin dissection.** *Comment: Review of 50 cases by Koh et al.[24] demonstrated median femoral vessel depth of 6.1 cm (range 2.0–18.5 cm); thus RT may have undertreated patients as dose was prescribed to 3 cm.*

Table 49.4 Results of GOG 88

	2-Yr OS	2-Yr PFS
Radical vulvectomy + groin RT	60%	65%
Radical vulvectomy + LND (with PORT if LN+)	85%	90%
p Value	.035	.033

■ Which resected patients benefit from adjuvant chemoRT?

Benefits are unclear given absence of prospective data. If done, weekly cisplatin is recommended concurrent CHT regimen.[20]

Gill, NCDB Analysis (*Gynecol Oncol* 2015, PMID 25868965): NCDB analysis from 1998 to 2011 of patients with SCC who underwent surgery with positive inguinal nodes. CHT used in 26% (41% in year 2006). CHT more common with greater number of nodes, stage IVA disease, and positive margins. CHT was associated with improved OS on propensity-adjusted modeling. **Conclusion: Adjuvant chemoRT may benefit node-positive patients.**

■ For whom is SLNB sufficient?

Per NCCN guidelines, SLNB is alternative standard of care to groin dissection for patients with negative physical exam, negative imaging, unifocal vulvar tumor <4 cm in diameter, and no previous vulvar surgery that may have altered lymph drainage. If only unilateral SLNB is performed and is positive, contralateral side should be considered for RT based on NCCN guidelines.[1] Preliminary data from GROINNS-V II study suggests RT may be beneficial for a single positive node (≤2 mm and no ENE) if inguinal dissection is omitted. Inguinal dissection is still recommended for macrometastasis (>2mm or ENE).

Levenback, GOG 173 (*JCO* 2012, PMID 22753905): Single-arm trial of 452 women with SCC of vulva with ≥1 mm of invasion, tumor size of 2 to 6 cm, and clinically negative groin. Patients underwent SLNB followed by inguinal dissection; 418 of 452 (92%) identified sentinel node. Incidence of nodal metastasis was 32%. False-negative rate was 8.3%. Sensitivity 91.7%, false-negative predictive value (1-negative predictive value) was 3.7% in all-comers and 2.0% in tumors <4 cm. **Conclusion: SLNB is reasonable alternative to inguinal dissection.**

Van der Zee, GROINSS-V (*JCO* 2008, PMID 18281661): Single-arm trial of 403 patients treated from 2000 to 2006 with unifocal vulvar SCC staged T1–2 with tumor size of <4 cm and depth of invasion >1 mm with clinically negative lymph nodes. Patients underwent radical excision with SLNB. If SLNB was negative, groin dissection was omitted. Postoperative RT to 50 Gy recommended if ≥2 nodes were positive or for ECE. 623 groins underwent SLNB. Rate of groin recurrence if SLNB was negative was 2.3% with 3-year OS of 97%. **Conclusion: Negative SLNB is associated with low rate of groin recurrence and should be standard.**

NEOADJUVANT/DEFINITIVE THERAPY FOR ADVANCED DISEASE

■ **Is neoadjuvant therapy feasible option for patients whose disease would require radical surgery?**

Multiple prospective trials and retrospective data[25] have demonstrated safety and feasibility of this approach for both unresectable vulvar primary tumors and unresectable adenopathy.

Moore, GOG 101 Unresectable Primary Cohort (*IJROBP* 1998, PMID 9747823): Multipart phase II study of 73 patients with stages III to IV vulvar SCC (T3–4 regardless of nodal status) requiring more than radical vulvectomy. This part required unresectable primary tumor; Montana report that follows required unresectable inguinal nodes. Patients (both parts) were treated with split-course RT via AP/PA fields to 47.6 Gy to primary and inguinal/pelvic nodes for N2 to 3 patients; 23.8 Gy with 1.7 Gy/fx BID for first 4 days during CHT (cisplatin 50 mg/m^2 and 4-day infusion of 5-FU 100 mg/m^2) and QD thereafter for total of 12 treatment days per course. Courses separated by 1.5 to 2.5 weeks. Surgery was performed 4 to 8 weeks later. Boost of 20 Gy was given for residual unresectable disease or 10 to 15 Gy to microscopically positive margins. Complete clinical response observed in 46.5%, 53.5% had gross residual cancer. Only two patients (2.8%) had residual unresectable disease and in three patients surgery required sacrificing bowel/bladder continence. **Conclusion: Preoperative chemoRT is feasible and may reduce rates of pelvic exenteration.**

Montana, GOG 101 Unresectable Lymph Node Cohort (*IJROBP* 2000, PMID 11072157): Second part of phase II study including 46 patients who underwent same treatment regimen per Moore except with fields including inguinal and pelvic nodes. Disease was resectable in 38/40 patients, and pCR rate was 40.5%. Control of lymphatic disease achieved in 36/37 patients (97%). **Conclusion: Preoperative chemoRT is feasible and high rates of control were achieved.**

Moore, GOG 205 (*Gynecol Oncol* 2012, PMID 22079361): Single-arm phase II trial of locally advanced primary tumors treated with chemoRT using 57.6 Gy/32 fx with weekly cisplatin 40 mg/m^2 followed by resection of residual disease. Fifty-eight evaluable patients, 69% completed treatment. Thirty-seven (64%) had complete clinical response and 29 (78% of 64%) had complete pathologic response. Of note, pathologic response rate overall was 50% in GOG 205 and 31% in GOG 101. **Conclusion: Cisplatin and RT induction yielded high response rates with acceptable toxicity.**

■ **What is the significance of *p16* and *p53* expression in vulvar squamous cell carcinoma?**

Recent meta-analysis found p16 overexpression to be associated with improved 5-year OS, possibly an independent prognostic factor. Women with p53-positive vulvar SCC were found to have lower OS compared with p53-negative, but p53 significance remains inconclusive.

Sand, Meta-Analysis (*Gynecol Oncol* 2018, PMID 30415992): A systematic review and meta-analysis of 18 studies analyzing the significance of *p16* and *p53* expression; 475 cases were used for *p16* OS analysis, 38% were *p16*-positive. *p16* expression is associated with improved 5-year OS (pooled HR:

0.40, 95% CI: 0.29–0.55) and remained significant on adjusted analysis. The analysis for p53 included 310 cases, 54% were *p53* positive. The 5-year OS pooled HR was 1.81 (95% CI: 1.22–2.68), with *p53* positive associated with a lower OS compared with *p53* negative. Unlike *p16*, *p53* was not significant on adjusted analysis, so the value remains inconclusive.

REFERENCES

1. Angervall L, Enzinger FM. Extraskeletal neoplasm resembling Ewing's sarcoma. *Cancer*. 1975;36:240–251. doi:10.1002/1097-0142(197507)36:1<240::AID-CNCR2820360127>3.0.CO;2-H

2. Daw NC, Laack NN, McIlvaine EJ, et al. Local control modality and outcome for ewing sarcoma of the femur: a report from the children's oncology group. *Ann Surg Oncol*. 2016;23(11):3541–3547. doi:10.1245/s10434-016-5269-1

3. Siegel RL, Miller KD, Jemal A. Cancer statistics, 2016. *CA Cancer J Clin*. 2016;66(1):7–30. doi:10.3322/caac.21387

4. Chino JP, Montana GS. *Carcinoma of the Vulva*. Lippincott Williams & Wilkins; 2013.

5. Alkatout I, Schubert M, Garbrecht N, et al. Vulvar cancer: epidemiology, clinical presentation, and management options. *Int J Womens Health*. 2015;7:305–313. doi:10.2147/IJWH.S68979

6. Chu CK, Zager JS, Marzban SS, et al. Routine biopsy of cloquet's node is of limited value in sentinel node positive melanoma patients. *J Surg Oncol*. 2010;102(4):315–320. doi:10.1002/jso.21635

7. Thaker NG, Klopp AH, Jhingran A, et al. Survival outcomes for patients with stage IVB vulvar cancer with grossly positive pelvic lymph nodes: time to reconsider the FIGO staging system? *Gynecol Oncol*. 2015;136(2):269–273. doi:10.1016/j.ygyno.2014.12.013

8. van der Linden M, Meeuwis KA, Bulten J, et al. Paget disease of the vulva. *Crit Rev Oncol Hematol*. 2016;101:60–74. doi:10.1016/j.critrevonc.2016.03.008

9. Homesley HD, Bundy BN, Sedlis A, et al. Prognostic factors for groin node metastasis in squamous cell carcinoma of the vulva (a gynecologic oncology group study). *Gynecol Oncol*. 1993;49(3):279–283. doi:10.1006/gyno.1993.1127

10. Kunos C, Simpkins F, Gibbons H, et al. Radiation therapy compared with pelvic node resection for node-positive vulvar cancer: a randomized controlled trial. *Obstet Gynecol*. 2009;114(3):537–546. doi:10.1097/AOG.0b013e3181b12f99

11. Kataoka MY, Sala E, Baldwin P, et al. The accuracy of magnetic resonance imaging in staging of vulvar cancer: a retrospective multi-centre study. *Gynecol Oncol*. 2010;117(1):82–87. doi:10.1016/j.ygyno.2009.12.017

12. Sand FL, Nielsen DMB, Frederiksen MH, et al. The prognostic value of p16 and p53 expression for survival after vulvar cancer: a systematic review and meta-analysis. *Gynecol Oncol*. 2019;152(1):208–217. doi:10.1016/j.ygyno.2018.10.015

13. Pecorelli S. Revised FIGO staging for carcinoma of the vulva, cervix, and endometrium. *Int J Gynaecol Obstet*. 2009;105(2):103–104. doi:10.1016/j.ijgo.2009.02.009

14. Heaps JM, Fu YS, Montz FJ, et al. Surgical-pathologic variables predictive of local recurrence in squamous cell carcinoma of the vulva. *Gynecol Oncol*. 1990;38(3):309–314. doi:10.1016/0090-8258(90)90064-R

15. Meads C, Sutton AJ, Rosenthal AN, et al. Sentinel lymph node biopsy in vulval cancer: systematic review and meta-analysis. *Br J Cancer*. 2014;110(12):2837–2846. doi:10.1038/bjc.2014.205

16. Gill BS, Bernard ME, Lin JF, et al. Impact of adjuvant chemotherapy with radiation for node-positive vulvar cancer: a national cancer data base (NCDB) analysis. *Gynecol Oncol*. 2015;137(3):365–372. doi:10.1016/j.ygyno.2015.03.056

17. Reade CJ, Eiriksson LR, Mackay H. Systemic therapy in squamous cell carcinoma of the vulva: current status and future directions. *Gynecol Oncol*. 2014;132(3):780–789. doi:10.1016/j.ygyno.2013.11.025

18. Faul CM, Mirmow D, Huang Q, et al. Adjuvant radiation for vulvar carcinoma: improved local control. *Int J Radiat Oncol, Biol, Phys*. 1997;38(2):381–389. doi:10.1016/S0360-3016(97)82500-X

19. Parthasarathy A, Cheung MK, Osann K, et al. The benefit of adjuvant radiation therapy in single-node-positive squamous cell vulvar carcinoma. *Gynecol Oncol*. 2006;103(3):1095–1099. doi:10.1016/j.ygyno.2006.06.030

20. Gaffney DK, King B, Viswanathan AN, et al. Consensus recommendations for radiation therapy contouring and treatment of vulvar carcinoma. *Int J Radiat Oncol Biol Phys*. 2016;95(4):1191–1200. doi:10.1016/j.ijrobp.2016.02.043

21. Chapman BV, Gill BS, Viswanathan AN, et al. Adjuvant radiation therapy for margin-positive vulvar squamous cell carcinoma: defining the ideal dose-response using the national cancer data base. *Int J Radiat Oncol Biol Phys*. 2017;97(1):107–117. doi:10.1016/j.ijrobp.2016.09.023

22. Videtic GMM, Woody N, Vassil AD. *Handbook of Treatment Planning in Radiation Oncology*. 3rd ed. Demos Medical; 2020. doi:10.1891/9780826168429

23. Ignatov T, Eggemann H, Burger E, et al. Adjuvant radiotherapy for vulvar cancer with close or positive surgical margins. *J Cancer Res Clin Oncol*. 2016;142(2):489–495. doi:10.1007/s00432-015-2060-9

24. Koh WJ, Chiu M, Stelzer KJ, et al. Femoral vessel depth and the implications for groin node radiation. *Int J Radiat Oncol, Biol, Phys*. 1993;27(4):969–974. doi:10.1016/0360-3016(93)90476-C

25. Beriwal S, Coon D, Heron DE, et al. Preoperative intensity-modulated radiotherapy and chemotherapy for locally advanced vulvar carcinoma. *Gynecol Oncol*. 2008;109(2):291–295. doi:10.1016/j.ygyno.2007.10.026

50 ■ VAGINAL CANCER

Camille A. Berriochoa and Sudha R. Amarnath

QUICK HIT ■ Vaginal cancer is a rare malignancy that arises as a primary in the vagina without involvement of the cervix or vulva. The majority (>80%) are squamous cell carcinomas, arise in the posterior aspect of the upper third of the vagina (60%–80%),[1,2] and are not amenable to organ-sparing surgical resection due to close proximity of the urethra, bladder, and rectum. Thus, treatment typically consists of definitive RT with or without CHT. Brachytherapy boost is often recommended, and choice of intracavitary cylinder vs. interstitial is based on depth of invasion (≤0.5 cm for cylinder vs. >0.5 cm for interstitial).

Table 50.1 General Treatment Paradigm for Vaginal Cancer[3,4]	
STAGE	**TREATMENT**
VAIN 1 to 2	Often addressed with close surveillance as ~80% of lesions will spontaneously regress.[5]
CIS (VAIN 3)	Surgery (local excision, partial or complete vaginectomy), topical 5-FU, or RT. RT usually delivered via intracavitary brachytherapy to 60 Gy* to entire vagina + boost to involved vaginal mucosa to 70 Gy.*
STAGE I	Surgery or RT. For lesions in the superior third of vagina, radical hysterectomy, pelvic lymphadenectomy, and partial vaginectomy may be performed. If located in the inferior two thirds, total vaginectomy (or vulvovaginectomy) with inguinal node dissection and reconstruction (e.g., split thickness skin graft) may be required. If surgery is not feasible, treat with RT. If lesion is ≤0.5 cm depth, use intracavitary brachytherapy alone to achieve vaginal surface dose of 60 to 65 Gy* (HDR 21–25 Gy, 5–7 Gy/week), with additional 20 to 30 Gy* (HDR = 14–18 Gy) prescribed to tumor + 2 cm margin using shielded vaginal cylinder. If lesion >0.5 cm depth, treat whole pelvis to 45 Gy with EBRT, then interstitial brachytherapy to a boost dose of 25 to 35 Gy* prescribed 0.5 cm beyond implant.
STAGE II (subvaginal infiltration only ≤0.5 cm depth)	Treat whole pelvis to 45 Gy, then boost with intracavitary implant of 25 to 35 Gy.*
STAGE II–IVA	Paravaginal/parametrial involvement: Treat whole pelvis to 45 Gy, then boost with interstitial implant 25 to 35 Gy* to achieve total dose of 75 to 80 Gy.* Surgical option is total exenteration with bilateral inguinal lymphadenectomy (though highly morbid surgery). For tumors involving lower third of the vagina, inguinal nodes should be treated 45 to 50.4 Gy. Boost clinically positive nodes to an additional 20 to 25 Gy. May need bolus to adequately cover inguinal nodes.

*Note that these doses refer to brachytherapy equivalents of 2 Gy EBRT per fraction assuming α/β of 10. When using LDR, available data suggest that achieving total dose of 70 to 85 Gy in 2 Gy EBRT equivalents should be utilized with preferred dose rate of 35 to 70 cGy/hour.[3] HDR approach is more variable; a common regimen is 7 Gy × 5 fractions.[6] Additional details regarding brachytherapy dose can be found in the following.

EPIDEMIOLOGY: Vaginal cancer is rare and accounts for less than 3% of all gynecologic cancers with about 6,000 cases in the United States annually.[7] The most common histology is squamous cell carcinoma (≥80%) followed by adenocarcinoma (~10%), with several other uncommon histologies including melanoma, small cell, lymphoid, and carcinoid comprising remaining subtypes.[8] Median age of diagnosis for SCC of vagina is 65.

ANATOMY: The vagina is a fibromuscular tube lined with mucous membrane and extends from uterus to vestibule. Urethra and bladder are located directly anterior to the vagina. Posteriorly, superoposterior vaginal wall is separated from rectum by fold of peritoneum called "rectouterine pouch" (pouch of Douglas). Extending caudally, the vagina runs adjacent to the rectum with the perineal body separating the two at their inferiormost location. Pelvic fascia, ureters, and levator ani run lateral to vagina. Posterior wall (~9 cm) is longer than anterior wall (~7 cm) because the vagina joins uterus at an angle of approximately 90 degrees. The cervix projects into the vaginal lumen, thus creating anterior, posterior, and lateral fornices. Layers of vagina are as follows: *inner mucosa* (nonkeratinizing, stratified squamous epithelium, no glands) → *lamina propria* (connective tissue) → *muscularis* (inner circular and outer longitudinal layers) → *adventitia* (thin, outer connective tissue). The vagina has two embryologic origins: upper third derives from uterine canal and lower two-thirds from urogenital sinus (implications for lymphatic drainage). Upper third drains in patterns similar to cervix (parametrial, obturator, and pelvic nodes). Lower third drains to inguinal nodes and then to external iliacs. Lesions in middle third can go either direction. Distant metastases can be seen in para-aortic LNs, lungs, liver, and bone.

PATHOLOGY[9]: See Table 50.2 for details.

Table 50.2 Summary of Pathologic Types of Vaginal Cancer		
Prevalence	Vaginal Cancer Subtype	Notes
Rare	CIS a.k.a. *VAIN3*	Most are multifocal and can involve all vaginal surfaces.
75%–95%	*Squamous cell carcinoma*	Most are nonkeratinizing and moderately differentiated.
5%–10%	*Adenocarcinoma (non–clear-cell)*	May be associated with another primary (ovarian, endometrial, renal, etc.). Otherwise, non–clear-cell adenocarcinoma of vagina has very poor prognosis.[10]
	Adenocarcinoma (clear cell)	Related to in utero DES exposure; 1/1,000 risk if exposed. Younger age. Preceded by vaginal adenosis in up to 95% of cases.
<5%	*Melanoma*	Projects into lumen, tends to involve the vaginal surface rather than invade into wall. Melanin differentiates this from sarcoma. Race: White more common than Black. OS <20%.
Rare	*Sarcoma botryoides* (embryonal rhabdomyosarcoma)	Most common vaginal neoplasm in infants and children. Characteristic "grape-like" exophytic mass. Aggressive. Treat with surgery, multiagent chemo, and XRT (OS 90%).
Rare	*Verrucous carcinoma* (variant of SCC), *serous papillary ACA, small cell, spindle cell epithelioma,* other *sarcoma,* and *lymphoma*	Verrucous CA presents as large, warty, fungating mass. Locally aggressive but rarely metastasizes and thus has overall favorable prognosis.

RISK FACTORS: Risk factors are similar to cervical cancer: current smoking, multiple lifetime sexual partners, and early age at first intercourse.[11,12] The latter two correlate with exposure to HPV, and multiple studies have shown that HPV DNA can be found in at least 75% of VAIN/invasive vaginal cancers, and specifically HPV 16 and 18 subtypes.[13,14] Additionally, previous gynecologic malignancy, DES exposure in utero (clear cell adenocarcinoma), and alcohol consumption have all been associated with vaginal cancer, with some controversy regarding exposure to prior pelvic RT.[11,15,16]

CLINICAL PRESENTATION: Vaginal bleeding, often postcoital, is the most common presenting symptom (~50%–60% of patients), though as many as 20% of patients may be asymptomatic.[1] Additional symptoms include vaginal discharge and dysuria. Frank vaginal and/or pelvic pain is often a late presenting symptom, suggestive of invasion to surrounding tissues.[1,2] If vaginal cancer is diagnosed <5 years after previous gynecologic malignancy, then new diagnosis should be categorized as recurrence. Differential diagnosis includes cervical cancer, vulvar cancer, and metastasis from ovarian, renal cell, or other primaries.

WORKUP: H&P including thorough abdominopelvic exam. Speculum exam can easily miss anterior and posterior lesions; to avoid this, rotate speculum upon exiting vault. Pelvic exam should include bimanual exam, rectovaginal exam, EUA with vaginal and cervical biopsies, and colposcopy (with acetic acid application first, lesions are white; can confirm with Schiller's test—Lugol's solution stains normal mucosal cells but not malignant cells). Perform cystoscopy and proctosigmoidoscopy for more advanced lesions.

Labs: CBC, CMP (with particular attention to creatinine and LFTs).

Imaging: CT chest/abdomen/pelvis, CXR. Recommend MRI and PET for more advanced presentations. MRI has excellent sensitivity (95%) and specificity (90%).[17]

PROGNOSTIC FACTORS: See Table 50.3 for details.

Table 50.3 Prognostic Factors for Vaginal Cancer	
Better	HPV+, SCC, involving less than one third length of vagina (*5-yr DFS 61% vs. 25%*),[18] location in upper third of vagina, >75 Gy total dose (*2-yr PFS 76% vs. 40%*).[19] Smaller size (<4–5 cm).[10,20,21] Prior hysterectomy also appears to be protective perhaps due to anatomy of tumor spread.[10,17,22]
Worse	Advanced clinical stage, larger size (≥4–5 cm), presence of symptoms, LN involvement, ACA, nonepithelial tumors, posterior wall, overexpression of *HER-2/neu* in SCC, mutated p53, longer treatment time, not being associated with DES exposure,[19] HIV.[23]

STAGING: AJCC 8th edition and FIGO staging system are outlined in Table 50.4.

Table 50.4 AJCC 8th Edition (2017) and FIGO Staging for Vaginal Cancer[8,20,24–26]		FIGO	Risk of LNs
AJCC			
T1	Confined to vagina, ≤2 cm	I	6%–14%
	b. Confined to vagina, >2 cm		
T2	**a.** Invades paravaginal tissues, but not pelvic wall, ≤2 cm*	II	23%–32%
	b. Invades paravaginal tissues, but not pelvic wall, >2 cm*		
T3	• Extends to pelvic side wall • Involves lower third of vagina • Hydronephrosis or nonfunctioning kidney*	III	78%
N1	• Pelvic or inguinal LNs		
T4	• Invasion into bladder, rectum, and/or extends beyond true pelvis**	IVA	83%
M1	• Distant metastasis	IVB	

AJCC Group Staging	
IA	T1aN0M0
IB	T1bN0M0
IIA	T2aN0M0
IIB	T2bN0M0
III	T3N0M0, T1–3N1M0
IVA	T4N0–1M0
IVB	M1

*Pelvic wall is muscle, fascia, neurovascular structures, or skeletal portions of bony pelvis.
**Bullous edema is not sufficient to classify tumor as T4.

TREATMENT PARADIGM[3,4,9]

Surgery: Wide local excision may be possible for VAIN 3/CIS. For superior lesions, hysterectomy with partial vaginectomy may be feasible. For distal one third lesions, excision with reconstruction may be possible but often exenteration (either total or anterior—including vagina and bladder only but sparing rectum) may be necessary. Multiple surgical series have demonstrated pathologic nodal involvement of approximately 10% for stage I lesions and 30% for stage II lesions.[24,25] Thus, pelvic LN dissection is often performed, and inguinofemoral nodes are also dissected if lesion is in distal vagina. Because of the extent of surgery often required in these cases, organ-sparing treatment with RT may improve quality of life.

Chemotherapy: Concurrent weekly cisplatin 40 mg/m^2 can be considered with other series using various multiagent combinations such as cisplatin/5-FU. This is extrapolating from cervical data (see retrospective data in the following section).

Radiation

Indications: RT delivered definitively typically for stages II to IVA lesions.

Dose: EBRT to whole pelvis to dose of 45 Gy/25 fx (50.4 Gy/28 fx also common). In postoperative or posthysterectomy setting or when treating inguinal lymph nodes, IMRT may be superior to four-field box. HDR brachytherapy is then given as boost, which may be intracavitary or interstitial depending on depth of invasion. One common dosing strategy for interstitial brachytherapy is 25 Gy/5 fx; see ABS guidelines for details.[3] If brachytherapy boost is not feasible, boost with EBRT to approximately 64 to 70 Gy to primary and 55 to 66 Gy to involved lymphadenopathy.

Toxicity: Acute: Vaginal irritation, pain, dysuria, proctitis. Chronic: vaginal stenosis, proctitis, fistulae, bleeding, bowel obstruction, incontinence, hemorrhagic cystitis, urethral stricture, sexual dysfunction. Risk factors include location, stage, and smoking.[19] Late RT toxicity is approximately 5% for bowel and bladder (each) with "vaginal morbidity" of 64%.[27]

Procedure: See *Handbook of Treatment Planning in Radiation Oncology*, Chapter 9.[28]

■ EVIDENCE-BASED Q&A

■ What evidence supports current treatment approaches and outcomes?

Most data for vaginal cancer treatment are retrospective; the two most commonly cited series are in the following.

Frank, MDACC (IJROBP 2005, PMID 15850914). RR of 193 patients with SCC of vagina, no prior gynecologic cancers. FIGO I (26%), II (50%), III (20%), and IVA (4%), treated from 1970 to 2000; 119 (62%) patients had EBRT + brachytherapy (median 85 Gy surface, 81 Gy to depth), 63 (32%) had EBRT alone (median 66 Gy), 11 (6%) had brachytherapy alone (median 65 Gy); 18 patients had gross excision. EBRT alone more likely for advanced lesions, bulky, or comorbid disease; 22% of advanced stage received CHT. In more recent years, EBRT was used in addition to brachytherapy even for stage I disease (see Table 50.5). Three of 9 patients w/ stage I treated with brachytherapy alone failed in regional lymph nodes. Four patients were treated with neoadjuvant CHT; all died of progressive disease. To the contrary, four of nine treated with concurrent CHT were NED. **Conclusion: Size was significantly associated with DSS (82% vs. 60% for <4 or >4 cm lesions, p = .027). Stage predictive of survival and toxicity. Predominant pattern of relapse was locoregional (I–II: 68%, III–IVA: 83%). Concurrent chemoRT reasonable for advanced disease.**

TABLE 50.5 Summary of MDACC Series on Vaginal Cancer				
FIGO Stage	5-Yr DSS	5-Yr Vaginal Control	5-Yr Pelvic Control	Severe Toxicity
I	85%	91%	86%	4%
II	78%		84%	9%
III	58%	83%	71%	21% (ss)
IVA				

Tran, Stanford (*Gynecol Oncol* 2007, PMID 17363046): RR of 78 patients with SCC of vagina treated with RT between 1959 and 2005. Median age 65 years. FIGO I (42%); II (29%); III (17%); and IVA/B (11%); 62% treated with EBRT and brachytherapy, 22% EBRT alone, 13% with brachytherapy alone. Intracavitary RT (46%) delivered to mean dose of 41 Gy; interstitial RT (31%) delivered to mean dose of 33 Gy; 62% treated with EBRT and brachytherapy to whole vagina. On MVA, stage, Hgb (<12.5 mg/dL), and prior hysterectomy were prognostic for DSS ($p < .02$). These three factors and tumor size (<4 cm) were all prognostic for LRC ($p = .01$). 26 patients failed: 13/26 local, 9/26 regional, 10/26 distant; 16/26 (62%) failed in pelvis only. MS after local failure 14 months. Of 35 patients with lower third vaginal involvement, 22 (63%) received elective inguinofemoral RT with no treatment failures in this group. Of 13 patients with lower third vaginal involvement who did *not* receive elective inguinofemoral RT, one patient failed. Toxicity: 14% grade 3/4 complications; tumor size (≥4 cm) and tumor dose (70 Gy) were independently predictive ($p < .05$). **Conclusion: RT is effective treatment for stage I/II disease. Advanced disease requires improved treatment. Most failures are local and most cancer-related deaths due to local failure not distant metastases. Hgb level at time of treatment appears to be clinically significant.** *Comment: Authors suggested that studies evaluating correction of anemia may be warranted; however, extrapolating from cervical cancer literature, transfusion may not be associated with improved prognosis for anemic patients.*[29]

Table 50.6 Stanford Vaginal Cancer Series			
FIGO Stage	5-Yr LRC	5-Yr DMFS	5-Yr DSS
I	83%	100%	92%
II	76%	95%	68%
III	62%	65%	44%
IVA	30%	18%	13%

■ Should concurrent CHT be utilized?

No prospective trials are available. Nevertheless, many argue that similarities between vaginal cancer and cervical cancer in terms of epidemiology, risk factors, histology, and anatomy warrant extrapolation from multiple randomized trials in cervical cancer showing improved PFS and OS with addition of concurrent CHT. In the absence of randomized data, the following retrospective reviews provide some support for use of concurrent CHT.

Rajagopalan, UPMC (*Gynecol Oncol* 2014, PMID 25281493): NCDB analysis of almost 14,000 patients reviewing treatment approach and outcomes in vaginal cancer patients treated between 1998 and 2011. Sixty percent of patients received RT. Of these, 48% received concurrent CHT, with increasing use from 1998 to 2011. Median survival was longer with use of concurrent CHT, improved from 41 to 56 months ($p < .0005$). On MVA, the following factors were independently prognostic for improved OS: younger age, higher facility volume, squamous histology, concurrent CHT, use of brachytherapy, and lower stage.

Miyamoto, Harvard (*PLoS One* 2013, PMID 23762284): Single-institution RR of 71 primary vaginal cancer patients treated with definitive RT ($n = 51$) or CRT ($n = 20$). MFU 3 years; 3-year OS improved from 56% with RT alone to 79% with CRT, $p = .037$. 3-year DFS also improved with CHT, from 43% w/ RT alone to 73% w/ CRT, $p = .011$. On MVA, use of concurrent CHT remained significant predictor of DFS (HR: 0.31, $p = .04$). **Conclusion: Concurrent CHT leads to improved outcomes in vaginal cancer patients.**

Samant, Ottawa (*IJROBP* 2007, PMID 17512130): Single-institution RR of all primary vaginal cancer patients ($n = 12$) treated with curative intent using concurrent cisplatin-based CRT. Median F/U 4 years. Ten patients had SCC, 2 patients had adenocarcinoma. Stage distribution: 6 stage II, 4 stage III, 2 stage IVA. All patients received pelvic EBRT to median dose of 45 Gy/25 fx followed by either interstitial brachytherapy (10 patients) or intracavitary brachytherapy (2 patients) to dose of 30 Gy; 5-year LRC was 92% and 5-year OS was 66%. Late toxicity necessitating surgery occurred in 2 patients. **Conclusion: Definitive CRT for management of vaginal cancer leads to excellent LC and acceptable toxicity.**

REFERENCES

1. Gallup DG, Talledo OE, Shah KJ, Hayes C. Invasive squamous cell carcinoma of the vagina: a 14-year study. *Obstet Gynecol*. 1987;69(5):782–785.

2. Rubin SC, Young J, Mikuta JJ. Squamous carcinoma of the vagina: treatment, complications, and long-term follow-up. *Gynecol Oncol*. 1985;20(3):346–353. doi:10.1016/0090-8258(85)90216-1

3. Beriwal S, Demanes DJ, Erickson B, et al. American brachytherapy society consensus guidelines for interstitial brachytherapy for vaginal cancer. *Brachytherapy*. 2012;11(1):68–75. doi:10.1016/j.brachy.2011.06.008

4. Lee LJ, Jhingran A, Kidd E, et al. ACR Appropriateness criteria management of vaginal cancer. *Oncology*. 2013;27(11):1166–1173.

5. Aho M, Vesterinen E, Meyer B, et al. Natural history of vaginal intraepithelial neoplasia. *Cancer*. 1991;68(1):195–197. doi:10.1002/1097-0142(19910701)68:1<195::AID-CNCR2820680135>3.0.CO;2-L

6. Mock U, Kucera H, Fellner C, et al. High-dose–rate (HDR) brachytherapy with or without external beam radiotherapy in the treatment of primary vaginal carcinoma: long-term results and side effects. *Int J Radiat Oncol Biol Phys*. 2003;56(4):950–957. doi:10.1016/S0360-3016(03)00217-7

7. Siegel RL, Miller KD, Jemal A. Cancer statistics, 2020. *CA Cancer J Clin*. 2020;70(1):7–30. doi:10.3322/caac.21387

8. Creasman WT, Phillips JL, Menck HR. The national cancer data base report on cancer of the vagina. *Cancer*. 1998;83(5):1033–1040. doi:10.1002/(SICI)1097-0142(19980901)83:5<1033::AID-CNCR30>3.0.CO;2-6

9. Perez CA, Brady LW, Halperin EC, Wazer DE. *Principles and Practice of Radiation Oncology*. 6th ed. Wulters Kluwer, Lippincott Williams & Williams; 2013.

10. Chyle V, Zagars GK, Wheeler JA, et al. Definitive radiotherapy for carcinoma of the vagina: outcome and prognostic factors. *Int J Radiat Oncol Biol Phys*. 1996;35(5):891–905. doi:10.1016/0360-3016(95)02394-1

11. Madsen BS, Jensen HL, van den Brule AJ, et al. Risk factors for invasive squamous cell carcinoma of the vulva and vagina: population-based case-control study in Denmark. *Int J Cancer*. 2008;122(12):2827–2834. doi:10.1002/ijc.23446

12. Daling JR, Madeleine MM, Schwartz SM, et al. A population-based study of squamous cell vaginal cancer: HPV and cofactors. *Gynecol Oncol*. 2002;84(2):263–270. doi:10.1006/gyno.2001.6502

13. Alemany L, Saunier M, Tinoco L, et al. Large contribution of human papillomavirus in vaginal neoplastic lesions: a worldwide study in 597 samples. *Eur J Cancer*. 2014;50(16):2846–2854. doi:10.1016/j.ejca.2014.07.018

14. Sinno AK, Saraiya M, Thompson TD, et al. Human papillomavirus genotype prevalence in invasive vaginal cancer from a registry-based population. *Obstet Gynecol*. 2014;123(4):817–821. doi:10.1097/AOG.0000000000000171

15. Lee JY, Perez CA, Ettinger N, Fineberg BB. The risk of second primaries subsequent to irradiation for cervix cancer. *Int J Radiat Oncol Biol Phys*. 1982;8(2):207–211. doi:10.1016/0360-3016(82)90515-6

16. Boice JD Jr, Engholm G, Kleinerman RA, et al. Radiation dose and second cancer risk in patients treated for cancer of the cervix. *Radiat Res*. 1988;116(1):3–55. doi:10.2307/3577477

17. Chang YC, Hricak H, Thurnher S, Lacey CG. Vagina: evaluation with MR imaging. Part II. Neoplasms. *Radiology*. 1988;169(1):175–179. doi:10.1148/radiology.169.1.3420257

18. Stock RG, Chen AS, Seski J. A 30-year experience in the management of primary carcinoma of the vagina: analysis of prognostic factors and treatment modalities. *Gynecol Oncol*. 1995;56(1):45–52. doi:10.1006/gyno.1995.1008

19. Frank SJ, Jhingran A, Levenback C, Eifel PJ. Definitive radiation therapy for squamous cell carcinoma of the vagina. *Int J Radiat Oncol Biol Phys*. 2005;62(1):138–147. doi:10.1016/j.ijrobp.2004.09.032

20. Shah CA, Goff BA, Lowe K, et al. Factors affecting risk of mortality in women with vaginal cancer. *Obstet Gynecol*. 2009;113(5):1038–1045. doi:10.1097/AOG.0b013e31819fe844

21. Rajagopalan MS, Xu KM, Lin JF, et al. Adoption and impact of concurrent chemoradiation therapy for vaginal cancer: a National Cancer Data Base (NCDB) study. *Gynecol Oncol*. 2014;135(3):495–502. doi:10.1016/j.ygyno.2014.09.018

22. Tran PT, Su Z, Lee P, et al. Prognostic factors for outcomes and complications for primary squamous cell carcinoma of the vagina treated with radiation. *Gynecol Oncol*. 2007;105(3):641–649. doi:10.1016/j.ygyno.2007.01.033

23. Merino MJ. Vaginal cancer: the role of infectious and environmental factors. *Am J Obstet Gynecol*. 1991;165(4 Pt 2):1255–1262. doi:10.1016/S0002-9378(12)90738-3

24. Al-Kurdi M, Monaghan JM. Thirty-two years' experience in management of primary tumours of the vagina. *Br J Obstet Gynaecol*. 1981;88(11):1145–1150. doi:10.1111/j.1471-0528.1981.tb01770.x

25. Davis KP, Stanhope CR, Garton GR, et al. Invasive vaginal carcinoma: analysis of early-stage disease. *Gynecol Oncol*. 1991;42(2):131–136. doi:10.1016/0090-8258(91)90332-Y

26. *AJCC Cancer Staging Manual*. 8th ed. Springer Publishing Company; 2017.

27. Lian J, Dundas G, Carlone M, et al. Twenty-year review of radiotherapy for vaginal cancer: an institutional experience. *Gynecol Oncol*. 2008;111(2):298–306. doi:10.1016/j.ygyno.2008.07.007

28. Videtic GMM, Woody N, Vassil AD. *Handbook of Treatment Planning in Radiation Oncology*. 3rd ed. Demos Medical; 2020. doi:10.1891/9780826168429

29. Bishop AJ, Allen PK, Klopp AH, et al. Relationship between low hemoglobin levels and outcomes after treatment with radiation or chemoradiation in patients with cervical cancer: has the impact of anemia been overstated? *Int J Radiat Oncol Biol Phys*. 2015;91(1):196–205. doi:10.1016/j.ijrobp.2014.09.023

IX ■ HEMATOLOGIC

51 ■ ADULT HODGKIN'S LYMPHOMA

Matthew C. Ward and Sheen Cherian

QUICK HIT ■ Hodgkin's lymphoma accounts for 10% of lymphomas in the United States and is broadly grouped into classical and nodular lymphocyte predominant types. Risk stratification of classical Hodgkin's determines treatment and includes early-stage favorable, early-stage unfavorable, and advanced (stages III–IV) disease. Each major study group (EORTC, German HSG, UK RAPID, Stanford) defines risk stratification differently. Most recent trials use PET response as judged by Deauville criteria to guide treatment. For early-stage favorable disease, despite multiple large trials, CHT alone is not noninferior to combined chemoRT (in terms of PFS). Despite this, many still favor CHT alone due to favorable salvage rates with autologous SCT and equivalent OS. Late effects with RT are of particular concern due to the disease's excellent prognosis. Although most trials delivered IFRT, ISRT is well accepted internationally and may reduce toxicity. Nodular lymphocyte predominant patients are treated similar to early stage low-grade non-Hodgkin's lymphoma. Treatment paradigms are different in children (age <21; see Chapter 64 for details).

Table 51.1: General Treatment Paradigm for Adult Hodgkin's Lymphoma

	Stage/Status	Example Treatment Options (see trials for specifics)[1]	Recent Trials Defining Paradigm
Classic HL	Stage IA/IIA Favorable	Combined chemoRT: ABVD ×2–4C and ISRT to 20 to 30 Gy or CHT Alone: ABVD ×3–4C (if PET-negative after 2–3C, i.e., Deauville 1–2) or Stanford V × 8 weeks + ISRT to 30 Gy	German HSG HD10, HD16, UK RAPID, EORTC H10F, Stanford G4
	Stage I/II Unfavorable	Combined chemoRT: ABVD ×4C and ISRT 30 Gy or ABVD × 6C or Stanford V × 12 weeks + ISRT 30 to 36 Gy	German HSG HD11, HD14, HD17, EORTC H10U
	Stages III to IV	ABVD ×6C (consider ISRT to initially bulky or select PET + sites) or Escalated BEACOPP × 6C	RATHL, German HSG HD15, ECOG 2496
NLPHL	Stage IA/IIA Stage IA/IIA bulky or IB/IIB Stages III to IV	ISRT alone to 30 Gy (consider + 6 Gy boost for bulky disease) CHT + rituximab + ISRT CHT + rituximab ± ISRT OR local RT for palliation only	

EPIDEMIOLOGY: Relatively uncommon; 0.6% of new cancer diagnoses, estimated 8,480 cases and 970 deaths in 2020.[2] Accounts for 10% of all lymphomas diagnosed in the United States. Slight male predominance, rare under age 10. Bimodal age distribution with peaks around 25 and 60 to 70 years of age.

RISK FACTORS: There is association between Hodgkin's lymphoma and EBV. EBV DNA has been isolated within RS cell and patients with history of infectious mononucleosis are at higher risk of developing Hodgkin's lymphoma. EBV tied most closely with mixed cellularity subtype and pediatric HD in developing countries.

ANATOMY: Primarily nodal disease with predictable spread. Extranodal spread is rare. Eighty percent of patients present with cervical nodes and >50% with mediastinal nodes. Most common site of extranodal disease is spleen; 13 individual lymphatic regions identified in 1965 now define Ann Arbor staging and include Waldeyer's ring, cervical/SCV/occipital/pre-auricular, infraclavicular, axillary/pectoral, mediastinal, hilar, para-aortic, spleen, mesenteric, iliac, inguinal/femoral, popliteal, and epitrochlear/brachial. Right and left hilar and cervical regions are counted as separate regions. Waldeyer's ring and spleen are considered lymphatic but extranodal regions for staging purposes. EORTC and German groups count differently than classic Ann Arbor system: EORTC includes axilla and infraclavicular as one site. German HSG includes cervical and infraclavicular regions as one site. Both EORTC and German HSG consider mediastinum and hilar areas as one site. These definitions have implications in risk stratification (see the following).

PATHOLOGY: Classic diagnostic cells are RS cells though these account for only 1% to 2% of tumor volume with rest being infiltration of lymphocytes, eosinophils, and plasma cells. RS cell classically binucleate with two prominent nucleoli, well-demarcated nuclear membrane, and eosinophilic cytoplasm with perinuclear halo. Likely origin is precursor B-cell. Monoclonal EBV DNA has been identified in RS cells in classical HL. Several subtypes of HL have slightly different pathologic and cytologic markers (Table 51.2).

Table 51.2: Histologic Characteristics of Hodgkin's Disease				
	Histology	Frequency	Clinicopathologic Features	Markers
CLASSICAL	NS	≥70%	Broad bands of birefringent collagen surrounding nodules of lymphocytes, eosinophils, plasma cells, and tissue histiocytes, intermixed w/ atypical mononuclear cells and RS cells. No gender predilection. Median age ~26. Mediastinum often involved. One-third have B symptoms.	CD15+, CD30+ Occasional CD20+
	MC	~20%	Less favorable than nodular sclerosis. Diffuse effacement of LNs by lymphocytes, eosinophils, plasma cells, and relatively abundant atypical mononuclear and RS cells. Males and older patients more common. Often have abdominal involvement or advanced dz. One-third with B symptoms.	
	LR	5%	Best prognosis. Occasional RS cell but mostly diffusely effaced with normal appearing lymphocytes. Male more common. Median age 30. Frequently stages I–II, <10% have B symptoms. Uncommon mediastinal/abdominal involvement.	
	LD	<5%	Worst prognosis. Paucity of normal-appearing cells and abundance of abnormal mononuclear cells, RS cells and variants. Difficult to differentiate from anaplastic large cell lymphoma. Males and older patients more common. Usually advanced disease. Two-thirds with B symptoms.	CD15+, CD30+ Occasional CD20+
	NLP	5%	Likely distinct entity from other HD with natural history similar to low-grade NHL. Lacks RS cells. Significant rate of transformation (to DLBCL) and frequent late relapse. Some response to rituximab. EBV negative.	CD19+, **CD20+,** Table 51.2 CD45+, **CD15–,** **CD30–**

CLINICAL PRESENTATION: Painless adenopathy most common. B symptoms: drenching night sweats, fever >38.0°C, weight loss >10% in 6 months (B symptoms present at diagnosis in one-third of patients; combination of weight loss and fever carries poor prognosis). Generalized pruritus/alcohol-induced pain in infiltrated tissues. Disease foci contiguous in 90% of patients (including connection of supraclavicular nodes to upper celiac/splenic nodes via thoracic duct). Visceral involvement is most frequently splenic and there is correlation between burden of splenic disease and likelihood of hematogenous spread. Marrow and liver involvement occur almost exclusively in setting of splenic disease. HL is not more common in HIV+ but can have a more aggressive course.

WORKUP: H&P with attention to LN regions, B symptoms, chest and abdominal (spleen/liver) exam.

Labs: Pregnancy test, HIV, CBC, ESR, albumin, BMP, LFT, LDH, PFTs including DLCO.

Imaging: CXR, PET/CT (≥90% sensitivity, changes treatment in 14%–25%), echocardiogram/MUGA (if doxorubicin CHT considered).

Biopsy: Excisional biopsy recommended vs. core needle biopsy (may be adequate if diagnostic of HL). FNA is inadequate. Bone marrow biopsy if PET is positive or cytopenias exist (overall frequency of bone marrow involvement 5% or less).[1]

PROGNOSTIC FACTORS: Several prognostic factors including stage, age, ESR, number of nodal sites involved, extranodal involvement, and lymph node bulk have been identified. In addition to Ann Arbor stage, these factors have defined risk stratification into early-stage favorable and early-stage unfavorable, which define treatment. For early-stage classic Hodgkin's disease (stages I–II), unfavorable factors vary by consensus statement and include:

- GHSG: ESR >50 with no B symptoms or >30 with B symptoms, mediastinal mass-intrathoracic diameter >0.33, >2 nodal sites, any extranodal lesion.
- EORTC: ESR >50 with no B symptoms or >30 with B symptoms, mass width at T5–6 >0.35, >3 nodal sites, ≥50 years of age.
- NCCN: ESR >50 or B symptoms, mediastinal mass-intrathoracic diameter >0.33, >3 nodal sites, >10 cm.

IPS: Prognostic scoring system for advanced Hodgkin's lymphoma composed of seven factors: albumin <4 g/dL, Hgb <10.5 g/dL, male gender, age ≥45, Ann Arbor stage IV, leukocytes ≥15,000, and lymphocytes <600/mm^3 or <8% of white count. Initial publication stratified PFS from 84% to 42% going from 0 to 7 points.[3] Scoring system was reanalyzed in 2012 and remained valid with PFS ranging between 88% and 69%.[4]

STAGING: See Table 51.3.

Table 51.3: Ann Arbor (Lugano Update) Staging System for Lymphoma[+s]		
I	One node or group of adjacent nodes OR single extranodal lesions without nodal involvement (IE)	**A:** No systemic symptoms **B:** Unexplained weight loss >10% in 6 mos before diagnosis. Unexplained fever with temperatures above 38°C. Drenching night sweats. **E*:** Extralymphatic involvement. **X*:** Bulky disease (≥10 cm or >1/3 of thoracic diameter)
II	≥2 nodal groups on same side of diaphragm OR stage I or II by nodal extent with limited contiguous extranodal involvement	
III	Nodes on both sides of diaphragm; nodes above diaphragm with spleen involvement	
IV	Additional noncontiguous extralymphatic involvement	

*Note that the 2014 Lugano update suggests "X" and "A/B" modifiers are necessary only for Hodgkin's lymphoma and "E" unnecessary for stage III to IV disease.[5]
†Number of involved regions may be designated with subscript (i.e., II3).

TREATMENT PARADIGM

Surgery: There is typically no role for surgery in treatment of adult Hodgkin's lymphoma. In children with NLPHL, resection followed by observation with CHT at progression has been investigated.[6]

Chemotherapy: Several CHT regimens have been used over history of Hodgkin's lymphoma. Historical regimen MOPP (mustard, vincristine, procarbazine, prednisone) resulted in sterility (80% of men, age-linked in women) and secondary acute nonlymphocytic leukemia. Modern regimens are associated with less sterility and secondary malignancy risk and include the following:

ABVD: (Adriamycin, bleomycin, vinblastine, dacarbazine). Toxicities include nausea, vomiting, hair loss, and marrow suppression. Long-term toxicities include cardiac and pulmonary toxicity. German HD13 study examined if bleomycin, dacarbazine, or both could be omitted (ABV, AVD, and AV arms) in early-stage HL. All alternative regimens were associated with inferior outcomes relative to ABVD.[7] Each cycle is generally one month with two infusions per cycle.

Stanford V: (nitrogen mustard, doxorubicin, vinblastine, vincristine, bleomycin, etoposide, prednisone) is quicker treatment (8–12 weeks vs. 16–24 weeks for 4–6 cycles of ABVD) and includes lower cumulative doses of doxorubicin and bleomycin. Designed as combined modality therapy with RT, which should not be omitted. Studies suggest similar outcomes as ABVD assuming RT is delivered.[8–10]

BEACOPP: Bleomycin, etoposide, doxorubicin, cyclophosphamide, vincristine, procarbazine, prednisone. Intensified treatment studied in setting of poor response or for unfavorable patients. Associated with higher response rates but also higher incidence of marrow suppression and alopecia.[11]

Brentuximab vedotin: Antibody–drug conjugate against CD30. Most common with relapsed and advanced disease.

Nivolumab: PD-1 inhibitors have demonstrated response in relapsed/refractory disease.[12,13] Further study is ongoing.

Number of cycles: Number of cycles delivered on trials varies by study group. Generally, risk group should be selected and treatment should proceed per trials evaluating response and outcomes in that risk group. Overall, in the PET era, Table 51.1 outlines common approaches and recent trials that defined each approach.

Response evaluation: Favorable (rapid/early) response to CHT has become an important predictor of outcome and is increasingly being used to determine treatment paradigm.[14–17] Deauville score (named after conference in Deauville, France) is standardized method of PET response (Table 51.4).

Table 51.4: Deauville (5-point) Score[18,19]	
Score	Definition
1	No uptake (background)
2	Uptake ≤ mediastinum
3	Uptake > mediastinum but ≤ liver
4	Uptake moderately > liver
5	Uptake markedly > liver and/or new lesions
X	Not attributable to lymphoma

Typically, trials consider early response of Deauville 1 to 2 to be favorable (CR), Deauville 3 to 4 to initiate adaptive treatment (PR), and Deauville 5 to define refractory disease. Of note, Deauville 3 is considered a favorable response in some trials.

Radiation: RT, once the only curative treatment for Hodgkin's lymphoma, continues to play an important role in the combined treatment of Hodgkin's lymphoma together with CHT. Thus far no randomized trial has identified population of early-stage Hodgkin's lymphoma where omission of RT did not result in significantly higher recurrence rate. NCDB study of utilization of RT in stage I/II HL between 1998 and 2011 revealed that RT use had declined from 55% to 44% and receipt of RT was associated with significant improvement in 5-year OS (94.5% vs. 88.9%).[20]

Indications: RT is used in combined modality treatment of early-stage patients and consolidation for select advanced-stage patients. Rationale for combined modality is to lower the intensity of CHT required for cure. For early-stage patients, RT use is defined by CHT paradigm set by accompanying clinical trial. RT is delivered after CHT to pre-CHT sites. Historically, large RT fields such as mantle, inverted-Y, or total nodal RT (mantle + inverted Y) were used alone to doses >40 Gy. Most recent trials used IFRT, but now ISRT is well accepted. ILROG guidelines guide ISRT or involved node RT (INRT, less common in the United States).[21] Studies have shown that appropriate use of these techniques results in equivalent outcomes.[22] For advanced (stages III–IV) disease, although controversial, RT can be considered for initially bulky or select sites which remain PET-positive after CHT.[1] If given, initiate RT within 3 to 6 weeks of completion of CHT.

Dose: RT dose should follow paradigm of clinical trial that applies based on PET response and number of CHT cycles given. Typically, for early-stage favorable disease following CHT, 20 to 30 Gy/10 to 15 fx is sufficient after PET CR. For early-stage unfavorable disease, 30 Gy is recommended and for bulky disease, 30 to 36 Gy/15 to 20 fx. For advanced disease residual on PET/CT or for consolidation of initially bulky disease, consider 30 to 36 Gy/15 to 20 fx.

Toxicity: Acute: Fatigue, RT dermatitis, esophagitis, odynophagia, cough, xerostomia, nausea, mucositis. Late: Site/age dependent but may include hypothyroidism, pneumonitis, cardiac disease, xerostomia, infertility. Second malignancy is of significant concern and may include leukemia (CHT related), breast cancer, lung cancer. Historical data show that cause of death in Hodgkin's lymphoma at 25 years is most commonly Hodgkin's (24% cumulative incidence), followed by second malignancy (13.5%) and cardiovascular disease (6.9%).[23] Note that late effects data are generally based on obsolete RT techniques and doses—late effects data in combined modality/ISRT era are evolving.

Procedure: See *Handbook of Treatment Planning in Radiation Oncology*, Chapter 10.[24]

■ EVIDENCE-BASED Q&A

EARLY-STAGE FAVORABLE HODGKIN'S LYMPHOMA

■ **What trials define current standard of care in early-stage favorable Hodgkin's lymphoma?**

Through much effort over many years, Hodgkin's has transitioned treatment from the 1950s' standard of large-field RT alone to modern PET-adapted combined-modality therapy.[25–32] The most recent trials define the current "standard" of care and have focused mainly on the role of PET and omission of IFRT from CHT. Most physicians prefer to pick an approach as defined by the following trials to guide treatment.

Omission of RT from ABVD remains controversial, but because of excellent OS results relating to effective salvage with autologous SCT, many argue that RT for all is overtreatment and may increase late effects, though this has not been validated with modern RT techniques, volumes, and doses.

Engert, German HD10 (*NEJM* 2010, PMID 20818855; Update Sasse *JCO* 2017, PMID 28418763): A total of 1,370 patients with early-stage favorable (by German criteria); 2×2 design randomized to ABVD × 4C vs. ABVD × 2C as well as IFRT 20 Gy vs. 30 Gy. Primary end point FFTF. PET was not used to assess response. MFU at update 98 months. No significant differences in initial or follow-up between either randomization. Noninferiority was confirmed for both (10-yr PFS of ABVD × 4C + 30 Gy vs. ABVD × 2C + 20 Gy was 87.4% vs. 87.2%). **Conclusion: ABVD for 2 cycles and IFRT to 20 Gy is standard as per German paradigm.**

Fuchs, German HD16 (*JCO* 2019, PMID 31498753): Randomized phase III trial, for early-stage favorable HL. Patients assigned to CMT with ABVD × 2C and 20 Gy consolidation RT or SMT omitting radiation with PET-guidance (Deauville score <3); 5-yr PFS 93.4% CMT vs. 86.1% SMT, HR 1.78 (95% CI 1.02-3.12). **Conclusion: In early-stage favorable HL, omitting RT results in loss of tumor control.**

Raemaekers, EORTC H10 (*JCO* 2014, PMID 24637998; Update André *JCO* 2017, PMID 28291393): PRT of PET-adapted therapy including both favorable (H10F stratum) and unfavorable (H10U stratum) early-stage Hodgkin's patients as defined by EORTC criteria earlier. Trial evaluated both ability to omit INRT in those with rapid PET response and utility of escalating to BEACOPP in patients not responding on early PET. In H10F, patients randomized to PET-adapted treatment vs. standard treatment, then received ABVD × 2C followed by PET. In standard arm, patients received 1 additional cycle of ABVD with INRT to 30 Gy (6 Gy boost allowed for residual disease). In experimental PET-adapted arm, patients received 2 additional cycles of ABVD (total 4) if PET negative (Deauville 1–2). If positive, patients received escalated BEACOPP × 2C and INRT to 30 Gy (6 Gy boost allowed for residual). See the following for H10U description/results. Primary end point PFS, designed as non-inferiority, powered to detect 5-year PFS decrease from 95% (H10F) to 85%. Randomization to PET-adapted therapy was stopped early as noninferiority was unlikely. In final report, 1,950 patients were recruited; 18.5% of PET scans were positive. Noninferiority of ABVD alone could not be established (H10F 5-yr PFS 99% vs. 87.1%, HR 15.8, 95% CI: 3.8–66.1, noninferiority margin was 3.2). Escalation to BEACOPP improved 5-year PFS from 77.4% (ABVD + INRT) to 90.6% (BEACOPP + INRT, $p = .002$). **Conclusion: Even in patients with excellent PET response, omission of INRT is associated with increased risk of progression (but no difference in OS).**

Radford, UK RAPID (*NEJM* 2015, PMID 25901426): Noninferiority trial of patients with classic Hodgkin's lymphoma stages IA to IIA (baseline PET not performed) without bulk (≥33% thoracic diameter at T5–6). Patients received three cycles of ABVD, then underwent PET and if negative (Deauville 1–2) randomized to 30 Gy IFRT or no further treatment. If positive, received total of four cycles of ABVD and 30 Gy IFRT. Primary end point PFS, noninferiority margin originally 10% decrease, then modified to 7%. Overall, 32% were unfavorable per German criteria and 31% had ≥3 nodal sites. MFU 60 months; 3-year PFS 94.6% in RT group and 90.8% in no additional therapy group, difference −3.8% (95% CI: −8.8%–1.3%). **Conclusion: ABVD alone is not noninferior to ABVD + IFRT although prognosis is excellent regardless.**

■ **What is Stanford V and how does it differ from other regimens?**

Stanford V CHT is the standard option consisting of abbreviated CHT with reduced anthracycline and bleo-mycin doses compared to ABVD. It was designed as a combined modality regimen and omission of RT is not recommended.

Advani, Stanford G4 (*Ann Oncol* 2013, PMID 23136225): Single-arm prospective trial of Stanford V CHT for nonbulky early-stage Hodgkin's lymphoma. CHT included mechlorethamine, doxorubicin, vinblastine, vincristine, bleomycin, and etoposide. In this trial, regimen was abbreviated to 8 weeks from 12 weeks (12 weeks remain standard option for early-stage unfavorable); 1 to 3 weeks after CHT, 30 to 30.6 Gy/17 to 20 fx of modified IFRT was delivered; 87 patients enrolled, MFU 10 years. FFP, DSS, and OS were 94%, 99%, and 94%, respectively. **Conclusion: Stanford V is well tolerated with excellent results and is comparable to other standard options.**

EARLY-STAGE UNFAVORABLE HODGKIN'S LYMPHOMA

The following trials are the most recent to define "standard" of care in early-stage unfavorable Hodgkin's lymphoma. Note that many trials define subsets of early-stage patients with other high-risk features such as bulk, B symptoms, or extranodal disease as advanced rather than early-stage unfavorable, so it is important to identify inclusion criteria for each paradigm when deciding treatment.

■ **What trials define current standard of care in early stage unfavorable Hodgkin's lymphoma?**

Eich, German HD11 (*JCO* 2010, PMID 20713848; Update Sasse *JCO* 2017, PMID 28418763): Precursor trial to the following HD14. PRT of patients with early-stage unfavorable (by German criteria) Hodgkin's lymphoma randomized in 2 × 2 fashion to either ABVD × 4C or BEACOPP × 4C as well as 20 Gy IFRT or 30 Gy IFRT; 1,395 patients included, FFTF primary end point, updated MFU 106 months. BEACOPP + 20 Gy was initially more effective than ABVD + 20 Gy, but not confirmed on long-term follow-up. No difference in FFTF between BEACOPP + 30 Gy and ABVD + 30 Gy. Similarly, after BEACOPP, 20 Gy was noninferior to 30 Gy but after ABVD 20 Gy was not noninferior to 30 Gy (10-yr PFS difference −8.3%, 95% CI: −15.2 to −1.3%). **Conclusion: ABVD × 4C + 30 Gy is standard for early-stage unfavorable Hodgkin's lymphoma.**

von Tresckow, German HD14 (*JCO* 2012, PMID 22271480): Follow-up to the preceding trial. Prospective superiority trial of patients <60 years of age with early-stage unfavorable (by German criteria) randomized to either ABVD × 4C or BEACOPP × 2C followed by ABVD × 2C ("2 + 2" regimen). No PET. Both arms received 30 Gy IFRT following CHT. Primary end point FFTF; 1,528 patients, MFU 43 months. FFTF improved with "2 + 2" regimen (FFTF HR 0.44, $p < .001$); 5-year difference in PFS 6.2% (95.4%–89.1%, $p < .001$). No difference in OS. **Conclusion: In patients <60 years of age, escalated "2 + 2" + 30 Gy is standard German HSG treatment for early-stage unfavorable patients.**

Borchmann, German HD17 (*Lancet Oncol* **2021, PMID 33539742):** 1,100 patients with early unfavorable disease randomized to BEACOPP x2c + ABVD x2c with 30 Gy (standard arm) vs. the same chemotherapy with 30 Gy only for pts with positive c4 PET (defined negative as Deauville 1-2, positive defined as 3-5). 5-yr PFS primary endpoint designed as non-inferiority with 8% margin. Results: 68% in the PET arm were negative at c4 and omitted RT. 5-yr PFS 97.3% (standard) vs. 95.1% (PET4 arm, 95% CI -0.9% to 5.3%), meeting criteria for non-inferiority. **Conclusions: PET4-negativity allowed omission of RT, essentially exchanging BEACOPP escalation for RT in about 2/3 of patients.**

Raemaekers, EORTC H10 (*JCO* **2014, PMID 24637998; Update André** *JCO* **2017, PMID 28291393):** Patients with unfavorable early-stage disease underwent total of four cycles of ABVD + INRT on standard arm and either six cycles of ABVD for PET-negative patients (Deauville 1–2) or two cycles of ABVD, two cycles of BEACOPP, and INRT if PET-positive.

H10U stratum powered to detect PFS decrease from 90% to 80%. Similar to favorable group, if PET was negative, 5-year PFS was not noninferior in ABVD alone group (ABVD + INRT 92.1% vs. ABVD alone 89.6%, HR 1.45, 95% CI: 0.8–2.5, noninferiority margin was 2.1). As noted previously, if PET was positive, escalation to BEACOPP improved 5-year PFS from 77.4% (ABVD + INRT) to 90.6% (BEACOPP + INRT, $p = .002$). **Conclusion: In both early-stage favorable and unfavorable Hodgkin's lymphoma, omission of INRT is associated with increased risk of recurrence even after excellent PET response (but no difference in OS).**

ADVANCED-STAGE HODGKIN'S LYMPHOMA

■ **What trials define current standard of care in advanced Hodgkin's lymphoma?**

The following trials are commonly cited to define treatment. Note that some unfavorable stages I to II patients were included in these trials.

Engert, German HD15 (*Lancet* **2012, PMID 22480758):** Prospective randomized noninferiority trial of patients with advanced stage Hodgkin's lymphoma with goal of reducing intensity of treatment. "Advanced" defined as stages III to IV or stage IIB with either extranodal lesions or mediastinal mass >33% maximum thoracic diameter. Patients randomized into three arms: BEACOPP × 8C, BEACOPP × 6C, or BEACOPP-14 (given over 14 instead of 21 days) × 8C. Patients with residual mass of ≥2.5 cm or positive PET received 30 Gy; 2,126 patients included, MFU 48 months; 5-year FFTF 84.4% for standard BEACOPP × 8C, 89.3% for BEACOPP × 6C, and 85.4% for BEACOPP-14. Mortality higher in intensified standard arm of BEACOPP × 8C; 11% received RT. **Conclusions: Treatment with BEACOPP × 6C followed by PET-guided RT should be standard for advanced Hodgkin's. PET post-CHT can guide need for additional RT.**

Johnson, UK RATHL (*NEJM* **2016, PMID 27332902):** Prospective randomized noninferiority study of patients with advanced classic Hodgkin's. "Advanced" defined as stages IIB to IV or IIA with ≥3 involved sites or bulky disease (>33% of transthoracic diameter or in other sites >10 cm). Goal was to omit bleomycin in patients with good PET response. All patients received ABVD × 2C, then PET/CT. If Deauville 1 to 3, randomized to ABVD or AVD (no bleomycin), both for four additional cycles (total of 6). Patients with Deauville 4 to 5 received BEACOPP. Noninferiority margin was 5% in 3-year PFS; 1,214 patients enrolled, MFU 41 months; 83.7% of interim PET scans were negative (Deauville 1–3); 3-year PFS (primary endpoint) was 85.7% (ABVD) vs. 84.4% (AVD), absolute difference 1.6 (95% CI: −3.2%–5.3%); 32 patients received consolidation RT (2.6% ABVD vs. 4.3% AVD). Rate of pulmonary events were less in AVD group (3% vs. 1%, $p < .05$). **Conclusion: AVD is not noninferior but results remain excellent and bleomycin omission may be reasonable (as accepted by NCCN 2021).**

Gordon, ECOG E2496 (*JCO* **2013, PMID 23182987):** PRT to assess superiority of Stanford V over ABVD. Patients with classical Hodgkin's stages III to IV or stages I to II with bulky adenopathy (mass >33% maximum intrathoracic diameter on PA chest x-ray) randomized to either ABVD × 6–8C vs. Stanford V for 12 weeks. Primary end point FFS. RT administered to all patients with bulky mediastinal adenopathy. Mediastinum, bilateral hila, and supraclavicular areas treated to 36 Gy. For Stanford V patients, any pretreatment site >5 cm and macroscopic splenic disease also treated to 36 Gy. 794 patients randomized, MFU 6.4 years. No difference in 5-year FFS for ABVD vs. Stanford V: 74% vs.

71% (p = .32). Subset analysis demonstrated improved FFS in patients with IPS of 3 to 7. Toxicity overall was no different. **Conclusion: ABVD, with consolidation RT to sites of pretreatment bulky disease, remains standard of care for advanced and locally extensive Hodgkin's lymphoma for patients treated in North America.**

■ What evidence specifically addresses the role of consolidative RT in the modern era?

Multiple trials have investigated this question directly. Older meta-analysis and trials in MOPP era suggested no benefit.[33–35] More recent trials in the ABVD/BEACOPP era have suggested improvement.[36,37] Overall, it seems that consolidative RT to sites not responding on PET/CT, or RT to initially bulky sites may be of value, although this is controversial and institution dependent.

Borchmann, German HD12 (*JCO* 2011, PMID 21990399): 2 × 2 PRT of advanced Hodgkin's defined as either stage III to IV or stage IIB with bulk (≥33% of maximal thoracic diameter) or extranodal lesions randomized 2 × 2 to escalated BEACOPP × 8C vs. escalated BEACOPP × 4C followed by reduced BEACOPP × 4C ("2 + 2") and to either consolidation RT vs. no further therapy. RT was 30 Gy to initially bulky sites or sites with residual tumor ≥1.5 cm. PET not used to assess response; 1,670 patients, MFU 78 months; 66% to 72% of patients in RT arm received RT compared to 11% in no RT arms. RT improved 5-year FFTF (difference −3.4, 95% CI: −6.6% to −0.2%) and PFS (95% CI: −6.6% to −0.2%). **Conclusion: BEACOPP × 8 cycles remained standard, and results support use of consolidation RT.** *Comment: This trial was performed in the pre-PET era, which may influence treatment selection process.*

Gallamini, Italian HD0607 Analysis (*JCO* 2020, PMID 32946355): PRT with substudy randomizing 296 advanced (IIB–IVB) Hodgkin's patients with nodal mass ≥5 cm and negative PET (at cycle 2 and 6) to either consolidation RT or no treatment after six cycles of ABVD. Median dose 30.6 Gy. Results showed no change in PFS regardless of nodal size. **Conclusion: Consolidation RT may not be necessary in patients with negative cycle 2 and 6 PETs.**

■ Is bentuximab useful in the initial treatment of advanced Hodgkin's?

Connors, ECHELON1 (*NEJM* 2018, PMID 29224502): PRT of 1,334 patients with advanced Hodgkin's randomized to ABVD vs. brentuximab along with doxorubicin, vinblastine and dacarbazine; 2-year PFS 82% vs. 77% favoring brentuximab. Pulmonary toxicity less with brentuximab, but neuropathy worse. Cost favors ABVD. **Conclusion: Brentuximab with AVD is FDA approved for advanced Hodgkin's, but cost and toxicity profile limit applicability.**

RELAPSED/REFRACTORY HODGKIN'S LYMPHOMA

■ Is there a role for adjuvant RT in refractory patients undergoing autologous SCT?

This is controversial and is without significant modern data. Some authors recommend consolidation RT prior to SCT to induce response if CR is not obtained on PET or consolidation RT after SCT for bulky disease but this is informed by small retrospective series.[38,39] See ILROG guidelines for details.[40]

REFERENCES

1. NCCN Clinical Practice Guidelines in Oncology: Hodgkin Lymphoma. 4.2021. 2021. https://www.nccn.org
2. Siegel RL, Miller KD, Jemal A. Cancer statistics, 2020. *Cancer J Clin*. 2020;70:7–30. doi:10.3322/caac.21590
3. Hasenclever D, Diehl V, Armitage JO, et al. Prognostic score for advanced Hodgkin's disease. *N Engl J Med*. 1998;339(21):1506–1514. doi:10.1056/NEJM199811193392104
4. Moccia AA, Donaldson J, Chhanabhai M, et al. International prognostic score in advanced-stage hodgkin's lymphoma: altered utility in modern era. *J Clin Oncol*. 2012;30(27):3383–3388. doi:10.1200/JCO.2011.41.0910
5. Cheson BD, Fisher RI, Barrington SF, et al. Recommendations for initial evaluation, staging, and response assessment of Hodgkin and non-Hodgkin lymphoma: Lugano classification. *J Clin Oncol*. 2014;32(27):3059–3068. doi:10.1200/JCO.2013.54.8800
6. Mauz-Körholz C, Gorde-Grosjean S, Hasenclever D, et al. Resection alone in 58 children with limited stage, lymphocyte-predominant Hodgkin lymphoma-experience from European Network Group on Pediatric Hodgkin Lymphoma. *Cancer*. 2007;110(1):179–185. doi:10.1002/cncr.22762

7. Behringer K, Goergen H, Hitz F, et al. Omission of dacarbazine or bleomycin, or both, from ABVD regimen in treatment of early-stage favourable Hodgkin's lymphoma (GHSG HD13): open-label, randomised, non-inferiority trial. *Lancet.* 2015;385(9976):1418–1427. doi:10.1016/S0140-6736(14)61469-0

8. Gobbi PG, Levis A, Chisesi T, et al. ABVD versus modified Stanford v versus MOPPEBVCAD with optional and limited RT in intermediate- and advanced-stage Hodgkin's lymphoma: final results of Multicenter Randomized Trial by Intergruppo Italiano Linfomi. *J Clin Oncol.* 2005;23(36):9198–9207. doi:10.1200/JCO.2005.02.907

9. Hoskin PJ, Lowry L, Horwich A, et al. Randomized comparison of Stanford v regimen and ABVD in treatment of advanced Hodgkin's lymphoma: United Kingdom national cancer research institute lymphoma group study ISRCTN 64141244. *J Clin Oncol.* 2009;27(32):5390–5396. doi:10.1200/JCO.2009.23.3239

10. Chisesi T, Bellei M, Luminari S, et al. Long-term follow-up analysis of HD9601 trial comparing ABVD versus stanford v versus MOPP/EBV/CAD in patients with newly diagnosed advanced-stage Hodgkin's lymphoma: study from Intergruppo Italiano Linfomi. *J Clin Oncol.* 2011;29(32):4227–4233. doi:10.1200/JCO.2010.30.9799

11. Federico M, Luminari S, Iannitto E, et al. ABVD compared with BEACOPP compared with CEC for initial treatment of patients with advanced Hodgkin's lymphoma: results from HD2000 gruppo italiano per lo studio dei linfomi trial. *J Clin Oncol.* 2009;27(5):805–811. doi:10.1200/JCO.2008.17.0910

12. Armad P, Engert A, Younes A, et al. Nivolumab for relapsed/refractory classic hodgkin lymphoma after failure of autologous hematopoietic cell transplantation: extended follow-up of the multicohort single-arm phase II checkmate 205 trial. *J Clin Oncol.* 2018;36(14):1428 to 1439. doi:10.1200/JCO.2017.76.0793

13. Ansell SM, Lesokhin AM, Borrello I, et al. PD-1 blockade with nivolumab in relapsed or refractory Hodgkin's lymphoma. *N Engl J Med.* 2015;372(4):311 to 9. doi:10.1056/NEJMoa1411087

14. Zittoun R, Audebert A, Hoerni B, et al. Extended versus involved fields irradiation combined with MOPP chemotherapy in early clinical stages of Hodgkin's disease. *J Clin Oncol.* 1985;3(2):207–214. doi:10.1200/JCO.1985.3.2.207

15. Raemaekers J, Burgers M, Henry-Amar M, et al. Patients with stage III/IV Hodgkin's disease in partial remission after MOPP/ABV chemotherapy have excellent prognosis after additional involved-field radiotherapy: interim results from ongoing EORTC-LCG and GPMC phase III trial. *Ann Oncol.* 1997;8(suppl 1):S111–S114. doi:10.1093/annonc/8.suppl_1.S111

16. Noordijk E, Carde P, Mandard A-M, et al. Preliminary results of EORTC-GPMC controlled clinical trial H7 in early-stage Hodgkin's disease. *Ann Oncol.* 1994;5(suppl 2):S107–S112. doi:10.1093/annonc/5.suppl_2.S107

17. Somers R, Carde P, Henry-Amar M, et al. Randomized study in stage IIIB and IV Hodgkin's disease comparing eight courses of MOPP with alteration of MOPP with ABVD: European organization for research and treatment of cancer lymphoma cooperative group and groupe pierre-et-marie-Curie controlled clinical trial. *J Clin Oncol.* 1994;12(2):279–287. doi:10.1200/JCO.1994.12.2.279

18. Gallamini A, Fiore F, Sorasio R, Meignan M. Interim positron emission tomography scan in Hodgkin lymphoma: definitions, interpretation rules, and clinical validation. *Leuk Lymphoma.* 2009;50(11):1761–1764. doi:10.3109/10428190903308072

19. Meignan M, Gallamini A, Meignan M, et al. Report on first international workshop on interim-PET scan in lymphoma. *Leuk Lymphoma.* 2009;50(8):1257–1260. doi:10.1080/10428190903040048

20. Parikh RR, Grossbard ML, Harrison LB, Yahalom J. Early-stage classic Hodgkin lymphoma: utilization of RT therapy and its impact on overall survival. *Int J Radiat Oncol Biol Phys.* 2015;93(3):684–693. doi:10.1016/j.ijrobp.2015.07.195

21. Specht L, Yahalom J, Illidge T, et al. Modern RT therapy for Hodgkin lymphoma: field and dose guidelines from international lymphoma radiation oncology group (ILROG). *Int J Radiat Oncol Biol Phys.* 2014;89(4):854–862. doi:10.1016/j.ijrobp.2013.05.005

22. Campbell BA, Voss N, Pickles T, et al. Involved-nodal RT therapy as component of combination therapy for limited-stage Hodgkin's lymphoma: question of field size. *J Clin Oncol.* 2008;26(32):5170–5174. doi:10.1200/JCO.2007.15.1001

23. Aleman BM, van den Belt-Dusebout AW, Klokman WJ, et al. Long-term cause-specific mortality of patients treated for Hodgkin's disease. *J Clin Oncol.* 2003;21(18):3431–3439. doi:10.1200/JCO.2003.07.131

24. Videtic GMM, Woody N, Vassil AD. "Lymphoma and myeloma radiotherapy." *Handbook of Treatment Planning in RT Oncology.* 3rd ed. Demos Medical; 2020:187.

25. Dühmke E, Franklin J, Pfreundschuh M, et al. Low-dose RT is sufficient for noninvolved extended-field treatment in favorable early-stage Hodgkin's disease: long-term results of randomized trial of RT alone. *J Clin Oncol.* 2001;19(11):2905–2914. doi:10.1200/JCO.2001.19.11.2905

26. Sasse S, Bröckelmann PJ, Goergen H, et al. Long-term follow-up of contemporary treatment in early-stage Hodgkin lymphoma: updated analyses of German Hodgkin study group HD7, HD8, HD10, and HD11 trials. *J Clin Oncol.* 2017;35(18):1999–2007. doi:10.1200/JCO.2016.70.9410

27. Noordijk EM, Carde P, Dupouy N, et al. Combined-modality therapy for clinical stage I or II Hodgkin's lymphoma: long-term results of European organisation for research and treatment of cancer H7 randomized controlled trials. *J Clin Oncol.* 2006;24(19):3128–3135. doi:10.1200/JCO.2005.05.2746

28. Fermé C, Eghbali H, Meerwaldt JH, et al. Chemotherapy plus involved-field radiotherapy in early-stage Hodgkin's disease. *N Engl J Med.* 2007;357(19):1916–1927. doi:10.1056/NEJMoa064601

29. Zittoun R, Audebert A, Hoerni B, et al. Extended versus involved fields irradiation combined with MOPP chemotherapy in early clinical stages of Hodgkin's disease. *J Clin Oncol.* 1985;3(2):207–214. doi:10.1200/JCO.1985.3.2.207

30. Hoskin PJ, Smith P, Maughan TS, et al. Long-term results of a randomised trial of involved field radiotherapy vs extended field radiotherapy in stage I and II Hodgkin lymphoma. *Clin Oncol (R Coll Radiol)*. 2005;17(1):47–53. doi:10.1016/j.clon.2004.07.004

31. Engert A, Schiller P, Josting A, et al. Involved-field radiotherapy is equally effective and less toxic compared with extended-field RT after four cycles of CHT in patients with early-stage unfavorable Hodgkin's lymphoma: results of HD8 trial of German Hodgkin's lymphoma study group. *J Clin Oncol*. 2003;21(19):3601–3608. doi:10.1200/JCO.2003.03.023

32. Arakelyan N, Jais JP, Delwail V, et al. Reduced versus full doses of irradiation after 3 cycles of combined doxorubicin, bleomycin, vinblastine, and dacarbazine in early stage Hodgkin lymphomas: results of randomized trial. *Cancer*. 2010;116(17):4054–4062. doi:10.1002/cncr.25295

33. Loeffler M, Brosteanu O, Hasenclever D, et al. Meta-analysis of chemotherapy versus combined modality treatment trials in Hodgkin's disease. International database on Hodgkin's disease overview study group. *J Clin Oncol*. 1998;16(3):818–829. doi:10.1200/JCO.1998.16.3.818

34. Aleman BM, Raemaekers JM, Tomisic R, et al. Involved-field RT for patients in partial remission after CHT for advanced Hodgkin's lymphoma. *Int J Radiat Oncol Biol Phys*. 2007;67(1):19–30. doi:10.1016/j.ijrobp.2006.08.041

35. Aleman BM, Raemaekers JM, Tirelli U, et al. Involved-field RT for advanced Hodgkin's lymphoma. *N Engl J Med*. 2003;348(24):2396–2406. doi:10.1056/NEJMoa022628

36. Laskar S, Gupta T, Vimal S, et al. Consolidation RT after complete remission in Hodgkin's disease following six cycles of doxorubicin, bleomycin, vinblastine, and dacarbazine chemotherapy: is there need? *J Clin Oncol*. 2004;22(1):62–68. doi:10.1200/JCO.2004.01.021

37. Borchmann P, Haverkamp H, Diehl V, et al. Eight cycles of escalated-dose BEACOPP compared with four cycles of escalated-dose BEACOPP followed by four cycles of baseline-dose BEACOPP with or without RT in patients with advanced-stage Hodgkin's lymphoma: final analysis of HD12 trial of German Hodgkin Study Group. *J Clin Oncol*. 2011;29(32):4234–4242. doi:10.1200/JCO.2010.33.9549

38. Poen JC, Hoppe RT, Horning SJ. High-dose therapy and autologous bone marrow transplantation for relapsed/refractory Hodgkin's disease: impact of involved field RT on patterns of failure and survival. *Int J Radiat Oncol Biol Phys*. 1996;36(1):3–12. doi:10.1016/S0360-3016(96)00277-5

39. Mundt AJ, Sibley G, Williams S, et al. Patterns of failure following high-dose CHT and autologous bone marrow transplantation with involved field RT for relapsed/refractory Hodgkin's disease. *Int J Radiat Oncol Biol Phys*. 1995;33(2):261–270. doi:10.1016/0360-3016(95)00180-7

40. Constine LS, Yahalom J, Ng AK, et al. The role of radiation therapy in patients with relapsed or refractory Hodgkin lymphoma: guidelines from the international lymphoma radiation oncology group. *Int J Radiat Oncol Biol Phys*. 2018;100(5):1000 to 1008. doi:10.1016/j.ijrobp.2018.01.011

James R. Broughman, Matthew C. Ward, and Chirag Shah

QUICK HIT ■ NHL is a heterogeneous disease. Aggressive NHL is a loosely defined group of B- and T-cell histologies with survival measured in months for those untreated. T-cell histologies are aggressive but uncommon. Multiagent CHT is indicated in almost all cases of aggressive NHL. DLBCL is the most common aggressive NHL and the subject of the majority of clinical data. Limited-stage DLBCL is typically treated with R-CHOP for either three cycles followed by ISRT to 30 to 36 Gy or R-CHOP for six cycles (Table 52.1). After six to eight cycles, the role for consolidative RT is controversial in the setting of a CR. Advanced-stage DLBCL can be treated with R-CHOP for six to eight cycles with consideration of consolidation RT. When selecting for consolidative RT, risk factors such as bulk (≥7.5 cm), skeletal involvement, inability to tolerate full CHT, residual disease after CHT on PET/CT, and perhaps genetic factors can be considered, although no clear standard exists. Relapsed or refractory DLBCL is typically managed with salvage chemoimmunotherapy followed by autologous stem cell transplant. Further relapse may be managed with CAR-T cell therapy or allogeneic stem cell transplant.

TABLE 52.1 General Overview of Treatment Paradigm for DLBCL	
Limited (Stage I–II)	R-CHOP × 3 cycles followed by 30–36 Gy for CR 40–50 Gy for PR or R-CHOP × 6–8 cycles
Advanced (Stages III–IV)	R-CHOP × 6–8 cycles ± ISRT 30–36 Gy
Relapsed/Refractory	High-dose CHT + autologous SCT ± RT pre- or posttransplant

EPIDEMIOLOGY: There are 77,240 cases of NHL expected in the United States in 2020, and 19,940 deaths with an incidence of approximately 1 in 50.[1] NHL is the seventh most common noncutaneous cancer and ninth most common cause of death. It is slightly more common in males (lifetime risk 1.26:1). Approximately 50% to 60% of NHLs are classified as aggressive. Most common NHLs are DLBCL (29%), follicular (26%), SLL/CLL (7%), MZL/MALT (9%), mantle cell (8%), MZL/nodal (3%), primary mediastinal DLBCL (2%) among others.[2,3] Aggressive NHL is more common in low–middle-income countries.

RISK FACTORS: NHL is a heterogeneous disease with a multitude of risk factors. Risk factors for any NHL[4]: older age, race, family history,[5] geographic region,[3] *viral infection* (EBV [NK-T-cell, Burkitt], HTLV-1, HHV8 [Kaposi sarcoma and various lymphomas in HIV+], hepatitis C [DLBCL and splenic MZL]), *bacterial infection* (*Helicobacter pylori* [gastric MALT], Chlamydia psittaci [orbital MALT], Borrelia burgdorferi [tick bite, mantle cell],[6] Campylobacter jejuni [intestinal MALT]), *autoimmune disease* (rheumatoid arthritis, Sjögren's syndrome, lupus), *immune suppression* (HIV, organ transplant), *medication* (immunosuppressants, alkylating agents), *chemicals* (hair dye, pesticides), previous CLL/hairy cell leukemia (Richter's transformation into DLBCL in 5%–10%).

ANATOMY: Thirteen individual nodal groups identified in 1965 now define staging and include: Waldeyer's ring, cervical/SCV/occipital/preauricular, infraclavicular, axillary/pectoral, mediastinal, hilar, para-aortic, spleen, mesenteric, iliac, inguinal/femoral, popliteal, and epitrochlear/brachial. Waldeyer's ring and the spleen are considered lymphatic but extranodal regions for staging purposes.

PATHOLOGY: NHL includes cancers originating from cells that normally differentiate into T or B lymphocytes, whether originating from the bone marrow or peripheral nodal tissues. Approximately 85% to 90% of NHLs derive from B-cell origins.[4] In contrast, leukemias derive from cells that differentiate into erythrocytes, monocytes, or granulocytes. Originally, it was thought that leukemia arose from the bone marrow and lymphoma from a mass lesion. Today, cell lineage, morphology, genetics, and immunotyping classify leukemia and lymphomas. Over 60 types of NHL are identified in the WHO 2016 classification, which does not attempt to differentiate into aggressive/indolent due to variable clinical behavior.[7] Many treat grade 3B follicular lymphoma similar to DLBCL.

GENETICS: See Table 52.2.

TABLE 52.2 Common Translocations, Immunotype, and Clinical Pearls for Select "Aggressive" Non-Hodgkin's Lymphomas

Histology		Classic Genetics and Implications	Classic Immunotype	Pearls
B-cell	DLBCL	t(14:18), BCL-2, BLC-6, ALK, many others	CD19+, CD20+, CD45+	Most common NHL. WHO 2016 subtypes: EBV+, germinal center, activated, primary cutaneous, ALK+, HHV8+, "double hit" (rearrangements of MYC and BCL2 or BCL6). Rare "triple-hit" subtype (MYC, BCL2 and BCL6) associated with dismal prognosis. Gray zone lymphoma is intermediate between DLBCL and Hodgkin's
	Primary mediastinal (thymic) DLBCL	No classic translocations	CD19+, CD20+, CD5−	Anterior mediastinal (thymic) mass most common in young women. Treatment different than DLBCL
	Mantle cell	t(11:14), cyclin D1	CD19+, CD20+, CD5+	Older age and advanced stage more common. Radiosensitive
	Burkitt	t(8:14) → C-MYC [transcription factor]	CD19+, CD20+, CD5−, CD10+	Classic "starry sky" appearance. Most common NHL in children, endemic type in Africa (jaw, EBV+). Also nonendemic (abdomen, visceral organs) and immune-deficient types
	Follicular, grade 3B	Grade 3B genetically distinct from grades 1–3A	CD19+, CD20+	High-grade FL (especially grade 3B) is often treated per DLBCL paradigm (grades 1–3A managed as per low-grade NHL paradigm)
T-cell	Peripheral T-cell, NOS (PTCL)	t(7:14), t(11:14) or t(14:14)	Variable T-cell (±CD 2, 3, 4, 5, 7)	Most common peripheral T-cell, older adults
	Anaplastic large cell	t(2:5) → ALK	CD30+, EMA+	More common in kids, good prognosis with ALK+. T-cell neoplasm
	Angioimmunoblastic	No classic translocations	CD4+	Older adults
	Extranodal NK-T-cell, nasal type	LOH 6q	CD2+, CD56+	More common in Asian males. EBV+ (EBER by FISH)
Either	Lymphoblastic lymphoma/ Leukemia	t(1:19), t(9:22)	TdT+	Nodal presentation of ALL and treated similarly. Can be T- or B-cell presentation

CLINICAL PRESENTATION: Most commonly presents with a painless enlarging LN. B symptoms (fever >38 °C, drenching night sweats, weight loss >10% in 6 months) or numerous other symptoms may be present (fatigue, anemia, pain, cord compression, SVC syndrome, etc.) depending on location and degree of involvement.

WORKUP: H&P with attention to constitutional symptoms (B symptoms), enlarged LNs, or hepatosplenomegaly.

Labs: CBC, CMP, β2 microglobulin, LDH, uric acid, hepatitis B testing (reactivation with rituximab), pregnancy test. Lumbar puncture with flow cytometry if symptomatic, testicular, double hit, HIV-associated, or epidural lymphoma (see CNS prognostic model for risk factors).[8]

Imaging: PET/CT is standard in almost all lymphoma histologies except certain low-grade histologies (extranodal MZL and SLL).[9–11] Uptake (SUV >10) in indolent lymphoma suggests transformation.[12,13] CT with contrast should also be obtained. Echocardiogram or MUGA if CHT dictates. EBV viral load for extranodal NK/T-cell, nasal type.

Biopsy: At least a core needle biopsy but preferably excisional biopsy should be performed for adequate pathologic evaluation including morphology, nodal architecture, genomic profiling and immuno-profiling. FNA is insufficient. A negative PET is usually sufficient at ruling out bone marrow involvement of DLBCL.[14,15] Bone marrow biopsy remains standard for most other NHLs (~20% risk of BM involvement for aggressive NHL vs. 50%–80% of indolent NHLs).

PROGNOSTIC FACTORS: Age, bulk (classically defined as ≥10 cm or >1/3 thoracic diameter, but more recently defined as ≥7.5 cm) and stage (see Table 52.5). Germinal center subtype more favorable than nongerminal center as defined by tissue microarray (combination of CD10, BCL6, and MUM1).[16] Multiple prognostic models exist for patients with aggressive NHL treated with CHT (Tables 52.3 and 52.4). The IPI[17] is classic (mnemonic "LEAPS": **L**DH, **e**xtranodal sites, **a**ge, **p**erformance status, and **s**tage). While the original IPI remains standard, modified indices such as the age-adjusted IPI, stage-adjusted IPI, and NCCN-IPI may have improved prognostic utility. Mantle cell may be best classified using the MIPI.[18] The Deauville (five-point) score is used to interpret PET scans and is prognostic, particularly at the end of treatment. This consists of five levels. Level 1 includes no uptake above background; level 2 is uptake less than or equal to mediastinal blood pool; level 3 is uptake above mediastinal blood pool but less than or equal to liver uptake; level 4 is uptake moderately above liver; and level 5 is uptake markedly greater than liver or new lesions.[19]

NATURAL HISTORY: Aggressive lymphoma, loosely defined, includes cancers with survival measured in months if untreated, as compared to indolent lymphoma, with survival measured in years. Compared to Hodgkin's disease, the pattern of spread is less predictable and can skip nodal levels/sites.

TABLE 52.3 Classic IPI Prognostic System (1993[17]) and NCCN-IPI (2014[20]) for Aggressive Non-Hodgkin's Lymphoma

	IPI		Age-Adjusted IPI		NCCN-IPI	
	Factor	*Score*	*Factor*	*Score*	*Factor*	*Score*
Age	>60	1	N/A	1	>40 to ≤60 >60 to <75 ≥75	1 2 3
LDH	High	1	High	1	>1× ULN but ≤3× ULN >3× ULN	1 2
Extranodal sites	≥2	1	N/A	1	Bone marrow, CNS, liver/GI tract, lung	1
Performance status (ECOG)	≥2	1	≥2	1	≥2	1
Stage (Ann Arbor)	III–IV	1	III–IV	1	I–II vs. III–IV	1

TABLE 52.4 Aggressive Non-Hodgkin's Lymphoma Outcome by IPI Score (See Table 52.3 for Risk Factors)													
Risk group	Original IPI (Prerituximab)[17]			Age-Adjusted IPI[17]				IPI in Rituximab Era[21]			NCCN-IPI[20]		
	Score	5-Yr OS	5-Yr RFS	Score	5-Yr OS (≤60 y/o)	5-Yr OS (>60 y/o)	5-Yr RFS	Score	3-Yr OS	3-Yr PFS	Score	5-Yr OS	5-Yr PFS
Low	0–1	73%	70%	0	83%	56%	86%	0–1	91%	87%	0–1	96%	91%
Low–intermediate	2	51%	50%	1	69%	44%	66%	2	81%	75%	2–3	82%	74%
High–intermediate	3	43%	49%	2	46%	37%	53%	3	65%	59%	4–5	64%	51%
High	4–5	26%	40%	3	32%	21%	58%	4–5	59%	56%	≥6	33%	30%

STAGING

TABLE 52.5 Ann Arbor (Lugano) Staging System for Lymphoma**		
I	One node or a group of adjacent nodes OR single extranodal lesions without nodal involvement (IE)	**A:** No systemic symptoms
II	≥2 nodal groups on the same side of the diaphragm OR stage I or II by nodal extent with limited contiguous extranodal involvement	**B:** Unexplained weight loss >10% in 6 mos before diagnosis. Unexplained fever with temperatures above 38 °C. Drenching night sweats
III	Nodes on both sides of the diaphragm; nodes above the diaphragm with spleen involvement	**E*:** Extranodal involvement
IV	Additional noncontiguous extralymphatic involvement	**X*:** Bulky disease (*Hodgkin's: >10 cm or mediastinal mass more than one third the maximum thoracic diameter at T5–6 on PA CXR*)

*Note that 2014 Lugano update suggests "X" and "A/B" modifiers are no longer necessary for NHL, and "E" is unnecessary for stages III–IV disease.[22]
**Number of involved regions may be designated with a subscript (i.e., II$_3$).

TREATMENT PARADIGM

Observation: Unlike indolent lymphomas, there is generally no role for observation of aggressive lymphomas. Notable exceptions may be mantle cell with a low tumor burden.[23]

Surgery: Generally the role for surgery is limited to excisional biopsy.

Chemotherapy: CHT is the backbone of treatment for NHL. See Table 52.6 for regimens. Rituximab is an anti-CD20 antibody consistently demonstrated in the early 2000s to improve 5-year OS for DLBCL by approximately 10% with minimal increase in toxicity.[24–26] R-CHOP: rituximab, cyclophosphamide, doxorubicin, vincristine, and prednisone, often given q21 days for six cycles. R-EPOCH consists of the same agents as R-CHOP but with etoposide and overall, across subtypes of DLBCL, did not demonstrate a benefit compared to R-CHOP in the CALGB/Alliance 50303 trial (although it is still an option in other subtypes, for example, primary mediastinal DLBCL or double-hit DLBCL). Consolidation with autologous SCT is not routinely recommended for DLBCL but can be considered for "double-hit" type.[27] CNS prophylaxis can be delivered to high-risk patients via systemic MTX, intrathecal MTX, or cytarabine.[8,9]

TABLE 52.6 Example Regimens for Aggressive Non-Hodgkin's Lymphoma		
Diagnosis	**Common/Example CHT Regimens**	**Notes**
DLBCL, germinal center type	R-CHOP × 6C ± RT	Good outcomes with standard R-CHOP
	R-CHOP × 3C + RT	
DLBCL, activated B-cell type	R-CHOP × 6-8C ± RT	Studies suggest inferior outcomes with standard R-CHOP, some intensify CHT
	R-ACVBP + MTX/Leukovorin[28]	
	R-CHOP + Lenalidomide[29]	
DLBCL, "double-hit" (MYC and BCL2 or BCL6) or "triple-hit" (MYC, BCL2, and BCL6)	R-EPOCH	Outcomes with standard R-CHOP are inferior, consider CNS prophylaxis or autologous SCT
	R-Hyper-CVAD	
DLBCL, transformed follicular	R-CHOP × 6C ± RT	Diagnosis: biopsy regions of PET SUV >10[13]
Follicular, grade 3B	R-CHOP ± RT	Per DLBCL paradigm
Primary mediastinal DLBCL	R-EPOCH × 6C ± RT[30]	
	R-CHOP × 6C + RT	
Mantle cell	R-CHOP + autologous SCT[31]	
	R-Hyper-CVAD/Cytarabine/MTX[32]	
	R-CHOP + RT	Select stages I–II patients
	R-CHOP	Not curative
	Bendamustine + rituximab	
	Many others	
Burkitt	CODOX-M[33]	
	CALGB regimen[34]	
	R-EPOCH[35]	
	Hyper-CVAD[36]	
Extranodal NK-T-cell, nasal type	SMILE + RT[37]	
	DeVIC + Concurrent RT[38]	
	GELOX + Sandwhich RT[39]	

Radiation

Indications: The role for RT in aggressive NHL is either for consolidation or for palliation. For select patients unable to receive CHT or in early-stage mantle cell lymphoma, definitive RT may be appropriate. RT decisions should be based on the CHT regimen chosen and response to induction therapy. Historical technique was IFRT; modern technique is now ISRT (when treated after CHT). ILROG guidelines delineate the technique for ISRT.[40] See Table 52.7 for RT dosing.

Dose

TABLE 52.7 NCCN RT Dose Guidelines for Aggressive Non-Hodgkin's Lymphoma[9,10]		
Mantle cell, stage I–II	RT alone	30–36 Gy
DLBCL*	Consolidation after CR	30–36 Gy
	Consolidation after PR	40–50 Gy
	Primary treatment (nonchemo candidate)	40–55 Gy
	Combined with SCT	20–36 Gy

(continued)

TABLE 52.7 NCCN RT Dose Guidelines for Aggressive Non-Hodgkin's Lymphoma[9,10] (*continued*)		
	Scrotal RT after CHT	25–30 Gy
Peripheral T-cell lymphoma	Consolidation	30–40 Gy
Extranodal NK-T-cell, nasal type	Concurrent with DeVIC	50 Gy
	Sequential after SMILE	45–50.4 Gy
	After GELOX	56 Gy
	RT alone	≥50 Gy

*Note that grade 3B follicular lymphoma is often managed according to DLBCL paradigm.
Source: From National Comprehensive Cancer Network. *NCCN Clinical Practice Guidelines in Oncology: B-Cell Lymphomas*; 2020. https://www.nccn.org; National Comprehensive Cancer Network. *NCCN Clinical Practice Guidelines in Oncology: T-Cell Lymphomas*; 2020. https://www.nccn.org

Toxicity: Acute: Fatigue, skin erythema, other sequelae are site-dependent. Late: Site-dependent but includes second malignancy, xerostomia, fibrosis, cardiotoxicity, and so on.

Procedure: See *Handbook of Treatment Planning in Radiation Oncology*, Chapter 10.[41]

■ **EVIDENCE-BASED Q&A**

■ **Historically, what data exist regarding the role of RT in DLBCL?**

Three cooperative groups (SWOG, ECOG, French GELA) investigated the role of consolidative IFRT after CHT with variable results in the prerituximab era. RT was effective at reducing in-field relapses but only improved OS in the initial results of one trial (SWOG), though these studies used higher doses and older RT techniques. Overall, it appears that less intense CHT with RT is comparable to intensive CHT alone. Toxicity is significant with intense CHT; therefore combined-modality treatment may be ideal for some patients.

Miller, SWOG 8736 (*NEJM* 1998, PMID 9647875, Update Stephens *JCO* 2016, PMID 27382104): PRT of 401 patients with localized intermediate- or high-grade NHL stage I, IE (including bulky, defined as ≥10 cm or >1/3 maximal chest diameter), nonbulky stage II or IIE disease were randomized to CHOP × 8C vs. CHOP × 3C followed by IFRT to 40 to 55 Gy. IFRT targeted any involved location pre-CHT. MFU 4.4 years. RT improved 5-year PFS (77% vs. 64%, *p* = .03) and OS (82% vs. 72%, *p* = .02) as compared to CHT alone with less life-threatening toxicity. Long-term follow-up of a subset of original population (MFU 17.7 years) suggested continuous treatment failure despite RT in patients receiving limited CHT. **Conclusion: Combined-modality treatment is superior to CHOP alone and less toxic although with long-term follow-up, this did not persist.**

Horning, ECOG 1484 (*JCO* 2004, PMID 15210738): PRT of 352 patients with early-stage diffuse aggressive lymphoma. Stage I with mediastinal or retroperitoneal involvement, bulky disease >10 cm, stage IE, II, or IIE included. Treatment was CHOP × 8C and then restaging by CT. PR received 40 Gy IFRT. Patients with CR randomized to observation vs. 30 Gy IFRT. MFU 12 years; 61% had CR; 31% of PR patients had CR after IFRT. See Table 52.8. **Conclusion: IFRT improved DFS but not OS.** *Comment: Powered for 20% OS difference.*

TABLE 52.8 Results of ECOG 1484 Non-Hodgkin's Lymphoma		
ECOG 1484	**6-Yr DFS**	**6-Yr OS**
CHOP × 8 → PR → RT	63%	69%
CHOP × 8 → CR → Obs	53%	67%
CHOP × 8 → CR → RT	69%	79%
p value	.05	.23

Reyes, GELA LNH 93-1 (*NEJM* 2005, PMID 15788496): PRT of 647 patients <61 years of age with localized stages I to IIE aggressive lymphoma and no IPI risk factors randomized to CHOP × 3C + IFRT vs. ACVBP alone (doxorubicin, cyclophosphamide, vindesine, bleomycin, prednisone) with MTX, etoposide, ifosfamide, and cytarabine consolidation. IFRT was 40 Gy/22 fx. MFU 7.7 years. ACVBP improved 5-year EFS (82% vs. 74%, p < .001) and OS (90% vs. 81%, p = .001). Grades 3 to 4 toxicity worse in the ACVBP arm (12% vs. 1%). Initial site relapse more common in ACVBP arm (41% vs. 23%) but out-of-field relapse more common in CHOP arm (72% vs. 38%). **Conclusion: In young patients, intensive CHT alone is superior to CHOP + IFRT. ACVBP is not a standard regimen in the United States.**

Bonnet, GELA LNH 93-4 (*JCO* 2007, PMID 17228021): PRT of 576 patients >60 years of age with localized stage I to IIE aggressive NHL and no IPI risk factors randomized to CHOP × 4C ± IFRT to 40 Gy. MFU 7 years. CR (89% vs. 91%), 5-year EFS (61% vs. 64%), 5-year OS (72% vs. 68%, p = .5) were no different with the addition of RT. **Conclusion: For older patients with favorable risk factors, CHOP alone appears adequate.**

■ **What was the impact of rituximab on outcomes with chemotherapy alone?**

The preceding historical trials were performed in the prerituximab era. The introduction of rituximab in the early 2000s markedly improved outcomes above CHOP alone, with approximately a 10% improvement in OS at 5 years.[24-26,42] Therefore, many argue consolidation with RT is unnecessary, though there is no level I evidence to support this conclusion at this time.

■ **How many cycles of R-CHOP are necessary for DLBCL?**

Trials performed either six or eight cycles for DLBCL given every 21 days. The RICOVER-60 trial directly addressed this question.

Pfreundschuh, RICOVER-60 (*Lancet Oncol* 2008, PMID 18226581): PRT of 1,222 patients, 61 to 80 years of age with aggressive B-cell lymphoma; 2 × 2 randomization: CHOP vs. R-CHOP and six vs. eight cycles (both q14 days, rather than conventional q21 days). IFRT to 36 Gy was recommended to sites initially ≥7.5 cm (bulky) or extranodal sites regardless of response. R-CHOP improved DFS and OS, but no difference between six vs. eight cycles. **Conclusion: Six cycles of R-CHOP is the preferred regimen for older adult patients.**

■ **Is consolidative RT necessary for early-stage DLBCL in the rituximab era?**

This is a controversial question and use of RT has been declining.[43] There may be some patients who benefit, but no high-quality data exist to guide decisions. The following retrospective and nonrandomized data support the role of RT. This includes at least three large databases (NCDB, SEER, NCCN) and multiple retrospective reviews.[43-50] Of note, the German UNFOLDER trial randomizing bulky or ENE patients to either RT or no RT closed its two arms omitting RT early due to inferior EFS.[51,52] It is likely that a subset of patients with DLBCL benefit from RT, although this has not been clearly defined. Risk factors such as bulk, skeletal involvement, inability to tolerate full CHT, residual disease after CHT on PET/CT, and perhaps genetic factors can be considered.[52]

Held, RICOVER-60 NoRTh (*JCO* 2014, PMID 24493716): After the completion of the RICOVER-60 trial, the protocol was amended and another 166 patients were accrued to the best arm of the RICOVER-60 trial (R-CHOP × 6C q14 days) but omitting RT. The arm from the original trial (RT arm) was compared to the no-RT cohort. MFU 39 months. MVA in the per-protocol population demonstrated worse EFS, PFS, and OS in those with bulky disease not treated with RT. **Conclusion: RT should be used in all patients with bulky disease, until PET-directed omission studies are completed. Further randomized trials are necessary.**

Held, German Pooled Analysis (*JCO* 2013, PMID 24062391): Pooled analysis of data from nine randomized trials including 3,840 patients with aggressive B-cell lymphoma; 7.6% had skeletal involvement. Skeletal involvement was associated with worse EFS after R-CHOP (EFS HR 1.5, p = .048).

Rituximab was not found to improve outcome for patients with skeletal involvement. RT did improve EFS for patients with skeletal involvement (EFS HR 0.3, p = .001; OS HR 0.5, p = .111). **Conclusion: RT may benefit those with skeletal involvement.**

Lamy, 02-03 Lysa/Goelams Group (*Blood* **2018, PMID: 29061568**): Patients with nonbulky (<7 cm) stage I–II DLBCL treated with R-CHOP for 4C (IPI of 0) or 6C (IPI >0) and then randomized to 40 Gy IFRT or observation. Patients with PR (PET-assessed) after 4C received 6C total and RT. At a median follow-up of 64 months, ITT analysis showed no difference in primary end point 5-year EFS (89% no RT vs. 92% with RT; p = .18). **Conclusion: Among patients with nonbulky stage I to II DLBCL who achieve CR after R-CHOP × 4–6C, observation is noninferior to consolidative RT.**

▪ Is there a role for consolidative RT for advanced-stage DLBCL?

This is also a controversial question with less data available. NCCN suggests R-CHOP for six cycles and if CR is confirmed on PET, to consider RT to initially bulky sites or areas of skeletal involvement. RICOVER-60 probably provides the best data for this, as it included all stages (60% in the no-RT cohort were stage III–IV). Retrospective data from MD Anderson,[53] Duke,[46] and observational data from the NCCN database also suggest a benefit.[50]

▪ What is the optimal radiation dose?

Classic trials often used doses >40 Gy, but modern doses are lower.

Lowry, UK (*Radiother Oncol* **2011, PMID 21664710**): PRT with any histologic subtype of NHL requiring RT for local control; 640 sites were randomized to either high-dose RT to 40–45 Gy/20–23 fx vs. low-dose RT (30 Gy/15 fx for aggressive histologies and 24 Gy/12 fx for indolent histologies). MFU 5.6 years. No difference in response rates, in-field progression, PFS, or OS. Toxicity was reduced (but not SS) in the low-dose arm. **Conclusion: 24 Gy and 30 Gy are sufficient for indolent and aggressive NHL, respectively.**

▪ How should response to treatment be evaluated for patients with NHL? Is interim PET predictive of outcome?

The updated Lugano classification[22] (named after Lugano, Switzerland, where the conference took place) defines both staging and response assessment. See the manuscript for details, but in brief, a CR should be defined as Deauville 1 to 3, without new lesions, no abnormal bone marrow uptake, regression of the nodal size to $\leq$1.5 cm in longest diameter, and no organomegaly. A Deauville 3 is usually sufficient but may be considered abnormal if reduced-intensity CHT is used. Of note, a midtreatment PET is not clearly predictive of outcome (as opposed to Hodgkin's), and it is not recommended that therapy be altered due to the midtreatment PET.[54]

▪ How is primary mediastinal DLBCL managed?

Primary mediastinal DLBCL is a different entity than other forms of DLBCL and has a natural history between NHL and Hodgkin's disease. It should be managed with either R-EPOCH CHT for six to eight cycles or R-CHOP for six cycles with RT.[9,30] There are minimal data investigating the omission of RT in these patients. Like Hodgkin's, midtreatment PET/CT is prognostic.[55]

▪ How is primary cutaneous B-cell lymphoma leg type managed?

PCLBCL leg type is a rare and highly aggressive form of cutaneous lymphoma and typically presents with nodules on one or both legs, though 10% to 15% may present outside of the lower extremities. Typical management for limited-stage disease includes R-CHOP × 3 to 6 cycles followed by 30 to 36 Gy for CR or 40 to 45 Gy for PR.

▪ How is testicular DLBCL managed?

Primary testicular DLBCL is an uncommon disease comprising just 1% to 2% of NHL cases. Though most patients present with early-stage disease, outcomes are generally poor. Relapse in extranodal sites including the CNS and contralateral testis remains a clinical challenge. The current treatment paradigm defined by the phase

II IELSG-10 trial consists of orchiectomy, R-CHOP, CNS prophylaxis, and prophylactic RT to the contralateral testis.[56] No testicular relapses were observed on trial. RT typically consists of 30 Gy to the entire scrotum.

How is primary bone DLBCL managed?

Primary lymphoma of the bone accounts for <2% of adult lymphomas and the vast majority are DLBCL of the germinal center subtype. Treatment historically consisted of multiagent CHT followed by RT, though the role of RT in the rituximab era is less clear. Typical management for limited-stage disease includes R-CHOP × 3 to 6 cycles followed by 30 to 36 Gy for CR or 40 to 45 Gy for PR.

REFERENCES

1. Siegel RL, Miller KD, Jemal A. Cancer statistics, 2020. *CA Cancer J Clin.* 2020;70(1):7–30. doi:10.3322/caac.21590
2. Armitage JO, Weisenburger DD. New approach to classifying non-Hodgkin's lymphomas: clinical features of the major histologic subtypes. Non-Hodgkin's Lymphoma Classification Project. *J Clin Oncol.* 1998;16(8):2780–2795. doi:10.1200/JCO.1998.16.8.278
3. Perry AM, Diebold J, Nathwani BN, et al. Non-Hodgkin lymphoma in the developing world: review of 4,539 cases from the International Non-Hodgkin Lymphoma Classification Project. *Haematologica.* 2016;101(10):1244–1250. doi:10.3324/haematol.2016.148809
4. Armitage JO, Gascoyne RD, Lunning MA, Cavalli F. Non-Hodgkin lymphoma. *Lancet.* 2017;390(10091):298–310. doi:10.1016/S0140-6736(16)32407-2
5. Cerhan JR, Slager SL. Familial predisposition and genetic risk factors for lymphoma. *Blood.* 2015;126(20):2265–2273. doi:10.1182/blood-2015-04-537498
6. Schöllkopf C, Melbye M, Munksgaard L, et al. Borrelia infection and risk of non-Hodgkin lymphoma. *Blood.* 2008;111(12):5524–5529. doi:10.1182/blood-2007-08-109611
7. Swerdlow SH, Campo E, Pileri SA, et al. The 2016 revision of the World Health Organization classification of lymphoid neoplasms. *Blood.* 2016;127(20):2375–2390. doi:10.1182/blood-2016-01-643569
8. Savage KJ, Zeynalova S, Kansara RR, et al. Validation of a prognostic model to assess the risk of CNS disease in patients with aggressive B-Cell lymphoma. *Blood.* 2014;124(21):394. doi:10.1182/blood.v124.21.394.394
9. National Comprehensive Cancer Network. *NCCN Clinical Practice Guidelines in Oncology: B-Cell Lymphomas*; 2020. https://www.nccn.org
10. National Comprehensive Cancer Network. *NCCN Clinical Practice Guidelines in Oncology: T-Cell Lymphomas*; 2020. https://www.nccn.org
11. Weiler-Sagie M, Bushelev O, Epelbaum R, et al. (18)F-FDG avidity in lymphoma readdressed: a study of 766 patients. *J Nucl Med.* 2010;51(1):25–30. doi:10.2967/jnumed.109.067892
12. Noy A, Schöder H, Gönen M, et al. The majority of transformed lymphomas have high standardized uptake values (SUVs) on positron emission tomography (PET) scanning similar to diffuse large B-cell lymphoma (DLBCL). *Ann Oncol.* 2009;20(3):508–512. doi:10.1093/annonc/mdn657
13. Schöder H, Noy A, Gönen M, et al. Intensity of ^{18}fluorodeoxyglucose uptake in positron emission tomography distinguishes between indolent and aggressive non-Hodgkin's lymphoma. *J Clin Oncol.* 2005;23(21):4643–4651. doi:10.1200/JCO.2005.12.072
14. Khan AB, Barrington SF, Mikhaeel NG, et al. PET-CT staging of DLBCL accurately identifies and provides new insight into the clinical significance of bone marrow involvement. *Blood.* 2013;122(1):61–67. doi:10.1182/blood-2012-12-473389
15. Alzahrani M, El-Galaly TC, Hutchings M, et al. The value of routine bone marrow biopsy in patients with diffuse large B-cell lymphoma staged with PET/CT: a Danish-Canadian study. *Ann Oncol.* 2016;27(6):1095–1099. doi:10.1093/annonc/mdw137
16. Hans CP, Weisenburger DD, Greiner TC, et al. Confirmation of the molecular classification of diffuse large B-cell lymphoma by immunohistochemistry using a tissue microarray. *Blood.* 2004;103(1):275–282. doi:10.1182/blood-2003-05-1545
17. International Non-Hodgkin's Lymphoma Prognostic Factors Project. A predictive model for aggressive non-Hodgkin's lymphoma. *N Engl J Med.* 1993;329(14):987–994. doi:10.1056/NEJM199309303291402
18. Hoster E, Dreyling M, Klapper W, et al. A new prognostic index (MIPI) for patients with advanced-stage mantle cell lymphoma. *Blood.* 2008;111(2):558–565. doi:10.1182/blood-2007-06-095331
19. Meignan M, Gallamini A, Haioun C. Report on the First International Workshop on Interim-PET-Scan in Lymphoma. *Leuk Lymphoma.* 2009;50(8):1257–1260. doi:10.1080/10428190903040048
20. Zhou Z, Sehn LH, Rademaker AW, et al. An enhanced International Prognostic Index (NCCN-IPI) for patients with diffuse large B-cell lymphoma treated in the rituximab era. *Blood.* 2014;123(6):837–842. doi:10.1182/blood-2013-09-524108
21. Ziepert M, Hasenclever D, Kuhnt E, et al. Standard International Prognostic Index remains a valid predictor of outcome for patients with aggressive CD20+ B-cell lymphoma in the rituximab era. *J Clin Oncol.* 2010;28(14):2373–2380. doi:10.1200/JCO.2009.26.2493

22. Cheson BD, Fisher RI, Barrington SF, et al. Recommendations for initial evaluation, staging, and response assessment of Hodgkin and non-Hodgkin lymphoma: the Lugano classification. *J Clin Oncol*. 2014;32(27):3059–3068. doi:10.1200/JCO.2013.54.8800

23. Martin P, Chadburn A, Christos P, et al. Outcome of deferred initial therapy in mantle-cell lymphoma. *J Clin Oncol*. 2009;27(8):1209–1213. doi:10.1200/JCO.2008.19.6121

24. Habermann TM, Weller EA, Morrison VA, et al. Rituximab-CHOP versus CHOP alone or with maintenance rituximab in older patients with diffuse large B-cell lymphoma. *J Clin Oncol*. 2006;24(19):3121–3127. doi:10.1200/JCO.2005.05.1003

25. Feugier P, Van Hoof A, Sebban C, et al. Long-term results of the R-CHOP study in the treatment of elderly patients with diffuse large B-cell lymphoma: a study by the Groupe d'Etude des Lymphomes de l'Adulte. *J Clin Oncol*. 2005;23(18):4117–4126. doi:10.1200/JCO.2005.09.131

26. Coiffier B, Lepage E, Briere J, et al. CHOP chemotherapy plus rituximab compared with CHOP alone in elderly patients with diffuse large B-cell lymphoma. *N Engl J Med*. 2002;346(4):235–242. doi:10.1056/NEJMoa011795

27. Greb A, Bohlius J, Schiefer D, et al. High-dose chemotherapy with autologous stem cell transplantation in the first line treatment of aggressive non-Hodgkin lymphoma (NHL) in adults. *Cochrane Database Syst Rev*. 2008;(1):CD004024. doi:10.1002/14651858.CD004024.pub2

28. Récher C, Coiffier B, Haioun C, et al. Intensified chemotherapy with ACVBP plus rituximab versus standard CHOP plus rituximab for the treatment of diffuse large B-cell lymphoma (LNH03-2B): an open-label randomised phase 3 trial. *Lancet*. 2011;378(9806):1858–1867. doi:10.1016/S0140-6736(11)61040-4

29. Vitolo U, Chiappella A, Franceschetti S, et al. Lenalidomide plus R-CHOP21 in elderly patients with untreated diffuse large B-cell lymphoma: results of the REAL07 open-label, multicentre, phase 2 trial. *Lancet Oncol*. 2014;15(7):730–737. doi:10.1016/S1470-2045(14)70191-3

30. Dunleavy K, Pittaluga S, Maeda LS, et al. Dose-adjusted EPOCH-rituximab therapy in primary mediastinal B-cell lymphoma. *N Engl J Med*. 2013;368(15):1408–1416. doi:10.1056/NEJMoa1214561

31. Fenske TS, Zhang MJ, Carreras J, et al. Autologous or reduced-intensity conditioning allogeneic hematopoietic cell transplantation for chemotherapy-sensitive mantle-cell lymphoma: analysis of transplantation timing and modality. *J Clin Oncol*. 2014;32(4):273–281. doi:10.1200/JCO.2013.49.2454

32. Khouri IF, Romaguera J, Kantarjian H, et al. Hyper-CVAD and high-dose methotrexate/cytarabine followed by stem-cell transplantation: an active regimen for aggressive mantle-cell lymphoma. *J Clin Oncol*. 1998;16(12):3803–3809. doi:10.1200/JCO.1998.16.12.3803

33. Evens AM, Carson KR, Kolesar J, et al. A multicenter phase II study incorporating high-dose rituximab and liposomal doxorubicin into the CODOX-M/IVAC regimen for untreated Burkitt's lymphoma. *Ann Oncol*. 2013;24(12):3076–3081. doi:10.1093/annonc/mdt414

34. Rizzieri DA, Johnson JL, Byrd JC, et al. Improved efficacy using rituximab and brief duration, high intensity chemotherapy with filgrastim support for Burkitt or aggressive lymphomas: Cancer and Leukemia Group B study 10 002. *Br J Haematol*. 2014;165(1):102–111. doi:10.1111/bjh.12736

35. Dunleavy K, Pittaluga S, Shovlin M, et al. Low-intensity therapy in adults with Burkitt's lymphoma. *N Engl J Med*. 2013;369(20):1915–1925. doi:10.1056/NEJMoa1308392

36. Thomas DA, Faderl S, O'Brien S, et al. Chemoimmunotherapy with hyper-CVAD plus rituximab for the treatment of adult Burkitt and Burkitt-type lymphoma or acute lymphoblastic leukemia. *Cancer*. 2006;106(7):1569–1580. doi:10.1002/cncr.21776

37. Yamaguchi M, Kwong YL, Kim WS, et al. Phase II study of SMILE chemotherapy for newly diagnosed stage IV, relapsed, or refractory extranodal natural killer (NK)/T-cell lymphoma, nasal type: the NK-Cell Tumor Study Group study. *J Clin Oncol*. 2011;29(33):4410–4416. doi:10.1200/JCO.2011.35.6287

38. Yamaguchi M, Tobinai K, Oguchi M, et al. Concurrent chemoradiotherapy for localized nasal natural killer/T-cell lymphoma: an updated analysis of the Japan Clinical Oncology Group study JCOG0211. *J Clin Oncol*. 2012;30(32):4044–4046. doi:10.1200/JCO.2012.45.6541

39. Bi XW, Xia Y, Zhang WW, et al. Radiotherapy and PGEMOX/GELOX regimen improved prognosis in elderly patients with early-stage extranodal NK/T-cell lymphoma. *Ann Hematol*. 2015;94(9):1525–1533. doi:10.1007/s00277-015-2395-y

40. Wirth A, Mikhaeel NG, Aleman BMP, et al. Involved site radiation therapy in adult lymphomas: an overview of international lymphoma radiation oncology group guidelines. *Int J Radiat Oncol Biol Phys*. 2020;107(5):909–933. doi:10.1016/j.ijrobp.2020.03.019

41. Videtic GMM, Woody N, Vassil AD. *Handbook of Treatment Planning in Radiation Oncology*. 3rd ed. Demos Medical; 2020.

42. Pfreundschuh M, Kuhnt E, Trümper L, et al. CHOP-like chemotherapy with or without rituximab in young patients with good-prognosis diffuse large B-cell lymphoma: 6-year results of an open-label randomised study of the MabThera International Trial (MInT) Group. *Lancet Oncol*. 2011;12(11):1013–1022. doi:10.1016/S1470-2045(11)70235-2

43. Vargo JA, Gill BS, Balasubramani GK, Beriwal S. Treatment selection and survival outcomes in early-stage diffuse large B-Cell lymphoma: do we still need consolidative radiotherapy? *J Clin Oncol*. 2015;33(32):3710–3717. doi:10.1200/JCO.2015.61.7654

44. Gill BS, Vargo JA, Pai SS, et al. Management trends and outcomes for stage I to II mantle cell lymphoma using the National Cancer Data Base: ascertaining the ideal treatment paradigm. *Int J Radiat Oncol Biol Phys*. 2015;93(3):668–676. doi:10.1016/j.ijrobp.2015.07.2265

45. Marcheselli L, Marcheselli R, Bari A, et al. Radiation therapy improves treatment outcome in patients with diffuse large B-cell lymphoma. *Leuk Lymphoma*. 2011;52(10):1867–1872. doi:10.3109/10428194.2011.585526

46. Dorth JA, Prosnitz LR, Broadwater G, et al. Impact of consolidation radiation therapy in stage III–IV diffuse large B-cell lymphoma with negative post-chemotherapy radiologic imaging. *Int J Radiat Oncol Biol Phys*. 2012;84(3):762–767. doi:10.1016/j.ijrobp.2011.12.067

47. Shi Z, Das S, Okwan-Duodu D, et al. Patterns of failure in advanced-stage diffuse large B-cell lymphoma patients after complete response to R-CHOP immunochemotherapy and the emerging role of consolidative radiation therapy. *Int J Radiat Oncol Biol Phys*. 2013;86(3):569–577. doi:10.1016/j.ijrobp.2013.02.007

48. Kwon J, Kim IH, Kim BH, et al. Additional survival benefit of involved-lesion radiation therapy after R-CHOP chemotherapy in limited stage diffuse large B-cell lymphoma. *Int J Radiat Oncol Biol Phys*. 2015;92(1):91–98. doi:10.1016/j.ijrobp.2014.12.042

49. Haque W, Dabaja B, Tann A, et al. Changes in treatment patterns and impact of radiotherapy for early-stage diffuse large B cell lymphoma after Rituximab: a population-based analysis. *Radiother Oncol*. 2016;120(1):150–155. doi:10.1016/j.radonc.2016.05.027

50. Dabaja BS, Vanderplas AM, Crosby-Thompson AL, et al. Radiation for diffuse large B-cell lymphoma in the rituximab era: analysis of the National Comprehensive Cancer Network lymphoma outcomes project. *Cancer*. 2015;121(7):1032–1039. doi:10.1002/cncr.29113

51. U.S. National Library of Medicine. *Rituximab and Combination Chemotherapy With or Without Radiation Therapy in Treating Patients With B-Cell Non-Hodgkin's Lymphoma*. https://clinicaltrials.gov/show/NCT00278408

52. Ng AK, Dabaja BS, Hoppe RT, et al. Re-examining the role of radiation therapy for diffuse large B-cell lymphoma in the modern era. *J Clin Oncol*. 2016;34(13):1443–1447. doi:10.1200/JCO.2015.64.9418

53. Phan J, Mazloom A, Medeiros LJ, et al. Benefit of consolidative radiation therapy in patients with diffuse large B-cell lymphoma treated with R-CHOP chemotherapy. *J Clin Oncol*. 2010;28(27):4170–4176. doi:10.1200/JCO.2009.27.3441

54. Moskowitz CH, Schöder H, Teruya-Feldstein J, et al. Risk-adapted dose-dense immunochemotherapy determined by interim FDG-PET in advanced-stage diffuse large B-Cell lymphoma. *J Clin Oncol*. 2010;28(11):1896–1903. doi:10.1200/JCO.2009.26.5942

55. Martelli M, Ceriani L, Zucca E, et al. [18F]fluorodeoxyglucose positron emission tomography predicts survival after chemoimmunotherapy for primary mediastinal large B-cell lymphoma: results of the International Extranodal Lymphoma Study Group IELSG-26 Study. *J Clin Oncol*. 2014;32(17):1769–1775. doi:10.1200/JCO.2013.51.7524

56. Vitolo U, Chiappella A, Ferreri AJ, et al. First-line treatment for primary testicular diffuse large B-cell lymphoma with rituximab-CHOP, CNS prophylaxis, and contralateral testis irradiation: final results of an international phase II trial. *J Clin Oncol*. 2011;29(20):2766–2772. doi:10.1200/JCO.2010.31.4187

53 ■ INDOLENT NON-HODGKIN'S LYMPHOMA

Christopher W. Fleming, Aryavarta M. S. Kumar, and Matthew C. Ward

> **QUICK HIT** ■ Indolent NHLs are a diverse group of diseases with survival measured in years to decades. Most common histologies are grade 1 to 2 follicular lymphoma and extranodal MALT lymphoma. Limited-stage disease (stages I–II) is typically treated with definitive RT alone. Advanced disease (stages III–IV) is typically treated with initial observation, with initiation of CHT for symptomatic disease and RT for palliation. ILROG guidelines are useful for treatment selection and field design (Table 53.1).

Table 53.1: General Treatment Paradigm for Indolent NHLs

	Treatment Options	Common RT Regimens
Stages I to II	Definitive RT	Follicular/other histologies: 24 Gy/12 fx
		Gastric MALT: 30 Gy/15 fx
Stages III to IV	Observation, CHT, and/or palliative RT	24–30 Gy/12–15 fx
		4 Gy/2 fx (i.e., "boom boom")

EPIDEMIOLOGY: A total of 77,240 cases annually with 19,940 deaths of all NHL subtypes, ninth-leading cause of death.[1] Indolent NHL is usually a disease of older adults; median age 65, peak incidence >70. More common in North America, Europe, and Australia.[2] Follicular type represents ~22% of all NHLs (second-most common NHL after DLBCL), SLL/CLL represents ~6%, and MALT/marginal zone is ~5%.[3] Other subtypes are less common.

RISK FACTORS: Four broad risk factors: immunosuppression, autoimmune diseases, infections, and environmental exposures. See Chapter 52 for details.

ANATOMY: Indolent NHLs can present as nodal or extranodal. Nodal anatomy is detailed further in Chapter 52. Extranodal presentation is more common among indolent NHL. Common extranodal lymphoid sites include thymus, spleen and tonsils, and adenoids (Waldeyer's ring). Extralymphatic sites include bone marrow, skin, CNS, ovary, testicle, ocular adnexae, liver, stomach, bowel, breast, and lung.

PATHOLOGY/GENETICS: B-cell indolent NHLs are more common than T cell. WHO 2016 classification defines subtypes.[4] System is complex, but a few pearls are as follows. *Follicular NHL:* Graded by number of centroblasts per high-powered field. Grade 1: 0 to 5/HPF, grade 2: 6 to 15/HPF, grade 3: >15, sometimes subdivided into 3A and 3B with 3B demonstrating sheets of centroblasts and often treated as DLBCL. t(14:18) is classic translocation, results in overexpression of BCL-2, blocking apoptosis. *Marginal zone NHL:* Both nodal and extranodal (i.e., MALT). See Table 53.2 for details.

CLINICAL PRESENTATION: Often presents only with slow-growing lymphadenopathy, hepatosplenomegaly, cytopenias, or nonspecific constitutional symptoms, such as fatigue, malaise, or low-grade fever. Most common in neck, inguinal, axilla, and abdominal lymphadenopathy. Less commonly involves skin, which manifests as rash or pruritus. Bone marrow involvement is common. Follicular NHLs commonly present as stage III to IV, whereas marginal zone NHL more commonly presents as localized disease. B symptoms are usually associated with aggressive histologies or extensive disease.

WORKUP: H&P with attention to lymphatic, liver, spleen, and/or skin exam. Lymph node biopsy of peripheral lymph node is ideal. Endoscopic biopsy for gastric MALT. FNA is insufficient for final diagnosis but may distinguish benign lymphadenopathy from clonal B-cell proliferation via flow cytometry. Bone marrow biopsy (unilateral generally sufficient) for most but not for extranodal MZL.[7] Lumbar puncture for testicular, paravertebral, parameningeal, positive bone marrow, HIV.

Table 53.2: Pathology, Immunophenotype, and Genetics of Common Indolent Non-Hodgkin's Lymphomas

Disease	Common Immunotype		Common Genetics	Notes
Follicular NHL	CD19+, CD20+	CD10+, CD21+, CD22+, CD79a+ CD5−, CD43−	t(14:18)	BCL-2 expression result of t(14:18), marrow involvement common, risk of transformation 28% at 10 years[5]
Nodal marginal zone (MZL)		CD22+, CD3 −, 5−, 10−, 23−	Trisomy 3, t(11:18)	Less common than extranodal
Extranodal MZL (MALT)				Frequently localized, t(11:18) associated with triple-antibiotic therapy failure for gastric MALT[6]
SLL/CLL		CD5+, 23+, HLA-DR CD22−	t(14:19), karyotype aberrations (trisomy 12) common but not diagnostic	SLL has morphology similar to CLL but with too low circulating leukemia cell count

Labs: CBC, peripheral smear, ESR, CMP, LDH, HIV, hepatitis B, hepatitis C, β-2 microglobulin (see the following FLIPI2 prognostic model), urea breath test for *Helicobacter pylori* (gastric MALT). Pregnancy test.

Imaging: Contrast-enhanced CT chest, abdomen, pelvis for peripheral lymphadenopathy. PET/CT in all nodal lymphomas (not CLL/SLL or MALT). PET SUV >10 in patients with indolent NHL may suggest transformation to high-grade histology and can be used to target biopsy (i.e., Richter transformation from CLL/hairy cell leukemia to DLBCL).[8] Obtain MRI brain/spine for symptoms. Obtain echocardiogram or MUGA scan if anthracycline CHT planned.

PROGNOSTIC FACTORS: FLIPI and updated FLIPI2 useful for prognostic assessment for follicular patients. FLIPI was designed pre-rituximab but remained prognostic in rituximab era.[9] See Table 53.3. Other prognostic factors include IRF4 gene rearrangement (follicular grade 3B), high Ki67 index (>30%, suggests rapid proliferation).

Table 53.3: FLIPI and FLIPI2 Risk Factors

Original FLIPI Risk Factors[9,10]		FLIPI2 Risk Factors[11]		
Hemoglobin < 12 ng/dL		Hemoglobin < 12 ng/dL		
Age > 60		Age > 60		
Stage III–IV		Serum β-2 microglobulin elevated		
Nodal sites > 4		Bone marrow involvement		
LDH elevated		Maximal diameter of lymph node > 6 cm		
		FLIPI Pre-Rituximab[10]		FLIPI2[11]
Score	Risk Group	5-Yr OS	10-Yr OS	Score	Risk Group	5-Yr PFS
0–1	Low	91%	71%	0	Low	80%
2	Intermediate	78%	51%	1–2	Intermediate	51%
≥3	High	52%	36%	3–5	High	19%

STAGING: See Chapter 52 for Ann Arbor Staging.

TREATMENT PARADIGM

Observation: Considered for older or asymptomatic patients with stage III/IV indolent NHLs; see CHT paradigm in the following for discussion on observation versus treatment.

Medical: Triple therapy often first line for *H. pylori*–positive gastric MALT and includes proton pump inhibitor, clarithromycin, and either amoxicillin or metronidazole. Give triple therapy as first line with endoscopic biopsy at 3 months to confirm resolution. If *H. pylori* negative and lymphoma negative, observation. If *H. pylori* positive and lymphoma negative, give second-line antibiotics. If *H. pylori* negative and lymphoma positive, can either continue observation with repeat biopsy or treat with RT for symptoms. If both remain positive, treat with second-line antibiotics with immediate or delayed RT. Response to doxycycline has been noted (65%) for ocular and cutaneous MZL.[12]

Surgery: Minimal role for NHL, used mostly for biopsy, but in small bowel can be therapeutic.

Chemotherapy: Used for later stage (stage III/IV typically). Note that grade 3B follicular NHL is often treated as per DLBCL regimens (see Chapter 52). When considering treatment for indolent stage III to IV NHL, factors such as rate of progression, symptoms, end-organ function, cytopenias, and bulk are considered. If none, then NCCN suggests observation.[13] If indications are present, treatment can be initiated and may consist of regimens such as bendamustine + rituximab, R-CHOP, R-CVP (rituximab, cyclophosphamide, vincristine, prednisone), or rituximab alone. Rituximab is chimeric monoclonal antibody against CD20; classic toxicities include infusion reactions, hepatitis B reactivation, and progressive multifocal leukoencephalopathy. Obinutuzumab is an alternative anti-CD20 monoclonal antibody with similar effects as rituximab but binds slightly different epitope of CD20.

Radiation

Indications: In limited-stage indolent NHLs (stage I–II), RT is treatment of choice for cure and is usually delivered to whole organ, particularly for gastric, thyroid, orbit (but not conjunctiva), breast, and salivary gland extranodal indolent NHL. In advanced disease, RT is typically used for focal palliation. ISRT is often appropriate when entire organ need not be treated. ILROG guidelines exist for both nodal and extranodal NHL.[14,15]

Dose: See Table 53.4 for NCCN dosing guidelines. Doses usually delivered at 1.8 to 2 Gy/fx. Some have advocated doses up to 36 Gy for bulky disease. Effective palliation can be provided via "boom boom" regimen of 4 Gy/2 fx (see the following data).

Table 53.4: NCCN Dosing Guidelines for Indolent Non-Hodgkin's Lymphomas	
Follicular	24–30 Gy
Gastric MALT	30 Gy
Other extranodal Sites (orbit, skin, thyroid, etc.)	24–30 Gy
Nodal MZL	24–30 Gy
Palliation of indolent lymphoma	4 Gy (i.e., "boom boom")

Toxicity: Generally, toxicity mild, given in low total doses. Fatigue is common; others are related to location of delivery.

Procedure: See *Handbook of Treatment Planning in Radiation Oncology*, Chapter 10.[16]

Unsealed sources: Y-90 ibritumomab tiuxetan (Zevalin®) and I-131 tositumomab (Bexxar®, now discontinued) are radiolabeled antibodies against CD20, indicated in use of previously untreated, relapsed, or refractory indolent NHL (primarily follicular) and often produce response in patients refractory to rituximab.

■ **EVIDENCE-BASED Q&A**

▨ **What data suggest that follicular NHL (grades 1–2) can be cured with RT alone?**

Multiple RRs are available, but one example is as follows.

Campbell, British Columbia (*Cancer* 2010, PMID 20564082): RR of 237 patients with stage I to II grade 1 to 3A follicular NHL treated with RT alone. Involved regional RT included LN group with

≥1 adjacent uninvolved LN group (60%), or INRT (40%). MFU 7.3 years; 10-year PFS 49%, OS 66%. Distant recurrence alone was the most common pattern of failure, occurring in 38% of involved regional RT and 32% of INRT. **Conclusion: Cure is possible with RT, and reducing field size does not compromise outcome.**

■ **For limited-stage follicular NHL, is there detriment to initial observation as compared to initial RT?**

Indolent lymphoma is slowly progressive, and no treatment may be a reasonable first approach. However, for early stage disease, this is not supported by observational data. Therefore, definitive treatment with RT should remain standard of care.

Pugh, SEER (*Cancer* 2010, PMID 20564102): SEER analysis of 6,568 patients with stage I to II, grade 1 to 2 follicular NHL diagnosed from 1973 to 2004; 34% received initial RT. Those observed were younger, stage I, and without extranodal disease. RT was associated with improved 20-year DSS (63% vs. 51%, HR 0.61, P < .0001) and OS (35% vs. 23%, HR 0.68, P < .0001). **Conclusion: Initial RT is standard for early-stage follicular NHL and deferring treatment until time of salvage is associated with worse outcomes. RT is greatly underused.**

Vargo, NCDB (*Cancer* 2015, PMID 26042364): NCDB analysis of 35,961 patients with stage I to II, grade 1 to 2 follicular NHL. RT use decreased from 37% to 24% between 1999 and 2012; 10-year OS was 68% for RT patients compared to 54% for no RT patients (p < .0001). **Conclusion: RT is significantly underutilized and is associated with improved survival in early stage follicular lymphoma. RT should remain standard.**

■ **What RT dose is optimal for indolent NHL?**

For definitive RT of early stage indolent lymphoma, 24 to 30 Gy is usually sufficient, with some advocating for 36 Gy in rare case of bulky disease. For palliation, 4 Gy/2 fx or 24 Gy/12 fx are both reasonable. Note that "boom boom" regimen of 4 Gy/2 fx was inferior for definitive treatment of limited-stage patients in FoRT trial and should not be extrapolated to aggressive NHL.

Lowry, British National Lymphoma Investigation (*Radiother Oncol* 2011, PMID 21664710): PRT including any subtype and stage of NHL requiring RT for local control. 361 sites of indolent NHL randomized to either 40 to 45 Gy/20 to 23 fx (standard) vs. 24 Gy/12 fx (low dose). For indolent patients, 59% were grade 1 to 2 follicular NHL, 19% MZL/MALT, and 69% were stage I to II. MFU 5.6 years. ORR no different: 93% vs. 92% in standard vs. low-dose groups, respectively. PFS and OS were also not significantly different. **Conclusion: 24 Gy is sufficient for indolent lymphomas.**

Hoskin, FoRT Trial (*Lancet Oncol* 2014, PMID 24572077; **Update Lancet Oncol 2021, PMID 33539729**): Noninferiority trial of patients with either follicular NHL or MZL requiring RT for either definitive or palliative treatment. Randomized between 4 Gy/2 fx (i.e., "boom boom") vs. 24 Gy/12 fx. Primary endpoint LC. Trial closed early with 548 patients, 614 sites, MFU 74 mos. 60% stage I to II. Response rate 81% vs. 74% in 24 Gy vs. 4 Gy arms, respectively. 5-year local progression-free rate was 89.9% for 24 Gy and 70.4% for 4 Gy (HR 3.46, p<0.0001). No difference in OS. **Conclusion: 24 Gy is more effective when durable local control is the goal. However, "boom boom" is useful in palliation and often induces response.**

■ **Is there benefit to adjuvant CHT after definitive RT for early-stage indolent NHL?**

Adjuvant CHT does not appear to improve OS based on results of at least five randomized trials from pre-rituximab era (Denmark, Milan, British, EORTC, MSKCC)[17-21] as well as the more recent TROG study outlined below.

MacManus, TROG 99.03 (*JCO* 2018, PMID 29975623): Multicenter PRT enrolling 150 patients with stage I to II low-grade follicular NHL after CT and bone marrow biopsies. PET was not mandatory. Patients randomized to 30 Gy IFRT alone vs. IFRT plus 6 cycles CVP. After 2006, rituximab was added to CVP (41% of CVP arm); 75% stage I. MFU 9.6 years; 10-year PFS superior with CVP (59% vs. 41%, HR 0.57, p = .033), and markedly improved with R-CVP (HR 0.26, p = .045). However, 10-year OS was not significantly different (87% vs. 95%, p = .40). **Conclusion: Systemic therapy with R-CVP after IFRT significantly improved PFS without benefit in OS.**

■ **What data inform treatment of gastric MALT?**

In addition to those summarized previously, few notable series are listed in Table 53.5. Study by Wündisch informs treatment of H. pylori–positive gastric MALT and supports observation when H. pylori is eradicated.

Table 53.5: Summary of Notable RR of Gastric MALT				
Institution	Year	N	RT Dose	LC
Dana Farber[22]	2007	21	30 Gy	21/21
PMH[23]	2010	25	25–30 Gy	15/15
Japan[24]	2010	8	30 Gy	8/8
MSKCC[25]	1998	17	30 Gy	17/17

Wirth, Multi-Center IELSG Study (*Ann Oncol* 2013, PMID 23293112): Multicenter RR of 102 gastric MALT patients treated with RT to median dose of 40 Gy. MFU 7.9 years; 10 and 15-year FFTF was 88%; 10-year OS 70%. Large cell component and exophytic growth pattern were risk factors for failure.

Wündisch, Germany (*JCO* 2005, PMID 16204012): Prospective trial tracking outcomes of *H. pylori*–positive gastric MALT; 120 patients, all with stage IE disease treated with antibiotics and observed after *H. pylori* eradication. MFU 75 months. Eighty percent achieved pCR, with 80% of those experiencing long-term pCR. Three percent relapsed and were referred for treatment, other 17% were observed, and all entered into CR. Fifteen percent positive for t(11:18). t(11:18) and ongoing monoclonality were associated with failure. **Conclusion: Cure of** *H. pylori* **results in continuous CR in most patients. Observation is appropriate for most patients when close follow-up is possible.**

■ **What data inform treatment of other MALT NHL?**

Tran, Australian Orbital MALT Series (*Leuk Lymphoma* 2013, PMID 23020137): A total of 27 orbits of 24 patients treated to 24 to 25 Gy. MFU 41 months. Fifty-nine percent conjunctival, 26% lacrimal, 4% eyelid, and 11% other; 100% CR, three failures, one local, one contralateral, one distant.

Teckie, MSKCC (*IJROBP* 2015, PMID 25863760): A total of 244 patients with stage IE or IIE MZL treated with RT alone. Ninety-two percent were stage IE. MFU 5.2 years. Stomach (50%), orbit (18%), nonthyroid head and neck (8%), skin (8%), and breast (5%). Median RT dose 30 Gy; 5-year OS 92%, RFS 74%. Most common relapse site was distant. Disease-specific death 1.1% at 5 years. All sites except H&N demonstrated worse RFS compared to gastric. Transformation to aggressive histology was rare (1.6%). **Conclusion: OS and DSS are high in early-stage extranodal MZL. Gastric MALT has improved prognosis compared to other sites.**

REFERENCES

1. Siegel RL, Miller KD, Jemal A. Cancer statistics, 2020. *CA Cancer J Clin.* 2020;70(1):7–30. doi:10.3322/caac.21590
2. Boffetta P. Epidemiology of adult non-Hodgkin lymphoma. *Ann Oncol.* 2011;22(Suppl 4): iv27–iv31. doi:10.1093/annonc/mdr167
3. Armitage JO, Weisenburger DD. New approach to classifying non-Hodgkin's lymphomas: clinical features of the major histologic subtypes. Non-Hodgkin's lymphoma classification project. *J Clin Oncol.* 1998;16(8):2780–2795. doi:10.1200/JCO.1998.16.8.2780
4. Swerdlow SH, Campo E, Pileri SA, et al. The 2016 revision of the World Health Organization classification of lymphoid neoplasms. *Blood.* 2016;127(20):2375–2390. doi:10.1182/blood-2016-01-643569
5. Montoto S, Davies AJ, Matthews J, et al. Risk and clinical implications of transformation of follicular lymphoma to diffuse large B-cell lymphoma. *J Clin Oncol.* 2007;25(17):2426–2433. doi:10.1200/JCO.2006.09.3260
6. Yepes S, Torres MM, Saavedra C, Andrade R. Gastric mucosa-associated lymphoid tissue lymphomas and Helicobacter pylori infection: a Colombian perspective. *World J Gastroenterol.* 2012;18(7):685–691. doi:10.3748/wjg.v18.i7.685
7. Ebie N, Loew JM, Gregory SA. Bilateral trephine bone marrow biopsy for staging non-Hodgkin's lymphoma: a second look. *Hematol Pathol.* 1989;3(1):29–33.

8. Noy A, Schöder H, Gönen M, et al. The majority of transformed lymphomas have high standardized uptake values (SUVs) on positron emission tomography (PET) scanning similar to diffuse large B-cell lymphoma (DLBCL). *Ann Oncol.* 2009;20(3):508–512. doi:10.1093/annonc/mdn657

9. Nooka AK, Nabhan C, Zhou X, et al. Examination of the follicular lymphoma international prognostic index (FLIPI) in the National LymphoCare study (NLCS): a prospective US patient cohort treated predominantly in community practices. *Ann Oncol.* 2013;24(2):441–448. doi:10.1093/annonc/mds429

10. Solal-Céligny P, Roy P, Colombat P, et al. Follicular lymphoma international prognostic index. *Blood.* 2004;104(5):1258–1265. doi:10.1182/blood-2003-12-4434

11. Federico M, Bellei M, Marcheselli L, et al. Follicular lymphoma international prognostic index 2: a new prognostic index for follicular lymphoma developed by the International Follicular Lymphoma Prognostic Factor project. *J Clin Oncol.* 2009;27(27):4555–4562. doi:10.1200/JCO.2008.21.3991

12. Ferreri AJ, Govi S, Pasini E, et al. Chlamydophila psittaci eradication with doxycycline as first-line targeted therapy for ocular adnexae lymphoma: final results of an international phase II trial. *J Clin Oncol.* 2012;30(24):2988–2994. doi:10.1200/JCO.2011.41.4466

13. NCCN clinical practice guidelines in oncology: B-Cell Lymphomas; 2020. https://www.nccn.org/professionals/physician_gls/pdf/b-cell.pdf

14. Yahalom J, Illidge T, Specht L, et al. Modern radiation therapy for extranodal lymphomas: field and dose guidelines from the International Lymphoma Radiation Oncology Group. *Int J Radiat Oncol Biol Phys.* 2015;92(1):11–31. doi:10.1016/j.ijrobp.2015.01.009

15. Illidge T, Specht L, Yahalom J, et al. Modern radiation therapy for nodal non-Hodgkin lymphoma-target definition and dose guidelines from the International Lymphoma Radiation Oncology Group. *Int J Radiat Oncol Biol Phys.* 2014;89(1):49–58. doi:10.1016/j.ijrobp.2014.01.006

16. Videtic GMM, Woody N, Vassil AD. *Handbook of Treatment Planning in Radiation Oncology* 3rd ed. Demos Medical; 2020. doi:10.1891/9780826168429

17. Monfardini S, Banfi A, Bonadonna G, et al. Improved five-year survival after combined radiotherapy-chemotherapy for stage I–II non-Hodgkin's lymphoma. *Int J Radiat Oncol Biol Phys.* 1980;6(2):125–134. doi:10.1016/0360-3016(80)90027-9

18. Nissen NI, Ersbøll J, Hansen HS, et al. A randomized study of radiotherapy versus radiotherapy plus chemotherapy in stage I–II non-Hodgkin's lymphomas. *Cancer.* 1983;52(1):1–7. doi:10.1002/1097-0142(19830701)52:1<1::AID-CNCR2820520102>3.0.CO;2-M

19. Carde P, Burgers JM, van Glabbeke M, et al. Combined radiotherapy-chemotherapy for early stages non-Hodgkin's lymphoma: the 1975–1980 EORTC controlled lymphoma trial. *Radiother Oncol.* 1984;2(4):301–312. doi:10.1016/S0167-8140(84)80072-9

20. Kelsey SM, Newland AC, Hudson GV, Jelliffe AM. A British National Lymphoma Investigation randomised trial of single agent chlorambucil plus radiotherapy versus radiotherapy alone in low grade, localised non-Hodgkins lymphoma. *Med Oncol.* 1994;11(1):19–25. doi:10.1007/BF02990087

21. Yahalom J, Varsos G, Fuks Z, et al. Adjuvant cyclophosphamide, doxorubicin, vincristine, and prednisone chemotherapy after radiation therapy in stage I low-grade and intermediate-grade non-Hodgkin lymphoma: results of a prospective randomized study. *Cancer.* 1993;71(7):2342–2350. doi:10.1002/1097-0142(19930401)71:7<2342::AID-CNCR2820710728>3.0.CO;2-I

22. Tsai HK, Li S, Ng AK, et al. Role of radiation therapy in the treatment of stage I/II mucosa-associated lymphoid tissue lymphoma. *Ann Oncol.* 2007;18(4):672–678. doi:10.1093/annonc/mdl468

23. Goda JS, Gospodarowicz M, Pintilie M, et al. Long-term outcome in localized extranodal mucosa-associated lymphoid tissue lymphomas treated with radiotherapy. *Cancer.* 2010;116(16):3815–3824. doi:10.1002/cncr.25226

24. Ono S, Kato M, Takagi K, et al. Long-term treatment of localized gastric marginal zone B-cell mucosa associated lymphoid tissue lymphoma including incidence of metachronous gastric cancer. *J Gastroenterol Hepatol.* 2010;25(4):804–809. doi:10.1111/j.1440-1746.2009.06204.x

25. Schechter NR, Portlock CS, Yahalom J. Treatment of mucosa-associated lymphoid tissue lymphoma of the stomach with radiation alone. *J Clin Oncol.* 1998;16(5):1916–1921. doi:10.1200/JCO.1998.16.5.1916

Kailin Yang and Sheen Cherian

QUICK HIT ■ Multiple myeloma is not considered curable with current treatment modalities. It is typically sensitive to a variety of cytotoxic drugs and treatment has been evolving rapidly due to emerging therapeutics such as thalidomide, lenalidomide, and bortezomib. The primary management of multiple myeloma is CHT ± autologous SCT. RT is reserved for symptomatic bone metastases, prevention of pathologic fractures, and spinal cord compression. Solitary plasmacytoma is a rare plasma cell dyscrasia that can occur locally in the bone (SBP) or soft tissue (SEP). Thorough work-up to exclude systemic disease is necessary. Definitive RT to a total dose of 35 to 50 Gy with 1.8 to 2 Gy daily fractions is the primary treatment for SBP and SEP (Table 54.1).

TABLE 54.1: Overview of Multiple Myeloma, SBP, and solitary SEP

Feature	Multiple Myeloma	SBP	SEP
Common location	Axial skeleton	Vertebral body and pelvic bone	Head and neck region
Progression to multiple myeloma	NA	>75%	10%–30%
Local control	Not curable	80–100%	90%–100%
Radiation	Palliative RT (25–30 Gy/10 fx, 17 to 20 Gy/5 fx, 8 Gy/1 fx). Primary treatment: CHT ± Autologous SCT	35–40 Gy (<5 cm) 40–50 Gy (≥5 cm)	40–50 Gy

EPIDEMIOLOGY: Multiple myeloma accounts for 1% of all cancer cases. In the United States, there are approximately 32,000 new diagnoses and 13,000 myeloma-related deaths per year.[1] Incidence in Blacks is 2 to 3 times higher than that seen in Caucasians. Incidence in men to women is 1.4:1. Median age at diagnosis is ~70 years.

RISK FACTORS: Risk of developing multiple myeloma is ~3.7-fold higher in those with a first-degree relative diagnosed with the disease. Other risk factors include older age, immunosuppression, and exposure to radiation, benzene, or herbicide.[2]

PATHOLOGY: Myeloma is caused by clonal proliferation of plasma cells, a type of terminally differentiated B lymphocytes. Myeloma cells appear in an ovoid shape with abundant blue cytoplasm and eccentric nucleus with coarse chromatin. Plasma cells can produce a large amount of monoclonal immunoglobulin (M protein), which can be detected with SPEP. For most patients, the increased immunoglobulin is either IgG (~70%) or IgA (~20%). A small fraction of patients (5%–10%) have light chain only disease, which can be detected using UPEP. Less than 2% of patients present with non-secretory myeloma.

GENETICS: Chromosomal abnormality is common in multiple myeloma.[3] Abnormalities associated with poor prognosis include 17p deletion, translocation 14:16, translocation 14:20, 1p deletion, translocation 4:14, and 1q gain.[4]

CLINICAL PRESENTATION: Symptoms include anemia, bone pain, elevated serum creatinine, fatigue, hypercalcemia, and weight loss. These presenting symptoms are typically associated with infiltration of myeloma cells into bone or other organs, or effect of excess light chains (such as kidney injury).

WORKUP: H&P

Labs: CBC with differential, peripheral blood smear (increased rouleaux formation), serum BUN/creatinine, albumin, calcium, LDH, and β_2 microglobulin. Serum quantitative immunoglobulin, SPEP, and free light chain ratio; 24-hour urine test for total protein and UPEP. Bone marrow biopsy with cytogenetics and FISH.

Imaging: Skeletal survey. PET/CT, MRI, and/or CT if bone pain or neurological symptoms concerning for spinal cord compression. For patients with suspected smoldering myeloma (presence of M protein but without myeloma defining events) or solitary plasmacytoma, PET/CT and MRI should be performed to confirm the absence of >1 focal lytic lesion.

PROGNOSTIC FACTORS: Age, performance status, comorbidity, albumin concentration, and high risk cytogenetic abnormalities (del[17p], t[4;14], t[14;16], t[14;20], 1q+) have been associated with prognosis.[5,6]

STAGING: Diagnosis of multiple myeloma requires clonal bone marrow plasma cells ($\geq$10%) with biopsy-proven bony or extramedullary plasmacytoma, and at least one of the myeloma-defining events, which include evidence of end-organ damage (hypercalcemia, renal insufficiency, anemia, or bone lesion) or biomarker of malignancy (clonal bone marrow plasma cells $\geq$60%, involved:uninvolved serum free light chain ratio $\geq$100, or >1 focal lesions on MRI studies). The ISS and R-ISS have been developed to stage multiple myeloma (Table 54.2).[6,7] OS for R-ISS stages I, II, and III is 82%, 62%, and 40% at 5 years, respectively.

TABLE 54.2: Staging for Multiple Myeloma		
Stage	ISS	R-ISS
I	Serum β2 microglobulin <3.5 mg/L and serum albumin $\geq$3.5 g/dL	ISS stage I and standard-risk cytogenetic abnormality such as no del(17p), t(4;14), or t(14;16)
II	Neither ISS stage I or III	Neither R-ISS stage I or III
III	Serum β2 microglobulin $\geq$5.5 mg/L	ISS stage III AND either serum LDH above normal limits or high-risk cytogenetic abnormality by FISH such as del(17p), t(4;14), or t(14;16)

TREATMENT PARADIGM

Surgery: Prophylactic internal fixation should be used for weight-bearing long bone lesions at risk for impending fracture. Vertebroplasty and kyphoplasty can also reduce pain and improve function for patients with compression fracture from lytic lesion in the vertebral body. See Chapter 67 for details.

Chemotherapy: High-dose CHT followed by autologous HCT is considered standard of care for eligible patients with newly diagnosed multiple myeloma. Autologous HCT is associated with improved OS, and therefore assessment for eligibility is critical for pretreatment evaluation.[8] Patients eligible for autologous HCT are typically treated with four cycles of induction CHT prior to transplantation. Early single or double HCT is preferred in high-risk patients after four cycles of CHT. Chemotherapeutic agents include bortezomib (proteasome inhibitor, side effects: herpes zoster, neuropathy, and GI disturbance), thalidomide (immunomodulatory), and lenalidomide (immunomodulatory). VRd (bortezomib, lenalidomide, and dexamethasone) is a commonly used regimen for induction, though Rd is an acceptable alternative for frail patients.[9] Patients who are ineligible for HCT typically receive 8 to 12 cycles of triplet induction therapy followed by maintenance therapy.

Radiation: For patients with multiple myeloma, radiation is indicated for palliative management of pain, prevention of pathologic fracture particularly for weight-bearing bones, or relief of spinal cord compression. Typical palliative doses such as 30 Gy/10 fx, 20 Gy/5 fx, or 8 Gy/1 fx are commonly used for bony metastasis and spinal cord compression. For large volume or retreatment, 20 to 30 Gy in 10 to 15 daily fractions may be preferred to reduce side effects on bone marrow and other critical structures.[10]

RT is the primary definitive management for SBP and SEP. For SBP, RT is commonly directed to the involved bone and areas of soft tissue involvement with a margin to 40 to 50 Gy in 1.8 to 2 Gy/fraction per NCCN. The ILROG consensus recommends 35 to 40 Gy for SBP <5 cm, and 40 to 50 Gy for SBP ≥5 cm.[10] RT dose is similar for SEP (40–50 Gy per ILROG consensus), though the treatment volume depends on the site of involvement.[10] For SEP of head and neck area, regional LNs can be considered though data of efficacy are limited. RT planning typically involves a GTV to CTV expansion based on tumor location: 0.5 to 1 cm for microscopic disease in soft tissue and 2 to 3 cm for long bones at proximal and distal expansions. When there is uncertainty regarding the extent of involvement and minimal additional toxicity, whole bone RT can be considered. SBP has a high risk to progress to multiple myeloma: 65% to 85% at 10 years and 100% at 15 years. The risk of progression to multiple myeloma for SEP is 10% to 30% at 10 years, though local failure can occur in ~20% of patients.[11]

■ EVIDENCE-BASED Q&A

▓ What is the role of combined CHT in addition to RT for solitary plasmacytoma?

The role of CHT for solitary plasmacytoma is controversial in general, though can be considered for SBP given high risk of progression to multiple myeloma. One historical prospective study of 53 patients demonstrated improved DFS and OS when adding combined melphalan and prednisone to RT.[12] Multiple retrospective studies using newer agents showed mixed results.[13-15] Ongoing phase III randomized clinical trials are investigating the efficacy of systemic therapy after RT for SBP.

REFERENCES

1. Siegel RL, Miller KD, Jemal A. Cancer statistics, 2020. *CA Cancer J Clin.* 2020;70(1):7–30. doi:10.3322/caac.21590
2. Dores GM, Landgren O, McGlynn KA, et al. Plasmacytoma of bone, extramedullary plasmacytoma, and multiple myeloma: incidence and survival in the united states, 1992–2004. *Br J Haematol.* 2009;144(1):86–94. doi:10.1111/j.1365-2141.2008.07421.x
3. Palumbo A, Anderson K. Multiple myeloma. *N Engl J Med.* 2011;364(11):1046–1060. doi:10.1056/NEJMra1011442
4. Rajan AM, Rajkumar SV. Interpretation of cytogenetic results in multiple myeloma for clinical practice. *Blood Cancer J.* 2015;5:e365. doi:10.1038/bcj.2015.92
5. Kyle RA, Gertz MA, Witzig TE, et al. Review of 1027 patients with newly diagnosed multiple myeloma. *Mayo Clin Proc.* 2003;78(1):21–33. doi:10.4065/78.1.21
6. Palumbo A, Avet-Loiseau H, Oliva S, et al. Revised international staging system for multiple myeloma: a report from International Myeloma Working Group. *J Clin Oncol.* 2015;33(26):2863–2869. doi:10.1200/JCO.2015.61.2267
7. Greipp PR, San Miguel J, Durie BG, et al. International staging system for multiple myeloma. *J Clin Oncol.* 2005;23(15):3412–3420. doi:10.1200/JCO.2005.04.242
8. Goldschmidt H, Lokhorst HM, Mai EK, et al. Bortezomib before and after high-dose therapy in myeloma: long-term results from the phase III HOVON-65/GMMG-HD4 trial. *Leukemia.* 2018;32(2):383–390. doi:10.1038/leu.2017.211
9. Palumbo A, Bringhen S, Mateos MV, et al. Geriatric assessment predicts survival and toxicities in elderly myeloma patients: an International Myeloma Working Group report. *Blood.* 2015;125(13):2068–2074.
10. Tsang RW, Campbell BA, Goda JS, et al. Radiation therapy for solitary plasmacytoma and multiple myeloma: guidelines from the International Lymphoma Radiation Oncology Group. *Int J Radiat Oncol Biol Phys.* 2018;101(4):794–808. doi:10.1016/j.ijrobp.2018.05.009
11. Ozsahin M, Tsang RW, Poortmans P, et al. Outcomes and patterns of failure in solitary plasmacytoma: a multicenter Rare Cancer Network study of 258 patients. *Int J Radiat Oncol Biol Phys.* 2006;64(1):210–217. doi:10.1016/j.ijrobp.2005.06.039
12. Aviles A, Huerta-Guzman J, Delgado S, et al. Improved outcome in solitary bone plasmacytomata with combined therapy. *Hematol Oncol.* 1996;14(3):111–117. doi:10.1002/(SICI)1099-1069(199609)14:3<111::AID-HON575>3.0.CO;2-G
13. Mignot F, Schernberg A, Arsene-Henry A, et al. Solitary plasmacytoma treated by lenalidomide-dexamethasone in combination with radiation therapy: clinical outcomes. *Int J Radiat Oncol Biol Phys.* 2020;106(3):589–596. doi:10.1016/j.ijrobp.2019.10.043
14. Le Ray E, Belin L, Plancher C, et al. Our experience of solitary plasmacytoma of the bone: improved PFS with a short-course treatment by IMiDs or proteasome inhibitors combined with intensity-modulated radiotherapy. *Leuk Lymphoma.* 2018;59(7):1756–1758. doi:10.1080/10428194.2017.1393667
15. Katodritou E, Terpos E, Symeonidis AS, et al. Clinical features, outcome, and prognostic factors for survival and evolution to multiple myeloma of solitary plasmacytomas: a report of the Greek myeloma study group in 97 patients. *Am J Hematol.* 2014;89(8):803–808. doi:10.1002/ajh.23745

X ■ SARCOMAS

55 ■ SOFT TISSUE SARCOMA

Shauna R. Campbell, Jonathan M. Sharrett, Jacob G. Scott, and Chirag Shah

QUICK HIT ■ STS are a heterogeneous group of tumors that together make up the most common sarcoma diagnosis. More than 100 histological subtypes have been identified, with the majority originating in the extremities. Core needle biopsy should be performed by the treating surgeon, preferably a surgical/orthopedic oncologist. Surgical resection is required for cure and the role of CHT is evolving in the targeted era. Positive margins and high grade confer worse LC with surgery alone. Role of RT is to improve outcomes for localized disease. General treatment paradigms are included in Table 55.1. For extremity STS, surgery alone may be considered for low-grade, stage I tumors resected with >1 cm negative margins. For stage II to III STS of the extremity that is resectable with reasonable functional outcomes (limb-sparing), RT is recommended and can be delivered either pre- or post-op. RT improves LC and may improve OS. RPS comprises 10% to 15% of STS and are most commonly LS. Surgical resection is standard and local recurrence following gross total resection is common. RT can be delivered preoperatively to improve LC, with consideration of IORT/brachytherapy boost.

Table 55.1: General Treatment Paradigm for Soft Tissue and Retroperitoneal Sarcoma[1]		
	Extremities/Superficial Trunk	**Retroperitoneal**
Stage I	Total en bloc excision alone. Add PORT if close (<1 cm), positive margins or high grade. PORT dose is 50 Gy/25 fx plus boost (60–66 Gy for close margins, 66–68 Gy for microscopic positive margins, and 70–76 Gy for gross residual)	Surgery alone OR Pre-op RT to 45–50.4 Gy/25 to 28 fx considered ±IORT boost (10–12 Gy)
Stage II to III	Pre-op RT (50 Gy/25 fx*). Post-op EBRT boost for positive/close margins of 16 Gy is controversial. OR PORT (50 Gy/25 fx plus boost as above) OR adjuvant brachytherapy alone (30–50 Gy given BID)	*PORT is not recommended for RPS. Consider when recurrence would be morbid and/or unresectable.*
Unresectable	Consider neoadjuvant RT, CHT, or chemoRT to facilitate surgery. Dose >70 Gy necessary for LC with RT alone.	Consider CHT or RT to facilitate surgery. If truly unresectable, treatment is palliative.
Desmoid	Observation may be reasonable. Primary management is surgical or medical. RT to 56 Gy if non-operative. PORT for positive margins is controversial; many reserve RT for recurrence or unresectable disease. Consider sorafenib, tamoxifen, sulindac, and imatinib for unresectable patients or those with FAP.	

*36 Gy/18 fx can be considered for myxoid liposarcoma[2]

EPIDEMIOLOGY: Sarcomas are rare, representing ~1% of malignancies, with 80% of these being STS and 20% originating in bone. Benign soft tissue masses are much more common than STS. In 2020, there were an estimated 13,130 cases of STS diagnosed in the United States, and an estimated 5,350 deaths.[3] Median age of diagnosis is 45 to 55 years with ~20% found before 40 years; 30% between 40 and 60 years; and 50% >60 years. Age by histology: FS (30–39), LMS (50–59), UPS (60–69) formerly known as MFH and LS (60–69).

RISK FACTORS: Male gender, genetic predisposition, prior exposure to RT or CHT, chemical carcinogens, chronic irritation or lymphedema, and HIV/HHV8 involvement in Kaposi's. In reported series from MSKCC, distribution of RT-induced sarcomas was osteosarcoma (21%), UPS (16%), and angiosarcoma (15%). These were seen most commonly following treatment of breast cancer (26%), lymphoma (25%), and cervical cancer (14%), with median latency of 10.3 years.[4] FAP, or more specifically Gardner syndrome, are a risk factor for desmoid tumors.

ANATOMY: STS arise from a mesenchymal cell of origin and can occur in all body sites; however, around two-thirds occur in extremities, most commonly in the lower extremity, above the knee. Remaining one-third is found in retroperitoneum and trunk or H&N region, with slightly more retroperitoneal cases. At diagnosis, 90% of extremity STS are localized to the muscle compartment of origin. Most common STS by site: extremities (LS, UPS, synovial, and FS); retroperitoneum (well-differentiated and dedifferentiated LS and LMS); visceral (GIST). The tumor is usually surrounded by a pseudocapsule (region of compressed reactive tissue) and reactive zone (high MRI T2 signal) that can harbor microscopic disease, which is important for resection assessment. In one series, infiltrating tumor cells were found up to 4 cm from pseudocapsule in 67% of patients, and all but one of which were found in "edema" region.[5]

PATHOLOGY: Greater than 100 histologic subtypes have been reported. Most common subtypes in decreasing order are LS, LMS, high-grade UPS, GIST, synovial sarcoma, myxofibrosarcoma, and MPNST. Certain subtypes have a propensity for metastasis, such as LMS. Histologic grade is determined by differentiation, mitotic count, and necrosis.[6] Of note, myogenic differentiation in pleomorphic sarcomas increases risk of DM and is prognostic for many subtypes. Grade is less prognostic for MPNST, angiosarcoma, extraskeletal myxoid chondrosarcoma, and clear cell sarcoma.

GENETICS: Simple karyotypes and reciprocal translocations may include alveolar rhabdomyosarcoma (t[2;13]), clear cell sarcoma (t[12;22]), myxoid LS (t[12;16]), synovial sarcoma (t[X;18]), dermatofibrosarcoma protuberans (ring [17;22]), and solitary fibrous tumor (fusion NAB2-STAT6). Characteristic amplifications: well-differentiation to undifferentiated LS (amplification of 12q, contains MDM2). Specific driver mutations: desmoid fibromatosis (CTNNB1), GIST (c-kit or PDGFRA), rhabdoid tumors (loss of INI1). Complex karyotypes may be found in some high-grade tumors. Some classic genetic syndromes with their specific mutations that increase risk of STS are characterized in Table 55.2.

Table 55.2: Genetic Syndromes Commonly Associated With Soft Tissue Sarcoma			
Syndrome	Clinical Findings	Gene	Chromosome
Neurofibromatosis Type 1 (NF1)	MPNST (5%), optic glioma, astrocytoma, neurofibromas, café au lait spots, Lisch nodules, axillary freckling	NF-1	17q11
Familial retinoblastoma (Rb)	STS, osteosarcoma, retinoblastoma	Rb-1	13q14
Li–Fraumeni	STS, osteosarcoma, leukemia, BC, CNS tumors, adrenal tumors	TP53	17p13
Werner's (adult progeria)	STS, osteosarcoma, meningioma	WRN	8p12
Gardner's (subset of FAP)	FS, intraabdominal desmoid, colon cancer	APC	5q21
Gorlin's (nevoid BCC)	FS, rhabdomyosarcoma, BCC, CNS tumors	PTC	9q22
Carney's triad	GIST, extra-adrenal paraganglioma, pulmonary chondroma	c-KIT	Unknown

CLINICAL PRESENTATION: Symptoms are generally site dependent. Typical presentation is enlarging, painless mass. Symptoms of compression may be reported including new onset edema and/or paresthesia. Constitutional symptoms including fever and weight loss are rare. Metastatic disease is present at initial diagnosis in 6%–10%, with increased risk in deep and high-grade tumors.[4]

WORKUP: As benign soft tissue disease is much more common, workup of painless enlarging mass should include thorough H&P with exam of mass and draining LN regions to assess for adenopathy and rule out benign causes.

Labs: CBC and CMP.

Imaging: CT and MRI with contrast of affected area. On MRI, the tumor is typically hypointense on T1 and hyperintense on T2. CT chest to evaluate for metastatic disease once STS is confirmed. Role of FDG PET/CT is evolving and according to NCCN may be useful in prognostication, grading, and determining response to neoadjuvant CHT.[1] It may also be helpful to distinguish MPNST from neurofibroma. PET/MR or at minimum MRI of the spine can be useful for primary spine sarcomas as well as for evaluation of spine metastases from myxoid LS and round cell sarcomas.

Procedures: Core needle biopsy is preferred to determine grade and histology. If necessary, open biopsy incisions should be placed longitudinally along extremity so scar can be resected at time of surgery. Ideally, surgeon performing biopsy should be surgeon performing resection, especially in complex anatomical locations, and be a trained surgical/orthopedic oncologist. May consider excisional biopsy for <3 cm superficial lesions. For RPS, use of CT-guided biopsy via RP approach can avoid seeding of peritoneum. FNA may be performed to detect recurrence or metastatic disease.

PROGNOSTIC FACTORS: Grade, size, and metastatic disease. Factors increasing risk of LF include age >50, recurrent disease, margins <1 cm, and poorly differentiated histology. Factors increasing risk of DM often include higher grade (G1: 5%–10%, G2: 25%–30%, G3: 50%–60%), size (>5 cm), deep seated tumor, recurrence, and histology.

NATURAL HISTORY: Most common route of DM is hematogenous, with lungs the most common site in 75% of patients, especially for STS of extremity/trunk region, with other less common sites in decreasing order including bone, other soft tissues (including bone marrow, for example, for myxoid/round cell LS), liver (e.g., from adjacent visceral sarcoma, RPS), and rarely brain metastasis (more commonly seen with LMS, angiosarcoma, and alveolar soft part sarcoma). If there are ≤4 lung metastases and long DFI w/o endobronchial invasion, approximately 25% can be cured with resection (3-year OS was 30%–50%).[7] This appears to be true regardless of ablative modality for metastasis.[8] LN involvement is rare (<5%), but more common in "CARE" histologies: **C**lear cell (27.7%), **A**ngiosarcoma (24.1%), **R**habdomyosarcoma (32.1%), and **E**pithelioid (31.8%).[5,9] Some histologies have unique natural histories, for example, dermal spread for superficial MFH; angiosarcoma; desmoid tumor with lack of pseudocapsule and poorly defined margins; and dermal nodules or skip metastases for epithelioid sarcoma. Specific subtypes primarily recurring locally include desmoid, MPNST, atypical lipomatous or well differentiation LS, and DMFSP. Those with local and intermediate risk for DM include myxoid LS, myxoid fibrosarcoma, and extraskeletal myxoid chondrosarcoma, and hemangiopericytoma. Those with local and high potential for DM include most other sarcomas, especially high grade. STS increase in size with direct local extension along tissue planes, which are not always superior/inferior, and may grow centrifugally. Myxoid LS are known to be the most radiosensitive. RPS of well-differentiated LS histology have long natural history and may not require aggressive treatment.[10]

STAGING: Emphasis in 8th edition placed on primary site of STS; thus multiple separate staging systems other than trunk/extremities are defined, including H&N, abdomen/thoracic visceral organs, GIST, and RPS.[6] Table 55.3 includes staging for STS of trunk and extremities.

Table 55.3: AJCC 8th Edition (2017): Staging for Soft Tissue Sarcoma of Trunk and Extremities (H&N, abdomen and thoracic, and retroperitoneal and GIST not included here)							
Tumor		**Node**		**Distant Metastasis**		**Grade**	
T1	• ≤5 cm	N0	• No regional LNs	M0	• No distant metastasis	G1	• Total differentiation, mitotic count, and necrosis score of 2 to 3
T2	• 5.1–10 cm	N1	• Regional LNs	M1	• Distant metastasis	G2	• Total differentiation, mitotic count, and necrosis score of 4–5

(continued)

Table 55.3: AJCC 8th Edition (2017): Staging for Soft Tissue Sarcoma of Trunk and Extremities (H&N, abdomen and thoracic, and retroperitoneal and GIST not included here) (*continued*)			
T3	• 10.1–15 cm	G3	• Total differentiation, mitotic count, and necrosis score of 6–8
T4	• >15 cm		

TNM	Grade	Group Stage
T1N0M0	G1	IA
T2-4N0M0	G1	IB
T1N0M0	G2 to 3	II
T2N0M0	G2 to 3	IIIA
T3–4N0M0	G2 to 3	IIIB
Any T, N1, M0	Any	IV
Any T, Any N, M1	Any	IV

TREATMENT PARADIGM

Surgery: Negative-margin resection with preservation of function is goal of treatment for localized disease. En bloc excision encompasses biopsy site, scar, and tumor achieving >1 to 2 cm margins ideally. Extent of surgical resection (originally described by Enneking[11]): (a) *intralesional*, (b) *marginal*: plane of resection through reactive tissue surrounding sarcoma, (c) *simple*: narrow margin (LR 60%–90%); (d) *wide*: plane of resection through normal tissue (~2–3 cm margin) and within compartment of STS origin (LR 30%–60%), (d) *radical/compartmental*: en bloc resection of anatomical compartment; includes amputation (LR 10%–20%). Margin status is the most important variable for LC. Violation of tumor is associated with higher LR rates. It is usually unnecessary to resect adjacent bone. About 75% of patients with LR after limb-sparing surgery and RT can be salvaged by subsequent amputation. Consider free or rotational flap closures for large wounds requiring PORT. Indication for amputation (~5% of cases): (a) involvement of major neurovascular structures or multiple compartments such that functional limb is not achievable; (b) RT dose and volume constraints; (c) recurrence not amenable to further surgery or RT; (d) severely compromised normal tissue (due to age, peripheral vascular disease, or other comorbidities). For distal extremity lesion, below knee amputation with prosthesis may be preferred to limb sparing. For RPS, en bloc resection of nearby organs (kidney, liver, spleen) may be required.

Chemotherapy: There are conflicting data regarding routine use of CHT in definitive management of STS, for which it has primarily been evaluated in extremity STS and less commonly in sites such as in RPS. For primary extremity STS, there appears to be the greatest benefit in LC, RFS, and OS when doxorubicin is combined with ifosfamide, and there is a trend to improved OS with single-agent doxorubicin based on an updated meta-analysis from the SMAC. Analysis of the US Sarcoma Collaborative database found that patients with extremity and trunk STS tumors >10 cm derive a benefit from neoadjuvant CHT, and just over half of patients in that analysis received RT.[12] Further trials are ongoing. Pazopanib, an oral multitarget TKI, improved PFS in the PALETTE trial for previously treated metastatic patients (median PFS 1.6 vs. 4.6 mos, $p < .0001$) and may be considered.[13] Other targeted agents are under investigation.

Radiation: EBRT for STS of Extremity: RT may be delivered pre-op or in the adjuvant setting and IORT can be considered as a boost when clinically indicated. *Pre-op RT:* For extremity sarcoma, dose is 50 Gy/25 fx. New data have emerged that myxoid LS of the trunk and extremity can be treated with 36 Gy/18 fx without a detriment in LC.[2] For close/positive margins after pre-op RT, utility of post-op EBRT boost of 10 to 16 Gy (total 60–66 Gy) is controversial but was performed on most trials. Other options for close margins include IORT (10–16 Gy) or brachytherapy (12–20 Gy).

PORT: If RT is given in the adjuvant setting, typical dosing and fractionation is 50 Gy/25 fx followed by a cone down to 60 to 66 Gy for negative margins, 66 to 68 Gy for microscopically positive margins, and 70 to 76 Gy for gross residual disease.

EBRT for RPS: Doses of 45 to 50.4 Gy/25 to 28 fx are recommended when treating pre-op, though indications for pre-op RT are controversial. PORT not generally recommended except when recurrence may be morbid or unresectable. Well-differentiated LS has long natural history and may not require RT (or aggressive surgery), though pre-op RT can be considered in the recurrent setting. Consensus statements exist for treatment selection and contouring for RPS.[10]

Brachytherapy: Advantages include conformal tumor bed irradiation, short overall tx time, less dose to surrounding normal tissue (may yield better functional outcome), and region well-oxygenated. Brachytherapy alone may be used as adjuvant for intermediate- to high-grade sarcomas of extremity or superficial trunk with negative margins and has been shown to improve LC.[14] ABS guidelines are available to guide dose and technique.[15] Brachytherapy implemented following primary wound closure should be delayed to post-op day 5 to decrease the risk of wound complications, but when using negative pressure wound therapy as a temporary closure, brachytherapy can be initiated immediately. Most commonly, HDR brachytherapy with Ir-192 is used as boost to dose of 12 to 20 Gy given twice daily (BID) over 2 to 3 days in conjunction with EBRT. Brachytherapy may also be utilized as adjuvant therapy alone (30–40 Gy given BID over 5 days) and often is preferred after resection of LR in previously irradiated patients.[15,16]

Procedure: See *Handbook of Treatment Planning in Radiation Oncology,* Chapter 11.[17]

■ EVIDENCE-BASED Q&A

PRIMARY EXTREMITY STS

▨ Can the addition of PORT to LSS avoid amputation?

Historically, high recurrence rates after local excision alone led to the use of radical compartment excisions or amputations. This generated the idea behind the Rosenberg NCI trial.

Rosenberg, NCI (*Ann Surg* 1982, PMID 7114936): PRT of 43 patients w/ extremity high-grade STS treated from 1975 to 1981 randomized to amputation (*n* = 16) vs. LSS + PORT (*n* = 27) consisting of 50 Gy with 10 to 20 Gy boost to tumor bed. All patients received post-op CHT with doxorubicin, cyclophosphamide, and methotrexate. LR was 15% in LSS arm vs. 0% (*p* = .06) in amputation arm; 5-year DFS (71% vs. 78%, NS) and OS (82% vs. 88%, NS) for LSS vs. amputation, respectively. QOL is reported elsewhere, but was same. Later analyses also showed no benefit to CHT. On MVA, only positive margins were correlated with LR, even in setting of PORT. **Conclusion: LSS + PORT is reasonable and effective; this has become standard of care.**

▨ With limited randomized data showing PORT with LSS is as effective as amputation, is it necessary in those who undergo LSS alone, and does grade matter?

Although LSS and PORT became standard after NCI study, morbidity with PORT is not trivial, and there were only historical comparisons to suggest it improved LR rates over LSS alone. This led to the NCI trial, which confirmed LC benefit with PORT, but no OS benefit was found. Additional large SEER meta-analysis suggests this benefit is limited to high-grade STS.

Yang, NCI (*JCO* 1998, PMID 9440743): Phase III PRT including 91 patients w/ high-grade extremity STS s/p LSS w/ negative or minimal microscopic margins randomized to post-op CHT alone (*n* = 44) vs. CHT + PORT (*n* = 47) to 63 Gy (45 Gy + 18 Gy boost at 1.8 Gy/fx) assessing LC, OS, and QOL. Additional 50 patients w/ low-grade sarcomas were enrolled to receive PORT (*n* = 26) vs. LSS alone (*n* = 24). MFU of 9.6 years. See Table 55.4. LC was significantly improved with addition of RT for both low- and high-grade patients, with no OS benefit. PORT resulted in significantly worse limb strength, edema, and range of motion, but these deficits were often transient and had little effect on ADLs or QOL. **Conclusion: Significant LC benefit with addition of PORT with no OS benefit.**

Table 55.4: Results of NCI Trial				
High Grade (*n* = 91)	10-Yr LC	10-Yr OS	Low Grade (*n* = 50)	10-Yr LC
Post-op CHT	78%	74%	No adjuvant tx	67%
Post-op ChemoRT	100%	75%	Post-op RT	96%
p value	.0028	.71	*p* value	.016

Koshy, SEER (*IJROBP* 2010, PMID 19679403): SEER retrospective analysis from 1988 to 2005 including 6,960 patients with both low-/high-grade extremity STS assessing OS benefit of RT after LSS; 47% of patients received RT, primarily post-op (86%). For high-grade STS, addition of RT was associated with 3-year OS benefit (73% vs. 63%, *p* < .001). There was no OS benefit for low-grade STS. **Conclusion: This large retrospective analysis showed higher OS with addition of RT in setting of LSS for high-grade STS, but not for low-grade STS.**

■ **Can the addition of adjuvant brachytherapy improve LC?**

Compared to surgery alone, there appears to be significant LC benefit, which is confined to high-grade histology, and there is no improvement in DSS or DM.

Pisters, MSKCC (*JCO* 1996, PMID 8622034): PRT of 164 patients w/ STS of extremity or superficial trunk, randomized intra-op to adjuvant brachytherapy vs. no further tx after R0 resection. Brachytherapy given via Ir-192 implant delivering 42 to 45 Gy over 4 to 6 days. MFU 76 months. Equivalent DSS and no difference in DM. Five-year actuarial LC was 82% vs. 69% (*p* = .04) in favor of brachytherapy. However, on further analysis, this improvement in LC was found to be for high-grade lesions, but not low-grade lesions as described in Table 55.5. There was no difference in wound complication rates among patients who were loaded after post-op day 5 (modified timing midtrial from loading <5 days to ≥6 days). **Conclusion: Brachytherapy improves LC for high-grade STS with no difference in DSS or DM, and no improvement for low-grade tumors.**

Table 55.5: Results of MSKCC Trial of Adjuvant Brachytherapy for Soft Tissue Sarcoma				
	5-Yr LC	5-Yr DSS	Low-Grade LC	High-Grade LC
No brachytherapy	69%	81%	72%	66%
Brachytherapy	82%	84%	73%	89%
p value	.04	.65	.49	.0025

■ **What is the optimal sequencing of RT when indicated for the management of STS?**

Both pre- and post-op EBRT are reasonable, with trade-offs. Pre-op RT allows for smaller field sizes and lower doses, which are generally associated with better long-term functional outcomes. This generally comes at expense of higher rates of acute wound complications.

O'Sullivan, NCIC SR2 (*Lancet* 2002, PMID 12103287; Davis, *Radiother Oncol* 2005, PMID 15948265): PRT of 190 patients w/ STS stratified by tumor size (≤10 cm vs. >10 cm) and randomized to pre-op RT (50 Gy/25 fx) vs. PORT (66–70 Gy; 50 Gy/25 fx to initial field + 16–20 Gy boost). Pre-op arm was treated w/ additional 16 to 20 Gy for positive margins (14 of 91 patients had positive margins, 10 treated w/ RT). Primary end point: Acute wound complications and erythema, with later analyses assessing 2-year late effects of grade 2 to 4 fibrosis, edema, and joint stiffness. Study terminated early at interim analysis. Updated at MFU 6.9 years. Median RT field size was smaller in pre-op arm. Complete results in Table 55.6. LC was identical between two arms. Initial trend toward improved OS in pre-op arm was lost at later FU. Tumor size and grade predicted for OS; grade predicted for RFS; margin status predicted for LC. Pre-op RT was associated with lower rates of acute skin erythema, late fibrosis, joint stiffness, and edema, albeit none were statistically significant. Pre-op RT had higher rates of acute wound complications (35% vs.

17%, highest in upper leg). **Conclusion: No difference in LC, RFS, or OS. Pre-op RT for extremity sarcomas may be preferred due to lower rates of irreversible late fibrosis, at the cost of higher, but generally reversible, acute wound complications.**

Table 55.6: Results of NCIC SR2 Trial of Preoperative vs. Postoperative RT for Soft Tissue Sarcoma									
	Acute Wound Complications	2-Yr Grade 2 to 4 Fibrosis	2-Yr Grade 2 to 4 Edema	2-Yr Joint Stiffness	5-Yr LC	5-Yr RFS	5-Yr Mets RFS	5-Yr OS	5-Yr CSS
Pre-op RT	35%	32%	15%	18%	93%	58%	67%	73%	78%
Post-op RT	17%	48%	23%	23%	92%	59%	69%	67%	73%
p value	.01	.07	.26	.51	NS	NS	NS	.47	.64

Al-Absi, Ontario (*Ann Surg Oncol* 2010, PMID 20217260): Systematic review and meta-analysis of five eligible studies of pre-op vs. PORT for localized, resectable STS including 1,098 patients. Significant improvement in LC with pre-op RT despite larger average tumor size in pre-op group with OR of 0.61 (95% CI: 0.42–0.89) by means of fixed-effects method, and OR of 0.67 (95% CI: 0.39–1.15) by means of random-effects method. Time-dependent survival averaged across all studies was 76% (range 62%–88%) pre-op vs. 67% (range 41%–83%) post-op, NS. **Conclusion: Findings must be interpreted with caution due to heterogeneity, but suggest that delay in surgery due to pre-op RT does not confer increased DM rate vs. PORT, and may provide superior LC.**

▓ **Can pre-op hypofractionated EBRT be given with comparable outcomes?**

Data are limited to single institution series, though it appears that neoadjuvant hypofractionated RT with or without CHT can be given prior to surgical resection; however, further investigation is needed.

Kosela-Paterczyk, Poland (*Eur J Surg Oncol* 2014, PMID 25282099): Prospective single-arm trial of 272 patients with locally advanced STS of trunk or extremities, grade 2 to 3 or deep seated (>10 cm) grade 1. Neoadjuvant RT 25 Gy/5 fx daily and surgery 3 to 7 days after RT. PORT of 30 Gy/15 fx for positive margin (7.7%). With MFU 35 months, 3-year LFRS 81% and OS 72%. Decreased LRFS associated with tumor size >10 cm, grade 3, positive margin and prior non-radical surgery. Early complication rate 32.4%, only 7% required re-operation for complications and none required amputation. **Conclusion: LC and OS similar to historical long course pre-op RT with acceptable rates of early toxicity, which is commonly reversible.**

Pennington, UCLA (*Am J Clin Oncol* 2018, PMID 29664796): RR of 116 patients from single institution treated 1990 to 2013 with neoadjuvant hypofractionated RT (28 Gy/8 fx daily) with ifosfamide-based chemotherapy. RT given concurrently with ifosfamide or sequentially with combined doxorubicin and ifosfamide. Resection 2 to 3 weeks after RT. MFU 5.9 years, actuarial LRR 11%, and 17% at 3- and 6-year, respectively. On MVA positive margin associated with increased risk of LR. Fifteen percent of patients experienced acute and long-term toxicity including 10% with acute and perioperative wound complications. **Conclusion: Ifosfamide-based NACT with hypofractionated RT provides acceptable tumor control with LF 17% at 6 years.**

Kalbasi, UCLA (*Clin Cancer Res* 2020, PMID 32054730): Phase II single-institution study of 52 patients evaluating safety of 5-day neoadjuvant RT (30 Gy/5 fx) with standard margins. Primary end point was grade ≥2 late-radiation toxicity. MFU 29 months with 7 of 44 (16%) evaluable patients developing grade ≥2 late-RT toxicity. Major wound complications in 50 patients (32%) associated with lower extremity tumor location and also a germline biomarker. **Conclusion: Five-day neoadjuvant RT demonstrates favorable rates of wound complications and late-toxicity, which may be predictive with germline biomarker if further validated.**

■ **Can dose-reduced dose pre-op EBRT be given for myxoid LS?**

A phase II non-randomized trial demonstrated that pre-op 36 Gy/18 fx had excellent LC with low risk of wound healing complications.

Lansu, DOREMY (*JAMA Oncol* 2020, PMID 33180100): International single-arm phase II trial of 79 patients with resectable extremity or trunk myxoid LS. Patients received 36 Gy/18 fx pre-op IMRT. Primary outcome was extensive pathological treatment response in definitive resection specimen, defined as <50% vital tumor cells with trial being positive if ≥70% of patients achieved this. Of 77 patients resected, 91% had extensive pathological response. Wound complications of any severity were observed in 22%, of which 17% needed any intervention. With MFU of 25 months, LC was 100% regardless of extent of pathological response. **Conclusion: Dose-reduced pre-op EBRT should be considered for myxoid LS tumors, which may lead to decreased wound complications without a detriment in LC.**

■ **What is the role of post-op boost with EBRT in patients who receive pre-op RT and undergo surgical resection with positive surgical margins?**

Data are limited to small RRs with no PRT to answer this question as of now. There is suggestion that EBRT boost may not be effective in preventing LR in patients with positive margins after pre-op RT.

Al Yami (*IJROBP* 2010, PMID 20056340): RR of 216 extremity STS patients treated from 1986 to 2003 who had positive surgical margin; 93 patients had been treated with pre-op RT (50 Gy), while 41 additionally received a postoperative boost (80% received boost dose of 16 Gy with EBRT to total dose of 66 Gy). No difference in tumor baseline characteristics. Five-year LRFS estimates were 90.4% for no boost vs. 73.8% for boost ($p = .13$). **Conclusion: Post-op boost with EBRT did not improve LRFS in this small retrospective analysis.**

■ **Can modern image-guided RT (3D or IMRT) improve morbidity?**

Part of rationale for pre-op RT is to decrease late effects by reducing irradiated volume. IGRT may be able to reduce volume even further without compromising tumor control.

Wang, RTOG 0630 (*JCO* 2015, PMID 25667281): Multi-institutional phase II trial assessing utility of IGRT (3DCRT or IMRT allowed) for reducing toxicity compared to O'Sullivan NCIC trial. Primary end point: 2-year grade ≥2 late RT morbidity; 98 patients were accrued to two cohorts: cohort A (12 patients; intermediate- to high-grade STS ≥8 cm who received CHT; results not reported) and cohort B (79 evaluable patients; all treated w/o CHT). RT: 50 Gy/25 fx with post-op boost suggested if positive margins (16 Gy/8 fx EBRT, 16 Gy LDR, 13.6 Gy/4 fx HDR, or 10 to 12.5 Gy IORT); 2 to 3 cm longitudinal CTV expansion and 1 or 1.5 cm radial (< or ≥8 cm) including suspicious edema with IGRT. MFU3.6 years. Most patients had UPS (22.8%), LS (21.5%), or myxoid FS (21.5%). Most common primary was upper thigh (41.8%); 74.7% were treated w/ IMRT. Five patients did not undergo surgery due to progression; 56 (76%) had R0 resection, and 11 (15%) received post-op boost. Five patients had in-field LF (three fifths with positive margins and two fifths treated with post-op boost). Overall rate of grade ≥2 late toxicity was significantly improved compared to O'Sullivan pre-op arm (10.5% vs. 37%, $p < .001$). Individual toxicities compared favorably: fibrosis (5.3% vs. 31.5%), joint stiffness (3.5% vs. 17.8%), edema (5.3% vs. 15.1%); 36.6% of patients experienced at least one wound complication, all in lower extremity tumors, and most commonly in proximal lower extremity. **Conclusion: Significant reduction of late toxicities and absence of marginal-field recurrences with IGRT suggest that smaller target volumes are appropriate for pre-op RT with IGRT for extremity STS.**

O'Sullivan, Canada (*Cancer* 2013, PMID 23423841): Single-arm phase II trial using IMRT with image guidance to deliver pre-op RT with primary end point of acute wound complications compared to NCIC trial: 70 patients, with 59 evaluable. RT dose/volumes: 50 Gy/25 fx without boost; 4-cm longitudinal and 1.5-cm radial expansions including edema with IGRT; dose restricted to "future surgical skin flaps" and bone. MFU of 49 months. Most patients had UPS (35.6%), myxoid LS (32.2%), or pleomorphic LS (10.2%). R1 resection in four patients. Buttock was most common site of wound complications (45%), followed by adductor (44%) and hamstring (44%). Overall rate of complications were not different from NCIC trial, but primary closure was more frequent (93.2% vs. 71.4%). Number of secondary operations was numerically less but not SS. Flap/PTV overlap was improved on MVA (<1% overlap, 14.3% vs. 39.5%). Four patients had LF (6.8%), none near surgical flaps, and two of four had positive margins. No grade >2 late toxicities in patients surviving longer than 2 years with no fractures. **Conclusion: Pre-op IMRT with IGRT significantly diminished need for tissue transfer, with NS reduction in acute wound complications, chronic morbidities, and need for subsequent secondary operations, while maintaining good limb function.**

■ **With respect to IMRT and brachytherapy, does one have a better therapeutic ratio compared to the other?**

Data are limited to RRs and comparisons of modern control rates of each separately, but there is suggestion of superior LC with IMRT.

Alektiar, MSKCC (*Cancer* 2011, PMID 21264834): RR of 134 patients with high-grade extremity STS who were treated with LSS and either brachytherapy (1995–2003) or IMRT (2002–2006). LDR brachytherapy (*n* = 71) was administered post-op with median dose 45 Gy. IMRT (*n* = 63) was delivered pre-op (*n* = 10) with mean dose of 50 Gy, and post-op (*n* = 53) to median dose of 63 Gy. MFU of 46 months for IMRT; 47 months for brachytherapy. There were statistically higher-risk tumors in IMRT cohort such as positive/close margins (<1 mm), large tumors (>10 cm), and requiring bone or nerve stripping/resection. Five-yr LC favored IMRT (92% vs. 81%, *p* = .04). On MVA, IMRT was only significant predictor of improved LC (*p* = .04). **Conclusion: LC with IMRT was significantly better than brachytherapy despite higher rates of adverse features for IMRT in this nonrandomized comparison. IMRT warrants further studies for this patient population.**

■ **Does the addition of adjuvant CHT improve outcomes for resected STS?**

This has been area of controversy based on risk vs. benefit of such therapy, but due to risk of local and distant failures, adjuvant CHT was often administered, typically with doxorubicin-based therapy. SMAC updated their meta-analysis in 2008 of RCTs including adjuvant CHT following surgical resection for STS confirming efficacy of doxorubicin-based CHT with greater benefit when given with ifosfamide.

Pervaiz, Sarcoma Meta-Analysis Collaboration (*Cancer* 2008, PMID 18521899): Comprehensive meta-analysis of 18 RCTs including 1,953 patients assessing failures and survival outcomes with doxorubicin-based adjuvant CHT in resectable STS. OR for LR was 0.73 (95% CI: 0.56–0.94; *p* = .02) favoring CHT. For DM and overall recurrence, OR was 0.67 (95% CI: 0.56–0.82, *p* = .0001) favoring CHT. On survival analysis, doxorubicin alone had OR of 0.84 (95% CI: 0.68–1.03, *p* = .09) while doxorubicin combined with ifosfamide was 0.56 (95% CI: 0.36–0.85; *p* = .01) favoring CHT. **Conclusion: This analysis confirms the benefit of CHT with respect to recurrence and metastasis for adjuvant doxorubicin, while addition of ifosfamide demonstrated significant survival benefit and further improved other outcomes.**

■ **In the pre-op setting, what is the role of the addition of CHT?**

DM continues to be a problem in STS. Previous small pilot studies of neoadjuvant CHT or CRT appeared promising, which led to RTOG 9514, which assessed the feasibility of neoadjuvant CHT interdigitated with RT prior to surgery followed by additional adjuvant CHT alone or following additional RT for + SM. Neoadjuvant CHT is not a standard of care approach at this time but can be considered for large, high-grade tumors.

Kraybill, RTOG 9514 (*JCO* 2006, PMID 16446334): Phase II trial evaluating neoadjuvant CHT with pre-op RT followed by CHT post-op in multi-institutional setting. High-grade extremity/body wall STS ≥8 cm were eligible. Sixty-six patients were enrolled. CHT consisted of MAID regimen (modified mesna, doxorubicin, ifosfamide, and dacarbazine), which was given for 3C, with interdigitated RT 44 Gy/22 fx split course (MAID→RT→MAID→RT→MAID) followed by resection 3 weeks later. Post-op therapy was based on margin status. If positive margins, additional 16 Gy/8 fx given to post-op bed + 1 cm margin, followed by MAID × 3C. If negative margins, MAID × 3C alone; 64 patients were analyzable; 79% completed pre-op CHT with only 59% receiving full CHT course due to toxicity, 5% experiencing grade 5 fatal toxicity, and 83% experiencing grade 4. Sixty-one patients underwent surgery, with 58 R0 resections (five amputations). At 3 years, estimated DFS was 56.6%, distant DFS 64.5%, and OS 75.1%. There were five amputations leading to 92% limb preservation rate. Estimated 3-year LRF of 18% if amputation considered failure, and 10% if not. **Conclusion: Just over half of 64 patients received planned treatment course due to substantial toxicity, but regimen does appear to show activity.**

Zaidi, U.S. Sarcoma Collaborative (*Ann Surg Oncol* **2019, PMID 31342400**): RR of 770 patients from U.S. Sarcoma Collaborative database treated from 2000 to 2016 with curative-intent resection of high-grade, primary truncal, and extremity STS ≥5 cm. Primary end points were RFS and OS. Most common histology was UPS (42%). A total of 216 patients (28%) received NACT, and had deeper and larger tumors (*p* < .001). For patients with tumors ≥10 cm, NACT improved 5-year RFS (51% vs. 40%; *p* = .053) and 5-year OS (58% vs. 47%; *p* = .043). When evaluating location, tumors ≥10 cm in the extremity had improved 5-year RFS (54% vs. 42%; *p*=0.042) and 5-year OS (61% vs. 47%; *p*=0.015) with NACT, but the truncal cohort did not; however, it was likely underpowered. **Conclusion: NACT improves RFS and OS for extremity tumors ≥10 cm, and further investigation is required to determine role in large truncal tumors.**

RETROPERITONEAL SARCOMA (RPS)

■ What is the general approach to managing RPS?

Primary management is based on achieving an R0 surgical resection. As with primary extremity STS, RPS data are limited mainly to small RRs; however, the recently completed EORTC STRASS trial failed to demonstrate a benefit of pre-op RT; however the LS subgroup may benefit. If RT is given, it is delivered in the preoperative setting as toxicity can be significant in the postoperative setting.

■ What current data suggest benefit, including OS, to addition of RT for RPS?

Based on SEER/NCDB datasets, there appears to be survival benefit with addition of RT, given either pre-op or post-op, with usual limitations of such nonrandomized registry studies; however, results of the randomized EORTC STRASS trial did not demonstrate a RFS benefit in all patients.

Zhou, SEER (*Arch Surg* **2010, PMID 20479339**): SEER analysis evaluating effect of surgical resection and RT for locoregional RPS and nonvisceral abdominal sarcoma from 1988 to 2005 including 1,901 patients; 81.8% underwent surgical resection and 23.5% received RT. Combined therapy was associated with improved OS vs. single modality therapy, and surgery or RT was better than no therapy (*p* < .001). Cox analysis demonstrated surgical resection (HR 0.24, *p* < .001) and RT (HR 0.78, 95% CI: 0.63–0.95, *p* = .01) independently predicted improved OS in locoregional disease only. In adjusted analyses stratified for stage, for stage I disease (*n* = 694), RT provided additional benefit (HR 0.49, *p* = .04) independent of that from resection (HR 0.35, *p* < .001). For stage II/III (*n* = 552), resection remained significant (HR 0.24, *p* < .001); however, RT was not associated with significant benefit (HR 0.78, 95% CI: 0.58–1.06, *p* = .11). **Conclusion: In this national cohort, surgical resection was associated with significant survival benefits for AJCC stage I to III RPS. RT provided additional benefit for patients with stage I disease.**

Nussbaum, NCDB Analysis (*Lancet Oncol* **2016, PMID 27210906**): Case–control, propensity score–matched analyses of 9,068 NCDB patients who were diagnosed with RPS from 2003 to 2011. Patients were included who had local RPS undergoing resection and either pre-op RT or PORT, but not both, and no additional therapy or IORT. Primary objective was OS for patients who received pre-op RT or PORT compared with those who received no RT within propensity score-matched datasets. A total of 563 patients received pre-op RT (MFU 42 months), 2,215 PORT (MFU 54 months), and 6,290 received no RT (MFU 43 months when compared to pre-op and 47 months for post-op cohort). Negligible differences in all demographic, clinic-pathological, and treatment-level variables. MS was 110 months for pre-op cohort vs. 66 months for matched no RT cohort comparator. MS was 89 months for post-op cohort vs. 64 months for matched no RT cohort. Both pre-op (HR 0.70, *p* < .0001) and PORT (HR 0.78, *p* < .0001) were significantly associated with higher OS compared with surgery alone. **Conclusion: RT is associated with higher OS compared with surgery alone when delivered either pre-op or post-op.**

Bonvalot, EORTC STRASS (*Lancet* **2020, PMID 32941794**): International phase III trial of 266 patients with RPS randomized to pre-op RT (50.4 Gy) vs. surgery alone. Primary endpoint of abdominal RFS defined as local relapse after complete resection, peritoneal carcinomatosis, progression during RT, or unresectable disease. Designed to demonstrate 20% increase in abdominal RFS at 5-year from 50% to 70%; 198 (74.5%) had LS. There was no significant increase in rate of inoperable tumors or re-operations in the RT plus surgery group. Twice as many LR observed in surgery alone group, specifically in LS group. Three-year abdominal RFS 60.4% in RT plus surgery vs. 58.7% surgery alone (NS). **Conclusion: There is no abdominal RFS benefit with pre-op RT in RPS; however, a subset of patients with LS may benefit and further follow up is needed.**

■ Does the addition of IORT to PORT improve outcomes following surgically resected RPS?

Retrospective data exist; however, only one small PRT has addressed this question. In that NCI trial, addition of IORT reduced LRR but did not translate into an OS benefit. Bowel toxicity may be reduced as well.

Sindelar, NCI (*Arch Surg* 1993, PMID 8457152): PRT of 35 patients with RPS treated with surgery and post-op high-dose EBRT (50–55 Gy) vs. low-dose EBRT (35–40 Gy) + IORT (20 Gy). MFU of 8 years. MS similar between groups. LRR improved in IORT cohort (40% vs. 80%). IORT cohort had less disabling enteritis but more peripheral neuropathy (60% vs. 5%).

■ Does preoperative RT improve outcomes compared to postoperative RT?

In theory, pre-op RT may reduce toxicity due to lower dose, smaller volumes of normal tissue in the irradiated volume due to better target delineation, normal tissue displacement, and subsequent smaller treatment fields. Additionally, it may be more effective from a radiobiological standpoint due to improved vascularity and oxygenation. Most do not recommend PORT for RPS.

Ballo, MDACC (*IJROBP* 2007, PMID 17084545): RR of 83 patients with localized RPS treated with complete surgical resection and RT; 60 patients presented with primary disease with remaining 23 having LR following previous surgery. MFU of 47 months. Actuarial overall DSS, LC, and DMFSP were 44%, 40%, and 67%, respectively. Of 38 deaths, local progression was only site of recurrence for 16 patients and was component of progression for another 11 patients. MVA indicated histologic grade was associated with 5-year rates of DSS (low grade, 92%; intermediate grade, 51%; high grade, 41%, $p = .006$), as well as inferior 5-year LC rate for patients presenting with recurrent disease, positive margins or uncertain margin status, and age >65 years. No improved LC with higher doses of RT, or with specific use of IORT. RT-related complications (10% at 5 years) developed in five patients, with all complications limited to those who received PORT (23%) vs. pre-op RT (0%). **Conclusion: Preoperative RT may be preferred over PORT.**

■ Is IORT combined with does-escalated IMRT safe and effective?

Roeder (*BMC Cancer* 2014, PMID 25163595): Unplanned interim analysis of phase I/II single-arm trial assessing feasibility of pre-op IMRT with IOERT in 27 patients with primary/recurrent RPS (>5 cm, M0, at least marginally resectable) from 2007 to 2013. Pre-op IMRT delivered using SIB with doses of 45 to 50 Gy to PTV and 50 to 56 Gy to GTV in 25 fx, followed by surgery and IOERT (10–12 Gy). Primary end point was 5-year LC. Majority of patients had high-grade lesions (82% grade 23), predominantly LS (70%), with median tumor size of 15 cm (6–31 cm). MFU 33 months. Pre-op IMRT performed as planned in 93%. GTR with contiguous-organ resection was feasible in 96%, with 22% achieving R0 and 74% R1 resections. IOERT was performed in 23 patients (85%) with median dose of 12 Gy (10–20 Gy). There were seven recurrences leading to estimated 3- and 5-year LC rates of 72%. Grade 3 acute toxicity in 4 patients (15%), and severe post-op complications in 9 patients (33%). Grade 3 late toxicity in 6% of surviving patients after 1 year and none after 2 years. **Conclusion: Combination pre-op IMRT, surgery, and IOERT is feasible with acceptable toxicity and yields good results in terms of LC and OS in patients with high-risk RPS. Long-term follow-up is needed.**

■ What are the current recommendations for unresectable disease?

According to NCCN, treatment may include CHT or RT alone or in combination to facilitate resection, if possible.[1]

Kepka, Poland (*IJROBP* 2005, PMID 16199316): RR of 112 patients treated with definitive RT for unresectable STS. Forty-three percent extremities, 26% retroperitoneal, 24% H&N, and 7% trunk, 89%

grade 2 to 3. Median RT dose 64 Gy (range, 25–87.5 Gy). CHT was given in 20%. MFU 139 months; 5-year LC, DFS, and OS 45%, 24%, 35%, respectively; 5-year LC affected by tumor size (51%, 45%, and 9% for tumors <5 cm, 5–10 cm, and >10 cm, respectively) and RT dose (<63 Gy, 22%; >63 Gy, 60%). Dose >68 Gy vs. <68 Gy was associated with higher risk of complications (27% vs. 8%). **Conclusion: Definitive RT for STS should be considered in inoperable setting, with consideration of higher RT dose to improve outcomes, though critical to find appropriate therapeutic window to reduce complications.**

REFERENCES

1. NCCN Clinical Practice Guidelines in Oncology: soft tissue sarcoma. 2020. https://www.nccn.org
2. Lansu J, Bovée J, Braam P, et al. Dose reduction of preoperative radiotherapy in myxoid liposarcoma: a nonrandomized controlled trial. *JAMA Oncol.* 2021;7(1):e205865. doi:10.1001/jamaoncol.2020.5865
3. Siegel RL, Miller KD, Jemal A. Cancer statistics, 2020. *CA Cancer J Clin.* 2020;70(1):7–30. doi:10.3322/caac.21590
4. Brady MS, Gaynor JJ, Brennan MF. Radiation-associated sarcoma of bone and soft tissue. *Arch Surg.* 1992;127(12):1379–1385. doi:10.1001/archsurg.1992.01420120013002
5. White LM, Wunder JS, Bell RS, et al. Histologic assessment of peritumoral edema in soft tissue sarcoma. *Int J Radiat Oncol, Biol, Phys.* 2005;61(5):1439–1445. doi:10.1016/j.ijrobp.2004.08.036
6. *AJCC Cancer Staging Manual.* 8th ed. Springer; 2017.
7. van Geel AN, Pastorino U, Jauch KW, et al. Surgical treatment of lung metastases: the European organization for research and treatment of cancer-soft tissue and bone sarcoma group study of 255 patients. *Cancer.* 1996;77(4):675–682. doi:10.1002/(SICI)1097-0142(19960215)77:4<675::AID-CNCR13>3.0.CO;2-Y
8. Falk AT, Moureau-Zabotto L, Ouali M, et al. Effect on survival of local ablative treatment of metastases from sarcomas: a study of the French sarcoma group. *Clin Oncol (R Coll Radiol).* 2015;27(1):48–55. doi:10.1016/j.clon.2014.09.010
9. Baratti D, Pennacchioli E, Casali PG, et al. Epithelioid sarcoma: prognostic factors and survival in a series of patients treated at a single institution. *Ann Surg Oncol.* 2007;14(12):3542–3551. doi:10.1245/s10434-007-9628-9
10. Baldini EH, Wang D, Haas RL, et al. Treatment guidelines for preoperative radiation therapy for retroperitoneal sarcoma: preliminary consensus of an international expert panel. *Int J Radiat Oncol Biol Phys.* 2015;92(3):602–612. doi:10.1016/j.ijrobp.2015.02.013
11. Enneking WF, Spanier SS, Goodman MA. A system for the surgical staging of musculoskeletal sarcoma. *Clin Orthop Relat Res.* 1980(153):106–120. doi:10.1097/00003086-198011000-00013
12. Zaidi MY, Ethun CG, Tran TB, et al. Assessing the role of neoadjuvant chemotherapy in primary high-risk truncal/extremity soft tissue sarcomas: an analysis of the multi-institutional U.S. sarcoma collaborative. *Ann Surg Oncol.* 2019;26(11):3542–3549. doi:10.1245/s10434-019-07639-7
13. van der Graaf WT, Blay JY, Chawla SP, et al. Pazopanib for metastatic soft-tissue sarcoma (PALETTE): a randomised, double-blind, placebo-controlled phase 3 trial. *Lancet.* 2012;379(9829):1879–1886. doi:10.1016/S0140-6736(12)60651-5
14. Pisters PW, Harrison LB, Leung DH, et al. Long-term results of a prospective randomized trial of adjuvant brachytherapy in soft tissue sarcoma. *J Clin Oncol.* 1996;14(3):859–868. doi:10.1200/JCO.1996.14.3.859
15. Campbell SR, Shah C, Scott JG, et al. American Brachytherapy Society (ABS) consensus statement for soft-tissue sarcoma brachytherapy. *Brachytherapy.* 2021 Jul 21:S1538-4721(21)00107-0. doi:10.1016/j.brachy.2021.05.011. Epub ahead of print. PMID: 34303600.
16. Pearlstone DB, Janjan NA, Feig BW, et al. Re-resection with brachytherapy for locally recurrent soft tissue sarcoma arising in a previously radiated field. *Cancer J Sci Am.* 1999;5(1):26–33.
17. Videtic GMM, Woody N, Vassil AD. *Handbook of Treatment Planning in Radiation Oncology.* 2nd ed. Demos Medical; 2015. doi:10.1891/9781617051975

56 ■ MEDULLOBLASTOMA

Timothy D. Smile, Camille A. Berriochoa, and Erin S. Murphy

QUICK HIT ■ Medulloblastoma (MB) is the most common malignant pediatric CNS tumor, accounting for 20% of all childhood brain cancers.[1] MB typically arises in the cerebellum, most commonly in the cerebellar vermis, leading to obstruction of CSF flow and hydrocephalus, with presenting symptoms related to increased ICP. Surgery alone leads to poor outcomes, with multiple studies showing an improvement with the use of RT and CHT.[2,3] Attempts to reduce CSI dose and its associated growth and neurocognitive toxicities have been facilitated by optimized CHT regimens.[4] The recommended treatment paradigm is determined by patients' risk status (average vs. high; see Table 56.1). In the average risk setting, clinicians are transitioning to CSI + involved field boost vs. historic standard of complete PF boost based on promising results from ACNS0331.[5] The role of molecular pathways and associated subgrouping is evolving, with Wnt/SHH groups conferring better prognosis with a worse prognosis seen for groups 3 and 4.

Table 56.1: General Treatment Paradigm for MB Following Maximal Safe Resection

	CSI	Posterior Fossa	Post-RT CHT	5-Yr OS
Average risk (Two-thirds of patients at presentation) • ≥3 years of age AND • M0 AND • ≤1.5 cm^2 of residual disease post-op • Favorable histology (classic; desmoplastic/nodular; extensive nodularity)	23.4 Gy/13 fx with weekly concurrent vincristine	Per recent ACNS 0331 results, boost IF (rather than entire PF) to 54 to 55.8 Gy	CDDP/ VCR/ CYC or CCNU	80%
High risk* (One-third of patients at presentation) • M + OR • >1.5 cm^2 residual disease post-op • Poor histology (large cell; anaplastic)	36 Gy/20 fx with weekly concurrent vincristine	Boost PF to 54 to 55.8 Gy**	CDDP/ VCR/ CYC	60%

*Infants <3 years old are considered high risk and warrant a risk-adapted approach combining maximal safe resection, CHT, second-look surgery with delayed CSI, or focal radiation given poor neurocognitive outcomes with standard CSI.
**For lesions of the spinal cord, boost to 45 Gy.

EPIDEMIOLOGY: MB accounts for 40% of all PF tumors and 20% of all pediatric CNS tumors with about 500 cases per year in the United States.[6] Most commonly present between 5 and 7 years of age with distribution as follows: 10% before age 1, 60% to 70% before age 9, 30% above age 10. When present in adults, the histology is typically desmoplastic. More common in males than females.

RISK FACTORS: The majority of MB cases arise sporadically but ~5% are thought to be secondary to familial syndromes.

■ *Gorlin syndrome* (also known as "nevoid basal cell carcinoma syndrome"): AD condition associated with basal cell carcinoma, skeletal anomalies, and macrocephaly; MB develops in about 5% of patients. Associated with a 9q22.3 germline mutation, which confers inactivation of PTCH1, a protein that functions as the receptor for sonic hedgehog whose pathway is important for development of the cerebellum.[7]
■ *Turcot syndrome:* AD; characterized by polyposis, colorectal cancers, gliomas, and MBs; 92-fold higher relative risk of developing MB than the unaffected population.[8] Associated with APC

mutation on chromosome 5q. The APC complex is in part responsible for degrading cytoplasmic β-catenin and is regulated by the Wingless pathway (Wnt). These molecular pathways help underpin the evolving biomolecular paradigm of MB.

- *Li–Fraumeni and NF-1:* both occasionally associated with MB.

ANATOMY: Most commonly presents in the PF with ~75% occurring in the midline vermis. Hemispheric location is associated with older age and desmoplastic histology. The boundaries of the PF are as follows: anterior—clivus and posterior clinoid; posterior—inion (bony prominence at confluence of straight and sagittal sinuses); inferior—occipital bone, lateral–temporal, occipital, and parietal bones; superior—tentorium cerebellum. CSF flows from the fourth ventricle into the subarachnoid space via the medial foramen of Magendie and the lateral foramina of Luschka. The tendency for MB to obstruct CSF efflux leads to symptoms associated with raised ICP.[6]

PATHOLOGY: The 2016 WHO classification subdivides MB into the four histologic subtypes in Table 56.2 (in addition to genetic differences discussed in the following).[6,9,10] IHC demonstrates neuronal markers (neurofilament, neuron-specific enolase, synaptophysin) in most cases, and occasionally stains positive for GFAP (glial fibrillary acidic protein). Rare subtypes: melanotic (<1%) and medullomyoblastoma (<1%; contains striated muscle differentiation).

GENETICS: Historically, risk stratification has relied primarily on clinicopathologic variables. However, in 2010, an international panel identified four main molecular subgroups (Table 56.3). A molecularly driven risk stratification system was established at a 2016 consensus, which supports the development of biomarker-driven clinical trials, described in Table 56.4.[11,12] Note that supratentorial PNET tumors are classically treated as high-risk MB. Bcl-2, ERBB2, and MIB-L1 are potential markers of aggressive behavior.[13] C-MYC amplification and alterations in chromosome 17 can be observed.[14]

CLINICAL PRESENTATION: Tumors usually grow into/fill the fourth ventricle with signs and symptoms related to increased ICP: headaches, morning emesis, papilledema, diplopia due to CN VI palsy; infants may manifest bulging anterior fontanelle and splitting of cranial sutures. Destruction of the vermis can cause truncal ataxia; other cerebellar symptoms include dysmetria, dysdiadochokinesia, or spasticity. Though most commonly seen in pineal gland tumors, Parinaud syndrome (upward gaze palsy, pseudo-Argyll Robertson pupils, convergence-retraction nystagmus, eyelid retraction) can be observed, as can the "setting sun sign" (conjugate down gaze). Extraneural metastases are uncommon (<5%) but most commonly involve bone. Differential diagnosis of a pediatric posterior fossa mass: BEAM (brainstem glioma, ependymoma, astrocytoma, medulloblastoma), hemangioblastoma, lymphoma, and dysplastic cerebellar ganglioglioma.

Table 56.2: Morphologic Classification of Medulloblastoma			
Histopathologic Subtype	Prognosis	Relative Frequency	Features
Desmoplastic/ Nodular	Good	15%–20%, more common in older patients	Biphasic w/ dense cellular areas surrounded by stromal component. Desmoplastic variant is associated with Gorlin syndrome and resultant inactivation of PTCH1.
Extensive nodularity	Good		Nodules dominate the histopathology and are typically large and irregularly shaped.
Classic	Intermediate	80%–90%	Densely cellular, undifferentiated small round blue cells. Classically associated with Homer Wright rosettes (rings of neuroblasts surrounding eosinophilic neuropil) but these are observed in the minority of cases.
Large cell/ anaplastic	Poor	~5%–10%, rare	Large cells w/ large nuclei, prominent nucleoli, many mitoses, and nuclear polymorphism. More cytoplasm than classic; associated w/ amplification of MYC, bulky spinal mets.

Table 56.3: Molecular Classification of Medulloblastoma

Molecular Subgroup[11]	Incidence	Age	5-Yr OS	Associated Histology	Pathogenesis
Wingless (Wnt)	10%	Older children and adults	95%	Classic	Mutation in *CTNNB1* gene upregulates the Wnt pathway, which increases accumulation of nuclear β-catenin and promotes cell division and proliferation.
Sonic hedgehog (Shh)	30%	Bimodal: <5 y/o, then adolescent/ young adults	75%	Desmoplastic/ nodular	Mutation in *PTCH1* gene, which upregulates Shh pathway and promotes DNA transcription, decrease in cell–cell adhesion, and increased angiogenesis.
Group 4*	35%	Median age 9 y/o	75%	Classic	Overexpression of histone methylases/acetylases. Oncogene *MYCN* amplification. Chromosome x loss in 80% of females with group 4 MB.
Group 3*	25%	Infants and young children	50%	Classic/large cell/anaplastic	Not well defined. Upregulation of OTX2 transcription factor upregulates *C-Myc* oncogene and associated overexpression.

*New evidence suggests that growth factor independent-1 (GFI1 and GFI1B) proto-oncogene activation is implicated in group 3 and 4 medulloblastoma.[15]

Table 56.4: Molecular-Based Risk Stratification: 2016 International Consensus[12]

	Survival Rates	Criteria	Clinical Significance
Low risk	>90%	• WNT subgroup • Nonmetastatic group 4 with whole chromosome 11 loss or whole chromosome 17 gain	May qualify for reduced intensity therapy
Average risk	75%–90%	Others	May warrant intensification of therapy
High risk	50%–75%	• MYCN amplified SHH tumors • Metastatic SHH tumors • Group 4 tumors	
Very high risk	<50%	• Group 3 with metastases • SHH with TP53 mutation	

WORKUP: H&P with detailed neurologic exam. Preoperatively, obtain MRI brain with contrast (MB appears as isointense/hypointense mass with patchy contrast enhancement on T1; isointense on FLAIR, and hyperintense on DWI) and establish baseline neuropsychiatric testing, neuroendocrine testing, growth curves, CBC, and audiologic evaluation. If imaging suggests MB or other brain tumor, up-front resection (not biopsy) is indicated. Obtain postoperative MRI brain with contrast *within* 72 hours (inflammation of the meninges and residual blood products in the CSF can become pronounced beyond 72 hours and falsely suggest M+ disease). Obtain MRI spinal axis 10 to 14 days post-op to avoid confounding due to artifactual changes that can be seen in the immediate post-op period. Lumbar puncture w/ cytology should be performed after MRI spinal axis is obtained to avoid confounding inflammation from the procedure. Usually, LP cannot be safely performed preoperatively due to increased ICP. False-positive LPs can occur within 10 days; this can be repeated if positive. Systemic staging not routinely performed.

PROGNOSTIC FACTORS: Factors associated with worse prognosis: age <3 years, M+ , STR (>1.5 cm² residual), group 3 or 4 molecular profile, anaplastic/large cell morphology.

STAGING: MB follows the Modified Chang system (Table 56.5), which is based on preoperative MRI, postoperative MRI, operative findings, and CSF analysis. Note: T stage is no longer thought to be prognostic.

TREATMENT PARADIGM

Multimodality therapy is currently the standard of care, as surgery alone confers dismal prognosis with only 1/61 patients surviving with single modality approach in Cushing's original paper.[16] Adjuvant RT was introduced in the 1950s with some improvement in survival though still poor compared to current standards. Improvements in outcome were finally observed with modern RT techniques and the addition of CHT.[17,18] Several cooperative trials have helped delineate the current treatment paradigm, which generally includes maximal safe resection followed by CSI + PF/IF boost with concurrent weekly vincristine followed by approximately eight cycles of CHT.

Surgery: Suboccipital craniotomy with maximal safe resection. The goal is to achieve GTR/NTR with <1.5 cm² residual on post-op MRI. Previous studies have indicated essentially equivalent outcomes between GTR and NTR.[19] Classically, PFS is improved with GTR/NTR vs. STR (~70% vs. 50%)[20] though this is evolving in the molecular era.[21] Stereotactic or open biopsy is rarely indicated. Preoperatively, vasogenic tumor edema may be managed with steroids. Obstructive hydrocephalus is typically relieved by removal of the tumor, but intraoperative ventriculostomy may be indicated to relieve pressure.

Table 56.5: Modified Chang Staging System for Medulloblastoma[22]	
Extent of tumor	
T1	≤3 cm diameter
T2	>3 cm diameter
T3a	>3 cm with extension into the aqueduct of Sylvius and/or foramen of Luschka
T3b	>3 cm with unequivocal extension into the brainstem
T4	> 3 cm with extension past the aqueduct of Sylvius and/or down past the foramen magnum (beyond posterior fossa)
Degree of metastasis	
M0	No CSF, cerebral, or spinal involvement
M1	Positive CSF cytology
M2	Gross nodular seeding along cerebellar/cerebral subarachnoid space or in the third or lateral ventricles
M3	Gross nodular seeding in the spinal subarachnoid space
M4	Metastasis outside the cerebrospinal axis

Complications: PF syndrome in up to 25% (also known as "cerebellar mutism": manifested by mutism, truncal ataxia, dysphagia, emotional lability; usually self-resolves over weeks to months and should not delay adjuvant treatment). Operative mortality is <2%.

Chemotherapy: MB is one of the most chemosensitive brain tumors. The incorporation of platinum agents is standard given their efficacy. Usually initiated ~4 weeks following CSI with eight to nine cycles delivered. Per the German HIT91 RCT, immediate postoperative CSI/vincristine followed by CHT became standard (as opposed to post-op CHT followed by CSI).[23] In young children, CHT is used to delay or avoid the use of radiation to decrease associated neurocognitive risks (treatment paradigm: induction CHT followed by surgery and then additional consolidation CHT, with RT offered only for salvage).[9] Complications: ototoxicity, infertility (related to cyclophosphamide; affects males more than females), myelosuppression, second malignancy.

Radiation: CSI indicated for all patients (aside from the very young, as noted previously) and should start within approximately 30 days of surgery. *Average risk*: After maximal safe resection: CSI to 23.4 Gy/13 fx with PF boost to 54 to 55.8 Gy, though with recent presentation of ACNS 0331, some clinicians have transitioned to involved field (tumor bed + margin) followed by adjuvant CHT.[5] Concurrent single agent vincristine is used at some institutions but considered too toxic at others. *High risk*: After maximal resection: CSI to 36 to 39.6 Gy/20 to 22 fx with PF boost to 55.8 Gy with concurrent vincristine followed by adjuvant CHT. If M+, boost metastatic disease as follows (per ACNS 0332): 50.4 Gy: intracranial mets or focal spinal mets below cord, 45 Gy: focal spine mets above cord terminus; 39.6 Gy: diffuse spinal disease. Both IMRT[24] and proton therapy[25] have been shown to reduce ototoxicity as compared to 3D-CRT regimens.

Complications of CSI: Acute: myelosuppression, nausea/vomiting, diarrhea, fatigue, hair loss, headaches, muffled hearing. Chronic: neurocognitive (mnemonic "I am able"/I M ABL—IQ, memory, attention, behavior, learning), neuroendocrine deficits (particularly GH deficiency, hypothyroidism, gonadal dysfunction), impaired soft tissue/bone growth, ototoxicity (RT and/or cisplatin), secondary neoplasms, Lhermitte's syndrome, cataract. Merchant et al. developed a model to predict for cognitive changes based on the dose and volume received by critical structures such as the temporal lobes.[26] Conventional CSI for low-risk MB has been observed to cause decline of full-scale IQ by 4.2 points per year from baseline,[27] while proton radiotherapy resulted in 1.5 point drop in IQ/year.[28] See Kahalley et al. for more information on CSI with protons vs. photons. There is evidence that proton plans facilitate decreased dose to the cochleae and temporal lobes compared to IMRT (~2% for protons, ~20% for IMRT) with essentially zero exit dose through the abdomen, chest, heart, and pelvis.[25,29] Additional data show that when administered to adults needing CSI, proton-based treatment was associated with essentially one-third the rates of nausea, vomiting, and weight loss, and 10-fold less esophagitis.[30] The risk for brainstem injury in patients treated with posterior fossa tumors treated with proton therapy has been shown to be roughly 2% at 5 years, which is roughly in line with the incidence reported for patients treated with photons; this evidence helps dispel prior concerns that the dose uncertainty associated with protons leads to higher rates of brainstem injury than seen with photons.[31] In a report of long-term survivors (adults who were treated as children) with a median follow-up of 10 years, 12 of 17 patients were able to live without assistance. The most common long-term side effects included executive dysfunction ($n = 15$), weakness/ataxia ($n = 14$), and depression/anxiety ($n = 9$).

Procedure: See *Handbook of Treatment Planning in Radiation Oncology,* Chapter 12[32]

■ **EVIDENCE-BASED Q&A**

STANDARD RISK MB

▥ **What did early studies show regarding the use of CHT?**

*CCG 942[33] and SIOP 1[34] were early studies evaluating the addition of post-RT CHT to CSI (at 36 Gy) in an unselected patient population. Both ultimately showed that CHT did **not** confer a survival benefit among all patients, though, on subset analysis, did show a benefit to those with T3–T4 disease and M1-3 disease as summarized below. Thus, several subsequent studies were performed without the incorporation of CHT as described in subsequent section.*

CCG 942, Evans (*J Neurosurg* 1990, PMID 2319316): PRT of 233 patients 2–16 years old w/ M0-3 MB enrolled after maximal surgical resection. Randomized to RT alone vs. RT w/ concurrent VCR followed by 8 cycles (q6 weeks) of VCR, CCNU, and prednisone. RT was 35–40 Gy CSI w/ PF boost to 50–55 Gy; 50 Gy boost to localized spinal metastases; 5-year EFS was 59% w/ CHT vs. 50% w/ RT alone (NS); 5-year OS was 65% for both groups. On unplanned subgroup analysis, patients w/ advanced disease (T3-4 and M1-3), 5-year EFS was 46% w/ CHT vs. 0% for RT alone ($p = .006$), and 5-year OS was 61% w/ CHT vs. 19% for RT alone ($p = .04$). Significant prognostic factors were M+, young age, and advanced T-stage. **Conclusion: Patients w/ T3–4 and M1–3 disease had the greatest benefit from CHT, whereas patients with T1–2 and M0 had no benefit.**

■ Since these results showed that CHT did not improve outcomes, can RT alone be modified to offer optimal EFS and OS while minimizing toxicity?

Acknowledging the neurocognitive toxicity of 36 Gy CSI, French investigators attempted to reduce RT volume by delivering RT to the infratentorium only; however, results were terrible, with <20% 6-yr EFS and 64% failure in the supratentorium.[32] With this study clearly demonstrating that RT should be delivered to both supratentorial and infratentorial regions, the POG/CCG collaborative group modified the dose rather than the volume with their RCT (POG 8631/CCG923) randomizing patients to a CSI dose of either 23.4 Gy or 36 Gy. The trial closed prematurely due to initial early relapses on the low-dose arm, though on longer FU 5-year PFS was not significantly different. A companion JCO publication by Mulhern et al. reported on neuropsychologic testing in long-term survivors (>6 years), finding significantly less neuropsychologic toxicity in those treated to 23.4 Gy rather than 36 Gy with the difference most pronounced in those <9 years old.[35]

Thomas, POG 8631/CCG 923 (JCO 2000, PMID 10944134): PRT of 126 patients 3 to 21 years old w/ T1-3aM0 maximally resected MB (residual ≤1.5 cm² on CT) randomized to 23.4 Gy vs. 36 Gy CSI, with all patients receiving a PF boost to 54 Gy. No CHT was given. (Note: This was the first PRT requiring extensive pre-randomization staging w/ myelography, LP, post-op CT w/ contrast, and first to assess neuropsychologic functioning.) Terminated early when interim analysis revealed an increased rate of any relapse or isolated neuraxis relapse in patients receiving reduced-dose RT. Final analysis revealed 5-year EFS rates of 67% and 52% in the standard- and reduced-dose cohorts, respectively ($p = .8$). **Conclusion: Reduced-dose CSI is associated with increased risk of early neuraxis relapse. The therapeutic gain of 36 Gy over 23.4 Gy CSI is at least partly offset by increased toxicity. This supports the rationale for reduced-dose CSI + CHT for future investigation; 5-year EFS of 67% serves as a benchmark for average-risk MB treated w/ surgery and best conventional RT.**

■ What trials ultimately led to the reincorporation of CHT in the management of MB?

Several trials continued to evaluate the role of CHT with a prospective multi-institutional study published in 1994 by Packer et al. showing promising results with the incorporation of concurrent weekly vincristine and adjuvant cisplatin/CCNS/vincristine.[36] Later, the PNET 3 PRT showed improved EFS with the addition of CHT, though with a reduction in health status (including hearing, speech, vision, ambulation, dexterity, emotion, cognition) in those who received CHT.[37,38]

Taylor, PNET-3 (JCO 2003, PMID 12697884): PRT of pre-RT CHT (four cycles of vincristine, etoposide, carboplatin, cyclophosphamide) vs. RT alone for M0 MB. RT was 35 Gy CSI followed by PF boost to 55 Gy; 217 patients, 179 evaluable; 3-year EFS improved with CHT (79% vs. 65% with RT alone), as did 5-year EFS (74% vs. 60%, both $p = .037$). There was no significant difference in 3- or 5-year OS. **Conclusion: First PRT to show improved EFS with the addition of CHT. Authors added that this non-cisplatin-containing regimen could also reduce ototoxicity and nephrotoxicity.**

■ What studies led to the use of reduced-dose CSI in average-risk disease?

The same Packer study referenced earlier treated standard-risk patients to 23.4 Gy with the use of concurrent weekly vincristine and found favorable outcomes.[36] This study was then expanded into CCG 9892 as outlined next.

Packer, CCG 9892 (JCO 1999, PMID 10561268): Phase II trial of 65 patients 3 to 10 years old w/ M0 MB enrolled following maximal surgical resection. Patients received RT within 28 days post-op with concurrent weekly VCR. RT was delivered as CSI to 23.4 Gy w/ PF boost to 55.8 Gy. Six weeks following RT, patients received CCNU, VCR, and CDDP for 8 cycles (q6 weeks). MFU 56 months. No prognostic factors identified; including ~33% RT protocol violation rate; 3-year PFS was 88% and 3-year OS was 85%. **Conclusion: These results suggest that reduced-dose CSI and adjuvant CDDP-based CHT during and after RT is feasible for M0 MB.**

■ Can cyclophosphamide replace CCNU in the adjuvant CHT portion of treatment?

COG A9961 was a large PRT randomizing average-risk MB patients (all of whom were post-op and received 23.4 Gy CSI) to two different adjuvant CHT regimens, one with cyclophosphamide and another with CCNU. The rationale was that data supporting the use of CCNU in pediatric tumors were scant whereas xenograft and early clinical data for the use of cyclophosphamide was more promising.[39] Ultimately, there was no significant difference between the two regimens, with 5-year OS about 85% in both arms. Authors concluded that though neither CHT regimen was superior, the favorable outcomes seen with both regimens offer additional support for the use of reduced-dose CSI.

■ **When treating average-risk MB, does hyperfractionation of CSI affect outcomes or reduce toxicity?**

MSFOP 98 was a phase I/II average risk trial using hyperfractionated therapy, 36 Gy CSI with boost to 68 Gy to the tumor bed at 1 Gy/fx BID.[40] It showed excellent long-term EFS in the absence of CHT and full-scale IQ drop was less pronounced compared to other standard RT reports. This led to HIT-SIOP PNET-4, which enrolled average-risk MB patients who were randomized to standard fractionation (23.4 Gy CSI with PF boost to 54 Gy at 1.8 Gy/fx) vs. hyperfractionation (36 Gy CSI with PF boost to 60 Gy and 68 Gy tumor bed at 1 Gy/fx BID with 8-hour interfx interval). Results showed equivalent outcomes for EFS and OS and no difference in ototoxicity; IQ measurements were not reported in their final publication. Based on these results, hyperfractionation is typically not employed in average-risk MB.[41]

■ **What is the optimal dose to deliver to the PF?**

This has never been prospectively studied, but a 1988 Harvard RR showed better LC if the PF dose was >50 Gy (LC 79% vs. 33% if less than 50 Gy; p < .02).[42]

■ **Can patients with average-risk MB who are most vulnerable to neurocognitive effects of CSI receive a lower dose? Can any average-risk patient receive IF boost rather than whole PF boost?**

ACNS0331 was developed to answer both questions. Multiple studies have shown that CSI doses >20 Gy can damage neurocognitive and growth outcomes, prompting investigators to determine whether lower doses could confer favorable outcomes with less toxicity.[43,44] In 1989, Goldwein et al. reported on their prospective cohort study of 10 MB patients delivering 18 Gy CSI with a PF boost of 50.4 to 55.8 Gy with weekly vincristine and subsequent CDDP/VCR/CCNU showing favorable cure rates.[45] Additionally, two retrospective studies showed that PF failure rate was ≤5% with the use of IF-directed boost, suggesting that IF boost may be appropriate.[46,47] These results help set the stage for ACNS 0331.

Michalski, COG ACNS0331 (*ASTRO 2016*, Abstract LBA2): Enrolled 464 patients ages 3 to 21 with average-risk MB with a primary end point of time to event (progression, recurrence, death from any cause, secondary malignant neoplasm). All patients underwent maximum safe resection followed by RT within 31 days delivered with weekly vincristine followed by cisplatin/vincristine and either CCNU or cyclophosphamide (alternating AABAAB pattern). Patients between 3 and 7 underwent two randomizations (CSI dose of 18 Gy vs. 23.4 Gy; and IF vs. PF boost). Patients from 8 to 21 were eligible only for the IF vs. PF question; all received CSI dose of 23.4 Gy. MFU 6.6 years. **Conclusion: IF boost is non-inferior to full PF boost for all standard risk patients 3 to 21 years old. However, reduced-dose CSI is associated with worse 5-year EFS and OS and thus average-risk MB patients should continue to receive 23.4 Gy as standard CSI dose unless enrolled on a clinical trial.**

Table 56.6: Preliminary Results of COG ACNS 0331 Medulloblastoma			
	5-Yr LF	**5-Yr EFS**	**5-Yr OS**
All patients 3–21 years of age			
IF boost	1.9%	82%	84%
PF boost	3.7%	81%	85%
	p = .178	p = .421; the 94% upper confidence limit on the HR was 1.3, lower than the prespecified limit of 1.6, and thus IFRT was deemed noninferior to PFRT	

(continued)

Table 56.6: Preliminary Results of COG ACNS 0331 Medulloblastoma (*continued*)			
	5-Yr LF	5-Yr EFS	5-Yr OS
Patients 3–7 years of age			
Low dose (18 Gy)		72%	78%
Standard dose (23.4 Gy)		83%	86%
			The 80% upper confidence limit of the HR was 1.9; this was higher than the prespecified limit of 1.6 and thus noninferiority of low-dose CSI was not established.

HIGH RISK MB

■ What data initially supported the use of CHT in high-risk disease?

CCG 942 (discussed earlier in the average-risk section) and SIOP I were both PRTs evaluating postoperative patients who received CSI and were then randomized to CHT or no CHT.[33,34] For both studies, there was no difference in outcomes between the two groups, but when limited to those with more advanced disease (T3–T4, M+, or STR), an improvement in EFS was observed.

■ Can outcomes be improved by intensifying the CHT regimen with additional agents?

CCG 921 was performed in patients with a variety of high-risk pediatric brain tumors to see if "8 in 1" CHT (eight types of CHT in 1 day: cisplatin, procarbazine, CCNU, vincristine, cyclophosphamide, methylprednisolone, hydroxyurea, cytarabine) was better than a combination of vincristine/CCNU/prednisone (VCP). A total of 421 children were enrolled, of which 203 had MB. Subset analysis of this group showed better outcomes with VCP than 8 in 1 CHT (5-year PFS 63% vs. 45%, p = .006).[20]

■ Is there a benefit to altering the sequence of CHT (e.g., delivering CHT immediately post-op followed by RT)?

Four PRTs have evaluated this question: SIOP II, SIOP III, POG 9031, and HIT 91 from Germany. All of them except for SIOP III showed no benefit to immediate post-op CHT; both POG 9031 and SIOP II showed 5-year EFS to be about 60% to 70% and 5-year OS about 75% in both groups with no significant difference between them, and HIT 91 actually showed an improvement in 3-year EFS with immediate RT (78% vs. 65%, p = .03).[4,23,48] SIOP III is the only exception, showing improved 3- and 5-year EFS with up-front CHT.[3] Therefore, with three of these four studies showing no benefit to up-front CHT, standard of care is to perform maximal safe resection followed by RT (with concurrent vincristine) followed by adjuvant CHT.

■ Is there any detriment to interrupting RT?

Interestingly, SIOP III also showed better 3-year OS when RT was delivered within 50 days, suggesting that avoiding RT interruption can lead to better outcomes.[3] These results confirm earlier findings from the University of Florida that prompt completion of RT confers better outcomes (used a cut point of 45 days).[49]

Table 56.7: SIOP III RT Duration Results	
RT Duration	3-Yr OS
<50 days	84.1%
>50 days	70.9%
p value	.0356

■ Does the use of carboplatin as a radiosensitizer during CSI lead to better outcomes?

This was addressed in COG 99701, a phase I/II trial that evaluated the role of adding carboplatin to vincristine during CSI.[50] Note that the adjuvant therapy offered changed slightly once the recommended dose of carboplatin was determined, but among all patients on this study, 5-year OS was approximately 75%. Authors concluded that CRT with vincristine + carboplatin followed by 6 months of maintenance CHT produced outcomes at least as good as (if not better than) other prior trials using higher dose CSI or higher dose alkylator-based therapy. This carboplatin-containing regimen is being tested in an ongoing phase III PRT, ACNS 0332 which is evaluating intensification of systemic therapy in high-risk MB (M+, STR and/or diffuse anaplasia) and is utilizing two randomizations: (a) concurrent carboplatin during RT and (b) isotretinoin during and after maintenance therapy.

■ Is there a role for re-irradiation?

Recurrent MB is rarely cured and has a dismal prognosis with 2-year OS historically <25%. However, a number of salvage treatments have been considered including surgical resection, brachytherapy, radiosurgery, high-dose CHT with autologous stem cell transplant and re-irradiation. Re-irradiation may be a reasonable option to consider in both standard- and high-risk patients.

Wetmore, St. Jude (*Cancer* 2014, PMID 25080363): RR of 38 patients with recurrent MB, 14 of whom received re-irradiation (8 repeat CSI, spinal only in 3, primary only in 3). For patients who initially had standard risk MB, 5-year OS with re-RT was 55% vs. 33% without; 10-year OS 46% with reRT vs. 0% without ($p = .003$). Median RT dose was 36.75 Gy (range 18–54) and median interval between RT courses was 39 months (range 10–107). Similarly, the high-risk individuals also benefited ($p = .003$). Re-irradiation did result in an increased rate of necrosis ($p = .0468$).

■ Is there a neurocognitive toxicity benefit to using proton RT?

Retrospective data suggest an intellect-sparing advantage with proton RT compared to photon RT.

Kahalley, Multi-institutional (*JCO* 2020, PMID 31774710): RR of 79 children with MB treated with either proton RT (PRT) or photon RT (XRT) at eight different cancer centers. Primary end points were various longitudinal intelligence composite scores. Demographic/clinical variables similar between patients except for boost dose ($p < .01$) and boost margin ($p = .01$). The PRT group exhibited superior long-term outcomes in global IQ, perceptual reasoning, and working memory (all $p < .05$). **Conclusion: Proton RT may significantly improve long-term neurocognitive toxicity from CSI.** *Comment: This study performed an unplanned comparison between non-randomized patients treated in different countries, had variable PF boost volume, and used whole brain fields that should have delivered equivalent biologic doses regardless of treatment modality.*

MB IN INFANTS

■ What is the recommended treatment for infants (<3 years)?

*The mainstay of treatment for MB involves maximal safe resection followed by CSI + boost. However, CSI can lead to significant neurocognitive toxicity, which is not only dose dependent but also age dependent (younger is worse).[27,51] Therefore, CHT has been evaluated as a stopgap to delay RT. Baby POG#1 showed this was possible with a 5-year OS of 40%. An unintended consequence of this study was complete parent refusal of radiation, which showed that in a select group of MB infants, there **may** not be a need for RT at all. As described earlier, the CCG group tried eight CHT drugs ("8-in-1") with worse outcomes but confirmed the approach of CHT before RT was feasible. Follow-up trials including the Head Start I and II for infant MB used intensive CHT and used RT only for salvage.[52] This approach eliminated CSI in 52% of patients and may preserve quality of life and intellectual function. However, the intense CHT is not without cost; 4 of 21 infants died of treatment-related toxicity. The findings of Baby POG#1 have been further bolstered by Rutkowski et al. using surgery and subsequent CHT, with 5-year OS for those s/p GTR of 93%, 56% if STR, and 38% for those with macroscopic metastases.[9]*

REFERENCES

1. Louis DN, Ohgaki H, Wiestler OD, et al. The 2007 WHO classification of tumours of the central nervous system. *Acta Neuropathol*. 2007;114(2):97–109. doi:10.1007/s00401-007-0243-4
2. Dhall G. Medulloblastoma. *J Child Neurol*. 2009;24(11):1418–1430. doi:10.1177/0883073809341668
3. Cuneo HM, Rand CW. *Brain Tumors of Childhood. Medulloblastoma*. Charles C. Thomas; 1952.
4. Taylor RE, Bailey CC, Robinson KJ, et al. Impact of radiotherapy parameters on outcome in the international society of paediatric oncology/United Kingdom children's cancer study Group PNET-3 study of preradiotherapy chemotherapy for M0–M1 medulloblastoma. *Int J Radiat Oncol Biol Phys*. 2004;58(4):1184–1193. doi:10.1016/j.ijrobp.2003.08.010
5. Bailey CC, Gnekow A, Wellek S, et al. Prospective randomised trial of chemotherapy given before radiotherapy in childhood medulloblastoma. international society of paediatric oncology (SIOP) and the (German) society of paediatric oncology (GPO): SIOP II. *Med Pediatr Oncol*. 1995;25(3):166–178. doi:10.1002/mpo.2950250303
6. Michalski J. Results of COG ACNS0331: A phase III trial of involved-field radiotherapy (IFRT) and low dose craniospinal irradiation (LD-CSI) with chemotherapy in average-risk medulloblastoma: a report from the children's oncology group. *Int J Radiat Oncol Biol Phys*. 2016;96(5):937. doi:10.1093/neuonc/now076.104
7. Stone DM, Hynes M, Armanini M, et al. The tumour-suppressor gene patched encodes a candidate receptor for sonic hedgehog. *Nature*. 1996;384(6605):129–134. doi:10.1038/384129a0
8. Hamilton SR, Liu B, Parsons RE, et al. The molecular basis of turcot's syndrome. *N Engl J Med*. 1995;332(13):839–847. doi:10.1056/NEJM199503303321302
9. Rutkowski S, Bode U, Deinlein F, et al. Treatment of early childhood medulloblastoma by postoperative chemotherapy alone. *N Engl J Med*. 2005;352(10):978–986. doi:10.1056/NEJMoa042176
10. Louis DN, Perry A, Reifenberger G, et al. The 2016 world health organization classification of tumors of the central nervous system: a summary. *Acta Neuropathol*. 2016;131(6):803–820. doi:10.1007/s00401-016-1545-1
11. Khatua S. Evolving molecular era of childhood medulloblastoma: time to revisit therapy. *Future Oncol*. 2016;12(1):107–117. doi:10.2217/fon.15.284
12. Ramaswamy V, Remke M, Bouffet E, et al. Risk stratification of childhood medulloblastoma in the molecular era: the current consensus. *Acta Neuropathol*. 2016;131(6):821–831. doi:10.2217/fon.15.284
13. Das P, Puri T, Suri V, et al. Medulloblastomas: a correlative study of MIB-1 proliferation index along with expression of c-Myc, ERBB2, and anti-apoptotic proteins along with histological typing and clinical outcome. *Childs Nerv Syst*. 2009;25(7):825–835. doi:10.1007/s00381-009-0884-9
14. Pan E, Pellarin M, Holmes E, et al. Isochromosome 17q is a negative prognostic factor in poor-risk childhood medulloblastoma patients. *Clin Cancer Res*. 2005;11(13):4733–4740. doi:10.1158/1078-0432.CCR-04-0465
15. Northcott PA, Lee C, Zichner T, et al. Enhancer hijacking activates GFI1 family oncogenes in medulloblastoma. *Nature*. 2014;511(7510):428–434.
16. Cushing H. Experiences with the cerebellar medulloblastomas: a critical review. *Acta Pathologica et Microbiologica Scandinavica*. 1930;7:1–86. doi:10.1111/j.1600-0463.1930.tb06503.x
17. Lampe I, Mac IR. Medulloblastoma of the cerebellum. *Arch Neurol Psychiatry*. 1949;62(3):322–329. doi:10.1001/archneurpsyc.1949.02310150069008
18. Tomlinson FH, Scheithauer BW, Meyer FB, et al. Medulloblastoma: I. Clinical, diagnostic, and therapeutic overview. *J Child Neurol*. 1992;7(2):142–155. doi:10.1177/088307389200700203
19. Gajjar A, Sanford RA, Bhargava R, et al. Medulloblastoma with brain stem involvement: the impact of gross total resection on outcome. *Pediatr Neurosurg*. 1996;25(4):182–187. doi:10.1159/000121121
20. Zeltzer PM, Boyett JM, Finlay JL, et al. Metastasis stage, adjuvant treatment, and residual tumor are prognostic factors for medulloblastoma in children: conclusions from the children's cancer group 921 randomized phase III study. *J Clin Oncol*. 1999;17(3):832–845. doi:10.1200/JCO.1999.17.3.832
21. Thompson EM, Hielscher T, Bouffet E, et al. Prognostic value of medulloblastoma extent of resection after accounting for molecular subgroup: a retrospective integrated clinical and molecular analysis. *Lancet Oncol*. 2016;17(4):484–495.
22. Chang CH, Housepian EM, Herbert C, Jr. An operative staging system and a megavoltage radiotherapeutic technic for cerebellar medulloblastomas. *Radiology*. 1969;93(6):1351–1359. doi:10.1148/93.6.1351
23. Kortmann RD, Kuhl J, Timmermann B, et al. Postoperative neoadjuvant chemotherapy before radiotherapy as compared to immediate radiotherapy followed by maintenance chemotherapy in the treatment of medulloblastoma in childhood: results of the German prospective randomized trial HIT '91. *Int J Radiat Oncol Biol Phys*. 2000;46(2):269–279. doi:10.1016/S0360-3016(99)00369-7
24. Packer RJ, Goldwein J, Nicholson HS, et al. Treatment of children with medulloblastomas with reduced-dose craniospinal radiation therapy and adjuvant chemotherapy: a children's cancer group study. *J Clin Oncol*. 1999;17(7):2127–2136. doi:10.1200/JCO.1999.17.7.2127
25. Huang E, Teh BS, Strother DR, et al. Intensity-modulated radiation therapy for pediatric medulloblastoma: early report on the reduction of ototoxicity. *Int J Radiat Oncol Biol Phys*. 2002;52(3):599–605. doi:10.1016/S0360-3016(01)02641-4
26. Moeller BJ, Chintagumpala M, Philip JJ, et al. Low early ototoxicity rates for pediatric medulloblastoma patients treated with proton radiotherapy. *Radiat Oncol*. 2011;6:58. doi:10.1186/1748-717X-6-58

27. Merchant TE, Schreiber JE, Wu S, et al. Critical combinations of radiation dose and volume predict intelligence quotient and academic achievement scores after craniospinal irradiation in children with medulloblastoma. *Int J Radiat Oncol Biol Phys*. 2014;90(3):554–561. doi:10.1016/j.ijrobp.2014.06.058

28. Ris MD, Packer R, Goldwein J, et al. Intellectual outcome after reduced-dose radiation therapy plus adjuvant chemotherapy for medulloblastoma: a children's cancer group study. *J Clin Oncol*. 2001;19(15):3470–3476. doi:10.1200/JCO.2001.19.15.3470

29. Yock TI, Yeap BY, Ebb DH, et al. Long-term toxic effects of proton radiotherapy for paediatric medulloblastoma: a phase 2 single-arm study. *Lancet Oncol*. 2016;17(3):287–298. doi:10.1016/S1470-2045(15)00167-9

30. Fossati P, Ricardi U, Orecchia R. Pediatric medulloblastoma: toxicity of current treatment and potential role of protontherapy. *Cancer Treat Rev*. 2009;35(1):79–96. doi:10.1016/j.ctrv.2008.09.002

31. Brown AP, Barney CL, Grosshans DR, et al. Proton beam craniospinal irradiation reduces acute toxicity for adults with medulloblastoma. *Int J Radiat Oncol Biol Phys*. 2013;86(2):277–284. doi:10.1016/j.ijrobp.2013.01.014

32. Gentile MS, Yeap BY, Paganetti H, et al. Brainstem injury in pediatric patients with posterior fossa tumors treated with proton beam therapy and associated dosimetric factors. *Int J Radiat Oncol Biol Phys*. 2018;100(3):719–729. doi:10.1016/j.ijrobp.2017.11.026

33. Videtic GM VA, Woody NM. *Handbook of Treatment Planning in Radiation Oncology*. 3rd ed. Springer Publishing; 2020.

34. Evans AE, Jenkin RD, Sposto R, et al. The treatment of medulloblastoma: results of a prospective randomized trial of radiation therapy with and without CCNU, vincristine, and prednisone. *J Neurosurg*. 1990;72(4):572–582. doi:10.3171/jns.1990.72.4.0572

35. Tait DM, Thornton-Jones H, Bloom HJ, et al. Adjuvant chemotherapy for medulloblastoma: the first multi-centre control trial of the international society of paediatric oncology (SIOP I). *Eur J Cancer*. 1990;26(4):464–469. doi:10.1016/0277-5379(90)90017-N

36. Mulhern RK, Kepner JL, Thomas PR, et al. Neuropsychologic functioning of survivors of childhood medulloblastoma randomized to receive conventional or reduced-dose craniospinal irradiation: a pediatric oncology group study. *J Clin Oncol*. 1998;16(5):1723–1728. doi:10.1200/JCO.1998.16.5.1723

37. Packer RJ, Sutton LN, Elterman R, et al. Outcome for children with medulloblastoma treated with radiation and cisplatin, CCNU, and vincristine chemotherapy. *J Neurosurg*. 1994;81(5):690–698. doi:10.3171/jns.1994.81.5.0690

38. Taylor RE, Bailey CC, Robinson K, et al. Results of a randomized study of preradiation chemotherapy versus radiotherapy alone for nonmetastatic medulloblastoma: the international society of paediatric oncology/United Kingdom children's cancer study group PNET-3 study. *J Clin Oncol*. 2003;21(8):1581–1591. doi:10.1200/JCO.2003.05.116

39. Bull KS, Spoudeas HA, Yadegarfar G, Kennedy CR, Cclg. Reduction of health status 7 years after addition of chemotherapy to craniospinal irradiation for medulloblastoma: a follow-up study in PNET 3 trial survivors on behalf of the CCLG (formerly UKCCSG). *J Clin Oncol*. 2007;25(27):4239–4245. doi:10.1200/JCO.2006.08.7684

40. Packer RJ, Gajjar A, Vezina G, et al. Phase III study of craniospinal radiation therapy followed by adjuvant chemotherapy for newly diagnosed average-risk medulloblastoma. *J Clin Oncol*. 2006;24(25):4202–4208. doi:10.1200/JCO.2006.06.4980

41. Carrie C, Grill J, Figarella-Branger D, et al. Online quality control, hyperfractionated radiotherapy alone and reduced boost volume for standard risk medulloblastoma: long-term results of MSFOP 98. *J Clin Oncol*. 2009;27(11):1879–1883. doi:10.1200/JCO.2008.18.6437

42. Lannering B, Rutkowski S, Doz F, et al. Hyperfractionated versus conventional radiotherapy followed by chemotherapy in standard-risk medulloblastoma: results from the randomized multicenter HIT-SIOP PNET 4 trial. *J Clin Oncol*. 2012;30(26):3187–3193. doi:10.1200/JCO.2011.39.8719

43. Hughes EN, Shillito J, Sallan SE, et al. Medulloblastoma at the joint center for radiation therapy between 1968 and 1984. The influence of radiation dose on the patterns of failure and survival. *Cancer*. 1988;61(10):1992–1998. doi:10.1002/1097-0142(19880515)61:10<1992::AID-CNCR2820611011>3.0.CO;2-J

44. Packer RJ, Sutton LN, Atkins TE, et al. A prospective study of cognitive function in children receiving whole-brain radiotherapy and chemotherapy: 2-year results. *J Neurosurg*. 1989;70(5):707–713. doi:10.3171/jns.1989.70.5.0707

45. Probert JC, Parker BR, Kaplan HS. Growth retardation in children after megavoltage irradiation of the spine. *Cancer*. 1973;32(3):634–639. doi:10.1002/1097-0142(197309)32:3<634::AID-CNCR2820320316>3.0.CO;2-A

46. Goldwein JW, Radcliffe J, Johnson J, et al. Updated results of a pilot study of low dose craniospinal irradiation plus chemotherapy for children under five with cerebellar primitive neuroectodermal tumors (medulloblastoma). *Int J Radiat Oncol Biol Phys*. 1996;34(4):899–904. doi:10.1016/0360-3016(95)02080-2

47. Wolden SL, Dunkel IJ, Souweidane MM, et al. Patterns of failure using a conformal radiation therapy tumor bed boost for medulloblastoma. *J Clin Oncol*. 2003;21(16):3079–3083. doi:10.1200/JCO.2003.11.140

48. Merchant TE, Kun LE, Krasin MJ, et al. Multi-institution prospective trial of reduced-dose craniospinal irradiation (23.4 Gy) followed by conformal posterior fossa (36 Gy) and primary site irradiation (55.8 Gy) and dose-intensive chemotherapy for average-risk medulloblastoma. *Int J Radiat Oncol Biol Phys*. 2008;70(3):782–787. doi:10.1016/j.ijrobp.2007.07.2342

49. Tarbell NJ, Friedman H, Polkinghorn WR, et al. High-risk medulloblastoma: a pediatric oncology group randomized trial of chemotherapy before or after radiation therapy (POG 9031). *J Clin Oncol*. 2013;31(23):2936–2941. doi:10.1200/JCO.2012.43.9984

50. del Charco JO, Bolek TW, McCollough WM, et al. Medulloblastoma: time-dose relationship based on a 30-year review. *Int J Radiat Oncol Biol Phys*. 1998;42(1):147–154. doi:10.1016/S0360-3016(98)00197-7

51. Jakacki RI, Burger PC, Zhou T, et al. Outcome of children with metastatic medulloblastoma treated with carboplatin during craniospinal radiotherapy: a children's oncology group phase I/II study. *J Clin Oncol*. 2012;30(21):2648–2653. doi:10.1200/JCO.2011.40.2792

52. Fouladi M, Gilger E, Kocak M, et al. Intellectual and functional outcome of children 3 years old or younger who have CNS malignancies. *J Clin Oncol*. 2005;23(28):7152–7160. doi:10.1200/JCO.2005.01.214

57 ■ EPENDYMOMA

Matthew C. Ward, John H. Suh, and Erin S. Murphy

> **QUICK HIT** ■ Uncommon CNS tumor originating from glial stem cells most commonly in the fourth ventricle (children) or filum terminale (myxopapillary type, adults); 10-year OS is ~80% in adults and ~65% in children. The treatment paradigm is maximal safe resection with attempt at GTR; the degree of resection classically represents the most important prognostic factor. RT should be given postoperatively to the resection bed and any remaining disease to 59.4 Gy in 33 fractions. For those 18 months old or younger, consider 54 Gy or CHT to delay RT. There is no clearly established role for CHT but may be used in select cases to delay RT or attempt second-look surgery.

EPIDEMIOLOGY: Uncommon tumor originating from glial stem cells that can occur in all age groups but are more common in children.[1] Represent about 6% of CNS tumors in children (150 cases per year) and 2% of CNS tumors in adults.[1–3]

RISK FACTORS: No risk factors have been clearly identified. NF2 patients may be at an increased risk for spinal ependymomas.[4]

ANATOMY: Can originate from anywhere in the CNS but most commonly originates from the ependymal lining of the fourth ventricle (a "tongue of tumor" often tracks caudally along the cervical spinal cord) or from the distal intramedullary spinal cord (adults). CSF enters the fourth ventricle from the cerebral aqueduct and exits via the foramen of Luschka laterally and foramen of Magendie medially. The obex is the most caudal aspect of the fourth ventricle. The spinal cord ends at approximately L3 in children and L1 to 2 in adults. The thecal sac (filum terminale) ends at approximately S2 in both children and adults.[5–7]

PATHOLOGY: WHO separates grade based on morphology; however, genetics may be more prognostic given the heterogeneity within various WHO grades (Table 57.1).[1] Perivascular pseudorosettes are the pathognomonic finding.

Table 57.1: 2016 WHO Update: Ependymoma Grades and Subtypes[8]		
Grade I	Myxopapillary ependymoma	Adults: conus/filum terminale
	Subependymoma	Adults: fourth ventricle most common
Grade II	Classic ependymoma (Variants: papillary, clear cell, tanycytic)	Variable clinical course
Grade III	Anaplastic ependymoma	Usually aggressive but again can be variable: studies ongoing to determine molecular subclassification
	Ependymoma, RELA fusion-positive	Distinct class recognized by the WHO 2016 update, represents majority of supratentorial tumors in children, poor prognosis[8,9]
Grade IV	Ependymoblastoma	Considered a PNET and treated as such.

GENETICS: RELA fusion: fusion between RELA (encodes a component of NF-κB, which is a complex regulating transcription, cytokine production, and cell survival) and a poorly understood gene C11orf95 (chromosome 11), which leads to an oncogene product that is independently prognostic. This led to the WHO recognizing this subtype as a separate classification.[8,9] Otherwise, ependymomas have a diverse and heterogeneous landscape of various genetic alterations. Methylation profiling and genomic profiling may lead to additional prognostic categories based on YAP1 and RELA fusions.[9] Currently, these evolving categories do not affect treatment.

CLINICAL PRESENTATION: Most common presenting symptoms are those of increased ICP (children; headache, nausea, ataxia, vertigo, papilledema) or back pain (adults), depending on location.

WORKUP: History and physical, MRI of the brain and entire spine (rule-out leptomeningeal dissemination) with and without contrast, consider ventriculostomy rather than shunt if symptomatic. Lumbar puncture for CSF preoperatively if concern for LMD or for grade II to III histology (contraindicated if increased ICP, in which case obtain 10–14 days post-op). Repeat MRI postoperatively to assess resection extent.

PROGNOSTIC FACTORS: Surgical resection is classically the most important prognostic factor.[10] Others may include younger age, high grade, male gender, and intracranial location.[11] Grade II and III tumors have a heterogeneous behavior and the prognostic significance of grade for these tumors is evolving.

NATURAL HISTORY: Grade I tumors have excellent outcomes, and failure is uncommon. For grade II to III tumors, local failure is usually more common than distant failure (12% vs. 8% in original phase II study by Merchant et al.).[12] Failure usually occurs within 2 years.[3] Event-free survival and overall survival for children at 7 years were 77% and 85% in the Merchant study, respectively.

TREATMENT PARADIGM

Surgery: Maximal safe resection with attempt at GTR is standard of care. Near-total resection is defined as ≤5 mm maximum diameter of residual disease while STR is defined as >5 mm on postop MRI.[12]

Chemotherapy: There is no clear role for the routine use of CHT. Various multidrug regimens (for example, vincristine, carboplatin, cyclophosphamide, and etoposide) have been used to delay RT for infants or to attempt a second-look surgery for those with an STR initially (see the following studies).

Radiation

Indications: RT is indicated for the postoperative treatment of ependymomas in essentially all cases. A spinal myxopapillary ependymoma after GTR is controversial with some recommending treatment to 54 Gy and others recommending observation.

Dose: For posterior fossa tumors treat to 59.4 Gy. For gross residual disease, there is no clear role for dose escalation (see the following studies). Spinal ependymomas typically treated to 50.4 to 54 Gy.

Toxicity: Acute: alopecia, fatigue, headache, nausea, and erythema. Late: Cognitive decline, hearing loss, endocrinopathies, and microcephaly.

Procedure: See *Handbook of Treatment Planning in Radiation Oncology*, Chapter 12.[13]

■ **EVIDENCE-BASED Q&A**

■ **Is there a role for craniospinal irradiation (CSI) for patients with limited disease at presentation?**

Historically, pediatric trials as recent as the early 1990s routinely delivered CSI to doses of 23.4 to 36 Gy with a boost to 54 to 55 Gy.[14,15] However, local relapse was the most common site of failure with distant CNS failure occurring in only 5% to 7% of patients. Subsequent protocols (see the following) demonstrated similar outcomes and patterns of failure treating only a CTV of GTV/postoperative bed +1 cm. Therefore, limited-field irradiation is now standard of care except in the uncommon situation of leptomeningeal spread at the time of diagnosis.

Merchant, St. Jude (*IJROBP* 2002, PMID 11872277; Update *JCO* 2004, PMID 15284268, Update *Lancet Oncol* 2009, PMID 19274783): Phase II trial of 153 children (2009 update) with ependymoma, 85 of whom were grade III. Evaluated the patterns of failure after conformal RT. The initial report included low-grade astrocytoma as well. CTV = GTV + 1 cm. GTV encompassed the postoperative bed and any residual tumor. PTV = CTV + 0.5 cm. Dose was 59.4 Gy except for those <18 months with a GTR who received 54 Gy. Spinal cord limited to approximately 57.8 Gy (54 Gy limit for first 30 fractions, then 70% of prescription for final three fractions). The 7-year rates of LC, EFS, and OS were 87%, 69%, and 81%, respectively. Negative prognostic factors included anaplastic histology, non-White race, STR, and pre-RT CHT. **Conclusion: Limited-volume irradiation allowed high rates of disease control and stable neurocognitive outcomes.**

■ How does the extent of resection affect outcome?

The extent of resection is a strong prognostic factor in nearly every study performed. On the more recent St. Jude studies, EFS/PFS ranged from 78% to 82% with GTR compared to 41% to 43% with subtotal resection.[3,12] One earlier retrospective study from Pittsburgh demonstrated an even more marked difference with 5-year PFS ranging from 68% with GTR to 9% without GTR.[16]

■ Is there a role for adjuvant CHT?

No trial has clearly demonstrated a benefit to the routine use of CHT. Two randomized trials prior to the 1990s showed no benefit to the routine use of CHT (CCG 942 initiated in 1975 and CCG 921 in 1986).[14,15,17] COG 9942 studied CHT for those with an STR and showed a 40% CR rate.[18] This gave consideration to the idea of CHT prior to second-look surgery for responders, which was studied in the modern ACNS0121 trial below.

■ How should we manage children who are too young for radiotherapy?

Patients <3 years of age experience worse neurocognitive outcomes with RT (particularly CSI) and may benefit from altered therapy. Patients on Dr. Merchant's study younger than 18 months old who underwent GTR were treated with focal radiation to 54 Gy rather than 59.4 Gy.[12] Other strategies include CHT to delay RT. Multiple studies (CCG 9921, HIT-SKK 87 & 92, UKCCSG/SIOP, and POG 9233) delayed or omitted RT with the use of CHT, with mixed results.[19-22] This was studied further on the modern ACNS 0121 study below.

Duffner, "Baby POG" (*NEJM* 1993, PMID 8388548; Update *Pediatr Neurosurg* 1998, PMID 9732252): Phase II trial for children <3 years old with malignant brain tumors (MB, ependymoma, PNET, brainstem glioma, and other gliomas). All patients were treated with cyclophosphamide, vincristine, cisplatin, and etoposide, which was continued until progression or for 2 years for patients <24 months old and for 1 year if 24 to 36 months old, at which time RT was delivered. RT was localized for ependymomas to 54 Gy but for anaplastic ependymomas was CSI to 35.2 Gy with a localized boost to 54 Gy. Forty-eight patients had ependymoma. The 5-year OS was 25% for those <23 months and 63% for those 24 to 36 months. **Conclusion: Delaying RT may lead to inferior survival for ependymomas.**

■ In the modern era, can a stratified approach lead to comparable outcomes while utilizing CHT and RT selectively?

The ACNS0121 study informs management in the modern era. The investigators utilized all data mentioned previously to conceive a logical stratification scheme that omitted RT for supratentorial grade II patients after GTR, utilized CHT to facilitate second-look surgery for STR patients, and delivered conformal RT alone for the rest.

Merchant, COG ACNS0121 (*JCO* 2019, PMID 30811284): Phase II trial of 356 children between 2003 and 2007. Enrolled into four strata based on degree of resection and histology. Stratum 1: grade II, supratentorial ependymoma with GTR (microscopic intraop and on postop MRI); stratum 2: STR, any grade; stratum 3: macroscopic GTR or NTR (defined as <5 mm thickness of gross disease remaining); and stratum 4: grade III supratentorial or grade II infratentorial after microscopic GTR. Stratum 1 patients were observed; stratum 2 received CHT (vincristine, carboplatin, cyclophosphamide, and etoposide) followed by optional second-look surgery then RT; strata 3 and 4 received immediate postoperative RT, which was 59.4 Gy except for those <18 months old (54 Gy). Stratum 1: 5-year EFS 61% (5 of 11 progressed). Stratum 2: 39% went to second-look surgery and 5-year EFS was 51% vs. 29% without second surgery. Stratum 3: EFS 67%. Stratum 4: EFS 69%. **Conclusion: Immediate conformal RT appeared beneficial in all strata (even children ages 1–3). Observation after GTR for grade II supratentorial ependymoma should not be standard of care.**

Massimino, AIEOP Italian Study (*Neuro Oncol* 2016, PMID 27194148): Prospective study stratifying by WHO grade and degree of resection. WHO grade II patients with a GTR received 59.4 Gy.

Grade III patients with a GTR received 59.4 Gy followed by vincristine, etoposide, and cyclophos-phamide. Patients with residual disease (either grade) received the same CHT for one to four cycles followed by second-look surgery, then 59.4 Gy with an 8-Gy boost if there was residual disease. A total of 160 children with an MFU of 67 months were enrolled. PFS and OS were 58% and 69% in the 40 patients with incomplete resection. **Conclusion: These results were comparable to the best single-institution results and the boost appeared effective.**

■ **Can dose-escalated hyperfractionation improve outcomes?**

None of three prospective trials (POG 9132, AIEOP, and SPO) performed in children clearly demonstrated a benefit to dose-escalated hyperfractionated RT.[23-25] The regimens included 69.6 Gy/58 fx at 1.2 Gy/fx (POG 9132), 70.4 Gy/64 fx at 1.1 Gy/fx BID (AIEOP), or 60–66 Gy/60–66 fx at 1 Gy/fx (SPO).

ADULT SPINAL EPENDYMOMA

■ **Can RT be omitted for select myxopapillary ependymomas?**

Although controversial, the adjuvant RT dose after GTR for myxopapillary ependymomas is to treat with at least 50.4 Gy, as omission of RT seems to confer increased local failure.

Pica, Switzerland (*IJROBP* 2009, PMID 19250760): RR of 85 patients with spinal myxopapillary ependymomas. Forty-five percent were treated with surgery alone, the median dose of RT for the others was 50.4 Gy. MFU 60 months. PFS was 74.8% with vs. 50.4% without RT. Approximately 20% of failures were elsewhere in the CNS. On MVA, a dose of 50.4 Gy or higher was an independent predictor of improved PFS. **Conclusion: 50.4 Gy or higher is recommended to reduce progression.**

Kotecha, Cleveland Clinic (*J Neurosurg Spine* 2020, PMID 32357340): RR of 59 patients with spinal myxopapillary ependymoma. Median age 34 years and MFU 6.2 years; 83% underwent initial surgery and 17% received postoperative RT to a median of 49 Gy (range 45–58 Gy). RFS was improved in the GTR group compared to STR: median 11.2 vs. 5.5 years, $p < .001$. RT did not improve RFS after GTR or STR. At time of salvage surgery, RT did improve RFS (9.5 vs. 1.6 years, $p = .006$). **Conclusion: Initial GTR is recommended when possible; the role for adjuvant RT is undetermined. Postsalvage RT appears to improve RFS.**

REFERENCES

1. Wu J, Armstrong TS, Gilbert MR. Biology and management of ependymomas. *Neuro Oncol.* 2016;18(7):902–913. doi:10.1093/neuonc/now016
2. Imbach P, Kühne T, Arceci R. *Pediatric Oncology: A Comprehensive Guide.* 2nd ed. Springer Publishing Company; 2011. doi:10.1007/978-3-642-20359-6
3. Merchant TE, Mulhern RK, Krasin MJ, et al. Preliminary results from a phase II trial of conformal radiation therapy and evaluation of radiation-related CNS effects for pediatric patients with localized ependymoma. *J Clin Oncol.* 2004;22:3156–3162. doi:10.1200/JCO.2004.11.142
4. Rubio MP, Correa KM, Ramesh V, et al. Analysis of the neurofibromatosis 2 gene in human ependymomas and astrocytomas. *Cancer Res.* 1994;54:45–47.
5. Binokay F, Akgul E, Bicakci K, et al. Determining the level of the dural sac tip: magnetic resonance imaging in an adult population. *Acta Radiol.* 2006;47:397–400. doi:10.1080/02841850600557158
6. Scharf CB, Paulino AC, Goldberg KN. Determination of the inferior border of the thecal sac using magnetic resonance imaging: implications on radiation therapy treatment planning. *Int J Radiat Oncol Biol Phys.* 1998;41:621–624. doi:10.1016/S0360-3016(97)00562-2
7. Dunbar SF, Barnes PD, Tarbell NJ. Radiologic determination of the caudal border of the spinal field in cranial spinal irradiation. *Int J Radiat Oncol Biol Phys.* 1993;26:669–673. doi:10.1016/0360-3016(93)90286-5
8. Louis DN, Perry A, Reifenberger G, et al. The 2016 World health organization classification of tumors of the central nervous system: a summary. *Acta Neuropathol.* 2016;131:803–820. doi:10.1007/s00401-016-1545-1
9. Pajtler KW, Witt H, Sill M, et al. Molecular classification of ependymal tumors across all CNS compartments, histopathological grades, and age groups. *Cancer Cell.* 2015;27:728–743. doi:10.1016/j.ccell.2015.04.002
10. Freeman CRF, Jean-Pierre T, Roger E. Central nervous system tumors in children. In: Halperin E, Wazer D, Perez C, Brady L, eds. *Principles & Practice of Radiation Oncology.* 6th ed. Lippincott & Williams; 2013:1632–1654.
11. Rodríguez D, Cheung MC, Housri N, et al. Outcomes of malignant CNS ependymomas: an examination of 2408 cases through the surveillance, epidemiology, and end results (SEER) database (1973–2005). *J Surg Res.* 2009;156:340–351. doi:10.1016/j.jss.2009.04.024

12. Merchant TE, Li C, Xiong X, et al. Conformal radiotherapy after surgery for paediatric ependymoma: a prospective study. *Lancet Oncol.* 2009;10:258–266. doi:10.1016/S1470-2045(08)70342-5

13. Videtic GMM, Woody N, Vassil AD. *Handbook of Treatment Planning in Radiation Oncology.* 3rd ed. Demos Medical; 2020. doi:10.1891/9780826168429

14. Robertson PL, Zeltzer PM, Boyett JM, et al. Survival and prognostic factors following radiation therapy and chemotherapy for ependymomas in children: a report of the children's cancer group. *J Neurosurg.* 1998;88:695–703. doi:10.3171/jns.1998.88.4.0695

15. Evans AE, Anderson JR, Lefkowitz-Boudreaux IB, et al. Adjuvant chemotherapy of childhood posterior fossa ependymoma: cranio-spinal irradiation with or without adjuvant CCNU, vincristine, and prednisone: a childrens cancer group study. *Med Pediatr Oncol.* 1996;27:8–14. doi:10.1002/(SICI)1096-911X(199607)27:1<8::AID-MPO3>3.0.CO;2-K

16. Pollack IF, Gerszten PC, Martinez AJ, et al. Intracranial ependymomas of childhood: long-term outcome and prognostic factors. *Neurosurgery.* 1995;37:655–666; discussion 666–667. doi:10.1097/00006123-199510000-00008

17. Gururangan S, Fangusaro J, Young Poussaint T, et al. Lack of efficacy of bevacizumab + irinotecan in cases of pediatric recurrent ependymoma–a pediatric brain tumor consortium study. *Neuro Oncol.* 2012;14(11):1404–1412. doi:10.1093/neuonc/nos213

18. Garvin JH, Selch MT, Holmes E, et al. Phase II study of pre-irradiation chemotherapy for childhood intracranial ependymoma. children's cancer group protocol 9942: a report from the children's oncology group. *Pediatr Blood Cancer.* 2012;59(7):1183–1189. doi:10.1002/pbc.24274

19. Geyer JR, Sposto R, Jennings M, et al. Multiagent chemotherapy and deferred radiotherapy in infants with malignant brain tumors: a report from the children's cancer group. *J Clin Oncol.* 2005;23(30):7621–7631. doi:10.1200/JCO.2005.09.095

20. Timmermann B, Kortmann RD, Kühl J, et al. Role of radiotherapy in anaplastic ependymoma in children under age of 3 years: results of the prospective German brain tumor trials HIT-SKK 87 and 92. *Radiother Oncol.* 2005;77(3):278–285. doi:10.1016/j.radonc.2005.10.016

21. Grundy RG, Wilne SA, Weston CL, et al. Primary postoperative chemotherapy without radiotherapy for intracranial ependymoma in children: the UKCCSG/SIOP prospective study. *Lancet Oncol.* 2007;8(8):696–705. doi:10.1016/S1470-2045(07)70208-5

22. Strother DR, Lafay-Cousin L, Boyett JM, et al. Benefit from prolonged dose-intensive chemotherapy for infants with malignant brain tumors is restricted to patients with ependymoma: a report of the pediatric oncology group randomized controlled trial 9233/34. *Neuro Oncol.* 2014;16(3):457–465. doi:10.1093/neuonc/not163

23. Kovnar E, Curran W, Tomato T, et al. Hyperfractionated irradiation for childhood ependymoma: improved local control in subtotally resected tumors. *Childs Nerv Syst.* 1998;14:489–490.

24. Massimino M, Gandola L, Giangaspero F, et al. Hyperfractionated radiotherapy and chemotherapy for childhood ependymoma: final results of the first prospective Associazione Italiana Di Ematologia-Oncologia Pediatrica (AIEOP) study. *Int J Radiat Oncol Biol Phys.* 2004;58:1336–1345. doi:10.1016/j.ijrobp.2003.08.030

25. Conter C, Carrie C, Bernier V, et al. Intracranial ependymomas in children: society of pediatric oncology experience with postoperative hyperfractionated local radiotherapy. *Int J Radiat Oncol Biol Phys.* 2009;74:1536–1542. doi:10.1016/j.ijrobp.2008.09.051

58 ■ BRAINSTEM GLIOMA

Sarah M. C. Sittenfeld, Jason W. D. Hearn, and John H. Suh

QUICK HIT ■ Brainstem gliomas (BSGs) are uncommon tumors arising predominantly in children. Prognosis varies between diffuse intrinsic tumors and more favorable types (focal, dorsally exophytic, or cervicomedullary). Diffuse intrinsic pontine glioma (DIPG) is most common and carries a poor prognosis, with MS of <1 year. Surgery is typically not feasible; therefore, standard treatment of unresectable tumors is often RT alone. Hyperfractionation, dose escalation, and CHT have generally not proven beneficial. For other subtypes, surgery may be feasible and prognosis is more favorable.

Table 58.1: General Treatment Paradigm for Brainstem Glioma

BSG Location/Subtype	Management
DIPG (most common)	RT alone, 54 Gy/30 fx. MS <1 yr
Focal, dorsally exophytic, cervicomedullary tumors	Surgery. RT for unresectable or recurrent disease
Focal tectal tumors	Indolent. CSF diversion and observation.[1] 5-yr OS >90%

EPIDEMIOLOGY: BSGs account for 10% to 15% of pediatric CNS tumors, with annual incidence of 300 to 400 in the United States, but constitute <2% of adult CNS tumors.[2,3] DIPG comprises 75% to 80% of pediatric BSGs and is most commonly diagnosed between 5 and 10 years of age.[4]

RISK FACTORS: NF1 confers increased risk of BSGs (second most common after optic-pathway glioma). Despite the increased incidence of BSGs in NF1 patients, these tumors tend to be relatively favorable compared to those in patients without NF1.[5]

ANATOMY: The brainstem comprises the midbrain, pons, and medulla oblongata. CN III to IV originate from the midbrain, CN V to VIII from the pons, and CN IX to XII from the medulla. The tectum (Latin for "roof"; also referred to as the "quadrigeminal plate") represents the dorsal midbrain, and includes the paired superior and inferior colliculi. The tegmentum forms the floor of the midbrain (region ventral to the ventricular system) and continues inferiorly through the pons and into the medulla. The tegmentum includes the nuclei of CN III and IV, the red nucleus, and the substantia nigra.

PATHOLOGY: Approximately 50% of BSGs are low grade (WHO I–II) and 50% are high grade (WHO III–IV); nearly all are astrocytic. BSGs may be intrinsic or exophytic, and if intrinsic they may be diffuse or focal. Focal tumors are generally defined as well-circumscribed lesions <2 cm without edema or infiltration.[1] Overall, BSGs are grouped into four categories based on imaging characteristics: diffusely infiltrating (typically pontine, a.k.a. DIPG), focal, dorsally exophytic, or cervicomedullary.[6] For pediatric DIPG there is generally no difference in outcome between tumors that are low grade vs. high grade at biopsy, perhaps due to a high tendency for malignant transformation as well as heterogeneity in grade within the tumor.[7] Focal tumors occur more frequently in the midbrain or medulla, and are typically low grade.[8] Dorsally exophytic gliomas are generally low grade and arise from subependymal glial tissue in the floor of the fourth ventricle, growing along the path of least resistance rather than infiltrating tissue. Cervicomedullary tumors also tend to be low grade, and in some cases may be infiltrative. These tumors can expand the medulla and upper cervical spinal cord, and may extend rostrally beyond the foramen magnum, since axial growth is limited ventrally by the pyramidal decussation.

GENETICS: Although the etiology is unknown, genomic studies have identified a number of alterations in *PDGFRA, MDM4, MYCN, EGFR, MET, KRAS, CDK4, H3F3A*, the Sonic Hedgehog (SHH) pathway, and others.[9-18] Approximately 80% of DIPGs harbor H3 K27M mutations and represent a distinct subset of midline gliomas; there is ongoing investigation of whether these tumors may be amenable to targeted therapies.[11,19]

CLINICAL PRESENTATION: CN palsies (e.g., diplopia, facial weakness, and difficulty with speech or swallowing), ataxia, long tract signs (motor weakness), or symptoms of elevated intracranial pressure (ICP) such as headache, nausea, and vomiting. Pontine CNs are most commonly affected, followed by medullary CNs, and then midbrain CNs. DIPG typically has rapid symptom onset (median 1 month before diagnosis), generally including bilateral cranial neuropathies, ataxia, and long tract signs. Focal tumors are usually more indolent and typically present with limited cranial neuropathies. Dorsally exophytic lesions present insidiously with failure to thrive and symptoms of elevated ICP; long tract signs are uncommon. Depending on the epicenter of the tumor, cervicomedullary lesions may present with predominantly medullary dysfunction (failure to thrive due to nausea, vomiting, dysphagia, chronic aspiration, sleep apnea, and head tilt) or cervical spinal cord dysfunction (facial or neck pain, progressive weakness, spasticity, hand preference, motor regression, and sensory deficits).[8] Tectal tumors often present with elevated ICP secondary to hydrocephalus from stenosis of the cerebral aqueduct.

WORKUP: H&P with careful neurological exam. MRI with gadolinium: DIPG is often hypointense on T1 with little enhancement (though variable), but hyperintense on T2. Diffusion tensor imaging can also be useful to evaluate the relationship of the tumor to white matter tracts, which can influence surgical candidacy and planning.[8] Up to 10% to 15% of BSGs have leptomeningeal involvement. Dorsally exophytic lesions often fill the fourth ventricle, causing obstruction and hydrocephalus. Such lesions are typically juvenile pilocytic astrocytomas (JPAs), which intensely enhance with gadolinium despite being low grade. Cervicomedullary tumors cause expansion of the medulla toward the fourth ventricle and/or expansion of the cervical cord. Biopsy is generally not indicated for lesions radiologically consistent with DIPG, since grade does not affect management. Since stereotactic biopsy techniques have reduced risks, biopsies may be done for research purposes and can be informative for cases with atypical radiologic or clinical features.[10,20,21] Notably, a biopsy may be more useful in adults, in whom histology appears to have more prognostic importance. Differential diagnosis includes primitive neuroectodermal tumor (PNET), atypical teratoid/rhabdoid tumor (ATRT), vascular malformation, demyelinating disorders (e.g., multiple sclerosis), ganglioglioma, hamartoma (especially in patients with neurofibromatosis), metastasis, abscess, encephalitis, and parasitic cysts, among others.

PROGNOSTIC FACTORS: Tumor location and type are the most important prognostic factors, with DIPG demonstrating worse outcomes than more favorable types (focal, dorsally exophytic, or cervicomedullary).

TREATMENT PARADIGM

DIPG: There is no therapeutic role for surgery and generally no benefit to systemic therapy. Studies investigating cytotoxic CHT, concurrent etanidazole (hypoxic cell radiosensitizer), high-dose tamoxifen, high-dose CHT with bone marrow transplant, blood–brain barrier disruption, p-glycoprotein inhibition (for multidrug resistance), and other strategies have generally not demonstrated significant benefit.[4] RT alone remains the standard treatment for DIPG, as it is the only modality proven to extend survival. Dose is 54 Gy/30 fx daily over 6 weeks. Other RT approaches, such as hyperfractionation, I-125 interstitial implants, and SRS, have been attempted with no clear benefit over standard RT. Most patients improve clinically after RT, though typical time to progression is 5 to 6 months, and MS in most studies is <9 to 12 months.

Focal: Surgical resection is indicated when feasible (e.g., for tumors that extend toward the surface of the brainstem laterally or at the floor of the fourth ventricle). Preservation of neurological function is important for these often indolent tumors and may require judicious use of subtotal resection. RT is useful for progression after surgery and for unresectable lesions.[1] As in the case of DIPG, RT dose is typically 54 Gy/30 fx, although smaller CTV margins are often appropriate.

Dorsally Exophytic or Cervicomedullary: Maximal safe resection is indicated when possible.[8,22,23] RT is a useful alternative for unresectable tumors and can be considered postoperatively for high-grade tumors or those with early progression after surgery. Those who have late progression may benefit from reoperation when feasible. CHT is occasionally a useful adjunct, and in some cases can yield tumor shrinkage followed by a more complete resection. CHT may produce disease stabilization or objective responses, although eventual progression is inevitable, with 5-year PFS in the range of 30% to 40%.[24] CHT is particularly helpful in very young children in order to delay RT, and thereby enable more physical and neurocognitive development.[8]

Tectal: Focal tectal tumors of the midbrain tend to be very indolent and may require only CSF diversion, such as with a third ventriculostomy or shunt.[25] The majority of patients with these tumors remain free from progression for extended periods without surgical resection (which is associated with substantial risk in this location) or RT.[26] Thus, definitive intervention is reserved for patients with evidence of progression.

Treatment-Related Complications: Complications of surgery may include impaired respiratory function (especially if medullary involvement), diplopia, facial palsy, dysphagia, vocal cord paralysis, loss of gag/cough reflexes, additional cranial neuropathies, long tract deficits, and death, among others. Complications of RT may include dermatitis (especially at the external auditory canal and retroauricular region), hearing loss, growth impairment, endocrine dysfunction, cognitive dysfunction, radiation necrosis, and radiation-induced tumors, among others.

■ EVIDENCE-BASED Q&A

■ Does RT dose escalation and/or altered fractionation improve outcomes?

No benefit to dose escalation or altered fractionation was observed across multiple studies (Table 58.2).

TABLE 58.2: Studies Evaluating Dose Escalation and/or Altered Fractionation in Brainstem Gliomas				
Author, institution/ group	**Study design**	**Radiation scheme**	**MS**	**Conclusion**
Freeman, POG 8495[27]	Phase I/II, dose escalation with hyperfractionation	66 Gy/60 fx BID 70.2 Gy/60 fx BID 75.6 Gy/60 fx BID	10 mos	No differences in PFS or OS across dose levels
Packer, CCG 9882[28]	Phase I/II, hyperfractionation	72 Gy/72 fx BID	1-yr OS 38%	No benefit with hyperfractionation
Lewis, UKCCSG[29]	Pilot study, hyperfractionation	48.6–50.4 Gy/27–28 fx BID	8.5 mos	No improvement with hyperfractionation
Mandell, POG 9239[30]	PRT, conventional vs. hyperfractionation with concurrent cisplatin	50.4 Gy/30 fx 70.2 Gy/60 fx BID	8.5 mos 8 mos	No significant improvement with hyperfractionation. Similar toxicity in both arms
Janssens, Netherlands[31]	Prospective, hypofractionation	39 Gy/13 fx or 33 Gy/6 fx, 4 days per week	8.6 mos	Shorter RT course is feasible, with similar toxicity. Note: only nine patients enrolled
Zaghloul, Egypt[32]	PRT, hypofractionation	39 Gy/13 fx 54 Gy/30 fx	7.8 mos 9.5 mos ($p = .59$)	Non-inferiority of hypofractionated RT could not be shown, conventional RT remains standard

▪ Is there a benefit from brachytherapy?

Dose escalation with brachytherapy does not appear to improve outcomes.

Chuba, Wayne State (*Childs Nerv Syst* 1998, PMID 9840381): RR of 28 pediatric patients with CNS tumors who had I-125 brachytherapy, 9 of whom had BSGs (8 with DIPG, 1 with a midbrain tumor). DIPG patients received EBRT (50 Gy) followed by a fractionated stereotactic boost of 3 Gy × 4 fx. After 4 to 6 weeks, patients were re-evaluated for stereotactic interstitial I-125 therapy. Planned implant dose was 82.9 Gy to the enhancing tumor (0.04 Gy per hour). Preliminary results showed no surgical complications associated with catheter placement. MS for the eight patients with DIPG was 8.4 months. The two patients who were alive at analysis had biopsy-proven persistent high-grade tumor. **Conclusion: Tumor control remained poor despite the combination of EBRT with a brachytherapy boost.**

▪ Does stereotactic radiosurgery (SRS) improve outcomes?

Data are very limited and do not imply any improvement relative to conventionally fractionated RT.

Fuchs, Austria (*Acta Neurochir Suppl* 2002, PMID 12379009): RR of 21 patients (8–56 years of age) treated with GKRS for BSG. Twelve lesions were located primarily in the pons, 2 in the medulla, and 7 in the midbrain. Median SRS dose 12 Gy (9–20 Gy) to the tumor margin by the median isodose of 45%. Prior to SRS, 4 patients had received conventional RT, 1 had RT and CHT, 1 underwent CHT, and 1 was shunted due to hydrocephalus. Of the 19 patients with follow-up imaging, tumor progression was seen in 2, stable disease in 10, and regression in 3 patients. MFU 29 months. Neurological status improved in 5 patients. Microsurgical cyst fenestration was performed in 1 patient after SRS and shunting was necessary for 2. Nine patients died unrelated to SRS at a median of 20.7 months. **Conclusion: SRS may be feasible in selected patients, but the very limited sample size and substantial heterogeneity in patients, tumors, and treatments limit interpretation.**

▪ Is there a role for re-irradiation?

Limited data show feasibility and suggest symptomatic benefit in selected patients.

Fontanilla, MDACC (*Am J Clin Oncol* 2012, PMID 21297433): RR of six patients who received re-irradiation for progressive DIPG. TTP after the first course of RT was 4 to 18 months, and all patients had further progression on salvage CHT. The interval between courses of RT was 8 to 28 months. Initial RT dose was 54 to 55.8 Gy. Re-irradiation was given with concurrent CHT, in 2 Gy fractions to 20 Gy (*n* = 4), 18 Gy (*n* = 1), and one patient withdrew care after a single fraction. Four patients had substantial clinical improvement in symptoms, and three patients showed renewed ability to ambulate after re-irradiation. Four patients had decreased tumor size on post-treatment MRI. Median clinical PFS was 5 months. Acute radiation-related toxicities were fatigue (*n* = 2), alopecia (*n* = 2), and decreased appetite (*n* = 1). No grade ≥3 toxicities were reported. **Conclusion: Re-irradiation with CHT is feasible and may improve symptoms with minimal toxicity. Those with prolonged response to initial therapy may be most suitable.**

▪ Is there a benefit from systemic therapy in diffuse intrinsic tumors?

The preponderance of evidence suggests that there is no benefit to systemic therapy (see Table 58.3). The most notable exception comes from the results of the French BSG 98 study, which suggested possible improvement in survival relative to historical controls; however, this regimen required protracted CHT, was quite toxic, and involved prolonged hospitalizations.

▪ Does histology have prognostic significance in adult diffuse intrinsic BSGs?

Adult BSGs appear to behave somewhat differently from those in children, particularly diffuse intrinsic low-grade gliomas, which carry a substantially better prognosis than those in children.

Guillamo, France (*Brain* 2001, PMID 11701605): French RR of 48 adult patients with BSG. Mean age 34 years (range 16–70). MRI demonstrated non-enhancing, diffusely infiltrative tumors (50%), contrast-enhancing localized masses (31%), isolated tectal tumors (8%), and other patterns (11%).

TABLE 58.3: Studies Evaluating Systemic Therapy in Diffuse Intrinsic Tumors

Author, institution/group	Study design	Systemic therapy	MS	Conclusion
Jenkin, CCSG[33]	PRT of 50–60 Gy RT ± adjuvant CHT	CCNU, vincristine, and prednisone	9 mos	No benefit with CHT
Freeman, Cross Trial Comparison of POG 9239/8495[34]	POG 9239: 70.2 Gy + CHT POG 8495: 70.2 Gy alone	Concurrent cisplatin No CHT	1-yr OS 28% 1-yr OS 40% (p = .723)	Cisplatin does not improve OS and may be detrimental
Marcus, Harvard[35]	63–66 Gy/42–44 fx + radiosensitizer	Etanidazole	8.5 mos	No benefit to etanidazole despite toxicity
Broniscer, St. Jude SJHG-98[36]	RT (median 55.8 Gy) + adjuvant CHT	Temozolomide (TMZ)	12 mos	No benefit to adjuvant TMZ
Frappaz, French BSG 98[37]	CHT given at 30-day intervals to delay RT (given at progression)	Tamoxifen, BCNU, cisplatin, followed by two cycles of HD-MTX	17 mos	Improved MS vs. historical controls but with significant toxicity and prolonged hospitalizations
Jalali, Tata Memorial[38]	54 Gy/30 fx + concurrent and adjuvant CHT	TMZ	9.2 mos	No benefit to concurrent and adjuvant TMZ

Treatments included subtotal resection (8%), RT (94%), and CHT (56%). MS 5.4 years. Significant prognostic factors on MVA included histologic grade, duration of symptoms, and the appearance of "necrosis" on MRI; 85% could be classified into one of the following three groups on the basis of clinical, histological, and radiological characteristics:

- Diffuse intrinsic low-grade gliomas (46%): In young adults with a long clinical history before diagnosis and a diffusely enlarged non-enhancing brainstem on MRI. Neurologic status improved with RT in 62% and MS was 7.3 years.
- Focal tectal gliomas (8%): In young adults, often presenting with isolated hydrocephalus. Indolent course with estimated MS >10 years (similar to children for this type of tumor).
- Malignant gliomas (31%): In older patients with short clinical history, as well as contrast enhancement and "necrosis" on MRI. Poor prognosis despite treatment: MS 11.2 months.

REFERENCES

1. Klimo P Jr, Pai Panandiker AS, Thompson CJ, et al. Management and outcome of focal low-grade brainstem tumors in pediatric patients: the st. jude experience. *J Neurosurg Pediatr.* 2013;11(3):274–281. doi:10.3171/2012.11.PEDS12317
2. Physician Data Query (PDQ) of the National Cancer Institute. 2020. https://www.cancer.gov/types/brain/hp/child-glioma-treatment-pdq
3. Hu J, Western S, Kesari S. Brainstem glioma in adults. *Front Oncol.* 2016;6:180. doi:10.3389/fonc.2016.00180
4. Warren KE. Diffuse intrinsic pontine glioma: poised for progress. *Front Oncol.* 2012;2:205. doi:10.3389/fonc.2012.00205
5. Mahdi J, Shah AC, Sato A, et al. A multi-institutional study of brainstem gliomas in children with neurofibromatosis type 1. *Neurology.* 2017;88(16):1584–1589. doi:10.1212/WNL.0000000000003881
6. Epstein FJ, Farmer JP. Brain-stem glioma growth patterns. *J Neurosurg.* 1993;78(3):408–412. doi:10.3171/jns.1993.78.3.0408
7. Hoffman LM, DeWire M, Ryall S, et al. Spatial genomic heterogeneity in diffuse intrinsic pontine and midline high-grade glioma: implications for diagnostic biopsy and targeted therapeutics. *Acta Neuropathol Commun.* 2016;4:1. doi:10.1186/s40478-016-0283-x

8. McAbee JH, Modica J, Thompson CJ, et al. Cervicomedullary tumors in children. *J Neurosurg Pediatr*. 2015;16(4):357–366. doi:10.3171/2015.5.PEDS14638

9. Barrow J, Adamowicz-Brice M, Cartmill M, et al. Homozygous loss of ADAM3A revealed by genome-wide analysis of pediatric high-grade glioma and diffuse intrinsic pontine gliomas. *Neuro Oncol*. 2011;13(2):212–222. doi:10.1093/neuonc/noq158

10. Grill J, Puget S, Andreiuolo F, et al. Critical oncogenic mutations in newly diagnosed pediatric diffuse intrinsic pontine glioma. *Pediatr Blood Cancer*. 2012;58(4):489–491. doi:10.1002/pbc.24060

11. Khuong-Quang DA, Buczkowicz P, Rakopoulos P, et al. K27M mutation in histone H3.3 defines clinically and biologically distinct subgroups of pediatric diffuse intrinsic pontine gliomas. *Acta Neuropathol*. 2012;124(3):439–447. doi:10.1007/s00401-012-0998-0

12. Li G, Mitra SS, Monje M, et al. Expression of epidermal growth factor variant III (EGFRvIII) in pediatric diffuse intrinsic pontine gliomas. *J Neurooncol*. 2012;108(3):395–402. doi:10.1007/s11060-012-0842-3

13. Paugh BS, Broniscer A, Qu C, et al. Genome-wide analyses identify recurrent amplifications of receptor tyrosine kinases and cell-cycle regulatory genes in diffuse intrinsic pontine glioma. *J Clin Oncol*. 2011;29(30):3999–4006. doi:10.1200/JCO.2011.35.5677

14. Paugh BS, Qu C, Jones C, et al. Integrated molecular genetic profiling of pediatric high-grade gliomas reveals key differences with the adult disease. *J Clin Oncol*. 2010;28(18):3061–3068. doi:10.1200/JCO.2009.26.7252

15. Warren KE, Killian K, Suuriniemi M, et al. Genomic aberrations in pediatric diffuse intrinsic pontine gliomas. *Neuro Oncol*. 2012;14(3):326–332. doi:10.1093/neuonc/nor190

16. Wu G, Broniscer A, McEachron TA, et al. Somatic histone H3 alterations in pediatric diffuse intrinsic pontine gliomas and non-brainstem glioblastomas. *Nat Genet*. 2012;44(3):251–253. doi:10.1038/ng.1102

17. Zarghooni M, Bartels U, Lee E, et al. Whole-genome profiling of pediatric diffuse intrinsic pontine gliomas highlights platelet-derived growth factor receptor alpha and poly (ADP-ribose) polymerase as potential therapeutic targets. *J Clin Oncol*. 2010;28(8):1337–1344. doi:10.1200/JCO.2009.25.5463

18. Puget S, Philippe C, Bax DA, et al. Mesenchymal transition and PDGFRA amplification/mutation are key distinct oncogenic events in pediatric diffuse intrinsic pontine gliomas. *PLoS One*. 2012;7(2):e30313. doi:10.1371/journal.pone.0030313

19. Himes BT, Zhang L, Daniels DJ. Treatment strategies in diffuse midline gliomas with the H3K27M Mmtation: the role of convection-enhanced delivery in overcoming anatomic challenges. *Front Oncol*. 2019;9:31. doi:10.3389/fonc.2019.00031

20. Cage TA, Samagh SP, Mueller S, et al. Feasibility, safety, and indications for surgical biopsy of intrinsic brainstem tumors in children. *Childs Nerv Syst*. 2013;29(8):1313–1319. doi:10.1007/s00381-013-2101-0

21. Puget S, Beccaria K, Blauwblomme T, et al. Biopsy in a series of 130 pediatric diffuse intrinsic pontine gliomas. *Childs Nerv Syst*. 2015;31(10):1773–1780. doi:10.1007/s00381-015-2832-1

22. Robertson PL, Allen JC, Abbott IR, et al. Cervicomedullary tumors in children: a distinct subset of brainstem gliomas. *Neurology*. 1994;44(10):1798–1803. doi:10.1212/WNL.44.10.1798

23. Di Maio S, Gul SM, Cochrane DD, et al. Clinical, radiologic and pathologic features and outcome following surgery for cervicomedullary gliomas in children. *Childs Nerv Syst*. 2009;25(11):1401–1410. doi:10.1007/s00381-009-0956-x

24. Raabe E, Kieran MW, Cohen KJ. New strategies in pediatric gliomas: molecular advances in pediatric low-grade gliomas as a model. *Clin Cancer Res*. 2013;19(17):4553–4558. doi:10.1158/1078-0432.CCR-13-0662

25. Daglioglu E, Cataltepe O, Akalan N. Tectal gliomas in children: the implications for natural history and management strategy. *Pediatr Neurosurg*. 2003;38(5):223–231. doi:10.1159/000069823

26. Griessenauer CJ, Rizk E, Miller JH, et al. Pediatric tectal plate gliomas: clinical and radiological progression, MR imaging characteristics, and management of hydrocephalus. *J Neurosurg Pediatr*. 2014;13(1):13–20. doi:10.3171/2013.9.PEDS13347

27. Freeman CR, Krischer J, Sanford RA, et al. Hyperfractionated radiation therapy in brain stem tumors: results of treatment at the 7020 cGy dose level of Pediatric Oncology Group study #8495. *Cancer*. 1991;68(3):474–481. doi:10.1002/1097-0142(19910801)68:3<474::AID-CNCR2820680305>3.0.CO;2-7

28. Packer RJ, Boyett JM, Zimmerman RA, et al. Hyperfractionated radiation therapy (72 Gy) for children with brain stem gliomas: a Children's Cancer Group Phase I/II Trial. *Cancer*. 1993;72(4):1414–1421. doi:10.1002/1097-0142(19930815)72:4<1414::AID-CNCR2820720442>3.0.CO;2-C

29. Lewis J, Lucraft H, Gholkar A. UKCCSG study of accelerated radiotherapy for pediatric brain stem gliomas. United Kingdom Childhood Cancer Study Group. *Int J Radiat Oncol Biol Phys*. 1997;38(5):925–929. doi:10.1016/S0360-3016(97)00134-X

30. Mandell LR, Kadota R, Freeman C, et al. There is no role for hyperfractionated radiotherapy in the management of children with newly diagnosed diffuse intrinsic brainstem tumors: results of a Pediatric Oncology Group phase III trial comparing conventional vs. hyperfractionated radiotherapy. *Int J Radiat Oncol Biol Phys*. 1999;43(5):959–964. doi:10.1016/S0360-3016(98)00501-X

31. Janssens GO, Gidding CE, Van Lindert EJ, et al. The role of hypofractionation radiotherapy for diffuse intrinsic brainstem glioma in children: a pilot study. *Int J Radiat Oncol Biol Phys*. 2009;73(3):722–726. doi:10.1016/j.ijrobp.2008.05.030

32. Zaghloul MS, Eldebawy E, Ahmed S, et al. Hypofractionated conformal radiotherapy for pediatric diffuse intrinsic pontine glioma (DIPG): a randomized controlled trial. *Radiother Oncol*. 2014;111(1):35–40. doi:10.1016/j.radonc.2014.01.013

33. Jenkin RD, Boesel C, Ertel I, et al. Brain-stem tumors in childhood: a prospective randomized trial of irradiation with and without adjuvant CCNU, VCR, and prednisone. a report of the childrens cancer study group. *J Neurosurg.* 1987;66(2):227–233. doi:10.3171/jns.1987.66.2.0227

34. Freeman CR, Kepner J, Kun LE, et al. A detrimental effect of a combined chemotherapy-radiotherapy approach in children with diffuse intrinsic brain stem gliomas? *Int J Radiat Oncol Biol Phys.* 2000;47(3):561–564. doi:10.1016/S0360-3016(00)00471-5

35. Marcus KJ, Dutton SC, Barnes P, et al. A phase I trial of etanidazole and hyperfractionated radiotherapy in children with diffuse brainstem glioma. *Int J Radiat Oncol Biol Phys.* 2003;55(5):1182–1185. doi:10.1016/S0360-3016(02)04391-2

36. Broniscer A, Iacono L, Chintagumpala M, et al. Role of temozolomide after radiotherapy for newly diagnosed diffuse brainstem glioma in children: results of a multiinstitutional study (SJHG-98). *Cancer.* 2005;103(1):133–139. doi:10.1002/cncr.20741

37. Frappaz D, Schell M, Thiesse P, et al. Preradiation chemotherapy may improve survival in pediatric diffuse intrinsic brainstem gliomas: final results of BSG 98 prospective trial. *Neuro Oncol.* 2008;10(4):599–607. doi:10.1215/15228517-2008-029

38. Jalali R, Raut N, Arora B, et al. Prospective evaluation of radiotherapy with concurrent and adjuvant temozolomide in children with newly diagnosed diffuse intrinsic pontine glioma. *Int J Radiat Oncol Biol Phys.* 2010;77(1):113–118. doi:10.1016/j.ijrobp.2009.04.031

59 ■ CRANIOPHARYNGIOMA

Martin C. Tom, Timothy D. Smile, and Erin S. Murphy

QUICK HIT ■ CP is a rare benign neoplasm arising from the hypophyseal duct (Rathke's pouch) most commonly in the suprasellar region in children and older adults. Presentation includes headache, visual disturbances, nausea/vomiting, and/or endocrine abnormalities, with imaging revealing a suprasellar solid and/or cystic (filled with classic "crankcase oil") enhancing mass with calcifications. Treatment typically consists of either gross total resection alone (can be morbid) or subtotal resection followed by adjuvant RT, which appear to have comparable long-term outcomes (PFS > 65%, OS > 90%). RT strategies include conventional EBRT, IMRT, or proton beam RT to 54 Gy with recommended on-treatment imaging to account for cyst volume fluctuation, or SRS.

EPIDEMIOLOGY: The incidence of CP is about 613 per year in the United States and is similar between genders, but slightly higher in Blacks.[1] CP represents 0.8% of all CNS tumors, 1.1% of all nonmalignant CNS tumors, and 3.4% of CNS tumors in children/adolescents (170 per year).[1] There is a bimodal age distribution between 5 to 14 and 50 to 75 years of age.[2] Among nonmalignant CNS tumors, 5-year OS was among the lowest at 86.1%.[1]

RISK FACTORS: No proven risk factors.

ANATOMY: CPs arise from the hypophyseal duct (Rathke's pouch), or its remnant in adults. They are typically suprasellar and can involve the optic chiasm, basal vasculature, hypothalamus, third ventricle, or pituitary stalk. They can appear grossly well encapsulated, but formation of multiple cysts is characteristic.[3]

PATHOLOGY: CPs are histologically benign epithelial tumors. The two major subtypes are adamantinomatous (85%–90%) and papillary (i.e., squamous papillary, 11%–14%). The adamantinomatous subtype is associated with children and appears solid and/or cystic with calcifications and dark brown/black fluid ("crankcase oil" appearance). They tend to be more adherent to surrounding structures, and on histology demonstrate wet keratin nodules, Rosenthal fibers, and a palisading basal layer of cells with intense gliosis.[4] The papillary subtype appears more similar to Rathke's cleft cysts with squamous differentiation and pseudopapillae, and is more likely to have calcification on imaging.[3,5]

GENETICS: The adamantinomatous subtype is related to WNT pathway activation and *CTNNB1* gene mutation, which codes for β-catenin.[6,7] The papillary subtype may harbor the *BRAF* (V600E) mutation.[8,9]

CLINICAL PRESENTATION: Typically includes headaches, visual deficits, nausea/vomiting, or hormonal abnormalities, such as GH insufficiency or hypothyroidism (growth failure), ADH insufficiency (central diabetes insipidus), impotence, amenorrhea, or galactorrhea. Can also include depression, lethargy/somnolence, coma, seizures, hyperphagia, diencephalic syndrome, and changes in cognitive function or personality.[10,11]

WORKUP: H&P with attention to endocrine symptoms and a detailed neurologic exam, including detailed visual field testing, memory, personality, psychological, and cognitive function testing.

Labs: Endocrine workup is indicated pretreatment to establish baseline function. Also consider electrolyte studies and urinalysis.

Imaging: MRI and/or CT revealing cystic (94%), calcified (92%, more common in papillary), enhancing, parasellar lesion, with hydrocephalus (67%).[9] MRI typically demonstrates a hyperintense abnormality on T1-weighted images, which differentiates craniopharyngioma from Rathke's cleft and tumor cysts. Upon contrast administration, both the solid and cystic components typically enhance. Diagnosis can be made based on radiographic appearance, cyst fluid analysis ("crankcase oil"), or otherwise histopathologically.

PROGNOSTIC FACTORS: Negative prognostic factors include >53 years of age in adults, >2 prior surgeries, tumor size >5 cm, STR alone (vs. with RT), hydrocephalus, and RT dose <54 to 55 Gy.[10,12-15] Close observation with on-treatment MRI to monitor for cyst expansion associated with improved control.[15]

TREATMENT PARADIGM

Surgery: Surgical resection is indicated for almost all patients for safe debulking. While some favor initial aggressive total resection, GTR can be morbid due to proximity to the hypothalamus and other surrounding structures. Therefore, others advocate for limited resection followed by RT (adjuvant or salvage). STR alone has poor LC rates. Intrasellar tumors can be removed transsphenoidally, while suprasellar tumors can be removed via an extended transsphenoidal approach using an endoscope.[16] Many utilize a pterional craniotomy. Tumors with large cysts may be aspirated prior to surgery. Ommaya reservoirs may be placed within cystic components, and the cysts can be accessed for draining if expansion occurs.

Chemotherapy: Intracystic CHT with either bleomycin or IFNα has been used, albeit with limited experience, for temporary tumor control with response rates of 62% to 100% and control rates of 59% to 71%. There is some suggestion that IFNα has fewer side effects than bleomycin.[16] Response to targeted therapy among those with a *BRAF* V600E mutation has been reported and is the subject of an ongoing trial.[17]

Radiation

Indications: RT is indicated following STR (adjuvant) or at tumor recurrence (salvage). Proton beam therapy alone or in conjunction with photon therapy has demonstrated efficacy in small retrospective series with limited follow-up.[18-20] An ongoing prospective phase II study utilizing proton beam RT reported similar incidence of severe complications compared to a historical cohort treated with conformal or intensity-modulated RT.[21] With fractionated conformal techniques, interfraction imaging every 1 to 2 weeks may be necessary to account for fluctuations in cyst volume.[16,22] For predominantly cystic lesions, intracavitary RT with rhenium-186, yttrium-90, or phosphorus-32 has demonstrated response rates of 50% to 100% and control rates of 67%, though data are limited.[16,23-26]

Dose: Conventional EBRT dose is typically 54 Gy/30 fx. Doses of 54 to 55.8 Gy or greater have demonstrated improved LC compared to lower doses.[13-15] Several series of Gamma Knife® SRS used doses of 10 to 14.5 Gy with long-term control rates of 66% to 80%.[27-30]

Procedure: See *Handbook of Treatment Planning in Radiation Oncology,* Chapter 12.[31]

■ EVIDENCE-BASED Q&A

■ Are clinical outcomes better with aggressive total resection or limited resection followed by RT?

This is controversial. Retrospective data and systematic reviews of the literature suggest GTR versus STR + adjuvant RT have similar OS and LC, but GTR may cause more endocrine dysfunction.[11,32-36]

Table 59.1: Yang et al. (2010): All CP				
n = 442	2-Yr PFS	5-Yr PFS	5-Yr OS	10-Yr OS
GTR	88%	67%	98%	98%
STR + RT	91%	69%	99%	95%
	All NS			

Source: From Yang I, Sughrue ME, Rutkowski MJ, et al. Craniopharyngioma: a comparison of tumor control with various treatment strategies. *Neurosurg Focus.* 2010;28(4):E5. doi:10.3171/2010.1.FOCUS09307

Table 59.2: Clark et al. (2013): Pediatric CP[33]		
n = 377	1-Yr PFS	5-Yr PFS
GTR	89%	77%
STR + RT	84%	73%
	All NS	

Source: From Clark AJ, Cage TA, Aranda D, et al. A systematic review of the results of surgery and radiotherapy on tumor control for pediatric craniopharyngioma. *Childs Nerv Syst*. 2013;29(2):231 to 238. doi:10.1007/s00381-012-1926-2

■ Can RT be reserved for salvage treatment?

Most likely. Retrospective data from the University of Pennsylvania found that LC was worse with surgery alone vs. surgery + adjuvant RT, but after accounting for the surgery alone patients who ultimately received salvage RT, LC, and OS were comparable.[37] Furthermore, retrospective data from the UK demonstrated similar outcomes among 87 patients treated with adjuvant RT vs. salvage RT.[38]

■ What are the late effects after treatment?

Craniopharyngioma originates in a highly sensitive area of the brain, particularly in children, and late effects are common, given the long natural history of the disease. Diabetes insipidus is common after aggressive surgical resection. Neuropsychological changes, including disinhibition, perseveration, attention, and memory deficits, are common. Endocrine effects including GH abnormalities are common in children. Additional effects of treatment near the hypothalamus include hypothalamic obesity, sleep disturbance, and defective thirst sensation. Visual impairment can occur from treatment or tumor progression. Stroke can occur due to proximity to the carotid artery and due to microvascular changes. Moyamoya syndrome (microvascular ischemia of the basal ganglia) is less common. Second malignancy (meningioma and others) can also occur.

REFERENCES

1. Ostrom QT, Gittleman H, Fulop J, et al. CBTRUS statistical report: primary brain and central nervous system tumors diagnosed in the United States in 2008-2012. *Neuro-oncology*. 2015;17 Suppl 4(Suppl 4):iv1–iv62. doi:10.1093/neuonc/nov189
2. Bunin GR, Surawicz TS, Witman PA, et al. The descriptive epidemiology of craniopharyngioma. *J Neurosurg*. 1998;89(4):547–551. doi:10.3171/jns.1998.89.4.0547
3. Gunderson LL TJ. *Clinical Radiation Oncology*, 4th ed. Elsevier; 2016.
4. Adamson TE, Wiestler OD, Kleihues P, Yasargil MG. Correlation of clinical and pathological features in surgically treated craniopharyngiomas. *J Neurosurg*. 1990;73(1):12–17. doi:10.3171/jns.1990.73.1.0012
5. Crotty TB, Scheithauer BW, Young WF, Jr., et al. Papillary craniopharyngioma: a clinicopathological study of 48 cases. *J Neurosurg*. 1995;83(2):206–214. doi:10.3171/jns.1995.83.2.0206
6. Gaston-Massuet C, Andoniadou CL, Signore M, et al. Increased Wingless (Wnt) signaling in pituitary progenitor/stem cells gives rise to pituitary tumors in mice and humans. *Proc Natl Acad Sci U S A*. 2011;108(28):11482–11487. doi:10.1073/pnas.1101553108
7. Hussain I, Eloy JA, Carmel PW, Liu JK. Molecular oncogenesis of craniopharyngioma: current and future strategies for the development of targeted therapies. *J Neurosurg*. 2013;119(1):106–112. doi:10.3171/2013.3.JNS122214
8. Brastianos PK, Taylor-Weiner A, Manley PE, et al. Exome sequencing identifies BRAF mutations in papillary craniopharyngiomas. *Nat Genet*. 2014;46(2):161–165. doi:10.1038/ng.2868
9. Larkin S, Karavitaki N. Recent advances in molecular pathology of craniopharyngioma. *F1000Research*. 2017;6:1202. doi:10.12688/f1000research.11549.1
10. Hetelekidis S, Barnes PD, Tao ML, et al. 20-year experience in childhood craniopharyngioma. *Int J Radiat Oncol Biol Phys*. 1993;27(2):189–195. doi:10.1016/0360-3016(93)90227-M
11. Merchant TE, Kiehna EN, Sanford RA, et al. Craniopharyngioma: the St. Jude Children's Research Hospital experience 1984-2001. *Int J Radiat Oncol Biol Phys*. 2002;53(3):533–542. doi:10.1016/S0360-3016(02)02799-2
12. Masson-Cote L, Masucci GL, Atenafu EG, et al. Long-term outcomes for adult craniopharyngioma following radiation therapy. *Acta Oncol*. 2013;52(1):153–158. doi:10.3109/0284186X.2012.685525
13. Regine WF, Kramer S. Pediatric craniopharyngiomas: long term results of combined treatment with surgery and radiation. *Int J Radiat Oncol Biol Phys*. 1992;24(4):611–617. doi:10.1016/0360-3016(92)90705-M

14. Habrand JL, Ganry O, Couanet D, et al. The role of radiation therapy in the management of craniopharyngioma: a 25-year experience and review of the literature. *Int J Radiat Oncol Biol Phys.* 1999;44(2):255–263. doi:10.1016/S0360-3016(99)00030-9

15. Varlotto JM, Flickinger JC, Kondziolka D, et al. External beam irradiation of craniopharyngiomas: long-term analysis of tumor control and morbidity. *Int J Radiat Oncol Biol Phys.* 2002;54(2):492–499. doi:10.1016/S0360-3016(02)02965-6

16. Steinbok P, Hukin J. Intracystic treatments for craniopharyngioma. *Neurosurg Focus.* 2010;28(4):E13. doi:10.3171/2010.1.FOCUS09315

17. Juratli TA, Jones PS, Wang N, et al. Targeted treatment of papillary craniopharyngiomas harboring BRAF V600E mutations. *Cancer.* 2019;125(17):2910–2914. doi:10.1002/cncr.32197

18. Luu QT, Loredo LN, Archambeau JO, et al. Fractionated proton radiation treatment for pediatric craniopharyngioma: preliminary report. *Cancer J.* 2006;12(2):155–159.

19. Fitzek MM, Linggood RM, Adams J, Munzenrider JE. Combined proton and photon irradiation for craniopharyngioma: long-term results of the early cohort of patients treated at Harvard Cyclotron Laboratory and Massachusetts General Hospital. *Int J Radiat Oncol Biol Phys.* 2006;64(5):1348–1354. doi:10.1016/j.ijrobp.2005.09.034

20. Rutenberg MS, Rotondo RL, Rao D, et al. Clinical outcomes following proton therapy for adult craniopharyngioma: a single-institution cohort study. *Neuro Oncol.* 2020;147(2):387–395. doi:10.1007/s11060-020-03432-9

21. Merchant TE, Hua CH, Sabin ND, et al. Necrosis, vasculopathy, and neurological complications after proton therapy for childhood craniopharyngioma: results from a prospective trial and a photon cohort comparison. *Int J Radiat Oncol Biol Phys.* 2016;96(2, Supplement):S120–S121. doi:10.1016/j.ijrobp.2016.06.294

22. Winkfield KM, Linsenmeier C, Yock TI, et al. Surveillance of craniopharyngioma cyst growth in children treated with proton radiotherapy. *Int J Radiat Oncol Biol Phys.* 2009;73(3):716–721. doi:10.1016/j.ijrobp.2008.05.010

23. Voges J, Sturm V, Lehrke R, et al. Cystic craniopharyngioma: long-term results after intracavitary irradiation with stereotactically applied colloidal beta-emitting radioactive sources. *Neurosurgery.* 1997;40(2):263–269: discussion 269–270. doi:10.1097/00006123-199702000-00006

24. Pollock BE, Lunsford LD, Kondziolka D, et al. Phosphorus-32 intracavitary irradiation of cystic craniopharyngiomas: current technique and long-term results. *Int J Radiat Oncol Biol Phys.* 1995;33(2):437–446. doi:10.1016/0360-3016(95)00175-X

25. Hasegawa T, Kondziolka D, Hadjipanayis CG, Lunsford LD. Management of cystic craniopharyngiomas with phosphorus-32 intracavitary irradiation. *Neurosurgery.* 2004;54(4):813–820; discussion 820-812. doi:10.1227/01.NEU.0000114262.30035.AF

26. Van den Berge JH, Blaauw G, Breeman WA, et al. Intracavitary brachytherapy of cystic craniopharyngiomas. *J Neurosurg.* 1992;77(4):545–550. doi:10.3171/jns.1992.77.4.0545

27. Niranjan A, Kano H, Mathieu D, et al. Radiosurgery for craniopharyngioma. *Int J Radiat Oncol Biol Phys.* 2010;78(1):64–71. doi:10.1016/j.ijrobp.2009.07.1693

28. Lee CC, Yang HC, Chen CJ, et al. Gamma knife surgery for craniopharyngioma: report on a 20-year experience. *J Neurosurg.* 2014;121 Suppl:167–178. doi:10.3171/2014.8.GKS141411

29. Kobayashi T. Long-term results of gamma knife radiosurgery for 100 consecutive cases of craniopharyngioma and a treatment strategy. *Prog Neurol Surg.* 2009;22:63–76. doi:10.1159/000163383

30. Xu Z, Yen CP, Schlesinger D, Sheehan J. Outcomes of Gamma knife surgery for craniopharyngiomas. *J Neurooncol.* 2011;104(1):305–313. doi:10.1007/s11060-010-0494-0

31. Videtic GMM VA, Woody NM. *Handbook of Treatment Planning in Radiation Oncology.* 3rd ed. Springer Publishing Company, LLC; 2020.

32. Clark AJ, Cage TA, Aranda D, et al. Treatment-related morbidity and the management of pediatric craniopharyngioma: a systematic review. *J Neurosurg Pediatr.* 2012;10(4):293–301. doi:10.3171/2012.7.PEDS11436

33. Clark AJ, Cage TA, Aranda D, et al. A systematic review of the results of surgery and radiotherapy on tumor control for pediatric craniopharyngioma. *Childs Nerv Syst.* 2013;29(2):231–238. doi:10.1007/s00381-012-1926-2

34. Yang I, Sughrue ME, Rutkowski MJ, et al. Craniopharyngioma: a comparison of tumor control with various treatment strategies. *Neurosurg Focus.* 2010;28(4):E5. doi:10.3171/2010.1.FOCUS09307

35. Schoenfeld A, Pekmezci M, Barnes MJ, et al. The superiority of conservative resection and adjuvant radiation for craniopharyngiomas. *J Neurooncol.* 2012;108(1):133–139. doi:10.1007/s11060-012-0806-7

36. Sughrue ME, Yang I, Kane AJ, et al. Endocrinologic, neurologic, and visual morbidity after treatment for craniopharyngioma. *J Neurooncol.* 2011;101(3):463–476. doi:10.1007/s11060-010-0265-y

37. Stripp DC, Maity A, Janss AJ, et al. Surgery with or without radiation therapy in the management of craniopharyngiomas in children and young adults. *Int J Radiat Oncol Biol Phys.* 2004;58(3):714–720. doi:10.1016/S0360-3016(03)01570-0

38. Pemberton LS, Dougal M, Magee B, Gattamaneni HR. Experience of external beam radiotherapy given adjuvantly or at relapse following surgery for craniopharyngioma. *Radiother Oncol.* 2005;77(1):99–104. doi:10.1016/j.radonc.2005.04.015

60 ■ RHABDOMYOSARCOMA

Shauna R. Campbell, Samuel T. Chao, and Erin S. Murphy

QUICK HIT ■ Rhabdomyosarcoma (RMS) is the most common malignant soft tissue tumor in children. Risk stratification is performed via preoperative staging, postoperative grouping, and histology to determine treatment. Presence of metastatic disease and PAX/FOX01 gene fusion are the two most important prognostic factors. All patients require multiagent CHT (usually VAC-based: vincristine, actinomycin D, and cyclophosphamide). General treatment paradigm is biopsy or non-morbid resection, followed by CHT, local therapy (surgery or RT), and more CHT for up to approximately 1 year. RT is indicated for all patients except those with embryonal histology after gross total resection without nodal involvement. The timing of RT varies by protocol and presentation. Patients with intracranial extension, vision loss, or cord compression should be considered for urgent RT, especially if not responding to CHT; those with CN palsies and base of skull erosion can receive delayed RT without a compromise in outcomes. Dosing guidelines are listed in Table 60.1.

Table 60.1: Summary of Radiation Dosing Guidelines for Rhabdomyosarcoma by Extent of Resection and Histology

Disease Status	Embryonal Histology	Alveolar Histology
Margin negative	No RT	36 Gy
Margin positive	36 Gy	36 Gy
Node positive	41.4 Gy	41.4 Gy
Gross disease*	50.4 Gy	50.4 Gy

*Gross disease in the orbit receives 45 Gy with VAC (although with lower cyclophosphamide dose and response <CR, 50.4 Gy should be considered) or 50.4 Gy with VA CHT.[1,2] Dose escalation to 59.4 Gy can be considered for patients with diffuse anaplasia or bulky disease (>5 cm) with < CR after CHT per ARST1431.

EPIDEMIOLOGY: RMS is the most common pediatric soft tissue sarcoma with 400 to 500 cases per year.[3] There is a slight male predominance, 1.4:1, and the peak incidence occurs at 3 to 5 years of age, with 70% of cases occurring before 10 years of age.[4,5]

RISK FACTORS: The majority of cases are sporadic, with no predisposing risk factor.[6] RMS has been associated with Li–Fraumeni,[6–8] NF-1,[9,10] Beckwith–Wiedemann syndrome,[11] Noonan syndrome,[12] and Costello syndrome.[13]

ANATOMY: RMS can arise anywhere in the body, with the most common locations being the GU and H&N sites (Table 60.2).[5] Locally invasive tumor with the potential to spread along fascial planes. Overall risk of regional lymphatic spread varies with site of primary lesion; GU, abdominal/pelvic, and extremity tumors more commonly involve regional lymph nodes, whereas H&N, trunk, and female genital organs rarely involve lymph nodes.[4] Distant metastases are present in 15% of cases at time of diagnosis with the lungs, bone, and bone marrow being most common.[14]

PATHOLOGY: There are three histologic subtypes: embryonal (includes botryoid and spindle cell variants), alveolar, and pleomorphic/undifferentiated (Table 60.3).

Table 60.2: Distribution of RMS by Anatomic Site		
Site[15]	Distribution (%)	Subdivisions
H&N (non-PM)	7	Cheek, hypopharynx, larynx, oral cavity, oropharynx, parotid, scalp, face, pinna, neck, masseter muscle
PM	25	Infratemporal fossa, mastoid, middle ear, nasal cavity, nasopharynx, paranasal sinus, parapharyngeal, pterygopalatine fossa
Orbit	9	*Note: Combined H&N (including PM and orbit) most common site*
GU	31	Bladder, paratesticular, prostate, urethra, uterus/ cervix, vagina, vulva
Extremity	13	
Trunk	5	Chest wall, paraspinal, abdominal wall
Retroperitoneum	7	
Other	3	Hepatobiliary tree, perineal, perianal

GENETICS[4]

Embryonal: Eighty percent are associated with LOH 11p15.5. Absence of N-myc amplification in most and 95% are PAX/FOX01 fusion negative.

Alveolar: Eighty percent are associated with PAX/FOXO1 gene fusion. N-myc amplification is found in 50% of cases. Two chromosomal translocations are identified: **t(2;13) (PAX3/FOX01 fusion)** in 60% of cases and **t(1;13) (PAX7/FOX01 fusion)** in 20% of cases. Genes are FKHR (on chr 13), PAX3 (chr 2), and PAX7 (chr 1). Twenty percent that do not have PAX/FOX01 gene fusion have prognosis similar to embryonal.

CLINICAL PRESENTATION: Often presents as asymptomatic mass but can have site-specific signs and symptoms (e.g., orbital tumors may cause proptosis and ophthalmoplegia, and GU tumors may cause hematuria or urinary obstruction).

WORKUP[14]: H&P with exam of affected area (H&N, pelvic exam under anesthesia as indicated).

Labs: CBC, BMP, LFTs, urinalysis.

Imaging: For all sites: CT or MRI of primary tumor area, PET/CT (can replace CT chest/abdomen/ pelvis and bone scan studies). Scrotal ultrasound is often first step for a paratesticular tumor. MRI spine is optional if CSF is positive or if patient is symptomatic.

Procedures: Bone marrow biopsy and aspirate. For H&N primary tumor with intracranial extension, a lumbar puncture with cytologic exam of CSF is indicated.

PROGNOSTIC FACTORS: For high-risk patients, Oberlin risk factors are predictive of outcome and include >10 years or <1 year of age, bone or bone marrow involvement, three or more metastatic sites, or unfavorable primary site. Patients with ≤1 Oberlin factor have a better outcome.[16] Table 60.4 compares favorable and unfavorable prognostic factors.

Table 60.3: Pathologic Subtypes of RMS[4,5]

Subtype	Frequency (%)	Common Site	Histologic Appearance	Age	Prognosis	5-yr OS (%)
Botryoid (grape-like appearance, embryonal variant)	6	Mucosa-lined organs: bladder, vagina, nasopharynx, nasal cavity, middle ear, biliary tree	Loose myxoid stroma w/ "cambium" tumor cell layer	Infants	Excellent	95
Spindle cell (embryonal variant)	3	Paratesticular	Spindled cells, often w/ storiform pattern	Childhood		88
Embryonal	60	Most commonly in H&N and GU tract	Small round cells on myxoid stroma	Childhood	Intermediate	66
Alveolar	20	Extremities, trunk, perianal, perineal region	Cords with pseudolining clefts, looks like lung alveoli	Adolescents	Poor	54
Undifferentiated	2	Extremity, trunk	Diffuse mesenchymal/ primitive cell population; diagnosis of exclusion	Adolescents		40
Other	9					

Table 60.4: Comparison of Favorable vs. Unfavorable Prognostic Factors in RMS

Variable	Favorable	Unfavorable
Metastases	None	Present
Primary site	Orbit, non-PM H&N, GU (nonbladder/prostate)	Extremity, trunk, PM, bladder, prostate
Histology	Botryoid, spindle cell, embryonal	Alveolar, undifferentiated
Lymph node metastasis	No	Yes
Resectability	Complete	Microscopic < gross residual
Age	2–10 y/o	<1 y/o, >10 y/o
DNA proliferation	Low S-phase	High S-phase
DNA ploidy	Hyperdiploid	Diploid
PAX/FOX01	Fusion negative	Fusion positive

STAGING: IRSG pretreatment staging system (Table 60.5). Pre-op based on "SSN" (site, size, nodes). If favorable site and nonmetastatic, all are stage I. If unfavorable site, must be BOTH <5 cm AND node-negative to be stage II.

Table 60.5: IRSG Staging System

Stage	Sites	Size	N	M	3-Yr Failure-Free Survival (%)[15]
I: Favorable site	Orbit H&N (non-PM) GU (nonbladder/prostate) Biliary tract	Any size	Any N	M0	86
II: Unfavorable site, N0 and ≤ 5 cm	Bladder/prostate Extremity Parameningeal Other (including RP, perineal, perianal, intrathoracic, GI) Liver (nonbiliary)	≤5 cm	N0 or Nx	M0	80
III: Unfavorable site, >5 cm or node-positive	Same as stage II	≤5 cm	N1	M0	68
		>5 cm	Any N	M0	
IV: Metastatic	All	Any size	Any N	M1	25

N0, Not clinically involved; N1, Clinically involved; Nx, Clinical status unknown; M0, No distant metastases; M1, Distant metastases.

Intergroup Rhabdomyosarcoma Study Clinical Grouping Classification[5]

Group is assessed at the time of diagnosis based on resectability (i.e., patient unresectable at diagnosis, treated with CHT, then undergoes GTR remains Group III).

Table 60.6: IRSG Grouping Classification

Group I	Localized disease, completely resected A: Confined to muscle or organ of origin B: Infiltration outside the muscle or organ of origin
Group II	Gross total resection with: A: Microscopic residual disease B: Regional LN spread, completely resected C: Regional LN resected with microscopic residual disease

(continued)

Table 60.6: IRSG Grouping Classification (*continued*)	
Group III	Incomplete resection with gross residual disease A: After biopsy only B: After major resection (>50%)
Group IV	Distant metastasis at diagnosis

Table 60.7: Risk Stratification Based on Pre-Op Staging + Post-Op Grouping	
Risk Group	**Involved Groups**
Low (~35%)	Favorable histology (embryonal) *and* PAX/FOX01 fusion negative *and* – Favorable site (stage I): groups I–III – Unfavorable site (stages II–III): groups I–II
Intermediate (~50%)	– Favorable histology (embryonal), PAX/FOX01 fusion negative, unfavorable site (stages II–III): groups III – Favorable histology (embryonal), PAX/FOX01 fusion positive, any site (stages I–III): groups I to III – Unfavorable histology (alveolar), PAX/FOX01 fusion positive or negative, any site (stages I–III): groups I–III – Stage IV, group IV, PAX/FOX01 fusion negative, <10 years old
High (~15%)	– Stage IV, group IV, PAX/FOX01 fusion negative, ≥10 years old – Stage IV, group IV, PAX/FOX01 fusion positive, any age

Source: Adapted from American Cancer Society. Rhabdomyosarcoma. 2020. https://www.cancer.org/cancer/rhabdomyosarcoma.html

TREATMENT PARADIGM

Surgery: Complete excision with 5-mm margin is preferable if functional and cosmetic outcomes are acceptable.[14] If not feasible (or if disease involves the orbit, vagina, bladder, or biliary tract), diagnostic incisional biopsy can be performed, followed by induction CHT and definitive local therapy. LC with organ preservation is the goal.[4] Delayed primary excision of group III patients after induction CHT permits reduced dose RT and has equivalent or improved outcomes.[18] Current COG studies require lymph node evaluation for all extremity tumors (SLNB acceptable if clinically negative), and all boys ≥10 years of age with a paratesticular RMS should undergo routine ipsilateral nerve-sparing retroperitoneal lymph node dissection. Consider ilioinguinal lymphadenectomy for perianal or anal tumors. In H&N primaries, neck dissection is not indicated, but suspicious nodes should be surgically evaluated.[4]

Chemotherapy: All patients require multiagent CHT, regardless of stage and group.[14] VAC (vincristine, actinomycin-D, cyclophosphamide) is standard regimen. In sequential IRS trials, the addition of many individually active agents (e.g., doxorubicin, cisplatin, etoposide, ifosfamide, topotecan, and melphalan) did not improve outcomes compared to VAC, in any subgroup. In IRS-IV, VA was equivalent to VAC in low-risk/excellent prognosis group. ARST0331 added modest-dose cyclophosphamide to VA while condensing therapy from 45 to 22 weeks with RT for low-risk patients, and there was no compromise in outcomes.[19] ARST 0531 compared VAC with VAC/VI alternating for intermediate-risk patients and found no improvement in EFS or OS, but less hematologic toxicity and cumulative cyclophosphamide dose making VAC/VI an alternative.[20] Vincristine ± irinotecan can be continued concurrently during RT per ARST0431.

Radiation: Per COG ARST trials, RT is indicated in all cases except group I embryonal. RT dosing is outlined in Table 60.1. Patients with pulmonary metastases and/or pleural effusion can be treated with whole lung irradiation (15 Gy/10 fx). Clinical trials, such as ARST1431, include consolidation RT to metastases in patients with intermediate-risk stage IV disease using standard dose fractionation for sites >5 cm and SBRT dose fractionation for sites ≤5 cm.

Procedures: See *Handbook of Treatment Planning in Radiation Oncology*, Chapter 12.[21]

■ **EVIDENCE-BASED Q&A**

▣ **What did the IRS studies show?**

The IRSG was formed in 1972 to investigate the biology and treatment of RMS; it was merged into the COG in 2000. They led a series of protocols (IRS I–V) that have dictated RMS management with a rise in OS seen for all patients from ~50% to >70%. Pertinent conclusions from the studies are summarized as follows:

Maurer, IRS-I (*Cancer* **1988, PMID 3275486):**

■ 5-year OS for all groups I to IV was 55%.
■ For FH group 1, RT was not needed if giving 2 years of VAC. However, benefit to RT for FFS and OS was seen in group I, UH.[22]
■ Primary tumors of orbit and GU tract had best prognosis compared to retroperitoneum with worst prognosis.
■ Limited RT volumes (GTV + 2 cm) had similar outcomes to big fields such as whole muscle bundle RT.

Maurer, IRS-II (*Cancer* **1993, PMID 8448756):**

■ 5-year OS for all groups I to IV was 63%, a significant improvement from IRS-I ($p < .001$).
■ 5-year OS for all nonmetastatic patients was improved from 63% (IRS-1) to 71%.
■ LC (93%) was improved with >40 Gy for orofacial and laryngopharyngeal sites.[23]
■ Cyclophosphamide was not needed in FH group I/II.

Crist, IRS-III (*JCO* **1995, PMID 7884423):**

■ 5-year OS for all groups I to IV was 71%, significantly better than IRS-II ($p < .001$).
■ Group 1, UH benefitted with addition of RT.
■ For PM H&N with CN palsy or BOS erosion, limited RT volumes was as good as WBRT (WBRT was still used for intracranial extension).

Breneman, IRS-IV (*JCO* **2003, PMID 12506174; Crist *JCO* 2001, PMID 11408506):**

■ For group III disease, no benefit to hyperfractionated regimen (59.4 Gy with 1.1 Gy BID) over conventional regimen of 50.4 Gy in 1.8 Gy/fx was found.
■ No benefit to VAI or VIE over VAC for nonmetastatic disease was found.
■ Group IV patients with ≤2 metastatic sites had improved 3-year OS and FFS on MVA ($p = .007$ and .006, respectively).

Raney, IRS-V (*JCO* **2011, PMID 21357783):**

■ Reduced RT dose (36 Gy for microscopic disease [stage 1/group IIa] and 45 Gy for group III orbit primaries if cyclophosphamide is included in systemic therapy) does not compromise local control.
■ Inclusion of an alkylating CHT agent (cyclophosphamide or ifosfamide) may be important for FFS.

▣ **What is the significance of the PAX/FOX01 gene fusion?**

Using clinical trial data from 6 COG trials, investigators evaluated the prognostic value of the PAX/FOX01 gene fusion as a stratification factor. The first factor important for stratification was localized vs. metastatic disease (EFS 52% vs. 78%; OS 84% vs. 42%), and the second factor was PAX/FOX01 status (positive vs. negative), which was found to be the most important factor for patients with RMS, improving risk stratification for patients with localized RMS (Table 60.8).[24]

Table 60.8: Prognostic Value of PAX/FOX01 Fusion From Pooled COG Trials		
	PAX/FOX01 Fusion Positive (%)	**PAX/FOX01 Fusion Negative (%)**
Localized disease EFS OS	 52 65	 78 88
Metastatic disease EFS OS	 6 19	 46 58

■ When should RT be initiated?

RT timing has varied by protocol and risk group through the years. On the most recent COG protocols, low-risk patients start RT at week 13, intermediate-risk week 4, and high-risk week 20. Metastatic sites may be treated at the end of CHT. Patients with cord compression, visual loss, or intracranial extension should be considered for urgent RT, on day 0 per high-risk COG ARST 0431. ARST 0531 moved RT earlier to week 4 for intermediate-risk patients with the hopes of improving LC, but results showed no advantage with this approach. Analysis from IRS II to IV[25] showed reduced LF if RT started within 2 weeks vs. >2 weeks for patients with meningeal impingement (18% vs. 33%, p = .03) and intracranial extension (16% vs. 37%, p = .07). A recent analysis from Spaulding et al. demonstrated similar clinical outcomes for patients with cranial nerve palsy or skull base erosion treated with immediate versus delayed RT[22]; thus, it is acceptable to treat patients with these high-risk features at a later date (week 20 per COG ARST 0431) but consider treating patients with intracranial extension on day 0.

■ What is the benefit of RT and in whom is RT required?

There are no good prospective randomized data. RT is currently indicated for all patients except embryonal tumors after gross total resection without lymph node involvement. Wolden et al. reviewed patients treated on IRS I to III and showed that patients with alveolar/undifferentiated histology after GTR (group I) have improved EFS and OS with the addition of RT.[23] Further, when comparing outcomes between IRS IV and MMT-89 (contemporary European International Society of Pediatric Oncology Malignant Mesenchymal Tumor study that attempted to avoid RT and radical surgery as much as possible by giving more CHT as necessary), RT appears to have significant benefits in LC, EFS, and OS.[23]

■ Is 45 Gy a sufficient dose for all orbital embryonal RMS?

Historically, patients with orbital embryonal RMS received VAC, followed by RT to 45 Gy. However, in a subset analysis of group III orbital embryonal RMS patients on ARST033, a higher risk of LR (16%) was seen in patients with less than a CR as compared with patients who achieved a CR (0%). This is a small subset of patients and thought provoking that local therapy may need to be changed, so for patients with a PR after VAC 50.4 Gy should be considered.

■ Is there a benefit to proton therapy in RMS?

The rationale is to reduce late effects and is permitted on ongoing RMS trials. Small series demonstrating dosimetric advantages have been published for orbit, parameningeal, and pelvic sites.[26–29]

REFERENCES

1. Ermoian RP, Breneman J, Walterhouse DO, et al. 45 Gy is not sufficient radiotherapy dose for Group III orbital embryonal rhabdomyosarcoma after less than complete response to 12 weeks of ARST0331 chemotherapy: a report from the Soft Tissue Sarcoma Committee of the Children's Oncology Group. *Pediatr Blood Cancer.* 2017;64(9):10.1002/pbc.26540. doi:10.1002/pbc.26540
2. Walterhouse DO, Pappo AS, Meza JL, et al. Reduction of cyclophosphamide dose for patients with subset 2 low-risk rhabdomyosarcoma is associated with an increased risk of recurrence: a report from the Soft Tissue Sarcoma Committee of the Children's Oncology Group. *Cancer.* 2017. doi:10.1002/cncr.30613
3. American Cancer Society. Rhabdomyosarcoma. 2020. https://www.cancer.org/cancer/rhabdomyosarcoma.html
4. Terezakis S, LM. Pediatric rhabdomyosarcoma. In: Merchant T, Kortmann R, eds. *Pediatric Radiation Oncology.* Springer Publishing Company; 2018. doi:10.1007/978-3-319-43545-9
5. Halperin EC, Constine LS, Tarbell NJ, Kun LE. *Pediatric Radiation Oncology.* Lippincott Williams & Wilkins; 2012.
6. Diller L, Sexsmith E, Gottlieb A, et al. Germline p53 mutations are frequently detected in young children with rhabdomyosarcoma. *J Clin Invest.* 1995;95(4):1606–1611. doi:10.1172/JCI117834
7. Li FP, Fraumeni JF, Jr. Rhabdomyosarcoma in children: epidemiologic study and identification of a familial cancer syndrome. *J Natl Cancer Inst.* 1969;43(6):1365–1373.
8. Trahair T, Andrews L, Cohn RJ. Recognition of Li Fraumeni syndrome at diagnosis of a locally advanced extremity rhabdomyosarcoma. *Pediatr Blood Cancer.* 2007;48(3):345–348. doi:10.1002/pbc.20795
9. Crucis A, Richer W, Brugieres L, et al. Rhabdomyosarcomas in children with neurofibromatosis type I: a national historical cohort. *Pediatr Blood Cancer.* 2015;62(10):1733–1738. doi:10.1002/pbc.25556
10. Ferrari A, Bisogno G, Macaluso A, et al. Soft-tissue sarcomas in children and adolescents with neurofibromatosis type 1. *Cancer.* 2007;109(7):1406–1412. doi:10.1002/cncr.22533

11. DeBaun MR, Tucker MA. Risk of cancer during the first four years of life in children from The Beckwith-Wiedemann Syndrome Registry. *J Pediatr*. 1998;132(3 Pt 1):398–400. doi:10.1016/S0022-3476(98)70008-3

12. Kratz CP, Rapisuwon S, Reed H, et al. Cancer in Noonan, Costello, cardiofaciocutaneous and LEOPARD syndromes. *Am J Med Genet C Semin Med Genet*. 2011;157C(2):83–89. doi:10.1002/ajmg.c.30300

13. Gripp KW. Tumor predisposition in Costello syndrome. *Am J Med Genet C Semin Med Genet*. 2005;137C(1):72–77. doi:10.1002/ajmg.c.30065

14. Breneman JC, Lyden E, Pappo AS, et al. Prognostic factors and clinical outcomes in children and adolescents with metastatic rhabdomyosarcoma: a report from the Intergroup Rhabdomyosarcoma Study IV. *J Clin Oncol*. 2003;21(1):78–84. doi:10.1200/JCO.2003.06.129

15. Crist WM, Anderson JR, Meza JL, et al. Intergroup rhabdomyosarcoma study-IV: results for patients with nonmetastatic disease. *J Clin Oncol*. 2001;19(12):3091–3102. doi:10.1200/JCO.2001.19.12.3091

16. Weigel BJ, Lyden E, Anderson JR, et al. Intensive multiagent therapy, including dose-compressed cycles of ifosfamide/etoposide and vincristine/doxorubicin/cyclophosphamide, irinotecan, and radiation, in patients with high-risk rhabdomyosarcoma: a report from the Children's Oncology Group. *J Clin Oncol*. 2016;34(2):117–122. doi:10.1200/JCO.2015.63.4048

17. Rodeberg DA, Garcia-Henriquez N, Lyden ER, et al. Prognostic significance and tumor biology of regional lymph node disease in patients with rhabdomyosarcoma: a report from the Children's Oncology Group. *J Clin Oncol*. 2011;29(10):1304–1311. doi:10.1200/JCO.2010.29.4611

18. Lautz TB, Chi YY, Li M, et al. Benefit of delayed primary excision in rhabdomyosarcoma: a report from the Children's Oncology Group (COG). *Cancer*. 2020. doi:10.1002/cncr.33275

19. Walterhouse DO, Pappo AS, Meza JL, et al. Shorter-duration therapy using vincristine, dactinomycin, and lower-dose cyclophosphamide with or without radiotherapy for patients with newly diagnosed low-risk rhabdomyosarcoma: a report from the Soft Tissue Sarcoma Committee of the Children's Oncology Group. *J Clin Oncol*. 2014;32(31):3547–3552. doi:10.1200/JCO.2014.55.6787

20. Hawkins DS, Chi YY, Anderson JR, et al. Addition of vincristine and irinotecan to vincristine, dactinomycin, and cyclophosphamide does not improve outcome for intermediate-risk rhabdomyosarcoma: a report from the Children's Oncology Group. *J Clin Oncol*. 2018;36(27):2770–2777. doi:10.1200/JCO.2018.77.9694

21. Videtic GMM, Woody N, Vassil AD. *Handbook of Treatment Planning in Radiation Oncology*. 2nd ed. Demos Medical; 2014. doi:10.1891/9781617051975

22. Spalding AC, Hawkins DS, Donaldson SS, et al. The effect of radiation timing on patients with high-risk features of parameningeal rhabdomyosarcoma: an analysis of IRS-IV and D9803. *Int J Radiat Oncol Biol Phys*. 2013;87(3):512–516. doi:10.1016/j.ijrobp.2013.07.003

23. Wolden SL, Anderson JR, Crist WM, et al. Indications for radiotherapy and chemotherapy after complete resection in rhabdomyosarcoma: a report from the Intergroup Rhabdomyosarcoma Studies I to III. *J Clin Oncol*. 1999;17(11):3468–3475. doi:10.1200/JCO.1999.17.11.3468

24. Hibbitts E, Chi YY, Hawkins DS, et al. Refinement of risk stratification for childhood rhabdomyosarcoma using FOXO1 fusion status in addition to established clinical outcome predictors: a report from the Children's Oncology Group. *Cancer Med*. 2019;8(14):6437–6448. doi:10.1002/cam4.2504

25. Michalski JM, Meza J, Breneman JC, et al. Influence of radiation therapy parameters on outcome in children treated with radiation therapy for localized parameningeal rhabdomyosarcoma in Intergroup Rhabdomyosarcoma Study Group trials II through IV. *Int J Radiat Oncol Biol Phys*. 2004;59(4):1027–1038. doi:10.1016/j.ijrobp.2004.02.064

26. Weber DC, Ares C, Albertini F, et al. Pencil beam scanning proton therapy for pediatric parameningeal rhabdomyosarcomas: clinical outcome of patients treated at the Paul Scherrer Institute. *Pediatr Blood Cancer*. 2016;63(10):1731–1736. doi:10.1002/pbc.25864

27. Leiser D, Calaminus G, Malyapa R, et al. Tumour control and Quality of Life in children with rhabdomyosarcoma treated with pencil beam scanning proton therapy. *Radiother Oncol*. 2016;120(1):163–168. doi:10.1016/j.radonc.2016.05.013

28. Fukushima H, Fukushima T, Sakai A, et al. Tailor-made treatment combined with proton beam therapy for children with genitourinary/pelvic rhabdomyosarcoma. *Rep Pract Oncol Radiother*. 2015;20(3):217–222. doi:10.1016/j.rpor.2014.12.003

29. Indelicato DJ, Rotondo RL, Krasin MJ, et al. Outcomes following proton therapy for Group III pelvic rhabdomyosarcoma. *Int J Radiat Oncol Biol Phys*. 2020;106(5):968–976. doi:10.1016/j.ijrobp.2019.12.036

61 ■ NEUROBLASTOMA

Charles Marc Leyrer and Erin S. Murphy

QUICK HIT ■ Neuroblastoma (NB) is a small round blue cell tumor arising from the neural crest cells of the sympathetic nervous system. NB is the most common malignancy in infants and the most common pediatric extracranial solid tumor. Workup includes H&P, labs including urinary catecholamines (VMA/HVA), CT/MRI of primary site, CT chest/abdomen/pelvis, MIBG scan, and bilateral bone marrow biopsy. Patients are stratified into risk groups based on stage, age, N-myc status, DNA ploidy, and Shimada classification. Risk group determines treatment.

Table 61.1: General Treatment Paradigm for Neuroblastoma		
INRG/Risk Group	**5-Yr OS[1-3]**	**General Treatment Paradigm**
INRG L1 or low risk	> 95%	Surgery alone. CHT for residual (if > 18 months or unfavorable factors), recurrent, or symptomatic disease.
INRG L2 or Intermediate Risk	90%–95%	Surgery followed by CHT. If initially unresectable: biopsy, CHT ± delayed surgery. RT if persistent/worsening symptoms despite other therapy (per ANBL0531).
High risk	30%–50%	Induction CHT, surgery, myeloablative CHT and tandem autologous SCT, consolidative RT, oral isotretinoin + anti-GD2 antibody (per ANBL0532). Ongoing investigation with the addition of I-131 MIBG or crizotinib for ALK-mutation. RT: Treat primary post-CHT and presurgical volume to 21.6 Gy/12 fx if GTR (no boost for residual). Treat metastatic sites active on post-CHT and pretransplant MIBG scan.

Note regarding spinal cord compression: Occurs in 5%–15% of patients. RT is reserved for those who fail initial CHT and/or surgery as RT is associated with late toxicity (e.g., scoliosis).

EPIDEMIOLOGY: Most common pediatric extracranial solid tumor, most common infant malignancy, third most common pediatric cancer overall (after leukemia, brain, lymphoma). Six percent to 10% of all childhood malignancies, 15% of deaths (most lethal pediatric solid tumor); 650 to 700 new cases per year, median age 17 to 20 months at diagnosis (90% < 5 y/o, 40% < 1 y/o). Incidence: higher in males than females and in Caucasians than Blacks.[3-5] Approximately 50% present with high-risk disease.[6]

RISK FACTORS: Poorly established. Increased incidence with maternal use of alcohol, diuretics, opioids/codeine, and paternal exposure to hydrocarbons/wood dust/solders.[7,8] There is suggestion of protective effect of vitamin/folic acid use and history of asthma/allergies. Majority of tumors are sporadic, hereditary in only 1% to 2% of cases. Associated with Hirschsprung disease and NF-1.[9]

ANATOMY: Can originate from anywhere along the sympathetic nervous system; most commonly along the paraspinal sympathetic ganglia (mediastinal or abdominal) or the adrenal glands.

PATHOLOGY: Spectrum that ranges from benign ganglioneuroma (well-differentiated, favorable prognosis), to ganglioneuroblastoma (moderately differentiated, unfavorable prognosis), to neuroblastoma (poorly differentiated, favorable to poor prognosis). Ninety-seven percent of neuroblastic tumors are NB.[10,11] Originates from neural crest cells of the sympathetic nervous system that migrate to form the adrenal medulla and spinal sympathetic ganglia. NB is a small round blue cell tumor with pathognomonic neuritic processes (neuropil) in almost all tumors except undifferentiated.

Homer Wright pseudorosettes are neuroblasts surrounding areas of eosinophilic neuropil (15%–50% of cases). IHC positive for neuron-specific enolase, chromogranin A, neurofilament protein, S100, and synaptophysin can aid distinction from other similar tumors (non-Hodgkin's lymphoma, Ewing's, sarcomas).[12–14] Negative for leukocyte common antigen, vimentin, myosin, desmin, and actin.

Shimada histopathologic system: Classifies tumors into favorable or unfavorable categories based on **S**tromal pattern, **A**ge, degree of neuroblastic **D**ifferentiation, **M**itosis-karyorrhexis index (MKI relating to fragmentation of the nucleus), a**n**d **N**odularity (mnemonic: SADMaN). Favorable Shimada: young age, low MKI, mature neuroblast differentiation, rich stroma with nonnodular pattern.[11]

GENETICS: N-myc protein amplification encoded by *MYCN* gene, proto-oncogene found on the short arm of chromosome 2 and identified by FISH. N-myc amplification found in 20% to 25% tumors: 0% to 10% early stage, 40% to 50% advanced stage.[15] Other poor prognostic factors include **deletion/loss of 1p or 11q, unbalanced gain of 17q, TERT** rearrangements, **ATRX** deletion, or **ALK** mutation (accounts for up to 15% of hereditary NB).[16–18] Favorable factors are tumor cell **hyperdiploidy** or **TRK-A amplification**.[15,19–21]

SCREENING: Currently not supported. Data from Japan, Canada, and Europe showed that screening urine for HVA/VMA at 3 weeks of age, 6 months of age, or 1 year of age increases detection overall; however, no change in detection of advanced-stage disease with unfavorable characteristics in older children.[22–24] It also failed to reduce the deaths from neuroblastoma in infants.[22–24] Earlier detection can identify a higher incidence of neuroblastomas in infants, but these tend to be more favorable, spontaneously regress in early infancy, and may not have been detected otherwise.[25]

CLINICAL PRESENTATION: Abdominal mass, abdominal pain, fever, malaise, weight loss, micturition, dyspnea, and dysphagia. Approximately one-third experience fatigue, anorexia, irritability, and pallor. Bone pain frequent in patients with skeletal mets (most often skull/posterior orbit). Excess catecholamines can produce flushing, sweating, and HTN (although rare). Can be confused with Wilms tumor (see Chapter 62, Table 62.3 comparing neuroblastoma and Wilms presentation). IVP classically shows renal displacement ("drooping lily sign") without pelvocaliceal disruption seen in Wilms tumor. See Table 61.2 for associated classic signs and symptoms.

Table 61.2: Clinical Eponyms for Neuroblastoma Presentation	
Dumbbell tumor	Paraspinal sympathetic ganglia tumors with invasion through neural foramina
Raccoon eyes	Proptosis and periorbital ecchymosis from retrobulbar/orbital bone metastases
Blueberry muffin	Cutaneous metastasis causing a blue skin discoloration (usually infants)
Pepper syndrome	Liver metastases with hepatomegaly leading to respiratory distress
Horner's syndrome	Ipsilateral ptosis, miosis, and anhidrosis due to cervical ganglion tumor
Hutchinson's sign	Limping and irritability due to bone or bone marrow metastases
Opsoclonus–myoclonus	Paraneoplastic syndrome (antineural antibodies) of myoclonic jerking, random eye movement, and truncal ataxia; can persist even after cure
Kerner–Morrison sign	Intractable secretory diarrhea, hypokalemia, dehydration due to VIP secretion

WORKUP: H&P with attention to child development and signs/symptoms as in the preceding text.

Labs: CBC, CMP, LDH, serum ferritin, urinary catecholamines. Elevated urinary catecholamines (including HVA or VMA) can be detected in 90% to 95% of patients.

Imaging: CT and/or MRI of the primary site, CT chest, abdomen, pelvis. PET/CT is not standard. MIBG scintigraphy labeled with I-123 is recommended for assessment of the primary and metastatic sites (sensitivity 90%, specificity ~ 100%).[26] MIBG is a norepinephrine analogue that is concentrated in cells of neural crest origin. MIBG may distinguish residual active tumor from necrotic tumor or scar tissue and is more sensitive than Tc-99 bone scans for assessing the response of cortical bone mets to treatment.[26] Bone scan not required unless primary tumor is not MIBG avid.

Pathology: Bilateral bone marrow biopsy. FNA is not adequate. Increased urinary HVA/VMA in conjunction with compatible tumor cells in the bone marrow is considered sufficient for establishing diagnosis without biopsy.[27]

PROGNOSTIC FACTORS: See Table 61.3.

Table 61.3: Neuroblastoma Prognostic Factors[11,28-36]	
Favorable	**Unfavorable**
Younger age (<1 y/o)	Older age (>5 y/o)
Low MKI	High MKI
Differentiated neuroblasts	Undifferentiated neuroblasts
Stromal pattern: rich and nonnodular	Stromal pattern: poor and nodular
1p intact	1p deleted
MYCN nonamplified (MYCN-NA)	MYCN amplified (MYCN-A)
Hypo/hyperdiploid (DNA index <1 or > 1)	Diploid (DNA index 1)
TRK amplification	17q gain; 11q LOH
Stage 1, 2, 4S	Stages 3, 4
Thorax primary, multifocal	H&N primary
Skin, liver, bone marrow mets	Bone, CNS, orbit, pleura, lung mets
Low NSE and ferritin	High NSE (> 100) or ferritin (> 143)

NATURAL HISTORY: Seventy percent of patients present with metastatic disease with bone marrow mets seen in 80% to 90%. LN+ in 35%. Abdomen is the most common primary site (50%–80%). Other common sites include adrenal gland (35%), low-thoracic or abdominal paraspinal ganglia (30%–35%), posterior mediastinum (20%), pelvis (2%), cervical spine (1%), and other sites (12%).[37] Spontaneous regression may occur, especially in infants with 4S disease[38]; 5-year OS is 71% in the modern era, but attributable mainly to increased cure rates in patients with less aggressive disease.[39] Relapsed patients can often be managed with chronic disease for years, but long-term DFS after relapse is rare.

STAGING: The INRGSS is a simplified staging system based on preoperative evaluation and extent of disease determined by image defined risk factors (IDRFs).[40] This is the staging system used in active protocols. The INSS can be used for staging but is included mostly for historical perspective (Tables 61.4 and 61.5).[27,40] The INSS staging system was further classified into low, intermediate, and high-risk groups by the COG, and treatment is determined by risk stratification (see protocols for details). Factors incorporated into the most recent COG risk grouping include **S**tage, **A**ge, **N**-myc, **D**NA ploidy, and **S**himada histology (mnemonic "SANDS": from trials ANBL00B1, ANBL0531, and ANBL0532). Patients with amplified N-myc are always high risk.

INRGSS Image-Defined Risk Factors[40]

- Ipsilateral tumor extension within two body compartments: neck and chest, chest and abdomen, abdomen and pelvis
- Infiltration of adjacent organs/structures: pericardium, diaphragm, kidney, liver, duodenopancreatic block, mesentery
- Encasement of major vessels by tumor: vertebral artery, internal jugular vein, subclavian vessels, carotid artery, aorta, vena cava, major thoracic vessels, iliac vessels, branches of the superior mesenteric artery at its root and the celiac axis
- Compression of trachea or central bronchi
- Encasement of brachial plexus
- Infiltration of porta hepatis or hepatoduodenal ligament
- Infiltration of the costovertebral junction between T9 and T12
- Tumor crossing the sciatic notch
- Tumor invading renal pedicle

- Extension of tumor to base of skull
- Intraspinal tumor extension with more than one third spinal canal invasion, leptomeningeal space obliteration, or abnormal spinal cord MRI signal

Table 61.4: Comparison of INSS[27] and More Recent INRGSS[40]

INSS (1993)		INRGSS (2009)	
1	Tumor on one side of the body. Complete resection (microscopic disease allowed). Ipsilateral LNs histologically negative (nodes adherent to and removed with the primary tumor may be positive).	L1	Localized tumor without vital structure involvement as defined by image-defined risk factor and limited to one body compartment (neck, chest, abdomen, pelvis)
2A	Same as stage I except residual disease after resection.	L2	Locoregional tumor with one or more image-defined risk factors
2B	Ipsilateral nonadherent lymph nodes contain tumor. Contralateral LNs must be negative microscopically. Residual disease after resection allowed.		
3	Unresectable unilateral tumor extending across midline (beyond opposite side of the vertebral body) with or without involved regional lymph nodes, OR unilateral tumor with contralateral regional LN involvement, OR midline tumor with bilateral extension by infiltration (unresectable) or by LN involvement.		
4	Dissemination to distant LNs, bone, bone marrow, liver, skin, and/or other organs (except as defined for 4S).	M	Distant metastatic disease (except stage MS)
4S	Localized primary tumor as in stage 1, 2A, or 2B, with dissemination limited to skin, liver, and/or bone marrow (< 10% of total nucleated cells on bone biopsy/aspirate). **Limited to infants <1 y/o.**	MS	Children <18 mos with metastatic disease limited to skin, liver, and/or bone marrow (no more than 10% marrow cells positive)

Table 61.5: Previous Staging Systems for Neuroblastoma

Evans/Children's Cancer Study Group (CCSG) Clinical Staging		St. Jude/POG Surgicopathologic Staging	
I	Tumor confined to organ or structure of origin	A	Gross total resection of primary, with or without microscopic residual. LN not adherent to primary tumor are negative and liver is histologically negative.
II	Tumor extending beyond organ or structure of origin but not crossing midline and/or involved ipsilateral lymph nodes	B	Grossly unresected primary tumor, nonadherent LN–, liver–
III	Tumor extending in continuity beyond the midline; regional LN may be involved bilaterally	C	Complete or incomplete resection of primary, nonadherent LN+, liver–
IV	Remote disease involving bone, bone marrow, soft tissue, or distant lymph nodes	D	Distant LN, bone, bone marrow, liver, or skin
IV–S	Stage I or II except for presence of mets confined to liver, skin, and/or marrow (does not include non-marrow bone mets)	D(S)	Infants <1 y/o with stage IV-S disease (as defined in CCSG system)

TREATMENT PARADIGM

Observation: Recommended initially for stage 4S, which may spontaneously resolve.

Surgery: Useful for diagnosis, staging, and treatment for local control. Goal is GTR of visible tumor, and regional lymph nodes with maintenance of function as organ preservation is key. Uninvolved contralateral lymph nodes should be sampled, and a liver biopsy should be obtained. Large tumors that encase regional organs or large vessels and "dumbbell" tumors that compress the spinal cord are considered unresectable. Intermediate- and high-risk patients with clinically unresectable disease should undergo initial biopsy/diagnostic surgery, induction CHT, and then delayed/second-look surgery. CR in 66% to 79% of patients after induction CHT. Piecemeal resection may be necessary and is acceptable. Subtotal resection can still be attempted after CHT. Titanium clips are recommended at sites of residual disease. Note that resection of the primary is no longer required for stage 4S, but a biopsy should be obtained.

Chemotherapy: CHT used in intermediate and high-risk patients to shrink primary tumors to facilitate delayed surgery. Generally no role for CHT in low-risk patients except for persistent/recurrent disease. Consider CHT for 4S with hepatomegaly. CHT regimen is dependent on protocol (no universal standard). Most common agents are cyclophosphamide, cisplatin, doxorubicin, and etoposide; others include (but are not limited to) carboplatin, vincristine, vindesine, ifosfamide, dacarbazine, topotecan, and melphalan. Intensive doses of combination CHT with short intervals between courses should be delivered in high-risk patients. In high-risk patients, myeloablative CHT with autologous SCT improved survival over CHT alone,[41] and tandem transplant improves EFS over single transplant.[42]

Differentiation Therapy: Neuroblastoma cell lines can be induced to terminally differentiate on exposure to retinoids. Risk of relapse is reduced in patients who receive isotretinoin, which is now part of standard therapy in high-risk patients.[43]

Immunotherapy: Neuroblastoma cells uniformly express disialoganglioside GD2 on their surface, which creates a target for immunotherapy. Dinutuximab, a chimeric anti-GD2 antibody (ch14.18), is FDA approved for adjuvant first-line therapy but is associated with significant acute toxicity in the form of capillary leak syndrome and pain. Human (rather than chimeric) forms are under evaluation and may improve tolerance.

Radiation

Indications: RT is delivered to the primary tumor and persistent metastatic sites in high-risk patients. In intermediate-risk patients, RT is delivered to recurrent or gross residual disease. Adjuvant RT is not indicated for low- or intermediate-risk disease unless urgent symptomatic (life/organ threatening) concerns without significant response to CHT (i.e., liver mets with respiratory compromise or cord compression). Emergency RT only if no response or unable to receive CHT. If >5 sites remain avid, repeat scan post-transplant.

Dose: A dose of 21.6 Gy/12 fx daily (COG). High-risk protocol ANBL0532 allowed a boost to 36 Gy for gross residual disease after surgery >1 cc (21.6 Gy to pre-op GTV, then 14.4 Gy boost); however, this did not improve the 5-year cumulative incidence of local progression.[42] Treatment volume is the *post-CHT GTV prior to attempted surgical resection.* If primary was grossly resected at diagnosis, GTV is the pre-op volume. Volume can be shaved out of normal tissues occupying space previously occupied by tumor (if the normal tissue was not infiltrated). CTV is the GTV + 1.5 cm margin (PTV is 0.5–1 cm). For hepatic metastases causing respiratory compromise: 4.5 Gy/3 fx (COG). For cord compression, CHT is preferred followed by surgical decompression. A recent study treated high-risk patients to 18 Gy at 1.5 Gy/fx BID and did not result in compromised LC or OS;[44] however, only 25 patients were enrolled and larger prospective studies for validation are warranted.

Toxicity: Acute: Diarrhea, nausea, vomiting, erythema, fatigue, myelosuppression. Late: Bony/soft tissue hypoplasia, scoliosis/kyphosis, slipped capital femoral epiphysis, short stature, second malignancy, renal impairment, renal insufficiency; others are location dependent.

Targeted Radionuclides: I-131 MIBG therapy has shown response rates of 30% to 40% in otherwise refractory patients and is being investigated before resection or in combination with SCT for consolidation.

Table 61.6: Neuroblastoma Treatment Overview by Risk Group
Low Risk (5-year OS > 95%): Patients with stage 4S disease may undergo spontaneous disease regression and can be observed (or given short-course CHT for hepatomegaly). No benefit from resection of primary (may biopsy skin nodule) for stage 4S. For other low-risk patients, *surgery alone* usually recommended.[1,29] Adjuvant RT has not improved outcomes after GTR and is not even indicated for STR or positive margins. CHT indicated for symptomatic patients or disease progression. RT reserved for CHT-resistant tumor.
Intermediate Risk (3-year OS 95%): Surgery and CHT (without RT) is standard. See Table 61.1 for RT indications. If primary is unresectable, biopsy → CHT → delayed surgery. CHT is typically given for approximately four cycles for favorable histology tumors and eight cycles for unfavorable histology.
High Risk (3-year OS 30%–50%): Paradigm includes combined modality therapy with intensive platinum-based multiagent induction CHT, delayed surgery, myeloablative CHT and autologous SCT (often twice, "tandem"), RT to primary site and residual mets, then isotretinoin and immunotherapy. CHT has a response rate of 70% to 80%. Exact timing of RT is not well established, but usually delivered after autologous SCT when disease burden is minimal. RT should be delivered to the primary site even if the patient has undergone GTR. RT should also be delivered to metastatic sites with persistent active disease (+ MIBG) after induction CHT. Adjuvant 13-cis-retinoic acid (isotretinoin) and anti-GD-2 monoclonal antibody improve EFS and OS, respectively, in those without progression.[41,43,45] Patients can have recurrent disease after completion of aggressive treatment.

■ **EVIDENCE-BASED Q&A**

LOW RISK

■ **What is the treatment paradigm for low-risk disease?**

Low-risk disease is the most common presentation of neuroblastoma. Surgery is the mainstay of therapy if the tumor is deemed resectable. Residual disease may be observed if ≤18 months old and favorable risk factors (favorable histology and nondiploid tumors).[46–48] CHT is reserved for unresectable, unfavorable, symptomatic, or progressive/recurrent disease.[1,49] There is no role for routine adjuvant RT in low-risk patients, given the outcomes with salvage therapy.

Strother, COG P9641 (*JCO* 2012, PMID 22529259): A total of 915 children with stage 2A and 2B disease underwent maximally safe resection with adjuvant CHT given if <50% resection at diagnosis, or with unresectable progressive disease after surgery; 5-year EFS and OS were 89% and 97%, respectively. Patients with 2B disease who were >18 months old had significantly lower OS. Patients with unfavorable histology or diploid tumors had significantly lower EFS and OS. **Conclusion: Patients with stage 2B disease and >18 months old or with unfavorable histology or diploid tumors have higher rates of recurrence with observation after surgery and adjuvant CHT may be warranted.**

STAGE 4S

■ **What are the outcomes for stage 4S disease?**

Patients <1 year of age presenting with abdominal tumors can still have excellent outcomes (3-year EFS and OS > 95%) if observed closely. Katzenstein et al.[50] showed that patients who may require intervention are those symptomatic from their disease (hepatomegaly), very young (<2 months), or have unfavorable histology. The concern with very young patients is that they have a higher risk of rapid clinical decline without intervention. If CHT is given for symptomatic disease, it is generally given until cessation of symptoms. Early results of COG-ANBL0531 for patients with 4S disappointingly showed a lower 2-year OS of 81%, which was thought to be due to inclusion of patients who could not undergo biopsy due to poor clinical factors previously excluded from prior trials (see intermediate risk later).

Katzenstein, POG Experience (*JCO* 1998, PMID 9626197): RR of 110 patients with stage D(S) NB registered on POG protocols; 3-year OS was 85%. OS was 71% for patients ≤2 months of age, 68% for patients with diploid tumors, 44% for patients with N-myc amplification, and 33% for patients with unfavorable histology. No difference in OS between those who received CHT (82%) vs. no CHT (93%, $p = .187$), or between those who underwent GTR of primary tumor (90%) vs. STR or bx (78%, $p = .083$). **Conclusion: Survival of infants with stage D(S) NB is good. However, prognosis is poor in those of very young age and with unfavorable biologic factors.**

Nickerson, CCG 3881 (*JCO* 2000, PMID 10653863): Prospective study of 77 patients with stage 4S NB treated with supportive care only (*n* = 44), CHT (cyclophosphamide 5 mg/kg/d × 5 days) + hepatic RT (4.5 Gy/3 fx; *n* = 22), CHT alone (*n* = 10), or RT alone (*n* = 1); 5-year EFS was 86% and 5-year OS was 92%. Of 44 patients undergoing supportive care only, OS was 100%, compared with 81% for those requiring CHT for symptoms (*p* = .005). Five of 6 deaths occurred in patients <2 months. Patients aged ≤3 months at diagnosis had decreased EFS. The only factor predictive for improved OS was favorable Shimada histopathologic classification. **Conclusion: Minimal treatment is appropriate for infants with stage 4S NB disease except those <2 months with progressive abdominal disease.**

Nutchtern, COG-ANBL00P2 (*Ann Surg* 2012, PMID 22964741): A total of 87 patients with small adrenal masses and <6 months of age whose parents elected for observation or surgical resection. Followed by abdominal ultrasound and VMA/HMA. Referred to surgery if >50% increase in mass volume OR >50% increase in urine catecholamine levels OR HMA:VMA ratio >2. 83 observed overall with 16 (19%) requiring surgery. Of those, 8 (50%) had stage I NB, 1 had stage 2B and 1 had 4S, 2 had low-grade adrenocortical neoplasm, and 4 were benign. MFU 3.2 years; 3-year EFS 97.7% and OS 100%. **Conclusion: Most infants <6 months with small adrenal masses can have excellent outcomes if closely observed without surgery.**

INTERMEDIATE RISK

▦ Is RT beneficial for intermediate-risk disease?

RT was shown to increase both EFS and OS when added to adjuvant CHT in the Castleberry study of POG C patients. However, in the modern era, additional genetic/biologic risk-stratification factors (such as N-myc status) are used to better risk-stratify patients. Thus, the current intermediate-risk patients (in whom RT is not a standard component of first-line therapy) are not the same group of patients as those in the Castleberry study. As in low-risk patients, RT is typically reserved for residual disease refractory to CHT, recurrent disease, or those who remain symptomatic.

Castleberry, POG (*JCO* 1991, PMID 2016621): PRT of 62 patients >1 year of age with POG stage C NB comparing surgery and CHT ± RT. All patients received AC CHT × 5 cycles. Patients randomized to RT received treatment to primary tumor and regional LNs. Age 12 to 24 months: total dose 18 to 24 Gy; age ≥ 24 months: total dose 24 to 30 Gy, with lower doses reserved for abdominal or thoracic paravertebral primary and SCV nodes. Second-look surgery was advised to evaluate response and to remove residual disease. Continuation CHT alternated AC with CDDP and teniposide for two courses each. **Conclusion: Stage C NB in children >1 year of age is a higher-risk group in whom the addition of RT to CHT provides superior initial and long-term control compared with CHT alone. Metastatic failures in both treatment groups suggest a need for more aggressive CHT.**

Table 61.7: Results of Castleberry Trial, RT for Intermediate Risk Neuroblastoma			
	CR	EFS	OS
RT	76%	59%	73%
No RT	46%	32%	41%
P value	.013	.009	.008

Twist, COG ANBL0531 (*JCO* 2019, PMID 31386611): Phase III trial of 404 intermediate-risk patients with neuroblastoma. Goal was to reduce therapy for subsets of patients using biology and response-based algorithm, while maintaining 3-year OS of ≥95%. MYCN-amplified tumors were excluded. Stratification based on age, INSS stage, INPC, N-myc status, LOH of 1p and/or 11q, and tumor ploidy. Treatment was CHT (± isotretinoin) × 2, 4, or 8 cycles and/or surgery based on prognostic markers. Prognostic markers included allelic status of 1p and 11q; 3-year EFS and OS were 83.2% and 94.9%, respectively, for the entire cohort. OS for patients with localized disease was 100%. Infants with stage 4 tumors with favorable biology had a superior 3-year EFS compared with patients with ≥1 unfavorable biologic features. **Conclusion: Excellent survival was achieved with this treatment algorithm, with reduction of therapy for subsets of patients. More effective treatment strategies are needed for infants with stage 4 unfavorable biology disease.**

HIGH RISK

■ **What is the role of autologous SCT and adjuvant isotretinoin in high-risk disease?**

Matthay, CCG 3891 (*NEJM* 1999, PMID 10519894; Update *JCO* 2009, PMID 19171716): Prospective study of 539 patients with high-risk NB. Induction CHT consisted of cisplatin, doxorubicin, etoposide, and cyclophosphamide × 5 cycles; then patients without progression underwent delayed primary surgery with nodal assessment, followed by RT to gross residual disease. RT dose was 20 Gy/10 fx to extra-abdominal disease and 10 Gy/5 fx to mediastinal and intra-abdominal tumors. Patients were subsequently randomized to consolidation CHT or myeloablative CHT + TBI with SCT. Consolidation CHT consisted of three cycles of cisplatin, etoposide, doxorubicin, and ifosfamide. Myeloablative CHT was carboplatin and etoposide. TBI was 10 Gy/3 fx daily. Following SCT or consolidation CHT, patients without disease progression were randomized to six cycles of 13-cis-retinoic acid (isotretinoin) or no further therapy; 5-year EFS and OS for all patients were 26% and 36%, respectively. The 5-year LRR was 51% for patients treated with CHT vs. 33% for patients treated with SCT ($p = .0044$); 3-year EFS with CHT was 22% vs. 34% with SCT; 3-year EFS after the second randomization was 46% among the 130 patients who received 13-cis-retinoic acid vs. 29% among the 128 who received no further therapy ($p = .027$). The 2009 update demonstrated 5-year EFS of 19% for patients treated with consolidation CHT vs. 30% for patients treated with SCT ($p = .04$); 5-year EFS from second randomization was higher for isotretinoin than no further therapy, although not significant (42% vs. 31%). **Conclusions: This study set the standard treatment regimen for high-risk neuroblastoma, which includes both autologous SCT and isotretinoin.**

Table 61.8: Initial Results of Matthay CCG 3891				
CCG 3891	**3-Yr EFS**	**5-Yr LRR**	**Second Randomization**	**3-Yr EFS**
CHT	22%	51%	**13-cis-RA**	46%
HDC + ABMT	34%	33%	**No therapy**	29%
p value	.034	.004	*p* value	.027

■ **Why are doses above 20 Gy recommended to control gross disease?**

There appeared to be a benefit to the addition of TBI when only 10 Gy was used.

Haas-Kogan, Secondary Analysis of CCG 3891/Matthay (*IJROBP* 2003, PMID 12694821): Secondary analysis of the Matthay CCG 3891 focusing on those who received 10 Gy to the primary (abdominal and mediastinal tumors with gross disease remaining postoperatively). For patients who received 10 Gy to the primary, the addition of 10 Gy of TBI and BMT decreased LR compared with those who received continuous CHT and no TBI (22% vs. 52%, $p = .022$). **Conclusion: There may be a dose–response relationship for EBRT (20 Gy better LC than 10 Gy), but cannot distinguish the impact of the high-dose CHT and BMT received with it.**

Wolden (*Pediatr Blood & Cancer* 2018, PMID 29469198): RR of high-risk patients who received consolidation RT after STR of primary to evaluate LC after 21 to 36 Gy; 19 patients evaluated; 5-year cumulative LF 17.2%, 30% for patients receiving < 30 Gy vs. 0% in those who received 30 to 36 Gy ($p = 0.12$). **Conclusion: A dose of 30 to 36 Gy likely needed for optimal control of gross residual disease during consolidation in high-risk disease.**

■ **Is there a benefit with a boost to gross residual tumor after induction therapy?**

Based on the early results of ANBL0532, there appears to be no benefit.

Liu, COG ANBL0532 (*JCO* 2020, PMID 32530765): PRT of children with high-risk neuroblastoma who received an increased local dose to residual primary tumor. Patients randomized to autologous SCT vs. tandem SCT after induction CHT. RT was then delivered to 21.6 Gy to preoperative tumor volume and an additional boost of 14.4 Gy to any gross residual disease for a total dose of 36 Gy. Primary end point of cumulative incidence of local progression (CILP), EFS, OS were compared with the historical control COG A3973, where only 21.6 Gy was delivered; 323 patients received RT; 5-year CILP, EFS, and OS rates of ANBL0532 and A3973 are shown in Table 61.9. **Conclusion: The presence of gross residual disease after induction therapy does not significantly improve 5-year CILP.**

Table 61.9: Comparative 5-Year Results of ANBL0532 vs. A3973					
Patients receiving RT (*n* = 323 for ANBL0532 and *n* = 328 for A3973)			**RT after incomplete resection** (*n* = 74 for ANBL0532 and *n* = 47 for A3973)		
	CILP	EFS	OS	CILP	EFS	OS
COG ANBL0532	11.2%	56.2%	68.4%	16.3%	50.9%	68.1%
COG A3973	7.1%	47%	57.4%	10.6%	48.9%	56.9%
p value	0.059	0.009	0.0088	.4126	.5084	.2835

■ Is there a benefit to tandem stem cell transplants?

Park, COG ANBL 0532 (*JAMA* 2019, PMID: 31454045): PRT of children with high-risk neuroblastoma randomized to single autologous SCT vs. tandem SCT; 355 patients, median age 3 years. Tandem SCT improved 3-year EFS from 48.4% to 61.6% (*p* = .006). Only 70% were able to receive subsequent immunotherapy, and had superior EFS than those not receiving immunotherapy. Improvement in EFS with tandem transplant persisted in subgroup receiving immunotherapy. There was no OS benefit to tandem transplant (69.1% vs. 75.9); however, if patients ultimately received immunotherapy, a survival advantage was observed with tandem transplant (84.0% vs. 73.5%). There was no significant difference in toxicity between the two regimens. **Conclusion: Tandem SCT improves EFS in patients with high-risk neuroblastoma, even in presence of immunotherapy.**

■ Is there a benefit to targeted immunotherapy in high-risk patients?

Dinutuximab (Ch14.18), a chimeric anti-GD2 antibody improves overall survival but at the cost of high acute toxicity in the form of pain and capillary leak syndrome.

Yu, COG ANBL0032 (*NEJM* 2010, PMID 20879881): PRT of 226 patients randomized to immunotherapy (ch14.18 with alternating GM-CSF and IL2) plus isotretinoin vs. isotretinoin alone after myeloablative therapy and stem cell rescue. Immunotherapy improved 2-year EFS (66% vs. 46%, *p* = .01) and improved 2-year OS (86% vs. 75%, *p* = .02). Grades 3 to 4 pain were higher in the immunotherapy arm, with 52% of patients having grade 3 or 4 pain. Additionally, 23% and 25% of patients in that arm had capillary leak syndrome and hypersensitivity reaction, respectively. Early in the study, two patients were inadvertently given an overdose of IL-2 (>20 times the intended dose), with one of these patients experiencing grade 5 toxicity in the form of capillary leak with pulmonary edema. **Conclusion: Immunotherapy with anti-GD2 monoclonal antibodies shows improved outcomes compared to standard therapy.** *Comment: Closed early due to highly favorable results. FDA approved dinutuximab in 2015 for use in combination with GM-CSF, IL-2, and isotretinoin for high-risk neuroblastoma patients who achieve at least a partial response to standard multimodality therapy.[51]*

■ Is there a benefit to MIBG with I-131 or crizotinib in high-risk neuroblastoma?

This is the question of the ongoing study COG ANBL1531. Iobenguane I-131 is essentially therapeutic MIBG including I-131 (diagnostic MIBG includes I-123) and has shown dramatic responses in relapsed/refractory cases. Crizotinib is active against ALK mutated tumors.[52]

REFERENCES

1. Strother DR, London WB, Schmidt ML, et al. Outcome after surgery alone or with restricted use of chemotherapy for patients with low-risk neuroblastoma: results of Children's Oncology Group study P9641. *J Clin Oncol.* 2012;30(15):1842–1848. doi:10.1200/JCO.2011.37.9990
2. Baker DL, Schmidt ML, Cohn SL, et al. Outcome after reduced chemotherapy for intermediate-risk neuroblastoma. *N Engl J Med.* 2010;363(14):1313–1323. doi:10.1056/NEJMoa1001527

3. American_Cancer_Society. Cancer Facts and Figures 2016. In: Atlanta GA. American Cancer Society; 2016: www.cancer.org/acs/groups/content/@research/documents/document/acspc-047079.pdf.

4. Maris JM. Recent advances in neuroblastoma. *N Engl J Med*. 2010;362(23):2202–2211. doi:10.1056/NEJMra0804577

5. Pizzo PA, Poplack DG. *Principles and Practice of Pediatric Oncology*. 6th ed. Wolters Kluwer/Lippincott Williams & Wilkins Health; 2011.

6. Maris JM, Hogarty MD, Bagatell R, Cohn SL. Neuroblastoma. *Lancet*. 2007;369(9579):2106–2120. doi:10.1016/S0140-6736(07)60983-0

7. Cook MN, Olshan AF, Guess HA, et al. Maternal medication use and neuroblastoma in offspring. *Am J Epidemiol*. 2004;159(8):721–731. doi:10.1093/aje/kwh108

8. Heck JE, Ritz B, Hung RJ, et al. The epidemiology of neuroblastoma: a review. *Paediatr Perinat Epidemiol*. 2009;23(2):125–143. doi:10.1111/j.1365-3016.2008.00983.x

9. Maris JM, Chatten J, Meadows AT, et al. Familial neuroblastoma: a three-generation pedigree and a further association with Hirschsprung disease. *Med Pediatr Oncol*. 1997;28(1):1–5. doi:10.1002/(SICI)1096-911X(199701)28:1<1::AID-MPO1>3.0.CO;2-P

10. Shimada H. Tumors of the neuroblastoma group. *Pathology (Phila)*. 1993;2(1):43–59.

11. Shimada H, Ambros IM, Dehner LP, et al. The International Neuroblastoma Pathology Classification (the Shimada system). *Cancer*. 1999;86(2):364–372. doi:10.1002/(SICI)1097-0142(19990715)86:2<364::AID-CNCR21>3.0.CO;2-7

12. Hachitanda Y, Tsuneyoshi M, Enjoji M. Expression of pan-neuroendocrine proteins in 53 neuroblastic tumors: an immunohistochemical study with neuron-specific enolase, chromogranin, and synaptophysin. *Arch Pathol Lab Med*. 1989;113(4):381–384.

13. Hachitanda Y, Tsuneyoshi M, Enjoji M. An ultrastructural and immunohistochemical evaluation of cytodifferentiation in neuroblastic tumors. *Mod Pathol*. 1989;2(1):13–19.

14. Sebire NJ, Gibson S, Rampling D, et al. Immunohistochemical findings in embryonal small round cell tumors with molecular diagnostic confirmation. *Appl Immunohistochem Mol Morphol*. 2005;13(1):1–5. doi:10.1097/00129039-200503000-00001

15. Brodeur GM, Seeger RC, Schwab M, et al. Amplification of N-myc in untreated human neuroblastomas correlates with advanced disease stage. *Science*. 1984;224(4653):1121–1124. doi:10.1126/science.6719137

16. Peifer M, Hertwig F, Roels F, et al. Telomerase activation by genomic rearrangements in high-risk neuroblastoma. *Nature*. 2015;526(7575):700–704. doi:10.1038/nature14980

17. Schleiermacher G, Javanmardi N, Bernard V, et al. Emergence of new ALK mutations at relapse of neuroblastoma. *J Clin Oncol*. 2014;32(25):2727–2734. doi:10.1200/JCO.2013.54.0674

18. Valentijn LJ, Koster J, Zwijnenburg DA, et al. TERT rearrangements are frequent in neuroblastoma and identify aggressive tumors. *Nat Genet*. 2015;47(12):1411–1414. doi:10.1038/ng.3438

19. Ambros PF, Ambros IM, Brodeur GM, et al. International consensus for neuroblastoma molecular diagnostics: report from the International Neuroblastoma Risk Group (INRG) Biology Committee. *Br J Cancer*. 2009;100(9):1471–1482. doi:10.1038/sj.bjc.6605014

20. Cheung NK, Dyer MA. Neuroblastoma: developmental biology, cancer genomics and immunotherapy. *Nat Rev Cancer*. 2013;13(6):397–411. doi:10.1038/nrc3526

21. Schwab M. Oncogene amplification in solid tumors. *Semin Cancer Biol*. 1999;9(4):319–325. doi:10.1006/scbi.1999.0126

22. Schilling FH, Spix C, Berthold F, et al. Neuroblastoma screening at one year of age. *N Engl J Med*. 2002;346(14):1047–1053. doi:10.1056/NEJMoa012277

23. Takeuchi LA, Hachitanda Y, Woods WG, et al. Screening for neuroblastoma in North America. Preliminary results of a pathology review from the Quebec Project. *Cancer*. 1995;76(11):2363–2371. doi:10.1002/1097-0142(19951201)76:11<2363::AID-CNCR2820761127>3.0.CO;2-P

24. Woods WG, Gao RN, Shuster JJ, et al. Screening of infants and mortality due to neuroblastoma. *N Engl J Med*. 2002;346(14):1041–1046. doi:10.1056/NEJMoa012387

25. Ikeda Y, Lister J, Bouton JM, Buyukpamukcu M. Congenital neuroblastoma, neuroblastoma in situ, and the normal fetal development of the adrenal. *J Pediatr Surg*. 1981;16(4 Suppl 1):636–644. doi:10.1016/0022-3468(81)90019-1

26. Brisse HJ, McCarville MB, Granata C, et al. Guidelines for imaging and staging of neuroblastic tumors: consensus report from the International Neuroblastoma Risk Group Project. *Radiology*. 2011;261(1):243–257. doi:10.1148/radiol.11101352

27. Brodeur GM, Pritchard J, Berthold F, et al. Revisions of the international criteria for neuroblastoma diagnosis, staging, and response to treatment. *J Clin Oncol*. 1993;11(8):1466–1477. doi:10.1200/JCO.1993.11.8.1466

28. Adams GA, Shochat SJ, Smith EI, et al. Thoracic neuroblastoma: a Pediatric Oncology Group study. *J Pediatr Surg*. 1993;28(3):372–377; discussion 377-378. doi:10.1016/0022-3468(93)90234-C

29. Castleberry RP, Shuster JJ, Altshuler G, et al. Infants with neuroblastoma and regional lymph node metastases have a favorable outlook after limited postoperative chemotherapy: a Pediatric Oncology Group study. *J Clin Oncol*. 1992;10(8):1299–1304. doi:10.1200/JCO.1992.10.8.1299

30. Cohn SL, Pearson AD, London WB, et al. The International Neuroblastoma Risk Group (INRG) classification system: an INRG Task Force report. *J Clin Oncol*. 2009;27(2):289–297. doi:10.1200/JCO.2008.16.6785

31. Cotterill SJ, Pearson AD, Pritchard J, et al. Clinical prognostic factors in 1277 patients with neuroblastoma: results of The European Neuroblastoma Study Group 'Survey' 1982–1992. *Eur J Cancer*. 2000;36(7):901–908. doi:10.1016/S0959-8049(00)00058-7

32. Evans AE, Albo V, D'Angio GJ, et al. Factors influencing survival of children with nonmetastatic neuroblastoma. *Cancer.* 1976;38(2):661–666. doi:10.1002/1097-0142(197608)38:2<661::AID-CNCR2820380206>3.0.CO;2-M

33. Hayes FA, Green A, Hustu HO, Kumar M. Surgicopathologic staging of neuroblastoma: prognostic significance of regional lymph node metastases. *J Pediatr.* 1983;102(1):59–62. doi:10.1016/S0022-3476(83)80287-X

34. Peuchmaur M, d'Amore ES, Joshi VV, et al. Revision of the International Neuroblastoma Pathology Classification: confirmation of favorable and unfavorable prognostic subsets in ganglioneuroblastoma, nodular. *Cancer.* 2003;98(10):2274–2281. doi:10.1002/cncr.11773

35. Yanik GA, Parisi MT, Shulkin BL, et al. Semiquantitative mIBG scoring as a prognostic indicator in patients with stage 4 neuroblastoma: a report from the Children's oncology group. *J Nucl Med.* 2013;54(4):541–548. doi:10.2967/jnumed.112.112334

36. Yoo SY, Kim JS, Sung KW, et al. The degree of tumor volume reduction during the early phase of induction chemotherapy is an independent prognostic factor in patients with high-risk neuroblastoma. *Cancer.* 2013;119(3):656–664. doi:10.1002/cncr.27775

37. Morris JA, Shcochat SJ, Smith EI, et al. Biological variables in thoracic neuroblastoma: a Pediatric Oncology Group study. *J Pediatr Surg.* 1995;30(2):296–302; discussion 302–293. doi:10.1016/0022-3468(95)90577-4

38. Nickerson HJ, Matthay KK, Seeger RC, et al. Favorable biology and outcome of stage IV-S neuroblastoma with supportive care or minimal therapy: a Children's Cancer Group study. *J Clin Oncol.* 2000;18(3):477–486. doi:10.1200/JCO.2000.18.3.477

39. Horner MJ RL, Krapcho M, Neyman N, et al. SEER Cancer Statistics Review, 1975–2006. 2009. http://seer.cancer.gov/csr/1975_2006/. Accessed 2016.

40. Monclair T, Brodeur GM, Ambros PF, et al. The International Neuroblastoma Risk Group (INRG) staging system: an INRG Task Force report. *J Clin Oncol.* 2009;27(2):298–303. doi:10.1200/JCO.2008.16.6876

41. Matthay KK, Villablanca JG, Seeger RC, et al. Treatment of high-risk neuroblastoma with intensive chemotherapy, radiotherapy, autologous bone marrow transplantation, and 13-cis-retinoic acid. Children's Cancer Group. *N Engl J Med.* 1999;341(16):1165–1173. doi:10.1056/NEJM199910143411601

42. Liu KX, Naranjo A, Zhang FF, et al. Prospective evaluation of radiation dose escalation in patients with high-risk neuroblastoma and gross residual disease after surgery: a report from the Children's Oncology Group ANBL0532 Study. *J Clin Oncol.* 2020;38(24):2741–2752. doi:10.1200/JCO.19.03316

43. Sidell N, Altman A, Haussler MR, Seeger RC. Effects of retinoic acid (RA) on the growth and phenotypic expression of several human neuroblastoma cell lines. *Exp Cell Res.* 1983;148(1):21–30. doi:10.1016/0014-4827(83)90184-2

44. Casey DL, Kushner BH, Cheung NV, et al. Reduced-dose radiation therapy to the primary site is effective for high-risk neuroblastoma: results from a prospective trial. *Int J Radiat Oncol Biol Phys.* 2019;104(2):409–414. doi:10.1016/j.ijrobp.2019.02.004

45. Ladenstein R, Potschger U, Gray J, et al. Toxicity and outcome of anti-GD2 antibody ch14.18/CHO in front-line, high-risk patients with neuroblastoma: final results of the phase III immunotherapy randomisation (HR-NBL1/SIOPEN trial). Paper presented at: ASCO2016; doi:10.1200/JCO.2016.34.15_suppl.10500

46. Nitschke R, Smith EI, Shochat S, et al. Localized neuroblastoma treated by surgery: a Pediatric Oncology Group Study. *J Clin Oncol.* 1988;6(8):1271–1279. doi:10.1200/JCO.1988.6.8.1271

47. Pérez-Manga G, Lluch A, Alba E, et al. Gemcitabine in combination with doxorubicin in advanced breast cancer: final results of a phase II pharmacokinetic trial. *J Clin Oncol.* 2000;18(13):2545–2552. doi:10.1200/JCO.2000.18.13.2545

48. Matthay KK, Sather HN, Seeger RC, et al. Excellent outcome of stage II neuroblastoma is independent of residual disease and radiation therapy. *J Clin Oncol.* 1989;7(2):236–244. doi:10.1200/JCO.1989.7.2.236

49. Nitschke R, Smith EI, Altshuler G, et al. Postoperative treatment of nonmetastatic visible residual neuroblastoma: a Pediatric Oncology Group study. *J Clin Oncol.* 1991;9(7):1181–1188. doi:10.1200/JCO.1991.9.7.1181

50. Katzenstein HM, Bowman LC, Brodeur GM, et al. Prognostic significance of age, MYCN oncogene amplification, tumor cell ploidy, and histology in 110 infants with stage D(S) neuroblastoma: the pediatric oncology group experience--a pediatric oncology group study. *J Clin Oncol.* 1998;16(6):2007–2017. doi:10.1200/JCO.1998.16.6.2007

51. Yang RK, Sondel PM. Anti-GD2 strategy in the treatment of neuroblastoma. *Drugs Future.* 2010;35(8):665. doi:10.1358/dof.2010.035.08.1513490

52. Chen Y, Takita J, Choi YL, et al. Oncogenic mutations of ALK kinase in neuroblastoma. *Nature.* 2008;455(7215):971–974. doi:10.1038/nature07399

62 ■ WILMS TUMOR

James R. Broughman and Erin S. Murphy

QUICK HIT ■ Wilms Tumor (WT) is the most common abdominal tumor in children. It is managed with initial resection, followed by risk-adapted CHT ± RT. CHT is variable and usually consists of vincristine, actinomycin-D, and Adriamycin (with carboplatin/etoposide/cyclophosphamide added on protocol for higher risk patients). RT is delivered based on pathologic findings as listed in Table 62.1 and should be delivered within 14 days post-op. For stage IV, RT can be directed to the abdomen and whole lung separately, based on indications.

Table 62.1: General Strategy of Postoperative RT for Wilms Tumor		
Indication	**Target**	**Dose**
Stage III, FH Stage IV, FH with hilar lymph nodes Stages I–IV, UH Recurrent disease Residual Flank disease	Flank	10.8 Gy/6 fx *(+ 9 Gy/5 fx boost for diffuse anaplasia)*
Surgical spillage Peritoneal seeding Malignant ascites Preoperative rupture	Whole abdomen	10.5 Gy/7 fx *(+9 Gy/6 fx boost for diffuse anaplasia age > 12 months or +10.5 Gy/7 fx boost for diffuse unresectable implants)*
Lung metastases on chest x-ray	Whole lung irradiation	12 Gy/8 fx *(10.5 Gy/7 fx if age < 1)*

EPIDEMIOLOGY: Accounts for 6% of childhood cancers with ~500 new cases per year in the United States. Most common abdominal tumor in children with a median age at diagnosis of 3 to 4 years for unilateral tumors. Bilateral cases occur in 4% to 8% at presentation and tend to present earlier at a median age of 2 to 3 years; 75% of patients present before age 5. Females are more commonly affected; F:M is 1.09:1 for unilateral tumors and 1.67:1 for bilateral tumors.[1]

RISK FACTORS: Paternal occupation as a machinist or a welder and maternal use of hair dye.[2] Also associated with congenital anomalies in 10% to 13% of cases:

■ **WAGR:** **W**ilms tumor, **A**niridia, **G**U malformations, mental **R**etardation. Caused by alteration of 11p13 with deletion of *WT1* gene (Wilms tumor suppressor gene, important for normal kidney/gonadal development) and *PAX6* (aniridia gene); 30% risk of developing WT.
■ **Beckwith–Wiedemann**: Macrosomia, hemihypertrophy, macroglossia, omphalocele, abdominal organomegaly, ear pits/creases. Caused by alteration of 11p15 locus, which causes loss of imprinting of genes. 5% risk of developing WT.
■ **Denys–Drash syndrome**: Renal disease (proteinuria during infancy, nephrotic syndrome, renal failure), male pseudohermaphroditism, and Wilms. Caused by alteration of 11p13 locus, causing point mutation in zinc-finger regions of *WT1* gene; 50% to 90% risk of developing WT.[3]

ANATOMY: Wilms tumor originates from the kidney parenchyma and drains to perinephric and para-aortic lymph nodes.

PATHOLOGY: WT is an embryonic kidney tumor, classically triphasic with blastemal, epithelial, and stromal elements. WT tends to be lobulated and solid, lacks calcifications, and may have soft and cystic areas. These tumors tend to be very large and often can compress adjacent structures, but only the minority of cases show pathologic evidence of organ invasion.[1]

Table 62.2: Pathologic Types of Renal Tumors in Children		
FH Wilms tumor	Typical features (blastemal, epithelial, and stromal elements) without anaplastic or sarcomatous components.	
UH Wilms tumor; anaplastic Wilms tumor	Anaplasia refers to enlargement of nuclei, hyperchromatism of nuclei, and increased mitotic figures.	Focal Anaplasia (FA): sharply localized in the primary tumor. Diffuse Anaplasia (DA): nonlocalized or localized with significant nuclear unrest in remainder of tumor or found outside tumor capsule, in metastases, or on random biopsy of the tumor.
RTK	Typically diagnosed before 2 years of age with eosinophilic cytoplasm and hyaline globular inclusions (+vimentin and cytokeratin), associated with primary CNS neoplasms (i.e., ATRT) and *INI1* mutations.	
CCSK	4% of all childhood renal tumors.[4] About 5% present with metastases and 40% to 60% with bone metastases compared to those with WT (2% incidence).[5] Tumor cells with abundant intracytoplasmic vesicles. No specific tumor markers but classically described as "chicken-wire" pattern with undifferentiated cells separated by fibrovascular septa.[6]	
Renal cell carcinoma	Approximately 6% of renal tumors in children, not included in classic studies; treatment is surgery alone, no clear role for adjuvant RT.	
All subtypes except FH are considered "high-risk" tumors.		

GENETICS: Poor prognosis associated with LOH of 1p and/or 16q (worse if both). Those with early stage disease and loss of 1p16q are treated more aggressively with three-drug regimen (as for stage III/IV).

- Gain of 1q is associated with inferior survival for unilateral FH WT.[7]
- Although Wilms is associated with inactivation of the *WT1* tumor suppressor gene in 5% to 10% of cases, about one-third of Wilms cases are associated with inactivation of a more recently described tumor suppressor gene *WTX* (unknown gene on X chromosome), which may be involved with normal kidney development. Tumors with *WTX* mutation lack *WT1* mutation. In contrast to *WT1*-associated Wilms, which required biallelic (two-hit) inactivation, *WTX* requires only one hit (i.e., the single X chromosome in males or the active X chromosome in females).[1]

SCREENING: If children present with worrisome physical exam findings that are associated with the predisposing genetic syndromes listed earlier, then screening may be appropriate with periodic abdominal ultrasounds.[1]

CLINICAL PRESENTATION: Abdominal mass (83%), fever (23%), hematuria (21%), abdominal pain (37%).[1] Can also have anemia (due to decreased EPO) and hypertension (from increased renin). See Table 62.3 for comparison between Wilms and neuroblastoma.

Table 62.3: Comparison Between Neuroblastoma and Wilms Tumor	
Neuroblastoma	Wilms
Classic eggshell calcifications on x-ray in 85%	No tumor calcifications (but may have calcifications from hemorrhage)
Displaces kidney ("drooping lily" sign) but does not distort renal architecture	Disrupts renal architecture
Mets to LNs, bone marrow, liver, skin (rarely to lung or brain)	Mets to lung, liver, bone
Frequently crosses midline	Rarely crosses midline

WORKUP: H&P (including assessment for congenital anomalies)

Labs: Urinalysis including urinary catecholamines (to rule out neuroblastoma)

Imaging: Abdominal ultrasound including contralateral kidney and evaluation of thrombosis/extension into renal vein or IVC. MRI, CT chest, abdomen, pelvis, and CXR (studies have relied on whether pulmonary metastases are visible on CXR; positive CT with a negative CXR can present controversy).

Biopsy: *Do not biopsy* unless unresectable or bilateral disease to avoid local tumor spillage. If biopsy is necessary, use posterior approach to avoid abdominal contamination and contain bleeding or spillage if they occur. Once pathology available, obtain further workup if CCSK (bone scan) or RTK (MRI brain).

PROGNOSTIC FACTORS: LOH 1p and/or 16q, gain of 1q, higher stage, unfavorable histology, and age > 24 months portend a worse prognosis.

STAGING: Two systems exist: NWTSG, often referred to as NWTS, versus Société Internationale d'Oncologie Pédiatrique (SIOP) staging. The NWTS system is used in the United States and Canada and emphasizes postsurgical, pre-CHT staging to obtain most "unadulterated" information (extent of primary, degree of anaplasia, presence of unusual histology, ± LN). The SIOP system is used in Europe and utilizes neoadjuvant treatment with CHT and/or RT in an effort to reduce extent of disease and increase en bloc resection, but at the expense of losing or obscuring some of the information listed earlier. NWTS staging is currently used by the COG and listed in Table 62.4.[1]

	TABLE 62.4: NWTS/COG Staging for Wilms Tumor[1]	
I	Completely excised tumor with negative margins of resection. Tumor limited to kidney with renal capsule intact, no renal sinus vessel involvement, and no rupture or biopsy prior to removal.	
II	Completely excised tumor with negative margins of resection. Tumor extends to renal capsule or soft tissue of the renal sinus or tumor is present in blood vessels within the nephrectomy specimen but outside the renal parenchyma (including the renal sinus).	
III	Residual tumor following surgery, confined to abdomen. Any one of the following criteria may be present: • Abdominal or pelvic lymph nodes involved by tumor • Tumor has penetrated through the peritoneal surface • Peritoneal implants are present • Gross or microscopic positive margins • Unresectable disease due to extension into vital structures • Tumor spillage either before or during surgery • Preoperative tumor biopsy (tru-cut, open, or fine-needle aspiration) • Piecemeal resection of tumor (including tumor cells found in separately removed adrenal gland or tumor thrombus in separately removed vessel).	**Helpful mnemonic for stage III Wilms (SLURPPIB):** **S:** STR/+margin **L:** LN (abdominal) **U:** Unresectable **R:** Rupture/Spillage **P:** Piecemeal resection (including thrombus not removed en bloc) **P:** Preoperative CHT required (unresectable) **I:** Implant (i.e., peritoneal involvement, including peritoneal penetration) **B:** Biopsy
IV	Distant metastases or lymph node metastases outside the abdomen or pelvis	
V	Bilateral renal involvement present at diagnosis	

Source: Data from Halperin EC, Constine LS, Tarbell NJ, Kun LE. *Pediatric radiation oncology.* Lippincott Williams & Wilkins; 2012.

TREATMENT PARADIGM

Surgery: Radical nephrectomy is the initial definitive treatment of choice for WT in the United States. Historically, nephrectomy alone (1930s) achieved cure in only 15% to 30% but may be appropriate in very low-risk patients (stage I FH, nephrectomy weight <550g, and <2y/o at time of diagnosis, 4-year EFS 90%).[8] About 90% to 95% of patients are resectable at diagnosis via wide transverse abdominal incision and radical nephrectomy with assessment of surgical margins and avoidance of spillage via a transperitoneal approach. Tumors that are marginally resectable or with large central necrosis, which may portend increased risk for spillage, may benefit from neoadjuvant therapy with CHT or RT. This is a complex surgery (10% tumors involve renal vein; 15% tumors involve IVC/atrium). Inspect/palpate abdominal cavity, liver, and LN for extent of tumor spread; examine and palpate opposite kidney; inspect and palpate renal vein to exclude tumor thrombus. Regional LN sampling for accurate staging. Tumor spillage incidence is 15% to 30%[1] and is significantly associated with abdominal recurrence and mortality.[9] Incidence of surgical complications with nephrectomy (as per NWTS-4) is 11%. Most common complications are hemorrhage and SBO. Quality of surgery has prognostic importance (e.g., degree of LN sampling, spillage, unnecessary biopsies), and QA among COG surgeons is underway.

Chemotherapy: CHT has improved overall results for WT in the past two decades via NWTS and SIOP studies. In Europe, CHT is typically given preoperatively. In North America, it is given adjuvantly following initial nephrectomy. Preoperative CHT may be required if there is bulky, unresectable disease, bilateral WT, WT in a solitary kidney, or tumor thrombus in IVC. The use of specific agents varies with stage. Stage I/II FH are typically treated with vincristine and actinomycin-D. Stage III/IV and UH are typically treated with three or more agents including Adriamycin.

Radiation: RT formerly played a much larger role in WT and was historically delivered postoperatively to the tumor bed at 2 Gy/day to 40 to 50 Gy. In the modern era, only ~25% of patients with WT are treated with RT (only 15% if metastatic disease is excluded). **Traditional start for RT is by day 10 after surgery**, no later than day 14, if surgery is designated day 0. A later RT start is linked to increased risk of abdominal recurrence in some studies. RT is given concurrently with vincristine and actinomycin-D.

Indications: See Table 62.1. Typically, at least flank RT is indicated for stage III disease, unfavorable histology, or positive margins. WAI indicated for mnemonic "SPAR" (**S**pillage during surgery, **P**eritoneal seeding, malignant **A**scites, or preoperative **R**upture).

Dose: Flank RT dose is 10.8 Gy/6 fx with boost to 21.6 Gy to gross residual disease. If ≥16 years old or stage III diffuse anaplasia or I-III rhabdoid, flank RT dose is 19.8 Gy (+ 10.8 Gy boost to gross disease; total 30.6 Gy). WAI typically 10.5 Gy/7 fx or 21 Gy/14 fx for diffuse unresectable peritoneal implants. WLI indicated for lung metastases on CXR (not if mets only visible on CT) at a dose of 12 Gy/8 fx (10.5 Gy if <1 year of age). If WLI and flank are both indicated, can treat flank to 10.5 Gy simultaneous with WLI to 12 Gy or at separate times (do not feather or block to adjust for overlap).

Procedure: See *Handbook of Treatment Planning in Radiation Oncology*, Chapter 12 for details.[10]

Toxicities

Renal: Approximately 1% of patients with unilateral WT will have end-stage renal disease from chronic renal failure 20 years from diagnosis; 3.1% for patients with bilateral WT.[11]

Premature mortality: Risk of death from all causes increased from 5.4% to 22.7% at 30 and 50 years of age, respectively, after WT diagnosis; 50% of excess deaths beyond 30 years from diagnosis were attributable to secondary neoplasms and 25% from cardiac diseases.[12]

Cardiac: The risk of CHF increases with increasing total dose of adriamycin received, increasing amount of RT received by the heart, and female gender; 1.7% of patients treated w/ ADR on NWTS-1-4 developed CHF compared to 5.4% in patients treated with WLI.[1,13]

Pulmonary: About 10% of patients with pulmonary mets treated on NWTS-3 developed "diffuse interstitial pneumonitis of unknown etiology" (possibly radiation pneumonitis) after WLI (using 14 Gy). There were four additional cases of diffuse pneumonitis secondary to *varicella* and PJP. Give trimethoprim/sulfamethoxazole for PJP prophylaxis with WLI. The incidence of pneumonitis has subsequently decreased by reducing the dose of Adriamycin and actinomycin-D given concurrently with RT, as well as reducing WLI dose to 12 Gy.

Hepatic: In SIOP-9, 8% of children developed hepatotoxicity consistent with veno-occlusive disease with the combination of CHT and RT.[14]

Reproductive: Females who receive RT or CHT during childhood for unilateral WT had an increased risk for hypertension complicating pregnancy, fetal malpositioning, and premature labor.[15]

Musculoskeletal: RT is associated with development of scoliosis and reduction in height with severity increasing with younger age and increasing dose to the spine.[16]

Second Malignancies: GI, soft tissue sarcomas, and breast cancers are the most frequent secondary neoplasms to develop after treatment.[17] Cumulative incidence of invasive breast cancer for survivors who received lung RT is almost 15% by 40 years of age.[18]

■ **EVIDENCE-BASED Q&A**

■ **What are the findings from the most recent National Wilms Tumor Study (NWTS) 5?**

The NWTS studies pooled patients with WT beginning in the 1970s with the goal of optimizing treatment outcomes. NWTS-5, along with AREN 0532, helped define the standard of care for very low risk patients (stage I FH, <2 years old, and tumors <550 g); both studies showed surgery alone is sufficient treatment in this patient population with excellent survival and effective salvage options.[8,19] NWTS-5 also aimed to further identify and incorporate histologic and genetic markers in order to guide treatment intensification for certain subgroups of patients.

Dome (*JCO* 2006, PMID 16710034): Single-arm study of stage II to IV WT with anaplasia treated with vincristine/adriamycin/cyclophosphamide/etoposide plus flank/abdominal RT (10.8 Gy plus 10.8 Gy boost to bulky residual tumor); 4-year EFS and OS for patients with diffuse anaplasia is worse than those with FH and treatment intensification is warranted.

Grundy (*JCO* 2005, PMID 16129848): Investigated prognostic significance of LOH 1p or 16q in patients with FH. For stages I to II FH, risk of relapse and death were increased with LOH at 1p, 16q, or both. For stages III to IV FH, risk of relapse and death were increased only with LOH for both 1p and 16q (RR = 2.4, p = .01 and RR = 2.7, p = .04).

■ **What is the impact of RT in the setting of tumor spillage?**

RT decreases abdominal tumor recurrence rates after tumor spillage.

Kalapurakal, NWTS 4 and 5 Pooled (*IJROBP* 2010 PMID 19395185): Analyzed influence of irradiation (flank and WAI) and CHT regimens on abdominal recurrence after intraoperative spillage of FH WT. OR for recurrence after RT vs. no RT was 0.35 (0.15–0.78) for 10 Gy and 0.08 (0.01–0.58) for 20 Gy. OR for CHT after adjusting for RT was not significant. For stage II patients (NWTS-4), 8-year RFS with and without spillage, respectively, was 79% vs. 87% (p = .07) and OS was 90% vs. 95% (p = .04). **Conclusion: RT (10 Gy or 20 Gy) reduced abdominal tumor recurrence rates after tumor spillage. Tumor spillage in stage II patients is associated with decreased RFS and significantly decreased OS.**

■ **What study helps guide treatment in stage III FH WT?**

The previous NWTS studies laid the foundation for the most recent AREN protocol, which incorporated previously identified prognostic factors. The results have helped define the standard of care for Wilms.

Fernandez, AREN 0532 (*JCO* 2018, PMID 29211618): A total of 535 stage III FH WT treated with DD4A and RT. MFU 5.2 years; 4-year EFS and OS estimates 88% and 97%, respectively; 58 of 66 relapses occurred in the first 2 years, predominately pulmonary (n = 36). Improved EFS was associated with negative LNs and absence of LOH 1p or 16q (p < .01 for both); 4-year EFS only 74% in those with both positive LNs and LOH 1p or 16q. **Conclusion: Overall favorable EFS and OS in stage III FH WT with DD4A and RT. Positive LNs and 1p or 16q LOH were highly predictive of worse EFS and should be considered a potential prognostic marker for future trials.**

■ **What is the role of WLI in patients with FH Wilms who have pulmonary metastases detected by CT only? What is the role of Adriamycin in this setting?**

In CT-detected lung metastases, there is no OS benefit with ADR or WLI, through EFS is improved with ADR.

Grundy, NWTS 4 and 5 Pooled (*Pediatr Blood Cancer* 2012, PMID 22422736): A total of 417 patients with FH WT and isolated lung metastases. Compared outcomes by method of detection (CXR vs. CT only), use of WLI, and 2- or 3-drug CHT (AMD and VCR ± ADR). For patients with CT-only lung mets (negative CXR), 5-year EFS was greater with three drugs (including Adriamycin) with or without WLI vs. only two drugs (80% vs. 56%; p = .004); OS was not impacted (87% vs. 86%; p = .91). In this group, WLI did not improve 5-year EFS when adjusting for CHT regimen used (p = .52). There was no difference in OS with or without WLI. **Conclusion: Patients with CT-only lung mets have improved EFS but not OS with the addition of ADR; they do not seem to benefit from WLI.**

■ **For which patients with lung metastases can WLI be omitted?**

WLI may not be necessary for patients with FH WT without 1p16q LOH, with CR of lung nodules after 6 weeks of CHT.

Dix, AREN 0533 (JCO 2018, PMID 29659330): A total of 292 patients with FH WT with isolated lung metastases who received DD4A × 6 weeks. If CR in the lungs, CHT continued without WLI. If PR in the lungs or 1p/16q LOH, they received WLI (12 Gy/8 fx) and 4c of intensified CHT (Regimen M); 133 had CR and 159 had PR. Among the 133 patients with CR, 4-year EFS and OS estimates were 79.5% and 96.1%, respectively. Among the 159 patients with PR, 4-year EFS and OS estimates were 88.5% and 95.4%, respectively. **Conclusion: Excellent OS even with omission of WLI in patients with CR after CHT, though more events than anticipated. Patients with PR benefit from WLI and CHT intensification with improvement in EFS and OS.**

REFERENCES

1. Halperin EC, Louis S. Constine, et al. Pediatric radiation oncology. Lippincott Williams & Wilkins; 2012.
2. Bunin GR, Nass CC, Kramer S, Meadows AT. Parental occupation and Wilms' tumor: results of a case-control study. *Cancer Res.* 1989;49(3):725–729. PMID: 2535965.
3. Dome JS, Coppes MJ. Recent advances in Wilms tumor genetics. Curr Opin Pediatr. 2002;14(1):5–11 doi:10.1097/00008480-200202000-00002.
4. Sebire NJ, Vujanic GM. Paediatric renal tumours: recent developments, new entities and pathological features. Histopathology. 2009;54(5):516–528. doi:10.1111/j.1365-2559.2008.03110.x
5. Miniati D, Gay AN, Parks KV, et al. Imaging accuracy and incidence of Wilms' and non-Wilms' renal tumors in children. J Pediatr Surg. 2008;43(7):1301–1307. doi:10.1016/j.jpedsurg.2008.02.077
6. Boo YJ, Fisher JC, Haley MJ, et al. Vascular characterization of clear cell sarcoma of the kidney in a child: a case report and review. J Pediatr Surg. 2009;44(10):2031–2036. doi:10.1016/j.jpedsurg.2009.06.023
7. Gratias EJ, Dome JS, Jennings LJ, et al. Association of chromosome 1q Gain with inferior survival in favorable-histology wilms tumor: a report from the Children's Oncology Group. *J Clin Oncol.* 2016;34(26):3189–3194. doi:10.1200/JCO.2015.66.1140
8. Fernandez CV, Perlman EJ, Mullen EA, et al. Clinical outcome and biological predictors of relapse after nephrectomy only for very low-risk wilms tumor: a report from Children's Oncology Group AREN0532. *Ann Surg.* 2017;265(4):835–840. doi:10.1097/SLA.0000000000001716
9. Shamberger RC, Guthrie KA, Ritchey ML, et al. Surgery-related factors and local recurrence of Wilms tumor in National Wilms Tumor Study 4. *Ann Surg.* 1999;229(2):292–297. doi:10.1097/00000658-199902000-00019
10. Videtic GMM, Woody N, Vassil AD. Handbook of treatment planning in radiation oncology. 3rd ed. Demos Medical; 2020. doi:10.1891/9780826168429
11. Lange J, Peterson SM, Takashima JR, et al. Risk factors for end stage renal disease in non-WT1-syndromic Wilms tumor. J Urol. 2011;186(2):378–386. doi:10.1016/j.juro.2011.03.110
12. Wong KF, Reulen RC, Winter DL, et al. Risk of adverse health and social outcomes up to 50 years after Wilms tumor: the British Childhood Cancer Survivor Study. *J Clin Oncol.* 2016;34(15):1772–1779. doi:10.1200/JCO.2015.64.4344
13. Green DM, Grigoriev YA, Nan B, et al. Congestive heart failure after treatment for Wilms' tumor: a report from the National Wilms' Tumor Study group. *Ann Surg.* 2001;19(7):1926–1934. doi:10.1200/JCO.2001.19.7.1926
14. Bisogno G, de Kraker J, Weirich A, et al. Veno-occlusive disease of the liver in children treated for Wilms tumor. Med Pediatr Oncol. 1997;29(4):245–251. doi:10.1002/(SICI)1096-911X(199710)29:4<245::AID-MPO2>3.0.CO;2-M
15. Green DM, Lange JM, Peabody EM, et al. Pregnancy outcome after treatment for Wilms tumor: a report from the national Wilms tumor long-term follow-up study. *J Clin Onco.* 2010;28(17):2824–2830. doi:10.1200/JCO.2009.27.2922
16. Hogeboom CJ, Grosser SC, Guthrie KA, et al. Stature loss following treatment for Wilms tumor. Med Pediatr Oncol. 2001;36(2):295–304. doi:10.1002/1096-911X(20010201)36:2<295::AID-MPO1068>3.0.CO;2-Y
17. Termuhlen AM, Tersak JM, Liu Q, et al. Twenty-five year follow-up of childhood Wilms tumor: a report from the Childhood Cancer Survivor Study. Pediatr Blood Cancer. 2011;57(7):1210–1216. doi:10.1002/pbc.23090
18. Lange JM, Takashima JR, Peterson SM, et al. Breast cancer in female survivors of Wilms tumor: a report from the national Wilms tumor late effects study. Cancer. 2014;120(23):3722–3730. doi:10.1002/cncr.28908
19. Shamberger RC, Anderson JR, Breslow NE, et al. Long-term outcomes for infants with very low risk Wilms tumor treated with surgery alone in National Wilms Tumor Study-5. *Ann Surg.* 2010;251(3):555–558. doi:10.1097/SLA.0b013e3181c0e5d7

63 ■ EWING'S SARCOMA

Kailin Yang, Ehsan H. Balagamwala, and Erin S. Murphy

QUICK HIT ■ Ewing's sarcoma is the second most common primary bone tumor in childhood. Males are affected more than females, and peak age is 10 to 15 years of age. Important genetic mutations include t(11;22) and t(21;22). Workup includes evaluation of primary site with CT/MRI, PET/CT, bilateral bone marrow biopsies, and biopsy of the primary tumor. The overall treatment paradigm is shown in Table 63.1.

Table 63.1: General Treatment Paradigm for Ewing's Sarcoma	
Induction (Weeks 1–12)	VAdriaC + IE × 6 cycles
Local control (Week 13)	Surgery or RT or combined modality (see Table 63.2)
Consolidation	VAdriaC + IE × 11 cycles, adjuvant RT (if indicated) starts cycle 1 of consolidation, ASAP after surgery

EPIDEMIOLOGY: Described in 1921 by James Ewing as an undifferentiated tumor involving the diaphysis of long bones that is radiation sensitive (in contrast to osteosarcoma).[1] Second most common primary bone tumor in children and the most lethal bone tumor. Approximately 200 cases per year (~3% of childhood cancers).[2] Peak age is ~15 years of age, with 30% each <10 years of age or >20 years of age.[2] More common in Caucasian boys (M:F ratio is 1.5:1).

RISK FACTORS: No known environmental or familial risk factors.[3] No convincing evidence of inheritance.

ANATOMY: Fifty percent originate in an extremity (20%–30% proximal and 30%–40% distal), and 50% central (45% pelvis, 35% chest wall, 10% spine, < 10% remainder). Long bone tumors are usually present in diaphysis, as opposed to osteosarcoma, which originates in the metaphysis.[4]

PATHOLOGY: Generally, sarcomas are divided into two categories: (a) tumors displaying complex karyotypic abnormalities with no distinct pattern and (b) tumors associated with particular chromosomal translocations that result in specific fusion genes. ESFT belongs to the second category. Although controversial, ESFT is thought to originate from the postganglionic parasympathetic neural cells as opposed to neuroblastoma, which originate from the sympathetic system. Microscopically, ESFT appears as monomorphic sheets of small, round blue cells usually with extensive necrosis, but morphology alone is insufficient for diagnosis. ESFT includes ESB, EOE, and primitive peripheral PNET (neuroepithelioma, adult neuroblastoma, Askin's tumor, and paravertebral small cell tumor). EOE has more favorable prognosis, and localized EOE is commonly managed with surgery alone. Staining: positive for MIC2 glycoprotein, PAS, vimentin. Negative for NSE and S100 (both positive in PNET). Types: typical (i.e., classic) versus atypical (lobular, alveolar, or organoid).[4]

GENETICS: ESFT is usually defined by a translocation in the *EWSR1* gene; 90% display t(11;22) (q24;q12). t(21;22)(q21;q12) is the second most common (~5%–10%) with a number of other less common translocations or structural aberrations in the remainder of cases (e.g., t[7;22], t[17;22], gain of chromosome 8 and 12, and deletion of 1p, del *CDKN2A*, mutation p53).[5] t(11;22) results in fusion of *FLI-1* gene (DNA-binding transcription factor) on 11q24 with the EWS gene (RNA-binding protein) on 22q12. EWS-FLI-1 is a transcription factor that impacts cell cycle regulation, apoptosis, and telomerase activity. t(21;22) results in EWS-ERG fusion product and phenotype is identical to EWS-FLI-1. FISH/PCR is used for detection of fusion transcripts. DSRCT and malignant melanoma of soft parts are also associated with EWS translocation. PNET that are positive for EWSR translocation

(CD99+) are classified and treated as pPNET; if negative for translocation they are cPNET and treated like an embryonal tumor

CLINICAL PRESENTATION: Pain (>90%), swelling or mass (65%), limitation in movement (25%), neurologic changes (15% overall, though 50% in central tumors), pathologic fracture (15%), fever (10%). Approximately 25% have overt metastases at presentation, most commonly in lung (40%) and bone (40%); 25% to 30% risk for overt metastases in pelvic primaries and <10% for extremity primaries. Micrometastases are assumed to be present at diagnosis in nearly all patients because of a high distant failure rate with local therapy alone. The risk of lymph node metastasis at diagnosis is low. Askin's tumor is a primary ES of the rib, associated with direct pleural extension and a large extraosseous soft tissue mass, and is more common in females.[4] Differential includes osteomyelitis, lymphoma of the bone, leukemia (chloroma), rhabdomyosarcoma, metastatic neuroblastoma, small cell osteosarcoma, eosinophilic granuloma, metastatic small cell lung cancer, or mesenchymal chondrosarcoma. Mnemonic for bone tumors "EG-MODE": **E**piphysis (**G**iant cell tumor), **M**etaphysis (**O**steosarcoma), **D**iaphysis (**E**wing's sarcoma). Differential for small round blue cell tumors (mnemonic LEMONS): **L**ymphoma, **E**wing's, **M**edulloblastoma, **O**ther (rhabdomyosarcoma, pineoblastoma, ependymoblastoma, etc.), **N**euroblastoma, **S**mall cell carcinoma.

WORKUP: H&P.

Labs: CBC, BMP, LDH.

Imaging: Plain x-ray, CT, and MRI of the involved bone, CT chest, PET/CT. Plain x-ray findings range from lytic (75%) to sclerotic (25%), "moth-eaten," "onion skinning" (layers of reactive bone), "Codman's triangle" (displaced periosteum with cortical destruction; also present in osteosarcoma), soft tissue mass in 50%. CT bone outlines bony destruction and soft tissue extent, enhances with contrast. MRI is 90% accurate for diagnosis with improved soft tissue definition. PET assesses tumor viability, evaluates for metastases (most helpful in lymph nodes and bone), and is the most sensitive test for follow-up after treatment. CT is more reliable for lung metastasis, compared to PET.[6] SUV > 5.8 associated with worse survival.[7]

Procedures: Bilateral bone marrow biopsy and biopsy of the tumor. Biopsy should be performed by the surgeon who will be resecting the tumor to avoid compromising later operation such as limb salvage. FNA is inadequate; CT-guided core needle biopsy is usually sufficient. Open biopsy should be done only if necrotic material on core. Always include biopsy site in predicted operative site.

PROGNOSTIC FACTORS: Presence of metastases is the most important (bone or liver worse than lung, multiple lung lesions worse than solitary). Other poor factors can be remembered with the mnemonic "**MASSS**ive **LD**H **R**esponse": **M**ale gender, **A**ge > 17, pelvic/axial **S**ite, **S**ize > 8 cm, **S**tage (+mets), high **LD**H, **R**esponse to CHT (> 90% is positive prognostic factor). Expression of p53 or deletion on INK4A also portends worse prognosis.

NATURAL HISTORY: Marked improvement in 5-year OS since 1975 (35%) to current 5-year OS (70%–80%) for nonmetastatic patients, principally due to addition of intensive CHT. Metastases are not uniformly fatal, with average 5-year OS of approximately 30% in modern era. Dominant pattern of failure for large tumors remains distant metastasis despite aggressive CHT.

STAGING: No formal staging. Stratification is by presence or absence of metastatic disease.

TREATMENT PARADIGM

Surgery: For local control, resection is preferred unless poor functional results are anticipated. Resection provides pathologic information post-CHT and avoids second malignancy and late effects of RT. Resection without reconstruction can be done in small bones such as rib, clavicle, proximal fibula, distal scapula, metatarsals, metacarpals, and small iliac wing or pubic bone lesions. Results are typically very good for these "dispensable bones."[8,9] Large lesions may require allograft or endoprosthetic reconstructions. In the metastatic setting, surgery may be helpful for limited pulmonary metastases, or palliation at primary site. A systematic review of local control options suggested that the optimal treatment approach should be individualized based on patient and disease characteristics, as well as patient preference.[9,10] Nodal dissection is not routinely indicated; however, if suggestion of nodal positivity on imaging, surgical pathology should be obtained since this would influence RT target.

Chemotherapy: Induction CHT is given to all patients. Compressed VAdriaC-IE (q2 week cycles) is the current standard. Agents: vincristine (neuropathy, constipation, myalgias, arthralgias, and cholestasis), cyclophosphamide (pancytopenia and dose-dependent hemorrhagic cystitis, infertility), doxorubicin (myocardial dysfunction and pancytopenia), ifosfamide (high incidence of hemorrhagic cystitis requiring use of Mesna and Fanconi syndrome of electrolyte wasting), etoposide (pancytopenia, anaphylactic reactions, and second malignancies such as AML). No role for further intensification with higher doses of cyclophosphamide, ifosfamide, and doxorubicin due to increased toxicity and risk of second malignancy without improvement in EFS and OS.[10]

Radiation: Potentially indicated pre-op, post-op, or definitively for the primary tumor and for treatment of pulmonary and skeletal metastases. Indications for postoperative RT include close margins (<1 cm), poor histologic response (<90% necrosis), or tumor spill.[11] Preoperative RT is considered when close/positive margins are expected. Treat pre-CHT volume due to high rate of local failure if limited to post-CHT volume.[12] Involved field rather than whole bone is sufficient. Adjuvant RT starts at the time of consolidation CHT (week 14) with VC-IE CHT given concurrently (doxorubicin held during RT). Dose as per AEWS 1031 in Table 63.2.

Table 63.2: Radiation Therapy Guidelines for Ewing's Sarcoma Summary per AEWS 1031			
Situation	Dose	Volumes	Concurrent Chemotherapy
Preoperative	36 Gy	Pre-CHT GTV	VC-IE (no doxorubicin when given concurrently)
Definitive	45 Gy CD to 55.8 Gy.	Pre-CHT GTV Gross residual/post-CHT	VC-IE
Postoperative (i.e., microscopic)	50.4 Gy (> 90% necrosis) 50.4 Gy (< 90% necrosis)	Post-CHT GTV Pre-CHT GTV	VC-IE
Lung metastases	15 Gy; 1.5 Gy/fx	Bilateral lungs (boost primary/lung nodules)	No doxorubicin or actinomycin D. CHT vs. RT being evaluated on AEWS1031
Bone metastasis	45 to 56 Gy (consider SBRT)		
Vertebral body	45 Gy Boost to 50.4 Gy	Pre-CHT GTV + 1 cm (entire VB + 0.5 cm) Post-CHT GTV + 0.5 to 1 cm	

Notes:
- Do not treat across a joint or encompass an extremity circumferentially (spare strip) unless absolutely necessary for tumor coverage.
- Reduce margins if there is no extension beyond joint space, but adjacent epiphysis is in volume.
- For diaphyseal lesion, exclude 1 epiphysis of affected bone, if possible. For intraoperative spill, boost pre-CHT volume.
- When using pre-op RT, if there is microscopic residual, evaluate necrosis; if > 90%, then 14.4 Gy boost to post-CHT GTV; if < 90%, then 14.4 Gy boost to pre-CHT GTV.
- If gross residual, cone down to 55.8 Gy to pre-CHT GTV.
- For metastatic lesions, SBRT to doses approximating 40 Gy/5 fx can be considered if TG 101 normal tissue constraints can be met (ongoing evaluation on current COG AEWS 1221).

Rib primary or Askin's tumor: Do not attempt resection prior to CHT. Preoperative CHT improves negative margins (50% vs. 77%) and decreases need for post-op RT (5-year EFS 56%).[13] Some treat entire ipsilateral hemithorax (15–18 Gy, 1.5 Gy/fx) before reducing field to complete dose schedule as noted previously, especially if lung metastasis or positive pleural cytology present.[14] Some have used intrapleural colloidal P32 in addition to EBRT to spare lung while treating pleura.

Metastatic disease: Low-dose bilateral lung RT (15 Gy/10 fx) can control gross metastatic disease in the lungs without significant pulmonary toxicity, and is usually recommended after CHT, despite paucity of data. Bone metastases can be controlled with doses from 45 to 56 Gy. If substantial amounts of marrow will be included in the RT field, consider delaying until the end of systemic therapy. SBRT for metastatic lesions is being evaluated on ongoing AEWS 1221.

Toxicity: May potentiate bladder and cardiotoxicity from CHT. Older studies demonstrated loss of 25% remaining growth in limb for > 50 Gy, particularly if including joint or epiphysis. May consider amputation and prosthesis in the very young as they recover function well.

Second malignancy: Rates reported from 6.5% to 9.2% at 20-year in recent studies. Risk is highest for doses > 60 Gy, and minimal for < 48 Gy. Most common second tumor is osteosarcoma. In a recent review of RT-induced osteosarcoma, most common primary was Ewing's (25%); median latency was 8 years.[15]

■ **EVIDENCE-BASED Q&A**

■ **What is the utility of chemotherapy in Ewing's sarcoma?**

CHT forms the cornerstone of therapy. Due to suboptimal outcomes with VAC-based CHT, efforts were made to add agents as well as intensify the regimens. VACA was found to be superior to VAC (IESS-1) and subsequently, high-dose intermittent VACA was found to be superior to standard-dose VACA (IESS-II).[16,17] Given the activity of IE in metastatic Ewing's sarcoma, VACA+IE was tested for both metastatic and nonmetastatic patients and was found to be superior to high-dose intermittent VACA for nonmetastatic patients (IESS-III).[18] Subsequently, dose intensification of 48 vs. 30 weeks of VAC+IE (IESS-IV) for local Ewing's sarcoma demonstrated no benefit to dose intensification, but showed that dropping actinomycin D was acceptable. Interval compression of q2wk vs. q3wk (AEWS0031) of VAdriaC+IE showed that VAdriaC+IE q2wk was superior and forms the current standard of care in the definitive setting.[19,20]

■ **What is the optimal local control modality: surgery or radiotherapy?**

Classically, surgery has been performed for tumors that are surgically resectable, and definitive RT has been reserved for tumors that are surgically unresectable. There are no prospective trials evaluating surgery vs. definitive RT, only retrospective reviews of either RCTs or institutional databases,[10] which suggest that surgery and definitive RT have similar outcomes (albeit with the inherent selection biases of retrospective institutional reviews). Furthermore, despite modern RT and surgical techniques, surgery + RT is associated with the lowest risk for local failure for pelvic tumors.[21] Surgery is generally preferred if possible but RT is preferred for patients who lack a function-preserving surgical option due to location (e.g., scapula, proximal humerus, skull, face, vertebrae) or extent.

Yock, INT 0091 (*JCO* 2006, PMID 16921035): PRT of 75 nonmetastatic pelvic Ewing's patients comparing VACA vs. VACA+IE to determine its influence on local control modality with respect to surgery, RT, or both (S+RT), which was chosen by the treating physicians. The effect of local control modality was assessed after adjusting for the size of tumor (<8 cm, ≥8 cm) and CHT type. Surgery was done in 12 patients, RT in 44, and S+RT in 19. The 5-year EFS and LF were 49% and 21% (16% LF only; 5% LF and distant failure). No significant difference in EFS or LF by tumor size (< 8 cm, > 8 cm), LC modality, or CHT. However, VACA-IE seems to confer a LC benefit (11% vs. 30%; P = .06). **Conclusion: VACA+ IE is superior for pelvic tumors. Surgery and RT produce comparable outcomes.**

Schuck, Review of CESS 81, CESS 86, and EICESS 92 Trials (*IJROBP* 2003, PMID 12504050): Review of 1,058 patients. Surgery as local therapy used when feasible, and adjuvant RT is given for poor histologic response or biopsy/STR. See Table 63.3. **Conclusion: Low rates of LF after induction CHT for resectable tumors. For incisional resection, definitive RT equivalent to surgery + post-op RT.** *Comment: RT patients were negatively selected, with unfavorable tumor sites.*

Table 63.3: Combined Analysis of CESS 81, 86, and EICESS 92 for Ewing's Sarcoma		
	5-Yr LF	5/10-Yr EFS
Surgery ± RT	7.5%	61%/55%
Pre-op RT	5.3%	59%/58%
RT alone	26.3%	47%/40%
	p = sig	p = sig

Daw, COG Trials (*Ann Surg Oncol*** 2016, PMID 27216741):** RR of 115 patients with Ewing's of the femur from three cooperative group trials; 84 underwent surgery alone, 17 had surgery + RT, and 14 had RT alone; 5-year EFS was 65% and 5-year OS was 70%. Tumor location and size did not influence patient outcomes. Treatment modality also did not lead to any statistically significant differences in EFS, OS, LF. **Conclusion: LC modality does not affect disease outcomes for Ewing's sarcoma of the femur.**

Ahmed, Mayo Clinic (*Pediatr Blood Cancer*** 2017, PMID 28244685):** RR of 73 patients, 48 pelvis and 25 spine. MFU 58.1 months. 52% pelvis patients presented with metastatic disease as compared to 24% spine patients. RT is alone utilized in 65% and 48%, surgery in 16.7% and 8%, and surgery + RT in 16.7% and 44% of pelvis and spine tumors, respectively. The 5-year OS and EFS for spine tumors were 73% and 54%, respectively. The 5-year OS and EFS for pelvic tumors were 73% and 65%, respectively. The 5-year EFS for local treatment of all metastases was 29% vs. 12% for untreated metastases (p = .02). **Conclusion: Excellent OS (73%) and LC (93%) for spine tumors (especially with dose ≥ 56 Gy). Pelvic tumors with inferior LC (81%) despite modern treatment. Surgery + RT and dose ≥56 Gy associated with the lowest LF rate and treatment of metastatic sites associated with improved OS and EFS.**

■ **Considering the bone marrow is one contiguous space, should RT volumes include the entire involved bone?**

Donaldson, POG-8346 (*IJROBP*** 1998, PMID 9747829):** A total of 178 patients with localized Ewing's. Adria/C × 12 weeks, followed by VAC × 50 weeks. Local therapy was surgery when possible without functional loss, otherwise RT. RT alone (n = 94), randomized to whole bone (39.6 Gy, boost to pre-CHT + 2 cm to 55.8 Gy) vs. tailored port (pre-CHT + 2 cm to 55.8 Gy). Results: 5-year EFS differed by site (distal extremity 65%, central 63%, proximal extremity 46%, pelvic/sacral 24%). LC for RT alone was 65%. No difference between whole bone and tailored port; 5-year LC differed by quality of RT (appropriate RT 80%, minor deviation 48%, major deviation 15%). LF 62% in RT volume, 24% outside RT volume, and 14% indeterminate. **Conclusion: Must treat adequate volumes. Tailored fields are reasonable.**

■ **Does the timing of RT (early versus delayed) impact outcome in metastatic patients?**

Cangir, IESS-MD-I and II (*Cancer*** 1990, PMID 2201433):** Reviewed IESS-MD-I (1975–1977, n = 53, VACA + concurrent RT) and IESS-MD-II (1980–1983, n = 69, VACA + 5-FU, RT at week 10). RT is given to areas of gross disease. No difference in overall response (73% vs. 70%), length of best response (3-year DFS 30% in both), > 5-year survivors (30% vs. 28%), and fatal toxicity (6% vs. 7%). Life-threatening toxicity worse in MD-I (30% vs. 9%, p = SS). **Conclusion: No survival advantage to early vs. delayed RT for metastatic disease. Less toxicity with delayed RT.**

■ **What is the role of SBRT for metastatic Ewing's sarcoma?**

Consolidation of metastatic sites of disease with SBRT is currently being evaluated on the COG AEWS 1221 trial. Previous retrospective series have demonstrated safety and feasibility of SBRT in this patient population, and further prospective validation is awaited.[22,23]

REFERENCES

1. Angervall L, Enzinger FM. Extraskeletal neoplasm resembling Ewing's sarcoma. *Cancer*. 1975;36:240–251. doi:10.1002/1097-0142(197507)36:1<240::AID-CNCR2820360127>3.0.CO;2-H

2. Glass AG, Fraumeni JF. Epidemiology of bone cancer in children. *J Natl Cancer Inst*. 1970;44:187–199.

3. Buckley JD, Pendergrass TW, Buckley CM, et al. Epidemiology of osteosarcoma and Ewing's sarcoma in childhood: a study of 305 cases by the Children's Cancer Group. *Cancer*. 1998;83:1440–1448. doi:10.1002/(SICI)1097-0142(19981001)83:7<1440::AID-CNCR23>3.0.CO;2-3

4. Halperin EC, Constine LS, Tarbell NJ, Kun LE. *Pediatric Radiation Oncology*. 5th ed. Lippincott Williams and Wilkins; 2010.

5. de Alava E, Gerald WL. Molecular biology of the Ewing's sarcoma/primitive neuroectodermal tumor family. *J Clin Oncol*. 2000;18:204–213. doi:10.1200/JCO.2000.18.1.204

6. Völker T, Denecke T, Steffen I, et al. Positron emission tomography for staging of pediatric sarcoma patients: results of a Prospective Multicenter Trial. *J Clin Oncol*. 2007;25:5435–5441. doi:10.1200/JCO.2007.12.2473

7. Hwang JP, Lim I, Kong C-B, et al. Prognostic value of SUVmax measured by pretreatment Fluorine-18 Fluorodeoxyglucose Positron Emission Tomography/Computed Tomography in patients with Ewing Sarcoma. *PLoS One*. 2016;11:e0153281. doi:10.1371/journal.pone.0153281

8. Sauer R, Jürgens H, Burgers JMV, et al. Prognostic factors in the treatment of Ewing's sarcoma. *Radiother Oncol*. 1987;10:101–110. doi:10.1016/S0167-8140(87)80052-X

9. Werier J, Yao X, Caudrelier J-M, et al. A systematic review of optimal treatment strategies for localized Ewing's sarcoma of bone after neo-adjuvant chemotherapy. *Surg Oncol*. 2016;25:16–23. doi:10.1016/j.suronc.2015.11.002

10. Miser JS, Goldsby RE, Chen Z, et al. Treatment of metastatic Ewing sarcoma/primitive neuroectodermal tumor of bone: evaluation of increasing the dose intensity of chemotherapy—a report from the Children's Oncology Group. *Pediatr Blood Cancer*. 2007;49:894–900. doi:10.1002/pbc.21233

11. Foulon S, Brennan B, Gaspar N, et al. Can postoperative radiotherapy be omitted in localised standard-risk Ewing sarcoma? An observational study of the Euro-E.W.I.N.G group. *Eur J Cancer*. 2016;61:128–136. doi:10.1016/j.ejca.2016.03.075

12. Donaldson SS. Ewing sarcoma: Radiation dose and target volume. *Pediatr Blood Cancer*. 2004;42:471–476. doi:10.1002/pbc.10472

13. Shamberger RC, LaQuaglia MP, Gebhardt MC, et al. Ewing sarcoma/primitive neuroectodermal tumor of the chest wall: impact of initial versus delayed resection on tumor margins, survival, and use of radiation therapy. *Ann Surg*. 2003;238:563–567; discussion 567–568. doi:10.1097/01.sla.0000089857.45191.52

14. Schuck A, Ahrens S, Konarzewska A, et al. Hemithorax irradiation for Ewing tumors of the chest wall. *Int J Radiat Oncol Biol Phys*. 2002;54:830–838. doi:10.1016/S0360-3016(02)02993-0

15. Koshy M, Paulino AC, Mai WY, Teh BS. Radiation-induced osteosarcomas in the pediatric population. *Int J Radiat Oncol Biol Phys*. 2005;63:1169–1174. doi:10.1016/j.ijrobp.2005.04.008

16. Nesbit ME, Gehan EA, Burgert EO, et al. Multimodal therapy for the management of primary, nonmetastatic Ewing's sarcoma of bone: a long-term follow-up of the First Intergroup study. *J Clin Oncol*. 1990;8:1664–1674. doi:10.1200/JCO.1990.8.10.1664

17. Burgert EO, Nesbit ME, Garnsey LA, et al. Multimodal therapy for the management of nonpelvic, localized Ewing's sarcoma of bone: intergroup study IESS-II. *J Clin Oncol*. 1990;8:1514–1524. doi:10.1200/JCO.1990.8.9.1514

18. Grier HE, Krailo MD, Tarbell NJ, et al. Addition of ifosfamide and etoposide to standard chemotherapy for Ewing's sarcoma and primitive neuroectodermal tumor of bone. *N Engl J Med*. 2003;348:694–701. doi:10.1056/NEJMoa020890

19. Granowetter L, Womer R, Devidas M, et al. Dose-intensified compared with standard chemotherapy for nonmetastatic Ewing sarcoma family of tumors: a Children's Oncology Group Study. *J Clin Oncol*. 2009;27:2536–2541. doi:10.1200/JCO.2008.19.1478

20. Womer RB, West DC, Krailo MD, et al. Randomized controlled trial of interval-compressed chemotherapy for the treatment of localized Ewing sarcoma: a report from the Children's Oncology Group. *J Clin Oncol*. 2012;30:4148–4154. doi:10.1200/JCO.2011.41.5703

21. Ahmed SK, Robinson SI, Arndt CAS, et al. Pelvis Ewing sarcoma: local control and survival in the modern era. *Pediatr Blood Cancer*. 2017;64(9). doi:10.1002/pbc.26504

22. Brown LC, Lester RA, Grams MP, et al. Stereotactic body radiotherapy for metastatic and recurrent ewing sarcoma and osteosarcoma. *Sarcoma*. 2014;2014:418270. doi:10.1155/2014/418270

23. Parsai S, Juloori A, Angelov L, et al. Spine radiosurgery in adolescents and young adults: early outcomes and toxicity in patients with metastatic Ewing sarcoma and osteosarcoma. *J Neurosurg Spine*. 2019;32(4):491–498. doi:10.3171/2019.9.SPINE19377

64 ■ PEDIATRIC HODGKIN'S LYMPHOMA

Sarah M. C. Sittenfeld and Erin S. Murphy

QUICK HIT ■ Pediatric Hodgkin's lymphoma accounts for ~7% of all childhood malignancies and is highly curable with survival rates >90% across risk groups. Nodular sclerosis is the most common histology (similar to adult Hodgkin's); however, mixed cellularity subtype is seen more frequently in pediatric Hodgkin's compared to other age groups. Given the excellent cure rates, trials in pediatric Hodgkin's have been designed to evaluate de-escalation of CHT and RT based on risk stratification. Generally, RT is delivered per protocol based on the selection of systemic therapy and response criteria specified. Table 64.1 presents some general principles, but specifics are determined by paradigms set forth by the trials listed.

Table 64.1: General Treatment Paradigm for Pediatric Hodgkin's Lymphoma	
Risk group	**Suggested Treatment Options**
Low risk	1. Two to four cycles of non-cross-resistant CHT + IFRT (15–25.5 Gy) a. Possible CHT regimens: AV-PC, ABVD, VAMP, OPPA, or OEPA 2. Four to six cycles of COPP/ABV alone 3. CHT + IFRT, response-adapted as per AHOD 0431

Intermediate risk	1. Four to six cycles of non–cross-resistant CHT + IFRT (15–25.5 Gy) (as per AHOD 0031)
	    a. Possible regimens: COPP/ABV, ABVE-PC, OPPA/COPP, or OEPA/COPDAC
	2. Six to eight cycles of non-cross-resistant CHT alone
	    a. Possible regimens: COPP/ABV

High risk	1. Six to eight cycles of non–cross-resistant CHT + IFRT (15–25.5 Gy)
	    a. Possible regimens: COPP/ABVD, OEPA/COPDAC
	2. Eight cycles of non–cross-resistant CHT alone
	    b. Possible regimens: COPP/ABVD
	3. CHT + response based ISRT per AHOD0831

EPIDEMIOLOGY: Of ~10,450 childhood cancer diagnoses per year, pediatric Hodgkin's (age up to 21) represents ~7% (~1,140 cases).[1] Bimodal age distribution. Pediatric Hodgkin's is rare before age 5, has a male predominance (M to F ratio 2–3:1), and is more likely than adult Hodgkin's to present as **mixed cellularity** (30%–35%) or **nodular lymphocyte predominant** (10%–20%) subtypes.[2] See Tables 64.2 and 64.3. The 5-year OS of all pediatric Hodgkin's lymphoma patients is 97%.[3]

RISK FACTORS

Pediatric Hodgkin's: Increasing family size, lower SES status, and early EBV exposure.[4] EBV exposure is associated with mixed cellularity Hodgkin's disease, and this disease tends to occur more in developing countries.

AYA Hodgkin's: Higher SES, early birth order, small family size, and delayed EBV exposure.

Adults: Immunosuppression (HIV, organ/bone marrow transplant), autoimmune disorders, or immune dysfunction (there is evidence to suggest adult Hodgkin's is biologically different and more aggressive compared to pediatric Hodgkin's).

ANATOMY AND PATHOLOGY: See Chapter 51 for details.

Table 64.2: Histologic Classification and Relative Frequency of Pediatric Hodgkin's Disease

	Histology	Pediatric Frequency	Adult Frequency	Markers
Classic Hodgkin's	• *Lymphocyte rich (LR)*	<5%	5%	CD15+, CD30+ Occ. CD20+
	• *Nodular sclerosis (NSHD)*	55%	≥70%	
	• *Mixed cellularity (MCHD)*	30%–35%	~20%	
	• *Lymphocyte depletion (LD)*	<5%	<5%	
Nodular lymphocyte predominance (NLPHD)		5%–10%	5%	CD19+, **CD20+**, CD45+, CD15-, CD30-

Source: Data from Halperin EC, Constine LS, Tarbell NJ, Kun LE. *Pediatric Radiation Oncology.* 5th ed. Lippincott Williams and Wilkins; 2010.

CLINICAL PRESENTATION[4]: Painless adenopathy is the most common presentation. Approximately 80% have cervical LN involvement at presentation and >50% have mediastinal disease. Approximately one third present with B symptoms: fevers (>38 °C), drenching night sweats, and weight loss (>10% in the past 6 months). May see **Pel–Ebstein fevers** (cyclical spiking fevers up to 40 °C, last ~1 week and remit for ~1 week; due to cytokine release), **generalized pruritus** or **alcohol-induced pain** in tissues infiltrated by HD.

Table 64.3: Comparison of Pediatric and Adolescent/Young Adult Hodgkin's Disease

	Pediatric (age <14 y/o)	AYA (age 15–35 y/o)
Gender (M:F)	2 to 3:1	1.1 to 1.3:1
Site of disease	More commonly have cervical (80%) LAD. Many also have mediastinal disease. Rare to have isolated mediastinal or subdiaphragmatic disease (<5%)	More commonly have mediastinal disease (75%)
Histology Nodular sclerosis Mixed cellularity Lymphocyte depleted NLPHL	 40%–45% 30%–45% 0%–3% 8%–20%	 65%–80% 10%–25% 1%–5% 2%–8%
EBV associated	27%–54%	20%–25%
Risk factors	Lower SES Increasing family size	Higher SES Smaller family size Early birth order
Stage at presentation B symptoms Stage III/IV	 25% 30%–35%	 30%–40% 40%
5-yr OS	>94%	90%

Source: From Halperin EC, Constine LS, Tarbell NJ, Kun LE. *Pediatric Radiation Oncology,* 5th ed. Lippincott Williams and Wilkins; 2010.

WORKUP AND STAGING: See Chapter 51.

PROGNOSTIC FACTORS: Poor prognostic factors include advanced stage, large mediastinal adenopathy, >4 subsites, B symptoms, poor histology, age (<10 y/o better than 11–16 y/o better than >20 y/o), male sex, slow response to CHT. Risk stratification for pediatric Hodgkin's lymphoma is per Table 64.4. CHIPS prognostic score for patients with COG Intermediate Risk (based on AHOD0031).[5] Stage IV disease, large mediastinal mass, albumin (<3.4), and fever were independent prognostic factors and were assigned one point each. EFS was 93.1% for patients with no points, 88.5% for patients with one point, 77.6% for patients with two points, and 69.2% for patients with three points.

Table 64.4: Risk Stratification Schemes for Pediatric Hodgkin's Lymphoma[4]			
Study group	Low Risk	Intermediate Risk	High Risk
COG	IA/IIA, no bulk	Everyone else	IIIB/IVB
German	IA/B or IIA	IIB, IIIEA, IIIB	IIEB, IIIEA/B, IIIB, IVA/B
St. Jude/Stanford/Dana Farber	IA/IIA, no bulk		Everyone else

TREATMENT PARADIGM

Historically, Hodgkin's disease was treated with large RT fields. Cure rates were found to be excellent, and long-term survivors of the disease were common. However, long-term sequelae of RT included profound musculoskeletal retardation, including intraclavicular narrowing, shortened sitting height, decreased mandibular growth, and decreased muscular development. Given the excellent control rates, less toxic treatments were desired and hence began the era of CHT as the primary treatment modality for Hodgkin's lymphoma (note must be made of issue of sterility with CHT and the modification of CHT regimens over the years to preserve fertility).

Surgery: There is no role for surgery in Hodgkin's disease beyond biopsy. The exception is favorable stage IA nodular lymphocyte predominant patients without risk factors who may be treated with complete excision followed by observation (one half to two thirds of patients can be cured with surgery alone), with 5-year OS approaching 100%.[6]

Chemotherapy: Initially, MOPP CHT was the backbone regimen used. However, due to significant impact on fertility (procarbazine is gonadotoxic), ABVD was introduced. In the modern era, all CHT regimens for Hodgkin's disease are a derivative of MOPP and/or ABVD, but more drugs are integrated to reduce total dose of any single drug (see Table 64.5).

Table 64.5: Common CHT Regimens in Pediatric Hodgkin's Lymphoma	
MOPP	Nitrogen mustard, vincristine, procarbazine, prednisone *Toxicities include sterility, secondary leukemia (latent period 3–7 yrs with risk of 3%–5% at 7–10 yrs). Historical regimen not used in the modern era.*
ABVD	Adriamycin, bleomycin, vinblastine, dacarbazine *Toxicities include pulmonary and cardiovascular*
OPPA	Vincristine, procarbazine, prednisone, adriamycin
COPP	Cyclophosphamide, vincristine, procarbazine, prednisone
AV-PC	Doxorubicin, vincristine, prednisone, cyclophosphamide
ABVE-PC	Doxorubicin, bleomycin, vincristine, etoposide, prednisone, cyclophosphamide
VAMP	Vincristine, adriamycin, methotrexate, prednisone

New treatment paradigms incorporate CHT response-based treatments using the following definitions:

Complete Response (CR): >80% reduction in the product of the perpendicular diameters (PPD)

Partial Response (PR): >50% reduction in PPD

Rapid Early Response (RER): CR after 3 cycles of AV-PC (low risk) or CR after 2 cycles of ABVE-PC (intermediate/high risk)

Slow early response (SER): <CR after 3 cycles of AV-PC (low risk) or CR after 2 cycles of ABVE-PC (intermediate/high risk)

Radiotherapy

Indications: Dosing and indications for pediatric Hodgkin's treatment are determined by the choice of CHT and should be followed per protocol. Involved field RT (IFRT) remains the standard approach in pediatrics. Involved site RT (ISRT) is an evolving paradigm and is currently being utilized on some clinical trials. Involved nodal RT (subset of ISRT) is not advised unless as a part of clinical trial. See ILROG guidelines on ISRT for details.[7,8]

Dose: Consolidative RT dose is determined by paradigm chosen but typically ranges from 15 to 25.5 Gy. Acute effects at common modern RT doses are minimal but may include fatigue, skin erythema, and esophagitis. Late effects drive protocol development and include second malignancy, heart disease, pulmonary fibrosis, skeletal hypoplasia, and infertility.

■ EVIDENCE-BASED Q&A

LOW-RISK/EARLY/FAVORABLE PEDIATRIC HODGKIN'S

■ Which early studies evaluated CHT deintensification in low-risk pediatric Hodgkin's disease?

ABVD and MOPP led to excellent cure rates (>90%); however, have significant associated toxicity. Initial trials focused on testing whether less-intensive CHT would lead to equivalent outcomes with improved toxicity. German HD-90[9] and French MDH-90[10] trials demonstrated excellent outcomes with CHT deintensification + ISRT.

■ Is it possible to omit RT in patients who have a complete response (CR) to CHT?

This question was evaluated in HD-95, POG 8625, and CCG 5942. HD-95 suggested that in patients who achieve CR after two cycles, RT can be omitted. However, POG 8625 showed that to omit RT, two additional cycles of CHT are required.[11] When CHT is further de-escalated from MOPP/ABVD, CCG 5942 showed that RT cannot be omitted (trial closed early).[12] Therefore, omitting RT in the setting of de-escalated CHT is not recommended.

Dorffel, HD-95 (*JCO* 2013, PMID 23509321): Prospective, nonrandomized trial of 925 patients divided into early stage (TG1), intermediate stage (TG2), and advanced stage (TG3). RT was given as follows: if CR (CT/MRI), no RT; if tumor reduction of >75%, IFRT to 25 Gy; and if residual tumors >50 cc (considered bulky), IFRT to 25 Gy with 10 to 15 Gy boost. IFRT was given to patients with poor CHT response; however, it was significantly associated with better EFS among intermediate- and high-risk patients but not among low-risk patients. No difference in OS. On QA, 2/17 relapses on RT arm due to poor quality RT; 4/14 patients with stage IIA, who failed, had prolonged delay between CHT and RT. **Conclusion: The omission of RT after CR results in increased risk of treatment failures, most notably in advanced-stage patients (note: a nonrandomized observation). May omit RT after CR in early-stage (low-risk) patients because no EFS benefit seen in this group.**

Metzger, St. Jude Favorable Risk PET-Adapted (*JAMA* 2012, PMID 22735430): Phase II trial of 88 children with low-risk HD. Patients who achieved CR after two cycles did not receive IFRT and those who achieved <CR received 25.5 Gy IFRT. Overall 2-year EFS was 90.8%. For those patients who did not require IFRT, the EFS was 89.4% compared to 92.5% for those who did require IFRT ($p = .61$). **Conclusion: In patients with low-risk pediatric HD who achieved a CR after two cycles of VAMP, omitting IFRT resulted in a high 2-year EFS.**

■ Can RT be omitted in patients who have a rapid early response?

This question was evaluated on the AHOD0431 trial, which demonstrated that rapid response (defined as CR after three cycles of AV-PC) does not adequately predict patients in which RT can be safely omitted (however, negative PET/CT after cycle 1 was prognostic). Of note, AV-PC is also de-escalated CHT. The next step in low-risk trials will evaluate whether CHT intensification can help eliminate the need for RT.

Keller, AHOD 0431 (*Cancer 2018, PMID 29738613*): Phase II trial of 287 patients with low-risk HD examining AV-PC × 3 cycles (doxorubicin, vincristine, prednisone, cyclophosphamide), and no IFRT for CR (> 80% reduction in PPD) after 3 cycles. Patients with PR (>50% PPD) receive IFRT 21 Gy/14 fx. Those who failed after initial CR, if failed as stage I/II, received IV/DECA (dexamethasone, etoposide, cisplatin, cytarabine) + IFRT 21 Gy. If failed as advanced stage, received high-dose CHT with autologous SCT. Study closed early due to higher risk for relapse in patients with CR who were PET+ after 1 cycle. CR after 3 cycles was achieved in 64%, PR in 35%, and stable disease in 2%. See Table 64.6 for additional results. Patients with mixed cellularity had significantly improved EFS compared to patients with nodular sclerosis histology (95% vs. 76%, $p = .008$). **Conclusion: Rapid response as defined in this trial does not adequately define a population in which RT can be avoided. PET response after 1 cycle is highly predictive of outcomes.**

Table 64.6: Results of AHOD 0431		
	4-Year EFS	4-Year EFS (−PET vs. +PET after 1C)
Entire cohort	· 80%	88% vs. 69% ($p = .0007$)
CR (no RT)	49%	85% vs. 60% ($p = .001$)
PR (+RT)	· 83%	96% vs. 70% ($p = .015$)

INTERMEDIATE-HIGH RISK/ADVANCED/FAVORABLE PEDIATRIC HODGKIN'S

▓ Can RT be avoided in patients with CR after CHT?

Several trials have evaluated whether RT can be eliminated for patients who have a CR to induction CHT. HD-95 and CCG 5942 studies showed that IFRT improved EFS, but no difference in OS.[12,13] TATA Memorial from India suggested that there was an OS benefit to IFRT after CR (caveat was that ~50% were AYA or adult HD).[14] However, POG 8725 trial (STNI) and CCG 521 (EFRT), both of which utilized large RT volumes, did not show an EFS or OS benefit to RT.[15,16] These trials together suggested that there may be patients in whom RT could be avoided without impacting oncologic outcome; however, it was unclear who those patients are.

▓ Since it is not clear which patients require titration of CHT and/or RT, is it possible to utilize response-based criteria to determine which intermediate-risk patients require escalation versus de-escalation of treatment?

Early response has been shown in previous studies to be predictive of long-term outcomes. Therefore, the AHOD0031 trial was initiated and demonstrated that rapid early responders (defined as CR after two cycles of ABVE-PC) have no benefit from IFRT. However, all others on the trial received IFRT.

Friedman, AHOD0031 (*JCO 2014, PMID 25311218*): PRT of 1,712 patients. All patients receive two cycles of ABVE-PC. CR defined as >80% PPD response, PR defined as >50% PPD response. Those with a rapid early response (CR or PR) after two cycles received two further cycles of ABVE-PC followed by repeat evaluation: if CR then IFRT vs. no IFRT (randomized); if <CR then IFRT. Those with slow early response (SER) randomized to [ABVE-PCx2C + IFRT] or [DECAx2C + ABVE-PCx2C + IFRT]. IFRT was 21 Gy/14 fx. The 4-year EFS was 85%; 87% for RER, and 77% for SER (SS). The 4-year OS was 98%; 99% for RER, 95% for SER. For RERs with CR, 4-year EFS with IFRT was 88% vs. 84% without IFRT (NS). For RERs with PET-negative at response assessment, 4-year EFS was 87% for patients who received IFRT vs. 87% for those who did not receive IFRT (NS). For SERs randomly assigned to DECA vs. no DECA, 4-year EFS was 79% vs. 75%, respectively, and 71% vs. 55% (NS) for SERs with PET+ at response assessment. **Conclusion: This trial was able to validate response-based therapeutic titration. For RERs with CR, IFRT could be safely omitted and for SERs with PET+ disease, CHT augmentation is recommended.**

Dharmarajan, AHOD0031 Patterns of Failure (*IJROBP 2015, PMID 25542311*): A subset analysis of 198 patients (out of 244) enrolled on AHOD0031, who had developed relapse. Of these patients, 30% were RER/no CR, 26% were SER, 26% RER/CR/no IFRT, 16% were RER/CR/IFRT, and 2%

remained uncategorized. Approximately three-fourths of relapses occurred at initially involved sites (bulky or nonbulky). First relapses rarely occurred at previously uninvolved or out-of-field sites. **Conclusion: Response-based therapy can help define treatment for selected RER patients; it has not proven beneficial for patients with SER, nor has facilitated refinement of IFRT treatment volumes. (Therefore, IFRT is standard of care currently.)** *Comment: A second subset analysis evaluated which patients who achieved RER and CR benefited from IFRT.[17] The results showed that most patients did not benefit from IFRT. However, those with anemia and bulky limited-stage disease had significantly improved 4-yr EFS with the addition of IFRT (89% vs. 78%, p = .019).*

■ Can response-adapted therapy be utilized in high-risk pediatric Hodgkin's?

High-risk patients were enrolled on AHOD0831 with the goal of treatment de-intensification to limit alkylator exposure and reduce RT volumes based on initial CHT response while maintaining comparable OS (the first COG trial to use response-based RT volumes and ISRT).

Kelly, AHOD0831 (*Br J Haematol* 2019, PMID 31180135): PRT of high-risk patients (stage IIIB/IVB) received ABVE-PC × 2C. RER received two additional cycles ABVE-PC and SER received ifosfamide/vinorelbine × 2C + ABVE-PC x 2C. IFRT given to sites of initial bulk (>2.5 cm) and/or SER (21Gy/14fx). The 4-year second EFS was 92%, which was below projected baseline of 95% (*p* = .038). The 5-year first EFS and OS rates were 79% and 95%. Persistent PET+ at the end of CHT was especially high risk for relapse/early progression (8/11 patients failed). **Conclusion: Despite not meeting pre-specified target, EFS and OS rates comparable with recent trials despite reduction in RT volumes.**

■ How are patients with relapsed or refractory disease managed?

Refractory disease is marked by failure to achieve CR or good PR with initial chemo (~6% overall). Salvage therapy in this setting may include high dose CHT ± RT with response rates of 50% to 70%, followed by autologous SCT. However, 5-year DFS is only ~20%. Relapsed disease is usually treated with high dose CHT (HDC) and ASCT. The most common HDC is CBV or BEAM. In general, autologous SCT is preferred over allogeneic SCT due to toxicity and overall lack of graft vs. lymphoma effect. An RR of 1,200 patients with HD who underwent transplant showed that treatment-related mortality was 65% for allogeneic transplant vs. 12% for autologous transplant and the 4-year OS was 25% vs. 37%, respectively (p = .005).[18] IFRT as part of salvage therapy has been shown to improve EFS and trend toward OS (especially in RT naïve patients) in several studies.[19]

*Whole lung irradiation: If treating lungs with RT, do RT **after** the transplant. Other than in the lung, consider RT **prior** to transplant (especially in the pelvis, RT prior to transplant prevents additional bone marrow toxicity to the new graft). Stem cells for transplant should be harvested prior to RT. Transplant has similar outcomes with or without TBI. If RT has been utilized prior to BMT, salvage RT may also be utilized to doses of 15 to 25 Gy.*

■ What is the risk for second malignancies in patients treated for Hodgkin's lymphoma?

The recently published observational study out of the Netherlands shows that the risk for second malignancies continues to increase even up to 40 years after treatment for Hodgkin's lymphoma.[20] The cumulative incidence of second cancers at 40 years was 48.5%. Compared to the general population, patients treated for Hodgkin's lymphoma had a standardized incident ratio of 4.6 for the development of second cancers (equivalent to 121.8 excess cancer diagnoses per 10,000 person-years). The risk for secondary hematological malignancies was lower in the more recent treatment years due to reduction in utilization of alkylating agents. However, reduction in solid tumors was not lower in more recent years (supradiaphragmatic RT was associated with lower second malignancies compared to mantle field RT). One study by O'Brien showed that all patients who developed secondary leukemias (usually due to CHT) had a fatal course, whereas those who developed secondary solid tumors (usually due to RT) had a 5-year OS of 85%.[21]

REFERENCES

1. Ward E, DeSantis C, Robbins A, et al. Childhood and adolescent cancer statistics, 2014. *CA Cancer J Clin.* 2014;64:83–103. doi:10.3322/caac.21219

2. Punnett A, Tsang RW, Hodgson DC. Hodgkin lymphoma across the age spectrum: epidemiology, therapy, and late effects. *Semin Radiat Oncol.* 2010;20:30–44. doi:10.1016/j.semradonc.2009.09.006

3. CureSearch for Children's Cancer Research—Home. CureSearch for Children's Cancer. https://curesearch.org

4. Halperin EC, Constine LS, Tarbell NJ, Kun LE. *Pediatric Radiation Oncology.* 5th ed. Lippincott Williams and Wilkins; 2010.

5. Schwartz CL, Chen L, McCarten K, et al. Childhood Hodgkin International Prognostic Score (CHIPS) Predicts event-free survival in Hodgkin Lymphoma: a Report from the Children's Oncology Group. *Pediatr Blood Cancer.* 2017;64:e26278. doi:10.1002/pbc.26278

6. Appel BE, Chen L, Buxton AB, et al. Minimal treatment of low-risk, pediatric lymphocyte-predominant Hodgkin Lymphoma: a report from the Children's Oncology Group. *J Clin Oncol.* 2016;34:2372–2379. doi:10.1200/JCO.2015.65.3469

7. Specht L, Yahalom J, Illidge T, et al. Modern radiation therapy for Hodgkin lymphoma: field and dose guidelines from the international lymphoma radiation oncology group (ILROG). *Int J Radiat Oncol Biol Phys.* 2014;89:854–862. doi:10.1016/j.ijrobp.2013.05.005

8. Hodgson DC, Dieckmann K, Terezakis S, et al. Implementation of contemporary radiation therapy planning concepts for pediatric Hodgkin lymphoma: Guidelines from the International Lymphoma Radiation Oncology Group. *Pract Radiat Oncol.* 2015;5:85–92. doi:10.1016/j.prro.2014.05.003

9. Schellong G, Pötter R, Brämswig J, et al. High cure rates and reduced long-term toxicity in pediatric Hodgkin's disease: the German-Austrian multicenter trial DAL-HD-90. The German-Austrian Pediatric Hodgkin's Disease Study Group. *J Clin Oncol.* 1999;17(12):3736–3744. doi:10.1200/JCO.1999.17.12.3736

10. Landman-Parker J, Pacquement H, Leblanc T, et al. Localized childhood Hodgkin's disease: response-adapted chemotherapy with etoposide, bleomycin, vinblastine, and prednisone before low-dose radiation therapy—results of the French Society of Pediatric Oncology Study MDH90. *J Clin Oncol.* 2000;18(7):1500–1507. doi:10.1200/JCO.2000.18.7.1500

11. Kung FH, Schwartz CL, Ferree CR, et al. POG 8625: a randomized trial comparing chemotherapy with chemoradiotherapy for children and adolescents with Stages I, IIA, IIIA1 Hodgkin Disease: a report from the Children's Oncology Group. *Pediatr Hematol Oncol.* 2006;28:362–368. doi:10.1097/00043426-200606000-00008

12. Wolden SL, Chen L, Kelly KM, et al. Long-term results of CCG 5942: a randomized comparison of chemotherapy with and without radiotherapy for children with Hodgkin's lymphoma: a report from the Children's Oncology Group. *J Clin Oncol.* 2012;30:3174–3180. doi:10.1200/JCO.2011.41.1819

13. Dörffel W, Rühl U, Lüders H, et al. Treatment of children and adolescents with Hodgkin lymphoma without radiotherapy for patients in complete remission after chemotherapy: final results of the multinational trial GPOH-HD95. *J Clin Oncol.* 2013;31(12):1562–1568. doi:10.1200/JCO.2012.45.3266

14. Laskar S, Gupta T, Vimal S, et al. Consolidation radiation after complete remission in Hodgkin's disease following six cycles of doxorubicin, bleomycin, vinblastine, and dacarbazine chemotherapy: is there a need? *J Clin Oncol.* 2004;22(1):62–68. doi:10.1200/JCO.2004.01.021

15. Weiner MA, Leventhal B, Brecher ML, et al. Randomized study of intensive MOPP-ABVD with or without low-dose total-nodal radiation therapy in the treatment of stages IIB, IIIA2, IIIB, and IV Hodgkin's disease in pediatric patients: a Pediatric Oncology Group study. *J Clin Oncol.* 1997;15:2769–2779. doi:10.1200/JCO.1997.15.8.2769

16. Hutchinson RJ, Fryer CJ, Davis PC, et al. MOPP or radiation in addition to ABVD in the treatment of pathologically staged advanced Hodgkin's disease in children: results of the Children's Cancer Group Phase III Trial. *J Clin Oncol.* 1998;16:897–906. doi:10.1200/JCO.1998.16.3.897

17. Charpentier A-M, Friedman DL, Wolden S, et al. Predictive factor analysis of response-adapted radiation therapy for chemotherapy-sensitive pediatric Hodgkin lymphoma: analysis of the Children's Oncology Group AHOD 0031 Trial. *Int J Radiat Oncol Biol Phys.* 2016;96:943–950. doi:10.1016/j.ijrobp.2016.07.015

18. Milpied N, Fielding AK, Pearce RM, et al. Allogeneic bone marrow transplant is not better than autologous transplant for patients with relapsed Hodgkin's disease. European Group for Blood and Bone Marrow Transplantation. *J Clin Oncol.* 1996;14:1291–1296. doi:10.1200/JCO.1996.14.4.1291

19. Poen JC, Hoppe RT, Horning SJ. High-dose therapy and autologous bone marrow transplantation for relapsed/refractory hodgkin's disease: the impact of involved field radiotherapy on patterns of failure and survival. *Int J Radiat Oncol Biol Phys.* 1996;36:3–12. doi:10.1016/S0360-3016(96)00277-5

20. Schaapveld M, Aleman BMP, van Eggermond AM, et al. Second cancer risk up to 40 years after treatment for Hodgkin's lymphoma. *N Engl J Med.* 2015;373:2499–2511.

21. O'Brien MM, Donaldson SS, Balise RR, et al. Second malignant neoplasms in survivors of pediatric Hodgkin's lymphoma treated with low-dose radiation and chemotherapy. *J Clin Oncol.* 2010;28:1232–1239. doi:10.1016/S0360-3016(96)00277-5

65 ■ MISCELLANEOUS CNS PEDIATRIC TUMORS

Shauna R. Campbell and Erin S. Murphy

QUICK HIT ■ There are a number of rare CNS tumors often presenting in childhood, which include ATRT, pineoblastoma, and intracranial GCT. Each compose <10% of childhood CNS malignancies and exhibit a wide variation in prognosis. Tumors that present in the very young tend to have a poor prognosis and the patient's young age complicates treatment decisions, particularly the role of RT. One similarity between these tumors is the propensity for dissemination within the neuroaxis; therefore, CSF sampling and MRI of the brain and complete spine are essential components of staging. Tumors of the pineal region can be accessed via neuroendoscopy, at which time third ventriculostomy can be performed to relieve obstruction, sample CSF, and biopsy the tumor.

ATYPICAL TERATOID/RHABDOID TUMOR

Epidemiology: Rare and aggressive malignancy often found in infants <3 years old. ATRT can present in the supratentorial or infratentorial brain, with infratentorial tumors more common in infants and patients >3 years of age and demonstrate more favorable survival. Disseminated disease, most commonly leptomeningeal involvement, is present in one-third of patients at diagnosis.[1,2]

Pathology/Genetics: ATRT is defined by loss of the SMARCB1 tumor suppressor gene on IHC. Germline mutations, rather than somatic, are associated with younger age at presentation and extracranial malignant rhabdoid tumors.[3]

Prognosis: The single prospective ATRT cooperative group trial, ACNS0333, demonstrated a significant improvement over historical controls with 4-year OS of 43%.[1] This phase III trial set intense multimodality treatment as the standard of care.

Treatment Paradigm: Defined by ACNS0333.[1] Surgery is first recommended with a maximal safe resection. Postoperatively, two cycles of induction CHT include vincristine, methotrexate, etoposide, cyclophosphamide, and cisplatin. If after induction CHT, there is persistent residual disease a second-look surgery is recommended. Consolidation CHT includes three cycles of carboplatin and thiotepa. RT follows consolidation CHT and consists of 50.4 Gy for patients <3 years of age and 54 Gy for those older. CSI to 23.4 to 36 Gy with a boost to gross disease can be considered for patients with metastatic disease. Historical reports found earlier RT was associated with improved outcomes,[4] but with the addition of intensive multimodality therapy, the delay of RT to after all CHT does not appear to be detrimental.[1]

PINEOBLASTOMA

Epidemiology: Pineoblastoma is the most aggressive (grade IV) primary pineal tumor, which is overall the second most common type of pineal gland tumor after GCT. It was previously categorized as a primary neuroectodermal tumor (PNET). Pineoblastoma is most common in children <5 years old and is associated with a poor prognosis, especially in younger children. Pineoblastoma commonly presents with elevated intracranial pressure with hydrocephalus and has a significant risk of leptomeningeal and extracranial dissemination.

Imaging: On MRI pineoblastomas are hyperdense and have no calcifications. The tumor often appears lobulated with poorly defined borders and heterogeneously contrast enhance.

Treatment Paradigm: Maximal safe resection is recommended, as it is possible extent of resection is associated with improved outcomes.[5–7] RT, most commonly CSI, is associated with improved OS; however, infants and young children are often treated with intensive CHT alone as investigated on the Head Start I–III protocols.[8] For older children, CSI of 18 to 36 Gy with boost to 50.4 to 54 Gy for gross disease is standard, and these children are eligible for the high-risk medulloblastoma COG trials (see Chapter 56). CHT can be delivered prior to CSI for young children or those with less than complete resection in which a second-look surgery after CHT could be beneficial.

INTRACRANIAL GERM CELL TUMOR

Epidemiology: Intracranial germ cell tumor is a heterogeneous group of tumors that represent 3% of childhood CNS malignancies. GCT are more commonly found in adolescents age 10 to 20 years old and spread through the subependymal lining and CSF, but rarely metastasize outside the CNS. Metastatic disease in the neuroaxis is present in 5% to 10% at diagnosis.

Pathology: GCT are categorized by WHO classification into pure germinoma and non-germinomatous germ cell tumor (NGGCT), which represent two-thirds and one-third of cases, respectively. NGGCT are further categorized as embryonal carcinoma, endodermal sinus/yolk sac tumor, choriocarcinoma, teratoma, and mixed tumors.

Tumor markers: Elevation of beta-human chorionic gonadotropin (β-hCG) and alpha-fetoprotein (AFP) in the serum and/or CSF are tumor markers associated with subtypes of NGGCT (Table 65.1). Included is the most recent COG trial cutoff for pure germinoma categorization, as syncytiotrophoblastic cells present in pure germinoma can cause a slight elevation of β-hCG.

Table 65.1: Tumor Markers		
	β-hCG (IU/L)	AFP (µg/L)
Pure germinoma	<100	<20 (or lab normal)
Immature teratoma Pure endodermal sinus/yolk sac Choriocarcinoma	100–1,000 >1,000 >1,000	20–50 >500 >500

Anatomy: Most commonly occur in the pineal gland, then the suprasellar region which can be associated with diabetes insipidus. Due to subependymal spread, patients may have plaque-like spread along ventricular lining that is not visible on MRI, but is an important factor guiding RT techniques. Pineal gland tumors can cause compression of the medial longitudinal fasciculus resulting in Parinaud's syndrome, a constellation of upward gaze palsy, convergence nystagmus, and impaired pupillary constriction but preserved accommodation.

Workup: May be delayed due to nonspecific symptoms such as pituitary dysfunction or increased intracranial pressure due to obstruction of the cerebral aqueduct.[9,10] *Imaging:* Includes contrast-enhanced MRI of the brain and entire spine. Occasionally, the primary tumor may be of subclinical size and not visible on imaging.[11] If GCT is found to involve both the suprasellar region and pineal gland the patient has bifocal disease, which is not metastatic. Bifocal disease is more commonly associated with pure germinoma. *Labs:* Serum and CSF tumor markers as above (CSF via LP if safe). *Pathology:* If safe, intracranial biopsy is necessary; complete resection rare due to risks (occasionally for teratoma). Occasionally, biopsy may obtain only a fraction of a mixed tumor and lead to inaccurate diagnosis.

Prognosis: Very favorable, with 95% 5-year OS for pure germinomas, which are treatment sensitive and require less intense therapy.[12] NGGCT are more aggressive but with multimodality treatment exhibit 5-year OS of 90%.[13] Given the excellent outcomes following therapy, decreasing treatment associated morbidity has been a focus of most clinical trials, specifically attempts to move away from CSI for nonmetastatic disease and decrease RT dose.

Treatment Paradigm: Defined by subtype and utilizes multimodality therapy. The role of up-front surgery at diagnosis is often restricted to biopsy as the morbidity and mortality of up-front surgical resection can near 20%.[14] Second-look surgery is recommended for patients with inadequate radiographic tumor reduction following CHT but with normalization of serum and CSF tumor markers.[15]

Pure germinoma: The current standard of care for nonmetastatic pure germinoma includes CHT with four cycles of carboplatin/etoposide, followed by 21 to 24 Gy WVI with 9 to 12 Gy per boost

ACNS1123. In prior studies of involved field RT alone, over 80% of failures were located in the periventricular region, supporting WVI as standard.[16] If CHT is not given, full dose CSI is an acceptable alternative. Metastatic patients should receive 21 to 24 Gy CSI with 9 to 12 Gy boost after CHT. The lower dose is often used for patients with a CR or PR to CHT. Two recently completed clinical trials, ACNS 1123 and SIOP CNS GCT II, will inform if 18 Gy WVI with 12 Gy boost and omission of tumor bed boost in the setting of a CR to CHT, respectively, are acceptable.

NGGCT: Nonmetastatic NGGCT is treated with six cycles of carboplatin/etoposide alternating with ifosfamide/etoposide prior to RT. CSI to 36 Gy with 18 Gy boost is the current RT standard; however, ACNS1123 investigated 30.6 Gy WVI with 23.4 Gy boost for patients with a CR or PR to CHT. The results demonstrated 3-year PFS of 88%; however, there was a unique pattern of failure in that all patients progressed in the spine.[17] Future investigations for the next NGGCT trial, ACNS 2021, includes WVI with full spine RT.

REFERENCES

1. Reddy AT, Strother DR, Judkins AR, et al. Efficacy of high-dose chemotherapy and three-dimensional conformal radiation for atypical teratoid/rhabdoid tumor: a report from the Children's Oncology Group Trial ACNS0333. *J Clin Oncol.* 2020;38(11):1175–1185. doi:10.1200/JCO.19.01776

2. Rorke LB, Packer R, Biegel J. Central nervous system atypical teratoid/rhabdoid tumors of infancy and childhood. *J Neurooncol.* 1995;24(1):21–28. doi:10.1007/BF01052653

3. Pawel BR. SMARCB1-deficient tumors of childhood: a practical guide. *Pediatr Dev Pathol.* 2018;21(1):6–28. doi:10.1177/1093526617749671

4. Pai Panandiker AS, Merchant TE, Beltran C, et al. Sequencing of local therapy affects the pattern of treatment failure and survival in children with atypical teratoid rhabdoid tumors of the central nervous system. *Int J Radiat Oncol Biol Phys.* 2012;82(5):1756–1763. doi:10.1016/j.ijrobp.2011.02.059

5. Hwang EI, Kool M, Burger PC, et al. Extensive molecular and clinical heterogeneity in patients with histologically diagnosed CNS-PNET treated as a single entity: a report from the Children's Oncology Group Randomized ACNS0332 Trial. *J Clin Oncol.* 2018;36(34):3388–3395. doi:10.1200/JCO.2017.76.4720

6. Jin MC, Prolo LM, Wu A, et al. Patterns of care and age-specific impact of extent of resection and Adjuvant Radiotherapy in Pediatric Pineoblastoma. *Neurosurgery.* 2020;86(5):E426–E435. doi:10.1093/neuros/nyaa023

7. Parikh KA, Venable GT, Orr BA, et al. Pineoblastoma-the experience at St. Jude children's research hospital. *Neurosurgery.* 2017;81(1):120–128. doi:10.1093/neuros/nyx005

8. Abdelbaki MS, Abu-Arja MH, Davidson TB, et al. Pineoblastoma in children less than six years of age: The Head Start I, II, and III experience. *Pediatr Blood Cancer.* 2020;67(6):e28252. doi:10.1002/pbc.28252

9. Sethi RV, Marino R, Niemierko A, et al. Delayed diagnosis in children with intracranial germ cell tumors. *J Pediatr.* 2013;163(5):1448–1453. doi:10.1016/j.jpeds.2013.06.024

10. Mootha SL, Barkovich AJ, Grumbach MM, et al. Idiopathic hypothalamic diabetes insipidus, pituitary stalk thickening, and the occult intracranial germinoma in children and adolescents. *J Clin Endocrinol Metab.* 1997;82(5):1362–1367. doi:10.1210/jc.82.5.1362

11. Liang L, Korogi Y, Sugahara T, et al. MRI of intracranial germ-cell tumours. *Neuroradiology.* 2002;44(5):382–388. doi:10.1007/s00234-001-0752-0

12. Calaminus G, Kortmann R, Worch J, et al. SIOP CNS GCT 96: final report of outcome of a prospective, multinational nonrandomized trial for children and adults with intracranial germinoma, comparing craniospinal irradiation alone with chemotherapy followed by focal primary site irradiation for patients with localized disease. *Neuro Oncol.* 2013;15(6):788–796. doi:10.1093/neuonc/not019

13. Goldman S, Bouffet E, Fisher PG, et al. Phase II trial assessing the ability of neoadjuvant chemotherapy with or without second-look surgery to eliminate measurable disease for nongerminomatous germ cell tumors: a Children's Oncology Group Study. *J Clin Oncol.* 2015;33(22):2464–2471. doi:10.1200/JCO.2014.59.5132

14. Calaminus G, Bamberg M, Jürgens H, et al. Impact of surgery, chemotherapy and irradiation on long term outcome of intracranial malignant non-germinomatous germ cell tumors: results of the German Cooperative Trial MAKEI 89. *Klin Padiatr.* 2004;216(3):141–149. doi:10.1055/s-2004-822626

15. Calaminus G, Bamberg M, Harms D, et al. AFP/beta-HCG secreting CNS germ cell tumors: long-term outcome with respect to initial symptoms and primary tumor resection. Results of the cooperative trial MAKEI 89. *Neuropediatrics.* 2005;36(2):71–77. doi:10.1055/s-2005-837582

16. Alapetite C, Brisse H, Patte C, et al. Pattern of relapse and outcome of non-metastatic germinoma patients treated with chemotherapy and limited field radiation: the SFOP experience. *Neuro-Oncol.* 2010;12(12):1318–1325.

17. Fangusaro J, Wu S, MacDonald S, et al. Phase II trial of response-based radiation therapy for patients with localized CNS nongerminomatous germ cell tumors: a Children's Oncology Group Study. *J Clin Oncol.* 2019;37(34):3283–3290. doi:10.1200/JCO.19.00701

66 ■ BRAIN METASTASES

Shauna R. Campbell, Martin C. Tom, and John H. Suh

QUICK HIT ■ Brain metastases are the most common intracranial tumor. Surgery, WBRT, HA-WBRT, and SRS are all treatment options and can be performed in many combinations based on careful patient selection.[1] Key factors for patient selection include performance status, number and size of lesions, histology, and status of extracranial disease. Typically, surgery is reserved for large or symptomatic lesions or when a tissue sample is required. SRS is preferred over WBRT due to less neurocognitive side effects and QOL benefit for patients with limited or intermediate volume intracranial disease.

EPIDEMIOLOGY: Most common intracranial tumor, with ~240,000 cases per year. Brain metastases occur in up to 30% of patients with cancer and are the direct cause of death in 30% to 50% of those. Incidence has increased in the MRI era due to the detection of smaller lesions as well as advances in cancer treatment allowing for longer patient survival.[2] Solitary brain metastasis is defined as a single lesion without evidence of extracranial disease; however, 80% of patients have multiple lesions.

ANATOMY: Most commonly occur at the gray–white matter junction due to decrease in diameter of blood vessels. Typically spherical, well-demarcated lesions with edema: 80% supratentorial, 15% cerebellum, and 5% brainstem.

PATHOLOGY: Most common histologies (overall prevalence) include lung (50%), breast (20%), melanoma (10%), and colon (5%).[2] Histologies with the highest predilection for the development of brain metastases (neurotropism) include SCLC, melanoma, choriocarcinoma, and germ cell. Hemorrhagic lesions are typically melanoma, choriocarcinoma, testicular, thyroid, and renal cell.

CLINICAL PRESENTATION: Variable but most commonly include impaired cognitive function (60%), hemiparesis (60%), headache (50%), aphasia (20%), and seizures (20%).[2]

WORKUP: H&P with detailed neurologic exam.

Imaging: Noncontrast head CT is often first-line test performed to rule out intracranial hemorrhage. MRI with and without contrast is best to detect and characterize small metastases. Biopsy may be necessary if the patient has no evidence of disease elsewhere. For patients presumed to have a single brain metastasis on imaging, up to 10% can be primary brain tumors,[3] although this is likely lower in the MRI era. For multiple lesions, >95% are metastatic rather than primary tumors and biopsy is not required.

PROGNOSTIC FACTORS: Numerous prognostic systems have been developed and updated to reflect contemporary outcomes. The initial RPA was developed by the RTOG, followed by the GPA (Table 66.1), then the diagnosis-specific GPA (Table 66.2), which was recently updated and is available at brainmetgpa.com.[4-6] Brain metastasis velocity (number of new brain metastases per year since initial SRS) ≥4 can help predict survival outcomes.[7]

Table 66.1: Original Graded Prognostic Assessment					
Graded prognostic assessment					
Characteristic	0	0.5	1.0	Grade	MS (mos)
Age	>60	50–59	<50	3.5–4	11.0
KPS	<70	70–80	90–100	3	6.9
# CNS metastases	>3	2–3	1	1.5–2.5	3.8
Extracranial metastases	Present	–	Absent	0–1	2.6

Source: From Sperduto PW, Berkey B, Gaspar LE, Mehta M, Curran W. A new prognostic index and comparison to three other indices for patients with brain metastases: an analysis of 1,960 patients in the RTOG database. *Int J Radiat Oncol Biol Phys.* 2008;70:510–514. doi:10.1016/j.ijrobp.2007.06.074. With permission from Elsevier.

Table 66.2: Diagnosis-Specific GPA					
Variable	0	0.5	1	1.5	2
	NSCLC				
Age	≥70	<70			
KPS	≤70	80	90–100		
Number of brain mets	≥5	1–4			
Extracranial mets	Present	–	Absent		
EGFR and ALK (adeno only)	Both negative or unknown	–	EGFR or ALK positive		
	Sum = MS (months) by GPA: Adenocarcinoma: 0–1 = 7; 1.5–2.0 = 13; 2.5–3.0 = 25; 3.5–4.0 = 46 Nonadenocarcinoma: 0–1 = 5; 1.5–2.0 = 10; 2.5–3.0 = 13; 3.5–4.0 = NA				
	Breast				
KPS	≤60	70–80	90–100		
Age	≥60	<60			
Number of brain mets	≥2	1			
Extracranial mets	Present	Absent			
Subtype	Triple negative	Luminal A (ER/PR+, HER2–)	–	HER2+ or Luminal B (triple +)	
	Sum = MS (months) by GPA: 0–1 = 6; 1.5–2.0 = 13; 2.5–3.0 = 24; 3.5–4.0 = 36				
	Renal				
KPS	≤70	–	80	–	90–100
Number of brain mets	≥5	1–4			
Extracranial mets	Present	Absent			
Hemoglobin	<11.1	11.1–12.5 or unknown	>12.5		
	Sum = MS (mos) by GPA: 0–1 = 4; 1.5–2.0 = 12; 2.5–3.0 = 17; 3.5–4.0 = 35				
	Melanoma				
Age	≥70	<70			
KPS	≤70	80	90–100		
Number of brain mets	≥5	2–4	1		

(continued)

Table 66.2: Diagnosis-Specific GPA (*continued*)					
Extracranial mets	Present	–	Absent		
BRAF	Negative or unknown	Positive			
	Sum = MS (months) by GPA: 0–1 = 5; 1.5–2.0 = 8; 2.5–3.0 = 16; 3.5–4.0 = 34				
	GI				
KPS	<70	–	80	–	90–100
Age	≥60	< 60			
Number brain mets	≥4	2–3	1		
Extracranial mets	Present	Absent			
	Sum = MS (months) by GPA: 0–1 = 3; 1.5–2.0 = 7; 2.5–3.0 = 11; 3.5–4.0 = 17				

Source: From Sperduto PW, Mesko S, Li J, et al. Survival in patients with brain metastases: summary report on the updated diagnosis-specific graded prognostic assessment and definition of the eligibility quotient. *J Clin Oncol*. 2020;38(32):3773–3784. doi:10.1200/JCO.20.01255

TREATMENT PARADIGM

Medical: Glucocorticoids such as dexamethasone are first-line medical therapy to improve symptoms in up to 75% within 1 to 3 days. Acute side effects include insomnia, hypergylcemia, irritability, and weight gain. Effects from long-term use include Cushingoid appearance, gastric ulcers (require GI prophylaxis), osteopenia, and proximal muscle weakness. Radiosensitizers such as motexafin gadolinium[8] and efaproxiral[9] have been studied with no demonstrable benefit.

Neurocognitive Protectant: Memantine is an NMDA receptor antagonist used for dementia and can be given with WBRT to minimize neurocognitive decline as demonstrated on RTOG 0614 (see following).

Surgery: Recommended for larger symptomatic lesions or when tissue diagnosis is necessary. A stereotactic approach with maximal safe resection is standard.

Systemic Therapy: Historically, there has been little role for CHT in the treatment of brain metastases due to the blood–brain barrier with the exception of metastatic germ cell tumors (e.g., testicular); however, with new targeted agents and immunotherapy, there is evidence of improved intracranial efficacy.[10,11] Brain metastases from EGFR and ALK mutant NSCLC, PD-L1 expressing NSCLC, HER2 amplified breast cancer, and melanoma all have approved agents with potential intracranial efficacy; however, these have not yet been proven to replace local therapy.[12]

Radiotherapy: RT is the cornerstone of treatment for brain metastases and is indicated in most patients except for those with exceptionally poor prognosis (see QUARTZ trial following). Options include SRS or WBRT.

Dose: For WBRT, dose options include 30 Gy/10 fx (most common), 37.5 Gy/15 fx (common on older RTOG trials but has not demonstrated improved outcomes),[13] 20 Gy/5 fx, and 10 Gy/1fx. HA-WBRT is delivered with 30 Gy/10 fx. The use of HA-WBRT with a simultaneous integrated boost to metastases is under evaluation.[14–16]

SRS: Traditionally, SRS delivers a single high-dose treatment using multiple converging beams.[17] Metastases are often ideal targets for SRS considering they are small, spherical, well-demarcated, and located at the gray–white matter junction away from critical structures. Dosing is performed per RTOG 9005 (see the following): 24 Gy for lesions ≤2 cm, 18 Gy for lesions 2.1 to 3.0 cm, and 15 Gy for those 3.1 to 4 cm. Lesions ≥2 cm may have worse LC and may be treated with fractionated SRS (common doses include 27 Gy/3 fx or 30 Gy/5 fx)[18–21] or staged SRS delivered 2 to 4 weeks apart.[22,23]

Postoperative SRS to the cavity of a resected brain metastasis decreases the risk of LR. Dose varies by institution but can be defined by the N107C study; 20 Gy if cavity volume <4.2 mL, 18 Gy if 4.2 to 7.9 mL, 17 Gy if 8.0 to 14.3 mL, 15 Gy if 14.4 to 19.9 mL, 14 Gy if 20.0 to 29.9 mL, and 12 Gy if ≥30.0 mL up to the maximal surgical cavity extent of 5 cm.[24] Preoperative SRS is currently being investigated, as it may address limitations of postoperative SRS including a higher incidence of LF, leptomeningeal disease, and radionecrosis compared with WBRT.[25] Phase III trials comparing pre- and postoperative SRS are currently being conducted (NCT03750227 and NCT03741673).

Of note, SCLC patients have historically been excluded from SRS studies, though recent retrospective data have shown potential for upfront SRS in this population[26] and phase II trials are currently ongoing (NCT03391362, NCT04516070, NCT03297788).

Toxicity: Side effects of SRS include fatigue, headache, nausea, radionecrosis, damage to nearby critical structures (optic nerve, chiasm, brainstem), and neurocognitive decline (less than WBRT). Side effects of WBRT include fatigue, hair loss, skin erythema, headache, nausea, temporary muffled hearing, and neurocognitive decline.

Procedure: See *Handbook of Treatment Planning in Radiation Oncology*, Chapters 3 and 13.[27]

■ EVIDENCE-BASED Q&A

▓ Is there a benefit to WBRT over best supportive care?

In poor performance patients with NSCLC not eligible for SRS or resection, the benefit of WBRT is questionable based on the QUARTZ study.

Mulvenna, QUARTZ (*Lancet* 2016, PMID 27604504): PRT (noninferiority) of optimal supportive care (OSC) vs. 20 Gy/5 fx WBRT for NSCLC. Primary end point was QALY (calculated using EQ-5D) with a noninferiority margin of 7 QALY days. Enrolled 538 patients, 83% were GPA 0 to 2 and 38% had a KPS <70. Did not demonstrate a difference in OS (HR 1.06, p = .81) or QALY days (mean QALYs 46.4 days WBRT vs. 41.7 days OSC, 4.7 QALY-day difference with 90% CI: −12.7– 3.3). Dexamethasone use was not significantly different. There were nonsignificant suggestions that WBRT may offer a survival benefit in patients with better prognoses. **Conclusion: Although OSC noninferiority was not met, WBRT may be unnecessary in poor performance patients.** *Comment: Patients selected for this trial were poor performance at baseline; results may not apply to patients with more favorable performance status.*

▓ Is there a benefit to dose escalation or hyperfractionation of WBRT?

There is no benefit to WBRT dose escalation with hyperfractionation.

Regine, RTOG 9104 (*IJROBP* 2001, PMID 9336134): PRT of 445 patients with a KPS ≥70 and NFS 1 to 2 randomized to either 30 Gy/10 fx or WBRT 32 Gy/20 fx with a boost to a total of 54.4 Gy/34 fx at 1.6 Gy BID. There was no difference in survival or grade 3 to 4 toxicity, but one fatal toxicity in the high-dose arm. **Conclusion: No benefit to dose escalation with hyperfractionation.**

▓ What is the role of surgery in patients with a single brain metastasis?

Surgery is beneficial for select patients and is typically reserved for patients with large and relatively few lesions in a resectable location. Three trials have looked at adding surgery to WBRT and two (Patchell I and Noordijk[28]) showed a survival benefit. The third did not show an OS benefit but enrolled poor-performance patients.[29]

Patchell I (*NEJM* 1990, PMID 2405271): PRT of 48 patients with single brain metastasis randomized to biopsy followed by WBRT vs. surgical resection with WBRT (36 Gy/12 fx). Of note, 6 of 54 patients (11%) were found to have a primary brain tumor or benign findings (pre-MRI era) (Results in Table 66.3). **Conclusion: Surgical resection + WBRT for a single brain metastasis improves OS compared to WBRT alone.**

Table 66.3: Patchell I Results

	LR	Time to LR	DM	MS	Time to Neurologic Death	Functional Independence
Biopsy + WBRT	52%	21 wk	13%	15 wk	26 wk	8 wk
Surgery + WBRT	20%	59 wk	20%	40 wk	62 wk	38 wk
p value	<.02	<.0001	.52	<.01	<.0009	<.005

■ **Does WBRT improve outcomes after surgery?**

Patchell II (*JAMA* **1998, PMID 9809728**): PRT of 95 patients with one brain metastasis and KPS ≥70 randomized to surgery alone vs. surgery with postoperative WBRT (50.4 Gy/28 fx). Nearly all outcomes were improved except survival; however, the trial was not powered for survival (Results in Table 66.4.). **Conclusion: WBRT after surgical resection of a single brain met improves local and distant brain control.**

Table 66.4: Patchell II Results

	Any Recurrence	Distant Recurrence	LR	MS	Neurologic Death	Functional Independence
Surgery	70%	37%	46%	43 wk	44%	35 wk
Surgery + RT	18%	14%	10%	48 wk	14%	37 wk
p value	<.001	<.01	<.001	.39	.003	.61

■ **What determines the dose of SRS?**

Dosing is based on tumor diameter as established by RTOG 9005. LC for larger metastases is suboptimal with single fx, and various attempts at improving outcomes for these patients are noted in the following.

Shaw, RTOG 9005 (*IJROBP* 2000, PMID 10802351): Phase I/II SRS dose escalation trial for patients with a recurrent primary brain tumor (36%) or metastases (64%) ≤4 cm after receiving previous brain RT ≥3 months prior. Treated to escalating dose levels. MTD was 15 Gy for tumors 3.1 to 4 cm and 18 Gy for tumors 2.1 to 3 cm. Investigators were unwilling to escalate above 24 Gy to tumors ≤2.0 cm even though MTD was not observed. A homogeneity index (ratio of max dose/prescription dose) of ≥2 was associated with increased toxicity. Incidence of radionecrosis was 11% at 2 years.

■ **When added to standard WBRT, does an SRS boost improve survival?**

SRS boost improves LC after WBRT, with no clear impact on OS.

Andrews, RTOG 9508 (*Lancet* 2004, PMID 15158627): Patients with one to three new brain metastases each ≤4 cm randomized to WBRT or WBRT + SRS boost. WBRT dose was 37.5 Gy/15 fx and boost was given 1 week after WBRT using RTOG 9005 SRS doses. While there was an improvement in LC, KPS, and steroid use in all patients, the primary endpoint of OS was not met (Table 66.5). Patients with a single metastasis did demonstrate a survival benefit (pre-planned stratification). On an unplanned subset analysis, patients in RPA class I, those with large metastases (>2 cm), squamous or NSCLC, or KPS 90 to 100 experienced a benefit that was not statistically significant after adjustment for unplanned subgroup analyses. **Conclusion: SRS boost improves LC after WBRT.**

Table 66.5: RTOG 9508 Results

RTOG 9508	Mean Survival (mos)						1-Yr LC	Stable/Improved KPS at 6 mos
	Overall	Single Met	*Tumor >2 cm	*RPA Class I	*Squamous/ NSCLC	*KPS 90–100		
WBRT alone	6.5	4.9	5.3	9.6	3.9	7.4	71%	25%
WBRT + SRS	5.7	6.5	6.5	11.6	5.9	10.2	82%	42%
p value	.136	.039	.045	.045	.051	.071	.013	.033

*Subset analysis, *p* value for significance = .0056

- **If SRS boost does not improve survival compared to WBRT alone, does WBRT improve survival when added to SRS?**

Aoyama (*JAMA* 2006, PMID 16757720): Randomized 132 patients with one to four brain metastases all ≤3 cm to WBRT (30 Gy/10 fx) with SRS vs. SRS alone. SRS doses alone were 22 to 25 Gy for tumors ≤2 cm, and 18 to 20 Gy for tumors >2 cm and reduced by 30% if given after WBRT. 49% had a single metastasis, 83% were RPA class II. Primary end point OS. Closed early on interim analysis because of higher than anticipated sample size needed to show a difference in OS. (Complete results in Table 66.6). Rate of LR and any recurrence were decreased significantly by WBRT. **Conclusion: The addition of WBRT does not confer a survival benefit when added to SRS, although not sufficiently powered for this endpoint.**

Table 66.6: Aoyama Trial Results

	MS	Neurologic Death	1-Yr Any Recurrence	1-Yr LR	1-Yr Distant Recurrence	Neurologic Preservation
SRS alone	8.0 m	19%	76%	27.5%	64%	70%
WBRT + SRS	7.5 m	23%	47%	11%	42%	72%
p value	.42	.64	<.001	.002	.003	.99

- **If survival is not improved by adding SRS to WBRT, do the neurocognitive risks of adding WBRT to SRS outweigh the benefits?**

The addition of WBRT to SRS leads to increased neurocognitive decline without a survival benefit compared to SRS alone in patients with limited brain metastases.

Chang, MD Anderson (*Lancet Oncol* 2009, PMID 19801201): PRT with one to three brain metastases to SRS with or without WBRT (similar arms to Aoyama) with primary endpoint of deterioration of HVLT-R-TR domain by five points at 4 months from treatment. Trial stopped early after 58 patients enrolled due to increased decline in WBRT arm. LC improved from 67% to 100% with WBRT and distant control by 45% to 73%. However, neurocognitive function declined in 23% of SRS patients vs. 49% of WBRT+SRS patients. **Conclusion: SRS + WBRT patients experienced a significant decline in neurocognitive function. SRS alone may be the preferred treatment strategy.** *Comment: MS was 15.2 months (SRS) vs. 5.7 months (WBRT+SRS), suggesting imbalance of patients in two arms.*

Kocher, EORTC 22952 (*JCO* 2011, PMID 21041710): PRT of 359 patients with one to three brain metastases randomized to observation or WBRT (30 Gy/10 fx) after either SRS or surgery. Primary end point was time to WHO PS >2. No difference in OS (10.7 vs. 10.9 months) and WBRT improved local failure (31% SRS, 59% surgery, 19% SRS+WBRT, and 27% surgery + WBRT) and any in-brain failure (42% surgery, 48% SRS, 33% SRS + WBRT, and 23% surgery +WBRT). No difference in the time to PS >2. **Conclusion: WBRT can be omitted in select patients with appropriate imaging follow-up.**

Sahgal, Meta-analysis (*IJROBP* 2015, PMID 25752382): Individual patient level meta-analysis of 359 patients from Aoyama, Chang, and Kocher trials, investigating SRS alone vs. WBRT + SRS in patients with one to four brain metastases. Age was a significant predictor of the effect of WBRT on OS and distant cranial failure. Younger patients treated with SRS alone had a lower hazard of mortality (MS for age ≤50: 13.6 months SRS alone vs. 8.2 months SRS+WBRT). Younger patients (≤50) also did not benefit in terms of distant brain failure, but patients >50 did benefit from the addition of WBRT. The addition of WBRT to SRS showed a local control benefit across all subgroups. **Conclusion: SRS alone may be the treatment of choice for patients ≤50 with one to four brain metastases.**

Brown, NCCTG N0574 (*JAMA* 2016, PMID 27458945): PRT of 213 patients with one to three brain metastases all <3 cm randomized to SRS or WBRT+SRS. Primary end point was declined in any of six cognitive tests (HVLT-R-IR, HVLT-R-DR, COWA, Trailmaking A & B, and Grooved Pegboard) at 3 months >1 standard deviation from baseline. 213 randomized, 111 included in primary endpoint analysis (63 in SRS arm, 48 in SRS+WBRT arm). Cognitive decline at 3 months was more common after WBRT+SRS than SRS alone (91.7% vs. 63.5%, $p < .001$). This was true across immediate recall, delayed recall, and verbal fluency. QOL was also improved in SRS group with no difference in functional independence. In-brain control was better in WBRT arm (93.7% vs. 75.3% at 3 months, $p < .001$) but survival was not different (10.4 months SRS vs. 7.4 months SRS+WBRT, $p = .92$). **Conclusion: WBRT does not improve survival despite better tumor control and is associated with more cognitive deterioration. SRS alone may be the preferred strategy.**

- **If WBRT is associated with a decline in neurocognitive function, what are some possible strategies to avoid this?**

Adding memantine and hippocampus sparing are two strategies to decrease the neurocognitive detriment associated with WBRT.

Brown, RTOG 0614 (*Neuro-Oncol* 2013, PMID 23956241): PRT of patients with KPS ≥70 and stable systemic disease randomized to receive 20 mg of memantine vs. placebo during and after WBRT for a total of 24 weeks. Dose was up-titrated by 5 mg weekly starting at 5 mg daily up to 10 mg BID for weeks 4 to 24. Primary endpoint was declined in HVLT-R-DR at 24 weeks compared to baseline, which trended toward improvement ($p = .059$) but statistical power was limited due to patient loss. The memantine arm did have statistically significant longer time to cognitive decline, lower probability of cognitive failure, and superior results for executive function, processing speed, and delayed recognition at 24 weeks. **Conclusion: Memantine is a well-tolerated medication and patients who received memantine compared with placebo had better cognitive function over time, although patient loss to follow-up limited significance of the primary endpoint.**

Brown, NRG CC001 (*JCO* 2020, PMID 32058845): Randomized phase III trial of 518 patients with brain metastases, stratified by RPA and prior SRS/surgery, randomized to WBRT (30 Gy/10 fx) + memantine vs. HA-WBRT + memantine. Primary end point was time to neurocognitive failure, defined as an established decline in one of the neurocognitive tests (HVLT, Trail Making, or COWA). No difference in OS, intracranial PFS, or toxicity between arms. Cognitive failure risk significantly lower in the HA-WBRT arm compared with the WBRT arm (HR 0.76; 95% CI 0.60–0.98; $p = .03$). The lower cognitive failure was secondary to statistically significantly less deterioration in executive functioning at 4 months and learning and memory at 6 months. On MVA age >61 years was also significant for time-to-cognitive failure (HR 0.635, $p = .0016$). HA-WBRT was also associated with less fatigue, difficulty remembering things, speaking, interference of neurologic symptoms with daily activities, and fewer cognitive symptoms (all $p < .05$). **Conclusion: HA-WBRT has comparable efficacy to standard WBRT, but better preserves neurocognitive function with the benefit first appreciated at 4 months pos treatment.**

- **How many metastases are necessary to warrant WBRT rather than SRS?**

The trend with modern planning systems is to treat with SRS alone to avoid WBRT but the specific number or volume remains unclear.

Yamamato, Japan (*Lancet Oncol* 2014, PMID 24621620): Prospective observational study of patients with 1 to 10 new metastases (maximum <3 cm) treated with SRS alone. Patients with 5 to 10 lesions were compared with patients with one tumor and patients with two to four tumors. Primary end point was OS. Results showed that OS did not differ between the 5 to 10 cohorts when compared to the 2 to 4 cohorts (noninferior). The rate of adverse events was also similar. **Conclusion: SRS may be suitable in patients with up to 10 brain metastases.**

Li, MDACC (ASTRO Abstract 2020): Phase III RCT of 72 patients with 4 to 15 untreated nonmelanoma brain metastases randomized to SRS ($n = 36$) or WBRT ($n = 36$). Prior SRS to one to three brain metastases with at least 3 months interval was permitted. Median number of brain metastases was 8, and 31 patients were evaluable for primary endpoint of HVLT-R-TR at 4 months. WBRT treated patients had greater decline in HVLT-R-TR compared with SRS patients ($p = .041$). MS 10.4 months for SRS and 8.4 months for WBRT ($p = .45$). **Conclusion: Nonmelanoma patients with 4 to 15 brain metastases can be treated with SRS without a detriment in OS based on abstract results.** *Note: Trial was closed early as HA-WBRT became standard.*

■ **What treatment options are there for large metastases who are not surgical candidates?**

Larger tumors treated with SRS have suboptimal LC using RTOG 9005 dosing.[30] *Strategies to improve LC include fractionated*[19–21,31] *and staged SRS*[22,23,32] *with the goal of dose escalation while limiting toxicity such as radionecrosis.*[17] Data from prospective studies investigating these SRS techniques to determine the optimal dose, fractionation, and timing for large brain metastases will be important to guide future standards.

■ **Is postoperative SRS to the resection cavity effective at reducing LF after complete resection?**

Mahajan, MDACC (*Lancet Oncol* 2017, PMID 28687375): Single-institution PRT of 132 patients randomized after complete resection of one to three metastases to either observation or postoperative SRS. MFU 11.1 months. Primary end point LR. At 12 months, freedom from LR was 43% in the observation group vs. 72% with SRS (*p* = .015). **Conclusion: Following complete resection of brain metastases, postoperative SRS reduces LR compared to observation.**

■ **Can SRS offer similar rates of control in the postoperative setting to WBRT but without the neurocognitive deficits?**

In an attempt to maintain control rates while decreasing neurocognitive changes, SRS can be given to the resection cavity, with initial retrospective data favoring a 2-mm margin around the cavity.[33] *Note that dosing to the resection cavity is often by volume rather than by diameter, but this varies by institution.*

Brown, N107C (*Lancet Oncol* 2017, PMID 28687377): PRT of 194 patients with ≤4 metastases (all <3 cm) with resection of a single lesion (cavity <5 cm), then randomized to WBRT (with SRS to unresected metastases) vs. SRS alone to the cavity and unresected lesions. Co-primary end points were OS and cognitive deterioration free survival (CDFS) at 6 months, defined as death or a drop by 1 standard deviation in one test (HVLT, COWA, Trailmaking A & B). Preferred sequencing was SRS to unresected metastases followed by WBRT within 14 days. Dosing to the surgical bed was 12 to 20 Gy depending on tumor volume (dosing to unresected lesions was 18 to 24 Gy depending on arm and diameter). No difference in OS (MS 12.2 months SRS vs. 11.6 months WBRT, *p* = .70). CDFS was improved in SRS arm: median 3.7 months vs. 3.0 months, *p* < .0001). **Conclusion: Postoperative SRS provides comparable OS with less neurocognitive deterioration as compared to WBRT and is thus preferred. This is an acceptable alternative to WBRT after resection of a brain metastasis with less cognitive deterioration.**

Kayama, JCOG 0504 (*JCO* 2018, PMID 29924704): PRT (noninferiority) of 271 patients with ≤4 lesions surgically resected with only one lesion >3 cm were randomized to SRS or WBRT after surgery. Primary end point was OS. MS 15.6 months on both arms, with HR of 1.05 (*p* = .027) meeting noninferiority criteria. Grades 2 to 4 cognitive dysfunction beyond 90 days was higher in WBRT arm (16.4% vs. 7.7%, *p* = .048) but the proportion of patients whose MMSE did not worsen were similar in both arms. **Conclusion: With respect to OS, postoperative salvage SRS is noninferior to WBRT.**

REFERENCES

1. Suh JH, Kotecha R, Chao ST, et al. Current approaches to the management of brain metastases. *Nat Rev Clin Oncol.* 2020;17(5):279–299. doi:10.1038/s41571-019-0320-3
2. Nichols EM, Patchell RA, Regine WF, et al. Palliation of brain and spinal cord metastases. In: Halperin EC, Wazer DE, Perez CA, Brady LW, eds. *Perez and Brady's Principles and Practice of Radiation Oncology.* 7th ed. Lippincott Williams & Wilkins; 2018.
3. Patchell RA, Tibbs PA, Walsh JW, et al. A randomized trial of surgery in the treatment of single metastases to the brain. *N Engl J Med.* 1990;322(8):494–500. doi:10.1056/NEJM199002223220802
4. Gaspar L, Scott C, Rotman M, et al. Recursive partitioning analysis (RPA) of prognostic factors in three Radiation Therapy Oncology Group (RTOG) brain metastases trials. *Int J Radiat Oncol Biol Phys.* 1997;37:745–751. doi:10.1016/S0360-3016(96)00619-0
5. Sperduto PW, Berkey B, Gaspar LE, et al. A new prognostic index and comparison to three other indices for patients with brain metastases: an analysis of 1,960 patients in the RTOG database. *Int J Radiat Oncol Biol Phys.* 2008;70:510–514. doi:10.1016/j.ijrobp.2007.06.074

6. Sperduto PW, Mesko S, Li J, et al. Survival in patients with brain metastases: summary report on the updated diagnosis-specific graded prognostic assessment and definition of the eligibility quotient. *J Clin Oncol.* 2020;38(32):3773–3784. doi:10.1200/JCO.20.01255

7. Farris M, McTyre ER, Cramer CK, et al. Brain metastasis velocity: a novel prognostic metric predictive of overall survival and freedom from whole-brain radiation therapy after distant brain failure following upfront radiosurgery alone. *Int J Radiat Oncol Biol Phys.* 2017;98(1):131–141. doi:10.1016/j.ijrobp.2017.01.201

8. Mehta MP, Rodrigus P, Terhaard CH, et al. Survival and neurologic outcomes in a randomized trial of motexafin gadolinium and whole-brain radiation therapy in brain metastases. *J Clin Oncol.* 2003;21(13):2529–2536. doi:10.1200/JCO.2003.12.122

9. Suh JH, Stea B, Nabid A, et al. Phase III study of efaproxiral as an adjunct to whole-brain radiation therapy for brain metastases. *J Clin Oncol.* 2006;24(1):106–114. doi:10.1200/JCO.2004.00.1768

10. Goldberg SB, Gettinger SN, Mahajan A, et al. Pembrolizumab for patients with melanoma or non-small-cell lung cancer and untreated brain metastases: early analysis of a non-randomised, open-label, phase 2 trial. *Lancet Oncol.* 2016;17(7):976–983. doi:10.1016/S1470-2045(16)30053-5

11. Goldberg SB, Schalper KA, Gettinger SN, et al. Pembrolizumab for management of patients with NSCLC and brain metastases: long-term results and biomarker analysis from a non-randomised, open-label, phase 2 trial. *Lancet Oncol.* 2020;21(5):655–663. doi:10.1016/S1470-2045(20)30111-X

12. Di Lorenzo R, Ahluwalia MS. Targeted therapy of brain metastases: latest evidence and clinical implications. *Ther Adv Med Oncol.* 2017;9(12):781–796. doi:10.1177/1758834017736252

13. Trifiletti DM, Ballman KV, Brown PD, et al. Optimizing whole brain radiation therapy dose and fractionation: results from a prospective phase 3 trial (NCCTG N107C [Alliance]/CEC.3). *Int J Radiat Oncol Biol Phys.* 2020;106(2):255–260. doi:10.1016/j.ijrobp.2020.01.012

14. Westover KD, Mendel JT, Dan T, et al. Phase II trial of hippocampal-sparing whole brain irradiation with simultaneous integrated boost for metastatic cancer. *Neuro Oncol.* 2020;22(12):1831–1839. doi:10.1093/neuonc/noaa092

15. Lebow ES, Hwang WL, Zieminski S, et al. Early experience with hippocampal avoidance whole brain radiation therapy and simultaneous integrated boost for brain metastases. *J Neurooncol.* 2020;148(1):81–88. doi:10.1007/s11060-020-03491-y

16. Chia BSH, Leong JY, Ong ALK, et al. Randomised prospective phase II trial in multiple brain metastases comparing outcomes between hippocampal avoidance whole brain radiotherapy with or without simultaneous integrated boost: HA-SIB-WBRT study protocol. *BMC Cancer.* 2020;20(1):1045. doi:10.1186/s12885-020-07565-y

17. Suh JH. Stereotactic radiosurgery for the management of brain metastases. *N Engl J Med.* 2010;362(12):1119–1127. doi:10.1056/NEJMct0806951

18. Minniti G, D'Angelillo RM, Scaringi C, et al. Fractionated stereotactic radiosurgery for patients with brain metastases. *J Neurooncol.* 2014;117(2):295–301. doi:10.1007/s11060-014-1388-3

19. Kim Y-J, Cho KH, Kim J-Y, et al. Single-dose versus fractionated stereotactic radiotherapy for brain metastases. *Int J Radiat Oncol Biol Phys.* 2011;81(2):483–489. doi:10.1016/j.ijrobp.2010.05.033

20. Remick JS, Kowalski E, Khairnar R, et al. A multi-center analysis of single-fraction versus hypofractionated stereotactic radiosurgery for the treatment of brain metastasis. *Radiat Oncol.* 2020;15(1):128. doi:10.1186/s13014-020-01522-6

21. Ernst-Stecken A, Ganslandt O, Lambrecht U, et al. Phase II trial of hypofractionated stereotactic radiotherapy for brain metastases: results and toxicity. *Radiother Oncol.* 2006;81(1):18–24. doi:10.1016/j.radonc.2006.08.024

22. Dohm A, McTyre ER, Okoukoni C, et al. Staged stereotactic radiosurgery for large brain metastases: local control and clinical outcomes of a one-two punch technique. *Neurosurgery.* 2018;83(1):114–121. doi:10.1093/neuros/nyx355

23. Angelov L, Mohammadi AM, Bennett EE, et al. Impact of 2-staged stereotactic radiosurgery for treatment of brain metastases ≥ 2 cm. *J Neurosurg.* 2018;129(2):366–382. doi:10.3171/2017.3.JNS162532

24. Brown PD, Ballman KV, Cerhan JH, et al. Postoperative stereotactic radiosurgery compared with whole brain radiotherapy for resected metastatic brain disease (NCCTG N107C/CEC·3): a multicentre, randomised, controlled, phase 3 trial. *Lancet Oncol.* 2017;18(8):1049–1060. doi:10.1016/S1470-2045(17)30441-2

25. Routman DM, Yan E, Vora S, et al. Preoperative stereotactic radiosurgery for brain metastases. *Front Neurol.* 2018;9:959. doi:10.3389/fneur.2018.00959

26. Rusthoven CG, Yamamoto M, Bernhardt D, et al. Evaluation of first-line radiosurgery vs whole-brain radiotherapy for small cell lung cancer brain metastases: The FIRE-SCLC Cohort Study. *JAMA Oncol.* 2020;6(7):1028–1037. doi:10.1001/jamaoncol.2020.1245

27. Videtic GMM, Woody N, Vassil AD. *Handbook of Treatment Planning in Radiation Oncology.* 3rd ed. Demos Medical; 2020. doi:10.1891/9780826168429

28. Noordijk E, Carde P, Mandard A-M, et al. Preliminary results of the EORTC-GPMC controlled clinical trial H7 in early-stage Hodgkin's disease. *Ann Oncol.* 1994;5(suppl 2):S107–S112. doi:10.1093/annonc/5.suppl_2.S107

29. Mintz AH, Kestle J, Rathbone MP, et al. A randomized trial to assess the efficacy of surgery in addition to radiotherapy in patients with a single cerebral metastasis. *Cancer.* 1996;78(7):1470–1476. doi:10.1002/(SICI)1097-0142(19961001)78:7<1470::AID-CNCR14>3.0.CO;2-X

30. Vogelbaum MA, Angelov L, Lee SY, et al. Local control of brain metastases by stereotactic radiosurgery in relation to dose to the tumor margin. *J Neurosurg.* 2006;104(6):907–912. doi:10.3171/jns.2006.104.6.907

31. Minniti G, Scaringi C, Paolini S, et al. Single-fraction versus multifraction (3 × 9 Gy) stereotactic radiosurgery for large (> 2 cm) brain metastases: a comparative analysis of local control and risk of radiation-induced brain necrosis. *Int J Radiat Oncol Biol Phys.* 2016;95(4):1142–1148. doi:10.1016/j.ijrobp.2016.03.013

32. Yomo S, Hayashi M, Nicholson C. A prospective pilot study of two-session Gamma Knife surgery for large metastatic brain tumors. *J Neurooncol.* 2012;109(1):159–165. doi:10.1007/s11060-012-0882-8

33. Choi CY, Chang SD, Gibbs IC, et al. Stereotactic radiosurgery of the postoperative resection cavity for brain metastases: prospective evaluation of target margin on tumor control. *Int J Radiat Oncol Biol Phys.* 2012;84(2):336–342. doi:10.1016/j.ijrobp.2011.12.009

67 ■ BONE AND SPINE METASTASIS

Ehsan H. Balagamwala, Samuel T. Chao, and Andrew D. Vassil

QUICK HIT ■ Up to 80% of advanced cancer patients develop bone metastases. RT is effective at palliation, with approximately two-thirds experiencing pain relief and up to one-third experiencing complete pain relief. The most common RT regimens include 8 Gy/1 fx, 20 Gy/5 fx, and 30 Gy/10 fx. Factors that influence treatment technique and dose/fractionation include performance status, logistics, tumor size, tumor location, soft tissue component, histology, previous surgery, neurologic deficits, impending fracture, prior RT, and physician preference. Per the Dutch Bone Metastasis study, RTOG 9714, and the Toronto meta-analysis, there is no difference in pain control between single- and multiple-fraction regimens for uncomplicated bone metastases; however, a higher retreatment rate noted with single fraction (perhaps due to physician bias). Pain flare may occur in up to one-third of patients and is treated using a short steroid taper. The precise role for SBRT/SRS is evolving; however, recent data show encouraging outcomes.

EPIDEMIOLOGY: Up to 80% of patients with advanced solid tumors develop bone metastasis to the spine, pelvis, or extremities[1] and over half of people who die of cancer are thought to have bone involvement.[2] Most common primary tumor sites are breast, prostate, lung, thyroid, and kidney. Metastases to bone most often occur in the red marrow, and thus follow red marrow distribution: spine (lumbar > thoracic) > pelvis > ribs > femur > skull.

ANATOMY: Axial skeleton includes the skull, spine, sternum, and ribs. Appendicular skeleton includes long bones and appendixes. Long bones consist of epiphysis (end), metaphysis, and diaphysis (shaft). Two types of bone: cortical and trabecular. Cortical bone is dense and compact, makes up 80% of skeletal mass, is found in diaphysis of long bones and surrounding cuboidal bones, and provides strength and protection; ~3% replaced per year. Trabecular bone is spongy; found inside long bones (concentrated at ends), throughout vertebral bodies, and the inner portions of pelvic bones and other large flat bones; and contains red marrow; ~25% replaced per year.

PATHOLOGY: Bone metastases occur via hematogenous spread, though bones can become involved via direct extension (e.g., oral cavity cancer invading the mandible). It is likely that a combination of tumor factors (cell adhesion molecules that bind to receptors on the cells of the marrow and bone matrix) and the bony microenvironment (growth factors released and activated during bone resorption) contributes to preferential metastasis to bone.[3] Normal bone is constantly remodeled over 3 to 6 months (remember: osteoblasts build bone and osteoclasts resorb bone). Bony metastasis causes a dysregulation of normal bone remodeling that can manifest as osteoblastic, osteolytic, or mixed lesions. Bone destruction by osteolytic metastasis is mediated by osteoclasts, which are activated by factors produced by tumor cells, such as TGF-β, PTH-rP, IL-1, and IL-6. Although classically certain cancers are thought to be primarily osteoblastic or osteolytic, the vast majority have components of both processes. *Osteoblastic*: prostate, SCLC, Hodgkin's lymphoma, and carcinoid. *Osteolytic*: renal cell, melanoma, multiple myeloma, NSCLC, thyroid, and NHL. *Mixed*: breast, GI, and squamous cell.

CLINICAL PRESENTATION: Most common presenting symptom is pain, reduced mobility (70%), pathological fractures (10%–20%), hypercalcemia (10%–15%), spinal cord/nerve compression (5%), and reduced marrow function.

WORKUP: H&P to assess for pain onset, sensory or motor dysfunction, walking ability, urinary retention or overflow incontinence, and bowel incontinence or constipation. On careful physical exam, palpate symptomatic site, extent of soft tissue extension, relationship to nearby neurovascular structures, functional status of the extremity, limb edema, muscle strength, range of motion, and evaluation for primary site.

Imaging: Appendicular skeletal metastases are best evaluated using x-ray of the entire involved bone from joint to joint (least sensitive but most specific): this allows one to evaluate bone structure, integrity, extent of involvement, evaluation of pathologic fracture, and impending fracture risk. Small lesions are difficult to assess on x-rays as 30% to 50% of bone mineral context must be lost to be visible, and metastases usually develop in the medulla and do not involve the cortex until later. Bone scan (Tc-99m) also considered first line, especially if prostate cancer is suspected; increased uptake is an indicator of osteoblastic activity (less effective when osteolysis dominates). Skeletal survey can be helpful in cases where osteolysis predominates such as multiple myeloma. CT is more sensitive than XR and may be useful in assessing pathologic fracture risk or guiding biopsies. MRI is most sensitive (91%–100% compared to 62%–85% for bone scan) and is most useful in evaluating neurovascular compression and assessing marrow involvement, particularly in vertebral bodies (best seen on T1 with contrast and STIR series). For those with lumbar spine metastasis, risk for concurrent asymptomatic metastasis in the C/T spine is significant and therefore, full spinal imaging is warranted. PET/CT is extremely sensitive and is useful in detecting osteolytic metastases. Neoplasms with lower metabolic rate (like prostate cancer) are not typically evident on FDG-PET; it is less sensitive than Tc-99m bone scan for detection of osteoblastic metastases.[4] Recent advances in prostate cancer imaging include fluciclovine (F-18) PET and PSMA-PET.[5]

Biopsy: Tissue diagnosis may not be needed for patients with a previous diagnosis of metastatic bone disease or pathologic fracture requiring repair. Tissue diagnosis is required in patients with solitary bone lesions without a history of cancer or as a first metastatic relapse. CT-guided FNA or core biopsy is preferred.

PROGNOSTIC FACTORS: Dependent on underlying histology and extent of metastatic disease.

TREATMENT PARADIGM

Surgery: Assessment of fracture risk is very important, and surgery is considered to prevent or treat pathologic fractures. Both lytic and blastic lesions reduce bone strength. Historically, ≥2 to 3 cm cortical involvement or lytic destruction of 50% of width of bone was concerning for impending fracture. Mirels scoring system is commonly utilized to predict risk for fracture and is based on a 12-point scale (Table 67.1).[6] Additional candidates for prophylactic fixation: all lesions with significant functionally limiting pain that is exacerbated by weight bearing or patients who have failed RT and have ongoing pain. Patients with spine metastases may also be at a risk for developing vertebral compression fracture (VCF). The Spinal Instability Neoplastic Score (SINS) is utilized to predict which patients will require surgical stabilization prior to RT.[7] Higher scores are assigned to patients with junction lesions (occiput-C2, C7-T2, T11-L1, and L5-S1), pain with movement or loading of the spine or relief with recumbency, subluxation/translation present, >50% vertebral body collapse, and/or bilateral posterolateral involvement of spinal elements.

Table 67.1: Mirels Nomogram for Pathologic Fracture Risk of Bone Metastases			
Site	Upper limb	Lower limb	Peritrochanteric
Degree of pain	Mild	Moderate	Severe
Radiographic nature	Blastic	Mixed	Lytic
Size of cortex	<1/3	1/3–2/3	>2/3
Some add 1 point if lesion in femur proximal to lesser trochanter, lesion in proximal half of humerus, breast cancer, no bisphosphonates, and osteoporosis present.			
≤7 points = <10% fracture risk → observe. 8 points = 15% fracture risk → consider fixation. 9 points = 33% fracture risk → prophylactic fixation. ≥10 points = >50% fracture risk → prophylactic fixation.			

Source: From Mirels H. Metastatic disease in long bones. A proposed scoring system for diagnosing impending pathologic fractures. *Clin Orthop.* 1989;(249):256–264.

Femoral metastases account for two thirds of pathologic fractures requiring intervention. Fractures of the femoral neck can be managed by total hip arthroplasty (replacing the femoral head and acetabulum) or proximal femoral endoprosthesis. Fractures of intertrochanteric region are managed by open reduction and internal fixation without prosthesis (better gait). Lytic disease below intertrochanteric area is treated with an intramedullary rod. Fractionated RT to the site of bone metastasis and surgical hardware is used to help ensure hardware integrity is not compromised by disease progression.

Percutaneous Procedures: Utilized in patients with VCF. Vertebroplasty is a procedure in which bone cement is injected into the vertebral body via a percutaneous approach. Kyphoplasty involves creating a cavity in the fractured vertebral body using a percutaneous placed balloon device followed by placement of bone cement in the cavity once the balloon is removed. The potential benefit of kyphoplasty is realignment of a kyphotic spine. The difference between the two procedures is that vertebroplasty does not restore the height of the vertebral body, whereas kyphoplasty potentially restores height and affects alignment. Vertebroplasty/kyphoplasty are not possible when the posterior wall of the vertebral body is fractured, with significant superior and inferior endplate fractures, significant kyphosis, or significant spinal canal narrowing. Stereotactic or fractionated RT may be used to control disease and maintain stability of vertebrae.

Medical Management

Bisphosphonates: Shown to decrease skeletal-related events (SRE) by inhibiting osteoclast-mediated bone resorption and promoting repair by stimulating osteoblast differentiation and bone formation.[8,9] Zoledronate and pamidronate are most common. Zoledronate also induces apoptosis and inhibits tumor cell adhesion to the extracellular matrix. Toxicities include osteonecrosis (1%–2%), hypocalcemia, and renal insufficiency.

RANK-L inhibitors: RANK/RANK-ligand/osteoprotegerin (RANK/RANK-L/OPG) pathway regulates osteoclast maturation, differentiation, and survival and is disrupted in the metastatic setting due to increased RANK expression.[10] Denosumab is a mAB that binds and inhibits RANK-L, and is FDA approved for prevention of SRE in patients with bone metastasis from solid tumors. A patient-level meta-analysis of three phase III trials comparing zoledronic acid vs. denosumab for metastatic bone disease in breast, prostate, or other solid tumors concluded that denosumab was superior to zoledronic acid in reducing the risk of a first-on-study SRE and in delaying the time to a first SRE or hypercalcemia of malignancy.[11] Bone-modifying agents are recommended by ASCO guidelines and approved for all solid tumors with bone metastases and multiple myeloma.[12–14]

Radiation: RT is the cornerstone of treatment for patients with bone metastases. EBRT is most frequently utilized; however, there is an increasing role of radiopharmaceuticals. The 2017 ASTRO guidelines suggest the following: 8 Gy/1 fx, 20 Gy/5 fx, 24 Gy/6 fx, 20 Gy/10 fx (for myeloma), or 30 Gy/10 fx as recommended doses.[15] Spine SRS or bone SBRT can be utilized for select cases. The clearest indication for spine SRS is in the retreatment setting (20 Gy/10 fx is also a common retreatment regimen). For spine SRS, the most common fractionation schemes include 16 to 18 Gy/1 fx or 24 Gy/1 to 2 fx. Doses of ≥20 Gy per fraction are associated with increased risk of VCF.[16] Guidelines are published for contouring of definitive spine SRS, postoperative spine SRS, and for response assessment (SPINO).[17–19] For nonspine osseous metastases, most common doses include 12 Gy/1 fx (size ≥4 cm), 16 Gy/1 fx (size <4 cm), or 30 Gy/3 fx.[20,21]

Procedure: See *Handbook of Treatment Planning in Radiation Oncology*, Chapter 13.

■ EVIDENCE-BASED Q&A

▦ Is there a benefit to longer fractionation schemes for uncomplicated bone metastases?

Several large prospective trials (Dutch Bone Metastasis Study, RTOG 9714) as well as the Toronto meta-analysis showed no difference in pain relief (~2/3) between single-fraction and multifraction regimens. Retreatment rates are higher after single-fraction RT, perhaps due to physician bias.[22] Note that complicated bone metastases (fractures, cord compression, previous RT) were excluded from these trials. When there is risk for pathologic fracture, fractionated RT is preferred (lower risk for fractures on the Dutch study[23]).

Steenland, Dutch Bone Metastasis Study (*Radiother Oncol* 1999, PMID 10577695): PRT of 1,171 patients randomized to receive either 8 Gy/1 fx or 24 Gy/6 fx. Weekly questionnaires used for self-assessment after treatment, and primary endpoint was pain score (0–10). Seventy-one percent experienced a response (median 3 weeks in both groups) and no differences between pain meds, QOL, or side effects between regimens. Twenty-five percent were retreated in the single-fraction group vs. 7% in the fractionated group (but time to retreat was shorter and pain score at time of retreatment was lower, likely suggesting doctors were more willing to retreat single fx patients). Of note, axial cortical involvement >30 mm ($p = .01$) and circumferential cortical involvement >50% ($p = .03$) were predictive of fracture, but not the Mirels nomogram score. If these high-risk patients are not candidates for surgery, offer fractionated RT.[24]

Hartsell, RTOG 9714 (*JNCI* 2005, PMID 15928300): PRT of 898 patients with breast or prostate cancer with one to three sites of painful bone metastases and moderate to severe pain randomized to 8 Gy/1 fx vs. 30 Gy/10 fx. No difference in overall RR (66%), CR (~15%), and PR (~50%). More frequent grade 2 to 4 acute toxicity (mostly GI related) in 30 Gy arm (17% vs. 10%, $p = .002$). No difference in late toxicity (4%), fracture rates (4%–5%), or narcotic use at 3 months. Higher rate of retreatment with single fraction (18% vs. 9%, $p < .001$). **Conclusion: A single fraction of 8 Gy provides similar efficacy in pain relief, with less acute toxicity but higher rates of retreatment than 30 Gy/10 fx.**

Chow, Toronto Meta-analysis (*JCO* 2007, PMID 17416863; Update *Clin Oncol* 2012, PMID 22130630): Meta-analysis of 25 PRT with over 5,600 patients comparing single- to multiple-fraction schedules. No difference in overall RR (60% vs. 61%), CR (23 vs. 24%), acute toxicity, or pathologic fracture risk (3.3% vs. 3.0%). Retreatment was more likely in the single-fraction group (20% vs. 8%, $p < .00001$).

■ **What is the best dose for single-fraction palliative RT?**

Based on a systematic review of 24 trials, a dose–response relationship was noted and 8 Gy/1 fx was found to be the optimal single-fraction dose.

Dennis, Toronto Meta-analysis on Dose (*Radiother Oncol* 2013, PMID 23321492): Systematic review of 24 trials with 3,233 patients randomized to 28 single-fraction arms, ranging from 4 to 15 Gy; 8 Gy was the most commonly used dose (84%), and higher doses produced better pain response rates. Trials that directly compared different single-fraction doses demonstrated that 8 Gy was statistically superior to 4 Gy.

■ **What is the expected time to pain response with EBRT? What about EBRT vs. SBRT?**

Median time to pain response is ~3 weeks with either single-fraction or multifraction EBRT regimens.[24,25] However, per the TROG 96.05 study, the durability of pain control appears to be lower for single-fraction compared to multifraction regimens (2.4 vs. 3.7 months, $p = .056$).[26] Newer data suggest that up to 40% of those treated will have pain reduction by 10 days suggesting palliative RT is effective even in those patients with poor expected survival.[27] For spine metastasis, the time to pain relief appears to be similar between EBRT and SRS, albeit a higher CR rate with SRS compared to EBRT (Sahgal et al, ASTRO 2020 Late Breaking Abstract).

■ **What are pain flares and what is the incidence? What about in spine SRS?**

A pain flare is a temporary worsening of bone pain in the irradiated site, usually in the first few days after RT and lasting 1 to 2 days; 80% of pain flares happen in the first 5 days following RT, with a minority happening between days 5 and 10. Up to 40% of patients treated with RT may develop a pain flare in the first 10 days after RT.[28] In spine SRS, the incidence of pain flare is variable and reported to be 15% to 70% depending on dose.[24] This can be treated (or possibly prevented) with a short course of steroids.[29]

■ **What is the role of RT after orthopedic stabilization?**

RT promotes remineralization and bone healing, alleviates pain, improves functional status, and reduces the risk for subsequent fracture or loss of fixation by treating residual metastatic disease. It also decreases need for second surgery and is associated with a prolonged survival.[30,31] Disadvantages include the potential effects on uninvolved bone and on postoperative wound healing. If an implant is placed, classically the entire implant is treated. RT is generally started within 2 to 4 weeks after surgery after wound healing. The optimal dose/fractionation is unclear as there is limited data regarding single-fraction treatments, so 30 Gy/10 fx is typically recommended.

■ What is the evidence for retreatment of bone metastasis?

About 20% will require retreatment of bone metastasis. Retreatment is feasible and can provide pain relief in 50% to 60%.[32,33] It is recommended to wait at least 4 weeks after initial RT before considering re-irradiation to allow for full response from initial course. Single fraction appears to have similar efficacy as multifraction regimens for uncomplicated metastases. Important to note that patients who respond favorably to prior RT have a higher chance of responding to reirradiation.

Chow, NCIC SC 20 (*Lancet Oncol*** 2014, PMID 24369114):** RCT of patients with painful (≥2 using brief pain inventory) bone metastases previously treated with RT randomized between 8 Gy/1 fx vs. 20 Gy in multiple fractions. Primary end point pain response at 2 months; 425 patients enrolled. Overall pain response at 2 months was 28% in the 8 Gy vs. 32% in the 20 Gy arm. Toxicity including lack of appetite and diarrhea was worse in the 20 Gy arm. **Conclusion: 8 Gy was noninferior and less toxic than 20 Gy for re-irradiation of painful bone metastases.**

■ What is the role of hemibody irradiation?

Hemibody irradiation may be indicated in those with extensive bony disease. Although single and multifraction regimens have been reported, they have not been compared in a randomized fashion. Hemibody irradiation is generally used when radiopharmaceuticals are not available or are contraindicated. An extended SSD technique is utilized and fields are matched at the umbilicus or L4/5. Lung blocks may be necessary to limit lung dose to 6 to 7 Gy. Typically, 6 Gy/1 fx is utilized for the upper body and 8 Gy/1 fx to the lower body. Alternate doses include 15 Gy/5 fx or 20 to 30 Gy/8 to 10 fx delivered three fractions weekly. Typically, the other half of the body is treated 6 to 8 weeks later.

■ What is the role of radiopharmaceuticals for the treatment of extensive bony metastases?

Radiopharmaceuticals are radioactive agents that are administered intravenously and localize to the site of osteoblastic activity, thereby delivering dose simultaneously at sites of disease. Most common isotopes used are beta-emitters (Sr-89, Sm-153, P-53) and alpha-emitters (Ra-223). Beta-emitters have a response rate of ~60% to 70% and a complete response of ~20%. The primary advantage of samarium (Sm-153) over strontium (Sr-89) is a significantly shorter half-life (1.5 vs. 50.5 days, respectively). Myelosuppression is the major toxicity, which can be prolonged with Sr-89 but generally nadirs at 3 to 4 weeks and recovers by 6 to 8 weeks with Sm-153. Recently, alpha-emitters (Ra-223) have gained favor (see the following) and offer the advantage of a high LET and short range (10 μm in bone and soft tissue).

Parker, ALSYMPCA (*NEJM*** 2013, PMID 23863050; Update Sartor *Lancet Oncol* 2014, PMID 24836273):** PRT of 921 patients with metastatic (>2 bony metastases and no known visceral metastases) castrate resistant prostate cancer (stratified by previous docetaxel use) randomized (2:1 ratio) to receive 6 IV injections of radium-223 (50 kBq/kg every 4 weeks) or placebo. OS was improved in the Ra-223 arm (14.9 vs. 11.3 months). They also evaluated time to first skeletal event, defined as RT use or development of spinal cord compression. Time to first skeletal event was improved with Ra-223 (15.6 vs. 9.8 months). Previous use of docetaxel was not associated with efficacy of Ra-223.[34] Incidence of adverse events was lower in the treatment arm than the placebo group, and there were very few grade 3 to 5 hematologic toxicities.

■ Does SBRT relieve pain from bone metastases more effectively than EBRT?

Nguyen, MDACC (*JAMA Oncol*** 2019, PMID: 31021390):** Phase II noninferiority (10% margin) RCT of 160 patients with painful bone metastases randomized to SBRT (12 Gy for ≥4 cm lesions, 16 Gy for <4 cm; prophylactic decadron recommended) vs. EBRT 30 Gy/10 fx (no prophylactic decadron). The SBRT group had more pain response (CR or PR; primary end point) at 2 weeks (62% vs. 36%, $p = .01$), 3 months (72% vs. 49%, $p = .03$), and 9 months (77% vs. 46%, $p = .03$). No difference in treatment toxicity. One year local-PFS 100% with SBRT vs. 91% with EBRT ($p = .01$). Subset analysis suggested 16 Gy group had highest rate of/most durable pain response. **Conclusions: SBRT is noninferior to EBRT for pain control and time to local progression, and SBRT had significantly higher pain response at 2 weeks, 3 months, and 9 months.** *Note: High attrition rate due to cancer deaths. Not all time points were significantly different (i.e., 1 month and 6 months).*

■ **What is the role of spine SRS for spine metastases?**

Spine SRS is a highly conformal treatment technique that allows for dose escalation within the treatment volume without exceeding spinal cord tolerance. Dose escalation is believed to improve pain response and durability of pain control. This is especially useful in patients with radioresistant histologies or recurrent disease after previous RT. Retrospective studies demonstrate local control rates >85% to 90% as well as excellent pain control rates.[35] The risk of pain flare after spine SBRT is ~15% and is adequately treated with a short course of steroids.[36] The risk of new or progressive VCF is also ~15% and increases with dose/fraction ≥20 Gy.[16] Preliminary results from RTOG 0631 and SC.24 show no difference in overall pain response rates with SRS compared to EBRT, however, do show higher rates of CR with spine SRS.

Ryu, RTOG 0631 (*ASTRO* 2019, Plenary Session PL-01): Randomized multi-institution phase II/III study of 339 patients with one to three sites of spinal metastatic disease randomized 2:1 to SBRT 16 or 18 Gy in 1 fx vs. EBRT 8 Gy in 1 fx to involved vertebral level plus one level above and below. Epidural extension permitted as long as ≥3 mm of separation from cord. Primary end point: pain control (3-point improvement on Numerical Rating Pain Scale [NRPS] at treated site 3 months post treatment). No significant difference in pain score between SRS group (−3.00 points) and EBRT group (−3.83 points), nor in proportion of patients with pain response (SBRT 40% vs. EBRT 58%, one-sided p = .99). **Conclusion: SBRT is not superior to EBRT for pain palliation in spine metastases.**

Sahgal, CCTG SC.24 (*ASTRO* 2020, Late Breaking Abstract 2): Randomized multi-institution phase II/III study of 229 patients with ≤3 consecutive spinal segments randomized 1:1 to SBRT 24 Gy/2 fx vs. EBRT 20 Gy/5 fx. Primary end point: CR rate at 3 months post treatment. MFU 6.7 months. At 3 months, pain CR rate was higher in SRS group compared to EBRT group (36% vs. 16%, p < .001). This difference was maintained at 6 months (33% vs. 16%, p = .004). **Conclusion: SRS offers higher pain CR rates compared to EBRT.**

REFERENCES

1. Nielsen OS. Palliative radiotherapy of bone metastases: there is now evidence for the use of single fractions. *Radiother Oncol J Eur Soc Ther Radiol Oncol.* 1999;52(2):95–96. doi:10.1016/s0167-8140(99)00109-7

2. Mundy GR. Metastasis to bone: causes, consequences and therapeutic opportunities. *Nat Rev Cancer.* 2002;2(8):584–593. doi:10.1038/nrc867

3. Barghash RF, Abdou WM. Pathophysiology of metastatic bone disease and the role of the second generation of bisphosphonates: from basic science to medicine. *Curr Pharm Des.* 2016;22(11):1546–1557. doi:10.2174/1381612822666160122093810

4. Kao CH, Hsieh JF, Tsai SC, et al. Comparison and discrepancy of 18F-2-deoxyglucose positron emission tomography and Tc-99m MDP bone scan to detect bone metastases. *Anticancer Res.* 2000;20(3B):2189–2192.

5. Turpin A, Girard E, Baillet C, et al. Imaging for metastasis in prostate cancer: a review of the literature. *Front Oncol.* 2020;10:55. doi:10.3389/fonc.2020.00055

6. Mirels H. Metastatic disease in long bones: a proposed scoring system for diagnosing impending pathologic fractures. *Clin Orthop.* 1989;(249):256–264.

7. Fisher CG, DiPaola CP, Ryken TC, et al. A novel classification system for spinal instability in neoplastic disease: an evidence-based approach and expert consensus from the Spine Oncology Study Group. *Spine.* 2010;35(22):E1221–1229. doi:10.1097/BRS.0b013e3181e16ae2

8. Ross JR, Saunders Y, Edmonds PM, et al. Systematic review of role of bisphosphonates on skeletal morbidity in metastatic cancer. *BMJ.* 2003;327(7413):469. doi:10.1136/bmj.327.7413.469

9. Berenson JR, Lichtenstein A, Porter L, et al. Long-term pamidronate treatment of advanced multiple myeloma patients reduces skeletal events. Myeloma Aredia Study Group. *J Clin Oncol Off J Am Soc Clin Oncol.* 1998;16(2):593–602. doi:10.1200/JCO.1998.16.2.593

10. Boyce BF, Xing L. Functions of RANKL/RANK/OPG in bone modeling and remodeling. *Arch Biochem Biophys.* 2008;473(2):139–146. doi:10.1016/j.abb.2008.03.018

11. Lipton A, Fizazi K, Stopeck AT, et al. Superiority of denosumab to zoledronic acid for prevention of skeletal-related events: a combined analysis of 3 pivotal, randomised, phase 3 trials. *Eur J Cancer Oxf Engl. 1990.* 2012;48(16):3082–3092. doi:10.1016/j.ejca.2012.08.002

12. Van Poznak C, Somerfield MR, Barlow WE, et al. Role of bone-modifying agents in metastatic breast cancer: an American Society of Clinical Oncology-Cancer care Ontario focused guideline update. *J Clin Oncol Off J Am Soc Clin Oncol.* 2017;35(35):3978–3986. doi:10.1200/JCO.2017.75.4614

13. Saylor PJ, Rumble RB, Tagawa S, et al. Bone health and bone-targeted therapies for prostate cancer: ASCO endorsement of a Cancer Care Ontario guideline. *J Clin Oncol Off J Am Soc Clin Oncol.* 2020;38(15):1736–1743. doi:10.1200/JCO.19.03148

14. Anderson K, Ismaila N, Flynn PJ, et al. Role of bone-modifying agents in multiple myeloma: American Society of Clinical Oncology Clinical Practice guideline update. *J Clin Oncol Off J Am Soc Clin Oncol*. 2018;36(8):812–818. doi:10.1200/JCO.2017.76.6402

15. Lutz S, Balboni T, Jones J, et al. Palliative radiation therapy for bone metastases: update of an ASTRO evidence-based guideline. *Pract Radiat Oncol*. 2017;7(1):4–12. doi:10.1016/j.prro.2016.08.001

16. Sahgal A, Atenafu EG, Chao S, et al. Vertebral compression fracture after spine stereotactic body radiotherapy: a multi-institutional analysis with a focus on radiation dose and the spinal instability neoplastic score. *J Clin Oncol Off J Am Soc Clin Oncol*. 2013;31(27):3426–3431. doi:10.1200/JCO.2013.50.1411

17. Thibault I, Chang EL, Sheehan J, et al. Response assessment after stereotactic body radiotherapy for spinal metastasis: a report from the SPIne response assessment in Neuro-Oncology (SPINO) group. *Lancet Oncol*. 2015;16(16):e595–603. doi:10.1016/S1470-2045(15)00166-7

18. Cox BW, Spratt DE, Lovelock M, et al. International Spine Radiosurgery Consortium consensus guidelines for target volume definition in spinal stereotactic radiosurgery. *Int J Radiat Oncol Biol Phys*. 2012;83(5):e597–605. doi:10.1016/j.ijrobp.2012.03.009

19. Redmond KJ, Robertson S, Lo SS, et al. Consensus contouring guidelines for postoperative stereotactic body radiation therapy for metastatic solid tumor malignancies to the spine. *Int J Radiat Oncol Biol Phys*. 2017;97(1):64–74. doi:10.1016/j.ijrobp.2016.09.014

20. Nguyen Q-N, Chun SG, Chow E, et al. Single-fraction stereotactic vs conventional multifraction radiotherapy for pain relief in patients with predominantly nonspine bone metastases: a randomized phase 2 trial. *JAMA Oncol*. 2019;5(6):872–878. doi:10.1001/jamaoncol.2019.0192

21. Chmura S. A phase 1 study of Stereotactic Body Radiotherapy (SBRT) for the treatment of multiple metastases. 2021. https://www.nrgoncology.org/Clinical-Trials/Protocol/nrg-br001?filter=nrg-br001

22. Nieder C. Repeat palliative radiotherapy for painful bone metastases. *Lancet Oncol*. 2014;15(2):126–128. doi:10.1016/S1470-2045(13)70581-3

23. van der Linden YM, Kroon HM, Dijkstra SPDS, et al. Simple radiographic parameter predicts fracturing in metastatic femoral bone lesions: results from a randomised trial. *Radiother Oncol J Eur Soc Ther Radiol Oncol*. 2003;69(1):21–31. doi:10.1016/s0167-8140(03)00232-9

24. Steenland E, Leer JW, van Houwelingen H, et al. The effect of a single fraction compared to multiple fractions on painful bone metastases: a global analysis of the Dutch Bone Metastasis Study. *Radiother Oncol J Eur Soc Ther Radiol Oncol*. 1999;52(2):101–109. doi:10.1016/s0167-8140(99)00110-3

25. Yarnold J. 8 Gy single fraction radiotherapy for the treatment of metastatic skeletal pain: randomised comparison with a multifraction schedule over 12 months of patient follow-up. Bone Pain Trial Working Party. *Radiother Oncol J Eur Soc Ther Radiol Oncol*. 1999;52(2):111–121.

26. Roos DE, Turner SL, O'Brien PC, et al. Randomized trial of 8 Gy in 1 versus 20 Gy in 5 fractions of radiotherapy for neuropathic pain due to bone metastases (Trans-Tasman Radiation Oncology Group, TROG 96.05). *Radiother Oncol J Eur Soc Ther Radiol Oncol*. 2005;75(1):54–63. doi:10.1016/j.radonc.2004.09.017

27. McDonald R, Ding K, Brundage M, et al. Effect of radiotherapy on painful bone metastases: a secondary analysis of the NCIC Clinical Trials Group Symptom Control Trial SC.23. *JAMA Oncol*. 2017;3(7):953–959. doi:10.1001/jamaoncol.2016.6770

28. Hird A, Chow E, Zhang L, et al. Determining the incidence of pain flare following palliative radiotherapy for symptomatic bone metastases: results from three Canadian cancer centers. *Int J Radiat Oncol Biol Phys*. 2009;75(1):193–197. doi:10.1016/j.ijrobp.2008.10.044

29. Chow E, Meyer RM, Ding K, et al. Dexamethasone in the prophylaxis of radiation-induced pain flare after palliative radiotherapy for bone metastases: a double-blind, randomised placebo-controlled, phase 3 trial. *Lancet Oncol*. 2015;16(15):1463–1472. doi:10.1016/S1470-2045(15)00199-0

30. Townsend PW, Smalley SR, Cozad SC, et al. Role of postoperative radiation therapy after stabilization of fractures caused by metastatic disease. *Int J Radiat Oncol Biol Phys*. 1995;31(1):43–49. doi:10.1016/0360-3016(94)E0310-G

31. Townsend PW, Rosenthal HG, Smalley SR, et al. Impact of postoperative radiation therapy and other perioperative factors on outcome after orthopedic stabilization of impending or pathologic fractures due to metastatic disease. *J Clin Oncol Off J Am Soc Clin Oncol*. 1994;12(11):2345–2350. doi:10.1200/JCO.1994.12.11.2345

32. Huisman M, van den Bosch MAAJ, Wijlemans JW, et al. Effectiveness of reirradiation for painful bone metastases: a systematic review and meta-analysis. *Int J Radiat Oncol Biol Phys*. 2012;84(1):8–14. doi:10.1016/j.ijrobp.2011.10.080

33. Chow E, van der Linden YM, Roos D, et al. Single versus multiple fractions of repeat radiation for painful bone metastases: a randomised, controlled, non-inferiority trial. *Lancet Oncol*. 2014;15(2):164–171. doi:10.1016/S1470-2045(13)70556-4

34. Hoskin P, Sartor O, O'Sullivan JM, et al. Efficacy and safety of radium-223 dichloride in patients with castration-resistant prostate cancer and symptomatic bone metastases, with or without previous docetaxel use: a prespecified subgroup analysis from the randomised, double-blind, phase 3 ALSYMPCA trial. *Lancet Oncol*. 2014;15(12):1397–1406. doi:10.1016/S1470-2045(14)70474-7

35. Vellayappan BA, Chao ST, Foote M, et al. The evolution and rise of stereotactic body radiotherapy (SBRT) for spinal metastases. *Expert Rev Anticancer Ther*. 2018;18(9):887–900. doi:10.1080/14737140.2018.1493381

36. Balagamwala EH, Naik M, Reddy CA, et al. Pain flare after stereotactic radiosurgery for spine metastases. *J Radiosurg SBRT*. 2018;5(2):99–105.

Camille A. Berriochoa and Bindu V. Manyam

QUICK HIT ■ Malignant spinal cord compression (mSCC) is considered an oncologic emergency and defined as any radiographic compression of the spinal cord or cauda equina secondary to an extradural or intramedullary malignancy. The most common presenting symptom is pain. Severity of symptoms can vary depending on the degree of compression, from asymptomatic to frank paraplegia, which may be reversible or irreversible. Initial treatment usually involves steroids (dexamethasone 10 mg loading dose, followed by 4 mg every 6 hours). Surgical evaluation should be obtained, and if surgical intervention is indicated, postoperative RT should follow, typically 30 Gy/10 fx about 2 to 4 weeks after surgery. If no surgical intervention is indicated, standard conventional fractionation is typically 30 Gy/10 fx or 20 Gy/5 fx. The use of SRS is established for re-irradiation and an evolving area for non-urgent treatment of spinal metastases in the absence of cord compression.

EPIDEMIOLOGY: Among patients with cancer, the annual incidence of mSCC is 2.5% to 3.4%, ranging from 0.2% in pancreatic cancer to 8% in multiple myeloma. Most cases are due to lung, breast, and prostate cancer. The highest proportional incidence is observed in multiple myeloma, lymphoma, and prostate cancer.[1,2] In pediatric patients, mSCC is observed in 5% of cancer patients, and is most commonly caused by Ewing's sarcoma and neuroblastoma.[3]

ANATOMY: The *spinal cord* extends from the foramen magnum to L1–L2 in adults. In children, the spinal cord extends more inferiorly (L2–L4). The *dural sac* surrounds the spinal cord and 31 nerve roots, which are cervical (8), thoracic (12), lumbar (5), sacral (5), and coccygeal (1). The sacral nerve roots S3 to S5 originate from the terminal segment of the spinal cord, called the *conus medullaris*. The *filum terminale* is a thin connective tissue filament that originates from the conus medullaris and is fused to the periosteum of the coccygeal bone. The *cauda equina* is defined as the lumbar and sacral spinal nerves located in the lumbar cistern from L1/L2 to S2.[4,5] The *spinal meninges*, from deep to superficial, are composed of the pia mater, arachnoid mater, and the dura mater. The *epidural space* is superficial to the dura mater and contains fat and a venous plexus. The *gray matter* of the spinal cord is composed of lower motor nuclei anteriorly and sensory nuclei posteriorly. The *white matter* of the spinal cord is composed of the dorsal columns (proprioception), lateral spinothalamic tract (pain, temperature), ventral spinothalamic tract (touch sensation), anterior corticospinal tract (axial musculature), and lateral corticospinal tract (extremities).

PATHOLOGY: mSCC occurs through two main mechanisms—external compression typically arising from the vertebral body (more common; due to arterial seeding of the bone) and internal compression due to intramedullary metastasis. Obstruction of the epidural venous plexus leads to the development of vasogenic edema of the white matter, and then the gray matter. Untreated, spinal cord infarction can ultimately develop.

CLINICAL PRESENTATION: Back pain is the most common presenting symptom, occurring in 83% to 95% of cases, typically most pronounced at night or early in the morning when adrenal steroid secretion is at its lowest.[6,7] Back pain often precedes neurologic symptoms by several weeks. An estimated 60% to 85% of patients present with weakness, with 48% to 77% non-ambulatory. Sensory symptoms present in about 50% and can be described as "band-like," ascending, or "saddle" anesthesia/paresthesias, depending on location.[8] Physical exam findings may include upper motor neuron signs of spasticity, hyperactive reflexes, Babinski sign, and lower motor neuron signs of atrophy, flaccidity, and loss of reflexes.

Spinal Cord Syndromes

Transection of the cord: Loss of all sensory modalities (proprioception, vibration, touch) with weakness below the level of transection and bowel/bladder dysfunction.

Ventral cord syndrome: Weakness and loss of pain and temperature sensation.

Dorsal cord syndrome: Loss of proprioception and vibration, weakness, ataxia.

Cauda equina: Radiculopathy, leg weakness and sensory loss, saddle anesthesia, bowel/bladder incontinence/retention. Bowel/bladder dysfunction is a late finding that can present in up to 50% of patients.[7]

WORKUP: Full H&P, focused on neurologic exam.

Imaging: MRI of entire spine with and without gadolinium. If MRI cannot be obtained, CT myelography is similar in terms of sensitivity and specificity for cord compression.[9]

Biopsy: Indicated for patients who are not surgical candidates and have an undiagnosed primary cancer, oligometastasis, or if there is discordance between the primary lesion and spinal lesion.

PROGNOSTIC FACTORS: A simple framework has been developed that incorporates the neurologic, oncologic, mechanical, and systemic status of the patient to determine the optimal management decision.[10] The epidural spinal cord compression scale is based on a 6-point grading system to quantify the degree of spinal cord or thecal sac compression to help determine management decisions. Grade 0: bone only disease; Grade 1a: epidural impingement, no deformation of thecal sac; Grade 1b: deformation of thecal sac, no spinal cord abutment; Grade 1c: deformation of thecal sac and spinal cord abutment, but no cord compression; Grade 2: spinal cord compression but visible CSF around cord; Grade 3: spinal cord compression with no visible CSF around cord.[11]

TREATMENT PARADIGM

Medical Treatment: Early initiation of high-dose corticosteroids is standard management of mSCC. Typically, patients are started on 10 mg dexamethasone, followed by 4 mg q6hr. Several studies have evaluated the benefit of steroid dose escalation with doses of 96 to 100 mg compared to 10 to 16 mg and have demonstrated no benefit with respect to pain control, ambulation rates, or neurologic outcomes, but have noted higher incidence of serious adverse effects, such as perforated gastric ulcer, psychosis, and death from infection.[12-14] Duration of steroid taper should be initiated based on severity of symptoms, clinical response, and definitive management. Initiation of CHT should be considered with CHT-sensitive disease (lymphoma, Ewing's sarcoma, germ cell tumors, neuroblastoma).

Surgical Treatment: Assessing spinal stability is an important decision-making point regarding whether or not to pursue surgery. In the event of spinal instability, the degree of spinal instability, neurologic symptoms, and location of disease dictate the management. Percutaneous vertebroplasty or kyphoplasty are minimally invasive procedures for patients without anterior extension of disease. The Spinal Instability Neoplastic Score (SINS) takes into account six different factors of clinical and radiographic findings, and a score of >7 warrants surgical consultation.[15] Surgery is also beneficial in providing immediate relief of compression, when a histological diagnosis is unknown, in a previously irradiated site of compression, and with progressive deterioration of neurologic status with poor response to steroids. Postsurgical ambulatory rates range between 70% and 90%, with surgical morbidity and mortality ranging from 5% to 10%.[16,17] Various surgical options are outlined in Table 68.1.

Radiation

EBRT: Indications include patients who are not surgical candidates, and in the postoperative setting (typically 2–4 weeks after surgery, except after corpectomy, which requires 6 weeks for fusion). The goal of RT is palliation of pain and LC for prevention or reduction of neurologic deficits. Studies have demonstrated a 70% improvement in pain and local control rates >75%.[19] Typical doses include 30 Gy/10 fx, 20 Gy/5 fx, and 8 Gy/1 fx. For radiosensitive histologies, such as multiple myeloma, 20 Gy/10 fx may be appropriate.[20] Several series demonstrated between 67% and 82% retention of ambulation following RT and about one-third of patients who were non-ambulatory regained the ability to walk following RT.[19,21] In the retreatment setting, consider lower doses or fraction sizes, 20

Table 68.1: Surgical Options in mSCC

	Corpectomy	Laminectomy	Separation Surgery	Vertebroplasty	Kyphoplasty
Procedure	Removal of vertebral body via thoracotomy or retroperitoneal approach. Delays RT for 6 weeks to allow for fusion.	Removal of posterior arch of vertebrae (unclear if it adds benefit compared to RT alone and may destabilize spine).[18]	Debulking and instrumentation to increase margin between tumor and spinal cord/thecal sac.	PMMA under fluoroscopy into a collapsed vertebral body	Inflatable bone tamps introduced into the vertebral body; once inflated, the bone tamps variably restore the height of the vertebral body, while creating a cavity to fill with viscous bone cement
Candidates	Good life expectancy and good-performing patients (see the Patchell trial)[17]	Anterior extension of posterior disease	Most commonly used to create adequate margin for adjuvant SRS	Patients with spinal instability, but without anterior extension	

Gy/10 fx, or SRS, in patients with extended life expectancy. Side effects are dependent on location and length of spine being treated and can include mucositis, dysphagia, nausea, diarrhea, or cytopenia.

SRS: Generally not indicated for spinal cord compression given tumor proximity to cord and time required to initiate therapy. The clearest indication for SRS is re-irradiation, but patients with radioresistant histologies with asymptomatic/minimally symptomatic disease or following separation surgery with gross residual disease may also benefit. Contraindications include significant epidural extension (a gap of >3 mm between the spinal cord and the edge of the lesion is ideal). A rate of >85% long-term pain control even in radioresistant patients has been observed.[22] SRS doses include, 16 to 18 Gy/1 fx, 24 Gy/1 fx, 30 Gy/5 fx.[23] Side effects include acute pain flare (15%), fatigue, nausea, diarrhea, vertebral fracture, myelopathy (<1%).[24]

Procedure: See Handbook of Treatment Planning in Radiation Oncology, Chapter 13.[25]

■ **EVIDENCE-BASED Q&A**

▪ **What is the value of surgical decompression in addition to radiotherapy?**

Addition of surgery (corpectomy) to RT improves median survival, ambulation rate, length of ambulation retention, ability to regain walking, and no change in hospitalization time in patients with a single site of cord compression with paraplegia <48 hours.

Patchell (*Lancet* 2005, PMID 16112300): PRT of 101 patients with confirmed cancer, life expectancy >3 months, single site of MRI-confirmed displaced cord, with at least one neurological sign or symptom, who were paraplegic <48 hours, randomized to surgery with post-op RT (30 Gy/10 fx) vs. RT alone. Surgery was primarily corpectomy. Lymphoma, myeloma, leukemia, and germ cell tumors were excluded. Primary end point was the ability to walk (at least four steps unassisted with or without a cane/walker). Secondary end points were urinary continence, muscle strength, functional status, need for steroids/opioids, OS. (Results are presented in Table 68.2.) Of note, 20% in the RT group clinically deteriorated and required surgery.

Table 68.2: Results of the Patchell Trial for mSCC				
	Ambulation Rate at the End of Treatment Primary End Point	Ambulation Retention Time Primary End Point	Median Survival Secondary End Point	Regained Ability to Walk	Length of Hospitalization
Surgery + RT	84%	122 d	126 d	62%	10 d
RT alone	57%	13 d	100 d	19%	10 d
p value	.001	.003	.03	.01	

Is there an ideal dose/fractionation regimen to use for mSCC?

Typical dose and fractionations include 20 Gy/5 fx and 30 Gy/10 fx; however, a superior dosing and fractionation schedule with regard to efficacy and toxicity has not been identified in prospective randomized trials and several trials support single fraction EBRT. Therefore, clinical decision-making should incorporate patient prognosis, functional status, disease burden, histology, future treatment plans, and patient convenience.

Thirion, ICORG 05-03 (*BJC* 2020, PMID 32157242): Phase III non-inferiority RCT of 73 patients comparing 10 Gy/1fx vs. 20 Gy/5 fx for mSCC with no surgical interventions performed. Hematologic/germ cell malignancies and prior treatment not eligible. Primary endpoint: change in mobility at 5 weeks by modified Tomita score (a mobility scale that had three possible scores: 1 = Unaided, 2 = With walking aid, and 3 = Bed-bound). Median age 69, KPS 70, 60% male; 34% prostate, 26% breast, 10% lung; 71% T-spine, 20% L-spine. MFU 5.6 months. Average change in mTomita score was −0.06 in single fx group, −0.3 in multi-fx group which met predefined noninferiority criterion. No difference in posttreatment bladder control or MS (6.6 months single fx vs. 6.0 months multifx). No difference in grade 2 to 3 acute or late AEs in multifx (26%) vs. single fx (11%) group (*p* = .069). **Conclusion: With respect to mobility preservation, 10 Gy/1 fx is non-inferior to 20 Gy/5 fx.**

Hoskin, SCORAD III (*JAMA* 2019, PMID 31794625): RCT of 686 patients comparing EBRT 8 Gy/1 fx vs. 20 Gy/5 fx. Spinal cord or cauda equina (C1–S2) compression confirmed by MRI/CT scan, treatable within a single radiation field, life expectancy >8 weeks, and no previous RT to the same area required. Primary end point was ambulatory status at 8 weeks graded from 1 to 4; grades 1 to 2 defined as ambulatory. Seventy-three percent male; median age 70 years; 44% prostate, 19% lung, 12% breast. Grade 1 to 2 at week 8: 69% of patients in single-dose group vs. 73% multi-fraction group (*p* = .06); 12-week OS 50% in single-fraction group, 55% in multi-fraction. **Conclusion: 8 Gy in 1 fx did not meet non-inferiority criterion for primary end point of ambulatory status at 8 weeks, with the caveat that lower bound of confidence interval overlapped with noninferiority margin, making the clinical relevance of this finding unclear.**

Rades (*JCO* 2016, PMID 26729431): PRT, non-inferiority study of 203 patients with mSCC and intermediate to poor life expectancy randomized to 20 Gy/5 fx vs. 30 Gy/10 fx. Primary end point was 1 month overall response, defined as improvement or no further progression of motor deficits. (Results are presented in Table 68.3). **Conclusion: 20 Gy/5 fx is not inferior to 30 Gy/10 fx in patients with intermediate to poor life expectancy.**

Maranzano (*JCO* 2005, PMID 15738534): PRT of 300 patients with mSCC randomized to 16 Gy/2 fx (given with a 6-day break in between fractions) vs. split-course RT (15 Gy/3 fx → 4 day rest → 15 Gy/5 fx; total of 30 Gy/8 fx over 2 weeks). Approximately 60% of patients in each arm had back pain relief, 70% in each arm were able to walk, and 90% had good bladder function. OS and toxicity were equivalent. **Conclusion: Both hypofractionated RT schedules are effective, with acceptable toxicity.**

Table 68.3: Results of Rades Randomized Trial				
	Overall Motor Function Response Rate	Ambulatory Rate (at 1 mos)	Local PFS (at 6 mos)	OS (at 6 mos)
20 Gy/5 fx	87.2%	71.8%	75.2%	42.3%
30 Gy/10 fx	89.6%	74.0%	81.8%	37.8%
p value	.73	.86	.51	.68

■ Is there a role for spine SRS as compared to fractionated RT?

With true cord compression, the role of SRS is limited, given the duration of planning required for SRS and the need for ≥3 mm separation for the cord/thecal sac. The literature currently suggests a local control benefit, though this is primarily retrospective. RTOG 0631 compared patient-reported pain outcomes between the two modalities; however, it excluded patients with <3 mm of separation from the cord/thecal sac. See Chapter 67 for details on spine SRS.

REFERENCES

1. Mak KS, Lee LK, Mak RH, et al. Incidence and treatment patterns in hospitalizations for malignant spinal cord compression in the United States, 1998–2006. *Int J Radiat Oncol Biol Phys.* 2011;80(3):824–831. doi:10.1016/j.ijrobp.2010.03.022
2. Loblaw DA, Laperriere NJ, Mackillop WJ. A population-based study of malignant spinal cord compression in Ontario. *Clin Oncol.* 2003;15(4):211–217. doi:10.1016/S0936-6555(02)00400-4
3. Klein SL, Sanford RA, Muhlbauer MS. Pediatric spinal epidural metastases. *J Neurosur.* 1991;74(1):70–75. doi:10.3171/jns.1991.74.1.0070
4. Binokay F, Akgul E, Bicakci K, et al. Determining the level of the dural sac tip: magnetic resonance imaging in an adult population. *Acta Radiol.* 2006;47(4):397–400. doi:10.1080/02841850600557158
5. Scharf CB, Paulino AC, Goldberg KN. Determination of the inferior border of the thecal sac using magnetic resonance imaging: implications on radiation therapy treatment planning. *Int J Radiat Oncol Biol Phys.* 1998;41(3):621–624. doi:10.1080/02841850600557158
6. Bach F, Larsen BH, Rohde K, et al. Metastatic spinal cord compression. Occurrence, sympatientoms, clinical presentations and prognosis in 398 patients with spinal cord compression. *Acta Neurochir.* 1990;107(1–2):37–43. doi:10.1016/S0360-3016(97)00562-2
7. Helweg-Larsen S, Sorensen PS. Sympatientoms and signs in metastatic spinal cord compression: a study of progression from first sympatientom until diagnosis in 153 patients. *Eur J Cancer.* 1994;30A(3):396–398. doi:.org/10.1016/0959-8049(94)90263-1
8. Bilsky MH. New therapeutics in spine metastases. *Expert Rev Neurother.* 2005;5(6):831–840. doi:10.1586/14737175.5.6.831
9. Loblaw DA, Perry J, Chambers A, Laperriere NJ. Systematic review of the diagnosis and management of malignant extradural spinal cord compression: the Cancer Care Ontario Practice Guidelines Initiative's Neuro-Oncology Disease Site Group. *J Clin Oncol.* 2005;23(9):2028–2037. doi:10.1200/JCO.2005.00.067
10. Laufer I, Rubin DG, Lis E, et al. The NOMS framework: approach to the treatment of spinal metastatic tumors. *Oncologist.* 2013;18(6):744–751. doi:10.1634/theoncologist.2012-0293
11. Bilsky MH, Laufer I, Fourney DR, et al. Reliability analysis of the epidural spinal cord compression scale. *J Neurosurg Spine.* 2010;13(3):324–328. doi:10.3171/2010.3.SPINE09459
12. George R, Jeba J, Ramkumar G, et al. Interventions for the treatment of metastatic extradural spinal cord compression in adults. *Cochrane Database Syst Rev.* 2008(4):CD006716. doi:10.1002/14651858.CD006716.pub2
13. Graham PH, Capp A, Delaney G, et al. A pilot randomised comparison of dexamethasone 96 mg vs 16 mg per day for malignant spinal-cord compression treated by radiotherapy: TROG 01.05 Superdex study. *Clin Oncol.* 2006;18(1):70–76. doi:10.1016/j.clon.2005.08.015
14. Vecht CJ, Haaxma-Reiche H, van Putten WL, et al. Initial bolus of conventional versus high-dose dexamethasone in metastatic spinal cord compression. *Neurology.* 1989;39(9):1255–1257. doi:10.1097/BRS.0b013e3181b77895
15. Mendel E, Bourekas E, Gerszten P, Golan JD. Percutaneous techniques in the treatment of spine tumors: what are the diagnostic and therapeutic indications and outcomes? *Spine.* 2009;34(22 Suppl):S93–S100. doi:10.1097/BRS.0b013e3181b77895

16. Rades D, Huttenlocher S, Dunst J, et al. Matched pair analysis comparing surgery followed by radiotherapy and radiotherapy alone for metastatic spinal cord compression. *J Clin Oncol*. 2010;28(22):3597–3604. doi:10.1200/JCO.2010.28.5635

17. Patchell RA, Tibbs PA, Regine WF, et al. Direct decompressive surgical resection in the treatment of spinal cord compression caused by metastatic cancer: a randomised trial. *Lancet*. 2005;366(9486):643–648. doi:10.3171/jns.1980.53.6.0741

18. Young RF, Post EM, King GA. Treatment of spinal epidural metastases: randomized prospective comparison of laminectomy and radiotherapy. *J Neurosurg*. 1980;53(6):741–748. doi:10.3171/jns.1980.53.6.0741

19. Maranzano E, Bellavita R, Rossi R, et al. Short-course versus split-course radiotherapy in metastatic spinal cord compression: results of a phase III, randomized, multicenter trial. *J Clin Oncol*. 2005;23(15):3358–3365. doi:10.1200/JCO.2005.08.193

20. Terpos E, Morgan G, Dimopoulos MA, et al. International Myeloma Working Group recommendations for the treatment of multiple myeloma-related bone disease. *J Clin Oncol*. 2013;31(18):2347–2357. doi:10.1200/JCO.2012.47.7901

21. Maranzano E, Latini P. Effectiveness of radiation therapy without surgery in metastatic spinal cord compression: final results from a prospective trial. *Int J Radiat Oncol Biol Phys*. 1995;32(4):959–967. doi:10.1016/0360-3016(95)00572-G

22. Jin R, Rock J, Jin JY, et al. Single fraction spine radiosurgery for myeloma epidural spinal cord compression. *J Exp Ther Oncol*. 2009;8(1):35–41.

23. Yamada Y, Bilsky MH, Lovelock DM, et al. High-dose, single-fraction image-guided intensity-modulated radiotherapy for metastatic spinal lesions. *Int J Radiat Oncol Biol Phys*. 2008;71(2):484–490. doi:10.1016/j.ijrobp.2007.11.046

24. Sahgal A, Atenafu EG, Chao S, et al. Vertebral compression fracture after spine stereotactic body radiotherapy: a multi-institutional analysis with a focus on radiation dose and the spinal instability neoplastic score. *J Clin Oncol*. 2013;31(27):3426–3431. doi:10.1200/JCO.2013.50.1411

25. Videtic GMM, Woody N, Vassil AD. *Handbook of Treatment Planning in Radiation Oncology*. 3rd ed. Demos Medical; 2020. doi:10.1891/9780826168429

69 ■ SUPERIOR VENA CAVA SYNDROME

Kailin Yang and Gregory M. M. Videtic

QUICK HIT ■ SVC syndrome is an urgent clinical scenario but not an emergency unless presenting with clinically severe airway, neurologic, or hemodynamic compromise. Treatment decision-making is best directed by patient performance, underlying tumor histology, and overall stage. Patients with SVC syndrome do not have worse prognosis than patients without it (for same stage and histologic diagnosis). In stable patients, pursue completion of staging and workup. When emergent intervention is required, intravascular stenting may provide most rapid relief. In the United States, the most common malignancies associated with SVC syndrome are NSCLC, SCLC, and lymphoma. Overall, about 60% to 80% respond to CHT or RT within 2 weeks (common treatment approaches are listed in Table 69.1).

Table 69.1: General Treatment Approaches for SVC Syndrome	
Supportive care	Head elevation with high-flow oxygen. Data unclear for use of steroids (may obscure diagnosis) and/or diuretics.
CHT	Consider as initial treatment for SCLC, lymphoma, germ cell tumors.
RT	Consider hypofractionated RT for urgent relief with initiation of definitive course if clinically appropriate. Palliative RT as initial treatment in advanced/emergent patients for histologies other than SCLC, lymphoma, or germ cell tumors.
Intravascular stenting	Consider if rapid relief is necessary, if unable to tolerate tumor-directed therapy, or symptoms refractory to prior to previous modalities.

EPIDEMIOLOGY: Approximately 15,000 cases per year in the United States with survival dependent on underlying etiology.[1]

ANATOMY: SVC carries about one-third of total venous return including drainage from head, arms, and upper torso including the mediastinum (Table 69.2). It contains low-pressure blood flow and is thus thin-walled and easily compressible. Brachiocephalic (innominate) veins join to form SVC beginning at sternal angle. SVC then extends inferiorly along right lateral side of ascending aorta, and inserts into right atrium. Azygos vein enters SVC posteriorly, just above pericardial reflection. When obstructed, blood flow is diverted through collateral vessels including internal mammary, intercostal, esophageal, lateral thoracic, paraspinal, and azygos veins ultimately to inferior vena cava.

Table 69.2: Anatomy of Mediastinum			
	Boundaries	**Contents**	**Etiology of Malignant SVC Syndrome**
Superior mediastinum	Below thoracic inlet at T1 to above plane between sternal angle and T4 to T5	Thymus, trachea, SVC, aortic arch, esophagus, lymph nodes	NHL, lung, thymoma, thymic, thyroid cancer, germ cell tumors
Anterior mediastinum	Between pericardium and sternum	Thymus, fat, lymph nodes	NHL, Hodgkin's, thyroid cancer, thymoma, germ cell tumors, metastasis
Middle mediastinum	Pericardium and its contents, from T5 to T8	Heart, lung, great vessels (including distal SVC), mainstem bronchi, lymph nodes	NHL, lung cancer, sarcoma, thymoma, teratoma, mesothelioma

(continued)

Table 69.2: Anatomy of Mediastinum (*continued*)			
	Boundaries	**Contents**	**Etiology of Malignant SVC Syndrome**
Posterior mediastinum	Between pericardium and vertebral column, down to T12	Esophagus, descending aorta, thoracic duct, azygos vein, lymph nodes	NHL, nerve sheath tumors, pheochromocytoma, ganglio/neuroblastoma

PATHOLOGY: SVC syndrome was previously associated with untreated infections such as tuberculosis, syphilis, or aortic aneurysms. With more advanced antibiotics, malignancy now accounts for 70% to 90% of cases.[1-3] Common malignant etiologies include NSCLC (50%) > SCLC (25%) > NHL (12%) > metastasis (9%) > germ cell tumors > thymoma > others. More common in SCLC at 10% compared to 2% of NSCLC patients. Overall, 2% to 4% of patients with primary lung malignancy will develop SVC syndrome during course of their disease.[1,4,5] Other benign causes include thrombosis (related to intravascular devices), thyroid goiter, postradiation fibrosis, CHF, and aortic aneurysm. Fibrosing mediastinitis, often associated with granulomatous disease, requires biopsy for confirmation.

CLINICAL PRESENTATION: Severity of symptoms related to degree and time frame of SVC obstruction with subsequent collateralization. Dyspnea and facial/neck swelling are most common presenting symptoms. Medical emergencies characterized by clinical symptoms including airway obstruction, neurologic compromise, or hemodynamic instability (see definition of grade 4 SVC syndrome in Table 69.3).[6] Symptoms are commonly exacerbated by leaning forward or lying supine. One third of patients develop symptoms over 2 weeks.[1] In most cases, symptoms gradually progress over several weeks and then get better over time due to development of collateral vessels.

Table 69.3: Proposed Grading System for Superior Vena Cava Syndrome[6]			
Grade	**Category**	**Incidence**	**Definition**
0	Asymptomatic	10%	Asymptomatic radiographic SVC obstruction
1	Mild	25%	Edema/vascular distention in head or neck, cyanosis, plethora
2	Moderate	50%	Edema in head or neck with associated symptoms (dysphagia; cough; mild or moderate movement impairment of head, jaw, or eyelid; visual disruption)
3	Severe	10%	Mild/moderate cerebral edema (HA, dizziness), laryngeal edema, or diminished cardiac reserve (syncope after bending)
4	Life-threatening	5%	Cerebral edema with associated confusion or obtundation; laryngeal edema with stridor, or significant hemodynamic compromise leading to syncope due to SVC obstruction
5	Life-threatening	<1%	Death

WORKUP: H&P with focus on previous malignancies, risk factors for coagulopathy, previous intravascular procedures, or risk factors for granulomatous disease.

Imaging: CXR, chest CT with contrast with attention to collateral vessels.[7,8] Ultrasound to assess for thrombus.

Procedures: Biopsy (bronchoscopic, CT-guided, mediastinoscopy/mediastinotomy, thoracentesis are options).[9,10] Further workup per histologic diagnosis.

PROGNOSTIC FACTORS: Prognosis determined by underlying histology. Negative factors specific to SVC include cerebral edema, laryngeal edema, hypotension, syncope, headache. SVC obstruction does not predict poor outcomes in patients with treatment-responsive tumors compared to those without SVC.[11-16]

NATURAL HISTORY: After obstruction of SVC, increased central venous pressure (from approximately 2 to 8 mmHg to >20 mmHg) diverts venous return through collateral circulation.[7,17,18] Obstruction above junction of azygos vein causes venous congestion of head, neck, and arms. Obstruction below azygos vein leads to distention of veins of thorax and abdomen. Laryngeal edema may lead to dyspnea, stridor, cough, dysphagia.[6] Symptoms are related to time of onset with protracted onset allowing time for collaterals to develop. Disruption of cardiac output is usually temporary due to subsequent collateral development.

TREATMENT PARADIGM

Supportive: Head elevation and supplemental oxygen. Dexamethasone may be helpful to reduce cerebral edema or for treatment of steroid-responsive malignancies (lymphoma), although data are unclear. Role of diuretics is unclear based on single retrospective study of 107 patients with similar symptomatic improvement (84%) regardless of use of steroids, diuretics, or neither.[19]

Surgery: There is no standard role for surgery in SVC syndrome but can be considered in definitive management of underlying malignancy. Resection or bypass grafting generally reserved for surgically managed tumors (e.g., thymoma) and progressive or persistent symptoms (>6 months). Common approach is sternotomy/thoracotomy with resection and/or reconstruction of SVC.[20-22]

Chemotherapy: For chemotherapy-responsive histologies such as SCLC, germ cell tumors, or lymphoma, CHT is often initial treatment of choice in order to allow time for staging and RT planning. CHT should be dosed according to underlying histology. In one systematic review of 46 studies, ~77% of SCLC patients had resolution of symptoms with average time of 7 to 14 days.

Radiation: For palliation, RT doses ranging from 10 Gy/1 fx to 30 Gy/10 fx may be reasonable depending on function of patient and disease status.[23] Urgent but still curable patients may benefit from higher dose per fraction up front (3–4 Gy/fx) to alleviate symptoms with dose-adapted definitive dose at standard 1.8 to 2 Gy/fx after 2 to 3 days, with total doses based on histology and for curative intent. Symptomatic relief can be apparent in 72 hours but can take up to 4 weeks.[5] Up to 20% of patients do not obtain symptomatic relief from RT. Among those who do respond, ~20% will have recurrent obstruction.[16] Symptomatic relief may occur without complete/partial SVC patency after treatment.[24] As per review of 24 CHT/RT studies, there were no reports of worsening symptoms with RT.[5,25]

Intravascular Stent: Intravascular stenting is the most rapid treatment for SVC syndrome.[5] Stent placement should be considered for severe symptoms (e.g., airway compromise or cerebral edema), inability to tolerate tumor-directed therapy, or low probability of response to CHT/RT (e.g., mesothelioma). Symptomatic improvement occurs in 75% to 100%, typically within 48 to 72 hours. Complication rate is 3% to 7%.[1,26,27] A small phase 3 study from Japan (32 patients) demonstrated significant superiority of stent placement compared to other management.[28] Early complications include infection, pulmonary embolus, stent migration, hematoma, bleeding, and perforation/rupture of SVC (rare). Late complications include bleeding (1%–14%) or death (1%–2%) from anticoagulation and stent failure with reocclusion.[29] Relative contraindications include patients without symptoms and inability to lie flat.

■ **EVIDENCE-BASED Q&A**

▧ **Is it safe to delay intervention to pursue workup?**

Yes, except when symptoms concerning for urgent treatment are present (e.g., airway compromise, cerebral edema). There have been three separate RRs of 107, 63, and 249 patients with SVC syndrome—there was no evidence of serious complications resulting from delay in treatment of SVC obstruction while diagnostic workup was completed.[2,19,30]

REFERENCES

1. Wilson LD, Detterbeck FC, Yahalom J. Clinical practice. Superior vena cava syndrome with malignant causes. *N Engl J Med.* 2007;356(18):1862–1869. doi:10.1056/NEJMcp067190

2.   Yellin A, Rosen A, Reichert N, Lieberman Y. Superior vena cava syndrome. The myth--the facts. *Am Rev Respir Dis.* 1990;141(5 Pt 1):1114–1118. doi:10.1164/ajrccm/141.5_Pt_1.1114

3.   Martins SJ, Pereira JR. Clinical factors and prognosis in non-small cell lung cancer. *Am J Clin Oncol.* 1999;22(5):453–457. doi:10.1097/00000421-199910000-00006

4.   Houman M, Ksontini I, Ben Ghorbel I, et al. Association of right heart thrombosis, endomyocardial fibrosis, and pulmonary artery aneurysm in Behcet's disease. *Eur J Intern Med.* 2002;13(7):455. doi:10.1016/S0953-6205(02)00134-6

5.   Rowell NP, Gleeson FV. Steroids, radiotherapy, chemotherapy and stents for superior vena caval obstruction in carcinoma of the bronchus: a systematic review. *Clin Oncol (R Coll Radiol).* 2002;14(5):338–351. doi:10.1053/clon.2002.0095

6.   Yu JB, Wilson LD, Detterbeck FC. Superior vena cava syndrome--a proposed classification system and algorithm for management. *J Thorac Oncol.* 2008;3(8):811–814. doi:10.1097/JTO.0b013e3181804791

7.   Kim HJ, Kim HS, Chung SH. CT diagnosis of superior vena cava syndrome: importance of collateral vessels. *AJR Am J Roentgenol.* 1993;161(3):539–542. doi:10.2214/ajr.161.3.8352099

8.   Parish JM, Marschke RF, Jr., Dines DE, Lee RE. Etiologic considerations in superior vena cava syndrome. *Mayo Clin Proc.* 1981;56(7):407–413.

9.   Mineo TC, Ambrogi V, Nofroni I, Pistolese C. Mediastinoscopy in superior vena cava obstruction: analysis of 80 consecutive patients. *Ann Thorac Surg.* 1999;68(1):223–226. doi:10.1016/S0003-4975(99)00455-5

10.   Dosios T, Theakos N, Chatziantoniou C. Cervical mediastinoscopy and anterior mediastinotomy in superior vena cava obstruction. *Chest.* 2005;128(3):1551–1556. doi:10.1378/chest.128.3.1551

11.   Urban T, Lebeau B, Chastang C, et al. Superior vena cava syndrome in small-cell lung cancer. *Arch Intern Med.* 1993;153(3):384–387. doi:10.1001/archinte.153.3.384

12.   Sculier JP, Evans WK, Feld R, et al. Superior vena caval obstruction syndrome in small cell lung cancer. *Cancer.* 1986;57(4):847–851. doi:10.1002/1097-0142(19860215)57:4<847::AID-CNCR2820570427>3.0.CO;2-H

13.   Dombernowsky P, Hansen HH. Combination chemotherapy in the management of superior vena caval obstruction in small-cell anaplastic carcinoma of the lung. *Acta Med Scand.* 1978;204(6):513–516. doi:10.1111/j.0954-6820.1978.tb08482.x

14.   Warde P, Payne D. Does thoracic irradiation improve survival and local control in limited-stage small-cell carcinoma of the lung? A meta-analysis. *J Clin Oncol.* 1992;10(6):890–895. doi:10.1200/JCO.1992.10.6.890

15.   Wurschmidt F, Bunemann H, Heilmann HP. Small cell lung cancer with and without superior vena cava syndrome: a multivariate analysis of prognostic factors in 408 cases. *Int J Radiat Oncol Biol Phys.* 1995;33(1):77–82. doi:10.1016/0360-3016(95)00094-F

16.   Spiro SG, Shah S, Harper PG, Tobias JS, Geddes DM, Souhami RL. Treatment of obstruction of the superior vena cava by combination chemotherapy with and without irradiation in small-cell carcinoma of the bronchus. *Thorax.* 1983;38(7):501–505. doi:10.1136/thx.38.7.501

17.   Trigaux JP, Van Beers B. Thoracic collateral venous channels: normal and pathologic CT findings. *J Comput Assist Tomogr.* 1990;14(5):769–773. doi:10.1097/00004728-199009000-00017

18.   Gonzalez-Fajardo JA, Garcia-Yuste M, Florez S, et al. Hemodynamic and cerebral repercussions arising from surgical interruption of the superior vena cava. Experimental model. *J Thorac Cardiovasc Surg.* 1994;107(4):1044–1049. doi:10.1016/S0022-5223(94)70379-5

19.   Schraufnagel DE, Hill R, Leech JA, Pare JA. Superior vena caval obstruction. Is it a medical emergency? *Am J Med.* 1981;70(6):1169–1174. doi:10.1016/0002-9343(81)90823-8

20.   Magnan PE, Thomas P, Giudicelli R, et al. Surgical reconstruction of the superior vena cava. *Cardiovasc Surg.* 1994;2(5):598–604. doi:10.1016/S0003-4975(98)00350-6

21.   Bacha EA, Chapelier AR, Macchiarini P, et al. Surgery for invasive primary mediastinal tumors. *Ann Thorac Surg.* 1998;66(1):234–239. doi:10.1016/S0003-4975(98)00350-6

22.   Chen KN, Xu SF, Gu ZD, et al. Surgical treatment of complex malignant anterior mediastinal tumors invading the superior vena cava. *World J Surg.* 2006;30(2):162–170. doi:10.1007/s00268-005-0009-x

23.   Straka C, Ying J, Kong FM, et al. Review of evolving etiologies, implications and treatment strategies for the superior vena cava syndrome. *Springerplus.* 2016;5:229. doi:10.1186/s40064-016-1900-7

24.   Ahmann FR. A reassessment of the clinical implications of the superior vena caval syndrome. *J Clin Oncol.* 1984;2(8):961–969. doi:10.1200/JCO.1984.2.8.961

25.   Egelmeers A, Goor C, van Meerbeeck J, et al. Palliative effectiveness of radiation therapy in the treatment of superior vena cava syndrome. *Bull Cancer Radiother.* 1996;83(3):153–157. doi:10.1016/0924-4212(96)81747-6

26.   Fagedet D, Thony F, Timsit JF, et al. Endovascular treatment of malignant superior vena cava syndrome: results and predictive factors of clinical efficacy. *Cardiovasc Intervent Radiol.* 2013;36(1):140–149. doi:10.1007/s00270-011-0310-z

27.   Sobrinho G, Aguiar P. Stent placement for the treatment of malignant superior vena cava syndrome: a single-center series of 56 patients. *Arch Bronconeumol.* 2014;50(4):135–140. doi:10.1016/j.arbr.2014.03.001

28.   Takeuchi Y, Arai Y, Sone M, et al. Evaluation of stent placement for vena cava syndrome: phase II trial and phase III randomized controlled trial. *Support Care Cancer.* 2019;27(3):1081–1088. doi:10.1007/s00520-018-4397-5

29.   Watkinson AF, Yeow TN, Fraser C. Endovascular stenting to treat obstruction of the superior vena cava. *BMJ.* 2008;336(7658):1434–1437. doi:10.1136/bmj.39562.512789.80

30.   Gauden SJ. Superior vena cava syndrome induced by bronchogenic carcinoma: is this an oncological emergency? *Australas Radiol.* 1993;37(4):363–366. doi:10.1111/j.1440-1673.1993.tb00096.x

Matthew C. Ward and Justin J. Juliano

The goal of palliative radiation therapy is to increase quality of life, and is most often applied when quantity of life cannot be reasonably improved. Palliative RT should be focused on the near term, be completed in a short time, in a convenient manner, without undue risks, and at minimal expense.[1] Deviation from these priorities risks an unnecessary burden on patients during a difficult time.

PALLIATION OF INCURABLE HEAD AND NECK CANCER

Locoregional disease can be distressing for patients even if poor performance status, advanced medical comorbidities, and/or metastatic disease precludes aggressive management. Symptoms of progressive disease warranting consideration of palliative RT include pain, odynophagia, otalgia, dysphagia, airway obstruction (cough, dyspnea) and ulceration/bleeding. Short courses of RT are available to minimize side-effects and reduce such symptoms (Table 70.1). Concurrent systemic therapy is typically avoided given the known increase in sequalae without a known benefit to quality of life.

Table 70.1: Selected Palliative Regimens for H&N Cancer

Regimen	Dose	Notes
Quad Shot[2-5]	14 Gy/4 fx BID over 2 days with ≥6 hour interval; repeat at 4-week intervals for up to 3–4 total cycles (42 Gy/12 fx)	Phase I–II trials did not enroll patients w/ previous RT or give concurrent CHT, but both appear safe
Hypo[6]	30 Gy/5 fx at least 3 days apart; additional 6 Gy boost to tumors ≤3 cm	No previous RT
Christie[7]	50 Gy/16 fx, 4 to 5 fx per week	
Italy[8]	50 Gy/20 fx with 2-week midtreatment break	
SCAHRT[9]	30 Gy/10 fx, 3- to 5-week break, if tolerated, then followed by additional 30–36 Gy/10 to 12 fx	
IHF2SQ[10]	6 Gy/2 fx, days 1 and 3 during first, third, and fifth weeks of platinum CHT	Concurrent CHT, no previous RT

SALVAGE OF LOCOREGIONALLY RECURRENT HEAD AND NECK CANCER

For patients with carcinoma of the H&N arising within or adjacent to a previous RT field, more aggressive options may be reasonable through the use of re-irradiation (loosely defined here as ≥100 Gy cumulative doses). Data for a survival benefit to re-irradiation over systemic therapy are lacking and limited primarily to retrospective outcomes. Absolute contraindications to aggressive re-irradiation include tumor adjacent to critical structures in which damage would be catastrophic such as the brainstem or spinal cord. Relative contraindications include poor performance status, distant metastatic disease, and short time interval since previous RT (≤6 months). Salvage surgery is optimal when possible.

Classic techniques for re-irradiation include hyperfractionated RT to doses of ~60 Gy with variable schedules including treatment breaks.[11,12] More modern techniques treat to 60 to 72 Gy without a break. Retrospective outcomes do not support elective nodal radiation.[13] Hyperfractionation may allow for dose escalation, but outcomes appear similar.[13] SBRT is an evolving option with doses of 35 to 44 Gy given in 5 fx every other day.[14] SBRT carries the advantage of convenience with more durable local control than other palliative regimens and late effects seem comparable.[15]

Our preference is to utilize an RPA model for patient selection.[16] In the post-surgical adjuvant re-irradiation setting, for RPA class I patients with risk factors according to the GORTEC trial,[17] we often recommend 60 to 66 Gy over 30 to 33 fx to the tumor bed alone. For non-operable class II patients, we often recommend 66 Gy in 33 fx with chemotherapy to the gross tumor plus margin. For RPA class III patients regardless of resection status, we consider short-course palliative re-treatment or SBRT, as long-term survival is not thought to be possible even with protracted regimens.

ADRENAL METASTASES PALLIATION

The adrenal gland is a common site of metastasis from other primary tumors (lung being most common), but with <5% of patients symptomatic at detection.[18] When symptomatic, pain (lower chest, abdomen, back, or flank) is most often reported. Other signs and symptoms include adrenal insufficiency, peritoneal hemorrhage, and inferior vena cava thrombosis. For symptomatic/palliative intent, RT is effective and standard regimens such as 20 Gy/5 fx, 30 Gy/10 fx, 36 Gy/20 fx, or 45 Gy/20 fx have been used.[19]

With increasing imaging surveillance of cancer patients, incidence of asymptomatic adrenal metastases is rising.[20] For patients with limited metastatic disease, adrenalectomy is the preferred treatment.[21] Other interventions include percutaneous ablation, conventional RT, and SBRT. While rare (and should be considered in context of bilateral adrenal metastases), adrenal insufficiency may be associated with weakness, weight loss, hypotension, hypoglycemia, hyponatremia, and hyperkalemia. Treatment is with glucocorticoids and mineralocorticoids. There are limited data for SBRT but ideally BED >100 Gy can be achieved while respecting normal tissue tolerance. See Table 70.2 for example regimens.

Table 70.2 :Selected Series of SBRT for Adrenal Metastases			
Series	N (patients)	Dose (Median/Mode)	Dose (Range)
Rochester[22]	30	40 Gy/10 fx	16 Gy/4 fx to 50 Gy/10 fx
Florence[23]	48	36 Gy/3 fx	30–54 Gy
Milan[24]	34	32 Gy/4 fx	20 Gy/4 fx to 45 Gy/18 fx
MDACC[25]	43	60 Gy/10 fx	50 Gy/4 fx to 63 Gy/9 fx

LIVER PALLIATION

The liver represents a common source of visceral metastatic disease. Patients with low volume and solitary metastatic disease may be considered for curative resection or SBRT (see Chapter 71). In colorectal cancer, 5- and 10-year OS of 40% and 25% are reported in such cases, respectively.[26]

Optimal candidates for ablative RT have preserved performance status, adequate liver function, solitary liver metastasis, and uninvolved liver volume >700 cc.[27] KRAS mutations carry a higher rate of local failure.[28] Both 3 and 5 fx regimens of SBRT have been used. For 3 fx regimens, prescription dose of ≥48 Gy (48–54 Gy) is recommended when safe.[29]

Other modalities such as RFA, cryotherapy, laser-induced thermotherapy, HIFU, TACE chemoembolization, or Y90 embolization have been employed as well.

In cases of advanced or refractory symptomatic hepatic metastases, RT to the whole liver can afford effective palliation of symptoms/signs such as pain (from capsule distention), nausea/anorexia, jaundice, and constitutional symptoms such as weight loss, fevers, or night sweats. Premedication with antinausea medication with or without dexamethasone is recommended when treating large volumes of liver. A number of regimens have safely been employed including: 8 Gy/1 fx,[30] 10 Gy/2 fx,[31] 21 Gy/7 fx,[32] and 30 Gy/15 fx.[27]

LUNG PALLIATION

Patients with primary lung cancer or progressive pulmonary metastases can present with symptoms including hemoptysis, cough, dyspnea, and chest pain. A definitive approach should be considered for those patients deemed nonmetastatic. For those in whom poor performance status and/or advanced medical comorbidities preclude aggressive management, a palliative approach is appropriate.

Treatment must be triaged according to urgency. In otherwise stable patients, locoregional control, relief of symptoms, limiting toxicity, maintaining quality of life, patient convenience, and cost of care are all important considerations. Early referral to a palliative care specialist is encouraged. Endoscopic interventions such as bronchoscopy with laser ablation ± endobronchial stenting may be helpful for rapid relief of central airway obstruction. Thoracentesis with drainage catheter placement can aid for pleural effusions. Endovascular stenting can aid for SVC syndrome (see Chapter 69).

Various RT fractionation schemes have been employed. ASTRO guidelines suggest protracted regimens (30 Gy/10 fx) for patients with a good performance status.[33] While survival and symptom scores are improved with higher dose schedules, the latter comes with the cost of higher treatment-related toxicity. Shorter courses are appropriate for patients with compromised performance status. Regimens to consider: 10 Gy/1 fx, 16 to 17 Gy/2 fx, 20 Gy/5 fx, 30 Gy/10 fx, 36 Gy/12 fx, 39 Gy/13 fx.[33,34]

PELVIC PALLIATION

RT is effective for palliation of pelvic progression of urogenital and anorectal malignancies. Most common symptoms include pain, bleeding, and obstruction (urinary or bowel). In addition to presenting symptoms, consideration should be given to the tumor burden (both at local level as well as systemic), prognosis, performance status, ongoing treatments, and personal preferences.

Palliative pelvic exenteration may be considered for select patients who are medically fit, are amenable to gross resection (no major peripheral nerve involvement, no direct invasion of common iliac vessels, or bony invasion at pelvic sidewall or sacrum), and have minimal extrapelvic disease.[35] Exenteration often requires both urinary and fecal diversion through ostomies.

For recurrent rectal cancer, experience exists for both definitive and peri-operative re-irradiation (see Chapter 36 for details). More limited experience exists for re-irradiation (e.g., 50 Gy/20–25 fx) of other malignancies.[36]

For those with metastatic, unresectable, or medically inoperable disease, RT is standard option for palliation. A wide variety of clinical scenarios mandate careful application of RT. Accepted regimens beyond standard doses of 20 Gy/5 fx or 30 Gy/10 fx are noted in Table 70.3. Other palliative modalities such as TAE and nerve blocks can be considered for bleeding and pain, respectively.

Table 70.3: Selected Palliative Regimens for Miscellaneous Pelvic Malignancies		
Regimen	Dose	Notes
Quad Shot/RTOG 8502[37,38]	14.8 Gy/4 fx BID over 2 days with ≥6-hr interval; repeat at 4-wk intervals for up to 3 total cycles (44.4 Gy/12 fx)	Break of 2 wk no different than 4-wk break (NS increase in acute effects)[39]
RTOG 7905[40]	10 Gy/1 fx once every 4 wks for up to 3 treatments	Abandoned due to Grade 3–4 late effects of 45%
MRC BA09 (UK)[41]	PRT 35 Gy/10 fx vs. 21 Gy/3 fx	Tested in bladder cancer only; no differences in efficacy or toxicity

REFERENCES

1. Lutz ST, Jones J, Chow E. Role of radiation therapy in palliative care of the patient with cancer. *J Clin Oncol.* 2014;32(26):2913–2919. doi:10.1200/JCO.2014.55.1143
2. Corry J, Peters LJ, D'Costa I, et al. The "QUAD SHOT" - A phase II study of palliative radiotherapy for incurable head and neck cancer. *Radiother Oncol.* 2005;77(2):137–142. doi:10.1016/j.radonc.2005.10.008

3. Paris KJ, Spanos WJ, Lindberg RD, Baby Jose AF. Phase I-II study of multiple daily fractions for palliation of advanced head and neck malignancies. *Int J Radiat Oncol Biol Phys*. 1993;25(4):657–660. doi:10.1016/0360-3016(93)90012-K

4. Lok BH, Jiang G, Gutiontov S, et al. Palliative head and neck radiotherapy with the RTOG 8502 regimen for incurable primary or metastatic cancers. *Oral Oncol*. 2015;51(10):957–962. doi:10.1016/j.oraloncology.2015.07.011

5. Gamez ME, Agarwal M, Hu KS, et al. Hypofractionated palliative radiotherapy with concurrent radiosensitizing chemotherapy for advanced head and neck cancer using the "QUAD-SHOT regimen." *Anticancer Res*. 2017;37(2):685–692. doi:10.21873/anticanres.11364

6. Porceddu SV, Rosser B, Burmeister BH, et al. Hypofractionated radiotherapy for the palliation of advanced head and neck cancer in patients unsuitable for curative treatment - "Hypo Trial." *Radiother Oncol*. 2007;85(3):456–462. doi:10.1016/j.radonc.2007.10.020

7. Al-Mamgani A, Tans L, van Rooij PHE, et al. Hypofractionated radiotherapy denoted as the "christie scheme": an effective means of palliating patients with head and neck cancers not suitable for curative treatment. *Acta Oncologica*. 2009;48(4):562–570. doi:10.1080/02841860902740899

8. Minatel E, Gigante M, Franchin G, et al. Combined radiotherapy and bleomycin in patients with inoperable head and neck cancer with unfavourable prognostic factors and severe symptoms. *Oral Oncol*. 1998;34(2):119–122. doi:10.1016/S1368-8375(97)00073-0

9. Bledsoe TJ, Noble AR, Reddy CA, et al. Split-course accelerated hypofractionated radiotherapy (scahrt): A safe and effective option for head and neck cancer in the elderly or infirm. Anticancer Research 2016;36(3):933–940.

10. Monnier L, Touboul E, Durdux C, et al. Hypofractionated palliative radiotherapy for advanced head and neck cancer: The IHF2SQ regimen. *Head and Neck* 2013;35(12):1683–1688. doi:.1002/hed.23219

11. Spencer SA, Harris J, Wheeler RH, et al. Final report of RTOG 9610, a multi-institutional trial of reirradiation and chemotherapy for unresectable recurrent squamous cell carcinoma of the head and neck. *Head and Neck* 2008;30(3):281–288. doi:10.1002/hed.20697

12. Langer CJ, Harris J, Horwitz EM, et al. Phase II study of low-dose paclitaxel and cisplatin in combination with split-course concomitant twice-daily reirradiation in recurrent squamous cell carcinoma of the head and neck: Results of Radiation Therapy Oncology Group protocol 9911. *J Clin Oncol*. 2007;25(30):4800–5. doi:10.1002/hed.20697

13. Caudell JJ, Ward MC, Riaz N, et al. Volume, dose, and fractionation considerations for IMRT-based reirradiation in head and neck cancer: a multi-institution analysis. *Int J Radiat Oncol Biol Phys*. 2018;100(3):606–17. Available from: doi:10.1016/j.ijrobp.2017.11.036

14. Vargo JA, Ferris RL, Ohr J, et al. A prospective phase 2 trial of reirradiation with stereotactic body radiation therapy plus cetuximab in patients with previously irradiated recurrent squamous cell carcinoma of the head and neck. *Int J Radiat Oncol Biol Phys*. 2015;91(3):480–488. doi:10.1016/j.ijrobp.2014.11.023

15. Vargo JA, Ward MC, Caudell JJ, et al. A multi-institutional comparison of SBRT and IMRT for definitive reirradiation of recurrent or second primary head and neck cancer. *Int J Radiat Oncol Biol Phys*. 2018;100(3):595–605. doi:10.1016/j.ijrobp.2017.04.017

16. Ward MC, Riaz N, Caudell JJ, et al. Refining patient selection for reirradiation of head and neck squamous carcinoma in the IMRT era: a multi-institution cohort study by the MIRI collaborative. *Int J Radiat Oncol Biol Phys*. 2017;100(3):586–594. doi:10.1016/j.ijrobp.2017.06.012

17. Janot F, de Raucourt D, Benhamou E, et al. Randomized trial of postoperative reirradiation combined with chemotherapy after salvage surgery compared with salvage surgery alone in head and neck carcinoma. *J Clin Oncol*. 2008;26(34):5518–5523. doi:10.1200/JCO.2007.15.0102

18. Shiue K, Song A, Teh BS, et al. Stereotactic body radiation therapy for metastasis to the adrenal glands. *Expert Rev Anticancer Ther*. 2012;12(12):1613–1620. doi:10.1200/JCO.2007.15.0102

19. Short S, Chaturvedi A, Leslie MD. Palliation of symptomatic adrenal gland metastases by radiotherapy. *Clin Oncol*. 1996;8(6):387–389. doi:10.1016/S0936-6555(96)80087-2

20. Mitchell IC, Nwariaku FE. Adrenal masses in the cancer patient: surveillance or excision. *Oncologist*. 2007;12(2):168–174. doi:10.1634/theoncologist.12-2-168

21. Sastry P, Tocock A, Coonar A. Adrenalectomy for isolated metastasis from operable non-small-cell lung cancer. *Interact Cardiovasc Thorac Surg*. 2014;18(4):495–497. doi:10.1093/icvts/ivt526

22. Chawla S, Chen Y, Katz AW, et al. Stereotactic body radiotherapy for treatment of adrenal metastases. *Int J Radiat Oncol Biol Phys*. 2009;75(1):71–75. doi:10.1016/j.ijrobp.2008.10.079

23. Casamassima F, Livi L, Masciullo S, et al. Stereotactic radiotherapy for adrenal gland metastases: University of Florence experience. *Int J Radiat Oncol Biol Phys*. 2012;82(2):919–923. doi:10.1016/j.ijrobp.2010.11.060

24. Scorsetti M, Alongi F, Filippi AR, et al. Long-term local control achieved after hypofractionated stereotactic body radiotherapy for adrenal gland metastases: a retrospective analysis of 34 patients. *Acta Oncologica*. 2012;51(5):618–623. doi:10.3109/0284186X.2011.652738

25. Chance WW, Nguyen QN, Mehran R, et al. Stereotactic ablative radiotherapy for adrenal gland metastases: factors influencing outcomes, patterns of failure, and dosimetric thresholds for toxicity. *Pract Oncol Radiother*. 2017;7(3):e195–203. doi:10.1016/j.prro.2016.09.005

26. Abdalla EK, Vauthey JN, Ellis LM, et al. Recurrence and outcomes following hepatic resection, radiofrequency ablation, and combined resection/ablation for colorectal liver metastases. *Ann Surg*. 2004;818–827. doi:10.1097/01.sla.0000128305.90650.71

27. Høyer M, Swaminath A, Bydder S, et al. Radiotherapy for liver metastases: a review of evidence. *Int J Radiat Oncol Biol Phys*. 2012;82(3):1047–1057. doi:10.1016/j.ijrobp.2011.07.020

28. Hong TS, Wo JY, Borger DR, et al. Phase II study of proton-based stereotactic body radiation therapy for liver metastases: importance of tumor genotype. *J Natl Cancer Inst.* 2017;109(9). doi:10.1093/jnci/djx031

29. Chang DT, Swaminath A, Kozak M, et al. Stereotactic body radiotherapy for colorectal liver metastases: a pooled analysis. *Cancer.* 2011;117(17):4060–4069. doi:10.1002/cncr.25997

30. Soliman H, Ringash J, Jiang H, et al. Phase II trial of palliative radiotherapy for hepatocellular carcinoma and liver metastases. *J Clin Oncol.* 2013;31(31):3980–3986. doi:10.1200/JCO.2013.49.9202

31. Bydder S, Spry NA, Christie DRH, et al. A prospective trial of short-fractionation radiotherapy for the palliation of liver metastases. *Australas. Radiol.* 2003;47(3):284–288. doi:10.1046/j.1440-1673.2003.01177.x

32. Leibel SA, Pajak TF, Massullo V, et al. A comparison of misonidazole sensitized radiation therapy to radiation therapy alone for the palliation of hepatic metastases: results of a radiation therapy oncology group randomized prospective trial. *Int J Radiat Oncol Biol Phys.* 1987;13(7):1057–1064. doi:10.1016/0360-3016(87)90045-9

33. Rodrigues G, Videtic GMM, Sur R, et al. Palliative thoracic radiotherapy in lung cancer: an American Society for Radiation Oncology evidence-based clinical practice guideline. *Pract Radiat Oncol.* 2011;1(2):60–71. doi:10.1016/j.prro.2011.01.005

34. Macbeth FR, Bolger JJ, Hopwood P, et al. Randomized trial of palliative two-fraction versus more intensive 13-fraction radiotherapy for patients with inoperable non-small cell lung cancer and good performance status. *Clin Oncol.* 1996;8(3):167–175. doi:10.1016/S0936-6555(96)80041-0

35. Finlayson C, Eisenberg B. Palliative pelvic exenteration: patient selection and results. *Oncology* (Williston Park). 1996;10(4):479–484.

36. Kamran SC, Harshman LC, Bhagwat MS, et al. Characterization of efficacy and toxicity after high-dose pelvic reirradiation with palliative intent for genitourinary second malignant neoplasms or local recurrences after full-dose radiation therapy in the pelvis: a high-volume cancer center experience. *Adv Radiat Oncol.* 2017;2(2):140–147. doi:10.1016/j.adro.2017.01.001

37. Spanos WT, Clery M, Perez CA, et al. Late effect of multiple daily fraction palliation schedule for advanced pelvic malignancies (RTOG 8502). International Journal of Radiation Oncology, Biology, Physics 1994;29(5):961–967. doi:10.1016/0360-3016(94)90389-1

38. Spanos W, Guse C, Perez C, et al. Phase II study of multiple daily fractionations in the palliation of advanced pelvic malignancies: Preliminary report of RTOG 8502. *Int J Radiat Oncol Biol Phys.* 1989;17(3):659–661. doi:10.1016/0360-3016(89)90120-X

39. Spanos WJ, Perez CA, Marcus S, et al. Effect of rest interval on tumor and normal tissue response-A report of phase III study of accelerated split course palliative radiation for advanced pelvic malignancies (RTOG-8502). *Int J Radiat Oncol Biol Phys.* 1993;25(3):399–403. doi:10.1016/0360-3016(93)90059-5

40. Spanos WJ, Wasserman T, Meoz R, et al. Palliation of advanced pelvic malignant disease with large fraction pelvic radiation and misonidazole: final report of RTOG phase I/II study. *Int J Radiat Oncol Biol Phys.* 1987;13(10):1479–1482. doi:10.1016/0360-3016(87)90314-2

41. Duchesne GM, Bolger JJ, Griffiths GO, et al. A randomized trial of hypofractionated schedules of palliative radiotherapy in the management of bladder carcinoma: Results of medical research council trial BA09. *Int J Radiat Oncol Biol Phys.* 2000;47(2):379–388. doi:10.1016/S0360-3016(00)00430-2

Ian W. Winter, Ehsan H. Balagamwala, and Martin C. Tom

QUICK HIT ■ OMD refers to a state between localized and widely metastatic cancer, wherein some patients may benefit from aggressive local therapy. OMD has been defined in several prospective trials as ≤3 to 5 lesions. Subgroups include synchronous, metachronous, oligoprogressive, and oligopersistent disease. Rationales for aggressive local treatment include a potential benefit in OS and/or PFS, as well as to spare patients from prolonged systemic therapy or a change in systemic therapy that is otherwise effective for the majority of their disease. SBRT is an attractive modality for MDT given that it is effective, noninvasive, and well tolerated. Multiple studies are ongoing to evaluate the role of local therapy for OMD. Phase II prospective trials have demonstrated favorable PFS, OS, and androgen deprivation-free survival with MDT for prostate cancer. Additionally, prostate-directed RT in low-volume metastatic prostate cancer improved OS in a randomized trial subset, and this is now included as an option in NCCN guidelines.

BACKGROUND: In 1995, Hellman and Weichselbaum noted that there exists a subset of patients with limited volume metastatic disease who not only have an improved prognosis, but in whom treatment of the oligometastatic site(s) may impact survival.[1] They described cancer as existing on a biologic spectrum extending from localized to systemic at presentation, but with many intermediate states. They hypothesized that some patients with metastatic disease could still benefit from local therapy and achieve a durable response or, in some cases, cure. Modern improvements in imaging to detect distant disease, systemic therapy to control metastatic disease, and less invasive treatment modalities (SBRT and minimally invasive surgery) have allowed further study of MDT to manage metastatic disease.

DEFINITIONS: Numerous definitions and subsets of OMD have emerged, with significant heterogeneity and likely differing prognosis. Disease burden is most commonly ≤3 or ≤5 metastatic lesions; however, some have argued that there is no biologically defined upper limit and that OMD should apply to any state where all sites of disease can be safely treated with MDT.[2] General terminology includes the following: (a) Synchronous: OMD at the time of initial diagnosis, with the primary tumor and limited number of metastases detected simultaneously. (b) Metachronous: Oligometastatic recurrence following primary therapy at least 3 to 6 months after the initial diagnosis, also referred to as oligorecurrence. (c) Oligoprogression: Few lesions progress on a background of otherwise stable metastatic disease. (d) Oligopersistence: Few lesions persist after systemic therapy.[2] A more comprehensive classification scheme has been proposed (Table 71.1).

EPIDEMIOLOGY: Oligometastatic states are not uncommon, but owing to the lack of a uniform definition the incidence/prevalence is difficult to quantify. In a series of patients at MSKCC with sarcoma, 19% of patients presented with isolated pulmonary metastasis as the first site of failure.[4] In a series of patients at British Columbia Cancer Agency with CRC, 46% of those with metastatic disease presented with isolated hepatic metastases, 38% of these had one to three sites of disease.[5] In a patterns of failure analysis of patients with recurrent locally advanced or metastatic lung cancer treated with first line systemic CHT, 53% of patients were considered eligible for consolidative SBRT at the time of first failure, with a median of three lesions.[6]

Table 71.1: EORTC and ESTRO Proposed OMD Classification[3]		
DE-NOVO OMD No history of OMD or polymetastatic disease	**REPEAT OMD** History of OMD, no polymetastatic disease	**INDUCED OMD** History of polymetastatic disease treated with systemic therapy

(continued)

Table 71.1: EORTC and ESTRO Proposed OMD Classification[3] *(continued)*		
Synchronous OMD OMD present at diagnosis or within ~6 months	**Repeat Oligorecurrence** OMD at diagnosis treated with local or systemic therapy → systemic therapy-free interval → new/growing OMD	**Induced Oligorecurrence** Polymetastatic disease treated with systemic therapy → systemic therapy-free interval → growing or regrowing OMD
Metachronous Oligorecurrence Primary treated in nonmetastatic state → systemic therapy-free interval → OMD at recurrence (>6 mo after first diagnosis)	**Repeat Oligoprogression** OMD at diagnosis treated with local or systemic therapy → on systemic therapy → growing or regrowing OMD	**Induced Oligoprogression** Polymetastatic disease treated with systemic therapy → on systemic therapy → growing or regrowing OMD
Metachronous Oligoprogression Primary treated in nonmetastatic state → on systemic therapy → OMD (>6 mos after first diagnosis)	**Repeat Oligopersistence** OMD at diagnosis treated with local or systemic therapy → on systemic therapy → persistent nonprogressive OMD	**Induced Oligopersistence** Polymetastatic disease treated with systemic therapy → on systemic therapy → persistent nonprogressive OMD

■ EVIDENCE-BASED Q&A

■ Are there any prospective studies assessing local therapy for OMD in NSCLC?

Two randomized phase II trials in patients with oligometastatic NSCLC after first line systemic therapy were closed early due to a PFS benefit with SBRT or MDT to all sites, one of which also demonstrated an OS benefit. These formed the basis of NRG LU002, an ongoing phase II/III RCT.

Gomez, "Oligomez" (*Lancet Oncol* 2016, PMID 27789196; Update *JCO* 2019, PMID 31067138): Phase II randomized multicenter study of 49 patients with ≤3 NSCLC oligometastases (not including primary lesion) after first line tx without PD randomized to local consolidative therapy (LCT; via RT [no standard dose] or surgery ± maintenance tx) vs. maintenance tx alone (or surveillance); 1° end-point PFS. Study was terminated early (49 of 74 patients accrued) because at 12.4 months, MFU the LCT arm had significantly improved PFS (median 12 vs. 4 mo, $p = .0054$). With updated 38.8-month MFU, PFS benefit persisted (median 14 vs. 4 mo, $p = .022$). Despite crossover to LCT arm, OS was improved in LCT arm (median 41 vs. 17 mo, $p = .017$). Grade 3 adverse events were similar in both arms with no grade 4+ toxicity. Exploratory analysis suggested that late LCT (after progression) may still improve OS. **Conclusion: In patients with oligometastatic NSCLC after first line systemic tx, LCT prolonged PFS and OS.** *Note: Study performed prior to immunotherapy era.*

Iyengar, UTSW NSCLC Oligomets (*JAMA Oncol* 2018, PMID 28973074): Phase II study of 29 patients with oligometastatic NSCLC (primary lesion and ≤5 metastases) without EGFR/ALK mutation following induction CHT without PD randomized to maintenance CHT vs. SBRT (various doses) to all sites and primary followed by maintenance CHT; 1° end-point PFS. Trial stopped early due to interim analysis showing significant improvement in PFS with SBRT plus maintenance CHT (9.7 vs 3.5 mo, $p = .01$). Similar toxicity. **Conclusion: In patients with oligometastatic NSCLC that did not progress after induction CHT, consolidative SBRT prior to maintenance CHT nearly triples PFS.**

■ Are there any prospective studies assessing local therapy for OMD outside of NSCLC?

SABR-COMET was a randomized phase II screening trial that included various-histology oligometastatic cancer and demonstrated SABR to all sites was associated with improved OS compared to standard therapy. Given the screening design of the study, results are to be confirmed in phase III studies. Other studies have demonstrated benefit in prostate cancer and CRC as detailed in the following.

Palma, SABR-COMET (*Lancet* 2019, PMID 30982687; Update *JCO* 2020, PMID 32484754): Phase II randomized screening trial ($p < .2$ considered significant) of 99 patients with oligometastatic cancer of various types (controlled primary and one to five lesions) randomized (1:2) to standard palliative treatment vs. SABR to all metastatic sites; 1° endpoint OS. SABR arm improved 5-year OS (42% vs. 18%, stratified log-rank $p = .006$). Three (4.5%) grade 5 toxicities in SABR arm. **Conclusion: SABR to all sites is associated with improved OS but with 4.5% treatment-related deaths. A phase III trial is needed to confirm results (SABR-COMET-3 and SABR-COMET-10 are ongoing).** *Comment: Ninety-three percent of patients had one to three lesions limiting extrapolation to four to five lesions. Higher proportion of patients in SABR arm had prostate cancer (21% vs. 6% in control arm); however, sensitivity analysis included in the update suggests the benefit of SABR holds true even in patients without prostate cancer.*

Phillips, ORIOLE (*JAMA Oncol* 2020, PMID 32215577): Phase II multicenter study of 54 men with oligorecurrent hormone-sensitive prostate cancer (previously treated with curative surgery or RT, and who had not received ADT within 6 mos) and ≤3 metastases detected by conventional imaging, randomized to observation vs. SABR (various doses) to all sites; 1° end point was 6 months rate of progression (by PSA, imaging, symptom progression, ADT initiation, or death), which was improved with SABR (19% vs. 61% with obs, $p = .005$). PFS also improved with SABR (NR vs. 5.8 mo with obs; HR 0.30; CI, 0.11–0.81; $p = .002$). Patients also received baseline PSMA PET (blinded to treatment team), and of the SABR group, those who had all PET-avid sites treated (20 of 36), 6-month progression was 5% vs. 38% ($p = .03$) in those who did not have all PET-avid sites treated; also with statistically significant improvements in PFS and DMFS. No grade ≥3 AEs with SABR. **Conclusion: Compared to observation, SABR improves outcomes for oligometastatic prostate cancer, which is enhanced by total consolidation of all PET-avid sites.**

Ost, STOMP (*JCO* 2018, PMID 29240541): Phase II multicenter study of 62 patients with metachronous asymptomatic oligometastatic (≤3 extracranial lesions by choline PET) prostate cancer with bF randomized to surveillance vs. MDT via SBRT (30 Gy/3 fx) or surgery. Indication to start ADT was symptomatic or disease progression; 1° end point ADT-free survival. At MFU of 3 years, MDT improved median ADT-free survival (21 vs. 13 mo, HR 0.60, 80% CI 0.40–0.90, $p = .11$; trial designed where $p < .2$ is significant). Quality of life was similar. No grade 2–5 toxicity was observed. **Conclusion: ADT-free survival was longer with MDT than with surveillance alone for metachronous oligometastatic PCa. MDT should be explored further in phase III trials.**

Ruers, EORTC 40004 (*Ann Oncol* 2012, PMID 22431703; Update *JNCI* 2017, PMID 28376151): Randomized phase II study of 119 patients with unresectable colorectal liver metastases (<10, no extrahepatic disease) randomized to systemic tx alone vs. systemic tx with RFA (± resection); 1° endpoint of 30-month OS was no different between arms, 62% for combined treatment vs. 58% for systemic treatment alone ($p = .22$); but mPFS was improved 17 months vs. 10 months ($p = .025$). Long-term outcomes at MFU 9.7 years showed improved MS of 46 months in combined tx vs. 41 months (HR 0.58, $p = .01$). **Conclusion: Aggressive local treatment can prolong OS in patients with unresectable colorectal liver metastases. However, the study did not meet its primary end point of 30-month OS as the control arm had a higher than anticipated survival.**

Gore, RTOG 0937 (*JTO* 2017, PMID 28648948): Phase II trial of oligometastatic ES-SCLC (1–4 extracranial mets) with PR/CR to CHT randomized to PCI ± consolidative RT (c-RT) to both chest and metastases. PCI 25 Gy/10 fx, consolidative RT 45 Gy/15 fx; 1° end point 1-year OS; 86 eligible patients with MFU 9 months. No difference in 1-year OS (60% PCI vs. 51% PCI + c-RT). Time to progression favored PCI + c-RT (HR 0.53, $p = .01$). One patient in each arm had grade 4 toxicity and one had grade 5 pneumonitis with PCI + c-RT. Trial closed at interim analysis for futility. **Conclusion: After PCI, consolidative RT to the chest and oligometastases (1–4) did not improve 1-year OS, but did delay progression.**

Treasure, PulMiCC (*Trials* 2019, PMID 31831062): Phase III study of 65 patients with CRC and oligometastatic pulmonary metastases (active disease limited to lungs, amenable to resection) randomized to active monitoring ± metastatectomy; 1° endpoint OS. No benefit to metastectomy, with a HR for death within 5 years of 0.82 (95% CI 0.43–1.56). No treatment-related deaths or major AEs. **Conclusion: Metastectomy for lung-only colorectal oligometastasis does not improve OS.** *Note: Study limited by poor recruitment and low sample size.*

■ **Does RT to the prostate improve outcomes in men with oligometastatic prostate cancer?**

Retrospective data suggested prostate RT may improve outcomes in metastatic prostate cancer. ADT ± prostate RT was then tested in two RCTs (HORRAD and STAMPEDE Arm H) and a meta-analysis of the two. Both trials ultimately demonstrated that for an unselected cohort, prostate RT does not improve OS. However, exploratory analysis HORRAD suggested there may be a benefit for those with low-volume metastatic disease. Subsequently, Arm H of the STAMPEDE trial was amended to test the hypothesis that prostate RT would benefit low-burden patients (using the CHAARTED definition). Results of the prespecified analysis showed an OS benefit with prostate RT only (compared to ADT alone) for low-volume patients, which was confirmed in the STOPCAP meta-analysis of both trials. NCCN has since added prostate RT as an option for those with low-burden metastatic prostate cancer. Note that neither trial included PET scans, pelvic LN RT, abiraterone/ enzalutamide/apalutamide, surgery, or MDT. Thus, multiple trials are ongoing to identify the role of each.

Boevé, HORRAD (*Eur Urol* 2019, PMID 30266309): Phase III RCT of 432 men with untreated prostate metastatic to bone (any amount detected on bone scan) and PSA ≥20 randomized to ADT ± prostate RT (70 Gy/35 fx daily or 57.76 Gy/19 fx 3 days/week). MFU 47 mo, 1° end point of OS was no different with RT (45 vs. 43 mos in control arm, $p = .4$). Time to PSA progression improved with RT (15 vs. 12 mos, $p = .02$). Exploratory subgroup analysis suggested men with ≤4 bone metastases may benefit (HR 0.68, 95% CI 0.42–1.1). **Conclusion: In an unselected group of men with metastatic prostate cancer, the addition of prostate RT does not improve OS compared to ADT alone. However, due to small sample size cannot exclude benefit for those with ≤4 bone metastases.** *Comment: No assessment of visceral or nodal disease.*

Parker, STAMPEDE Arm H (*Lancet* 2018, PMID 30355464): Phase III RCT of 2,061 men with untreated metastatic prostate cancer (assessed by bone scan and CT or MRI) randomized to lifelong ADT (later allowed docetaxel) ± prostate RT (55 Gy/20 fx daily in 4 weeks or 36 Gy/6 fx weekly over 6 weeks). MFU 37 mos; 1° endpoint of OS was no different for entire cohort with RT (median 48 vs. 46 mo in control, $p = .266$), but it improved FFS (median 17 vs. 13 mo in control, HR 0.76, $p < .0001$). Prespecified subgroup analysis was stratified by metastatic burden (per CHAARTED definition: High burden—[1] ≥ 4 bone metastases with ≥1 outside the vertebral bodies or pelvis, or [2] visceral metastases. All others were considered to have low metastatic burden [e.g., patient could have multiple pelvic LN+ and innumerable bone lesions in spine/pelvis only, and still be "low burden"]). In those with low metastatic burden, RT improved OS (3-yr OS 81% vs. 73% in control, HR 0.68, $p = .007$). No difference in high metastatic burden group. **Conclusion: Although prostate RT did not improve OS in an unselected cohort of men with metastatic prostate cancer, it significantly improved OS over ADT alone among those with low metastatic burden in a prespecified subgroup analysis.** *Comment: No MDT was given.*

Burdett, STOPCAP Meta-analysis (*Eur Urol* 2019, PMID 30826218): Meta-analysis of HORRAD and STAMPEDE trials noted previously. Overall, the addition of prostate RT to ADT showed no overall improvement in OS or PFS, but did improve biochemical progression and FFS by ~10% at 3 years. Among those with ≤4 bone metastases, prostate RT improved OS by ~7% at 3 years ($p = .007$). **Conclusion: Prostate RT should be considered for men with ≤4 bone metastases at presentation.** *Comment: Unable to use STAMPEDE/CHAARTED metastatic burden definition because HORRAD did not collect data on visceral metastases.*

■ **Does RT to the nasopharynx improve outcomes in patients with metastatic nasopharyngeal cancer?**

You, China (*JAMA Oncol* 2020, PMID 32701129): Phase III trial of 126 patients with metastatic nasopharyngeal carcinoma (not limited to OMD) with PR/CR following three cycles cisplatin + 5-FU randomized to CHT ± locoregional IMRT (70 Gy/35 fx + risk-adapted nodal volumes) to primary site; 1° endpoint OS. The addition of locoregional RT was associated with improved 2-year OS, 76% vs. 55% ($p = .004$). RT was associated with greater risk of >grade 3 dermatitis, mucositis, xerostomia, and late effects including hearing loss and trismus. **Conclusion: The addition of locoregional RT to palliative CHT in patients with CHT-sensitive synchronous metastatic nasopharyngeal carcinoma is associated with improved OS.**

■ **Are there any data regarding SBRT in combination with immunotherapy to stimulate the abscopal effect?**

Two phase I prospective studies suggest SBRT concurrent or sequential with checkpoint inhibitors appears safe.[7,8] Response rate outside of the irradiated field was modest and it is unclear whether the response was a result of checkpoint inhibition alone or due to combination with SBRT. A phase II study of 62 patients with metastatic SCC of the head and neck randomized to nivolumab ± SBRT to a single lesion (21 Gy/3 fx) demonstrated no difference in response rates with the addition of RT.[9] The phase II PEMBRO-RT study randomized patients with metastatic NSCLC to pembrolizumab ± SBRT to a single site. Overall response rate was higher with SBRT (36% vs. 18%, p = .07) but did not meet the study's criteria for meaningful clinical benefit. The PD-L1-negative subgroup seemed to derive the greatest benefit with SBRT.[10]

■ **Are there any large series describing outcomes of SBRT for extracranial oligometastatic disease?**

Chalkidou, UK (*Lancet Oncol* 2021, PMID 33387498): Prospective observational registry of 1,422 adults in 17 hospitals in England with one to three extracranial lesions and a disease-free interval from primary tumor development to metastases of ≥6 months (except for synchronous colorectal liver mets), WHO PS ≤2, and life expectancy >6 months. Patients were treated with 24 to 60 Gy in 3 to 8 fx. Primary end point was OS. The most common primary sites were prostate (29%), colorectal (28%), and renal (10%). At MFU 13 months, 1-year OS was 92 and 2-year OS was 79. LC was 87% and 72% at 1 and 2 years, respectively. MFS was 84% and 52% at 1 and 2 years, respectively. Treatment was well tolerated, and there were no treatment-related deaths. **Conclusion: SBRT for patients with one to three extracranial oligometastatic lesions, with a disease-free interval of at least 6 months, and good performance status, was well tolerated and associated with favorable LC and MFS.**

■ **What is the optimal dose of SBRT for treatment of oligometastatic lesions?**

The optimal dose of SBRT for OMD is unknown. The majority of studies have used doses previously studied in the non-metastatic setting, and studies are ongoing to further refine the doses used for oligometastatic lesions in order to best balance safety and efficacy.

Zelefsky, MSKCC (*IJROBP* 2021, PMID 33422612): Phase III PRT of 117 patients, each with ≤5 oligometastatic bone or lymph node metastases, ≤6 cm in size, KPS ≥80, randomized to SDRT 24 Gy/1 fx vs. SBRT 27 Gy/3 fx, with adjuvant systemic therapy at the discretion of the treating physician. The primary end point was LC. At MFU 52 months, cumulative incidence of LR was 5.8% (95% CI 0–11.1%) at 3 years with SDRT vs. 22% (95% CI 11.9–32.1%) with SBRT. Cumulative incidence of DM at 3 years was 5.3% (95% CI 0–11.1%) with SDRT vs. 22.5% (95% CI: 11.1–33.9%) with SBRT. **Conclusion: Treatment with 24 Gy/1 fx was associated with improved LC and reduced DM compared with 27 Gy/3 fx.**

REFERENCES

1. Hellman S, Weichselbaum RR. Oligometastases. *J Clin Oncol.* 1995;13(1):8–10. doi:10.1200/JCO.1995.13.1.8
2. Lievens Y, Guckenberger M, Gomez D, et al. Defining oligometastatic disease from a radiation oncology perspective: an ESTRO-ASTRO consensus document. *Radiother Oncol.* 2020;148:157–166. doi:10.1016/j.radonc.2020.04.003
3. Guckenberger M, Lievens Y, Bouma AB, et al. Characterisation and classification of oligometastatic disease: a European Society for Radiotherapy and Oncology and European Organisation for Research and Treatment of Cancer consensus recommendation. *Lancet Oncol.* 2020;21(1):e18–e28. doi:10.1016/S1470-2045(19)30718-1
4. Gadd MA, Casper ES, Woodruff JM, et al. Development and treatment of pulmonary metastases in adult patients with extremity soft tissue sarcoma. *Ann. Surg.* 1993;218(6):705–712. doi:10.1097/00000658-199312000-00002
5. Ksienski D, Woods R, Speers C, Kennecke H. Patterns of referral and resection among patients with liver-only metastatic colorectal cancer (MCRC). *Ann Surg Oncol.* 2010;17(12):3085–3093. doi:10.1245/s10434-010-1304-9
6. Rusthoven KE, Hammerman SF, Kavanagh BD, et al. Is there a role for consolidative stereotactic body radiation therapy following first-line systemic therapy for metastatic lung cancer? A patterns-of-failure analysis. *Acta Oncol.* 2009;48(4):578–583. doi:10.1080/02841860802662722
7. Tang C, Welsh JW, de Groot P, et al. Ipilimumab with stereotactic ablative radiation therapy: phase I results and immunologic correlates from peripheral T cells. *Clin Cancer Res.* 2017;23(6):1388–1396. doi:10.1158/1078-0432. CCR-16-1432
8. Luke JJ, Lemons JM, Karrison TG, et al. Safety and clinical activity of pembrolizumab and multisite stereotactic body radiotherapy in patients with advanced solid tumors. *J Clin Oncol.* 2018;36(16):1611–1618. doi:10.1200/JCO.2017.76.2229
9. McBride S, Sherman E, Tsai CJ, et al. Randomized phase II trial of nivolumab with stereotactic body radiotherapy versus nivolumab alone in metastatic head and neck squamous cell carcinoma. *J Clin Oncol.* 2020:JCO2000290.
10. Theelen W, Peulen HMU, Lalezari F, et al. Effect of pembrolizumab after stereotactic body radiotherapy vs pembrolizumab alone on tumor response in patients with advanced non-small cell lung cancer: results of the PEMBRO-RT Phase 2 Randomized Clinical Trial. *JAMA Oncol. JAMA Oncol.* 2019;5(9):1276-1282.

XIII ■ BENIGN DISEASES

Ahmed Halima and Chirag Shah

Table 72.1: QuickHit Radiation Treatment for Benign Diseases	
Disease	**Radiation Treatment**
Heterotopic ossification	7 Gy/1 fx AP/PA <24 hrs before surgery or within 72–96 hrs after surgery.
Keloids	21 Gy/3 fx for most locations and 18 Gy/3 fx for earlobe 24–72 hrs after surgical excision. 37.5 Gy/5 fx if RT is used definitively.
Graves' ophthalmopathy	Treat underlying thyroid disease first. 20 Gy/10 fx.
Desmoid tumors	50 Gy for microscopic disease and 55–58 Gy to gross disease.
Pterygium	Use Sr-90 or Y-90 (β-emitter), giving 8–10 Gy on days 0 (<8 hrs post-op), 7, and 14 after surgery. EBRT dose 24 to 60 Gy/3 to 6 fx.
AVM	SRS, usually 15–30 Gy. Dose can be estimated according to volume using $27/\sqrt[3]{Volume}$.[1]
Coronary restenosis	15–20 Gy/1 fx using intravascular brachytherapy, typically with Sr-90 source, at 2 mm depth, 5 cm active length.
Glomus tumor	Embolization and surgery ± post-op RT, or RT alone: 45–50 Gy; or SRS 14–16 Gy.
Juvenile nasopharyngeal angiofibroma	30 to 36 Gy/10 to 12 fx, up to 50 Gy/25 fx if inoperable.
Langerhans cell histiocytosis	6–8 Gy as prophylaxis against bone fracture.
Gynecomastia	Prophylactic RT effective if given before ADT, using 9 Gy/1 fx or 12 to 15 Gy/3 fx with 9–12 MeV electrons. 20 Gy/5 fx has 90% pain relief for mammalgia after DES.
Orbital pseudotumor	20 Gy/10 fx.
Pigmented villonodular synovitis	30–50 Gy, local control >80%.
Peyronie's disease	8–36 Gy at 2–3 Gy/fx. Penis positioned upright in tube, using 4–8 MeV electrons or 4–6 MV photons.
Splenomegaly	Variety of RT doses can be used for palliation, most commonly 10 Gy/10 fx over 2 weeks but lower doses can be used (5 Gy/5 fx). Monitor blood counts on treatment.
Plantar warts	10 Gy/1 fx may be considered for refractory cases.
Dupuytren's disease/plantar fibromas	RT can be used for palmar/plantar nodules and mild-moderate contractures. Typical dose regimens include 30 Gy/10 fx split course with an 8- 12-wk break, or 21 Gy/7 fx.
Refractory ventricular tachycardia	SBRT 25 Gy/1 fx delivered to the arrhythmogenic ventricular scar identified with cardiac MRI/SPECT/CT and electrophysiologic mapping for target delineation.
Choroidal hemangioma	20 Gy/10 fx or brachytherapy with I-125 plaques. Higher dose (30 Gy) can be used for diffuse type.

HETEROTOPIC OSSIFICATION: Formation of mature bone in periarticular soft tissue occurs in 30% to 40% of patients beginning 3 to 6 weeks after total hip arthroplasty (60%–80% incidence if high risk).[2] Graded per Brooker Classification (Table 72.2).[3] Risk factors: prior HO, trauma, burns, acetabular fracture, ankylosing spondylitis, Paget's disease, skeletal hyperostosis, hypertrophic osteoarthritis. RT dose is 7 Gy/1 fx AP/PA, given within 24 hours pre-op or within 72 to 96 hours post-op (before mesenchymal cell differentiation).[4,5] Pre-op RT effectiveness equivalent to post-op RT;[6] 10% rate of HO recurrence following RT.[4-6] Other tx options include indomethacin.[7,8]

Table 72.2: Brooker's Classification	
I	Isolated bone islands in the soft tissue.
II	Bone spurs originating from two adjacent articulating bones at least 1 cm apart
III	Bone spurs originating from two adjacent articulating bones decreasing the space between the two bones to <1 cm
IV	Bony ankylosis between proximal femur and pelvis.

KELOIDS: Excess scar tissue after stressors including skin incision, piercing, burn, acne, skin tension, or infection.[9] LR >50% after surgery alone. RT given within 24 to 72 hours after surgical excision: 21 Gy/3 fx for most locations and 18 Gy/3 fx if on the earlobe.[10] LC 75%.[10-12] Definitive RT dose is 37.5 Gy/5 fx.[11] Other options include steroid injection, cryotherapy, pulsed-dye laser, interferon, or topical agents.

GRAVES OPHTHALMOPATHY: Presents with proptosis, altered vision, periorbital edema, and extraocular muscle dysfunction. Pathology shows lymphocytic infiltration of retro-orbital fat due to T-cell invasion and glycosaminoglycan production by fibroblasts. Must first treat underlying thyroid disease if possible. RT dose is 20 Gy/10 fx with 5 × 5 cm lateral fields using 6 MV photons and 5° posterior tilt or half-beam block.[13-15] Usually given after failed trial of steroids. Response rate of RT is 50% to 70%.[13-17] Other options include surgical decompression.

DESMOID TUMORS (I.E., FIBROMATOSIS): Nonencapsulated, locally invasive tumor that rarely metastasizes. Associated with familial adenomatous polyposis, Gardner's syndrome (mutation *CTNNB1* gene, B-catenin), prior trauma. Extra-abdominal types are less destructive and occur in shoulder, chest, back, thigh, and head and neck. Abdominal type arises from rectus muscle, often in young peri- or postpartum women; may regress with antiestrogen therapy. Intra-abdominal type arises in iliac fossa, pelvis, or mesentery (associated with Gardner's syndrome, may be >10 cm), in young women unrelated to gestation. Treatment is surgery with wide margins.[18,19] RT indicated for unresectable, close margins or gross disease not amenable to re-resection.[18,19] Treat microscopic disease to 50 Gy, gross disease to 55 to 58 Gy, with large margins.[20] LC is 70% to 85% for RT of either gross or microscopic disease. Regression is slow. Alternative options include sulindac, tamoxifen, and systemic therapy.[20-24] Sorafenib, an oral mutikinase inhibitor, is associated with increased PFS and can be used for progressive, refractory, or symptomatic tumors.[25]

PTERYGIUM: Wig-shaped, benign fibrovascular growth at cornea/conjunctiva junction, located nasally. Risk factors: fair skin, UV light, or dust exposure. Surgery alone has 30% to 70% recurrence rate. Adjuvant RT decreases recurrence to 15%. Use Sr-90 or Y-90 (β-emitter), giving 8 to 10 Gy on days 0 (<8 hours post-op), 7, and 14 after surgery. EBRT dose 24–60 Gy/3 to 6 fx. Avoid 20 Gy/1 fx as it has a 5% risk of scleromalacia or corneal ulceration.[26,27]

ARTERIOVENOUS MALFORMATION: Untreated, annual risk of spontaneous hemorrhage is 1% to 4%, and mortality 1%. Grading system is Spetzler–Martin on scale of 1 to 5 (size: 0–3 cm vs. 3–6 cm vs. >6 cm; eloquent brain region: yes vs. no; venous drainage: deep vs. superficial), which predicts for operative mortality (not risk of hemorrhage). Low risk: may treat with observation or surgery. High-risk lesions can be treated with SRS, dose ~15–30 Gy to margin of nidus. Dose can be estimated according to AVM volume using 27/Volume.[1] Control rate 45% at 1 year, 80% at 2 years, depending on size. Risk of bleeding (5%–10%) persists after SRS during latency period of approximately 2 years until obliteration. Risk of permanent injury 3% to 4%.[28]

CORONARY RESTENOSIS: Intravascular brachytherapy is an option to prevent coronary restenosis. Typically source is Sr-90, although Ir-192, P-32, or I-125 have been used. RT dose 15–20 Gy/1 fx at 2 mm depth, 5 cm active length. RT improves restenosis rates compared to placebo 15% to 20% vs. 50%. Drug-eluting stents (paclitaxel, sirolimus) were found to have better outcomes, but intravascular brachytherapy may be option for select patients after failure of drug-eluting stents.[29]

GLOMUS TUMOR: Also known as chemodectoma/nonchromaffin paraganglioma/carotid body tumor (chromaffin-producing). Generally benign (only 1%–5% malignant). Usually presents as painless mass; may also present w/ ear pain, pulsation, tinnitus, bone destruction, or CN palsies. Rare LN or distant mets (<5%). Origin is neural crest (chief cells of paraganglia in adventitia of dome in jugular bulb). Occurs in carotid body (60%–70%), temporal bone (along internal jugular vein = glomus jugulare; along tympanic branch of CN IX = glomus tympanicum). Can present with bluish mass behind tympanic membrane. Staged by Glasscock–Jackson or McCabe–Fletcher classifications.[30] Contrast-enhancing (hypervascular) with areas of low attenuation (necrosis and hemorrhage). Treatment options include (a) embolization and surgery ± post-op RT (surgery plus post-op RT leads to tumor control of >90%)[31]; (b) RT alone 45 to 50 Gy; or (c) SRS 14 to 16 Gy. LC >90% at 10 years.[32]

JUVENILE NASOPHARYNGEAL ANGIOFIBROMA: Red vascular mass in nasopharynx of young boys ~12 to 15 years of age, presenting w/ epistaxis or nasal obstruction. Can have bone destruction, spreading into paranasal sinuses, infratemporal fossa, orbit, or middle cranial fossa. May have androgynous hormone receptors (rarely spontaneously regresses after puberty). Often associated with hemorrhage, so biopsy is contraindicated. Treatment is embolization and surgery if limited to NP or nasal cavity. RT 30 to 36 Gy/10 to 12 fx, up to 50 Gy/25 fx if inoperable w/ intracranial spread. LC 80% to 90%, but tumors regress slowly.[33,34]

LANGERHANS CELL HISTIOCYTOSIS: Previously known as histiocytosis X. Common sites of single eosinophilic granulomas are bone, skin, and lymph nodes; multiple sites include liver, spleen, marrow, GI, CNS. Can involve single organ (older children/adults) or diffuse multisystem disease (young children). Heterogeneous prognosis. Electron microscopy shows Birbeck granules. Associated diseases include solitary eosinophilic granuloma (<2 y/o, excellent prognosis), Hans–Schuller–Christian (>2 y/o, good prognosis, triad of exophthalmos, diabetes insipidus, and skull lesions), and Letterer–Siwe (<2 y/o, wasting, rash, otitis, lymphadenopathy, bleeding, fulminant, acute, fatal). Treatment options include steroids, etoposide, and vinblastine. RT is used for prophylaxis against bone fracture with doses of 6 to 8 Gy.[35]

GYNECOMASTIA: Incidence of up to 90% of patients on anti-androgens or estrogens. Prophylactic RT effective if given before androgen deprivation, using 9 Gy/1 fx or 12–15 Gy/3 fx with 9 to 12 MeV electrons, or tangential Co-60 or 4 MV photons; 20 Gy/5 fx has 90% pain relief for mammalgia after DES. Tamoxifen represents another alternative with increasing use.[36]

ORBITAL PSEUDOTUMOR (AKA ORBITAL PSEUDOLYMPHOMA): Typically unilateral inflammation, but may be bilateral. Diagnosis of exclusion: differential includes Graves', lymphoma, and lymphoid hyperplasia. Up to 30% progress to lymphoma. About 50% respond to steroids. Consider surgery or immunosuppression. RT dose 20 Gy/10 fx (technique as per Graves).[37]

PEYRONIE'S DISEASE: Inflammation of tunica albuginea in corpus cavernosa that progresses to hard plaques or bands on dorsum of penis, causing painful upward angulation. Up to 50% spontaneously resolve in 12 to 18 months. Treatment includes surgery, steroid injections, verapamil, and RT (if early). RT dose 8 to 36 Gy at 2 to 3 Gy/fx. Penis positioned upright in tube, using 4 to 8 MeV electrons or 4 to 6 MV photons.[38]

PIGMENTED VILLONODULAR SYNOVITIS: Proliferation in synovial cells of tendon sheaths and joint capsules. LR after synovectomy in 45%. RT dose 30–50 Gy, local control >80%.[39,40]

SPLENOMEGALY: Associated with myeloproliferative disorders or CLL. Variety of RT doses can be used for palliation, most common 10 Gy/10 fx over 2 weeks but lower doses can be used (5 Gy/5 fx). Monitor blood counts on treatment. 85% to 90% response rate.[41]

PLANTAR WARTS: Treatment options include surgery, salicylic ointment, liquid nitrogen cryotherapy, or bleomycin injection. Superficial RT can be used in refractory cases, dose 10 Gy/1 fx.[42]

DUPUYTREN'S DISEASE: Relatively common condition caused by progressive fibrosis of the palmar fascia resulting in fascial thickening and nodule formation. Staged using the Tubiana staging (Table 72.3).[43] Some lesions regress spontaneously. Glucocorticoid injection may be helpful in patients with nodules.[44] Fasciotomy or fasciectomy for severe functional impairment. RT can be used to prevent progression and provide symptomatic relief in mild to moderate disease (nodules only, or with contractures up to 10 degrees). Regression of contractures in over 50% of patients, and only rarely is surgery needed within 1 year after RT. Typical dose regimens include 30 Gy/10 fx split course with a 8- to 12-week break, or 21 Gy/7 fx.[45]

Table 72.3: Tubiana Staging of Dupuytren's Contracture[43]	
0	No deficit in the joint extension
N	Nodule but without contracture
1	Contracture 0–45°
2	Contracture 45–90°
3	Contracture 90–135°
4	Contracture >135°

PLANTAR FIBROMAS: Also known as Ledderhose disease. Similar to Dupuytren's disease but with nodules arising in the arch of the foot, with RT used in a similar fashion. In one series after treatment with 30 Gy/10 fx split course, 71% of patients experienced regression and the rest had stable disease in 1 to 4 years.[46]

VENTRICULAR TACHYCARDIA: Refractory ventricular tachycardia can be treated with electrophysiology-guided radioablation with SBRT (25 Gy/1 fx) to the arrhythmogenic scar identified by cardiac MRI, SPECT or Cardiac CT. Electrophysiologic planning is incorporated for delineation of PTV.[47]

CHOROIDAL HEMANGIOMA: Two types: diffuse and circumscribed. If progressive, can lead to visual loss depending on the location. Diffuse type occurs in children and is almost always associated with Sturge–Weber syndrome. Circumscribed type occurs in adults. Localized disease is treated with EBRT with 18 to 20 Gy with 2 Gy/fx with 64% rate of reattachment of the retina.[48] Brachytherapy is also an option in localized hemangiomas using I-125 plaques, with average dose of 30 Gy with excellent outcomes.[49,50] Diffuse type can be treated with 30 Gy/15 fx with photons or protons.

REFERENCES

1. Missios S, Bekelis K, Al-Shyal G, et al. Stereotactic radiosurgery of intracranial arteriovenous malformations and the use of the K index in determining treatment dose. *Neurosurg Focus*. 2014;37(3):E15. doi:10.3171/2014.7.FOCUS14157
2. Neal B, Gray H, MacMahon S, Dunn L. Incidence of heterotopic bone formation after major hip surgery. *ANZ J Surg*. 2002;72(11):808–821. doi:10.1046/j.1445-2197.2002.02549.x
3. Hug KT, Alton TB, Gee AO. Classifications in brief: Brooker classification of heterotopic ossification after total hip arthroplasty. *Clin Orthop Relat Res*. 2015;473(6):2154–2157. doi:10.1007/s11999-014-4076-x
4. Gregoritch SJ, Chadha M, Pellegrini VD, Rubin P, Kantorowitz DA. Randomized trial comparing preoperative versus postoperative irradiation for prevention of heterotopic ossification following prosthetic total hip replacement: preliminary results. *Int J Radiat Oncol Biol Phys*. 1994;30(1):55–62. doi:10.1016/0360-3016(94)90519-3
5. Seegenschmiedt MH, Makoski HB, Micke O. Radiation prophylaxis for heterotopic ossification about the hip joint: a multicenter study. *Int J Radiat Oncol Biol Phys*. 2001;51(3):756–765. doi:10.1016/S0360-3016(01)01640-6
6. Konski A, Pellegrini V, Poulter C, et al. Randomized trial comparing single dose versus fractionated irradiation for prevention of heterotopic bone: a preliminary report. *Int J Radiat Oncol Biol Phys*. 1990;18(5):1139–1142. doi:10.1016/0360-3016(90)90450-X
7. Kölbl O, Knelles D, Barthel T, Kraus U, Flentje M, Eulert J. Randomized trial comparing early postoperative irradiation vs. the use of nonsteroidal antiinflammatory drugs for prevention of heterotopic ossification following prosthetic total hip replacement. *Int J Radiat Oncol Biol Phys*. 1997;39(5):961–966. doi:10.1016/S0360-3016(97)00496-3
8. Pakos EE, Ioannidis JP. Radiotherapy vs. nonsteroidal anti-inflammatory drugs for the prevention of heterotopic ossification after major hip procedures: a meta-analysis of randomized trials. *Int J Radiat Oncol Biol Phys*. 2004;60(3):888–895. doi:10.1016/j.ijrobp.2003.11.015
9. Berman B, Maderal A, Raphael B. Keloids and hypertrophic scars: pathophysiology, classification, and treatment. *Dermatol Surg*. 2017;43 Suppl 1:S3–S18. doi:10.1097/DSS.0000000000000819
10. Renz P, Hasan S, Gresswell S, Hajjar RT, Trombetta M, Fontanesi J. Dose effect in adjuvant radiation therapy for the treatment of resected keloids. *Int J Radiat Oncol Biol Phys*. 2018;102(1):149–154. doi:10.1016/j.ijrobp.2018.05.027
11. Mankowski P, Kanevsky J, Tomlinson J, Dyachenko A, Luc M. Optimizing radiotherapy for keloids: a meta-analysis systematic review comparing recurrence rates between different radiation modalities. *Ann Plast Surg*. 2017;78(4):403–411. doi:10.1097/SAP.0000000000000989

12. Ogawa R, Miyashita T, Hyakusoku H, Akaishi S, Kuribayashi S, Tateno A. Postoperative radiation protocol for keloids and hypertrophic scars: statistical analysis of 370 sites followed for over 18 months. *Ann Plast Surg.* 2007;59(6):688–691. doi:10.1097/SAP.0b013e3180423b32

13. Prummel MF, Terwee CB, Gerding MN, et al. A randomized controlled trial of orbital radiotherapy versus sham irradiation in patients with mild Graves' ophthalmopathy. *J Clin Endocrinol Metab.* 2004;89(1):15–20. doi:10.1210/jc.2003-030809

14. Mourits MP, van Kempen-Harteveld ML, García MB, Koppeschaar HP, Tick L, Terwee CB. Radiotherapy for Graves' orbitopathy: randomised placebo-controlled study. *Lancet.* 2000;355(9214):1505–1509. doi:10.1016/S0140-6736(00)02165-6

15. Petersen IA, Kriss JP, McDougall IR, Donaldson SS. Prognostic factors in the radiotherapy of Graves' ophthalmopathy. *Int J Radiat Oncol Biol Phys.* 1990;19(2):259–264. doi:10.1016/0360-3016(90)90532-O

16. Bradley EA, Gower EW, Bradley DJ, et al. Orbital radiation for graves ophthalmopathy: a report by the American Academy of Ophthalmology. *Ophthalmology.* 2008;115(2):398–409. doi:10.1016/j.ophtha.2007.10.028

17. Prummel MF, Mourits MP, Blank L, Berghout A, Koornneef L, Wiersinga WM. Randomized double-blind trial of prednisone versus radiotherapy in Graves' ophthalmopathy. *Lancet.* 1993;342(8877):949–954. doi:10.1016/0140-6736(93)92001-A

18. Cates JM, Stricker TP. Surgical resection margins in desmoid-type fibromatosis: a critical reassessment. *Am J Surg Pathol.* 2014;38(12):1707–1714. doi:10.1097/PAS.0000000000000276

19. Janssen ML, van Broekhoven DL, Cates JM, et al. Meta-analysis of the influence of surgical margin and adjuvant radiotherapy on local recurrence after resection of sporadic desmoid-type fibromatosis. *Br J Surg.* 2017;104(4):347–357. doi:10.1002/bjs.10477

20. Donaldson SS, Torrey M, Link MP, et al. A multidisciplinary study investigating radiotherapy in Ewing's sarcoma: end results of POG #8346. Pediatric Oncology Group. *Int J Radiat Oncol Biol Phys.* 1998;42:125–135. doi:10.1016/S0360-3016(98)00191-6

21. Tsukada K, Church JM, Jagelman DG, et al. Noncytotoxic drug therapy for intra-abdominal desmoid tumor in patients with familial adenomatous polyposis. *Dis Colon Rectum.* 1992;35(1):29–33. doi:10.1007/BF02053335

22. Quast DR, Schneider R, Burdzik E, Hoppe S, Möslein G. Long-term outcome of sporadic and FAP-associated desmoid tumors treated with high-dose selective estrogen receptor modulators and sulindac: a single-center long-term observational study in 134 patients. *Fam Cancer.* 2016;15(1):31–40. doi:10.1007/s10689-015-9830-z

23. Desurmont T, Lefèvre JH, Shields C, Colas C, Tiret E, Parc Y. Desmoid tumour in familial adenomatous polyposis patients: responses to treatments. *Fam Cancer.* 2015;14(1):31–39. doi:10.1007/s10689-014-9760-1

24. Hansmann A, Adolph C, Vogel T, Unger A, Moeslein G. High-dose tamoxifen and sulindac as first-line treatment for desmoid tumors. *Cancer.* 2004;100(3):612–620. doi:10.1002/cncr.11937

25. Gounder MM, Mahoney MR, Van Tine BA, et al. Sorafenib for advanced and refractory desmoid tumors. *N Engl J Med.* 2018;379(25):2417–2428. doi:10.1056/NEJMoa1805052

26. Ali AM, Thariat J, Bensadoun RJ, et al. The role of radiotherapy in the treatment of pterygium: a review of the literature including more than 6000 treated lesions. *Cancer Radiother.* 2011;15(2):140–147. doi:10.1016/j.canrad.2010.03.020

27. Nishimura Y, Nakai A, Yoshimasu T, et al. Long-term results of fractionated strontium-90 radiation therapy for pterygia. *Int J Radiat Oncol Biol Phys.* 2000;46(1):137–141. doi:10.1016/S0360-3016(99)00419-8

28. Joshi NP, Shah C, Kotecha R, et al. Contemporary management of large-volume arteriovenous malformations: a clinician's review. *J Radiat Oncol.* 2016;5(3):239–248. doi:10.1016/S0360-3016(99)00419-8

29. Benjo A, Cardoso RN, Collins T, et al. Vascular brachytherapy versus drug-eluting stents in the treatment of in-stent restenosis: a meta-analysis of long-term outcomes. *Catheter Cardiovasc Interv.* 2016;87(2):200–208. doi:10.1016/S0360-3016(99)00419-8

30. Perez CA, Thorstad WL. Glomus tumors. In: Brady LW, Yaeger TE, eds. *Encyclopedia of Radiation Oncology.* Springer Berlin Heidelberg; 2013:298–303.

31. Manzoor NF, Yancey KL, Aulino JM, et al. Contemporary management of jugular paragangliomas with neural preservation. *Otolaryngol Head Neck Surg.* 2020:194599820938660. doi:10.1177/0194599820938660

32. Jacob JT, Pollock BE, Carlson ML, Driscoll CL, Link MJ. Stereotactic radiosurgery in the management of vestibular schwannoma and glomus jugulare: indications, techniques, and results. *Otolaryngol Clin North Am.* 2015;48(3):515–526. doi:10.1016/j.otc.2015.02.010

33. Lee JT, Chen P, Safa A, et al. The role of radiation in the treatment of advanced juvenile angiofibroma. *Laryngoscope.* 2002;112(7 Pt 1):1213–1220. doi:10.1097/00005537-200207000-00014

34. López F, Triantafyllou A, Snyderman CH, et al. Nasal juvenile angiofibroma: current perspectives with emphasis on management. *Head Neck.* 2017;39(5):1033–1045. doi:10.1002/hed.24696

35. Lian C, Lu Y, Shen S. Langerhans cell histiocytosis in adults: a case report and review of the literature. *Oncotarget.* 2016;7(14). doi:10.18632/oncotarget.7892

36. Viani GA, Bernardes da Silva LG, Stefano EJ. Prevention of gynecomastia and breast pain caused by androgen deprivation therapy in prostate cancer: tamoxifen or radiotherapy? *Int J Radiat Oncol Biol Phys.* 2012;83(4):e519–524. doi:10.1016/j.ijrobp.2012.01.036

37. Mendenhall WM, Lessner AM. Orbital pseudotumor. *Am J Clin Oncol.* 2010;33(3):304–306. doi:10.1097/COC.0b013e3181a07567

38. Seegenschmiedt M-H, Micke O, Niewald M, et al. DEGRO guidelines for the radiotherapy of non-malignant disorders: Part III: Hyperproliferative disorders. *Strahlentherapie und Onkologie: Organ der Deutschen Rontgengesellschaft [et al]*. 2015;191. doi:10.1007/s00066-015-0818-2

39. Heyd R, Micke O, Berger B, Eich HT, Ackermann H, Seegenschmiedt MH. Radiation therapy for treatment of pigmented villonodular synovitis: results of a national patterns of care study. *Int J Radiat Oncol Biol Phys*. 2010;78(1):199–204. doi:10.1016/j.ijrobp.2009.07.1747

40. Heyd R, Seegenschmiedt MH, Micke O. The role of external beam radiation therapy in the adjuvant treatment of pigmented villonodular synovitis. *Z Orthop Unfall*. 2011;149(6):677–682. doi:10.1055/s-0030-1250687

41. Zaorsky NG, Williams GR, Barta SK, et al. Splenic irradiation for splenomegaly: a systematic review. *Cancer Treat Rev*. 2017;53:47–52. doi:10.1016/j.ctrv.2016.11.016

42. Perez CA, Lockctt MA, Young G. Radiation therapy for keloids and plantar warts. *Front Radiat Ther Oncol*. 2001;35:135–146. doi:10.1159/000061273

43. Hindocha S, Stanley JK, Watson JS, Bayat A. Revised Tubiana's staging system for assessment of disease severity in Dupuytren's disease-preliminary clinical findings. *Hand (N Y)*. 2008;3(2):80–86. doi:10.1007/s11552-007-9071-1

44. Ketchum LD, Donahue TK. The injection of nodules of Dupuytren's disease with triamcinolone acetonide. *J Hand Surg Am*. 2000;25(6):1157–1162. doi:10.1053/jhsu.2000.18493

45. Seegenschmiedt MH, Olschewski T, Guntrum F. Radiotherapy optimization in early-stage Dupuytren's contracture: first results of a randomized clinical study. *Int J Radiat Oncol Biol Phys*. 2001;49(3):785–798. doi:10.1016/S0360-3016(00)00745-8

46. Attassi M, Seegenschmiedt HM. Radiotherapy is effective in the treatment of progressive plantar fibromatosis (morbus ledderhose). *Int J Radiat Oncol Biol Phys*. 2001;51(3, Supplement 1):47. doi:10.1016/S0360-3016(01)01908-3

47. Cuculich PS, Schill MR, Kashani R, et al. Noninvasive Cardiac Radiation for Ablation of Ventricular Tachycardia. *N Engl J Med*. 2017;377(24):2325–2336. doi:10.1056/NEJMoa1613773

48. Schilling H, Sauerwein W, Lommatzsch A, et al. Long-term results after low dose ocular irradiation for choroidal haemangiomas. *Br J Ophthalmol*. 1997;81(4):267–273. doi:10.1136/bjo.81.4.267

49. Lewis GD, Li HK, Quan EM, Scarboro SB, Teh BS. The role of eye plaque brachytherapy and MR imaging in the management of diffuse choroidal hemangioma: an illustrative case report and literature review. *Pract Radiat Oncol*. 2019;9(5):e452–e456. doi:10.1016/j.prro.2019.05.007

50. Augsburger JJ, Freire J, Brady LW. Radiation therapy for choroidal and retinal hemangiomas. *Front Radiat Ther Oncol*. 1997;30:265–280. doi:10.1159/000425713

ABBREVIATIONS

^{106}Ru	ruthenium 106
3D-CRT	3D conformal radiation therapy
5-FU	5-fluorouracil
AA	anaplastic astrocytoma
AAD	American Academy of Dermatology
AASLD	American Association of Liver Diseases
Ab	antibody
ABR	auditory brainstem response
ABS	American Brachytherapy Society
ABVD	Adriamycin, bleomycin, vinblastine, dacarbazine
AC	Adriamycin, cyclophosphamide
ACA	adenocarcinoma
ACM	all-cause mortality
ACOG	American Congress of Obstetricians and Gynecologists
ACOSOG	American College of Surgeons Oncology Group
ACR	American College of Radiology
ACS	American Cancer Society
ACTH	adrenocorticotropic hormone
ACVBP	Adriamycin, cyclophosphamide, vindesine, bleomycin, prednisone
AD	autosomal dominant
ADH	antidiuretic hormone
ADT	androgen deprivation therapy
AE	adverse event
AF	altered fractionation
AFP	alpha fetoprotein
AG	anaplastic glioma
AHT	adjuvant hormone therapy
AI	aromatase inhibitor
AJCC	American Joint Committee on Cancer

AK	actinic keratosis
ALARA	as low as reasonably achievable
ALH	atypical lobular hyperplasia
ALK	anaplastic lymphoma kinase
Alkphos	alkaline phosphatase
ALL	acute lymphocytic leukemia
ALN	axillary lymph node
ALND	axillary lymph node dissection
AM	active monitoring
AMA	American Medical Association
ANZMTG	ANZ Melanoma Trials Group
AO	anaplastic oligodendroglioma
AOA	anaplastic oligoastrocytoma
AP	doxorubicin and cisplatin
AP/PA	anterior–posterior/posterior–anterior
APBI	accelerated partial breast irradiation
APC	argon plasma coagulation
APR	abdominoperineal resection
AR	autosomal recessive
Ara-C	cytarabine
ARR	absolute risk reduction
AS	active surveillance
ASBS	American Society of Breast Surgeons
ASC-H	atypical squamous cells, cannot exclude HSIL
ASCO	American Society of Clinical Oncology
ASCT	autologous stem cell transplant
ASCUS	atypical squamous cells of undetermined significance
ASTRO	American Society for Radiation Oncology
ATA	American Thyroid Association
ATC	anaplastic thyroid cancer
ATEM	analytical transmission electro microscopy
ATRT	typical teratoid/rhabdoid tumor
ATRX	alpha thalassemia/mental retardation syndrome X-linked

AUA	American Urologic Association
AUC	area under the curve
AV	Adriamycin, vinblastine
AVD	Adriamycin, vinblastine, dacarbazine
AVM	arteriovenous malformation
AV-PC	Adriamycin, vincristine, prednisone, cyclophosphamide
AYA	adolescent/young adult
BAER	brainstem auditory evoked response
BC	breast cancer
BCC	basal cell carcinoma
BCFI	breast cancer free interval
BCG	bacillus Calmette-Guerin therapy
BCLC	Barcelona Clinic Liver Cancer
BCM	breast cancer mortality
BCNU	1,3-bis(2-chloroethyl)-1-nitrosourea
BCS	breast-conservation surgery
BCSM	breast cancer specific mortality
BCT	breast-conservation therapy
bDFS	biochemical disease free survival
BEAM	carmustine, etoposide, cytarabine, melphalan
BED	biologically equivalent dose
BEP	bleomycin, etoposide, cisplatin
bF	biochemical failure
BID	twice daily
BI-RADS	Breast Imaging Reporting and Data System
BM	bone marrow
BMI	body mass index
BMP	basic metabolic panel
bNED	biochemical no evidence of disease
BNI	Barrow Neurologic Institute
BOS	base of skull
BOT	base of tongue
bPFS	biochemical progression free survival

BPH	benign prostatic hypertrophy
bRFS	biochemical relapse-free survival
BSO	bilateral salpingo-oophorectomy
C	cyclophosphamide
CALGB	cancer and leukemia group B
CaP	cancer of the prostate
CAP	cyclophosphamide–doxorubicin–cisplatin
CAPS	International Cancer of Pancreas Screening
CAR-T	chimeric antigen receptor T
CAV	cyclophosphamide, Adriamycin, vincristine
CBC	complete blood count
CBTR	contralateral breast tumor recurrence
CBV	cyclophosphamide, carmustine, etoposide
CC	cholangiocarcinoma
CCG	Children's Cancer Group
CCNU	lomustine
cCR	clinical complete response
CCSG	Children's Cancer Study Group
CDC	Centers for Disease Control and Prevention
CDDP	cisplatin
CECT	contrast-enhanced CT head/neck
CExP	carcinoma ex pleomorphic adenoma
CF	conventional fractionation
CFS	colostomy-free survival
CGE	cobalt gray equivalent
ChemoRT	concurrent chemoradiation
CHEP	cricohyoidoepiglottopexy
CHIPS	Childhood Hodgkin International Prognostic Score
CHOP	cyclophosphamide, Adriamycin, vincristine, prednisone
CHT	chemotherapy
CI	confidence interval
CIS	carcinoma in situ
CKC	cold knife conization

CLL	chronic lymphocytic leukemia
CMF	cyclophosphamide, methotrexate, 5-FU
CMP	complete metabolic profile
CMT	combined modality therapy
CN	cranial nerve
CNS	central nervous system
CODOX-M	cyclophosphamide, vincristine, doxorubicin, methotrexate
COG	Children's Oncology Group
COMS	Collaborative Ocular Melanoma Study
CP	craniopharyngioma
CPA	cerebellopontine angle
CPM	cyclophosphamide
CPT	charged-particle therapy
CR	complete response
DD4A	vincristine, doxorubicin, dactinomycin
DD-MVAC	dose-dense methotrexate, vinblastine, doxorubicin, cisplatin
DEB	drug-eluting beads
DES	diethylstilbestrol
DeVIC	dexamethasone, etoposide, ifosfamide, carboplatin
DF	distant failure
DFI	disease-free interval
DFS	disease-free survival
DHEA	dehydroepiandrosterone
DHT	dihydrotestosterone
DIBH	deep inspiration breath hold
DIPG	diffuse intrinsic pontine glioma
DLBCL	diffuse large B-cell lymphoma
DLCO	diffusion capacity for carbon monoxide
DLT	dose-limiting toxicity
DM	distant metastasis
DMFS	distant metastatis-free survival
DMFSP	dermatofibrosarcoma protuberans
DOI	depth of invasion

DRE	digital rectal examination
DSM	disease-specific mortality
DSS	disease-specific survival
DVT	deep vein thrombosis
EBCTCG	Early Breast Cancer Trialists' Collaborative Group
EBER	EBV encoded RNA
EBRT	external beam radiotherapy
EBUS	endobronchial ultrasound
EBV	Epstein–Barr virus
ECE	extracapsular extension
ECF	epirubicin, cisplatin, and 5-Fu
ECOG	Eastern Cooperative Oncology Group
EEG	electroencephalogram
EFRT	extended field radiation therapy
EFS	event free survival
EGD	esophagogastroduodenoscopy
EGFR	epidermal growth factor receptor
EIC	extensive intraductal component
EIN	endometrial intraepithelial neoplasia
EMR	endoscopic mucosal resection
ENE	extranodal extension
ENI	elective nodal irradiation
EOE	extraosseous Ewing's
EORTC	European Organization for Research and Treatment of Cancer
EP	etoposide/cisplatin
EPE	extraprostatic extenstion
EPOCH	etoposide, vincristine, doxorubicin, cyclophosphamide, prednisolone
EPP	extra-pleural pneumonectomy
EQ-5D	EuroQol Five Dimensions Quality of Life Questionnaire
EQD2	equivalent dose 2 Gy
ER	estrogen receptor
ERCP	endoscopic retrograde cholangiopancreatography
ERSPC	European Randomized Study of Screening for Prostate Cancer

ESB	Ewing's sarcoma of bone
ESD	endoscopic submucosal dissection
ESFT	Ewing's sarcoma family of tumors
ESR	erythrocyte sedimentation rate
ESS	endometrial stromal sarcoma
ES-SCLC	extensive-stage small cell lung cancer
EUA	exam under anesthesia
EUS	endoscopic ultrasound
FAMMM	familial atypical multiple mole melanoma
FAP	familial adenomatous polyposis
FDA	Food and Drug Administration
FEV1	forced expiratory volume in 1 second
FFBF	freedom from biochemical failure
FFDP	freedom from disease progression
FFLP	freedom from local progression
FFLR	freedom from locoregional recurrence
FFR	freedom from recurrence
FFS	failure-free survival
FFTF	freedom from treatment failure
FH	favorable histology
FIGC	familial intestinal gastric cancer
FIGO	International Federation of Gynecologic and Obstetrics
FIR	favorable intermediate risk
FISH	fluorescence in situ hybridization
FIT	fecal immunochemical
FL	follicular lymphoma
FLAIR	fluid attenuated inversion recovery
FLOT	5-FU, leucovorin, oxaliplatin and docetaxel
FNA	fine needle aspiration
FOM	floor of mouth
FS	fibrosarcoma
FSH	follicle stimulating hormone
FSRT	fractionated stereotactic radiation therapy

FTC	follicular thyroid cancer
FU	follow up
FVC	forced vital capacity
Fx	fractions
GAPPS	gastric adenocarcinoma and proximal polyposis of stomach
GBM	glioblastoma multiforme
GC	gemcitabine, cisplatin
GCT	germ cell tumor
GEJ	gastroesophageal junction
GELOX	gemcitabine, oxaliplatin, L-asparaginase
GERD	gastrointestinal reflux disease
GFAP	glial fibrillary acidic protein
GGT	gamma-glutamyl transferase
GH	growth hormone
GHSG	German Hodgkin Study Group
GI	gastrointestinal
GIST	gastrointestinal stromal tumor
GITSG	Gastrointestinal Tumor Study Group
GKRS	gamma knife radiosurgery
GnRH	gonadotropin-releasing hormone
GOG	Gynecologic Oncology Group
GPA	graded prognostic assessment
GS	Gleason score
GTR	gross total resection
GTV	gross tumor volume
GU	genitourinary
Gy	gray
H&N	head and neck
H&P	history and physical exam
HAART	highly active antiretroviral therapy
HA-WBRT	hippocampal avoidance whole brain radiation therapy
HBV	hepatitis B virus
HCC	hepatocellular carcinoma

hCG	human chorionic gonadotropin
HCRC	hereditary clear cell renal carcinoma
HCT	hematopoietic cell transplantation
HCV	hepatitis C virus
HD	Hodgkin's disease
HDGC	hereditary diffuse gastric cancer
HDR	high dose rate
HIFU	high-intensity focused ultrasound
HIR	high intermediate risk
HMSC	HPV-related multiphenotypic sinonasal carcinoma
HNCUP	head and neck cancer of unknown primary
HNPCC	hereditary nonpolyposis colorectal carcinoma
HNSCC	head and neck squamous cell carcinoma
HO	heterotopic ossification
HPF	high-powered field
HPRC	hereditary papillary cell renal carcinoma
HPV	human papillomavirus
HR	hazard ratio
HR-QOL	health-related quality of life
HT	hyperthermia
HTLV	human T-lymphotrophic virus
HU	Hounsfield unit
HVA	homovanillic acid
HVLT-R	Hopkins Verbal Learning Test-Revised
HVLT-R-DR	Hopkins Verbal Learning Test-Revised for Delayed Recall
HVLT-R-TR	Hopkins Verbal Learning Test-Revised for Total Recall
I-125	iodine-125
IASLC	International Association for the Study of Lung Cancer
IBC	inflammatory breast cancer
IBCSG	International Breast Cancer Study Group
IBD	inflammatory bowel disease
IBE	ipsilateral breast events
IBTR	in-breast tumor recurrence

ICHD-3	International Classification of Headache Disorders, 3rd Edition
ICP	intracranial pressure
IDC	invasive ductal carcinoma
IDH	isocitrate dehydrogenase
IDL	isodose line
IDRF	image-defined risk factor
IELSG	International Extranodal Lymphoma Study Group
IF	involved fossa
IFI	involved-field irradiation
IFRT	involved-field radiation therapy
IHC	immunohistochemistry
IJ	internal jugular
ILC	invasive lobular carcinoma
ILROG	International Lymphoma Radiation Oncology Group
ILRR	ipsilateral LRR
IM	internal mammary
IMA	inferior mesenteric artery
IMN	internal mammary nodes
IMNI	internal mammary irradiation
IMRT	intensity modulated radiation therapy
INR	international normalized ratio
INRG	International Neuroblastoma Risk Group
INRT	involved nodal radiation therapy
INSS	International Neuroblastoma Staging System
IO	immunotherapy
IOERT	intraoperative electron RT
IORT	intraoperative radiation therapy
IPI	International Prognostic Index
IPS	International Prognostic Score
IPSS	International Prostate Symptom Score
IR	intermediate risk
ISCL	International Society for Cutaneous Lymphomas
ISRT	involved-site radiation therapy

ITMIG	International Thymic Malignancy Interest Group
ITT	intention to treat
IV	intravenous
IV/DECA	ifosfamide, vinorelbine, decadron, etoposide, cisplatin, cytarabine (dose-reduced chemo)
IVC	inferior vena cava
IVP	intravenous pyelogram
JART	Japanese Association for Research on the Thymus
JNA	juvenile nasopharyngeal angiofibroma
JRSGC	Japanese Research Society for Gastric Cancer
KPS	Karnofsky Performance Status
LABC	locally advanced breast cancer
LAD	lymphadenopathy
LAP	locally advanced pancreatic cancer
LAR	low anterior resection
LC	local control
LCIS	lobular carcinoma in situ
LCNEC	large-cell neuroendocrine carcinoma
LCT	local consolidative therapy
LCV	leucovorin
LD	lymphocyte depleted
LDCT	low dose computed tomography scan
LDH	lactate dehydrogenase
LDHD	lymphocyte depleted HD
LDR	low dose rate
LE	local excision
LF	local failure
LFT	liver function tests
LGG	low-grade glioma
LH	luteinizing hormone
LIQ	lower inner quadrant
LIR	low intermediate risk
LMA	large mediastinal adenopathy
LMD	leptomeningeal disease

LMS	leiomyosarcoma
LN	lymph node
LND	lymph node dissection
LOH	loss of heterozygosity
LOQ	lower outer quadrant
LP	lumbar puncture
LR	local recurrence
LRBC	locally recurrent breast cancer
LRC	locoregional control
LRF	locoregional failure
LRFS	local recurrence free survival
LRR	locoregional recurrence
LSIL/HSIL	low-grade squamous intraepithelial lesion/high-grade squamous intraepithelial lesion
LSS	limb sparing surgery
LS-SCLC	limited-stage small cell lung cancer
LUTS	lower urinary tract symptoms
LVEF	left ventricular ejection fraction
LVSI	lymphovascular invasion
M	melphalan
mAB	monoclonal antibody
MALT	mucosa-associated lymphoid tissue
MB	medulloblastoma
MC	mixed cellularity
MCB	multicatheter brachytherapy
MCC	Merkel cell carcinoma
MCE	major coronary events
MCHD	mixed cellularity HD
MCV	methotrexate, cisplatin, vinblastine
MD	maximum dose
MDACC	MD Anderson Cancer Center
MDADI	MD Anderson Dysphagia Inventory
MDT	metastasis directed therapy
MELD	model for end-stage liver disease

MEN	multiple endocrine neoplasia
MEN2	multiple endocrine neoplasia type 2
MF	mycosis fungoides
MFH	malignant fibrous histiocytoma
mFOLFOX	modified folinic acid (leucovorin), 5-FU, oxaliplatin
MFS	metastasis free survival
MFU	median follow-up
MG	myasthenia gravis
MGH	Massachusetts General Hospital
MGMT	O-6-methylguanine-DNA methyltransferase
MHD	mean heart dose
MI	myometrial invasion
MIBC	muscle invasive bladder cancer
MIBG	metaiodobenzylguanidine
MIPI	Mantle Cell Lymphoma International Prognostic Index
MMC	mitomycin C
MMP	matrix metalloproteinases
MMR	mismatch repair genes
MMSE	Mini-Mental Status Exam
MMT	multimodality therapy
MOA	mechanism of action
MPEC	multipolar electrocoagulation
MPM	malignant pleural mesothelioma
MPNST	malignant peripheral nerve sheath tumor
MPV	methotrexate, procarbazine, vincristine
MRC	Medical Research Council
MRCP	magnetic resonance cholangiopancreatography
MRI	magnetic resonance imaging
MRM	modified radical mastectomy
MRND	modified radical neck dissection
MS	median overall survival
mSCC	malignant spinal cord compression
MSKCC	Memorial Sloan Kettering Cancer Center

MTD	maximum tolerated dose
MSLT	multi-institutional selective lymphadenectomy
MTC	medullary thyroid cancer
MTD	metastasis directed therapy
MTIC	3-methyl-(triazen-1-yl)imidazole-4-carboximide
MTX	methotrexate
MUGA	multigated acquisition scan
MVA	multivariable analysis
MZL	marginal zone lymphoma
NACT	neoadjuvant chemotherapy
NASH	non-alcoholic steatohepatitis
NCAM	neural cell adhesion molecule
NCCN	National Comprehensive Cancer Network
NCCTG	North Central Cancer Treatment Group
NCDB	National Cancer Database
NCI	National Cancer Institute
NCIC	National Cancer Institute Of Canada
NF1	neurofibromatosis type 1
NF2	neurofibromatosis type 2
NFS	neurologic function score
NHL	non-Hodgkin's lymphoma
NHT	neoadjuvant/concurrent ADT
NLP	nodular lymphocyte predominant
NNS	number needed to screen
NNT	number needed to treat
NOS	not otherwise specified
NP	new primaries
NPC	nasopharynx carcinoma
NPVM	nonpulmonary visceral metastasis
NPX	nasopharynx
NS	not statistically significant
NSABP	National Surgical Adjuvant Breast And Bowel Project
NSAID	nonsteroidal anti-inflammatory drug

NSCLC	non-small cell lung cancer
NSE	neuron specific enolase
NSGCT	non-seminomatous germ cell tumor
NSHD	nodular sclerosis HD
NSS	nephron-sparing surgery
NTE	normal tissue effect
NTR	near total resection
OA	oligoastrocytoma
OAR	organ at risk
Obs	observation
OCOG	Ontario Cooperative Oncology Group
OCP	oral contraceptive pills
OC-SCC	oral cavity squamous cell carcinoma
OLT	orthotopic liver transplant
OM	overall mortality
OMD	oligometastatic disease
OPC	oropharyngeal cancer
OPX	oropharynx
OR	odds ratio
ORR	overall response rate
OS	overall survival
OSHA	Occupational Safety and Health Administration
OTT	overall treatment time
P/D	pleurectomy and decortication
PA	posterior–anterior
PAB	posterior axillary boost
PALNS	para-aortic lymph node sampling
PAS	para-aortic strip
PBI	partial breast irradiation
PBT	proton beam therapy
PCa	prostate cancer
PCA3	prostate cancer antigen 3
PCI	prophylactic cranial irradiation

PCLBCL	primary cutaneous large B-cell lymphoma
PCM	prostate cancer mortality
PCNSL	primary central nervous system lymphoma
pCR	pathologic complete response
PCSM	prostate cancer specific mortality
PCSS	prostate cancer–specific survival
PCV	procarbazine, lomustine (CCNU), vincristine
PD-1	programmed cell death-1 receptor
PDL	programmed cell death ligand
PDR	pulsed dose rate
PDT	photodynamic therapy
PET	positron emission tomography
PET-CT	positron emission tomography with computerized tomography
PF	posterior fossa
PFS	progression-free survival
PFT	pulmonary function test
PLCO	Prostate, Lung, Colorectal, and Ovarian Cancer Screening Trial
PLND	pelvic lymph node dissection
PMH	Princess Margaret Hospital, Toronto, Canada
PMID	PubMed ID number
PMMA	percutaneous injection of bone cement
PMRT	postmastectomy radiation therapy
PN	partial nephrectomy
PNET	primitive neuroectodermal tumor
PNI	perineural invasion
POC	postoperative complication
POG	Pediatric Oncology Group
PORT	postoperative radiotherapy
PPD	product of perpendicular diameters
PPI	proton pump inhibitor
PPT	pineal parenchymal tumor
PPV	positive predictive value
PPW	posterior pharyngeal wall

PR	partial response; progesterone receptor
PRL	prolactin
PRT	prospective randomized trial
PS	performance status
PSA	prostate specific antigen
PSADT	PSA doubling time
PSC	primary sclerosing cholangitis
PSMA	prostate specific membrane antigen
PTC	papillary thyroid cancer
PTCH	patched tumor suppressor gene
PTHC	percutaneous transhepatic cholangiography
PTV	planning target volume
PUVA	psoralen plus ultraviolet A
PVE	preoperative portal vein embolization
PVI	protracted venous infusion
Q	quadrantectomy
QA	quality assurance
QALY	quality-adjusted life years
QD	once daily
QOL	quality of life
RAI	radioactive iodine
RBE	relative biological effectiveness
RCC	renal cell carcinoma
R-CHOP	rituximab, cyclophosphamide, doxorubicin, vincristine, prednisone
RCT	randomized controlled trial
rdWBRT	reduced dose whole brain radiation therapy
R-EPOCH	rituximab, etoposide, prednisone, vincristine, cyclophosphamide, doxorubicin
RER	rapid early response
reRT	re-irradiation
RF	risk factor(s)
RFA	radiofrequency ablation
RFS	recurrence free survival
RILD	radiation-induced liver disease

RM	radical mastectomy
RMH/GOC	UK Royal Marsden Hospital/Gloucestershire Oncology Centre
R-MPV	rituximab, methotrexate, procarbazine, vincristine, leucovorin
R-MPV-A	rituximab, methotrexate, procarbazine, vincristine, leucovorin, and consolidation cytarabine
RMS	rhabdomyosarcoma
RNI	regional nodal irradiation
RP	radical prostatectomy
RPA	recursive partitioning analysis
RPLND	retroperitoneal lymph node dissection
RPN	retropharyngeal nodes
RPS	retroperitoneal sarcoma
RR	retrospective review
RS	Reed–Sternberg cells
RT	radiation therapy
RTK	rhabdoid tumor of the kidney
rTNM	recurrent TNM
RTOG	Radiation Therapy Oncology Group
RT-PCR	reverse transcription polymerase chain reaction
RUQ	right upper quadrant
s/p	status post
SABR	stereotactic ablative body radiotherapy
SBP	selective bladder preservation
SBRT	stereotactic body radiotherapy
SC/GC	small cell/germ cell
SCC	squamous cell carcinoma
SCCHN	squamous cell carcinoma of the head and neck
SCCUP	squamous cancers remaining as "unknown primary"
SCLC	small cell lung cancer
SCM	sternocleidomastoid muscle
SCPL–CHEP	supracricoid partial laryngectomy
SCT	stem cell transplant
SCV	supraclavicular

SDRT	single-dose RT
SEER	surveillance, epidemiology, and end results
SER	slow early responder
SES	socioeconomic status
SGL	supraglottic laryngectomy
SHH	sonic hedgehog
SHIM	Sexual Health Inventory for Men
SIB	simultaneous integrated boost
SINS	Spine Instability Neoplastic Score
SJHG	St. Jude High-Grade (Study)
SLL	small lymphocytic lymphoma
SLL/CLL	small lymphocytic lymphoma/chronic lymphocytic leukemia
SLN	sentinel lymph node
SLNB	sentinel lymph node biopsy
SM	surgical margin
SMA	superior mesenteric artery
SMAC	sarcoma meta-analysis collaboration
SMILE	steroid, methotrexate, ifosfamide, L-asparaginase, etoposide
SMT	single modality therapy
SMV	superior mesenteric vein
SND	selective neck dissection
SNUC	sinonasal undifferentiated carcinoma
SPECT	single photon emission computed tomography
SPN	solitary pulmonary nodules
SRE	skeletal-related event
SRS	stereotactic radiosurgery
SS	statistically significant
SSM	skin-sparing mastectomy
SSO	Society for Surgical Oncology
START	Standardisation of Breast Radiotherapy
STD	sexually transmitted disease
STNI	subtotal nodal irradiation
STR	subtotal resection

STS	soft tissue sarcoma
SUV	standardized uptake value
SV	seminal vesicle
SVC	superior vena cava
SVI	seminal vesicle invasion
SWOG	Southwest Oncology Group
Sx	symptoms
TACE	transarterial chemoembolization
TAE	transcutaneous arterial embolization
TAH	total abdominal hysterectomy
Tam	tamoxifen
TCC	transitional cell carcinoma
TCR	T-cell receptor
TKI	tyrosine kinase inhibitor
TL	total laryngectomy
TLM	transoral laser microsurgery
TM	total mastectomy
TME	total mesenteric excision
TMZ	temozolomide
TNBC	triple negative breast cancer
TNM	tumor, node, metastasis
TNMB	tumor, node, metastasis, blood
TNT	total neoadjuvant treatment
TORS	transoral robotic surgery
TPF	cisplatin, docetaxel, and 5-Fu
TR	true recurrences
TROG	Trans Tasman Radiation Oncology Group
TRUS	transrectal ultrasound
TSEBT	total skin electron beam therapy
TSH	thyroid stimulating hormone
TSS	transsphenoidal surgery
TTB	total toxicity burden
TTF	tumor treating fields

TTF-1	thyroid transcription factor 1
TTP	time to progression
TURBT	transurethral resection of bladder tumor
TURP	transurethral resection of prostate
TV	tumor volume
TVUS	transvaginal ultrasound
tx	treatment
UCLA	University of California Los Angeles
UCSF	University of California San Francisco
UES	upper esophageal sphincter
UH	unfavorable histology
UIQ	upper inner quadrant
UIR	unfavorable intermediate risk
UKCCSG	United Kingdom Childhood Cancer Study Group
ULN	upper limit of normal
UM	uveal melanoma
UOQ	upper outer quadrant
UPS	undifferentiated pleomorphic sarcoma
US	ultrasound
USPSTF	United States Preventative Services Task Force
UTI	urinary tract infection
UVA1	ultraviolet A1
UVB	ultraviolet B
VAC	vincristine, actinomycin D, cyclophosphamide
VACA	vincristine, actinomycin D, cyclophosphamide, Adriamycin
VAdriaC-IE	vincristine, Adriamycin, cyclophosphamide, irinotecan, etoposide
VAIA	vincristine, actinomycin D, irinotecan, adriamycin
VAIA+E	vincristine, actinomycin D, irinotecan, Adriamycin, etoposide
VATS	video assisted thoracoscopic surgery
VBT	vaginal brachytherapy
VCB	vaginal cuff brachytherapy
VCF	vertebral compression fracture
VCR	vincristine

VEGF	vascular endothelial growth factor
VHL	Von Hippel Lindau
VHR	very high risk
VIP	vasoactive intestinal peptide
VMA	vanillylmandelic acid
VNPI	Van Nuys Prognostic Index
VP-16	etoposide
VS	vestibular schwannoma
VTE	venous thromboembolism
WAI	whole abdominal irradiation
WART	whole abdomen radiation therapy
WBI	whole breast irradiation
WBRT	whole brain radiation therapy
WE	wide excision
WHO	World Health Organization
WLE	wide local excision
WLI	whole lung irradiation
WNL	within normal limits
WPRT	whole pelvis radiation therapy
WT	Wilms tumor
WW	watchful waiting
XP	xeroderma pigmentosum

INDEX

AA. *See* anaplastic astrocytoma
abdominal pain, 326
abdominoperineal resection (APR), 327
accelerated partial breast irradiation (APBI)
    ductal carcinoma in situ, 221, 226
    early-stage breast cancer, 198–201
    techniques, 201
acinic cell carcinoma, 116
acoustic neuroma. *See* vestibular schwannoma
acral lentiginous melanoma, 168
acromegaly (GH), 40
active surveillance
    intermediate-and high-risk prostate cancer, 374
    seminoma, 406
adaptive replanning, nasopharyngeal cancer, 103
adenocarcinoma
    cervical cancer, 430
    non-small-cell lung cancer, 239
adenohypophysis, 39
adenoid cystic carcinoma, 116
adjuvant chemotherapy
    advanced endometrial cancer, 447
    cervical cancer, 432
    cholangiocarcinoma (CC), 349
    colorectal cancer (CRC), 328
    early-stage indolent NHL, 496
    ependymoma, 533
    nasopharyngeal cancer, 101
adjuvant hysterectomy, cervical cancer, 431
adjuvant radiation
    advanced endometrial cancer, 447
    bladder cancer, 400
    cervical cancer, 433
    cholangiocarcinoma (CC), 350
    endometrial cancer, 443
    postoperative prostate cancer, 388
    renal cell carcinoma, 425
    urethral cancer, 421, 422
    vulvar cancer, 458
adrenal metastases palliation, 626
adriamycin
    breast cancer, 188, 189
    Wilms tumor, 573
aggressive non-Hodgkin's lymphoma (NHLs)
    biopsy, 483
    clinical presentation, 483
    epidemiology, 481
    imaging, 483
    natural history, 483
    pathology, 482
    prognostic factors, 483
    risk factors, 481
    staging, 484
    translocations and immunotype, 482
    treatment paradigm, 484–485
    workup, 483

alpha-thalassemia/mental retardation syndrome
    x-linked gene (ATRX) mutation
    glioblastoma, 3
    low-grade gliomas (LGGs), 19
alveolar rhabdomyosarcoma (RMS), 550
American Joint Committee on Cancer (AJCC) staging
    system
    anal cancer, 340
    bladder cancer, 396
    cervical cancer, 430–431
    cholangiocarcinoma (CC), 348
    esophageal cancer, 284–285
    gastric cancer, 295
    hepatocellular carcinoma (HCC), 304, 305
    low-risk prostate cancer, 359
    lung cancer (NSCLC), 240
    malignant pleural mesothelioma, 270
    pancreatic adenocarcinoma, 313
    penile cancer, 412
    rectal cancer, 327
    renal cell carcinoma, 424
    soft tissue sarcoma (STS), 507–508
    thymoma, 276
    urethral cancer, 420
    uterine cancer, 440
    uterine sarcoma, 451
    vaginal cancer, 465
    vulvar cancer, 456
anal canal, 339
anal cancer
    clinical presentation, 340
    epidemiology, 339
    histology, 339
    imaging, 340
    lymphatics, 339
    pathology, 339
    prognostic factors, 340
    risk factors, 339
    staging, 340
    treatment paradigm, 339, 340–341
    workup, 340
anal verge, 339
anaplastic astrocytoma (AA), 11–12
anaplastic gliomas
    anatomy, 11
    epidemiology, 11
    genetics, 11
    imaging, 11
    natural history, 12
    pathology, 12
    prognostic factors, 12
    risk factors, 11
    treatment, 12, 13
anaplastic oligodendroglioma (AO), 11–12
anaplastic thyroid cancer (ATC)
    epidemiology, 131

anaplastic thyroid cancer (ATC) (*cont.*)
  staging, 140–141
  standard treatment regimen, 143
  treatment paradigm, 143
  workup, 140
anastrozole
  ductal carcinoma in situ (DCIS), 224
  early-stage breast cancer, 189
androgen deprivation therapy medications
  hormone therapy, 380
  intermediate-and high-risk prostate cancer,
    374–377
  postoperative prostate cancer, 388
Ann Arbor (Lugano) staging system
  aggressive non-Hodgkin's lymphoma, 484
  Hodgkin's lymphoma, 473
anorectal ring, 326
antiepileptic drugs, trigeminal neuralgia, 48
APBI. *See* accelerated partial breast irradiation
appendicular skeleton, 607
arteriovenous malformation, 640
Askin's tumor, 577
ATC. *See* anaplastic thyroid cancer
ATRT. *See* atypical teratoid/rhabdoid tumor
atypical teratoid/rhabdoid tumor (ATRT)
  epidemiology, 589
  pathology/genetics, 589
  prognosis, 589
  treatment paradigm, 589
axial skeleton, 607
axillary lymph node dissection, 188

balloon compression, trigeminal neuralgia, 48
barrel cervix, 430
Bartholin glands, 445
basal cell adenoma, 116
basal cell carcinoma (BCC)
  clinical presentation, 156
  definitive RT, 161
  epidemiology, 155
  genetics, 156
  pathology, 156
  risk factors, 155
  screening, 156
  staging, 157–158
  surgical resection, 158–159
  systemic therapy, 160
  treatment paradigm, 155
basal cell nevus syndrome, 156
basaloid carcinoma, 456
base of tongue, 79
Bazex–Dupré–Christol syndrome, 156
BCC. *See* basal cell carcinoma
Beckwith–Wiedemann syndrome, 569
bentuximab, Hodgkin's lymphoma, 478
bevacizumab, recurrent/progressive glioblastoma, 8
bilateral nerve-sparing procedure, low-risk prostate
    cancer, 360
bisphosphonate, bone and spine metastasis, 609
bladder, anatomy, 395
bladder cancer
  clinical presentation, 396
  epidemiology, 395
  imaging, 396
  pathology, 395
  prognostic factors, 396
  risk factors, 395
  staging, 396
  treatment paradigm, 395–398
bone and spine metastasis
  biopsy, 608
  clinical presentation, 607
  epidemiology, 607
  hemibody irradiation, 611
  imaging, 608
  Mirels Nomogram, 608
  pathology, 607
  prognostic factors, 608
  retreatment, 611
  treatment paradigm, 608–609
  workup, 607–608
bone marrow biopsy
  Hodgkin's lymphoma, 473
  primary central nervous system lymphoma, 34
Bormann classification, gastric cancer, 294
Bowen's disease, 156
brachytherapy, 201
  brainstem gliomas (BSGs), 540
  cervical cancer, 432
  endoscopic therapy, 290
  oral cavity squamous cell carcinoma (OC-SCC), 94
  penile cancer, 414–415
  soft tissue sarcoma (STS), 509
brachyury, 70
BRAF V600E mutation
  glioblastoma, 3
  low-grade gliomas (LGGs), 19
  melanoma, 168
brain metastases
  clinical presentation, 595
  epidemiology, 595
  imaging, 595
  pathology, 595
  prognostic factors, 595–597
  treatment paradigm, 597–598
  workup, 595
brainstem, 537
brainstem gliomas (BSGs)
  adult diffuse intrinsic, 540–541
  clinical presentation, 538
  epidemiology, 537
  genetics, 538
  pathology, 537
  prognostic factors, 538
  re-irradiation, 540
  risk factors, 537
  stereotactic radiosurgery (SRS), 540
  systemic therapy, 540
  treatment paradigm, 537, 538–539
  workup, 538
breast cancer
  ductal carcinoma in situ, 219–227
  early-stage, 183–201
  locally advanced, 207–217
  recurrent, 229–234
breast-conservation therapy (BCT), 190, 221
Brigham and Women's Hospital Staging System,
    cutaneous SCC, 158

bronchioloalveolar carcinoma, 239
Brooker's classification, 640
BSGs. *See* brainstem gliomas

CALGB 9343 (Hughes) Trial, 197
carbamazepine, 48
carbon ion therapy, salivary gland tumors, 120–121
carcinosarcoma, 441, 450
cauda equina, 615, 616
CC. *See* cholangiocarcinoma
CDKN2A/B homozygous deletion, low-grade
    gliomas, 19
celiac axis, 293
cervical cancer
    clinical presentation, 430
    definitive management, 434–436
    epidemiology, 429
    imaging, 430
    pathology, 430
    prognostic factors, 430
    risk factors, 429–430
    screening guidelines, 430
    staging, 430–431
    surgical management, 433–434
    treatment paradigm, 431–433
    workup, 430
cervical tumors, 285
cervix, 430, 464
cetuximab
    locally advanced laryngeal cancer, 113
    oropharynx cancer, 84–85
charged particle RT
    sinonasal cancer, 148
    uveal melanoma (UM), 64, 66
chemoradiation (chemoRT)
    advanced endometrial cancer, 448–449
    anal cancer, 341
    colorectal cancer (CRC), 328–333
    esophageal cancer, 288–289
    locally advanced unresectable pancreatic cancer,
        318–319
    nasopharyngeal cancer (NPC), 100–101
    pancreatic adenocarcinoma, 315–317
    sinonasal tumors, 148
    thymoma, 279
chemotherapy (CHT)
    aggressive non-Hodgkin's lymphoma, 484–485
    anaplastic gliomas, 12
    bladder cancer, 397
    breast cancer, 188–189
    cervical cancer, 431–432
    cholangiocarcinoma (CC), 349
    chondrosarcoma and chordoma, 72
    colorectal cancer (CRC), 328
    craniopharyngioma, 546
    ductal carcinoma in situ (DCIS), 221
    ependymoma, 532
    esophageal cancer, 286
    Ewing's sarcoma, 577, 578
    gastric cancer, 296
    glioblastoma, 4
    head and neck carcinoma, 135
    head and neck carcinoma of unknown primary
        (HNCUP), 126

hepatocellular carcinoma (HCC), 305
Hodgkin's lymphoma, 474
indolent non-Hodgkin's lymphoma (NHLs), 495
laryngeal cancer, 110
locally advanced breast cancer (LABC), 208
locoregionally recurrent breast cancer, 230
low-grade gliomas (LGGs), 20, 23
medulloblastoma, 522
meningioma, 27
multiple myeloma, 500
mycosis fungoides (MF), 177
nasopharyngeal cancer (NPC), 100–102
neuroblastoma (NB), 561
non-small-cell lung cancer (NSCLC), 241
oral cavity squamous cell carcinoma (OC-SCC),
    94
oropharynx cancer, 82
pancreatic adenocarcinoma, 314
pediatric Hodgkin's lymphoma, 583–584
penile cancer, 414
postoperative prostate cancer, 388
primary central nervous system lymphoma, 34–35
rhabdomyosarcoma (RMS), 553
salivary gland tumors, 118
seminoma, 406
sinonasal tumors, 147–148
sinonasal undifferentiated carcinoma (SNUC), 149
small-cell lung carcinoma (SCLC), 259
soft tissue sarcoma (STS), 508
thymoma, 277
urethral cancer, 421
uterine cancer, 442
uveal melanoma (UM), 64
vaginal cancer, 466
vestibular schwannoma, 55
vulvar cancer, 457
Wilms tumor (WT), 572
Child–Pugh Functional Status, chronic liver disease,
    304
cholangiocarcinoma (CC)
    clinical presentation, 347
    epidemiology, 347
    imaging, 348
    incidence, 347
    pathology, 347
    prognostic factors, 348
    risk factors, 347
    screening, 347
    staging, 348
    treatment paradigm, 348–349
    workup, 347–348
chondrosarcoma
    anatomy, 70
    biopsy, 71
    clinical presentation, 70
    epidemiology, 69
    genetics, 70
    imaging, 71
    pathology, 70
    prognostic factors, 71
    risk factors, 69
    staging, 71–72
    treatment paradigm, 69, 72–73
    workup, 71

chordoma
  anatomy, 70
  biopsy, 71
  clinical presentation, 70
  epidemiology, 69
  genetics, 70
  imaging, 71
  pathology, 70
  prognostic factors, 71
  risk factors, 69
  staging, 71–72
  treatment paradigm, 69, 72–73
  workup, 71
choroidal hemangioma, 642
chromosomal abnormality, multiple myeloma,
    499
CHT. *See* chemotherapy
cisplatin
  anal cancer, 342
  bladder cancer, 397
  head and neck cancer, 135
  mesothelioma, 271
  oropharynx cancer, 82
  sinonasal tumors, 147–148
  small-cell lung carcinoma (SCLC), 259
  uterine cancer, 442
Cloquet's/Rosenmüller's node, 445
CN palsies, 538
Codman's triangle, 576
colorectal cancer (CRC)
  clinical presentation, 326
  epidemiology, 325
  imaging, 327
  incidence, 325
  long-course RT, 328–333
  pathology, 326
  prognostic factors, 327
  risk factors, 326, 326
  screening, 326
  short-course RT, 333–335
  treatment paradigm, 325, 327–328
  workup, 327
colposcopy, 430
conus medullaris, 615
Cooper's ligaments, 183
coronary restenosis, 640
corpus uteri carcinoma, 441
cortical bone, 607
craniopharyngioma
  adamantinomatous subtype, 545
  clinical presentation, 545
  epidemiology, 545
  genetics, 545
  imaging, 545
  papillary subtype, 545
  pathology, 545
  prognostic factors, 546
  treatment paradigm, 546
  workup, 545–546
craniospinal irradiation (CSI)
  ependymoma, 532
  medulloblastoma, 524, 525
CRC. *See* colorectal cancer
cryoablation, renal cell carcinoma, 425

cryotherapy, 159
Cushing's disease (ACTH), 40
cutaneous SCC
  clinical and microscopic PNI, 163
  clinical presentation, 156
  concurrent chemoRT, 163
  definitive RT, 161
  epidemiology, 155
  immunotherapy, 160
  local therapies, 159–160
  pathology, 156
  risk factors, 155
  screening, 156
  staging system, 158
  surgical resection, 158–159
cystectomy, bladder cancer, 396–397
cystosarcoma phyllodes, 184

DCIS. *See* ductal carcinoma in situ
Deauville (5-point) Score, 474
Denys–Drash syndrome, 569
dermis, 167
dermis, 156
desmoid tumors, 640
dexamethasone, 623
diffuse astrocytoma
  IDH-mutant, 18
  IDH-wild-type, 18
diffuse intrinsic pontine glioma (DIPG), 538
diffuse large B-cell lymphoma (DLBCL)
  consolidative RT, 488
  primary bone, 489
  primary mediastinal, 488
  radiation, 486–487
  R-CHOP, 487
  rituximab, 487–488
  testicular, 488–489
  treatment paradigm, 481
dinutuximab, 561
diplopia, 100
distal esophagogastrectomy, 285
diuretics, 623
DLBCL. *See* diffuse large B-cell lymphoma
dorsal cord syndrome, 616
ductal carcinoma in situ (DCIS)
  biopsy technique, 220
  clinical presentation, 220
  epidemiology, 219
  genetics, 219
  genomic assays, 226
  imaging, 220
  vs. lobular carcinoma in situ, 227
  optimal dose and fractionation, 224
  pathology, 219
  prognostic factors, 220
  recurrence, 225
  risk factors, 219
  screening, 219–220
  staging, 220
  surgical margins, 225
  treatment paradigm, 220
  workup, 220
Dupuytren's disease, 641–642
dural sac, 615

early aggressive therapy
    mycosis fungoides (MF), 177
Early Breast Cancer Trialists' Collaborative Group
        Meta-Analysis, 211–212
early-stage breast cancer
    adjuvant WBI, 191–193
    cardiac-sparing RT techniques, 195–196
    clinical presentation, 185
    differential diagnosis, 185
    epidemiology, 183
    estrogen exposure, 183
    genetics, 184
    hormone therapy, 189
    hypofractionation, 193–195
    IMRT, 195
    IORT, 197–198
    lifestyle/exposure, 183
    pathology, 184
    personal history, 183
    prognostic factors, 186
    rarer subtypes, 184
    regional nodal irradiation, 193
    risk factors, 183
    screening, 184–185
    staging, 186–187
    treatment paradigm, 187–189
    workup, 186
EBRT. *See* external beam radiotherapy
ectocervix, 430
EGFRv3 variant, glioblastoma, 3
elective neck dissection, OC-SCC, 95
embryonal rhabdomyosarcoma, 549
enchondromatosis, 69
endocervical canal, 430
endocrine therapy, breast conservation, 196–197
endometrial biopsy, 441
endometrial cancer
    advanced, 447–450
    categories, 442
    early-stage, 442–446
    nodal involvement, 442–443
endoscopic therapy
    brachytherapy, 290
    esophageal cancer, 286
    gastric cancer, 295
    proton therapy, 290
    resectable/operable, 287–289
    sinonasal tumors, 146
    sinonasal tumors, 147
    unresectable/inoperable, 286–287
enucleation
    choroidal melanomas, 65
    uveal melanoma (UM), 64
ependymoma
    adult spinal, 534
    clinical presentation, 532
    epidemiology, 531
    genetics, 531–532
    natural history, 532
    pathology, 531
    prognostic factors, 532
    risk factors, 531
    treatment paradigm, 532
    workup, 532

epidermis, 167
epidermis, 156
epidural spinal cord compression scale, 616
episcleral brachytherapy, uveal melanoma, 64, 64
esophageal cancer
    clinical presentation, 284
    epidemiology, 283
    imaging, 283
    natural history, 284
    pathology, 284
    prognostic factors, 284
    risk factors, 283
    staging, 284–285
    treatment paradigm, 283, 285–286
    workup, 283
esophagectomy, 285
esophagus, 283–284
esthesioneuroblastoma, 150
ethmoid sinus, 145
ethmoid sinus tumors
    biopsy, 146
    epidemiology, 145
    staging, 147
Evans/Children's Cancer Study Group (CCSG)
        Clinical Staging, 560
Ewing's sarcoma
    clinical presentation, 576
    epidemiology, 575
    genetics, 575–576
    imaging, 576
    natural history, 576
    pathology, 575
    prognostic factors, 576
    risk factors, 575
    treatment paradigm, 575, 576–578
Ewing's Sarcoma Family of Tumors, 575
excisional biopsy
    aggressive non-Hodgkin's lymphoma, 483
    head and neck carcinoma of unknown primary
        (HNCUP), 124
    Hodgkin's lymphoma, 473
extensive stage small-cell lung carcinoma (ES-SCLC),
        263–265
external beam radiotherapy (EBRT)
    bone and spine metastasis, 610
    cervical cancer, 432
    differentiated thyroid cancer, 143
    low-risk prostate cancer, 364
    malignant spinal cord compression, 616–617
    penile cancer, 414
    soft tissue sarcoma (STS), 509
extramammary Paget's disease of vulva, 456
extra-pleural pneumonectomy (EPP), 271, 272

facial nerve, 115
facial nerve (CN VII), 53
familial colorectal cancer syndromes, 326
fibroadenoma, 185
fibromatosis, 640
fibromuscular stroma, 357
FIGO staging system. *See* International Federation
        of Gynecologic and Obstetrics staging
        system
filum terminale, 615

fine needle aspiration (FNA)
    ductal carcinoma in situ (DCIS), 220
    head and neck cancer, 132
follicular non-Hodgkin's lymphoma (NHLs), 495–496
follicular thyroid cancer (FTC)
    epidemiology, 131
    staging, 140–141
    treatment paradigm, 141–142
    workup, 140
fractionated radiation
    oropharynx cancer, 83–84
    pituitary adenoma, 42, 43
    vestibular schwannoma, 57
fractionated stereotactic radiation therapy (FSRT), 55
Frey's syndrome, 116
frontal sinus, 145
FTC. *See* follicular thyroid cancer

ganglioglioma, 19
Gardner–Robertson Hearing Loss Scale, 54
Gardner's syndrome, 640
gastrectomy, 295
gastric cancer
    clinical presentation, 294
    epidemiology, 293
    genetics, 294
    imaging, 294
    natural history, 295
    pathology, 294
    prognostic factors, 295
    risk factors, 294
    screening, 294
    staging, 295
    treatment paradigm, 293, 295–297
gastric MALT, 497
GBM. *See* glioblastoma
GCT. *See* germ cell tumor
gemistocytic astrocytoma, IDH-mutant, 18
genetic syndromes
    anaplastic gliomas, 11
    low-grade gliomas (LGGs), 17
    soft tissue sarcoma, 506
genomic classifiers, postoperative prostate cancer,
    391
germ cell tumor (GCT), 404
    histologies, 404
    pathology, 404
glandular tissue, 183
glioblastoma (GBM)
    anatomy, 3
    biopsy, 4
    clinical presentation, 4
    epidemiology, 3
    genetics, 3
    imaging, 4
    pathology, 3
    prognostic factors, 4
    recurrent/progressive, 8
    treatment, 4
Glisson's capsule, 303
glomus tumor, 641
glottic cancers
    clinical presentation, 108
    radiation, 100–101
    staging, 109
    surgery, 109–110
glottis, 107
glycerol rhizolysis, trigeminal neuralgia, 48
Gorlin syndrome, 156, 519
graves ophthalmopathy, 640
gray matter, 615
gynecomastia, 641

H3 G34 mutation, 19
H3 K27M mutation, 19
HCC. *See* hepatocellular carcinoma
head and neck carcinoma of unknown primary
    (HNCUP)
    biopsy, 124
    clinical presentation, 124
    HPV-associated, 127
    imaging, 125
    lymph node levels, 124
    natural history, 125
    pathology, 124
    prognostic factors, 125
    risk factors, 123
    staging, 125
    treatment paradigm, 123, 125–126
    workup, 124–125
hearing loss, 53
hematochezia, 326
hemivulvectomy, 457
hepatocellular carcinoma (HCC)
    biopsy, 304
    clinical presentation, 303–304
    epidemiology, 303
    imaging, 304
    pathology, 303
    prognostic factors, 304
    risk factors, 303
    screening, 303
    treatment paradigm, 304–306
    workup, 303–304
HNCUP. *See* head and neck carcinoma of unknown
    primary
Hodgkin's lymphoma
    advanced, 477–478
    biopsy, 473
    clinical presentation, 473
    early-stage, 475–476
    early-stage unfavorable, 476–477
    epidemiology, 471
    histologic characteristics, 472
    imaging, 473
    prognostic factors, 473
    relapsed/refractory, 478
    risk factors, 471, 472
    treatment paradigm, 471, 473–475
    workup, 473
hormone therapy
    ductal carcinoma in situ (DCIS), 221
    early-stage breast cancer, 189
    intermediate-and high-risk prostate cancer,
    379–380
House–Brackmann Facial Paralysis Scale, 54
HPV-related multi-phenotypic sinonasal carcinoma,
    149

Hurthle cell, 140–141
Hyams histologic grading system,
    esthesioneuroblastoma, 150
hyperdiploidy, neuroblastoma, 558
hyperfractionation
    bladder cancer, 400
    early-stage laryngeal cancer, 111
    glioblastoma management, 6
hyperplasia, 441
hyperthermia (HT), 230
hyperthyroidism (TSHoma), 40
hypodermis, 167
hypofractionation
    bladder cancer, 400
    low-risk prostate cancer, 364–366
hypopituitarism, 42

IDH1 and IDH2 mutations, 19
IDH1 mutation, 3
image defined risk factors (IDRFs), 559
immunotherapy
    melanoma, 170–171
    neuroblastoma (NB), 561
    renal cell carcinoma, 425
    stage III non-small-cell lung cancer, 250
IMRT. *See* intensity modulated radiation therapy
incidentally appreciated meningiomas, 28
indolent non-Hodgkin's lymphoma
    clinical presentation, 493
    imaging, 494
    pathology/genetics, 493
    prognostic factors, 494
    risk factors, 493
    treatment paradigm, 493, 494–495
    workup, 493
INRGSS, neuroblastoma, 559–560
intensity modulated radiation therapy (IMRT)
    anal cancer, 343
    cervical cancer, 435
    early-stage breast cancer, 195
    early-stage laryngeal cancer, 112
    esophageal cancer, 289
    oropharynx cancer, 87
    rectal cancer, 335
intermediate-and high-risk prostate cancer
    imaging, 374
    natural history, 374
    risk factors, 373–374
    treatment paradigm, 373, 374–375
    workup, 374
International Federation of Gynecologic and
    Obstetrics (FIGO) staging system
    uterine cancer, 440
    uterine sarcoma, 451
    vaginal cancer, 465
    vulvar cancer, 456
intracranial germ cell tumor, 590–591
intraoperative radiation therapy (IORT)
    ductal carcinoma in situ (DCIS), 221, 226
    early-stage breast cancer, 197–198
intraoral cone radiation, OC-SCC, 94
intravascular stent, superior vena cava syndrome,
    623
intravesical therapy, bladder cancer, 397

invasive ductal carcinoma, 184
invasive lobular carcinoma, 184
involved field RT (IFRT), 584
involved site RT (ISRT), 584
iobenguane I-131, 565
Ivor Lewis esophagogastrectomy, 286

juvenile nasopharyngeal angiofibroma, 641

Kadish staging system, esthesioneuroblastoma, 150
keloids, 640
keratinizing squamous cell carcinoma, 99
Klatskin tumors, 347
Koos Grading Scale, 54
kyphoplasty, 500, 609

LABC. *See* locally advanced breast cancer
langerhans cell histiocytosis, 641
laryngeal cancer
    clinical presentation, 108
    early-stage disease, 110–112
    epidemiology, 107
    imaging, 108
    locally advanced disease, 112–113
    pathology, 108
    risk factors, 107
    staging, 108–109
    treatment paradigm, 107, 109–110
    workup, 108
larynx, anatomy, 107–108
Lauren histological classification, gastric cancer, 294
Ledderhose disease, 642
lentigo maligna, 168
leukoplakia, 92
LGGs. *See* low-grade gliomas
limited stage small-cell lung carcinoma (LC-SCLC),
    260–263
linear-accelerator-based radiosurgery, trigeminal
    neuralgia, 49
lingual tonsillectomy, 125
liver, 312
lobular carcinoma in situ (LCIS), 227
locally advanced breast cancer (LABC)
    clinical presentation, 207
    epidemiology, 207
    imaging, 207–208
    prognostic factors, 208
    recurrence, 212
    T3N0 tumors, 212–213
    treatment paradigm, 207, 208–209
    workup, 207
locoregionally recurrent breast cancer
    after mastectomy, 232–234
    clinical presentation, 229
    epidemiology, 229
    imaging, 229
    interstitial brachytherapy, 232
    prognostic factors, 230
    re-irradiation, 232
    risk factors, 229
    staging, 230
    treatment paradigm, 229, 230
    workup, 229
long bones, 607

low anterior resection, colorectal cancer, 327
low-grade gliomas (LGGs)
    anatomy, 17
    clinical presentation, 19
    epidemiology, 17
    genetics, 19
    natural history, 19
    pathology, 17–19
    postoperative treatment paradigm, 17
    prognostic factors, 19
    risk factors, 17
    treatment paradigm, 20
    WHO 2016 glioma classification, 18
    workup, 19
low-risk prostate cancer
    active surveillance, 362–364
    biopsy, 358
    clinical presentation, 358
    epidemiology, 356
    genetics, 357
    imaging, 358
    natural history, 358
    pathology, 357
    prevention, 361–362
    prognostic factors, 358
    risk factors, 356
    risk stratification, 360
    screening, 357–358, 361–362
    staging, 359
    treatment paradigm, 355–356, 360–361
lumpectomy, 188
lymph node dissection (LND)
    gastric cancer, 295–297
    low-risk prostate cancer, 361
lymph node involvement
    oropharynx cancer, 92
    sinonasal tumors, 148
lymph node-positive prostate cancer, 383
lymphadenectomy, uterine cancer, 441
lymphatics, uterine, 440

Maffucci syndrome, 70
magnetic resonance imaging (MRI)
    anaplastic glioma, 11
    early-stage breast cancer, 186
    low-grade glioma, 19
    postoperative prostate cancer, 388
    soft tissue sarcoma (STS), 507
    uterine cancer, 440
malignant melanoma
    adjuvant RT, 171–172
    axillary nodal RT, 172
    epidemiology, 167
    imaging, 168
    incidence, 167
    lentigo maligna, 168
    mucosal, 168
    nodular, 167–168
    pathology, 167–168
    prognostic factors, 168
    risk factors, 167
    screening, 168
    staging, 169
    treatment paradigm, 168, 170–171

    workup, 168
malignant spinal cord compression (mSCC)
    biopsy, 616
    clinical presentation, 615–616
    epidemiology, 615
    imaging, 616
    pathology, 615
    prognostic factors, 616
    treatment paradigm, 616–617
    workup, 616
mammography
    ductal carcinoma in situ (DCIS), 220
    early-stage breast cancer, 186
mandibular nerve (V3), 47
Masaoka–Koga staging system, thymoma, 276
mastectomy
    early-stage breast cancer, 188, 190
    locoregionally recurrent breast cancer, 232–234
maxillary nerve (V2), 47
maxillary sinus, 145
maxillary sinus tumors, 131, 146
MCC. *See* Merkel cell carcinoma
McKeown esophagogastrectomy, 286
mediastinoscopy, non-small-cell lung cancer, 240
mediastinum, 621–622
medical therapy
    bone and spine metastasis, 609
    brain metastases, 597
    indolent non-Hodgkin's lymphoma (NHLs), 495
    malignant spinal cord compression, 616
    mycosis fungoides (MF), 176–177
    trigeminal neuralgia, 48
medullary thyroid cancer (MTC)
    radiation, 142
    surgery, 142
    systemic therapy, 142
    thyroid hormone replacement, 142
    workup, 141
medulloblastoma
    clinical presentation, 520
    epidemiology, 519
    genetics, 520
    high risk, 526–527
    infants, 527
    molecular-based risk stratification, 521
    morphologic classification, 520–521
    pathology, 520
    prognostic factors, 521
    risk factors, 519–520
    staging, 521
    standard risk, 523–526
    treatment paradigm, 519, 522–523
    workup, 521
melanocytes, 167
meningiomas
    anatomy, 25
    asymptomatic grade I, 25
    clinical presentation, 26
    epidemiology, 25
    genetics, 26
    grade II, 25
    natural history, 26, 27
    pathology, 26
    prognostic factors, 26

recurrent, 25
risk factors, 25
RT dose guidelines, 25
unresectable, 25
workup, 27
meningiomatosis, 29
Merkel cell carcinoma (MCC)
    biopsy, 157
    clinical presentation, 156
    early-stage, 163–164
    epidemiology, 155
    immunotherapy, 165
    pathology, 156
    prognostic factors, 157
    risk factors, 155
    staging, 159
    surgical resection, 158–159
    treatment paradigm, 155
Merkel cells, 156
mesothelioma
    biopsy, 270
    clinical presentation, 269–270
    dose-escalated RT, 274
    epidemiology, 269
    imaging, 270
    natural history, 270
    pathology, 269
    prognostic factors, 270
    risk factors, 269
    staging, 270
    treatment paradigm, 270–271
    unresectable, 274
    workup, 270
metaiodobenzylguanidine (MIBG), 558, 561, 565
methotrexate
    primary central nervous system lymphoma, 34
MF. *See* mycosis fungoides
microcystic, elongated, and fragmented (MELF)
    pattern, 440
microvascular decompression, trigeminal neuralgia,
    48–49
Milan criteria, hepatocellular carcinoma (HCC), 305
mitotic index, endothelial proliferation, nuclear
    atypia, or necrosis (MEAN), 11
modified Chang staging system, medulloblastoma,
    522
Mohs surgery, 161
mSCC. *See* malignant spinal cord compression
MTC. *See* medullary thyroid cancer
mucosal melanoma, 168
multiple myeloma
    clinical presentation, 499
    epidemiology, 499
    genetics, 499
    imaging, 500
    pathology, 499
    prognostic factors, 500
    risk factors, 499
    staging, 500
    treatment paradigm, 500–501
mycosis fungoides (MF)
    clinical presentation, 175
    epidemiology, 175
    pathogenesis, 175

prognostic factors, 176
staging, 176
treatment paradigm, 175, 176–177
workup, 175–176
myxopapillary ependymoma, 534

nasopharyngeal cancer (NPC)
    clinical presentation, 100
    epidemiology, 99
    imaging, 100
    pathology, 99
    pediatric, 103–104
    prognostic factors, 100
    risk factors, 99
    screening, 100
    staging, 100
    treatment paradigm, 100–101
    workup, 100
nasopharynx, anatomy, 99
National Wilms Tumor Study (NWTS), 573
NB. *See* neuroblastoma
NCCN Criteria for Resectability, 314
NCCN dosing guidelines, indolent non-Hodgkin's
    lymphoma, 495
neuroblastoma (NB)
    clinical eponyms, 558
    clinical presentation, 558
    epidemiology, 557
    genetics, 558
    high-risk, 564–565
    imaging, 558
    intermediate-risk disease, 563
    low-risk, 562
    natural history, 559
    pathology, 557–558, 559
    prognostic factors, 559
    risk factors, 557
    screening, 558
    stage 4S disease, 562–563
    staging, 559
    treatment paradigm, 557, 561
    workup, 558–559
neutron therapy, salivary gland tumors, 120
nevoid basal cell carcinoma syndrome, 519
nipple-sparing mastectomy, 188
N-myc protein amplification, neuroblastoma (NB),
    558
nodular melanoma, 167–168
nodular sclerosis, 581
non-Hodgkin's lymphoma (NHLs)
    aggressive (*see* aggressive non-Hodgkin's
        lymphoma)
    indolent non-Hodgkin's lymphoma, 493–495
nonkeratinizing carcinoma, 99
nonmelanomatous skin cancer
    clinical presentation, 156
    early-stage, 163
    epidemiology, 155
    genetics, 156
    imaging, 157
    pathology, 156
    prevalence, 155
    prognostic factors, 157
    risk factors, 155

nonmelanomatous skin cancer (*cont.*)
  screening, 156
  staging, 158
  treatment paradigms, 155, 158–161
  workup, 156–157
non-small-cell lung cancer (NSCLC)
  clinical presentation, 240
  epidemiology, 239
  genetics, 239
  imaging, 240
  medically inoperable, 243–247
  medically operable patients, 242–243
  pathology, 239
  radiographic screening, 241–242
  risk factors, 239
  screening, 240
  stage III, 249–255
  treatment paradigm, 239, 241
  workup, 240
NPC. *See* nasopharyngeal cancer
NSCLC. *See* non-small-cell lung cancer
NSGCTs, 404
  histologies, 404
  imaging, 405
  pathology, 404
  prognostic factors, 405
NUT-midline carcinoma, 150

observation
  cervical cancer, 431
  indolent non-Hodgkin's lymphoma (NHLs), 494
  meningiomas, 27
  neuroblastoma (NB), 561
  non-small-cell lung cancer (NSCLC), 241
  salivary gland tumors, 117
  uveal melanoma (UM), 64
  vestibular schwannoma, 55
OC-SCC. *See* oral cavity squamous cell carcinoma
ocular biopsy, primary central nervous system
     lymphoma, 34
ocular tumors, 67
Ohngren's line, 131
olfactory neuroblastoma, 150
oligodendroglioma, IDH-Mutant and 1p19q
     codeleted, 18
oligodendrogliomas, 11
oligometastatic disease (OMD)
  definitions and subsets, 631
  epidemiology, 631
  nasopharyngeal cancer, 634
  in NSCLC, 631–632
  prostate cancer, 633–634
  SBRT, 634
Ollier disease, 70
OMD. *See* oligometastatic disease
O-6-methylguanine-DNA methyltransferase
     (MGMT) gene methylation
  glioblastoma, 3
  low-grade gliomas (LGGs), 19
Oncotype DX 21-gene Recurrence Score, 208
Ontario Cooperative Oncology Group 93-010
     Hypofractionation Trial, 194
oophorectomy, early-stage breast cancer, 188
ophthalmic nerve (V1), 47

oral cavity
  anatomy, 91–92
oral cavity squamous cell carcinoma (OC-SCC)
  biopsy, 92
  clinical presentation, 92
  epidemiology, 91
  genetics, 92
  imaging, 92
  natural history, 92
  pathology, 92
  postoperative RT, 95–96
  prognostic factors, 92
  risk factors, 91
  screening, 92
  staging, 93
  treatment paradigm, 93–94
  workup, 92
orbital embryonal rhabdomyosarcoma, 555
orbital exenteration
  sinonasal tumors, 147
  uveal melanoma (UM), 64
orbital pseudotumor, 641
organ-preservation, urethral cancer, 421
oropharynx borders, 79
oropharynx cancer
  anatomy, 79
  clinical presentation, 80
  epidemiology, 79
  imaging, 80
  natural history, 80–81
  pathology, 80
  prognostic factors, 80
  risk factors, 79
  treatment paradigm, 79, 81–82
  workup, 80
osteochondromas, 69
otalgia, 108
oviducts, 439

Paget's disease, 184
palatine tonsillectomy, 125
palliative nephrectomy, 425
palliative radiotherapy
  adrenal metastases, 626
  bladder cancer, 401
  head and neck cancer, 625–626
  liver palliation, 626
  lung palliation, 627
  pterygium, 640
  urethral cancer, 421
pancreas, 312
pancreatic adenocarcinoma
  biopsy, 313
  borderline resectable, 317–318
  clinical presentation, 312
  epidemiology, 311
  genetics, 312
  imaging, 312
  incidence, 311
  locally advanced/unresectable, 318–320
  lymphatics/patterns of spread, 312
  pathology, 312
  prognostic factors, 313
  resectable, 315–317

risk factors, 311
screening, 312
staging, 313
treatment paradigm, 313–315
workup, 312–313
panendoscopy, head and neck carcinoma of
unknown primary, 125
panhypopituitarism, 42
papillary thyroid cancer (PTC)
epidemiology, 131
risk factors, 131
staging, 140–141
treatment paradigm, 141–142
workup, 140
paraneoplastic syndromes, 258, 276
parinaud syndrome, 520
parotid, 115
partial nephrectomy (PN), 424
pazopanib, 508
PCNSL. *See* primary central nervous system
lymphoma
pediatric Hodgkin's lymphoma
vs. adolescent/young adult Hodgkin's disease, 582
clinical presentation, 582
epidemiology, 581
histologic classification, 582
intermediate-high risk/advanced/favorable,
585–586
low-risk/early/favorable, 584–585
prognostic factors, 582–583
relative frequency, 582
risk factors, 581
risk stratification scheme, 583
treatment paradigm, 581, 583–584
pediatric tumors
atypical teratoid/rhabdoid tumor, 589
ependymoma, 531–534
intracranial germ cell tumor, 590–591
medulloblastoma, 519–527
pineoblastoma, 589–590
Pel–Ebstein fevers, 582
pelvic nodal dissection, early-stage endometrial
cancer, 443
penile cancer
biopsy, 412
clinical presentation, 411–412
early-stage lesions, 415–416
epidemiology, 411
historical outcomes, 415
imaging, 412
limited excision, 415
pathology, 411
prognostic factors, 412
risk factors, 411
staging, 412
treatment paradigm, 411, 412–415
workup, 412
penis, 411
perihilar CC
clinical presentation, 347
diagnosis criteria, 348
Mayo Clinic transplant protocol, 349
pathology, 347
surgery, 348

perihilar tumors, 347
perilesional edema, meningiomas, 27
Peyronie's disease, 641
phototherapy, mycosis fungoides (MF), 177
pigmented villonodular synovitis, 641
pilocytic astrocytoma, 18
pineoblastoma, 589–590
pituitary adenoma
anatomy, 39
clinical presentation, 40
epidemiology, 39
imaging, 40
pathology, 39
risk factors, 39
treatment paradigm, 39, 41–42
workup, 40
pituitary carcinoma, 40
plantar warts, 640
plaque brachytherapy, uveal melanoma (UM), 66
pleomorphic adenoma, 116
pleomorphic xanthoastrocytoma, 18
pleura, 269
pleurodesis, 271
pontine CNs, 538
PORT. *See* postoperative radiation therapy
Posterior uvea, 61
posterior uvea, 61
postmastectomy radiation therapy (PMRT)
implant-related complications, 215
locally advanced breast cancer (LABC), 208–209,
214
postoperative prostate cancer
epidemiology, 387
genetics, 387
imaging, 388
natural history, 388
prognostic factors, 388
treatment paradigm, 387, 388–389
workup, 387–388
postoperative radiation therapy (PORT)
current standard dosing, 133
head and neck cancer
clinical presentation, 132
epidemiology, 131
genetics, 131
natural history, 132
pathology, 131
preoperative radiation, 133
prognostic factors, 132
risk factors, 131
screening, 131
treatment paradigm, 132–133
workup, 132
indications and dosing summary, 131
low-risk patients, 136–137
risk-adapted approach, 134
soft tissue sarcoma (STS), 509
1p19q codeletion, low-grade gliomas (LGGs), 19
primary central nervous system lymphoma (PCNSL)
anatomy, 33
clinical presentation, 33, 34
epidemiology, 33
imaging, 34
prognostic factors, 34, 40

primary central nervous system lymphoma (PCNSL)
(*cont.*)
   risk factors, 33
   treatment paradigm, 33–35
   workup, 34
primary cutaneous B-cell lymphoma (PCLBCL) leg
   type, 488
PRIME II Trial, 197
prolactinoma, 40
prophylactic cranial irradiation (PCI), 265–266
prostate, 356–357
proton therapy
   chondrosarcoma and chordoma, 74
   endoscopic therapy, 290
   hepatocellular carcinoma (HCC), 309
   medulloblastoma, 527
   pituitary adenoma, 43
   rhabdomyosarcoma, 555
   sinonasal tumors, 148
proximal femur, 70
PTC. *See* papillary thyroid cancer
pterygium, 640
pure germinoma, 590–591

radiation therapy
   aggressive non-Hodgkin's lymphoma, 485–486
   anaplastic gliomas, 12
   arteriovenous malformation, 640
   bladder cancer, 397–398
   brain metastases, 597–598
   cervical cancer, 432–433
   cholangiocarcinoma (CC), 349
   chondrosarcoma and chordoma, 73
   choroidal hemangioma, 642
   colorectal cancer (CRC), 328
   coronary restenosis, 640
   craniopharyngioma, 546
   desmoid tumors, 640
   ductal carcinoma in situ (DCIS), 221
   Dupuytren's disease, 641–642
   early-stage breast cancer, 189
   ependymoma, 532
   esophageal cancer, 286
   Ewing's sarcoma, 577, 578
   gastric cancer, 296
   glioblastoma, 4
   glomus tumor, 641
   graves ophthalmopathy, 640
   gynecomastia, 641
   head and neck carcinoma of unknown primary
      (HNCUP), 126
   hepatocellular carcinoma (HCC), 306
   heterotopic ossification, 639–640
   Hodgkin's lymphoma, 474–475
   indolent non-Hodgkin's lymphoma (NHLs), 495
   intermediate-and high-risk prostate cancer,
      374–375
   juvenile nasopharyngeal angiofibroma, 639, 641
   keloids, 640
   langerhans cell histiocytosis, 641
   locally advanced breast cancer (LABC), 208–209
   locoregionally recurrent breast cancer, 230
   low-grade gliomas (LGGs), 20, 21
   low-risk prostate cancer, 361

malignant spinal cord compression, 616–617
medullary thyroid cancer (MTC), 142
medulloblastoma, 523
melanoma, 171
meningioma, 27
mesothelioma, 271
multiple myeloma, 500–501
mycosis fungoides (MF), 177
nasopharyngeal cancer (NPC), 100–101, 101
neuroblastoma (NB), 561
non-small-cell lung cancer (NSCLC), 241
oral cavity squamous cell carcinoma (OC-SCC), 94
orbital pseudotumor, 641
oropharynx cancer, 82
pancreatic adenocarcinoma, 314
pediatric Hodgkin's lymphoma, 584
penile cancer, 414
Peyronie's disease, 641
pigmented villonodular synovitis, 641
pituitary adenoma, 42
plantar warts, 640
primary central nervous system lymphoma, 35
renal cell carcinoma, 425
rhabdomyosarcoma (RMS), 553, 555
salivary gland tumors, 118, 120
seminoma, 406
sinonasal tumors, 148
small-cell lung carcinoma (SCLC), 259
soft tissue sarcoma (STS), 508–509
splenomegaly, 640
stage III non-small-cell lung cancer, 250
superior vena cava syndrome, 623
thymoma, 277
urethral cancer, 421
uterine cancer, 442
uveal melanoma (UM), 64
vaginal cancer, 466
ventricular tachycardia, 642
vestibular schwannoma, 55
vulvar cancer, 457
well-differentiated thyroid cancer, 142
Wilms tumor (WT), 572
radical cystectomy, bladder cancer, 396–397
radical hysterectomy, uterine cancer, 441
radical mastectomy, 188, 190
radical neck dissection
   medullary thyroid cancer (MTC), 142
   oropharynx cancer, 81
radical nephrectomy (RN), 424, 571
radical prostatectomy
   intermediate-and high-risk prostate cancer, 374
radical trachelectomy, 431
radioembolization, 306
radiofrequency ablation (RFA), 306
   non-small-cell lung cancer (NSCLC), 241
   renal cell carcinoma, 425
radiofrequency rhizotomy, 48
radiopharmaceuticals, 611
radiosurgery, glioblastoma, 6
raloxifene, 188
RCC. *See* renal cell carcinoma
rectal cancer, 326. *See also* colorectal cancer
re-irradiation
   medulloblastoma, 527

pituitary adenoma, 42
recurrent/progressive glioblastoma, 8
renal cell carcinoma (RCC)
    biopsy, 424
    clinical presentation, 423
    epidemiology, 423
    genetics, 423
    imaging, 424
    pathology, 423
    prognostic factors, 424
    risk factors, 423
    staging, 424
    treatment paradigm, 424–425
    workup, 424
retromandibular vein, 115
retroperitoneal sarcoma (RPS), 514–516
    chemotherapy, 508
    en bloc resection, 508
    natural history, 507
    radiation, 509
    treatment paradigm, 505
RFA. *See* radiofrequency ablation
rhabdomyosarcoma (RMS)
    alveolar, 550
    classification, 552–553
    clinical presentation, 550
    embryonal, 550
    epidemiology, 549
    genetics, 549
    imaging, 550
    orbital embryonal, 555
    pathologic subtypes, 551
    pathology, 549
    PAX/FOX01 gene fusion, 554
    prognostic factors, 550, 552
    proton therapy, 555
    radiation dosing guidelines, 549
    risk factors, 549
    risk stratification, 553
    staging, 552
    treatment paradigm, 553
    workup, 550
RMS. *See* rhabdomyosarcoma
robotic surgery, low-risk prostate cancer, 360
Rotter's nodes, 183
RPS. *See* retroperitoneal sarcoma

sacral nerve roots, 615
salivary gland anatomy, 115–116
salivary gland tumors
    benign, 116
    characteristics, 116
    clinical presentation, 117
    epidemiology, 115
    genetics, 117
    histology, 115
    malignant, 116–117
    nodal metastasis, 119–120
    pathology, 116
    prognostic factors, 117
    risk factors, 115
    staging, 117
    treatment paradigm, 117–118
    workup, 117

sarcomas, 575
SCLC. *See* small-cell lung carcinoma
SCPL–CHEP
    glottic cancers, 110
    supraglottic cancers, 110
seminiferous tubules, 403
seminomas
    histologies, 404
    imaging, 405
    pathology, 404
    prognostic factors, 405
    stage I, 406–408
    stage II, 408
    treatment paradigm, 406
sentinel lymph node biopsy (SLNB)
    breast cancer, 188
    locally advanced breast cancer (LABC), 208
    locoregionally recurrent breast cancer, 230
    melanoma, 168, 170, 172–173
    Merkel cell carcinoma (MCC), 157, 159
    vulvar cancer, 457, 459
Shimada histopathologic system, neuroblastoma
        (NB), 558
Siewert classification. gastric cancer, 294
Simpson Grading System, meningioma resection,
        27
sinonasal tumors
    biopsy, 146
    clinical presentation, 146
    epidemiology, 145
    imaging, 146
    lymph node involvement, 148
    pathology, 145–146
    prognostic factors, 146
    risk factors, 145
    sinonasal undifferentiated carcinoma, 149
    staging, 146–147
    subtypes, 149–150
    treatment paradigms, 147–148
    workup, 146
sinonasal undifferentiated carcinoma (SNUC), 149
SINS. *See* Spinal Instability Neoplastic Score
skene glands, 445
skin anatomy, 156, 167
skin-sparing mastectomy, 188
skull base chordoma, 70, 71
SLNB. *See* sentinel lymph node biopsy
small choroidal melanomas, 65
small-cell lung carcinoma (SCLC)
    biopsy, 258
    clinical presentation, 258
    epidemiology, 257
    extensive stage, 263–265
    genetics, 258
    imaging, 258
    limited stage, 260–263
    natural history, 258
    pathology, 257
    prognostic factors, 258
    prophylactic cranial irradiation, 265–266
    risk factors, 257
    staging, 258
    treatment paradigm, 257, 258–259
    workup, 258

SMARCB1 (INI-1)-deficient sinonasal carcinom, 150
soft tissue sarcoma (STS)
    clinical presentation, 506
    epidemiology, 505
    genetics, 506
    imaging, 507
    natural history, 507
    pathology, 506
    primary extremity, 509–514
    prognostic factors, 507
    risk factors, 505
    staging, 507–508
    treatment paradigm, 505, 508–509
    workup, 506
solitary enchondromas, 69
solitary plasmacytoma, 500, 501
solitary pulmonary nodule, 241
sphenoid sinus, 145
spinal cord, 615
Spinal Instability Neoplastic Score (SINS), 608, 616
spinal meninges, 615
spine tumors. *See* chondrosarcoma; *chordoma*
splenomegaly, 641
squamous cell carcinoma
    oral cavity squamous cell carcinoma, 91–96
    oropharynx cancer, 79–82
SRS. *See* stereotactic radiosurgery
St. Jude/POG Surgicopathologic Staging, 560
stage III non-small-cell lung cancer (NSCLC)
    clinical presentation, 249
    imaging, 249–250
    medically operable, 251–252
    nonoperative management, 252–255
    prognostic factors, 250
    superior sulcus tumors, 255
    treatment paradigm, 249, 250
    workup, 249
stereotactic needle biopsy
    early-stage breast cancer, 186
    primary central nervous system lymphoma, 34
stereotactic body radiotherapy (SBRT)
    Ewing's sarcoma, 579
    extracranial oligometastatic disease, 635
    hepatocellular carcinoma (HCC), 306–308
    locally advanced pancreatic cancer, 319–320
    low-risk prostate cancer, 366–367
    lung tumors, 244–247
    pancreatic adenocarcinoma, 314
    renal cell carcinoma, 425
stereotactic radiosurgery (SRS)
    brain metastases, 597–603
    brainstem gliomas (BSGs), 540
    chondrosarcoma and chordoma, 73
    malignant spinal cord compression, 617
    meningioma, 29
    pituitary adenoma, 42
    spine metastasis, 610, 612
    trigeminal neuralgia, 48, 49
    vestibular schwannoma, 55–57
stomach
    anatomy, 293
    vascular supply, 293–294
STS. *See* soft tissue sarcoma
subependymal giant cell astrocytoma, 19

subglottis, 108
sunitinib, 425
superior sulcus tumors, 255
superior vena cava (SVC) syndrome
    clinical presentation, 622
    epidemiology, 621
    grading system, 622
    imaging, 622
    natural history, 623
    pathology, 622
    prognostic factors, 622
    treatment approaches, 621
    treatment paradigm, 623
    workup, 622
supraglottic cancers
    clinical presentation, 108
    staging, 109
    surgery, 110
    voice-preserving options, 110
supraglottis, 107
surgical resection
    aggressive non-Hodgkin's lymphoma, 484
    bladder cancer, 396–397
    bone and spine metastasis, 608–609
    brain metastases, 597
    cervical cancer, 431
    cholangiocarcinoma (CC), 348–349
    chondrosarcoma and chordoma, 72
    colorectal cancer (CRC), 327–328
    craniopharyngioma, 546
    early-stage breast cancer, 188
    ependymoma, 532
    Ewing's sarcoma, 576–577
    gastric cancer, 295
    head and neck carcinoma of unknown primary
        (HNCUP), 124–127
    hepatocellular carcinoma (HCC), 305
    Hodgkin's lymphoma, 473
    indolent non-Hodgkin's lymphoma (NHLs), 495
    intermediate-and high-risk prostate cancer, 374
    locally advanced breast cancer (LABC), 208
    locoregionally recurrent breast cancer, 230
    low-grade gliomas (LGGs), 20
    low-risk prostate cancer, 360–361
    malignant spinal cord compression, 616
    medulloblastoma, 522
    melanoma, 167, 170
    meningiomas, 27
    mesothelioma, 270–271
    multiple myeloma, 500
    nasopharyngeal cancer (NPC), 100
    neuroblastoma (NB), 561
    nonmelanomatous skin cancer, 160–161
    non-small-cell lung cancer (NSCLC), 241
    oral cavity squamous cell carcinoma (OC-SCC), 93
    oropharynx cancer, 81–82
    pancreatic adenocarcinoma, 313
    pediatric Hodgkin's lymphoma, 583
    penile cancer, 412–413
    pituitary adenoma, 41
    primary central nervous system lymphoma, 34
    renal cell carcinoma, 424–425
    rhabdomyosarcoma (RMS), 553
    salivary gland tumors, 117

seminoma, 406
sinonasal tumors, 147
small-cell lung carcinoma (SCLC), 258–259
soft tissue sarcoma (STS), 508
stage III non-small-cell lung cancer, 250
superior vena cava syndrome, 623
trigeminal neuralgia, 48
urethral cancer, 420–421
uveal melanoma (UM), 64
vaginal cancer, 466
vestibular schwannoma, 55
vulvar cancer, 457
well-differentiated thyroid cancer, 141–142
Wilms tumor (WT), 571–572
SVC syndrome. *See* superior vena cava syndrome
systemic therapy
    brain metastases, 597
    brainstem gliomas (BSGs), 540
    melanoma, 170
    mesothelioma, 271
    nonmelanomatous skin cancer, 160
    renal cell carcinoma, 425

tamoxifen
    ductal carcinoma in situ (DCIS), 223
    early-stage breast cancer, 188
targeted therapy
    neuroblastoma (NB), 561
    stage III non-small-cell lung cancer, 250
tectal tumors, 538, 539
temozolomide (TMZ)
    anaplastic gliomas, 14
    glioblastoma, 4
    low-grade gliomas (LGGs), 22
    primary central nervous system lymphoma, 36
TERT promoter mutation, low-grade gliomas, 19
testicular arteries, 403
testicular cancer
    clinical presentation, 404
    differential diagnosis, 404
    epidemiology, 403
    histologies, 404
    imaging, 405
    natural history, 405
    pathology, 404
    risk factors, 403
    secondary malignancy risk, 408–409
    staging, 405–406
    treatment paradigm, 403, 406
    workup, 404
thymectomy, 277
thymic carcinoma, 278
thymoma
    chemoRT, 279
    clinical presentation, 276
    epidemiology, 275
    imaging, 276
    pathology, 275
    staging, 276
    treatment paradigm, 275, 277
    unresectable/inoperable, 278–279
    workup, 276
thyroid cancer
    clinical presentation, 139

epidemiology, 139
follow-up, 143
genetics, 139
pathology, 139, 140
prognostic factors, 140
risk factors, 139
staging, 140–141
subtypes, 140
treatment paradigm, 141–143
workup, 140
thyroid gland, 139
thyroid hormone replacement, MTC, 142
tic douloureux. *See* trigeminal neuralgia
tinnitus, 53
TMZ. *See* temozolomide
tongue base mucosectomy, 125
tonsil tumors, 86
total mastectomy, 188
total mesorectal excision, colorectal cancer, 328
total skin electron beam therapy (TSEBT), mycosis
        fungoides (MF), 177, 178
TP53 mutation, low-grade gliomas (LGGs), 19
trabecular bone, 607
transarterial chemoembolization (TACE), 306
transcranial approach, pituitary adenoma, 41
transhiatal esophagogastrectomy, 285
transoral lingual tonsillectomy, 127
transpupillary thermotherapy, 65
trans-scrotal biopsy, 405
transsphenoidal surgery (TSS), 41
trastuzumab, 188
trigeminal nerve (CN V), 47
trigeminal neuralgia
    anatomy, 47
    clinical presentation, 47
    epidemiology, 47
    etiologies, 47
    etiology, 47
    risk factors, 47
    treatment paradigm, 48
    workup, 47
Tubiana Staging, Dupuytren's Contracture, 642
tumor spillage, 573
Turcot syndrome, 519–520

UM. *See* uveal melanoma
unilateral neck treatment, 127–128
urethra, 411, 419
urethral cancer
    clinical presentation, 419
    early-stage, 421
    epidemiology, 419
    imaging, 419
    locally advanced, 421–422
    organ-preservation approach, 421
    pathology, 419
    prognostic factors, 419
    risk factors, 419
    staging, 420
    treatment paradigm, 419–421
    workup, 419
urinary diversions, 397
uterine cancer
    clinical presentation, 440

uterine cancer (*cont.*)
    endometrial biopsy, 441
    epidemiology, 439
    genetics, 440
    imaging, 440
    natural history, 441
    pathologic types, 440
    prognostic factors, 441
    risk factors, 439
    screening, 440
    staging, 441
    treatment paradigm, 439, 441–442
    workup, 440
uterine corpus, 439
uterine sarcoma, 440, 451–452
uterosacral ligament, 430
uveal melanocytes, 61
uveal melanoma (UM)
    anatomy, 61
    clinical presentation, 62
    epidemiology, 61
    genetics, 61
    globe-conserving therapy, 67
    large tumors, 66
    medium tumors, 65–66
    natural history, 62
    pathology, 61
    prognostic factors, 62
    risk factors, 61
    small tumors, 65
    staging, 62–64
    treatment paradigm, 61, 64–65
    workup, 62

vagina, 463
vaginal cancer
    clinical presentation, 464
    current treatment approaches, 466–467
    epidemiology, 463
    imaging, 465
    pathologic types, 464
    prognostic factors, 465
    risk factors, 464
    staging, 465
    treatment paradigm, 463, 466
    workup, 465
ventral cord syndrome, 616
ventricular tachycardia, 642
verrucous carcinoma, 456
vertebroplasty, 500, 609
vertical hemilaryngectomy, 109
vestibular schwannoma
    anatomy, 53
    clinical presentation, 53, 54
    epidemiology, 53

genetics, 53
imaging, 53
Koos Grading Scale, 54
pathology, 53
prognostic factors, 54
risk factors, 53
treatment paradigm, 54–55
workup, 53
Villaret's syndrome, 100
vulva, 445
vulvar cancer
    adjuvant therapy, 458–460
    clinical presentation, 456
    epidemiology, 455
    imaging, 456
    neoadjuvant/definitive therapy for, 460–461
    pathology, 456
    prognostic factors, 456
    risk factors, 455
    staging, 456
    treatment paradigm, 455, 457
    workup, 456
vulvectomy, 457

Warthin's tumor, 116
WBRT. *See* whole brain radiation therapy
white matter, spinal cord, 615
WHO classification
    anaplastic gliomas, 11
    low-grade gliomas (LGGs), 17
    medulloblastoma, 520
    meningiomas, 26
    nasopharyngeal cancer (NPC), 99
    thymoma, 275
whole brain radiation therapy (WBRT)
    brain metastases, 597, 598–603
    glioblastoma, 6
    primary central nervous system lymphoma, 35–37
whole breast irradiation (WBI)
    ductal carcinoma in situ (DCIS), 221
    early-stage breast cancer, 191, 194
Wilms tumor (WT)
    biopsy, 571
    clinical presentation, 570
    genetics, 570
    imaging, 571
    lung metastases, 574
    National Wilms Tumor Study, 573
    postoperative RT, 569
    prognostic factors, 571
    risk factors, 569
    screening, 570
    treatment paradigm, 571–573
Wilms tumor, Aniridia, GU malformations, mental
    Retardation (WAGR), 569

Printed in the United States
by Baker & Taylor Publisher Services